American Cancer Society

Atlas of Clinical Oncology

Series Volumes

Blumgart, Fong, Jarnagin	*Hepatobiliary Cancer*
Cameron	*Pancreatic Cancer*
Carroll, Grossfeld, Reese	*Prostate Cancer*
Char	*Tumors of the Eye and Ocular Adnexa*
Clark, Duh, Jahan, Perrier	*Endocrine Tumors*
Eifel, Levenback	*Cervical, Vulvar and Vaginal Cancer*
Ginsberg	*Lung Cancer*
Grossbard	*Malignant Lymphomas*
Ozols	*Ovarian Cancer*
Pollock	*Soft Tissue Sarcomas*
Posner, Vokes, Weichselbaum	*Cancer of the Upper Gastrointestinal Tract*
Prados	*Brain Cancer*
Raghavan	*Germ Cell Tumors*
Shah	*Head and Neck Cancer*
Silverman	*Oral Cancer*
Sober, Haluska	*Skin Cancer*
Steele, Richie	*Kidney Tumors*
Volberding	*Viral Causes of Cancer*
Wiernik	*Adult Leukemias*
Willett	*Cancer of the Lower Gastrointestinal Tract*
Winchester, Winchester	*Breast Cancer*
Yasko	*Bone Tumors*

American Cancer Society

Atlas of Clinical Oncology

Editors

Glenn D. Steele Jr, MD
University of Chicago

Theodore L. Phillips, MD
University of California

Bruce A. Chabner, MD
Harvard Medical School

Managing Editor

Ted S. Gansler, MD, MBA
Director of Health Content, American Cancer Society

American Cancer Society

Atlas of

Clinical Oncology

Tumors of the Eye and Ocular Adnexa

Devron H. Char, MD

Director, The Tumori Foundation
Ophthalmic Oncology and Orbital Surgery
San Francisco, California
Clinical Professor
Department of Ophthalmology
Stanford University Medical School

2001
BC Decker Inc
Hamilton • London

BC Decker Inc
20 Hughson Street South
P.O. Box 620, L.C.D. 1
Hamilton, Ontario L8N 3K7
Tel: 905-522-7017; 1-800-568-7281
Fax: 905-522-7839
E-mail: info@bcdecker.com
Website: www.bcdecker.com

00 01 / UTP / 9 8 7 6 5 4 3 2 1

ISBN 1–55009–144–1
Printed in Canada

Sales and Distribution

United States
BC Decker Inc
P.O. Box 785
Lewiston, NY 14092-0785
Tel: 905-522-7017; 1-800-568-7281
Fax: 905-522-7839
E-mail: info@bcdecker.com
Website: www.bcdecker.com

Canada
BC Decker Inc
20 Hughson Street South
P.O. Box 620, L.C.D. 1
Hamilton, Ontario L8N 3K7
Tel: 905-522-7017; 1-800-568-7281
Fax: 905-522-7839
E-mail: info@bcdecker.com
Website: www.bcdecker.com

Foreign Rights
John Scott & Company
International Publishers' Agency
P.O. Box 878
Kimberton, PA 19442
Tel: 610-827-1640
Fax: 610-827-1671

U.K., Europe, Scandinavia, Middle East
Harcourt Publishers Limited
Customer Service Department
Foots Cray High Street
Sidcup, Kent
DA14 5HP, UK
Tel: 44 (0) 208 308 5760
Fax: 44 (0) 181 308 5702
E-mail: cservice@harcourt_brace.com

Australia, New Zealand
Harcourt Australia Pry. Limited
Customer Service Department
STM Division
Locked Bag 16
St. Peters, New South Wales, 2044
Australia
Tel: (02) 9517-8999
Fax: (02) 9517-2249
E-mail: stmp@harcourt.com.au
Website: www.harcourt.com.au

Japan
Igaku-Shoin Ltd.
Foreign Publications Department
3-24-17 Hongo
Bunkyo-ku,Tokyo, Japan 113-8719
Tel: 3 3817 5680
Fax: 3 3815 6776
E-mail: fd@igaku.shoin.co.jp

Singapore, Malaysia, Thailand, Philippines, Indonesia, Vietnam, Pacific Rim
Harcourt Asia Pte Limited
583 Orchard Road
#09/01, Forum
Singapore 238884
Tel: 65-737-3593
Fax: 65-753-2145

Notice: The authors and publisher have made every effort to ensure that the patient care recommended herein, including choice of drugs and drug dosages, is in accord with the accepted standard and practice at the time of publication. However, since research and regulation constantly change clinical standards, the reader is urged to check the product information sheet included in the package of each drug, which includes recommended doses, warnings, and contraindications. This is particularly important with new or infrequently used drugs.

Contributing Author

J. William Harbour, MD
Assistant Professor of Ophthalmology and Molecular Oncology
Washington University School of Medicine
Staff Surgeon,
Barnes-Jewish Hospital
St. Louis, Missouri

Contents

ORBITAL TUMORS

Preface

It is a daunting challenge to write another textbook of ophthalmic oncology at the millennium. Several issues combine to make this undertaking difficult. First, paradoxically obtaining inclusive literature searches has become harder over the last 10 years. A generation ago, I was confident that I could survey the entire world's literature in an area. Several factors have coalesced to make this an almost impossible challenge. One, there has been a virtual revolution in the number of publications in ophthalmology and cancer. Almost 20,000 biomedical journals exist. Two, library budgets have been severely restricted. In some cases, it has taken up to 2 months to get an interlibrary loan of an article I wish to review. Three, although we have come to rely on computer searching, the relative explosion in the number of publications has resulted in many of those journals not being indexed. Some studies estimate that "inclusivity" of a thorough computerized library search is approximately 75%.[1] Even occasionally in a journal that is indexed, differences in spelling between "countries separated by a common language" have occasionally provided an interesting challenge in obtaining articles.

Second, we are in the midst of a molecular biology revolution regarding medicine. Unfortunately for a book author with a significant interval between writing and publication, this presents several potential quagmires. Our understanding of the molecular biology of oncogenesis and tumor progression is becoming more clear cut, and there are some shared central pathways in most malignancies (Figure 1). In several tumors, the abnormalities in the p53 pathway are important in tumor development and in response to radiation. p53 has been termed the guardian of the genome. Its role is to determine if there is significant DNA damage. When DNA damage occurs, p53 either shuts down the cell cycle until repair can be accomplished or shunts the cell to an apoptotic programmed cell death pathway. The retinoblastoma gene abnormality (Rb1), although first described in the intraocular tumor, is also present in many systemic neoplasms. Loss of the RB protein with subsequent increased activation of the transcription factor E2F occurs in a number of human malignancies and may be a central component of malignant transformation (see Figure 1). In melanomas and other neoplasms, alterations in the cdk-4 inhibitor p161NK4A occurs and impacts the central cell cycle control pathway. This area is discussed in the first chapter on retinoblastoma.

In any new research area, progress is uneven. For some tumors, such as retinoblastoma, our understanding of many of the important molecular events is well understood. In other areas, there have been many false starts. As an example, in neuroblastoma,

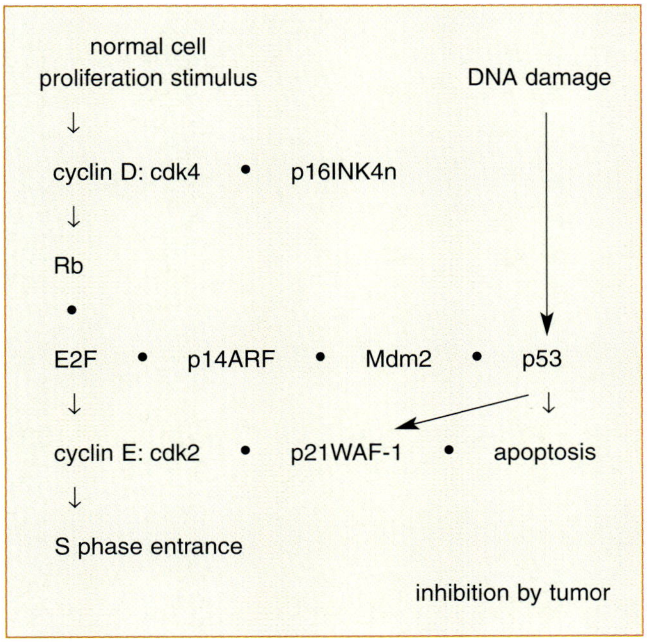

Figure 1. Normal cell cycle components. Note both positive (→) and suppressor (•) influences that have been demonstrated in many tumors.

it was thought that the expression of N-mye was one of the early examples in which molecular biologic tests would have great clinical import. Patients whose tumors expressed this oncogene had an adverse outcome. A recent article has demonstrated that a more primitive analysis, gain in a portion of the 17th chromosome, actually has a better correlation with prognosis in multivariate analysis.[2] As with any rapidly evolving field, I suspect that some of the chapters on oncogenesis and pathophysiology will be out of date shortly after they have been finished. A good example is molecular therapy. Although these approaches have been used for various hematologic abnormalities for a number of years, there is a paucity of phase III clinical trial data. I suspect that it will be another 3 to 4 years before important data on the use of gene therapy for ophthalmic malignancy become available. At the time of writing this book, a proposed gene therapy trial for retinoblastoma was rejected by one of the governing agencies.[3]

As always in writing a large book, I want to thank my collaborators, the editorial staff, and the support staff who have allowed this to happen, and my teachers and mentors who have helped me attain the knowledge I have.

REFERENCES

1. Kleijen J, Knipschild P. The comprehensiveness of MEDLINE and Embase computer searches. Searches for controlled trials of homeopathy, ascorbic acid for common cold and gingko biloba for cerebral insufficiency and intermittent claudication. Pharm Weekbl Sci 1992;14:316–20.
2. Brown N, Cotterill S, Lastowska M, O'Neill S, Pearson AD, Plantaz D, Meddeb M, Danglot G, Brinkschmidt C, Christiansen H, Laureys G, Speleman F. Gain of chromosome arm 17q and adverse outcome in patients with neuroblastoma. N Engl J Med 1999; 340:1954–61.
3. Graber K. RAC nixes plan to treat retinoblastoma. Science 1999;284:2006.

Dedication

I would like to dedicate this book to my family,
Valerie Charlton Char, MD and Danton S. Char,
as well as to my long time editor, O.E.E. Anderson

I wish to thank the Tumori Foundation
for support of ophthalmic research,
clinical studies, and publications

1

Diagnosis of Lid Tumors

Lid malignancies are quite common and most often develop in sun-exposed older males. Approximately half of all malignancies involve the skin, and 9 to 15 percent of cutaneous malignancies involve the lid. About 1,300,000 basal cell carcinomas and squamous cell carcinomas are diagnosed yearly in the United States.[1] It is estimated that 60,000 cases of eyelid malignancies are diagnosed yearly.[2–8] Forty percent of skin neoplasms are basal cell carcinomas; in the periorbital region, basal cell carcinoma is the most common cutaneous malignancy and accounts for 85 to 95 percent of lid tumors.[2,3]

The frequency of various types of tumors depends on the geographic location. In contrast to the above figures, in China, the basal cell carcinomas accounted for only 38 percent of 3,510 cases.[9] Even among the Asian populations, however, there are variations. For example, a study from Singapore noted that basal cell carcinomas accounted for 84 percent of eyelid tumors.[3] In a small population-based study from Florida of non–basal cell or squamous cell carcinomas, the incidence of other eyelid tumors was 1.8 per million Caucasians over the age 20 years; in contrast, it was less than 0.3 in African American patients.[10]

Increased solar exposure is considered to be responsible for the increased incidence of cutaneous tumors.[11,12] In a small area of England, the diagnosis of cutaneous basal cell carcinoma, squamous cell carcinoma, and melanoma increased from 153 to 235 percent over the last 10 to 15 years.[13]

EYELID TUMORS: PATHOPHYSIOLOGY

The pathogeneses and pathophysiologies of eyelid malignancies are varied. The etiology of rarer malignancies are poorly understood. In contrast, the events leading to the induction and development of Kaposi's sarcoma (KS), squamous cell carcinoma, sebaceous cell carcinoma, basal cell carcinoma, and malignant melanoma are beginning to be understood on a molecular level as well as from epidemiologic data that have been known, in some of these tumors, for over 100 years.

Solar radiation, especially the ultraviolet B (UV-B) spectrum (290 to 320nm) is crucial in the development of squamous cell carcinoma, basal cell carcinoma, and melanoma. Both epidemiologic and laboratory data demonstrate different patterns in each of these neoplasms. Shorter wave length UV light is blocked by ozone. Sun exposure and latitude have been shown to be important in all three skin cancers, as have lighter skin color, poor tanning, and blue eyes.[8,14,15]

While both squamous cell carcinoma and basal cell carcinoma are associated with cumulative sun exposure, the correlation is not as strong with the latter neoplasm; similarly, other epidemiologic features, such as proximity to the equator, exposure to UV-B, and increased patient age, are not as tightly correlated with basal cell carcinoma, compared with squamous cell carcinoma.[14–17] While the incidence of squamous cell carcinoma is increased 20- to 30-fold in immunosuppressed patients, it is only modestly increased for basal cell carcinoma.[18] In cutaneous malignant melanoma, intermittent intense UV exposure (as opposed to cumulative exposure for basal cell and squamous cell carcinomas) is a principal epidemiologic parameter.[19] As a result melanomas arise more often in indoor workers and in skin areas that are only intermittently exposed to the sun.

That solar-induced DNA damage was important in the etiology of skin cancer was initially demonstrated by Cleaver, who showed that there was deficient DNA repair in patients with xeroderma pigmentosum who have > 1,000-fold increased incidence of skin malignancies.[20] Probably, UV-B interaction with epithelial DNA is the initiating event in the induction of skin malignancies. Solar radiation is absorbed into proteins, purines, and pyrimidines that have unsaturated chemical bonds. The frequencies of these DNA damaging events and alterations in DNA repair are both important in tumor induction.[21,22] Cellular cytotoxicity secondary to UV radiation does not result in mutation, but a lower level of nonlethal damage often does. The most prevalent DNA damage is the induction of dimerizations between adjacent pyrimidines, termed cyclobutane pyrimidine dimers; other pyrimidine (6 to 4) pyrimidone photoproducts are probably less important in the induction of human epithelial malignancies.[23] The relative importance of various sites of UV mutations in the DNA of epithelial cells is uncertain. Tumors could develop under either positive influences of oncogenes or loss of normal tumor-suppressor genes. As an example, *p53*, which has been demonstrated to be altered in almost 50 percent of epithelial tumors, has been termed the guardian of the genome. Its role is to assess intracellular DNA damage and prevent faulty DNA replication. If there is grave alteration of the cellular DNA, normal *p53* routes that cell into apoptosis (programmed cell death). In cells with reparable DNA defects, *p53*, through a series of other gene interactions, temporarily shuts down the DNA cell cycle until the defect is repaired. Several groups have demonstrated UV alterations in the *p53* tumor suppresser gene in skin cancers.[22] Other workers have also shown UV-induced alterations in Ha-*ras* and N-*ras* oncogenes.[24,25]

The relative importance and role of alterations in DNA repair function for the development of skin cancers is not clear. As patients age, there is diminution of DNA repair capacity and increased mutations.[26,27] Decreased DNA repair is noted in young patients who develop basal cell carcinomas, compared with age-matched controls.[26] Several pathways of DNA repair exist. Two major pathways are nucleotide and base excision repair; the former is responsible for removal of pyrimidine dimers and has been well characterized.[28] As mentioned, nucleotide excision repair is abnormal in several syndromes associated with skin malignancies, including xeroderma pigmentosum.[20]

Apparently, unique to basal cell carcinoma pathogenesis, in contrast to other eyelid malignancies, is an abnormal increased expression of the *PTCH2* gene, termed the human patched gene. This gene was first noted in basal cell nevus syndrome (Gorlin's syndrome). Mutations disrupt its regulation, with resultant overexpression, which seems to be a necessary component for the development of basal cell carcinoma.[29,30]

The estimated incidence of malignant eyelid tumors is approximately 19.6 per 100,000 per year for males, and 13.3 for females in a study reported from a predominantly Caucasian population in Minnesota.[31] Basal cell and squamous cell carcinomas have a propensity for the lower eyelid, although the reason for this is uncertain.[32] Lindgren and associates were unable to demonstrate a gradient UV exposure between the lower and the upper eyelids.[33]

There is a paucity of data on the pathogenesis of sebaceous gland carcinomas. This tumor accounts for between 1 and 6 percent of eyelid tumors. It is much more common in the Chinese population.[34] In a small study of seven women with this tumor from Virginia, those with invasive disease had abnormalities of *p53*, and at least in one case, the molecular form of the *p53* abnormality with G:C/T:A transversion was observed which is often associated with bulky carcinogens.[34]

In squamous cell carcinoma of various body sites, UV damage to *p53* has been documented.[35] There are several other alterations that may be important in the development of squamous cell carcinoma. A cytoplasmic factor, which translocates the nucleus, Rel/NF-kB is activated by UV-B and suppresses apoptosis. In a transgenic mouse model, the inhibition of Rel/NF-kB signaling resulted in increased development of squamous cell carcinomas.[36]

As discussed in the next chapter, with the development and widespread use of protease inhibitors, the incidence of KS has markedly decreased in patients with acquired immunodeficiency disease. Several early studies demonstrated that KS had an epidemiology suggestive of an infectious agent independent of the human immunodeficiency virus (HIV).[37] A number of investigations have now shown that human herpes virus-8 (HHV-8) is important in the classic form of KS as well as in that associated with immunodeficiency.[38] There are several enigmas regarding KS—whether these cells are truly neoplastic or result from a chronic inflammatory response, and to what degree HHV-8 is the transforming virus for this process.[39]

The incidence of cutaneous melanoma in the United States has been projected to be 1 in 75 by the year 2000;[40] it rose by approximately 120 percent between 1973 and 1994.[41] Several investigations have demonstrated alterations in both familial and sporadic melanoma. As discussed in the introduction to this book, *p16* ^{INK4a} is coded in the area of chromosome 9q21. This factor, which is important in the control of cell cycling, has been demonstrated to be abnormal in both in the familial and sporadic cutaneous melanomas.[42,43]

In cutaneous and uveal melanomas, as well as in most other human malignancies, the relative importance and order of the genomic changes that have been described, and at what phase during malignant transformation and tumor progression each genomic change affects the neoplasm's development, are uncertain. Using a variety of techniques, a number of chromosomal gains and losses have been demonstrated in cutaneous melanomas.[44] When melanomas progress from the radial to the vertical growth phase, there appears to be clonal derivation of those more malignant cells. It appears that alterations on chromosome 9 and chromosome 10 occur early on in melanoma progression, whereas increases on chromosome 7 are a later event.

Clinical Diagnosis of Eyelid Tumors

Malignant lid lesions can mimic a number of benign conditions, and growing lid tumors usually require biopsies to classify their nature. As a general rule, any growing lid lesion, recurrent sty in the same location, or chronic rodent ulcer should be biopsied. Other clinical signs suggestive of lid malignancy include localized loss of eye lashes, a pearly telangiectatic change in an area of cutaneous disturbance, an area of diffuse induration, or rarely a scirrhous, retracted area.

Table 1–1. SIMULATING LID LESIONS

Inclusion cyst
Papilloma
Senile keratosis
Keratoacanthoma
Inverted follicular keratosis
Benign keratosis
Pseudoepitheliomatous hyperplasia
Dermoid cyst
Malherbe's calcifying epithelioma (pilomatrixoma)
Sebaceous adenoma
Benign sweat gland tumors (syringoma, porosyringoma, myoepithelioma, mixed tumors)
Amyloidosis
Intravenous pyogenic granuloma of the ocular adnexa
Necrobiotic xanthogranuloma
Malacoplakia

Table 1–1 lists a number of benign simulating lid lesions. Clinically typical benign lesions, such as a seborrheic keratosis, can usually be merely watched. However, when a probable benign simulating lesion shows growth, a biopsy should be done to establish the histologic diagnosis. Often, even expert clinicians cannot make a correct diagnosis without a biopsy. Two excellent examples of these problems are typified by the cases shown in Figures 1–1 through 1–3. The patient in Figure 1–1 had rapid onset and growth of his lower lid lesion over a 6-week period. The time course is most consistent with a keratoacanthoma, but this benign lesion can occur in association with either local or distant malignancy and requires histologic data to differentiate it from a squamous cell carcinoma.[45,46] Histologically, this was a benign keratoacanthoma and regressed rapidly after biopsy. The patient in Figure 1–2A showed a similar time course and was clinically followed up

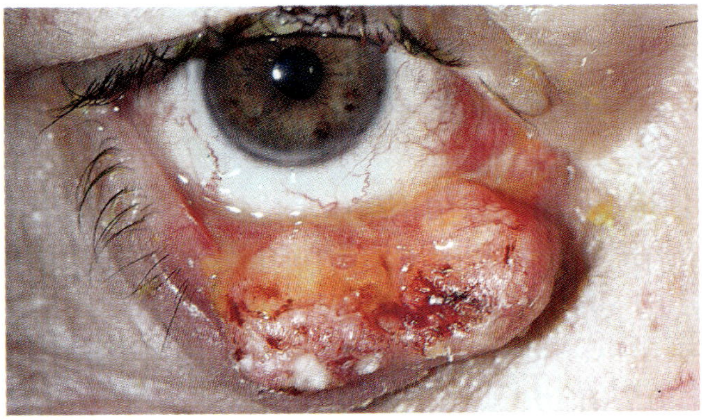

Figure 1–1. Biopsy proven keratoacanthoma; lesion enlarged to size shown in approximately 6 weeks.

elsewhere. The lesion continued to expand (see Figures 1–2B and 1–2C) and, on biopsy, was found to be a squamous cell carcinoma. Sometimes, the clinical behavior is in contrast to the histologic features. Grossniklaus and colleagues reported three such cases of apparent keratoacanthomas, in which all were invasive and one later invaded the central nervous system.[47] Some keratoacanthomas behave as a variant of a squamous cell carcinoma.

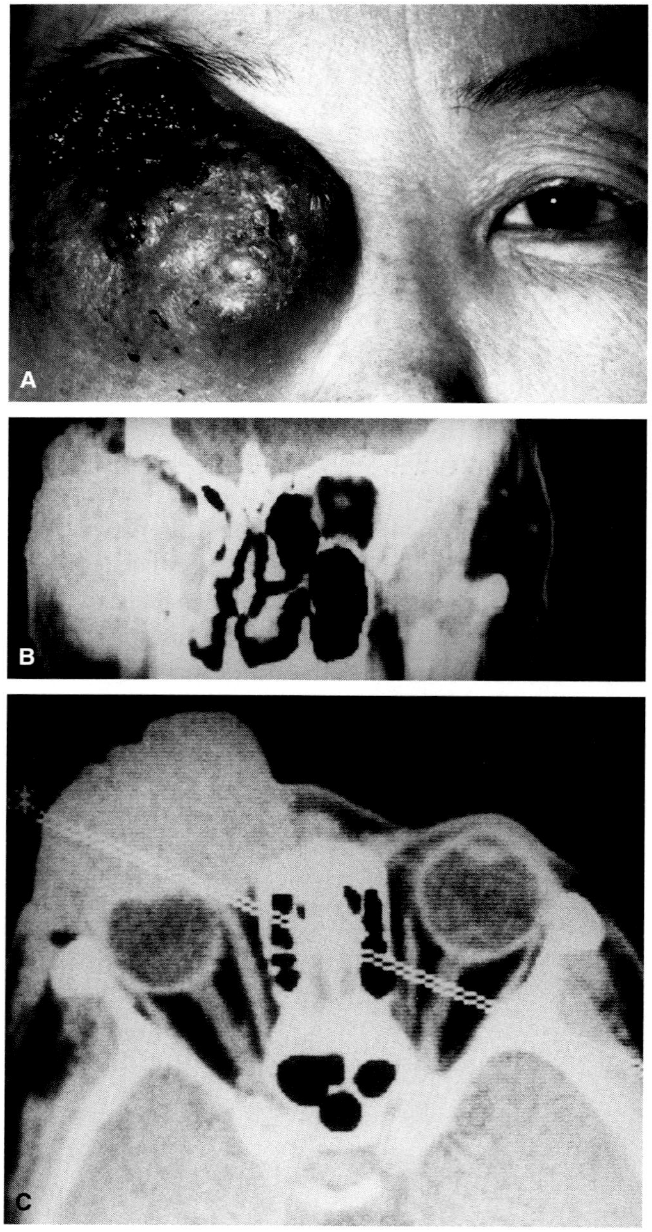

Figure 1–2. *A,* Squamous cell carcinoma, initially thought to be a keratoacanthoma. *B* and *C,* Axial CT with computer reformatting demonstrates an invasive carcinoma initially believed to be a keratoacanthoma.

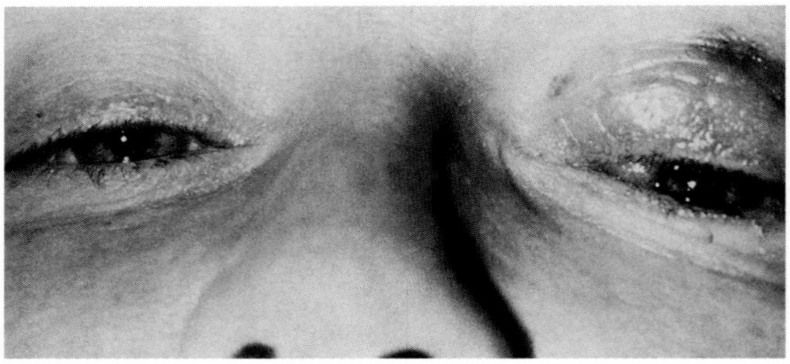

Figure 1–3. Diffuse amyloid infiltration of the upper lid.

Figure 1–3 demonstrates diffuse upper lid infiltration due to amyloid. Figure 1–4 shows a cutaneous horn, histologically, due to a benign papilloma. A number of other benign lesions can clinically simulate a malignant neoplasm.[48] More often, rare benign lesions have been present for many years and have a tenuous history of growth.[49–51] Rarely, an inflammatory process can simulate malignant epithelial tumor, and cases of nodular fascitis, Kamura's disease, isolated Langerhan's cell histiocytosis, and discoid lupus in the eyelid have been described.[52–56]

Similarly, some malignant lesions can appear relatively innocuous. The lesion in Figure 1–5 was the first manifestation of systemic lymphoma. Figure 1–6 shows minimal lower lid signs in a diffuse sebaceous gland carcinoma. Alternatively, the clinical pattern of some malignancies can simulate other neoplasms. Figure 1–7 demonstrates a pigmented basal cell carcinoma. Pigmented lid neoplasms are much more frequently basal cell carcinomas than malignant melanomas.

Table 1–2 lists the most frequent lid malignancies. There is essentially no morbidity with a small, superficial, incisional biopsy.[57–59] Several generations of ophthlamic surgeons have reported on false-

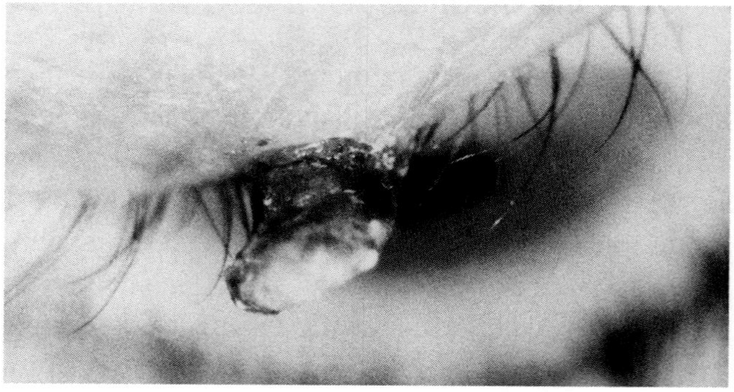

Figure 1–4. Cutaneous horn part of a benign papilloma.

Table 1–2. LID MALIGNANCIES
(in order of frequency in the author's experience)
Basal cell carcinoma
Sebaceous gland carcinoma
Squamous cell carcinoma (or its variant, adenoid squamous cell carcinoma)
Malignant melanoma
Kaposi's sarcoma
Adnexal carcinoma
Metastatic tumors
Lymphoma
Mycosis fungoides
Malignant sweat gland tumors (mucinous sweat gland adenocarcinoma, malignant syringoma)
Malignant Merkel cell neoplasm

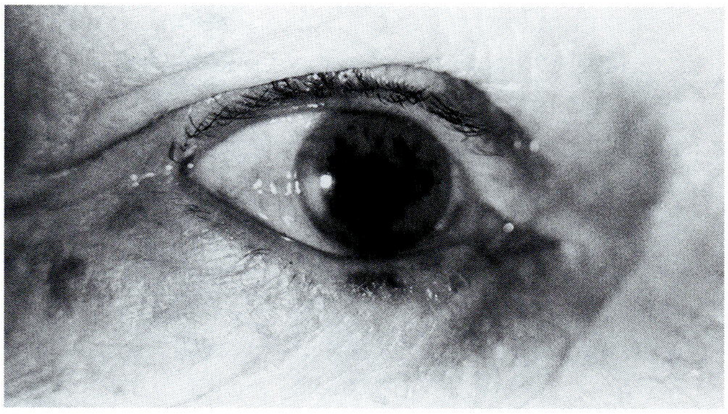

Figure 1–6. Minimal clinical findings in a diffuse lower lid sebaceous gland carcinoma.

positive and false-negative diagnostic rates in cutaneous eyelid lesions. In a study from Cincinnati, these authors noted that of 864 lesions, there was a false-positive diagnosis rate of malignancy of 8.5 percent and a false-negative rate (in lesions that were thought to be benign and turned out to be malignant) of approximately 2 percent.[60] As discussed in Chapter 3, even much larger areas of the lid removed with a "laissez faire" technique often have a reasonable cosmetic appearance, and an incisional biopsy with forceps and scissors or scalpel should not produce a cosmetic deformity. Small cytology series with the diagnostic use of hematoporphyrin-induced fluorescence and Doppler laser have been reported, but results have not yet shown great clinical utility.[61,62]

BASAL CELL CARCINOMA

Basal cell carcinoma is the most common malignancy of the lid. The first reported case was in 1827. Over 60 percent occur on the lower lids, and in descending order of frequency, the medial canthus, upper lid, and lateral canthal areas may be involved.[63] This neoplasm can present as a nodular, diffuse (morpheaform), ulcerative, or multicentric lesion.[64] Typically, nodular tumors account for approximately 60 percent of basal cell carcinomas of the lid and present as a chronic, indurated, nontender, raised, pearly, telangiectatic, well-circumscribed lesion with an elevated surround and a depressed, crater-like center (Figures 1–8A through 1–8D). Unfortunately, in 10 to 40 percent of basal cell carcinomas of the lid, clinically indistinct margins are noted.[3,63] Often these morpheaform or multicentric basal cell carcinomas present with either an ulcerative pattern (Figures 1–9A through 1–9C) or demonstrate a relatively uniform area of induration with lash loss (Figure 1–10). In addition to being more likely to have clinically nonapparent spread, morpheaform lesions are more likely to have deep invasion than other types of basal cell carcinomas.[65] Occasionally, basal

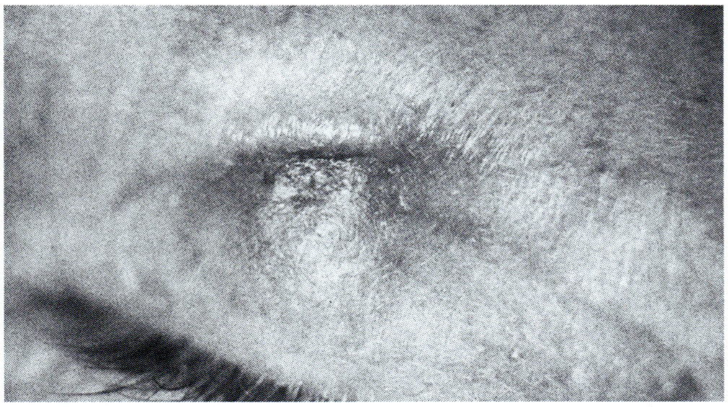

Figure 1–5. Systemic lymphoma first presenting as an innocuous-appearing lid tumor.

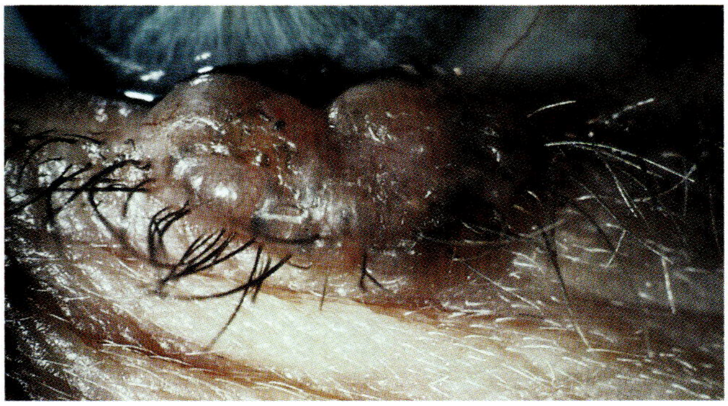

Figure 1–7. Pigmented lid tumors are most commonly basal cell carcinomas; these often simulate a malignant melanoma.

cell carcinomas can have a mixed pattern, and that was noted in one series in approximately 12 percent of the cases.[66] Figure 1–11 shows medial canthal basal cell carcinomas with orbital invasion. Orbital involvement is manifested clinically as a fixed nonmobile tumor and/or a frozen globe. A rarer form of basal cell carcinoma is a cystic lesion which can cause clinical confusion.[65]

The management of basal cell carcinomas is discussed in Chapters 2 and 3. The majority of tumors can be eradicated with preservation of ocular function and good cosmesis. Rarely, some may regress spontaneously; however, there is little data on this feature that can be used to make a decision on the management of a primary lesion.[67] The basal cell carcinomas most difficult to manage are morpheaform tumors, neoplasms that are not freely moveable (that finding is suggestive of underlying bone invasion), medial canthal tumors (since they have a greater tendency for orbital invasion), and tumors with orbital extension. Treated basal cell carcinomas require long-term follow-up.[68] Only 50 percent of recurrences are detected within 2 years of treatment; in a large meta-analysis, even after 5 years, there was an 8.7 percent recurrence rate. In addition, as many as 20 percent of patients who were previously treated for a basal cell carcinoma develop a new primary within 1 year of initial therapy.[49,68] Patients with a nonmelanomatous skin cancer are also at increased risk of cancer mortality, although the mechanism is uncertain.[69]

Overall, approximately 2 to 4 percent of basal cell carcinomas are sufficiently advanced to require orbital exenteration.[70] Howard and co-workers noted that only 13 of 622 eyelid epithelial carcinomas had orbital invasion at the time of initial presentation.[71] In the subgroup of basal cell carcinomas, the mean

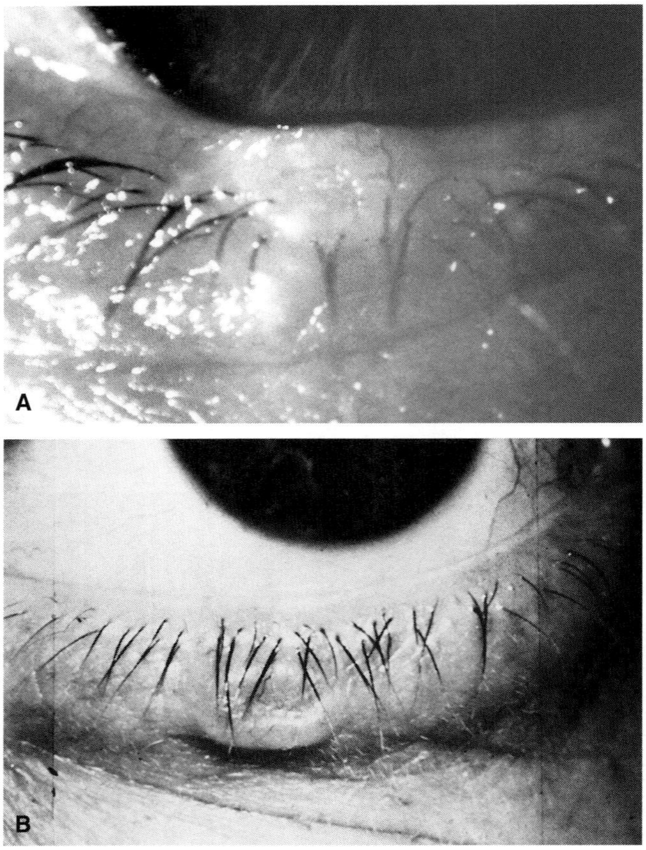

Figures 1–8. *A* and *B,* Typical nodular basal cell carcinomas with nontender, raised, pearly, telangiectatic border and crater-like center.

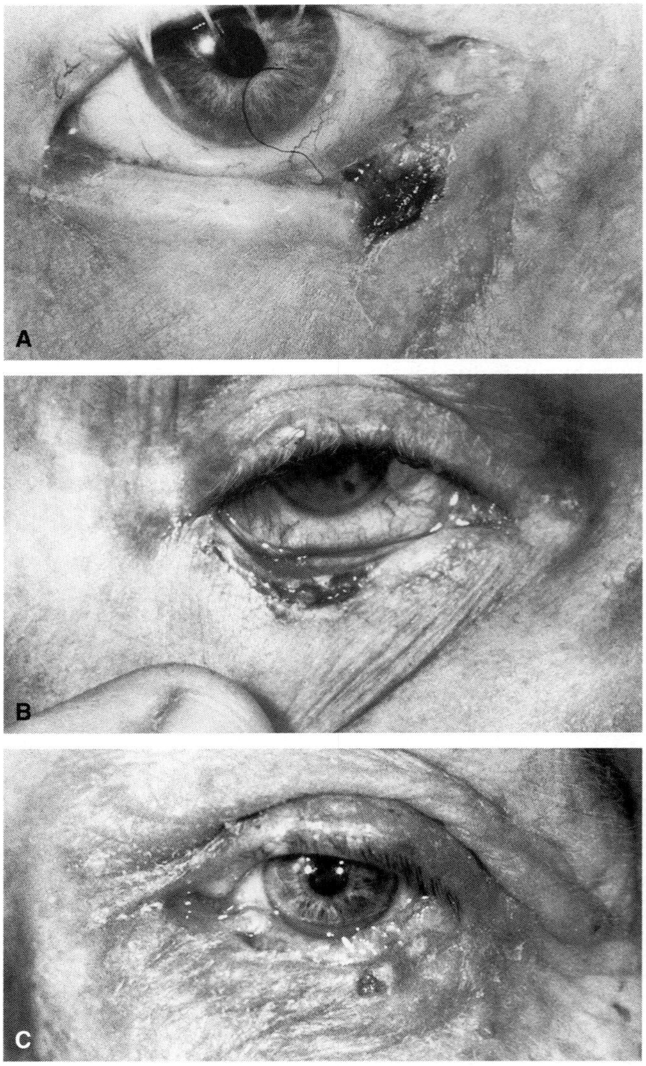

Figures 1–9. *A* to *C,* Ulcerative basal cell carcinomas with diffuse involvement of lid.

duration of the eyelid lesion prior to discovery of orbital involvement was almost 10 years, and most were recurrent tumors with a morpheaform pattern.[71] Rarely, intraocular invasion can occur in basal cell carcinoma.[72,73]

Metastases from basal cell carcinomas are exceedingly rare. The first report was in 1894; approximately 130 cases have been described.[74–76] Metastases are associated with tumors that have deep invasion, usually spreading to the lymph nodes, lung, and bones. In one report of 5 cases, 3 originated from the lid area.[75] The risk of basal cell carcinoma metastases is < 1 percent.[77] Overall, three-quarters of cutaneous cancer deaths are due to melanoma; in one study, only a third of the remaining quarter was due to basal cell carcinoma.[78] In the group of patients who died from basal cell carcinoma, the mean age was 85 years, and 40 percent had refused surgery.[78]

SEBACEOUS GLAND CARCINOMA

Sebaceous gland carcinoma is one of the most dangerous eyelid tumors for five reasons. (1) It often masquerades as a recurrent chalazion, sty, or chronic blepharoconjunctivitis, and the correct diagnosis may be delayed until the tumor has metastasized. (2) The incidence of metastases is as high as 41 percent, although earlier diagnosis has resulted in decreased tumor-related mortality.[79–81] (3) Because it may have intraepithelial pagetoid spread and/or multicentric pattern, delineation of tumor margins, even with excellent paraffin-embedded sections, can be difficult[79,82–86] (4) Even histologically, the tumor can be misdiagnosed, especially if lipid stains (such as oil-red-O) or monoclonal antibodies are not used or if tissue is improperly prepared.[81] A recent study by Sinard showed that a combination of antibodies, including those to EMA, BRST-1, and Cam 5.2, were useful to distinguish sebaceous gland carcinoma from other eyelid malignancies.[87,88] (5) Frozen-section control of tumor margins has an error in this malignancy of up to 25 percent, especially if there is a pagetoid component.[89]

The cell of origin in these tumors is not certain in 50 to 60 percent of cases; the remainder arise most commonly from the meibomian gland, anterior to the gray line from the glands of Zeis or Moll.[79] This

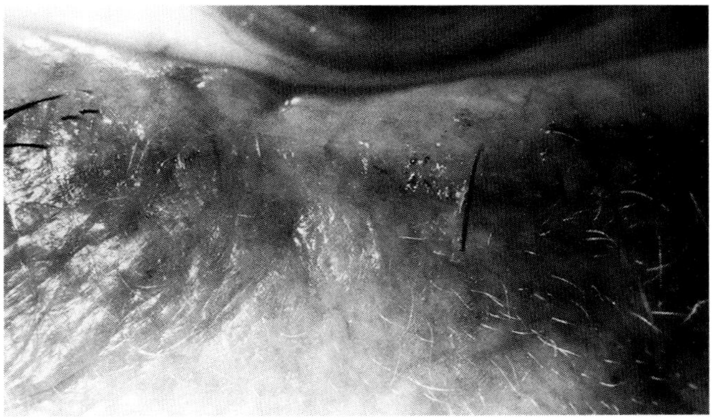

Figure 1–10. Morpheaform basal cell carcinoma diffusely involving lower lid; note telangiectasia and lash loss.

tumor is more common in the Asian than in the western races. Ginsberg found only 142 cases in the entire western literature prior to 1968.[90] In the United States, the reported incidence is approximately 0.5 to 5 percent of lid tumors, while in China, it accounts for over 10 percent of lid carcinomas.[80,91] In most series, female patients outnumber males.[89] It is most common in older patients, with a mean age at diagnosis in the mid-60s, although it has been described even in children as young as 3.5 years old.[92]

Unlike basal cell carcinoma, sebaceous cell carcinoma has a predilection for the upper lid. This location is affected two to three times more frequently than the lower lid.[80,84] In contrast to basal cell and squamous cell carcinomas, which usually arise from a more superficial portion of the cutis, sebaceous gland carcinomas that arise most commonly from the meibomian gland are less prone to ulcerate. In over 50 percent of cases, the tumor presents as either a pseudochalazion or a chronic blepharoconjunctivitis.[93–95] The tumor can present as a focal mass, a multicentric tumor, or a diffuse lesion

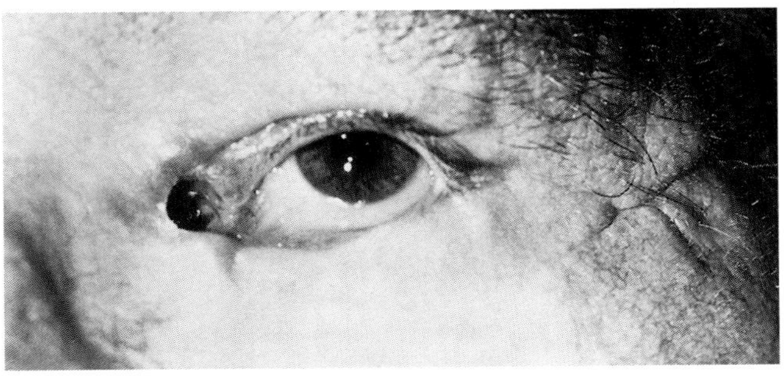

Figure 1–11. Medial canthal basal cell carcinoma invading orbit. The globe is frozen.

Table 1–3. POOR PROGNOSTIC FACTORS IN SEBACEOUS GLAND CARCINOMA

Invasion: vascular-lymphatic (8 of 9)*, or orbital (13 of 17)*
Diffuse involvement of both lids (5 of 6)*
Multicentric origin
Tumor diameter > 10 mm (No deaths in 25 cases with tumors < 6 mm)
> 6 months symptoms (38% mortality)

*Tumor-related mortality/number of cases with this pattern

with pagetoid spread.[80,83,95] The latter two types of sebaceous carcinomas are associated with a poorer prognosis (Table 1–3). Typically, these tumors may have a superficial and yellowish appearance due to their origin and lipid content.

Figure 1–12 demonstrates a typical presentation of a sebaceous carcinoma, and this clinical pattern accounts for almost 50 percent of cases. The patient was believed to have four recurrent chalazia in the same location of the lower lid. A small sebaceous gland carcinoma, unsuspected before a cautious ophthalmologist biopsied a chalazion, is shown in Figure 1–13. In the pagetoid pattern, there is often involvement of both lids as well as the conjunctiva.[83,96] Figure 1–14 shows another small tumor arising from the lower eyelid. Figure 1–15 illustrates a case initially believed to be chronic keratoconjunctivitis and then felt to be a squamous cell carcinoma of the conjunctiva, until histologic data were available. The patient shown in Figure 1–16 was initially referred to the author by a head and neck surgeon; the patient presented with a parotid mass and a history of four recurrent chalazia in the same location in the lower lid. Figure 1–17 demonstrates a large sebaceous carcinoma of the upper lid.

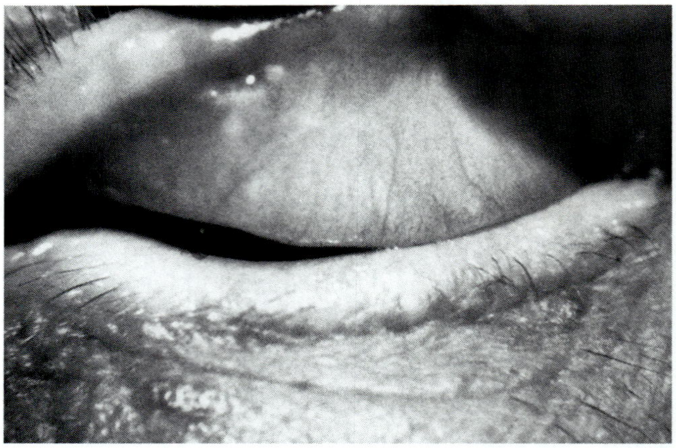

Figure 1–13. Very small sebaceous gland carcinoma diagnosed when a cautious ophthalmologist biopsied an apparent chalazion.

The prognosis with sebaceous gland carcinomas is dependent on multiple factors (see Table 1–3). As mentioned above, some of the recent decrease in tumor-related mortality is due to earlier diagnosis. In the author's experience, patients with recurrent chalazia who have had metastases at initial presentation had been observed for over 4 years. In most series with long-term follow-up, almost 30 percent of cases eventually metastasized; as shown in Table 1–3, risk factors have been relatively well delineated, and this author has personally not seen a small sebaceous gland carcinoma metastasize after surgical resection. Tumors < 6 mm in diameter generally have an excellent prognosis. Lower survival rates are observed in tumors > 20 mm in diameter, and tumors less histologically differentiated with highly infiltrative growth, pagetoid spread, or multicentricity.[84] This latter factor may result in tumor recurrence, even with histologic evidence of clear mar-

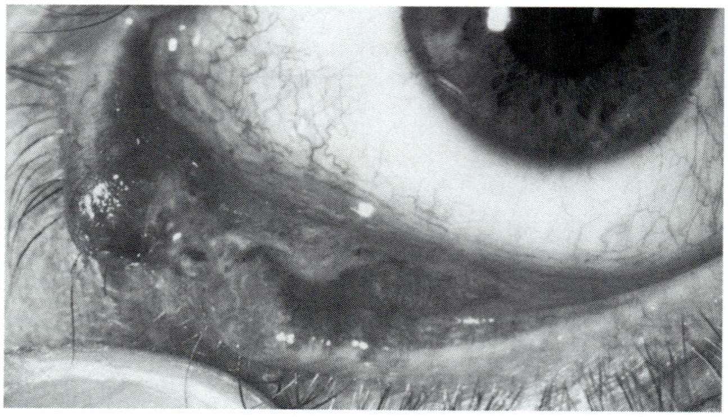

Figure 1–12. Sebaceous carcinoma simulating a recurrent chalazion.

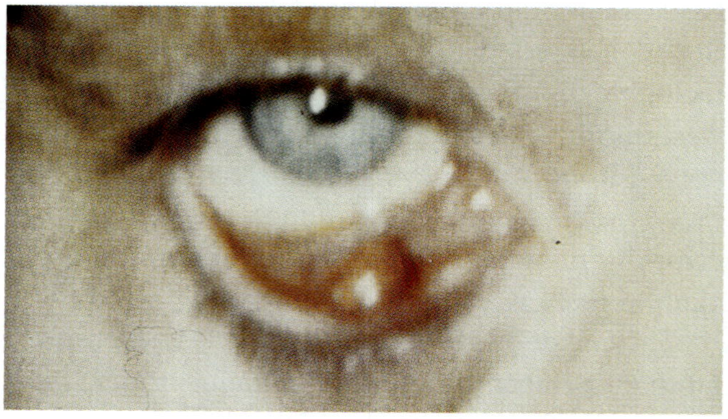

Figure 1–14. Small sebaceous gland carcinoma of the lower lid. Lower eyelid involvement is less common in this malignancy.

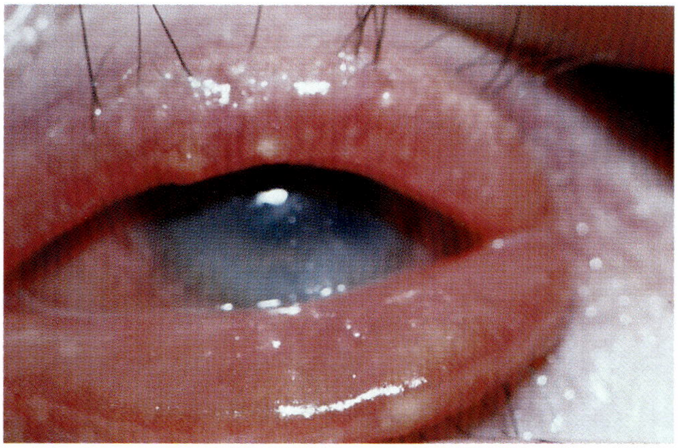

Figure 1–15. Sebaceous gland carcinoma simulating keratoconjunctivitis or squamous cell carcinoma of the conjunctiva.

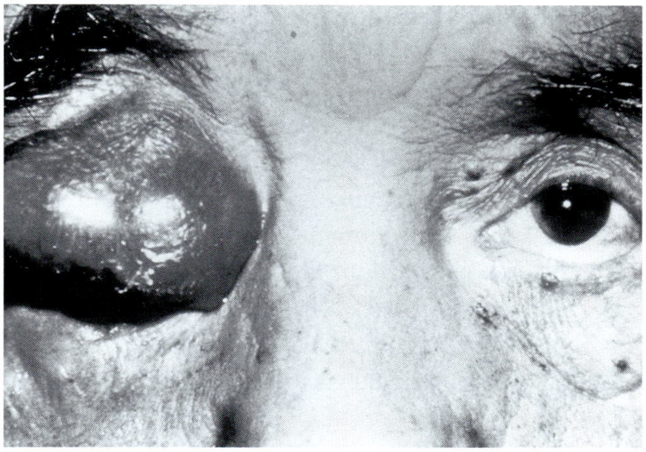

Figure 1–17. Large sebaceous carcinoma of the upper lid.

gins. Approximately 30 percent of sebaceous gland carcinomas recur after resection.[90,97]

Systemic extension of a sebaceous gland carcinoma of the eyelid occurs by contiguous growth, lymphatic spread, and hematogenous seeding. Most commonly, these lesions spread into the orbit, to the preauricular or submandibular nodes, or the parotid gland. Less commonly, there is involvement of the cervical node,[5] lung, pleura, liver, brain, pericardium, lip, ethmoid sinus, or skull.[79,80,84,90,98] Some patients with regional nodal metastases remain alive for long periods of time, and radical neck dissection for isolated cervical node disease is often indicated.[84]

Sebaceous gland tumors can be associated with the Muir-Torre syndrome.[99] This is an autosomal-dominant disease with either a benign or malignant sebaceous gland tumor in association with an internal malignancy, generally of the gastrointestinal tract. Usually, the sebaceous tumor precedes the internal malignancy by several years.[99] A few cases of Muir-Torre syndrome with ocular involvement have been reported.[100,101]

SQUAMOUS CELL CARCINOMA

Squamous cell carcinoma of the lid is relatively uncommon. It accounts for approximately 1 percent of lid malignancies in Caucasians, although in the Chinese, the incidence of this tumor was approximately 19 percent.[102] In a series of 5,392 lid tumors examined at the Wilmer Institute, 31 (0.5 percent) were squamous cell carcinomas.[103] Some series have noted a slightly higher incidence—up to 4 percent—of eyelid tumors in Caucasians.[104] The ratio of basal cell carcinoma to squamous cell carcinoma of the lid is approximately 39:1, except in transplant recipients.[105,106] There is no pathognomonic clinical pre-

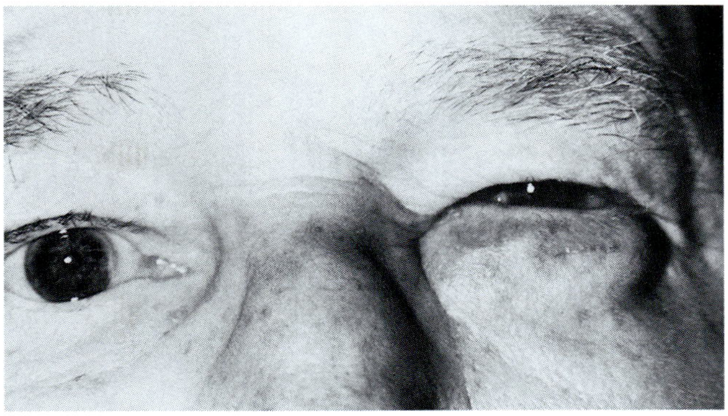

Figure 1–16. Sebaceous gland carcinoma initially diagnosed as a parotid mass.

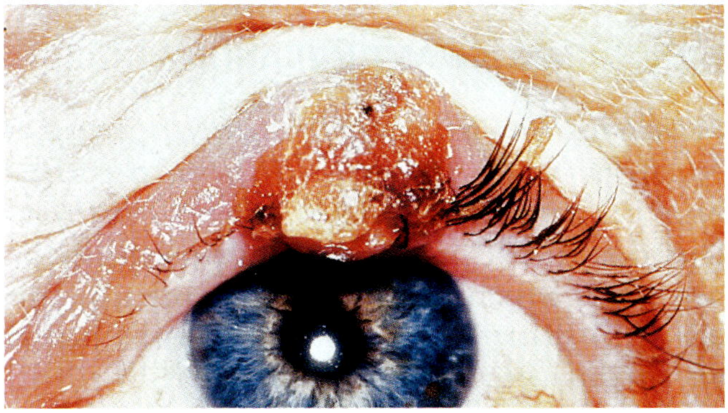

Figure 1–18. Squamous carcinoma of the upper lid; keratinization is more common with tumor.

sentation; however, the appearance of a cutaneous horn or extensive keratinization is most consistent for this neoplasm (Figure 1–18). Histologic diagnosis can also be difficult; in one series, only 12 of 115 tumors initially diagnosed as squamous cell carcinomas retained that diagnosis on re-evaluation.[105] As discussed under "treatment", squamous cell carcinoma has a slightly more malignant course than has basal cell carcinoma.[107–110] Often, extension to the regional nodes, direct invasion, or perineural progression can occur; the last was first described in 1909. Most of the patients with perineural progression have had a resection of the tumor in the past and present with recent onset diplopia (Figure 1–19). On a direct coronal scan of the patient shown in Figure 1–19, perineural invasion is seen in the superior orbit (Figure 1–20).[111,112] Most commonly, direct perineural invasion into the central nervous system is the cause of death.[10,107–110,112] The patient with perineural extension from an undiagnosed squamous cell carcinoma of the face (often the history is removal of a facial lesion without histologic confirmation of its nature) usually presents to the neurophthalmologist with either paraesthesias, numbness, or paresis of the extraocular muscles. If a primary is known, the median time between its diagnosis and the development of orbital involvement is usually less than 2 years, but an interval as long as 10 years has been reported.[113]

The biology of keratoacanthoma is uncertain. Some immunologic data would be consistent with the hypothesis that keratoacanthomas are a "forme fruste" of regressed squamous cell carcinoma.[114,115] As previously noted, biologically, these can progress to squamous cell carcinomas.[48]

MALIGNANT MELANOMA

Melanomas account for approximately 1 percent of eyelid tumors.[116] As discussed above, pigmented basal cell carcinoma is almost 10 times more common than melanoma as a cause of a pigmented lid neoplasm. Several studies have shown that the annual incidence of melanoma has at least tripled in the last four decades in all age groups.[116,117]

Probably the majority of melanomas arise from malignant degeneration of pre-existing nevi.[118] There are four types of cutaneous melanomas: lentigo maligna, acral lentiginous, nodular melanomas, and superficial spreading melanomas. All melanomas, with the exception of the nodular subgroup, have a radial growth-phase component.[119] Approximately 50 percent of eyelid melanomas are nodular melanomas, and 40 percent are superficial spreading melanomas.[116] Signs suggestive of a melanoma are variegated pigmented tumors, often with inflammation, the new development or spread of pigment, or increase in tumor thickness.[120] The histologic diagnosis of a cutaneous melanoma can be difficult. Several studies have shown discordance between expert pathologists in the diagnoses of benign and malignant cutaneous pigmented lesions.[120,121] About 40 percent of lid melanomas are nonpigmented. Typical lid melanomas are shown in Figures 1–21 through

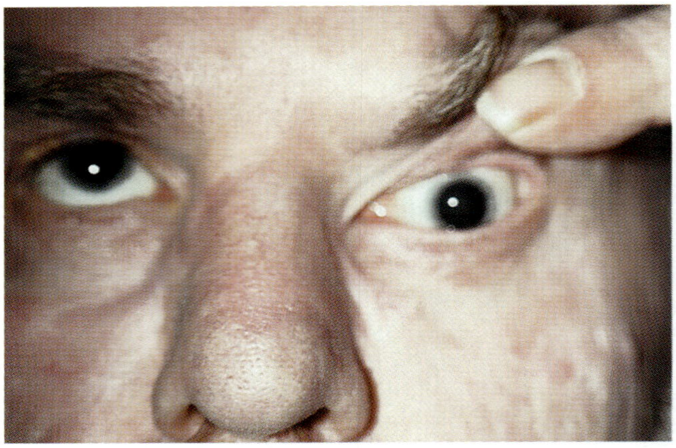

Figure 1–19. Patient with perineural invasion of the superior orbit from a squamous cell carcinoma producing diplopia in upgaze.

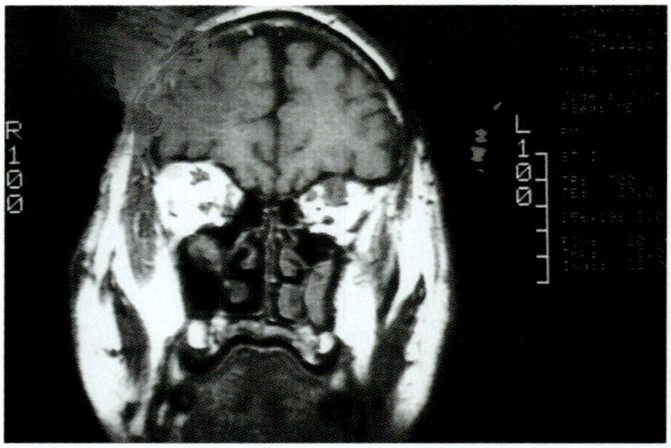

Figure 1–20. The direct coronal MR image from the patient shown in Figure 1–19 demonstrates perineural invasion into the superior orbit.

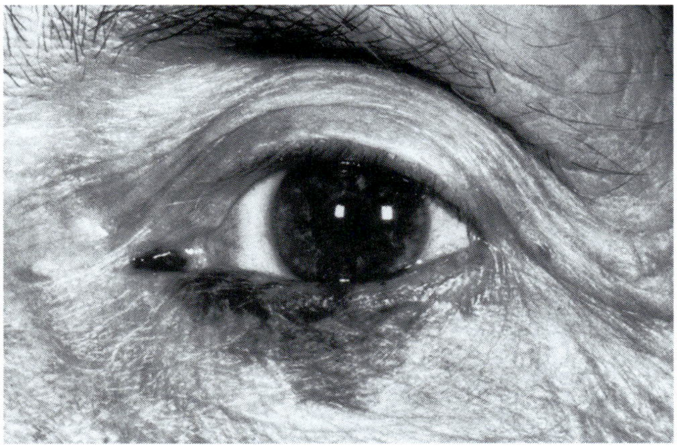

Figure 1–21. Lentigo maligna lid melanoma.

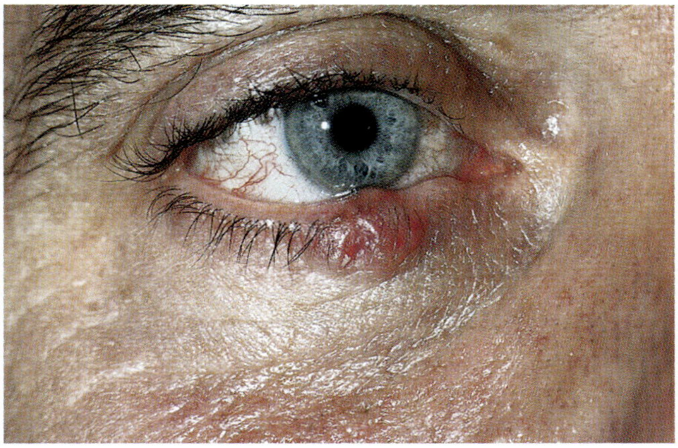

Figure 1–23. Amelanotic lid melanoma.

1–23. Occasionally, the eyelid may be secondarily involved by a conjunctival melanoma (Figure 1–24).

Early diagnosis of melanomas, when the tumor is relatively thin, has resulted in improved prognosis. While other factors, including gender, age, site, ulceration, regression, and mitotic index are correlated with prognosis, tumor thickness remains the most important predictor of prognosis.[122–124] In melanomas of < 0.85 mm thickness, there is < 1 percent tumor-related mortality, while lesions > 3.65 mm thick have 8-year survival rates of < 38 percent.[125] Further, for cutaneous melanomas, the average time to metastasize varies according to tumor thickness. In thin melanomas, tumor-related mortality peaked at 6 years, while thicker tumors had a mortality peak at approximately 40 months.[126] The reason for the better prognosis in women is uncertain; hypotheses advanced include a difference in anatomic sites, differences in tumor thickness, and hormonal factors.[123]

Unlike uveal melanomas, in which it is not uncommon to develop metastases more than 10 years after diagnosis, late onset of widespread disease is rare with cutaneous melanomas, and over 80 percent of late metastases have occurred with uveal melanomas.[127–131]

There have been several staging systems for cutaneous melanoma since one of the earliest in 1947 by Ackerman and Del Regato.

Table 1–4 shows a truncated revision of the 1997 Joint Committee on the cancer staging system for melanoma. It is very rare to see melanomas of the lid present with nodal involvement. "Level" in Table 1–4 refers to the earlier Clark classification, while "thickness" is derived from the work of Breslow.[132] In a large retrospective study by Volmer, he noted that in

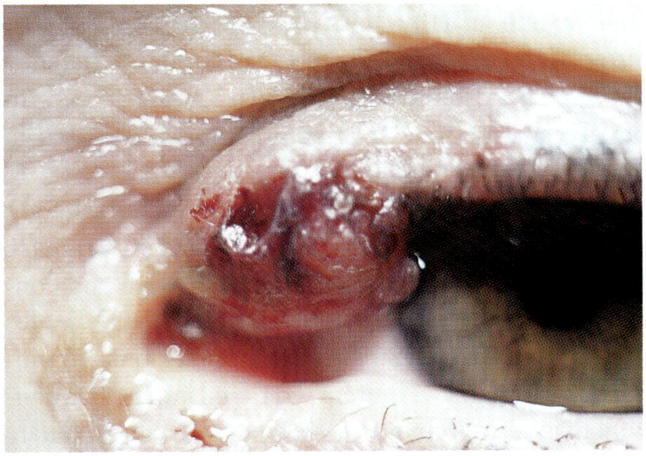

Figure 1–22. Sparsely pigmented lid melanoma.

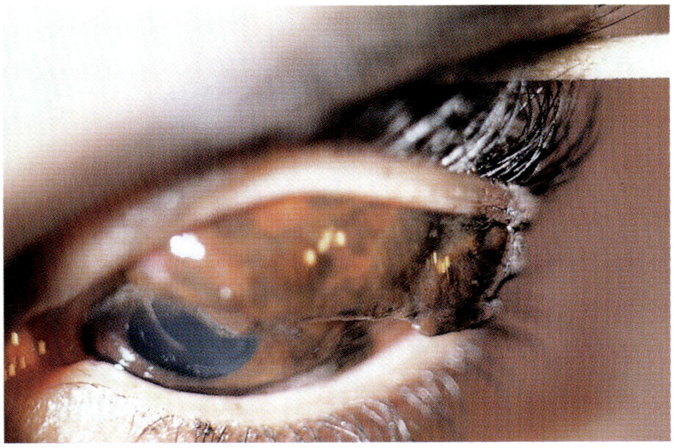

Figure 1–24. Palpebral conjunctival melanoma involving the entire upper lid.

Table 1–4. TRUNCATED REVISION OF THE 1997 JOINT COMMITTEE ON CANCER STAGING SYSTEM FOR MELANOMA

Stage	Criterion Stage
IApT1	< 0.75 mm thickness or level II
IBpT2	> 0.75 to 1.50 mm thick or level III
IIApT3	> 1.50 to 4.00 mm thick or level IV
IIBpT4	> 4 mm thick or level V

a vast majority of cases, thickness is a more important prognostic parameter than level.[133] In cases where there appears to be a difference in the level and thickness criteria, the recommendation has been to use the finding with the worst prognostic significance to stage the tumor. In patients with lid tumors < 1 mm thick, it is probably not cost effective to do a metastatic work-up, unless they are symptomatic.[133]

TUMORS METASTATIC TO THE LIDS

Tumors metastatic to the lids are very rare. In a review of 1,502 lid biopsies, Foos and colleagues noted only one such lesion.[134] Similarly, < 1 percent of 892 consecutive lid biopsies were metastatic in Aurora and Blodi's series.[3] Approximately 60 cases have been reported, some with both lid and orbital involvement. The vast majority have other known metastases at the time of presentation.[135–143] As is the case for uveal metastases, lung and breast carcinomas account for approximately 80 percent of lesions that metastasize to the lid; however, rare malignancies, such as carcinoid and Merkel cell carcinomas, have also been reported.[134,144,145]

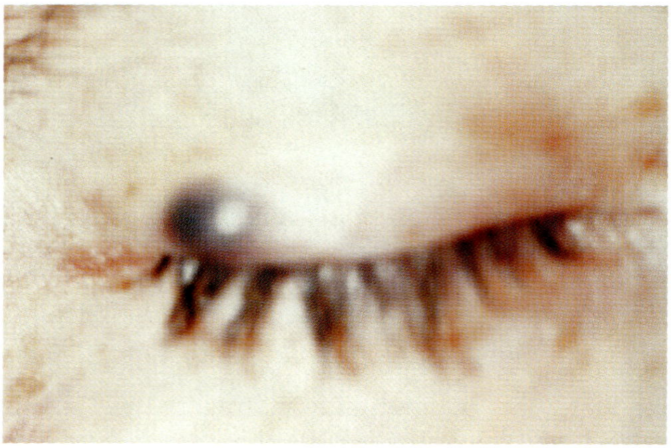

Figure 1–25. Cutaneous melanoma metastatic to lid.

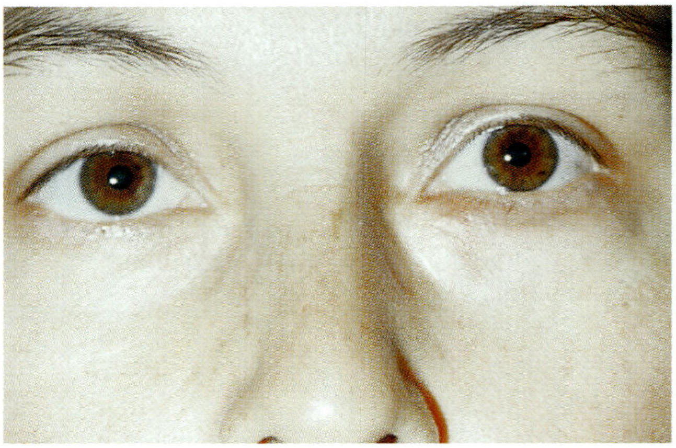

Figure 1–26. Metastatic breast carcinoma diffusely involving the lower eye lid.

The clinical pattern of lid metastases is not pathognomonic. Usually, these lesions occur as a nodular or diffuse indurated area. The former presentation, as shown in Figure 1–25, is typical for a metastatic cutaneous melanoma, although occasional lid metastases can simulate a chalazion.[120,136] Figure 1–26 shows metastasis of a diffuse breast carcinoma to the left lower eye lid, which responded completely to chemotherapy. In most cases, other evidence of metastasis are present at the time the lid lesion is diagnosed. As with uveal metastases, once the lid metastases are noted, survival is usually < 1 year.

KAPOSI'S SARCOMA

KS was first described in 1872, although prior to 1981, most of the cases of KS occurred in elderly Italian or Jewish males or African children.[146,147] This vascular sarcoma had an indolent disease course and usually involved the extremities. KS, prior to the outbreak of acquired immunodeficiency disease syndrome (AIDS), was rarely noted to involve the periocular structures. Only 30 cases in the lids or conjunctiva were described prior to 1982.[147–151] KS is now a less common manifestation of AIDS, since the use of multiple protease inhibitors. Lid KS or, more commonly, lid and conjunctival KS can develop in homosexual males known to have AIDS. Usually, these lesions are violaceous in color (Figure 1–27), and often, the conjunctival involvement is diffuse and can simulate inflammation (see Chapter 4, Figure 4–36).

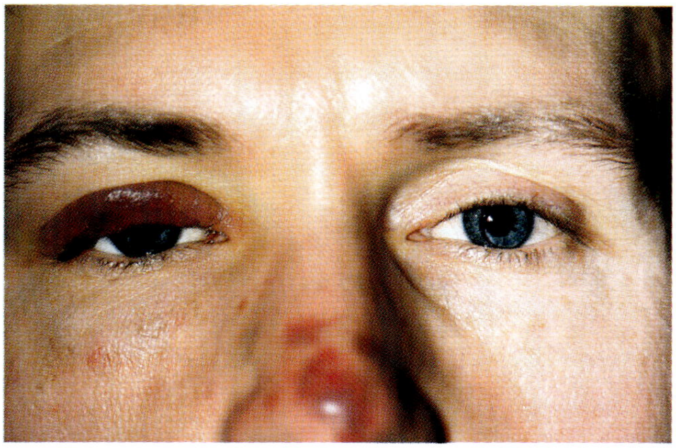

Figure 1–27. Kaposi's sarcoma in a patient with AIDS.

Unfortunately, while local control is easily achieved with low-dose radiation therapy, the systemic disease process has been rapidly fatal.[102] As mentioned above, with the newer generation of drugs, KS is much less common, and it is uncertain if this statement regarding mortality is still relevant.

RARE LID MALIGNANCIES

There are a number of rare lid malignant tumors that are only diagnosed on histologic examination. As discussed above, these tumors, like other malignant lesions, show growth, inflammation, or other signs of invasive behavior; but none have a pathognomonic appearance.[152–161] An adnexal malignancy is shown in Figure 1–28; as in a basal cell carcinoma, there is loss of lashes, but the author has not observed ulceration with these lesions.

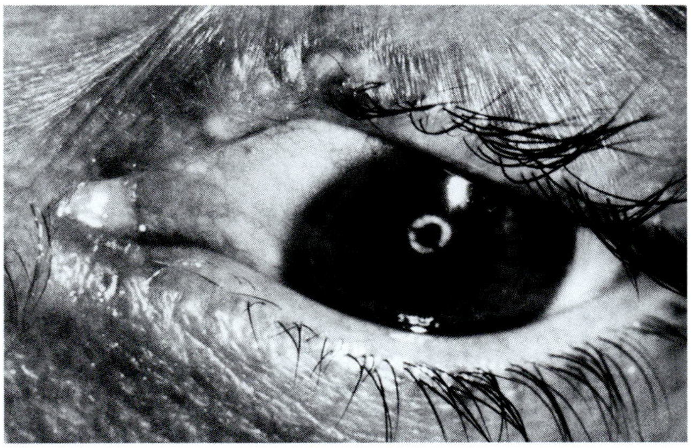

Figure 1–28. Adnexal malignant tumor with loss of lashes.

Merkel cell carcinomas are derived from neuroendocrine cells that are present in the basal layer of the epidermis and outer root sheath of hair follicles, and function as mechanoreceptors. These neoplasms typically involve the upper lid and are usually violaceous and have overlying telangiectasia;[120,162–165] rarely, these lesions can be multiple.[166] They occur more commonly in females, and often express both cytokeratin-20 and neurofilament protein.[167] They often have a typical pattern; in the one Merkel cell tumor that this author managed, the diagnosis was not made prior to biopsy.[168,169] Some of the rarer lid malignancies are listed in Table 1–2.[170] Several case reports document such rare lesions as mucinous eccrine carcinomas, signet ring carcinomas of the eccrine gland, syringomatous carcinomas, and procarcinoma, all simulating more common tumors.[171–177]

In contrast to most lymphoid lesions that more commonly involve either the conjunctiva or the orbit, mycosis fungoides, an uncommon T-cell lymphoma, has a predilection for the eyelids when it involves the ocular structures.[164–179] More commonly, T-cell lymphomas, when they involve the eye, produce other findings. In a large Mayo Clinic series, a cicatricial ectropion was the most common finding in 17 of 42 (40 percent) patients.[180]

PEDIATRIC LID TUMORS

Infantile Hemangioma

Capillary hemangiomas that involve the lid, conjunctiva, orbit, or a combination of these sites, most commonly present either at birth or in the first few months of life and are the most frequent ophthalmic neoplasm of infancy. There has been recent investigation in the molecular pathogenesis of this entity, although it currently does not have clinical application.[5]

A number of different terms have been used to describe this tumor, including juvenile hemangioma, cellular hemangioma, and benign hemangioendothelioma. These lesions usually present as a swelling of the eyelid, often involving the contiguous conjunctiva and the orbit (Figure 1–29). The mass is easily compressible and often has a reddish tint, although it may be bluish when the child cries (Figures 1–29 and 1–30). Figure 1–31 shows a parasagittal T_1-weighted

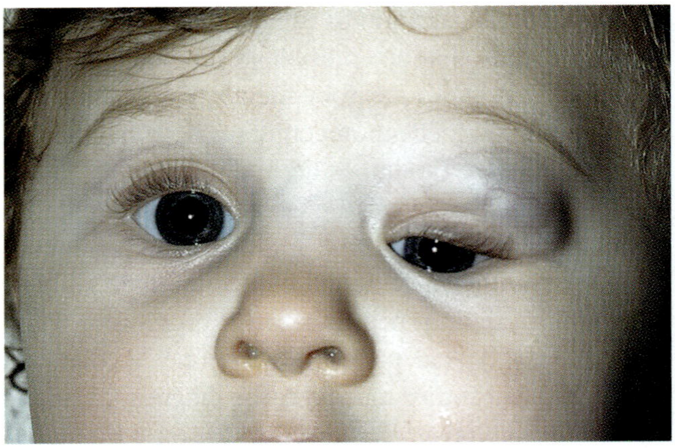

Figure 1–29. Capillary hemangioma involves the lid, conjunctiva, and anterior orbit.

magnetic resonance imaging (MRI) scan of such a lesion. In contradiction to nonvascular tumors, capillary hemangiomas are dark on T_1 -weighted images and hyperintense to brain on T_2-weighted images (Figures 1–32 and 1–33). On the T_2-weighted image, this mass is hyperintense to brain. Ninety-five percent of capillary hemangiomas are evident before age 6 months, and occasionally, they are noted in the first week of life. Usually, the growth in the first year is rapid, and then slow regression occurs.[181] An example is shown in Figures 1–34 and 1–35. Figure 1–34 is a child the day after birth; the same child 1 year later is shown in Figure 1–35. Involution is usually complete by 5 years. Initial clinical findings of involution are a central loss of the bright color of the mass.[182] Most series have noted more females than males, often in a 3:1 ratio. Similarly, it appears that women who have undergone chorionic villus sampling have over a 10-fold increased chance of developing this problem.[183]

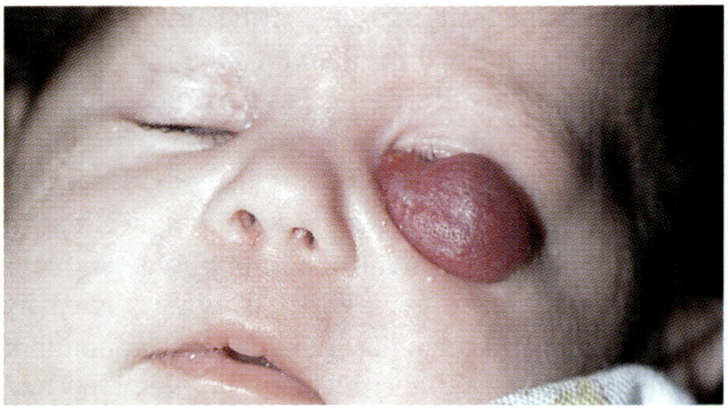

Figure 1–30. Typical color of lid hemangioma.

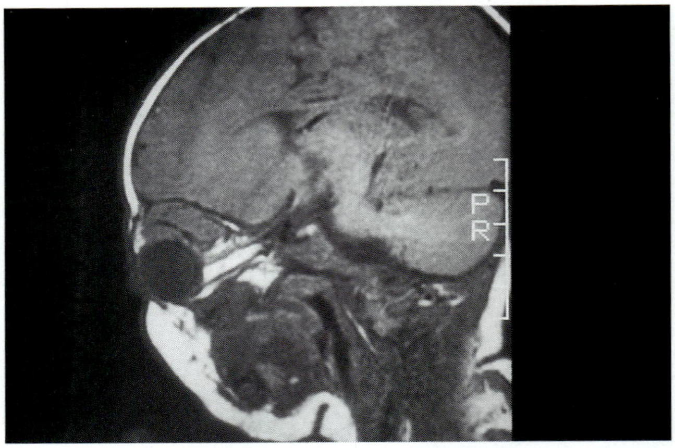

Figure 1–31. T_1-weighted parasagittal MR image of a capillary hemangioma. On T_2–weighted scans the lesion is hyperintense to brain.

The clinical course of these lesions is extremely variable. Often, they will show growth in the first 3 to 9 months of life, remain stationary, and then slowly resolve. Stigmar and colleagues noted that approximately 60 percent of cases resolved by age 4 years and 75 percent by age 7 years.[184]

Unfortunately, a number of major complications can occur; most commonly, these include strabismus,

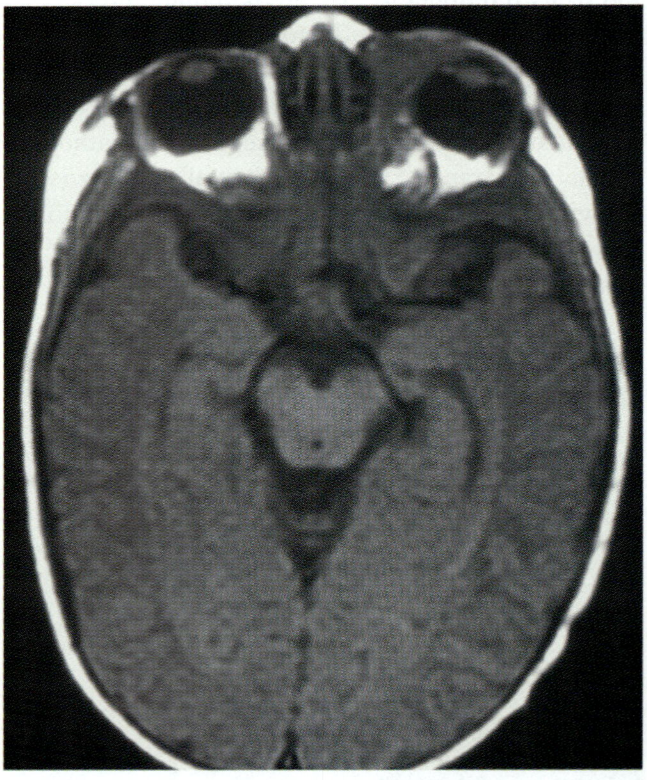

Figure 1–32. T_1-weighted axial MR images. The tumor is hypointense in respect to brain.

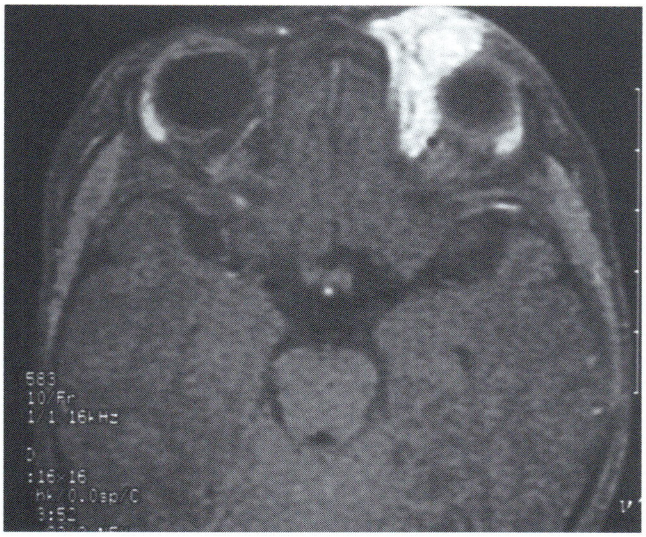

Figure 1–33. T_2-weighted MR image. The capillary hemangioma is hyperintense with respect to brain.

anisometropic amblyopia, proptosis, and compression of the optic nerve. Haik and colleagues reviewed 101 cases of capillary hemangioma and found an 80 percent complication rate, with 60 percent of patients having amblyopia.[185] In a study of 51 cases, Stigmar and associates noted that 27 developed amblyopia, and 17 had strabismus.[123] Robb found that 46 percent of 37 patients had refractive errors, with both myopia and astigmatism.[186] Amblyopia occurred most commonly when the eyelid occluded the pupil.

The author conservatively monitors most infants with capillary hemangiomas, unless a biopsy is needed to exclude the diagnosis of a possible malignant tumor or, more commonly, enlargement of the mass makes the development of amblyopia likely.

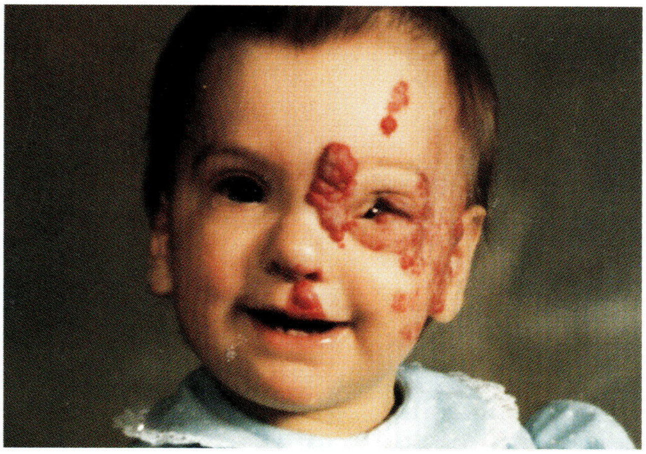

Figure 1–35. Patient shown in Figure 1-34 at age 1 year.

Generally, if the visual axis is not occluded, the author has opted for serial observation, since these children are at much less risk for developing amblyopia, although pressure of the tumor may alter the refractive status of the globe. If the mass grows and the visual axis is obstructed, then intervention is mandated.

There have been a number of therapeutic options, including injection of sclerosing agents, radiotherapy, systemic steroids, local steroid injection, diathermy, and surgical excision.[187] Most clinicians have abandoned the use of radiation, diathermy, or sclerosing agents. Certainly, the use of radon seeds is no longer advisable, given the public health safety problems with that particular isotope. In some of the experimental models, therapy with angiogenesis inhibitors has shown some promise.[188]

Intralesional steroid injection has been used in a number of infantile hemangiomas. Fost and Esterly

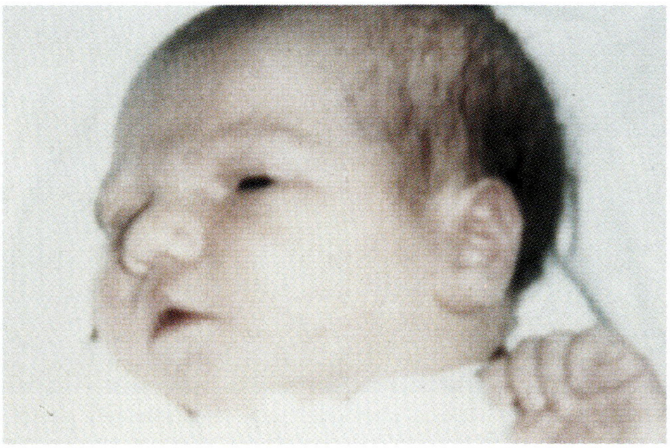

Figure 1–34. Neonate prior to appearance of hemangioma.

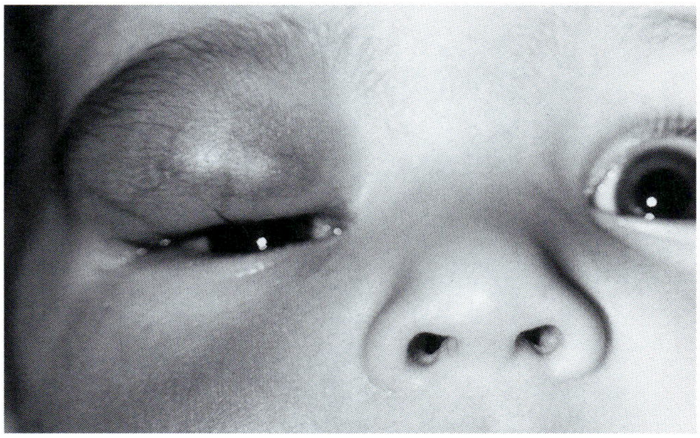

Figure 1–36. Growing capillary hemangioma of the lid with amblyopia.

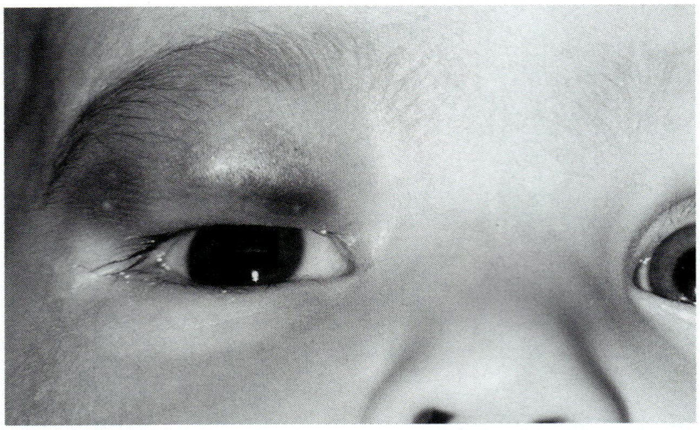

Figure 1–37. Three days after intralesional steroid injection with shrinkage.

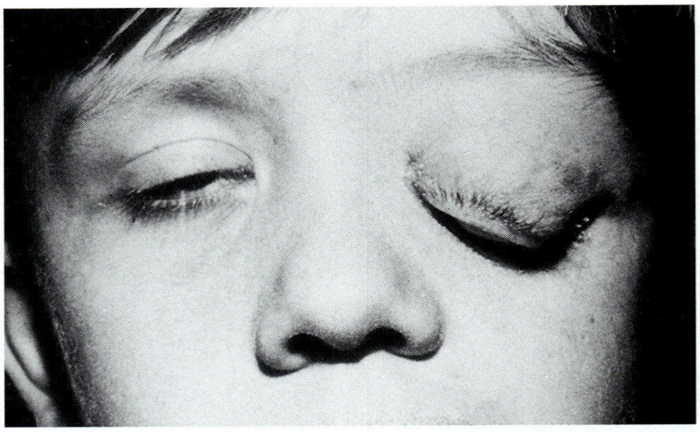

Figure 1–39. Plexiform lid neurofibroma in Von Recklinghaus neurofibromatosis.

first described this technique in nonophthalmic cases in 1968.[189] Hiles and Plichard first described its use in the management of ophthalmic cases, and Kushner popularized this technique.[190,191] Kushner described good resolution in most patients with intralesional steroids.[191,192] In growing lesions or in those that occlude the peripapillary axis on initial examination, approximately 1.0 cc of 40 mg/mL of methylprednisolone sodium succinate (Solu-Medrol) is injected into multiple sites of the lesion. Usually, there is blanching of the vascular pattern with rapid regression of tumor size within 48 hours after injection. In lesions that respond, involution is quite rapid over the first 2 weeks but may continue over a 2-month period. Some lesions have not responded to steroid injection, and if no response occurs in the first 2 weeks, a second injection is given. The author has never seen a patient who has not responded to two injections respond to further steroids. Figures 1–36 and 1–37 demonstrate a patient with a growing capillary hemangioma of the lid prior to and 3 days after intralesional steroids. Two injections of intralesional steroids have

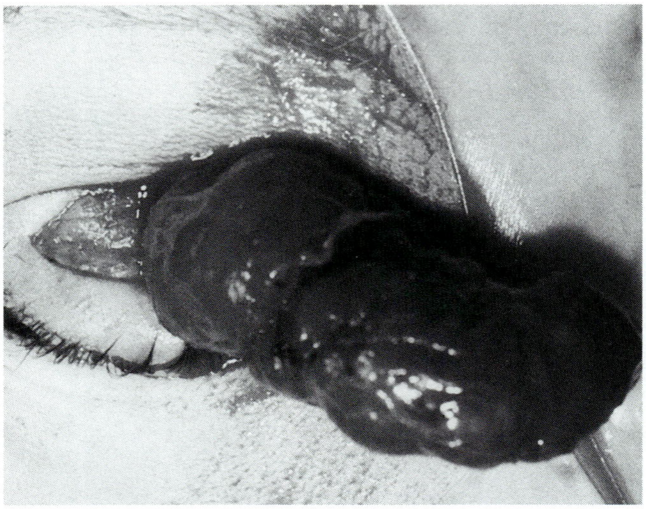

Figure 1–38. Resections of capillary hemangioma after failure to respond to intralesional corticosteroids.

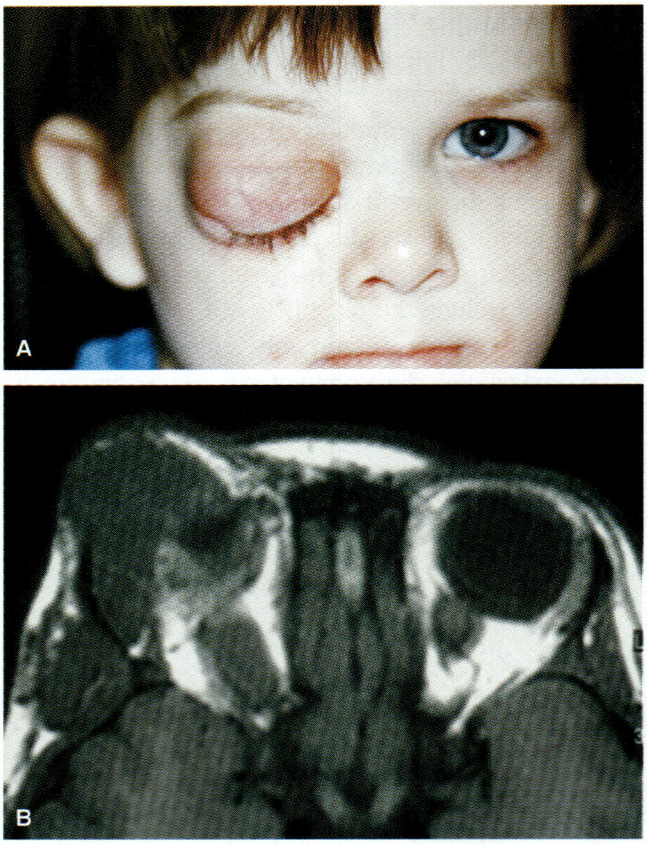

Figure 1–40. *A,* Clinical photograph of a large plexiform neurofibroma. *B,* T1-weighted axial MR scan of the NF-1 patient shown in 1–40A.

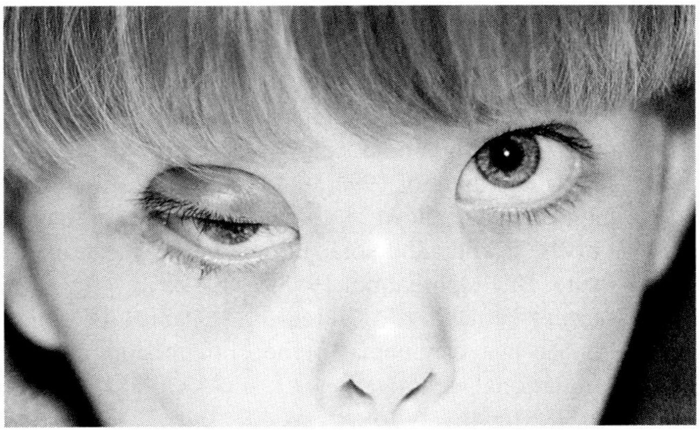

Figure 1–41. One day after excision of neurofibroma shown in Figure 1–40.

little systemic morbidity, but there have been isolated reports of other complications. Sutula and Glover noted eyelid necrosis after steroid injection in a young female.[193] Other case reports have noted other corticosteroid complications, such as linear fat atrophy, pigmentation, subcutaneous atrophy, adrenal suppression, and occlusion of the central retinal artery.[194–196] Neither Kushner nor this author have had these complications occur.[192] Oral steroids (oral prednisone) are also used, generally in a dose of 3 to 5 mg/kg daily. Most investigators have noted about a 30 percent complete resolution rate, 30 percent stabilization, and 40 percent failure rate with this technique.[197] Many pediatric ophthalmologists prefer this approach. This author has generally found intralesional injection more efficacious; however, the opposite response has been noted in a few cases. There have been a few reports of interferon use in this tumor; however, interferon-associated retinopathy has also been described; therefore, the relative safety and efficacy of that approach are uncertain.[198,199]

If these approaches are not effective, the author has debulked tumors that produce significant ocular morbidity (Figure 1–38). Care is taken to avoid damage to the levator and extraocular muscles, since these capillary hemangiomas are quite diffuse. In this author's experience, surprisingly, there have not been problems with hemostasis, although in a couple of cases, the author used the CO_2 laser to debulk a lesion, with hemostasis. Two series of 5 and 12 cases have used a similar approach, as we have, with good results.[196,200] Rarely, a similar process can develop in an adult.[200,201]

Lid Neurofibromas

Plexiform neurofibromas are often observed on the lid of patients with neurofibromatosis. The systemic disease and newer molecular genetics are discussed under "Pediatric Orbital Tumors." A typical lid neurofibroma is shown in Figure 1–39.[167] Often, there is congenital localized hypertrichosis.[202] The management of these lesions is difficult. Usually, in large tumors, only incomplete excision is possible, and over time, other eyelid and orbital neurofibromas become clinically detectable. Figures 1–40 and 1–41 show a patient with a large tumor prior to and 1 day after a partial excision.

REFERENCES

1. Preston DS, Stern RS. Nonmelanoma cancers of the skin. N Engl J Med 1992;327:1649–62.
2. Hollander L, Krugh FJ. Cancer of the eyelid. Am J Ophthalmol 1944;27:244–53.
3. Aurora AL, Blodi FC. Lesions of the eyelids. A clinicopathologic study. Surv Ophthalmol 1974;15:94–104.
4. Stetson CG, Schultz MD. Carcinoma of the eyelids: analysis of 301 cases and review of the literature. N Engl J Med 1949;241:725–32.
5. Smith AG, Brockman JL. Epithelial tumors of the eyelids. Am J Ophthalmol 1955;40:522–8.
6. Welch RB, Duke JR. Lesions of the lids: a statistical note. Am J Ophthalmol 1958;45:415–6.
7. Fayos JV, Wildermuth O. Carcinomas of the skin of the eyelids. Arch Ophthalmol 1962;67:298–301.
8. Kopf AW. Computer analysis of 3,500 basal cell carcinomas of the skin. J Dermatol 1979;6:267–81.
9. Ni Z. Histopathological classification of 3,510 cases with eyelid tumors. Chung Hua Yen Ko Tsa Chih 1996;32:435–7.
10. Margo CE, Mulla ZD. Malignant tumors of the eyelid: a population-based study of non-basal cell and non-squamous cell malignant neoplasms. Arch Ophthalmol 1998;116:195–8.
11. Miller SJ. Biology of basal cell carcinoma (part II). J Am Acad Dermatol 1991;24:161–75.
12. Kwa RE, Campana K, Moy RL. Biology of cutaneous squamous cell carcinoma. J Am Acad Dermatol 1992;26:1–26.
13. Ko CB, Walton S, Keczkes K, et al. The emerging epidemic of skin cancer. Br J Dermatol 1994;130: 269–72.
14. Green A, Battistutta D. Incidence of determinants of skin cancer in high-risk Australian population. Int J Cancer 1990;46:356–61.

15. Fitzpatrick TB, Sober AJ. Sunlight and skin cancer. N Engl J Med 1985;313:818–20.
16. Scotto J, Fears TR, Fraumeni JF. Incidence of non-melanoma skin cancer in the United States. Bethesda: National Cancer Institute (Publication No. NIH 82-2433)1981;1–14.
17. Magnus K. The Nordic profile of skin cancer incidence: a comparative epidemiological study of the three main types of skin cancer. Int J Cancer 1991;47:12–19.
18. Gupta AK, Cardella CJ, Haberman HF. Cutaneous malignant neoplasms in patients with renal transplants. Arch Dermatol 1986;122:1288–93.
19. Gilchrest BA, Eller MS, Geller AC, Yaar M. The pathogenesis of melanoma induced by ultraviolet radiation. N Engl J Med 1999;340:1341–8.
20. Cleaver JE. Defective repair replication of DNA in xeroderma pigmentosum. Nature 1968;218:652–6.
21. Gao S, Drouin R, Holmquist GP. DNA repair rates mapped along the human PGK 1 gene at nucleotide resolution. Science 1994;263:1438–40.
22. Tornaletti S, Pfeifer GP. Slow repair of pyrimidine dimers at *p53* mutation hotspots in skin cancer. Science 1994;263:1436–8.
23. Brash DE, Seetharam S, Kraemer K, et al. Photoproduct frequency is not the major determinant of UV base substitution hot spots or cold spots in human cells. Proc Natl Acad Sci USA 1987;84:3782–6.
24. Anathaswamy HN, Price JE, Goldberg LH, Bales ES. Detection and identification of activated oncogenes in human skin cancers occurring on sun-exposed body sites. Cancer Res 1998;48:3341–6.
25. Suarez HG, Daya-Grosjean L, Schlaifer D, et al. Activated oncogenes in human skin tumors from a repair-deficient syndrome, xeroderma pigmentosum. Cancer Res 1989;49:1223–8.
26. Wei Q, Matanoski GM, Farmer ER, et al. DNA repair and aging in basal cell carcinoma: a molecular epidemiology study. Proc Natl Acad Sci, USA 1993; 90:1614–8.
27. Moriwaki S, Ray S, Tarone RE, et al. The effect of donor age on the processing of UV damaged DNA by cultured human cells: reduced DNA repair capacity and increased DNA mutability. Mutat Res 1996;364:117–26.
28. Cleaver JE, Mitchell DL. UV radiation carcinogenesis. In: Holland JF, Bast RC Jr., Morton DL, et al., editors. Cancer Medicine, 4th edition, Vol. 1. Baltimore: Williamsen & Hickens;1997.
29. Kallassy M, Toftgard R, Ueda M, et al. Patched (*ptch*)-associated preferential expression of smoothened (smoh) in human basal cell carcinoma of the skin. Cancer Res 1997;57:4731–35.
30. Zaphiropoulos PG, Unden AB, Rahnama F, et al. *PTCH2*, a novel human patched gene, undergoing alternative splicing and up-regulated in basal cell carcinomas. Cancer Res 1999;59:787–92.
31. Cook BE Jr, Bartley GB. Epidemiologic characteristics and clinical course of patients with malignant eyelid tumors in an incidence cohort in Olmsted County, Minnesota. Ophthalmology 1999;106:746–50.
32. Reifler DM. Squamous cell carcinoma of the eyelid. Surv Ophthalmol 1996;30:349–65.
33. Lindgren G, Diffey BL, Larko O. Basal cell carcinoma of the eyelids and solar ultraviolet radiation exposure. Br J Ophthalmol 1998;82:1412–5.
34. Gonzalez-Fernandez F, Kaltreider SA, Patnaik BD, et al. Sebaceous carcinoma. Tumor progression through mutational inactivation of *p53*. Ophthalmology 1998;105:467–506.
35. Einspahr J, Alberts DS, Aickin M, et al. Expression of *p53* protein in actinic keratosis, adjacent, normal-appearing, and non-sun-exposed human skin. Cancer Epidemiol Biomarkers Prev 1997;6:583–7.
36. von Hogerlinden M, Rozell BL, Ahrlund-Richter L, Toftgard R. Squamous cell carcinomas and increased apoptosis in skin with inhibited rel/nuclear factor-kb signaling. Cancer Res 1999;59:3299–3303.
37. Fife K, Bower M. Recent insights into the pathogenesis of Kaposi's sarcoma. Br J Cancer 1996;73:1317–22.
38. Jaffe HW, Pellett PE. Human herpes virus 8 and Kaposi's sarcoma—some answers, more questions. N Engl J Med 1999;340:1912–3.
39. Gallo RC. The enigmas of Kaposi's sarcoma. Science 1998;282:1837–9.
40. Rigel DS, Fiedman RJ, Kopt AW. Lifetime risk for develomental skin cancer in US population: current estimate is now 1 in 5. J Am Acad Dermatol 1996; 35:1012–3.
41. Hall HI, Miller DR, Rogers JD, Bewerse B. Update on the incidence and mortality from melanoma in the United States. J Am Acad Dermatol 1999;40:35–42.
42. Borg A, Johannsson O, Hakansson S, et al. Novel germline *p16* mutation in familial malignant melanoma in southern Sweden. Cancer Res 1996; 56:2497–500.
43. Flores JF, Walker GJU, Glendening JM, et al. Loss of the p16INK4a and p15INK4b genes, as well as neighboring 9p21 markers, in sporadic melanoma. Cancer Res 1996;56:5023–32.
44. Bastain BC, LeBoit PE, Hamm H, et al. Chromosomal gains and losses in primary cutaneous melanomas detected by comparative genomic hybridization. Cancer Res 1998;58:2170–5.
45. Rook A, Whimster I. Keratoacanthoma—a thirty year retrospective. Br J Dermatol 1979;100:41–7.
46. Kingman J, Callen JP. Keratoacanthoma: a clinical study. Arch Dermatol 1984;120:736–40.
47. Grossniklaus HE, Wojno TH, Yanoff M, Font RL. Invasive keratoacanthoma of the eyelid and ocular adnexa. Opthalmology 1996;103:(6):937–41.
48. Amann J, Spaul CW, Mattfeld T, Lang GK. Eccrine spi-

radenoma of the eyelid. Klin Monatsbl Augenheilkd 1999;214:53–4.
49. Mawn LA, Jordan DR, Olberg B. Spindle-cell lipoma of the preseptal eyelid. Ophthal Plast Reconstr Surg 1998;14:174–7.
50. Sharara N, Lee WR, Weir C. Myolipoma of the eyelid. Graefes Arch Clin Exp Ophthalmol 1998;236:630–4.
51. Sandinha T, Lee WR, Reid R. Pleomorphic fibroma of the eyelid. Graefes Arch Clin Exp Ophthalmol 1998; 236:333–8.
52. Huey C, Jakobiec F, Iwamoto T, et al. Discoid lupus erythematosus of the eyelid. Ophthalmology 1983;90: 1389–98.
53. Tosti A, Tosti G, Giovannini A. Discoid lupus erythematosus solely involving the eyelids: report of three cases. J Am Acad Dermatol 1987;16:259–60.
54. Chikama T, Yoshino H, Nishida T, et al. Langerhans cell histiocytosis localized in the eyelid. Arch Opthalmol 1998;280(10):910–2.
55. Meffert JJ, Kennard CD, Davis TL, Quinn BD. Intradermal nodular fasciitis presenting as an eyelid mass. Int J Dermatol 1996;35:548–52.
56. Kang MC, Chang CH, Su MY, et al. Kimura's disease of bilateral upper eyelids: a case report. Kao Hsiung I Hsueh Ko Hsueh Tsa Chih 1999;15:239–43.
57. Batasakis JG. Melanoma (cutaneous and mucosal) of the head and neck. In: Barsakis JG, editor. Tumors of the head and neck. Baltimore, MD: Williams & Wilkins; 1974.
58. Breslow A, Macht SD. Evaluation and prognosis in stage I cutaneous melanoma. Plast Reconstr Surg 1978;61:342–6.
59. Callen JP, Chanda JJ, Stawiski MA. Malignant melanoma. Arch Dermatol 1978;114:369–70.
60. Kersten RC, Ewing-Chow D, Kulwin DR, Gallon M. Accuracy of clinical diagnosis of cutaneous eyelid lesions. Ophthalmology 1997;104:479–84.
61. Mannor GE, Wardell K, Wolfley DE, Nilsson GE. Laser doppler perfusion imaging of eyelid skin. Ophthal Plast Reconstr Surg 1996;12:178–85.
62. Bargon K, Curling OM, Paridaens ADA, Hungerford JL. The role of cytology in the diagnosis of periocular basal cell carcinomas. Ophthal Plast Reconstr Surg 1996;12:190–5.
63. Milverton EJ. A survey of basal cell carcinoma of the eyelid. Austral J Ophthalmol 1997;5:106–8.
64. Lund HZ. Tumors of the skin. Washington DC: Armed Forces Institute of Pathology; 1957. Sect I, Fasc 2: p. 205–34.
65. Karcioglu ZA, al-Hussain H, Svedberg AH. Cystic basal cell carcinoma of the orbit and eyelids. Ophthal Plast Reconstr Surg 1998;14:134–40.
66. Bonner PK, Bergman DK, McLean IW, LaPiana FG. Mixed type basal cell carcinoma of the eyelid. Ophthal Plast Reconstr Surg 1998;14:216–21.
67. Hunt MJ, Halliday GM, Weedon D, et al. Regression in basal cell carcinomas: an immunohistochemical analysis. Br J Dermatol 1994;130:1–8.
68. Rowe DE, Carroll RJ, Day CL Jr. Long-term recurrence rates in previously untreated (primary) basal cell carcinoma: implications for patient follow-up. J Dermatol Surg Oncol 1989;15:315–28.
69. Kahn HS, Tatham LM, Patel AV, et al. Increased cancer mortality following a history of nonmelanoma skin cancer. JAMA 1998;280:910–2.
70. Payne JW, Duke JR, Butner R, Elfrig DE. Basal cell carcinoma of the eyelids: a long-term follow-up study. Arch Ophthalmol 1969;81:553–8.
71. Howard GR, Nerad JA, Carter KD, Whitaker DC. Clinical characteristics associated with orbital invasion of cutaneous basal cell and squamous cell tumors of the eyelid. Am J Ophthalmol 1992;113:123–33.
72. Aldred WV, Ramierez VG, Nicholson DH. Intraocular invasion by basal cell carcinoma of the lid. Arch Ophthalmol 1980;98:1821–2.
73. Moro F, De Caro R, De Caro G, Ninfo V. Eyelid basal cell carcinoma with intracranial extension. Ophthal Plast Reconstr Surg 1998;14:56–76.
74. Beadles CF. Rodent ulcer. Trans Pathol Soc London 1984;45:176–81.
75. Conley J, Sachs ME, Romo T, et al. Metastatic basal cell carcinoma of the head and neck. Otolaryngol Head Neck Surg 1985;93:78–85.
76. Wieman TJ, Shively EH, Woodcock TM. Responsiveness of metastatic basal cell carcinoma to chemotherapy. A case report. Cancer 1983;52:1583–85.
77. Lo JS, Snow SN, Reizner GT, et al. Metastatic basal cell carcinoma: report of twelve cases with a review of the literature. J Am Acad Dermatol 1991;24:715–9.
78. Weinstock MA, Bogaars HA, Ashley M, et al. Nonmelanoma skin cancer mortality, a population based study. Arch Dermatol 1991;127:1194–7.
79. Boniuk M, Zimmerman LE. Sebaceous carcinoma of the eyelid, eyebrow, caruncle, and orbit. Trans Am Acad Ophthalmol Otolaryngol 1968;72:619–42.
80. Ni C, Kuo PK. Meibomian gland carcinoma: a clinicopathologic study of 156 cases with long-period follow-up of 100 cases. Jpn J Ophthalmol 1979;23:388–401.
81. Doxanas MT, Green WR. Sebaceous gland carcinoma. Review of 40 cases. Arch Ophthalmol 1984;102: 245–9.
82. Cavanagh HD, Green WR, Goldberg HK. Multicentric sebaceous adenocarcinoma of the meibomian gland. Am J Ophthalmol 1974;77:326-32.
83. Russell WG, Page DL, Hough AJ, Rogers LW. Sebaceous carcinoma of meibomian gland origin: the diagnostic importance of pagetoid spread of neoplastic cells. Am J Clin Pathol 1980;73:504–11.
84. Rao N, Hidayat AA, McLean IW, Zimmerman LE. Sebaceous carcinomas of the ocular adnexa: a clin-

icopathologic study of 104 cases with five-year follow-up data. Hum Pathol 1982;13:113–22.
85. Wolfe JT III, Yeatts RP, Wick MR, et al. Sebaceous carcioma of the eyelid. Errors in clinical and pathologic diagnosis. Am J Surg Pathol 1984;8:597–606.
86. Lee SC, Roth LM. Sebaceous carcinoma of the eyelid with pagetoid involvement of the bulbar and palpebral conjunctiva. J Cutan Pathol 1977;4:134–45.
87. Sinard JH. Immunohistochemical distinction of ocular sebaceous carcinoma from basal cell and squamous cell carcinoma. Arch Ophthalmol 1999;117:776–83.
88. Sugiki H, Ansai S, Imaizumi T, et al. Ocular sebaceous carcinoma. Two unusual cases and their histochemical and immunohistochemical findings. Dermatology 1996;192:364–7.
89. Khan JA, Doane JF, Grove AS Jr. Sebaceous and meibomian carcinomas of the eyelid: recognition, diagnosis and management. Ophthal Plast Reconstr Surg 1991;7:61–6.
90. Ginsberg J. Present status of meibomian gland carcinoma. Arch Ophthalmol 1965;73:271–7.
91. Khalil MK, Lorenzetti HD. Sebaceous gland carcinoma of the lid. Can J Ophthalmol 1980;15:117–21.
92. Straatsma BR. Meibomian gland tumors. Arch Ophthalmol 1956;56:71–93.
93. Scheie HG, Yanoff M, Frayer WC. Carcinoma of sebaceous glands of the eyelid. Arch Ophthalmol 1964; 72:800–3.
94. Foster CS, Allansmith MR. Chronic unilateral blepharoconjunctivitis caused by sebaceous carcinoma. Am J Ophthalmol 1978;86:218–20.
95. Sweebe EC, Cogan DG. Adenocarcinoma of the meibomian gland: a pseudochalazion entity. Arch Ophthalmol 1959;61:282–90.
96. Condon GP, Brownstein S, Codere F. Sebaceous carcinoma of the eyelid masquerading as superior limbic keratoconjunctivitis. Arch Ophthalmol 1985;103: 1525–9.
97. Epstein GA, Putterman AM. Sebaceous adenocarcinoma of the eyelid. Ophthal Surg 1983;11:935–40.
98. Mashburn MA, Chonkich GD, Chase DR. Meibomian gland adenocarcinomas of the eyelid with preauricular lymph node metastasis. Laryngoscope 1985;95: 1141–3.
99. Cohen PR, Kohn SR, Kurzrock R. Association of sebaceous gland tumors and internal malignancy: the Muir-Torre syndrome. Am J Med 1991;90:606–13.
100. Finan MC, Connally SM. Sebaceous gland tumors and systemic disease: a clinicopathologic analysis. Medicine 1984;78:323–42.
101. Jakobiec FA, Zimmerman LE, La Piana F, et al. Unusual eyelid tumors with sebaceous differentiation in the Muir-Torre syndrome. Rapid clinical regrowth and frank squamous transformation after biopsy. Ophthalmology 1988;95:1543–48.
102. Lee SB, Saw SB, Eong KG, Chan TK, et al. Incidence of eyelid cancers in Singapore from 1968 to 1995. Br J Ophthalmol 1999;83:595-7.
103. Doxanas MT, Iliff WJ, Iliff NT, Green WR. Squamous cell carcinoma of the eyelids. Ophthalmology 1987; 94:538–41.
104. Dailey JR, Kennedy RH, Flaharty PM, et al. Squamous cell carcinoma of the eyelid. Ophthal Plast Reconstr Surg 1994;10:153–9.
105. Kwitko ML, Boniuk M, Zimmerman LE. Eyelid tumors with reference to lesions confused with squamous cell carcinoma. Incidence and errors in diagnosis. Arch Ophthalmol 1963;63:693–7.
106. Rao NA, Dunn SA, Romero JL, Stout W. Bilateral carcinomas of the eyelid. Am J Ophthalmol 1986;101: 480–2.
107. Baclesse F, Dollfus MA. The roentgenotherapy of cancers of the eyelids. Arch Ophthal (Par) 1960;20: 473–89.
108. Szymanski FJ. Keratoacanthoma. In: Graham JH, Johnson WC, Helwig EG, editors. Dermal pathology. Hagerstown: Harper & Row; 1972. p. 625.
109. Lund HZ. How often does squamous cell carcinoma of the skin metastasize? Arch Dermatol 1965;92:635–7.
110. Epstein E, Epstein NN, Bragg K, Linden G. Metastases from squamous cell carcinomas of the skin. Arch Dermatol 1968;97:245–51.
111. Csaky KG, Custer P. Perineural invasion of the orbit by squamous cell carcinoma. Ophthal Surg 1993;21: 218–20.
112. Shulman J. Treatment of malignant tumours of the eyelids by plastic surgery. Br J Plast Surg 1962;15:37–47.
113. McNab AA, Francis IC, Benger R, Crompton JL. Perineural spread of cutaneous squamous cell carcinoma via the orbit: clinical features and outcome in 21 cases. Ophthalmology 1997;104:1457–62.
114. Patel A, Halliday JM, Cooke BE, Barnetson RS. Evidence that regression in keratoacanthoma is immunologically mediated: a comparison with squamous cell carcinoma. Br J Dermatol 1994;131:789–98.
115. Farmer ER, Gonin R, Hanna MP. Discordance in the histopathologic diagnosis of melanoma and melanocytic nevi between expert pathologists. Hum Pathol 1996;27:528–31.
116. Garner A, Koornneff L, Levene A, Collin JRO. Malignant melanoma of the eyelid skin: histopathology and behavior. Br J Ophthalmol 1985;69:180–6.
117. Berg P, Lindelof B. Difference in malignant melanoma between children and adolescents. Arch Dermatol 1997;133:295–7.
118. Koh HK. Cutaneous melanoma. N Engl J Med 1991; 325:171–92.
119. Clark WH Jr, Elder DE, Van Horn M. The biologic forms of malignant melanoma. Hum Pathol 1986; 17:443–50.

120. Hartstein ME, Biesman B, Kincaid MC. Cutaneous malignant melanoma metastatic to the eyelid. Ophthal Surg Lasers 1998;29:993–5.
121. Corona R, Mele A, Amini M, et al. Interobserver variability on the histopathologic diagnosis of cutaneous melanoma and other pigmented skin lesions. J Clin Oncol 1996;14:1218–23.
122. Koh HK. Prognosis in melanoma — what have we learned? Arch Dermatol 1986;122:993–4.
123. Worth AJ, Gallagher RP, Elwood JM, et al. Pathologic prognostic factors for cutaneous malignant melanoma. The Western Canada Melanoma Study. Int J Cancer 1989;43:370–5.
124. Karakousis CP, Emrich LJ, Rao K. Tumor thickness and prognosis in clinical stage I malignant melanoma. Cancer 1989;64:1432–6.
125. Day CL Jr, Mihm MC Jr, Sober AJ, et al. Narrower margins for clinical stage I malignant melanoma. N Engl J Med 1982;306:479–82.
126. Rogers GS, Kopf AW, Rigel DS, et al. Hazard-rate analysis in stage I malignant melanoma. Arch Dermatol 1986;122:999–1002.
127. Gatchell FC, Minor D. Malignant melanoma of the eye, metastatic after twenty-nine years: a case report. J Okla State Med Assoc 1972;65:211–3.
128. Hall WE. Malignant melanoma of the uveal tract: report of a case with death 30 years after enucleation. Arch Ophthalmol 1950;44:381–94.
129. Kirk HA. Delayed metastasis from choroidal melanoma. Surg Ophthalmol 1966;11:651–6.
130. Rosenkranz ZL, Schroeder C. Recurrent malignant melanoma following a 46 year disease-free interval. NY State J Med 1985;85:95.
131. Fournier GA, Albert DM, Arrigg CA, et al. Resection of solitary metastasis: an approach to palliative treatment of hepatic involvement with choroidal melanoma. Arch Ophthalmol 1984;102:80–2.
132. Gershenwald JE, Buzaid AC, Ross MI. Classification and staging of melanoma. Hematol Oncol Clin North Am 1998;12:737–65.
133. Volmer R. Malignant melanoma. A multivariate analysis of prognostic factors. Pathol Ann 1989;24:383–475.
134. Arnold AC, Bullock JD, Foos RY. Metastatic eyelid carcinoma. Ophthalmology 1985;92:114–9.
135. Riley FC. Metastatic tumors of the eyelids. Am J Ophthalmol 1970;69:259–64.
136. Weinstein GW, Goldman JN. Metastatic adenocarcinoma of the breast masquerading as chalazion. Am J Ophthalmol 1963;56:960–3.
137. Rodrigues MM, Font RL, Shannon GM. Metastatic mucus-secreting mammary carcinoma in the eyelid. A report of two cases. Br J Ophthalmol 1974;58:877–81.
138. Mottow-Lippa L, Jakobiec FA, Iwamoto T. Pseudoinflammatory metastatic breast carcinoma of the orbit and lids. Ophthalmology 1981;88:575–80.
139. Cowan TW: Adenocarcinoma of the lid, secondary to adenocarcinoma of the stomach. Arch Ophthalmol 1952;48:496–7.
140. Hart WM. Metastatic carcinoma to the eye and orbit. Int Ophthalmol Clin 1962;1:465–82.
141. Brownstein MH, Helwig EB. Patterns of cutaneous metastasis. Arch Dermatol 1972;105:862–8.
142. Reingold IM. Cutaneous metastases from internal carcinoma. Cancer 1966;19:162–8.
143. Muenzler WS, Olson JR, Eubank MD. Metastatic tumors of the eyelid: a report of two cases and review of the literature. Am J Ophthalmol 1963;55:791–4.
144. Purgason PA, Hornblass A, Harrison W. Metastatic Merkel cell carcinoma to the eye. Ophthalmology 1991;98:1432–4.
145. Gritz DC, Rao NA. Metastatic carcinoid tumor diagnosis from a caruncular mass. Am J Ophthalmol 1991;112:470–1.
146. Kaposi M. Idiopathisches mutiples Pigmentsarkom der Haut. Arch Dermatol Syph (Berlin) 1872;4:265–73.
147. Kalinske M, Leone CR Jr. Kaposi's sarcoma involving the eye lids and conjunctiva. Ann Ophthalmol 1982;14:497–9.
148. Graham T. Idiopathic multiple hemorrhagic sarcoma. Arch Ophthalmol 1942;27:1188.
149. Sacks I. Kaposi's disease manifesting in the eye. Br J Ophthalmol 1956;40:574.
150. Quere MA, Basset A, Camain R. Les localisations oculaires de l'angioreticulosarcomatose de Kaposi. Ophthalmologica 1963;146:23.
151. Weiter JJ, Jakobiec FA, Iwamoto T. The clinical and morphologic characteristics of Kaposi's sarcoma of the conjunctiva. Am J Ophthalmol 1980;89:546–52.
152. Lahav M, Albert DM, Bahr R, Craft J. Eyelid tumors of sweat gland origin. Albrecht von Graefe Klin Ophthalmol 1981;216:301–11.
153. Cohen KL, Peiffer RL, Lipper S. Mucinous sweat gland adenocarcinoma of the eye. Am J Ophthalmol 1981;92:183–8.
154. Gardner TW, O'Grady RB. Mucinous adenocarcinoma of the eyelid. A case report. Arch Ophthalmol 1984;102:912.
155. Addison DJ. Malacoplakia of the eyelid. Ophthalmology 1986;93:1064–7.
156. Caya JG, Hidayat AA, Weiner JM. A clinicopathologic study of 21 cases of adenoid squamous cell carcinoma of the eyelid and periorbital region. Am J Ophthalmol 1985;99:291–7.
157. Perez RC, Nicholson DH. Malherbe's calcifying epithelioma (pilomatrixoma) of the eyelid. Arch Ophthalmol 1979;97:314–5.
158. Glatt HJ, Proia AD, Tsoy EA, et al. Malignant syringoma of the eyelid. Ophthalmology 1984;91:970–90.
159. Seregard S. Apocrine adenocarcinoma arising in Moll gland cystadenoma. Ophthalmology 1993;100:1716–9.

160. Dailey JR, Helm KF, Goldberg SH. Tricholemmal carcinoma of the eyelid. Am J Ophthalmol 1993;115: 118–9.
161. Robinson ML, Knibbe MA, Roberson JB. Microcystic adnexal carcinoma: report of a case. J Oral Maxillofac Surg 1995;53:846–9.
162. Searl SS, Boynton JR, Markowitch W, DiSant'Agnese PA. Malignant Merkel cell neoplasm of the eyelid. Arch Ophthalmol 1984;102:907–11.
163. Kirham N, Cole MD. Merkel cell carcinoma: a malignant neuroendocrine tumour of the eye lid. Br J Ophthalmol 1983;67:600–3.
164. Lins ME, Wirtschafter JD. Polymorphic B-cell lymphoma of the eyelid. Am J Ophthalmol 1984;98: 634–5.
165. Stenson S, Ramsay DL. Ocular findings in mycosis fungoides. Arch Ophthalmol 1981;99:272–7.
166. Marshmann WE, McNab AA. Merkel cell tumor occurring simultaneously in the upper and lower eyelids. Austral NZ Ophthalmol 1996;24:377–80.
167. Metz KA, Jacob M, Schmidt U, et al. Merkel cell carcinoma of the eyelid: histological and immunohistochemical features with special respect to differential diagnosis. Graefes Arch Clin Exp Ophthalmol 1998; 236:561–6.
168. Soltau JB, Smith ME, Custer PL. Merkel cell carcinoma of the eyelid. Am J Ophthalmol 1996;121:331–2.
169. Dini M, Lo Russo G. Merkel cell carcinoma of the eyelid. Eur J Ophthalmol 1997;7:108–12.
170. Lee SB, Saw SM, Eong KG, et al. Incidence of eyelid cancers in Singapore from 1968 to 1995. Br J Ophthalmol 1999;83:595–7.
171. Boynton JR, Markowitch W Jr. Mucinous eccrine carcinoma of the eyelid. Arch Ophthalmol 1998;116: 1130–1.
172. Wollensak G, Witschel H, Bohm N. Signet ring cell carcinoma of the eccrine sweat glands in the eyelid. Ophthalmology 1996;103(11):1788–93.
173. Hoppenreijs VP, Reuser TT, Mooy CM, et al. Syringomatous carcinoma of the eyelid and orbit: a clinical and histopathological challenge. Br J Ophthalmol 1997;81:668–72.
174. Esmaeli B, Ramseay J, Chorney KA, et al. Sclerosing sweat-duct carcinoma (malignant syringoma) of the upper eyelid. A patient report with immunohistochemical and ultrastructural analysis. Ophthal Plast Reconstr Surg 1998;14:441–5.
175. Boynton JR, Markowitch W Jr. Porocarcinoma of the eyelid. Ophthalmology 1997;104:1626–8.
176. Sudesh R, Siddique S, Pace L. Primary eyelid mucinous adenocarcinoma of eccrine orgin. Ophthal Surg Lasers 1999;30:394–5.
177. Lapidus CS, Sutula FC, Stadecker MJ, et al. Angiosarcoma of the eyelid: yellow plaques causing ptosis. J Am Acad Dermatol 1996;34:308–10.
178. Kirsch LS, Brownstein S, Codere F. Immunoblastic T-cell lymphoma presenting as an eyelid tumor. Ophthalmology 1990;97:1352–7.
179. Tanzi E, Edelman M, Rosenbaum PS. Ki-1 positive anaplastic large-cell lymphoma of the eyelid. Arch Ophthalmol 1999;117:955–8.
180. Cooke BE Jr, Bartley GB, Pittelkow MR. Ophthalmic abnormalities in patients with cutaneous T-cell lymphoma. Trans Am Ophthalmol Soc 1998;96:309–24.
181. Smith SW, Carruthers JD. Intractable periocular hemangioma of infancy. Can J Ophthalmol 1985;20:220–4.
182. Haik BG, Karcioglu ZA, Gordon RA, Pechous BP. Capillary hemangioma (infantile periocular hemangioma). Survey Ophthalmol 1994;38:339–426.
183. Drolet BA, Esterly NB, Frieden IJ. Hemangiomas in children. N Engl J Med 1999;341:173–81.
184. Stigmar G, Crawford JS, Ward CM, Thomson HG. Ophthalmic sequelae of infantile hemangiomas of the eyelids and orbit. Am J Ophthalmol 1978;85:806–13.
185. Haik BG, Jakobiec FA, Ellsworth RM, Jones IS. Capillary hemangioma of the lid and orbit. An analysis of the clinical features and therapeutic results in 101 cases. Ophthalmology 1979;86:760–92.
186. Robb RM. Refractive errors associated with hemangiomas of the eyelids and orbit in infancy. Am J Ophthalmol 1977;83:52–8.
187. Thierfelder S, Hagen R, Sold-Darseff JE, Uhlmann A. Magnesium seeding in therapy of pediatric hemangioma of the temporal region, lower eyelid and orbit. Klin Monatsbl Augenheilkd 1996;208:243–5.
188. Liekens S, Verbeken E, Vandeputte M, et al. A novel animal model for hemangiomas: inhibition of hemangioma development by the angiogenesis inhibitor TNP-470. Cancer Res 1999;59:2376–83.
189. Fost NC, Esterly NB. Successful treatment of juvenile hemangiomas with prednisone. J Pediatr 1968;72: 351–7.
190. Hiles DA, Plichard WA. Corticosteroid control of neonatal hemangiomas of the orbit and ocular adnexa. Am J Ophthalmol 1971;71:1003–8.
191. Kushner BJ. Local steroid therapy in adnexal hemangioma. Ann Ophthalmol 1979;11:1005–9.
192. Kushner BJ. Hemangioma. Arch Ophthalmol 2000; 118:835–6.
193. Sutula FC, Glover AT. Eyelid necrosis following intralesional corticosteroid injection for a capillary hemangioma. Ophthalmic Surg 1987;18: 103–5.
194. Ruttum MS, Abrams GW, Harris GJ, Ellis MK. Bilateral retinal embolization associated with intralesional corticosteroid injection for capillary hemangioma of infancy. J Pediatr Ophthalmol Strabismus, 1993;30:4–7.

195. Walker RS, Custer PL, Nerad JA. Surgical excision of periorbital capillary hemangiomas. Ophthalmology 1994;101:1333–40.
196. Droste PJ, Ellis FD, Sondhi N, Helveston EM. Linear subcutaneous fat atrophy after corticosteroid injection of periocular hemangiomas. Am J Ophthalmol 1988;105:65–9.
197. Loughnan MS, Elder J, Kemp A. Treatment of a massive orbital-capillary hemangioma with interferon alpha-2b: short term results. Arch Ophthalmol 1992;110:1366–7.
198. Guyer DR, Tiedeman J, Yannuzzi LA, et al. Interferon-associated retinopathy. Arch Ophthalmol 1993;111: 350–6.
199. Deans RM, Harris GJ, Kivlin JD. Surgical dissection of capillary hemangiomas. Arch Ophthalmol 1992;110: 1743–7.
200. Murphy BA, Dawood GS, Margo CE. Acquired capillary hemangioma of the eyelid in an adult. Am J Ophthalmol 1997;124:403–4.
201. Rumelt S, You TT, Remulla HD, et al. Prepartum mixed type cavernous-capillary hemangioma arising in nevus flammeus. Ophthalmology 1999;106: 219–22.
202. Ettl A, Marinkovic M, Koorneef L. Localized hypertrichosis associated with periorbital neurofibroma: clinical findings and differential diagnosis. Ophthalmology 1996;103:942–8.

2

Nonsurgical Treatment of Lid Tumors

Optimum management of all eyelid malignancies depends on correct histologic diagnosis, assessment of tumor margins, and the delineation of the extent of systemic spread. In many eyelid cancers, the choice of therapy is not critical and is partially predicated on the surgical skill and expertise available with other therapeutic modalities. A focal malignancy can be successfully treated with surgery, radiation, or cryotherapy. In at least four clinical settings, the choice of optimal therapy is crucial: (1) in either morpheaform basal cell carcinoma or sebaceous carcinoma, especially with pagetoid spread, it is almost impossible to assess tumor margins without histologic evaluation. In such cases cryotherapy is contraindicated. Unfortunately, as many as 40 percent of basal cell carcinomas are relatively diffuse, and this fact is responsible for most of the 10 percent failure rate noted with cryotherapy;[1] (2) in tumors that have extended into the orbit, bones, or sinuses, the ability to determine tumor margins, even with frozen sections, is limited. If an attempt is made to salvage these eyes, usually either very wide field excision or the use of adjuvant therapy (either chemotherapy or radiation) is required (see below); (3) there is very little data on immunotherapy and chemotherapy for eyelid tumors, and as discussed below, these modalities have a significantly lower control rate than surgery, radiation, or cryotherapy. The author limits the use of chemotherapy and immunotherapy to patients with advanced tumors; often those with a cancer diathesis (such as xeroderma pigmentosum and basal cell nevus syndrome) or those who have recurrent or refractory tumors after multiple other therapies; and (4) if there is a lack of local expertise with a given therapeutic modality, that treatment should not be used. Especially with radiation, we have seen a number of complications that occurred as a result of either poor treatment planning or delivery.

In all patients referred with a lid malignancy, except Kaposi's sarcoma (KS) in acquired immunodeficiency syndrome (AIDS) (see below), we either review the outside biopsy slides or obtain a small incisional biopsy prior to definitive therapy. This author has seen two disasters that resulted from the attending surgeon relying on an outside interpretation of pathology slides. In both cases, inappropriate management occurred, and the author strongly believes that the surgeon should review all slides prior to therapy, with an ophthalmic pathologist or dermatopathologist.

As part of our initial evaluation of all lid tumor patients, a complete review of systems is obtained to determine if metastatic disease is present (weight loss, adenopathy, respiratory or liver symptomatology). Regional lymph nodes (preauricular, submandibular, cervical) are palpated to detect gross evidence of local tumor spread.

In patients with large, diffuse malignancies, in whom orbital exenteration is likely to be necessary, extensive sinus, central nervous system, and systemic evaluations are indicated. Orbit, sinus, and brain magnetic resonance imaging (MRI) scans with contrast should be obtained. Figure 2–1 shows a very small focus of cutaneous melanoma that has tracked back into the orbit along a superior orbital nerve; this neoplasm was not detectable with high resolution, thin-section computerized tomography (CT). We have also managed several cases of squamous cell carcinomas of the face, some removed without histiologic evaluation where "the first sign of malignancy" was orbital invasion with neurologic dysfunc-

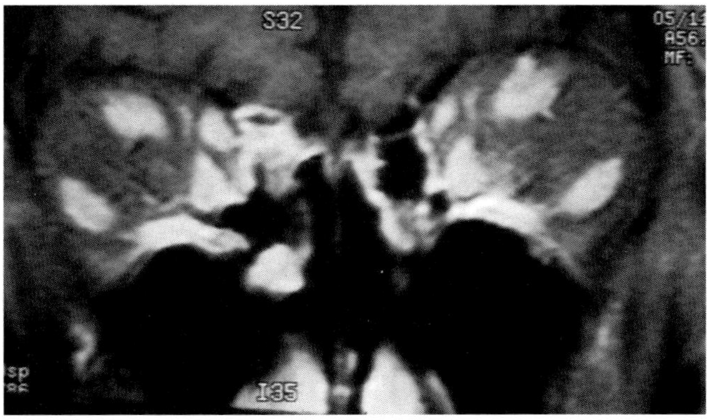

Figure 2–1. MRI demonstrates a small focus of cutaneous melanoma that has tracked back into the left orbit along the superior orbital nerve. This lesion was not detectable on thin-section CT.

tion. In epithelial malignancies or eyelid melanomas with possible systemic spread, chest-abdominal scans and serum liver function tests (lactic dehydrogenase, glutamyl transpeptidase, and alkaline phosphatase) are obtained prior to surgery. If metastatic disease is documented, palliation, instead of definitive surgery, is the treatment of choice.

If orbital invasion is suspected, as when the lid is adherent to underlying bone, or when there are unilateral abnormalities of ocular motility, thin-section, high-resolution CT or MRI scans are obtained. Often, the degree of orbital involvement may be subtle, but with modern imaging equipment, orbital invasion can often be documented. Figure 2–2A shows the clinical appearance and Figure 2–2B the CT pattern of a medial canthal basal cell carcinoma that has invaded the orbit. The choice of therapy for most eyelid malignancies is based on the tumor's size and location and the clinician's relative expertise with surgery and other therapeutic modalities. Almost all rare eyelid malignancies have been managed surgically.

To simplify the organization of this chapter, the management of each of the more common eyelid malignancies has been overviewed and then nonsurgical treatment data for each modality have been summarized.

BASAL CELL CARCINOMA

Focal basal cell carcinomas can be cured with a number of modalities, including cryotherapy, radiation, or surgery, with histologic monitoring of tumor edges.[2] Locally aggressive malignancies with extensive orbital invasion or bone involvement often require exenteration, although some can be cured with ocular preservation. In basal cell carcinomas with medial canthal penetration into the orbit, not involving the sinus or affecting the medial rectus, the author has removed the area from the medial periosteum to the edge of the medial rectus, en bloc, with long-term cure. If a more diffuse tumor is noted, but is contained in a portion of the orbit, adjuvant chemotherapy or radiation followed by aggressive local resection can sometimes be effective. Occasionally, such tumors are sufficiently advanced to require multimodality surgical and radiation treatment (Figure 2–3). The surgical management of all lid tumors, including basal cell carcinoma, is discussed in Chapter 3. Other therapeutic modalities are discussed below.

More than 95 percent of all eyelid basal cell carcinomas not involving the orbit or bone and < 20 mm in diameter, can be cured.[3,4] Larger tumors, espe-

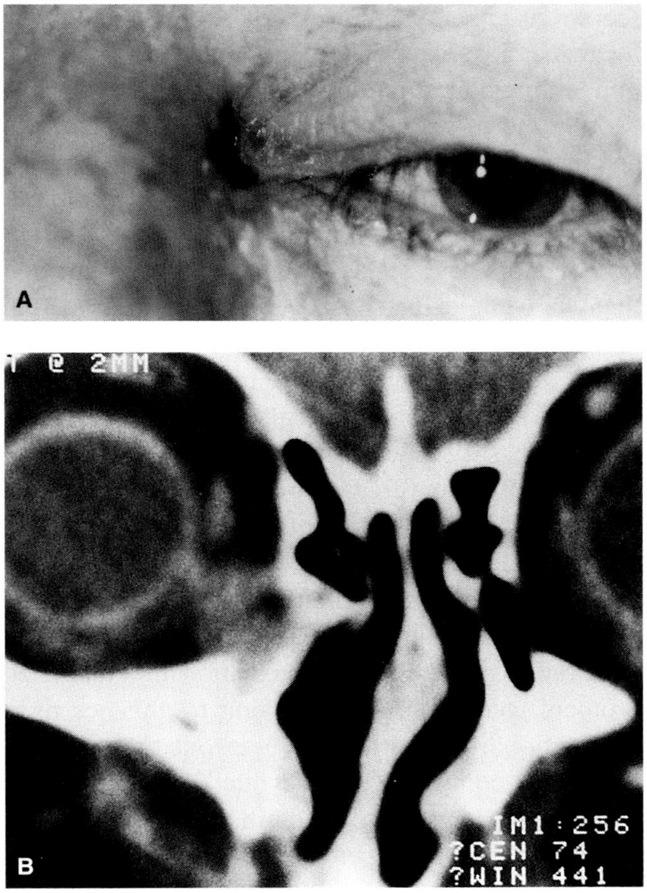

Figure 2–2. *A*, Clinical photograph of medial canthal basal cell carcinoma with erosion into orbit. *B*, Reformatted coronal CT demonstrates anterior orbital extension of basal cell carcinoma.

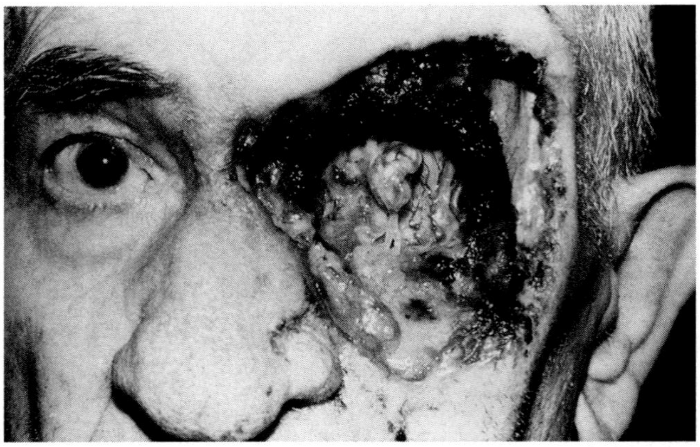

Figure 2–3. Far advanced basal cell carcinoma requiring multimodality therapy to preserve life.

cially if there is bone involvement, have an approximately 50 percent cure rate even with multimodality therapy.[4] In almost all series, tumors that have failed locally after treatment have a lower cure rate with repeat or second therapy, as would be expected.

There is a paucity of data on the use of chemotherapy as either an adjuvant or a single modality for localized, advanced epithelial eyelid tumors. In the ophthalmic literature, Luxenburg and colleagues and Morley and co-workers have reported a few basal cell carcinoma patients in whom chemotherapy has been used for this purpose.[5,6] Others have noted similar positive results in isolated case reports.[7,8] Other investigators have stressed caution and documented that while clinically a basal cell carcinoma treated in this manner may appear to have undergone complete regression, biopsy can demonstrate residual tumor.[5,9] In a trial of 28 patients with advanced squamous or basal cell carcinoma, 5 of which involved periocular structures, complete response to chemotherapy was noted in 28 percent of cases. In the 13 of those cases in which chemotherapy was used as an adjuvant with either radiation or surgery for advanced, localized disease, 12 maintained long-term regression.[10] Similarly, results with a modified protocol using an electric current to enhance drug penetration into a variety of cutaneous tumors had a 56 percent complete response rate.[11]

Several groups have used other chemotherapy or immunotherapy treatments either for carcinomas in situ or frank malignancy. Topical 5-fluorouracil has been used for many years to treat in situ lesions with recurrence rates between 20 and 50 percent.[12] Retinoids and beta carotenes have been tried with marginal results.[13,14] Various interferons that affect tumor cell cycling have also been used, with response rates reported between 20 and 70 percent.[15,16] Chang and co-workers reported on a modified topical use of chemotherapy with iontophoresis to deliver cisplatin in 15 tumors, with complete response in 4 and a partial response in 7 tumors.[17] Orenberg and colleagues used a sustained-release intralesional 5-fluorouracil implant in 20 patients with nonocular disease.[18] Wang and colleagues used a protoporphyrin derivative and photosensitization in 19 basal cell carcinomas, with complete resolution in 8 (42%).[19]

There is some controversy regarding the recurrence rates of basal cell carcinoma after treatment.[20–21] In large series, recurrences have been observed many years after treatment, and most dermatopathologists have noted that very late recurrences, even 5 or more years after treatment, are not rare.[18] In a meta-analysis, only two-thirds of recurrences were detected within 3 years of initial treatment.[18] In addition, in a patient with either a basal cell or squamous cell carcinoma, the risk for developing another new skin malignancy is as high as 20 percent at 18 months and 36 percent in 5 years.[22,23]

Rarely, basal cell carcinomas metastasize. Metastatic basal cell carcinoma usually goes to the local lymph nodes and then to the lung. As mentioned previously, < 1 percent of far advanced cases develop clinically detectable metastases; approximately 270 cases have been reported worldwide.[24] Most patients survive less than 1 year, although long-term response to chemotherapy has been reported.[24–27]

SEBACEOUS GLAND AND SQUAMOUS CELL CARCINOMA

Sebaceous gland and squamous cell carcinomas are managed by local excision, orbital exenteration, radical neck dissection, radiation, or chemotherapy, depending on their stage at presentation. The surgical resection for a focal sebaceous or squamous gland carcinoma is relatively straightforward. We routinely examine the patient carefully for evidence of pagetoid spread or multicentric tumor origins. The lids are double-everted, and if there are any areas of conjunctival alteration, such as telangiectasia, papillary change, or a mass, conjunctival punch biopsies are taken in addition to the surgical resection of the lid lesion.[28] In some cases, the degree of tumor involvement is not clinically apparent. Figure 2–4 shows a patient referred as a candidate for resection of a third to a half of the upper eyelid. As shown, both eyelids were removed to obtain tumor-free margins. Extensive orbital involvement mandates exenteration. In a few cases with only superficial, intraepithelial pagetoid spread of sebaceous carcinoma, cryotherapy has been reported to have good results.[29] In our experience, however, with long-term follow-up, most of these eyes with superficial sebaceous carcinoma have not done well.

If there is local nodal disease without distant metastases, chemotherapy, radiation, or radical neck dissection may be indicated.[30–33]

Radiation has been used to treat some sebaceous gland carcinomas, but there is a paucity of data, and results have not been uniformly excellent.[28,34,35] Pardo and co-workers reported excellent results in a mixed series of 10 sebaceous carcinoma patients, in whom radiation was used as sole treatment, as an adjuvant to surgery, or for local lymph node spread, with good results.[33] Most ocular oncologists use this therapeutic modality in patients who are not surgical candidates, in cases with widespread disease where palliation is the goal, or in patients who refuse exenteration for advanced local disease. Fewer than 30 cases have been reported where radiation was used as a single modality to cure primary tumor.[33] An example of a sebaceous carcinoma prior to and after 45 gray (Gy) of electron irradiation is shown in Figure 2–5A, B.

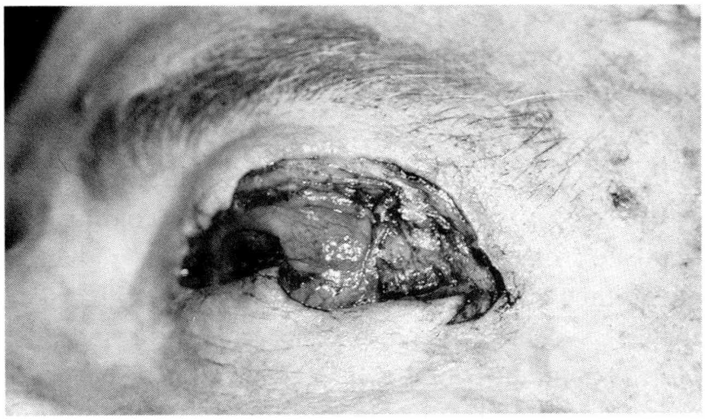

Figure 2–4. Case referred for what was thought to be candidate for resection of one-third to one-half of upper eyelid. Both eyelids were removed to obtain tumor-free margins.

LID MELANOMA

Generally, cutaneous melanomas that involve the eyelids are surgically managed. In contrast to earlier ideas, as Day and co-workers have emphasized, there is a poor correlation between the size of tumor-free clear margins and survival.[36] Some general surgeons remove melanomas with < 10 mm of margins.[33] We tend to resect lid melanomas that involve only the eyelid in this manner, using smaller margins so that we may retain the globe. While most dermatopathologists correctly point out the problems of frozen section control of melanomas, we use that technique, since if an eye is to be preserved, smaller margins are necessary than in most other body sites.[34]

If the melanoma is > 1.5 mm thick, we obtain a complete metastatic evaluation as outlined above. Lid melanomas that involve the orbit are usually treated with exenteration, if no evidence of metastatic disease is present. Melanomas have a variable behavior; we have treated some very large tumors

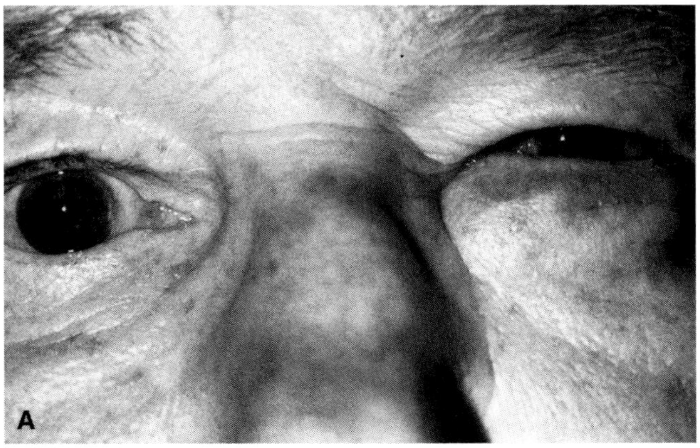

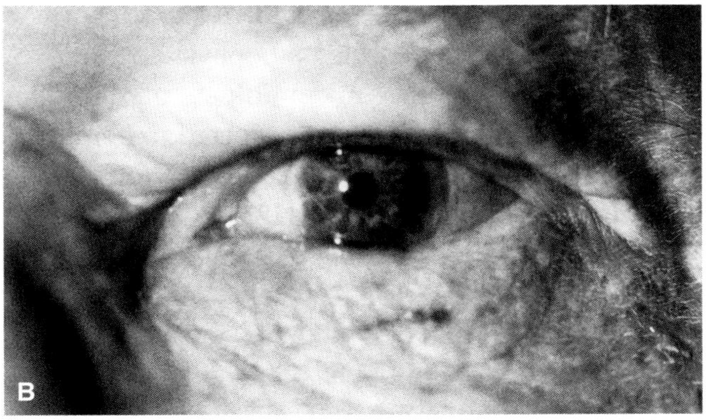

Figure 2–5. *A,* Sebaceous gland carcinoma with metastases prior to local irradiation. *B,* After 45 Gy of photon irradiation, tumor shows marked regression.

with local excision, and some of these patients who refused exenteration have remained tumor free 5 years after surgery.[37] Similarly, some patients with lid melanoma and localized nodal disease have apparently been cured with both local lid excision and radical neck dissection (personal experience). We have also seen a few patients with spontaneous complete regression.[38]

The most important prognostic factors in lid melanoma are tumor thickness, tumor ulceration, gender, and patient age. Women have better survival rates than men. Patients with tumors < 1 mm in thickness have 8-year tumor-related mortality of < 10 percent, while those > 3.5 mm thick have 8-year survival of < 40 percent.[36]

Radiation is rarely used for lid melanomas.[39,40] Radiation-induced destruction of a large, diffuse melanoma which involves the lid, conjunctiva, and orbit produces sufficient damage to the lacrimal gland and goblet cells to usually necessitate an anterior exenteration, even though the melanoma was eradicated.

In poor-risk cutaneous melanomas, there was preliminary evidence that adjunctive therapy with interferon-alpha 2a was lengthening the disease-free interval; however, longer follow-up has shown that it is less effective in preventing metastatic disease.[39] The management of metastatic melanoma is not within the scope of this book, although a small section under uveal melanoma therapy covers some of its aspects.

KAPOSI'S SARCOMA

As discussed in Chapter 1, human herpes virus-8 (HHV-8) is important in the pathophysiology of KS, helping to explain the epidemiology of this neoplasm where most cases have occurred in homosexual males with AIDS.[41]

The clinical appearance of KS and its occurrence in either homosexual males or intravenous drug abusers is so characteristic that we do not biopsy these lesions. Fortunately, the use of a new generation of protease inhibitors has markedly reduced the incidence of this disease. The choice of therapy depends on the patient's status, the morbidity of the lesion, and its rate of growth. We have observed some of these lesions in which no growth occurred for many months. We have treated others either because of ocular morbidity or cosmetic defect. As discussed below, these tumors are exceedingly sensitive to ionizing radiation. In a few patients with multiple lesions on all four eyelids, chemosensitization and laser therapy has been effective.

METASTATIC AND RARE PRIMARY LID TUMORS

Metastatic lid tumors are treated with chemotherapy, if it is indicated for other body sites, or with ionizing radiation. Virtually all rare primary lid malignancies are treated surgically.

NONSURGICAL TREATMENTS

Ionizing Radiation

There are different types of radiation that have been used in the management of lid tumors. Unlike intraocular or orbital neoplasms, lid carcinomas are superficial, and radiation delivery systems should deposit a maximum dose to the skin, while sparing deeper structures. Brachytherapy with either radon seeds or iridium wires has been described. The former is of historic interest only, since the risk of radon gas leaks has resulted in its total abandonment. Most lid malignancies that are treated with radiation are sufficiently large to obviate the advantages of brachytherapy, although a few cases have been managed in this manner.[42] A few small periocular basal cell carcinomas have been managed with radiation with good results.[43]

Two external beams most commonly used to treat lid neoplasms are orthovoltage (approximately 250-k photons) or megavoltage (MeV) electrons. Both deliver maximum energy to the skin surface, although with higher energy electrons, more energy is deposited distally.[44] The vast majority of radiation experience with lid malignancies has been with orthovoltage systems, which are more plentiful and cost less to operate; 6 or 8 MeV electrons can be more sharply focused both laterally and distally to the skin surface (Figure 2–6), although, as Amdur and colleagues point out, electrons deliver more radiation to the lens and retina even with shielding, compared with orthovoltage.[44] Significant problems with lens doses errors as much as 27 percent can occur when lead shields and electrons are used so that several modifications are necessary to minimize complications.[45,46]

It is difficult to compare the treatment results from radiation and surgical series; there are no prospective data, and often tumor sizes are either not stipulated or discrepant.[47] Some series have a high enough incidence of loss to follow-up as to make evaluation difficult.[48] Generally, large radiation series have been reported from institutions without a strong interest in oculoplastics, and some reports have been from centers with relatively unsophisticated radiation oncology.

In the management of basal cell carcinoma, most centers treat patients with 300-cGy (300-rad) daily fractions of either orthovoltage photons or electrons to a total dose of 45 to 50 Gy. One centimeter of apparently normal lid margin is included in the treatment field to avoid a marginal miss; however, the recurrence rates cited, usually between 2.5 and 10 percent, are most likely due to either failure to include the entire tumor in the treatment field, especially with morpheaform lesions, or the combination of biologic aggressiveness and radioresistance noted when basal cell carcinoma invades orbital bones.[40,49–54] If a patient has orbit or bone involvement noted prior to radiation, a combination of ortho- and megavoltage photons can be used to maximize tumor coverage. In all lid radiation, a field cut-out and a lead shield are placed over the cornea to protect the intraocular contents (Figures 2–7A, B). As discussed earlier, tumors that recur after radiation may be more difficult to control locally.[47,55,56]

In a large series of over 1,000 eyelid basal cell carcinomas reported by Fitzpatrick and co-workers, there was a 5-year control rate of 95 percent.[56] Similarly, Schlienger and colleagues noted a 5-year level control rate of 97.5 percent in 850 cases.[40] In that report, radiation appeared equally effective as either primary treatment or therapy after tumor recurrence following management by another modality.[55] In

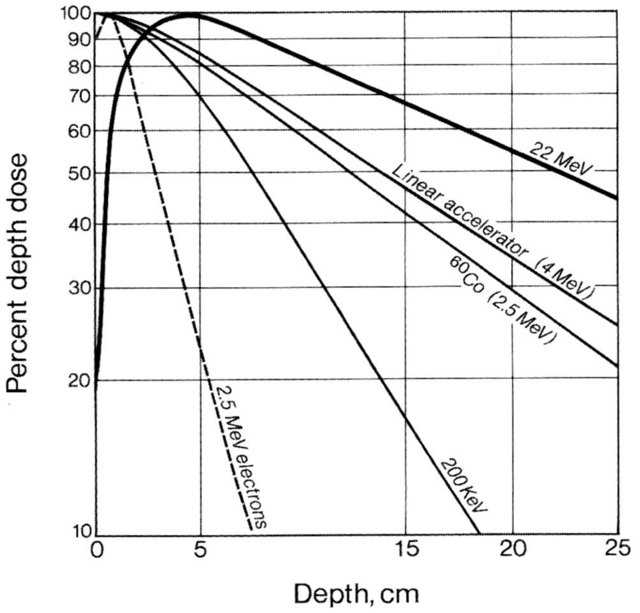

Figure 2–6. Comparison of megavoltage electron therapy versus orthovoltage irradiation for treatment of lid tumors.

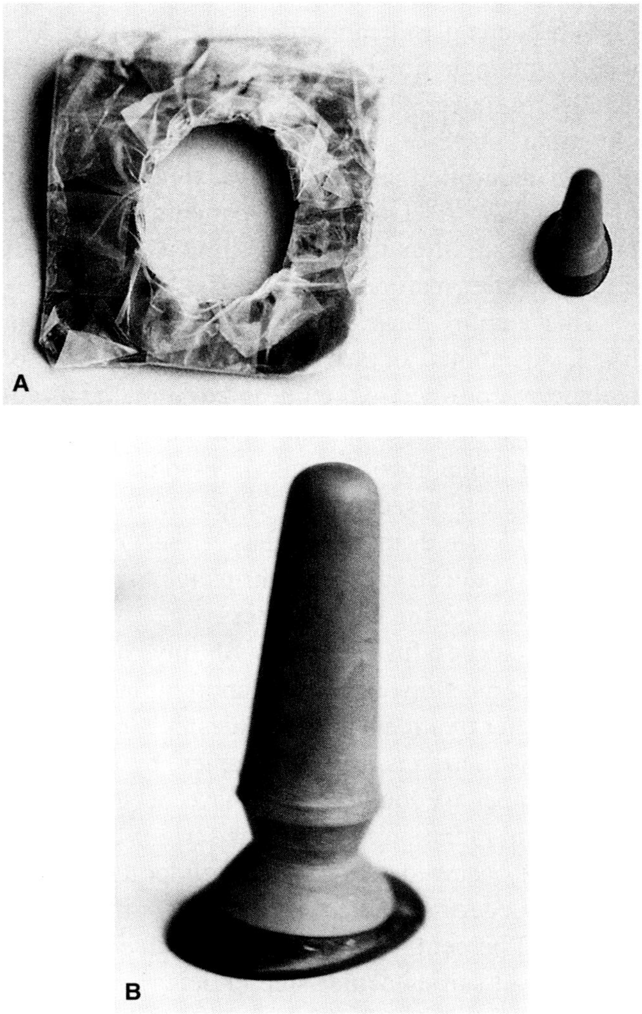

Figure 2–7. *A,* Lead cut-out. *B,* Corneal lead shield used for irradiation therapy.

squamous cell carcinoma, slightly lower tumor control rates have been achieved; Fitzpatrick and colleagues noted a 5-year control rate of 93 percent.[56]

In our limited experience with KS, approximately 90 percent of lesions responded to a single 800-cGy fraction of orthovoltage or electrons, and results appeared to be as good as with fractionated doses totalling 1,500 to 3,600 cGy.[57] Lid or conjunctival KS lesions are usually more diffuse than evident on clinical examination; they should be treated with a relatively wide surround. An example of a lid and conjunctival KS prior to and after irradiation is shown in Chapter 4, Figures 4–42 and 4–43. While other options, including intralesional vinblastine sulfate (Velban), cryotherapy, and surgical resection, have been reported, single-fraction radiation seems to be the most effective with the least morbidity.[58,59]

We have not used radiation as a primary therapy for sebaceous gland carcinomas of the eyelids. The results with radiation in the literature have been variable. Some early failures were due to insufficient radiation; however, some recurrences have been described despite treatment with as much as 119 Gy of radiation.[32,34,60] One of three patients treated with primary radiation developed nodal metastases 6 months after treatment.[61]

This author's bias has been to use surgery for basal, squamous, or sebaceous cell carcinoma or melanoma confined to the lid, and to limit the use of radiation to diffuse tumors that have sufficient orbital or bone involvement to preclude conventional surgical resection. In some of these latter cases, wide-field radiation has either cured the tumor or produced sufficient shrinkage to allow surgical removal of the residual mass.

After successful radiation of any lid tumor, epitheliitis develops and peaks approximately 10 to 20 days after treatment and subsides in 2 to 4 weeks. Tumor destruction is usually complete by 2 months.

A number of complications have been reported after eyelid radiation. Most of the serious complications have occurred after treatment of large upper lid tumors. Lederman noted an overall complication rate of 10 percent.[53,54] In a large French series, < 4 percent had serous ocular side effects.[40] Almost all irradiated lids develop keratinization of the palpebral conjunctiva (Figure 2–8). Patients radiated for tumors in the middle of the upper lid are more prone to develop ocular complications, even when the cornea is shielded. Radiation complications include lid atrophy, skin necrosis, ectropion, lid telangiectasia (Figure 2–9), epiphora, lash loss (Figures 2–9, 2–10), keratitis, and cataract.[52,53,62] An example of a disastrous complication after an appropriate dose and fractionation of radiation for a basal cell carcinoma of the upper lid is shown in Figure 2–11. Anterior exenteration was eventually required in this case. A lower incidence of significant complications occurs with external beam technique versus iridium wire technique, and most complications occur in patients with large tumors.[51,56,63,64]

Cryotherapy

Cryotherapy is an effective alternative treatment for small, localized basal cell carcinomas.[65–68] It is especially useful in debilitated patients or others in whom there are systemic contraindications to surgery.[56–59] An advantage of cryotherapy, compared with radiation, for the treatment of small basal cell carcinomas is that cryotherapy can be performed in one session versus the 3- to 5-week course needed for external beam radiation. Overall, there is about a 10 percent recurrence rate after cryotherapy, mostly due to inadvertent inclusion of morpheaform, diffuse, or multicentric lesions in the treatment session. In addition to diffuse tumors, other contraindications to this technique include conjunctival fornix involvement, bone involvement, denervated lid, or tumors in dark-skinned patients.[60]

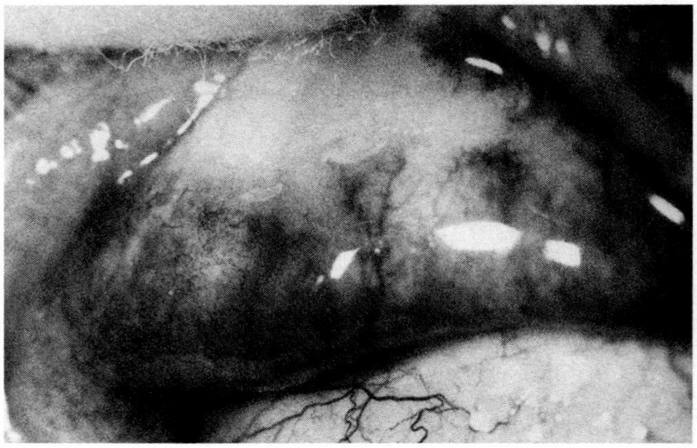

Figure 2–8. Keratinization of the palpebral conjunctiva after radiation of a lid tumor.

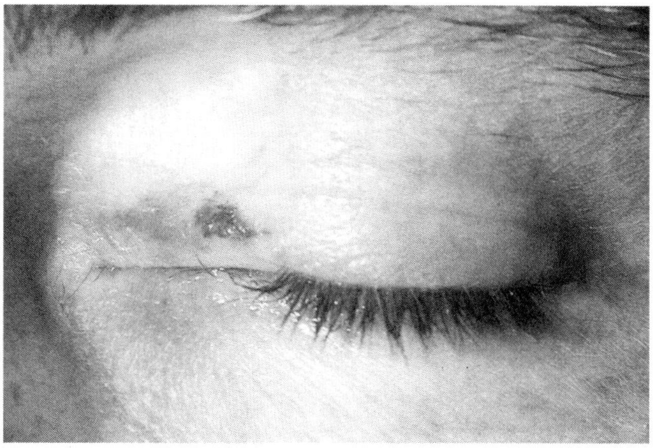

Figure 2–9. Lid telangiectasia after photon radiation of a lid tumor.

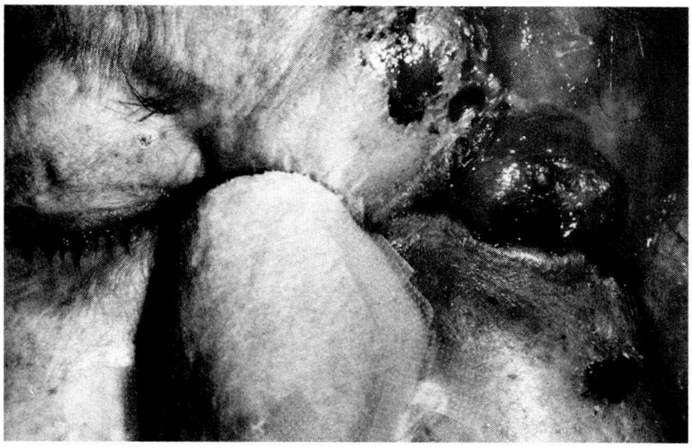

Figure 2–11. Slough of the entire lid after radiation of a diffuse upper lid basal cell carcinoma.

To effectively treat a basal cell carcinoma, the entire tumor must be frozen to –30°C. Liquid nitrogen is the most effective freezing agent to obtain this temperature, especially in thick tumors. It is necessary to monitor intratumor temperature with a thermocouple or similar device (Figure 2–12). While some investigators rely on visual appearance to gauge temperature, it has been the experience of the group at the University of California, San Francisco, that only with a thermocouple can one be certain that adequate freezing has occurred, and that excessive morbidity from an unnecessarily low temperature is limited.

A typical cryotherapy treatment apparatus is shown in Figure 2–13A, B. Lesions can be treated with either a direct liquid nitrogen spray or an applicator tip that has liquid nitrogen circulating through it. Prior to treatment, the treatment area is injected with a 1:1 mixture of 0.5 percent marcaine and 1 percent lidocaine (Xylocaine) with 1:100,000 epinephrine. The lateral and medial aspects of the field are masked off with tape if the liquid nitrogen spray is used. We place a plastic retractor between the lid and the bulbar conjunctiva to avoid inadvertent ocular freezing. A thermocouple in a 22-gauge needle is placed in the center of the tumor (Figure 2–14). Treatment is performed to reach a –30°C temperature through the entire malignancy and a cycle of freeze-thaw-freeze-thaw is used. As with any type of thermal injury, there is transient redness, swelling, and usually ulceration. These changes subside in 10 to 21 days. Often, there is permanent depigmentation, not noticeable in light-skinned patients.

Fraunfelder and colleagues reported a 5-year control rate of 97 percent for basal cell carcinomas, with

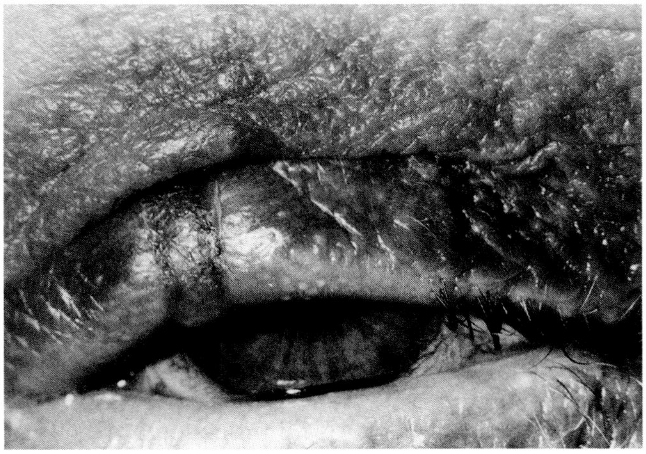

Figure 2–10. Eyelash loss after radiation of a lid tumor.

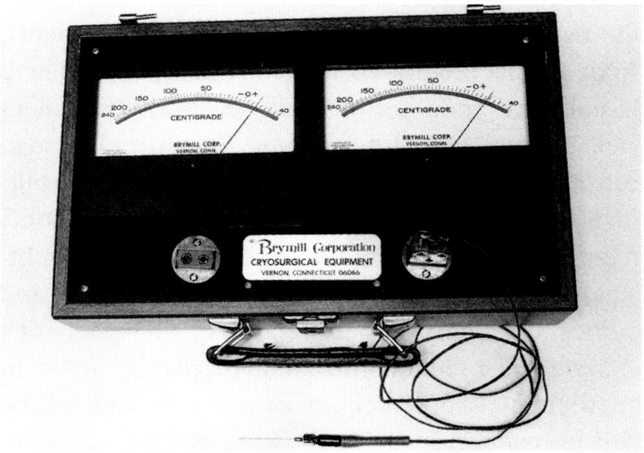

Figure 2–12. Thermocouple for use in cryotherapy of lid tumors.

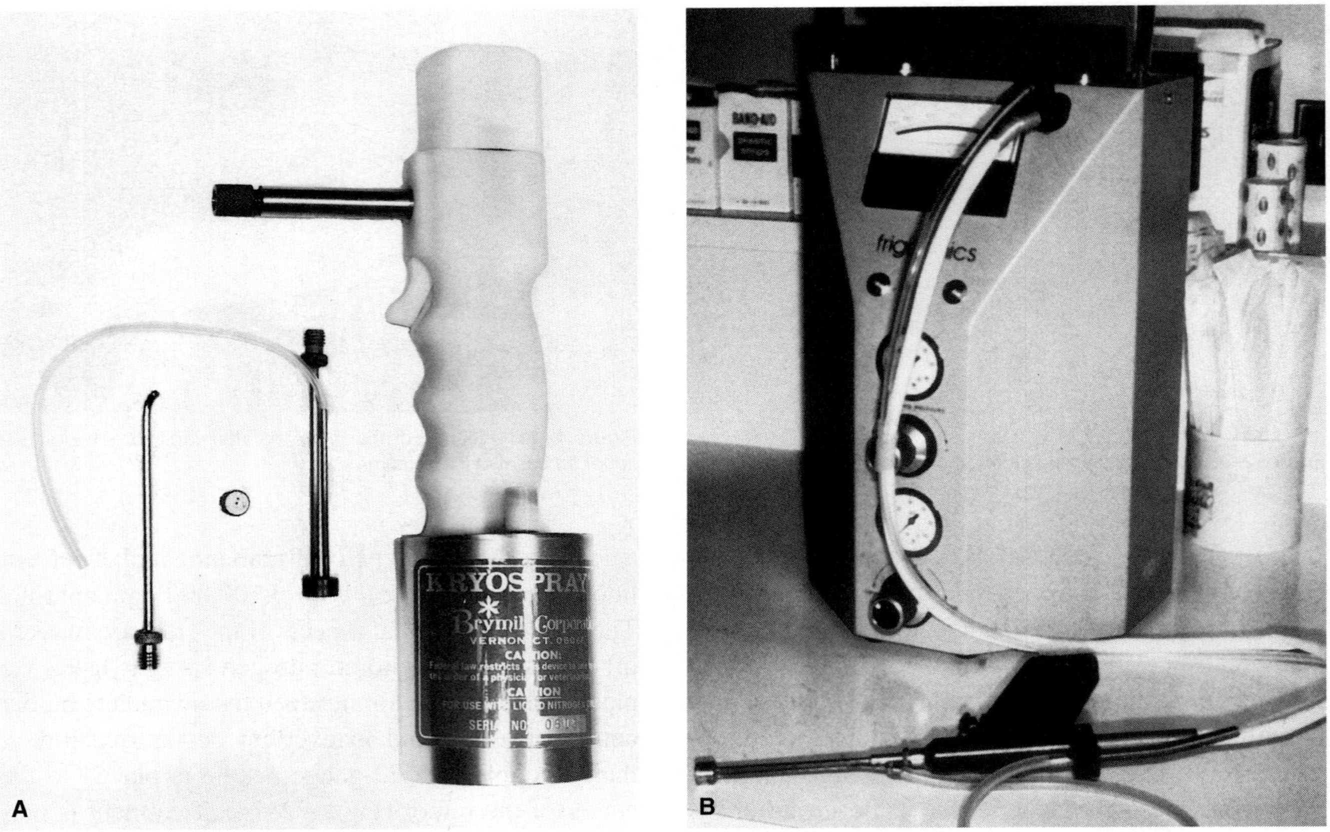

Figure 2–13. *A,* Liquid nitrogen cryoapparatus for treatment of malignant lid tumors. A spray device shown with different nozzles. *B,* A device with liquid nitrogen circulation through the tip.

nodular lesions $<$ 10 mm in diameter. A similarly high control rate was noted in a Swedish series of 222 tumors.[69] However, with lesions larger than this, approximately 15 to 17 percent of tumors recurred.[70]

A number of complications have been observed with cryotherapy, and overall, approximately 25 percent of cases have some type of complication.[71] Depigmentation of the treated area severely limits the use of this technique in dark-skinned patients, since results are not cosmetically acceptable. There is universal epilation of eyelashes in the treatment field. Visual loss, lid notching, hypertrophic scar, ectropion, pseudoepithelial hyperplasia, hyperpigmentation, chronic granulation, devitalized bone, rectus paresis, lacrimal drainage obstruction, trichiasis, symblepharon, activation of herpes, and corneal ulcer have all been reported.[71] In the author's experience, pseudoepithelial hyperplasia, noted in approximately 5 percent of cases, is the most difficult to manage, in that only with repeat biopsy can one exclude recurrent tumor, especially if the patient was treated for a squamous cell carcinoma. In one of the author's patients, this complication developed 4 years after cryotherapy. Repeat biopsies were negative for malignancy, but eventually the author reconstructed the lid to repair the cosmetic defect. As Visnes has stressed, there may be recurrences, and so patients require careful monitoring after treatment. Some investigators have used cryotherapy for recurrent tumors, although we have preferred surgical resection in that setting.[72]

Experimental Therapies

Many other approaches have been used to treat eyelid tumors. Three additional modalities discussed below have limited use. The author has used these treatments in the management of patients who have a cancer diathesis, such as xeroderma pigmentosum or basal cell nevus syndrome, and have recurrent lid tumors after multiple surgical procedures, radiation, and cryotherapy.

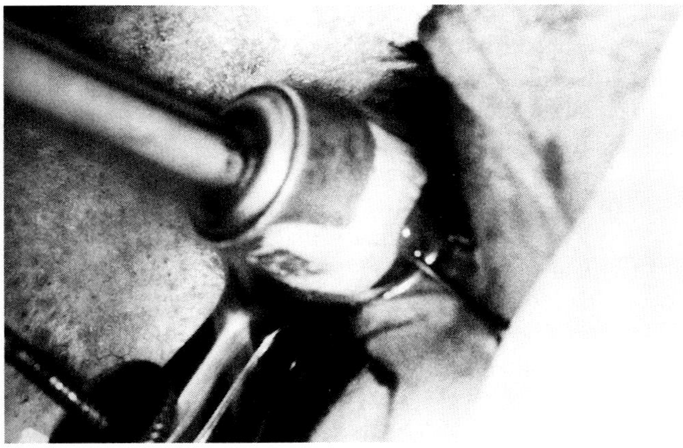

Figure 2–14. The lid carcinoma and the contiguous normal structures are draped prior to treatment of a lid tumor with cryotherapy. The thermocouple is in place, and the tape is used to try to limit the spread of the freeze to normal structures.

Hematoporphyrin derivative (HpD) photochemotherapy has been used to successfully treat a number of bladder and lung malignancies. As discussed under basal cell carcinomas, few patients with lid carcinomas have been treated with reasonable results.[19,73] Preliminary results with newer sensitizers have suggested that there may be less morbidity, but there is a paucity of controlled trial data.[19] Dermatologists have noted the beneficial effects of vitamin A for over 40 years. Since 1978, retinoids have been used to treat some malignancies, including basal cell, squamous cell, and adnexal carcinomas.[74–76] In patients with high risk of multiple eyelid tumors, these approaches may afford some prevention. Immunotherapy has similarly been used to treat some of these disparate lid cancers, with occasional success.[77,78] These approaches are not routinely used for lid tumors and are well discussed in the references listed.

Two other newer experimental treatments should be briefly discussed. As mentioned in Chapter 1, the standard treatment of pediatric capillary hemangiomas is steroid injection; if this is not effective, local surgical debulking is sometimes indicated. In large capillary hemangiomas, especially around the airway, the use of systemic interferon-alpha 2b has been tried with good success. One case with orbital involvement has been treated in this manner; significant morbidity precludes the routine use of this agent.[79,80] Hyperthermia is being used to treat a number of tumors, and some centers are using it for superficial malignancies.[81]

REFERENCES

1. Fraunfelder FT, Zacarian SA, Limmer BL, Wingfield D. Cryosurgery for malignancies of theeyelid. Ophthalmology 1980;87:461–5.
2. Payne JW, Duke JR, Butner R, Eifrig DE. Basal cell carcinoma of the eyelids. A long-term follow-up study. Arch Ophthalmol 1969;81:553–8.
3. Mohs FE. Micrographic surgery for the microscopically controlled excision of eyelid cancers. Arch Ophthalmol 1986;104:901–9.
4. Kopf AW. Computer analysis of 3531 basal-cell carcinomas of the skin. J Dermatol 1979;6:267–81.
5. Luxenberg MN, Guthrie TH Jr. Chemotherapy of basal cell and squamous cell carcinoma of the eyelids and periorbital tissues. Ophthalmology 1986;93:504–10.
6. Morley M, Finger PT, Perlin M, et al. Cis-platinum chemotherapy for ocular basal cell carcinoma. Br J Ophthalmol 1991;75:407–10.
7. Neudorfer M, Merimsky O, Lazar M, Geyer O. Cisplatin and doxorubicin for invasive basal cell carcinoma of the eyelids. Ann Ophthalmol 1993;25:11–3.
8. Morley M, Finger PT, Perlin M, et al. Cis-platinum chemotherapy for ocular basal cell carcinoma. Br J Ophthalmol 1991;75:407–10.
9. Baxter DL Jr, Joyce AP, Feldman BD, Lynch JW Jr. Cisplatin chemotherapy for basal cell carcinoma: The need for posttreatment biopsy—report of a case. J Am Acad Dermatol 1990;23:1167–8.
10. Guthrie TH Jr, Porubsky ES, Luxenberg MN, et al. Cisplatin-based chemotherapy in advanced basal and squamous cell carcinomas of the skin: results in 28 patients including 13 patients receiving multimodality therapy. J Clin Oncol 1990;8:342–6.
11. Mir LM, Glass LF, Sersa G, et al. Effective treatment of cutaneous and subcutaneous malignant tumours by electrochemotherapy. Br J Cancer 1998;77:2336–42.
12. Olbricht SM. Treatment of malignant cutaneous tumors. Clin Plast Surg 1993;20:167–80.
13. Greenberg ER, Baron JA, Stukel TA, et al. A clinical trial of beta carotene to prevent basal-cell and squamous-cell cancers of the skin. N Engl J Med 1990; 323:789–95.
14. Hughes BR, Marks R, Pearse AD, Gaskell SA. Clinical response and tissue effects of etretinate treatment of patients with solar keratoses and basal cell carcinoma. J Am Acad Dermatol 1988;18:522–9.
15. Greenway HT Jr, Cornell RC. Interferon. Coming of age. Arch Dermatol 1990;126:1080–2.
16. Baron S, Tyring SK, Fleischmann WR Jr, et al. The interferons. Mechanisms of action and clinical applications. JAMA 1991;266:1375–83.
17. Chang BK, Guthrie TH Jr, Hayakawa K, Gangarosa LP. A pilot study of iontophoretic cisplatin chemotherapy of basal and squamous cell carcinomas of the skin. Arch Dermatol 1993;129:425–7.
18. Orenberg EK, Miller BH, Greenway HT, et al. The

effect of intralesional 5-fluorouracil therapeutic implant (MPI 5003) for treatment of basal cell carcinoma. J Am Acad Dermatol 1992;27:723–8.
19. Wang I, Bauer B, Andersson-Engels S, et al. Photodynamic therapy utilising topical delta-aminolevulinic acid in non-melanoma skin malignancies of the eyelid and the periocular skin. Acta Ophthalmol Scand 1999;77:182–8.
20. Tijl JWM, Koornneff L. The optimal follow-up time for a basal cell carcinoma of the eyelid. Doc Ophthalmol 1990;75:275–9.
21. Rowe DE, Carroll RJ, Day CL Jr. Long-term recurrence rates in previously untreated (primary) basal cell carcinoma: implications for patient follow-up. J Dermatol Surg Oncol 1989;15:315–28.
22. Bergstresser PR, Halprin KM. Multiple sequential skin cancers: the risk of skin cancer in patients with previous skin cancer. Arch Dermatol 1975;111:995–6.
23. Robinson JK. Risk of developing another basal cell carcinoma. A 5 year-prospective study. Cancer 1987; 60:118–20.
24. Lo JS, Snow SN, Reizner GT, et al. Metastatic basal cell carcinoma: report of twelve cases with a review of the literature. J Am Acad Dermatol 1991;24:715–9.
25. Conley J, Sachs ME, Romo T, et al. Metastatic basal cell carcinoma of the head and neck. Otolaryngol Head Neck Surg 1985;93:78–85.
26. Wieman TJ, Shively EH, Woodcock TM. Responsiveness of metastatic basal-cell carcinoma to chemotherapy. A case report. Cancer 1983;52:1583–5.
27. Khandekar JD. Complete response of metastatic basal cell carcinoma to cisplatin chemotherapy: a report on two patients. Arch Dermatol 1990;126:1660.
28. Putterman AM. Conjunctival map biopsy to determine pagetoid spread. Am J Ophthalmol 1986;102:87–90.
29. Kass LG. Role of cryotherapy in treating sebaceous carcinoma of the eyelid. Ophthalmology 1990;97:2–4.
30. Mashburn MA, Chonkich GD, Chase DR. Meibomian gland adenocarcinoma of the eyelid with preauricular lymph node metastasis. Laryngoscope 1985;95: 1441–3.
31. Ginsberg J. Present status of meibomian gland carcinoma. Arch Ophthalmol 1965;73:271–7.
32. Doxanas MT, Green WR. Sebaceous gland carcinoma. Review of 40 cases. Arch Ophthalmol 1984;102: 245–9.
33. Pardo FS, Wang CC, Albert D, Stracher MA. Sebaceous carcinoma of the ocular adnexa: radiotherapeutic management. Int J Radiat Oncol Biol Phys 1989;17:643–7.
34. Nunery WR, Welsh MG, McCord CD Jr. Recurrence of sebaceous carcinoma of the eyelid after radiation therapy. Am J Ophthalmol 1983;96:10–5.
35. Matsumoto C, Nakatsuka K, Matsuo K, et al. Sebaceous carcinoma responds to radiation therapy. Ophthalmologica 1995;209:280–3.
36. Day CL Jr, Mihm MC Jr, Sober AJ, et al. Narrower margins for clinical stage I malignant melanoma. N Engl J Med 1982;306:479.
37. Urist MM, Balch CM, Soong S, et al. The influence of surgical margins and prognostic factors predicting the risk of local recurrence in 3445 patients with primary cutaneous melanoma. Cancer 1985;55:1398–402.
38. Avril MF, Charpentier P, Margulis A, Guillaume JC. Regression of primary melanoma with metastases. Cancer 1992;69:1377–81.
39. Kirkwood JM, Ibrahim JG, Sondak VK, et al. High- and low-dose interferon alfa-2b in high-risk melamoma: first analysis intergroup trial E1690/S9111/C9190. J Clin Oncol 2000;18(12):2444–58.
40. Schlienger P, Brunin F, Desjardins L, et al. External radiotherapy for carcinoma of the eyelid. Report of 850 cases treated. Int J Radiat Oncol Biol Phys 1996;34:277–87.
41. Moore PS, Chang Y. Detection of herpes virus-like DNA sequences in Kaposi's sarcoma in patients with and without HIV infection. N Engl J Med 1995;332: 1181–5.
42. Stanowsky A, Krey HF, Kopp J, et al. Irradiation of malignant eyelid melanoma with iodine 125 plaque. Am J Ophthalmol 1990;100:44–8.
43. Buatois F, Coquard R, Pica A, et al. Treatment of eyelid carcinomas of 2cmm or less by contact radiotherapy. J Fr Ophthalmol 1996;19:405–9.
44. Amdur RJ, Kalbaugh KJ, Ewald LM, et al. Radiation therapy for skin cancer near the eye: kilovoltage X-rays versus electrons. Int J Radiat Oncol Biol Phys 1992;23:769–79.
45. Kishi K, Shirai S, Sonomura T, et al. Lead contact lens for crystalline lens shielding in electron therapy for eyelid tumors. Radiat Med 1996;14:107–9.
46. Shiu AS, Tung SS, Gastorf RJ, et al. Dosimetric evaluation of lead and tungsten eye shields in electron beam treatment. Int J Radiat Oncol Biol Phys 1996; 35:599–604.
47. Rodriguez-Sains RS, Robins P, Smith B, Bosniak SL. Radiotherapy of periocular basal cell carcinomas: recurrence rates and treatment with special attention to the medial canthus. Br J Ophthalmol 1988;72: 134–8.
48. Leshin B, Yeatts P, Anscher M, et al. Management of periocular basal cell carcinoma: Mohs' micrographic surgery versus radiotherapy. Surv Ophthalmol 1993;38:193–212.
49. Cobb GM, Thompson GA, Allt WE. Treatment of basal cell carcinoma of the eyelids by radiotherapy. Can Med Assoc J 1964;91:743–8.
50. Fayos JV, Wildermuth O. Carcinoma of the skin of the eyelids. Arch Ophthalmol 1962;67:298–302.
51. Fitzpatrick PJ, Jamieson DM, Thompson GA, Allt WE. Tumors of the eyelids and their treatment by radiotherapy. Radiology 1972;104:661–5.
52. Lederman M. Discussion of carcinomas of the conjunctiva and eyelid. In: Boniuk M, editor. Ocular

and adnexal tumors. St. Louis, MO: CV Mosby; 1964. p. 104.
53. Lederman M. Radiation treatment of cancer of the eyelids. Br J Ophthalmol 1976;60:794–805.
54. Nordman EM, Nordman LE. Treatment of basal cell carcinoma of the eyelid. Acta Ophthalmol 1978;56: 349–56.
55. Hirshowitz B, Mahler D. Incurable recurrences of basal cell carcinoma of the mid-face following radiation therapy. Br J Plast Surg 1971;24:205–11.
56. Fitzpatrick PJ, Thompson GA, Easterbrook WM, et al. Basal and squamous cell carcinoma of the eyelids and their treatment by radiotherapy. Int J Radiat Oncol Biol Phys 1984;10:449–54.
57. Ghabrial R, Quivey JM, Dunn JP Jr, Char DH. Radiation therapy of acquired immunodeficiency syndrome-related Kaposi's sarcoma of the eyelids and conjunctiva. Arch Ophthalmol 1992;110:1423–6.
58. Dugel PU, Gill PS, Frangieh GT, Rao NA. Treatment of ocular adnexal Kaposi's sarcoma in acquired immune deficiency syndrome. Ophthalmology 1992; 99:1127–32.
59. Heinemann MH. Medical management of AIDS patients. Ophthalmic problems. Med Clin North Am 1992;76:83–97.
60. Ide CH, Ridings GR, Yamashita T, Buesseler JA. Radiotherapy of a recurrent adenocarcinoma of the meibomian gland. Arch Ophthalmology 1968;79: 540–4.
61. Hendley RL, Rieser JC, Cavanagh HD, et al. Primary radiation therapy for meibomian gland carcinoma. Am J Ophthalmol 1979;87:206–9.
62. Levitt SH, Bogardus CR Jr, Brandt EN Jr. Complications and late changes following radiation therapy for carcinoma of the eyelid and canthi. Radiology 1966;87:340–7.
63. Call NB, Welham RAN. Epiphora after irradiation of medial eyelid tumors. Am J Ophthalmol 1981;92: 842–5.
64. Daly NJ, de Lafontan B, Combes PF. Results of the treatment of 165 lid carcinomas by iridium wire implant. Int J Radiat Oncol Biol Phys 1984;10: 455–9.
65. Bullock JD, Beard C, Sullivan JH. Cryotherapy of basal cell carcinoma in oculoplastic surgery. Am J Ophthalmol 1976;82:841–7.
66. Zacarian SA. Cryosurgery of tumors of the skin and oral cavity. Springfield, IL: Charles C. Thomas; 1973.
67. Matthaus W, Lange G, Roitzch E. Cryotherapy of eyelid conjunctival tumors. Ophthalmologica 1976; 173:53–62.
68. Fraunfelder FT, Wingfield D. Therapy of intraepithelial epitheliomas and squamous cell carcinoma of the limbus. Trans Am Ophthalmol Soc 1980;78: 290–300.
69. Lindgren G, Larko O. Long-term follow-up of cryosurgery of basal cell carcinoma of the eyelid. J Am Acad Dermatol 1997;36:742–6.
70. Fraunfelder FT, Zacarian SA, Wingfield DL, Limmer BL. Results of cryotherapy for eyelid malignancies. Am J Ophthalmol 1984;97:184–8.
71. Wood JR, Anderson RL. Complications of cryosurgery. Arch Ophthalmol 1981;99:460–3.
72. Kuflik EG, Gage AA. Recurrent basal cell carcinoma treated with cryosurgery. J Am Acad Dermatol 1997;37:82–4.
73. Tse DT, Kersten RC, Anderson RL. Hematoporphyrin derivative photoradiation therapy in managing nevoid basal-cell carcinoma syndrome. A preliminary report. Arch Ophthalmol 1984;102:990–4.
74. Peck GL. Chemoprevention and treatment of skin cancer with retinoids. Cancer Surv 1983;2:315–26.
75. Roach M III. A malignant eccrine poroma responds to isotretinoin (13-cis-retinoic acid). Ann Intern Med 1983;99:486–8.
76. Meyskens FL Jr, Goodman GE, Alberts DS. 13-cis-retinoic acid: pharmacology, toxicology, and clinical applications for the prevention and treatment of human cancer. Crit Rev Oncol Hematol 1985;3: 75–101.
77. Char DH, Beard C. Immunotherapy in ocular malignancy. In: Hornblass A, editor. Tumors of the ocular adnexa and orbit. St. Louis, MO: CV Mosby; 1979. p. 300.
78. Hoffmann D, Jennings PA, Spradbrow PB. Immunotherapy of bovine ocular squamous cell carcinomas with phenol-saline extracts of allogenic carcinomas. Austr Vet J 1981;57:159–62.
79. Loughnan MS, Elder J, Kemp A. Treatment of a massive orbital-capillary hemangioma with interferon alpha-2b: short term results. Arch Ophthalmol 1992;110:1366–7.
80. Guyer DR, Tiedeman J, Yannuzzi LA, et al. Interferon-associated retinopathy. Arch Ophthalmol 1993;111: 350–6.
81. Engin, K, Leeper, DB, Tupcong, L, Waterman, FM. Thermoradiotherapy in the management of superficial malignant tumors. Clin Cancer Res 1995;1:139–45.

3

Surgical Treatment of Lid Tumors

SURGICAL TECHNIQUES

Regardless of surgical technique, the removal of a tumor must be carefully monitored. The inclusion of the entire tumor in the treatment field and the histologic control of the tumor edges are crucial to the success of any surgical strategy. There are two options for surgical resection of eyelid tumors: Mohs' micrographic technique and standard surgery with frozen section control of tumor margins. There are advantages and disadvantages with each approach.

Standard Resection with Frozen Section Control

The major advantages of standard resection with frozen section control are its good control of tumor margins, its availability in almost all hospitals, and its high cure rate.[1] There are, however, three major disadvantages of standard frozen section control: (1) it is a more time-consuming procedure than the Mohs' micrographic procedure for the ophthalmic surgeon; (2) Especially in a teaching institution (ie, where residents perform frozen sections), the level of pathologic expertise is generally less than if tumor resection is monitored by a trained Mohs' surgeon; and (3) in many cases, a larger amount of normal tissue must be sacrificed to obtain free margins, especially if the tumor has areas of small islands or pseudopod extensions of malignant cells.

A number of publications have reported that lid tumor resections without frozen section control, but with an arbitrary 3- to 5-mm margin, have between a 23 and 50 percent incidence of incomplete tumor removal.[2–7] In cases of incomplete resection, approximately 35 percent of basal cell carcinomas have been reported to recur.[7] These numbers vary markedly; Frank noted that 18 of 21 "incompletely excised tumors" had no residual neoplasm on repeat excision.[8]

In an institution with excellent pathologists, the incidence of tumor recurrence with frozen section control is less than 2 percent.[5,9] If a tumor is to be excised under standard frozen section control, orientation is vital. We routinely orient all specimens on a sterile tissue map (Figure 3–1). Even an experienced pathologist is often confused regarding small lid tumor resection margins. This confusion can be decreased if the main tumor mass is sent to the pathologist separately from carefully oriented small marginal sections that represent the presumably normal tissue margins surrounding the malignancy. As a further precaution, placing a 5-0 marker suture in one edge of each margin specimen and listing its location on the map are useful for orientation. Finally, this author often uses a blue surgical marking pen to highlight the side of the margin away from the neoplasm so that it can be optimally oriented to make frozen sections. Occasionally, it is important to accompany the material to the pathology laboratory.

It is difficult to be certain that the histologic material is processed correctly, and failure to do so can result in an incorrect assessment of tumor extension. For example, at UCSF we have had a case in which the pathology resident used a transverse section through the lateral margin instead of sampling the entire length of the horizontal and both vertical resection margins. He thought erroneously that the margins were clear, when, in fact, they were involved with tumor. This case illustrates the need for close communication with the pathologist. Similarly, a tissue block can be inadvertently reversed so that the lateral free margin is thought to be the margin closest to the tumor and is not studied, while the margin closest to the tumor was sampled as the "free margin" and thought to be contaminated by tumor. When the correctly oriented tissue was analyzed, the distal margin was tumor free. Finally, tangentially cut sections can result in confusion between hair follicle epithelium, rete ridges, and carcinoma.

Regardless of the pathologist's experience, the delineation of a sebaceous cell carcinoma margin, given its propensity for both pagetoid spread and multicentricity, is difficult.[10] Similarly, frozen section control for cutaneous melanomas has a significant false-negative rate.[11]

Mohs' Micrographic Technique

In 1941, Mohs described a different approach to monitor skin tumor resection.[12] A number of alternative terms have been used to describe his procedure, but the current nomenclature is "Mohs' micrographic technique." Previous terms include chemosurgery, microsurgery, Mohs' microsurgery, and Mohs' technique.[13,14] Three major advantages to Mohs' technique are the use of two different teams to separately resect and reconstruct the eyelid to avoid inadequate tumor resection margins, the sparing of the ophthalmic surgeon's time by not having to wait in the operating room until tumor-free margins are obtained, and the low incidence of tumor recurrence. The major disadvantages of this technique are cost to the patient for two separate procedures, the need for a trained Mohs' surgeon, and the possibility of excess lid resection.

The goal of the micrographic technique is to accurately delineate the tumor margins, while sparing normal tissue. As in an archeologic excavation of an elevated mound, once the major tumor mass is removed, a layer-by-layer approach is used by the Mohs' chemosurgeon to carefully outline the position of the remaining tumor and remove it. As shown in Figure 3–2, the undersurface of tangential small sections of each tissue layer is histologically studied for residual tumor, and further dissection and micrographic survey are carried out only in those areas where tumor is found. These tissue blocks are approximately 5 to 10 mm in diameter and 2 to 4 mm in thickness. The Mohs' procedure is probably more accurate than frozen section control in detecting small pseudopod extensions of tumor, but the technique may be less conservative in sparing tumor-free tissue. Unlike standard frozen sections that are perpendicular to skin, Mohs' technique is, by definition, tangential. Tangential sections obtained through either normal hair follicle epithelium or rete ridges can often simulate basal cell carcinoma. It has been the impression of many dermatopathologists that

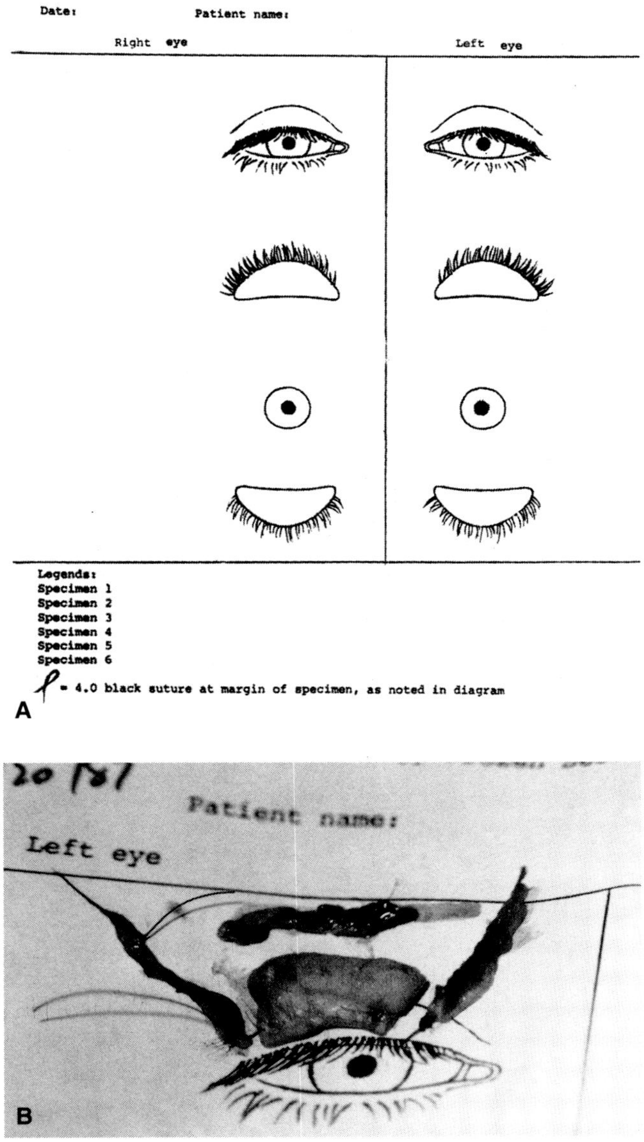

Figure 3–1. *A*, Sterile tissue map used for specimen orientation during standard tumor lid surgery. *B*, Example of specimen oriented on the sterile tissue map.

some patients treated with the Mohs' technique have more tissue sacrificed than is necessary. Conversely, in other cases, Mohs' technique does limit the area of neoplastic resection, since only tumor-containing areas are removed, instead of straight cuts through both involved and uninvolved lid structures.

The initial micrographic technique was based on in situ tissue fixation, followed by removal and histologic examination of successive tissue layers,[12–15] although lid tumor micrographic surgery is now performed using a fresh tissue technique.[16] Local anesthesia is used, minor hemostasis is achieved with oxidized cellulose, and larger vessels are electrocoagulated. Thin, precisely oriented specimens are examined, with the sides of each specimen color coded with red or blue dyes. A technician cuts the flat undersurface of each specimen with a frozen section. Further sections are taken only in areas in which residual tumor is found.

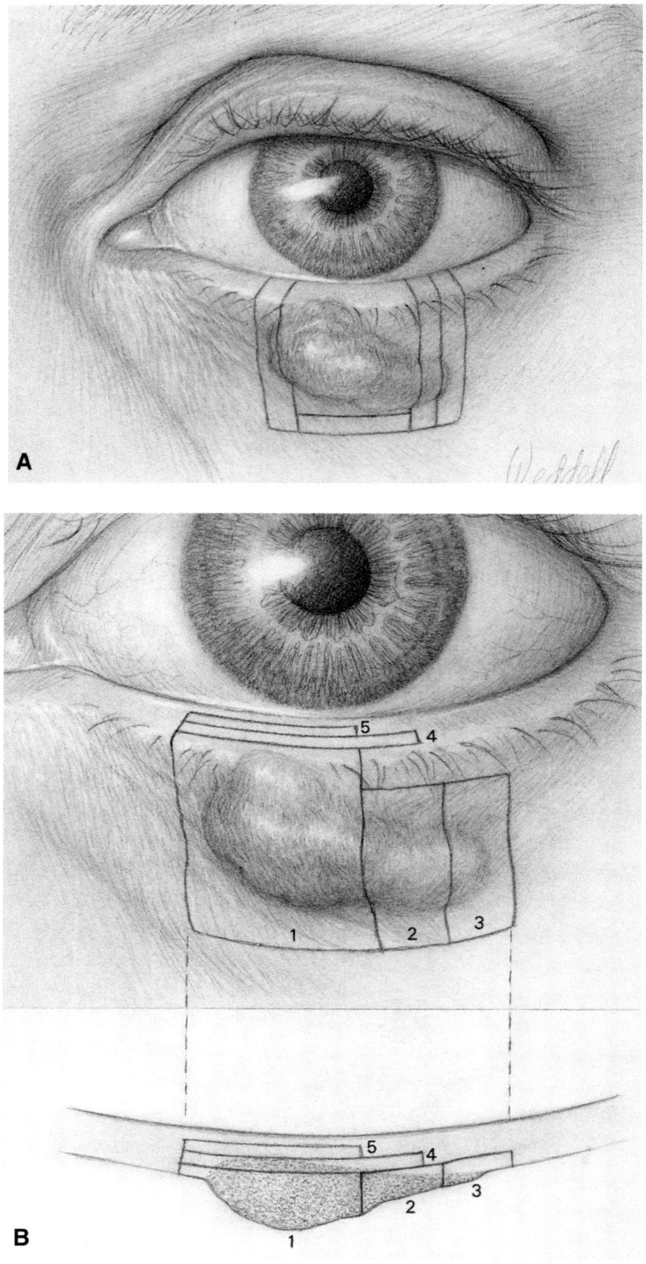

Figure 3–2. *A*, Schematic representation of standard frozen section control. *B*, Mohs' micrographic technique of histologic analysis.

The fixed tissue technique is used for two types of ophthalmic adnexal tumors: (1) in the management of malignant melanoma, Mohs felt that in situ fixation was less likely to spread viable melanoma cells;[15] and (2) better anatomic detail is obtained with tissue fixed in situ, and tumors that extend into the deep orbit or that involve bone are more accurately resected with the fixed tissue technique.[15,17]

Mohs advocated granulation (secondary intention healing) after tumor resection.[18] While this laissez-faire reconstruction technique is adequate, especially in large medial canthal lesions, most ophthalmic surgeons reconstruct eyelid defects created by the Mohs' approach.[1,19–22] Overall, in Mohs' personal experience with the micrographic approach, > 98 percent of eyelid squamous cell or basal cell carcinomas have no noted recurrence 5 years after resection. Lateral canthal lesions have a lower cure rate (91% for basal cell, 87.5% for squamous cell) than tumors in other locations. Similarly, recurrent tumors have a slightly lower success rate (92.4% for basal cell, 98.5% for squamous cell). Tumors > 30 mm in size have only a 50 percent cure rate.[16] Smaller series, presumably in centers with less voluminous experience, have reported slightly lower control rates.[23,24]

GENERAL PRINCIPLES OF LID RECONSTRUCTION

There are many operations that have been created to repair surgical lid defects. As in most areas of medicine, many procedures have been re-invented or are very slight modifications of procedures described previously and therefore they have not been discussed here. The anatomy is altered differently by every lid tumor resection, and each reconstructive procedure is unique. It is almost impossible to

describe the judgment on which subtleties of repair of lid and canthal tumors is based.

There are four general principles that guide surgical lid defect reconstruction: (1) the lid consists of two components, an anterior and posterior lamella; both must be present or be replaced to have a competent lid repair. The anterior lamella consists of myocutaneous tissue. The posterior lamella requires a mucous membrane on a stiff cartilaginous material to prevent the lid from turning in or out; (2) if one lamella is replaced with a free graft, the other layer must have a good vascular supply and therefore requires a transpositional, rotation, advancement, or bridge pedicle flap; (3) there are limited sources of good graft tissue. The anterior lamella of either lid can be best matched for color and texture with skin from the contralateral or vertically opposite lid; next in order of preference is skin from the retroauricular and supraclavicular areas. Myocutaneous tissue can be obtained as a free graft; a bridge, pedicle, advancement, or rotational flap; or a myocutaneous island.[25] The blood supply to the underside of the skin in the periocular region is good enough that a flap of just subcutaneous tissue attached to overlying skin is usually moveable with adequate vascular support; and (4) the posterior lid lamella can be obtained from a pedicle or advancement flap of tarsus and conjunctiva, a free nasal-septal graft, a free tarsoconjunctival (posterior composite) graft, or a hard palate graft (for lower eyelids only). All combinations of these anterior and posterior lamella reconstruction options, with the exclusion of free grafts for both lid layers, have been used to repair lid defects.

Those surgical procedures that the author has found to be both simple and effective in the reconstruction of over 90 percent of lids after complete tumor resection have been described here. Undoubtedly, this choice reflects the bias of the author's training and experience. A number of other procedures could be substituted with similar results. The heroic multispecialty surgeries for tumors that extend outside of usual ophthalmic boundaries have not been addressed here deliberately.

LOWER LID RECONSTRUCTION

Four procedures can be used to reconstruct almost all lower lid defects: (1) primarily, apposition of the resected lid margins, (2) a lateral cantholysis with a lateral advancement flap (Tenzel and Reese procedures),[26–28] (3) a tarsoconjunctival pedicle flap (Hewes-Beard procedure),[29] or (4) an upper lid tarsoconjunctival advancement flap (Hughes procedure).[30] The choice of procedure depends on the size of the defect and the patient's age. Patients under 40 years of age generally have little skin laxity, and less of the lid can be resected and closed primarily.

After the tumor has been completely removed with adequate margins, two Bishop-Harmon toothed forceps are used to grasp the medial and lateral lid remnants to determine if the lid defect can be closed either primarily or with lateral cantholysis and a mucocutaneous advancement flap (Figure 3–3A). If the ends of the lid defect cannot be brought together without too much pressure (Figure 3–3B), even after lateral cantholysis, then a tarsoconjunctival pedicle flap, an upper lid tarsoconjunctival advancement procedure or a free posterior lamellar graft with a pedicle skin graft must be considered.

Primary Closure of Lower Lid Defects

While historically halving procedures were used to approximate the lid margins, most surgeons now align the tarsus with either a single vertical suture, as shown in Figure 3–3B, or with two horizontal sutures. The ends of the tarsus must be perpendicular and its margins aligned to obtain a good cosmetic closure. The choice of suture material is not critical. Tarsal or periosteal sutures must retain strength for over 14 days, while conjunctival sutures only require 5 to 7 days of integrity. The materials normally used in our procedures are given below, but others could be used with equal results.

A 4-0 or 5-0 chromic gut suture is placed in the tarsus so that the knot is distal to the lid margin. Prior to tying this tarsal suture, a running 6-0 plain gut conjunctival suture is fashioned; it is necessary to bury the knots so they do not contact the surface of the mucous membrane. We generally close the subcuticular lid in two layers, with deeper 5-0 chromic gut sutures horizontally bolstering the tarsal closure. The skin is closed with interrupted 7-0 silk (Figure 3–3C). The cut ends of interrupted sutures at the gray line and lash margin are deliberately left long, and the ends of these sutures are then tied into the first and second interrupted sutures along the anterior edge of the lid skin to avoid abrading the cornea (see Figure 3–3C).

A number of complications can occur with primary lid closure. As in any surgical procedure, infection or untoward reaction to suture material may be a problem. Most commonly, incorrect apposition of the tarsal margins results in lid notch (Figure 3–4). This problem cannot be overstressed. Probably, if only the tarsal sutures were used to close an eyelid defect, cosmesis would be excellent. In contrast, a poorly aligned tarsus almost guarantees a poor cosmetic result. If the lid defect is too large for primary closure, wound breakdown or entropion is likely to occur. It is not uncommon for conjunctival edema to occur from an overly tight lid, especially in the first 2 weeks after surgery.

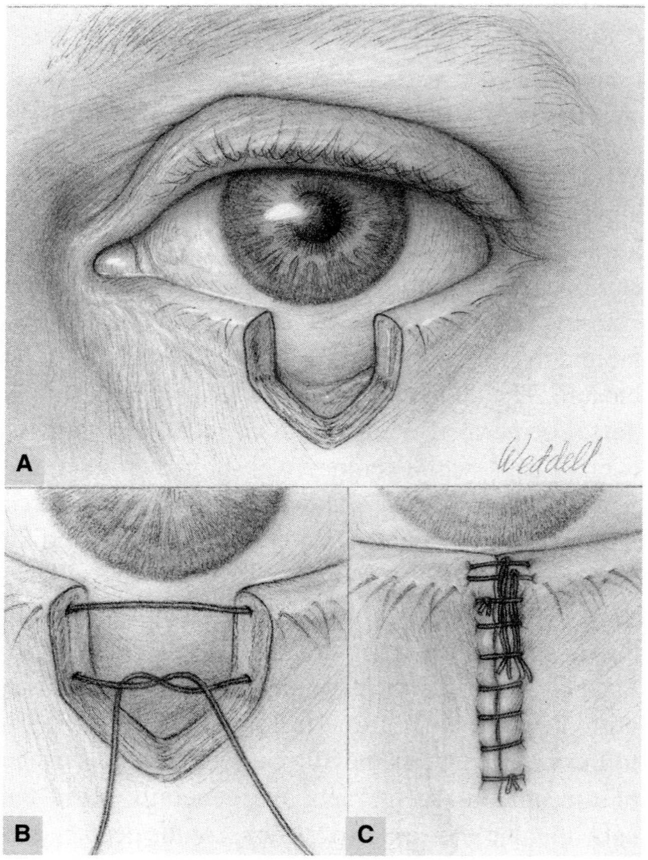

Figure 3–3. *A,* Primary lower lid closure — initial surgical defect. *B,* The tarsus is approximated with a 4-0 chromic gut suture. *C,* The suturing material is left long at the gray line and lash margins, and it is tied into the stitches lower on the lid margins to prevent the ends from abrading the cornea. (See discussion in text)

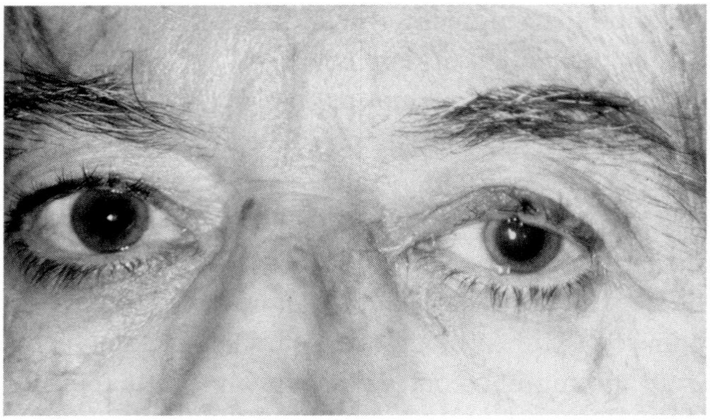

Figure 3–4. Lid notch resulting from an incorrect apposition of tarsal margins.

Lateral Cantholysis and a Lateral Advancement Flap (Tenzel and Reese Procedures)

Generally, lesions involving 33 to 60 percent of the lower lid cannot be closed primarily; a lateral myocutaneous advancement flap with cantholysis is advised in these cases. Two variations of this procedure have been widely used. The initial procedure, by Reese, was a straight lateral horizontal incision.[28] The author has used it with good results.

Figure 3–5 shows a 6-month postoperative view of a Reese procedure to correct resection of 60 percent of the lower lid. Tenzel modified this approach by making a highly curved incision with the convex apex running laterally above the brow.[26,27] The rationale for the latter approach is to decrease the likelihood of lower lid ectropion by bringing a correctly oriented flap into the lower lid.[31] This procedure is shown in Figure 3–6A.

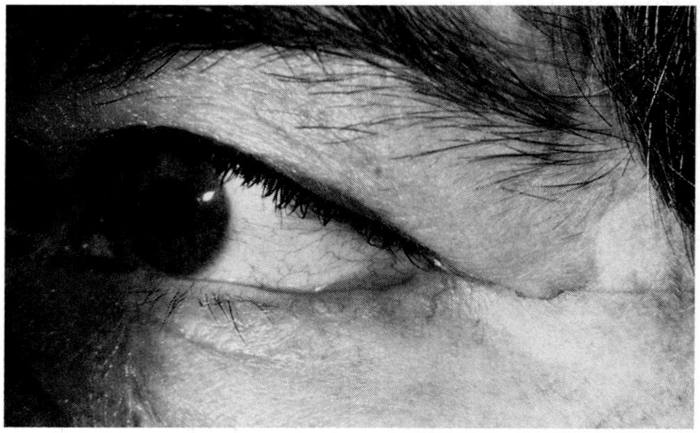

Figure 3–5. Postoperative view of a 60 percent lower lid resection and repair using a Reese procedure.

The inferior crus of the lateral canthal tendon is palpated and cut through the lateral conjunctival fornix (Figure 3–6B). After the tendon is severed, the lateral inferior lid remnant should be easily mobilized. A curvilinear incision arched upward is created, and the ends of the lid remnants are apposed, as in primary lid closure. In closing the lateral aspect of this incision, it is important to first reconstruct the lateral canthus (Figure 3–6C) and correctly place the lateral conjunctival fornix in relation to the posterior edge of the new canthal skin area. This avoids both symblepharon formation and rounding of the canthus. Interrupted 5-0 chromic sutures are used to close the subcutaneous layers (Figure 3–6D). A length of 7-0 running silk is used to close much of the lateral defect after a few interrupted 7-0 silk sutures are placed to approximate the medial lid position (Figure 3–6E). If the lateral canthal tendon has been sacrificed, the posterior aspect of the lateral lid is either sutured to the periosteum inside the entrance to the lateral orbit, or, if that has also been resected, the lid is sutured with wire to a hole drilled into bone. Failure to anchor the lateral lid posteriorly may result in lid sag or lateral ectropion. The two most common complications with this procedure are failure to completely sever the inferior

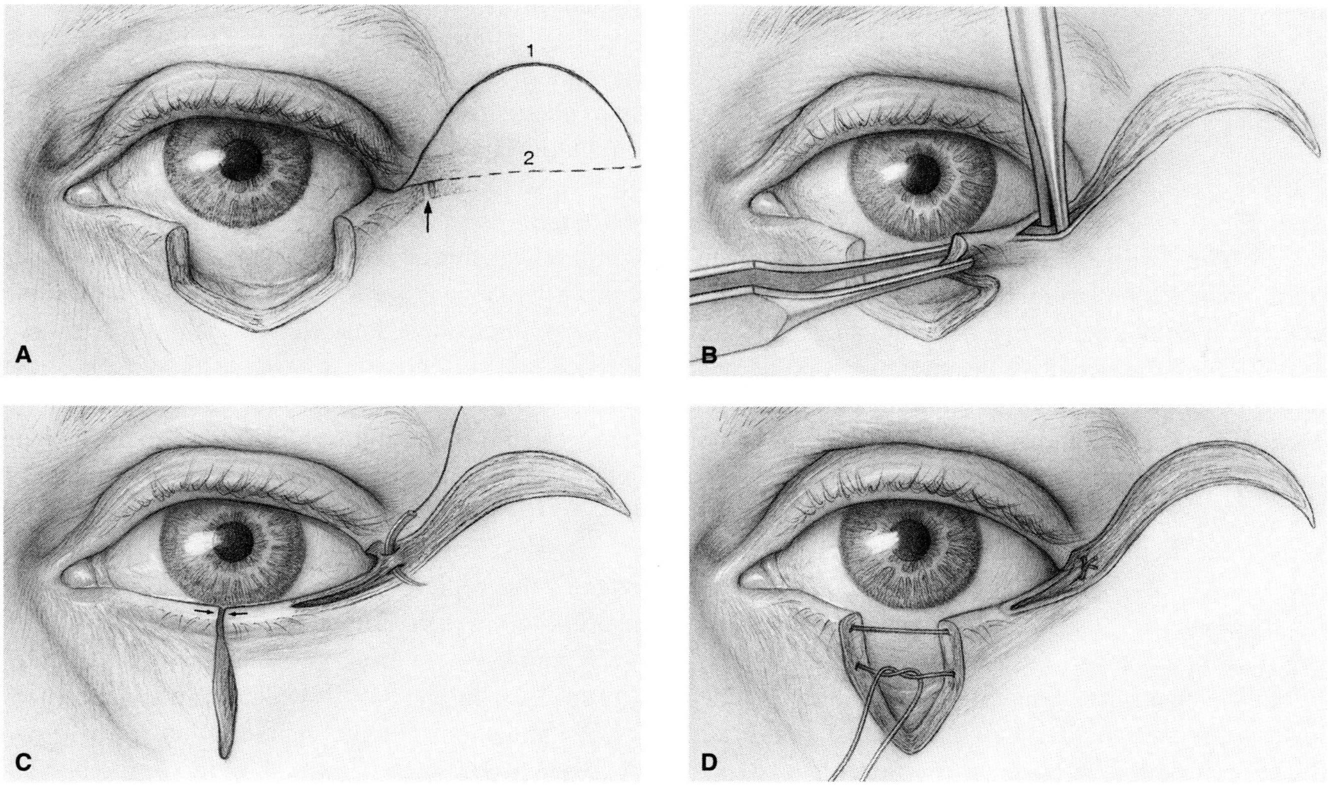

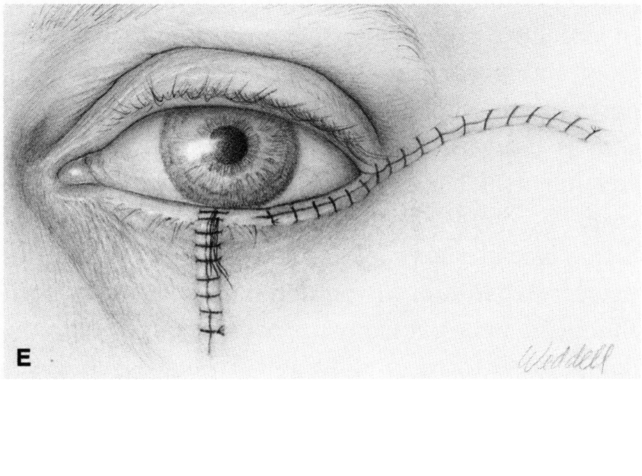

Figure 3–6. *A,* Tenzel (1) and Reese (2) procedures. Incision lines for lower lid reconstruction. *B,* The inferior crus of the lateral canthal tendon is severed. Forceps are used to determine if the lid can be closed primarily with cantholysis, or if a tarsoconjunctival flap is needed. *C,* In closing a Tenzel procedure, first the lateral canthus is reconstructed. *D,* Then, the tarsal defect is closed. *E,* Finally, the skin incisions are closed.

lateral canthal tendon and poor reconstruction of the lateral canthus. In the former situation, the lateral lid remnant cannot be adequately mobilized. If the inferior crus has not been cut, tension remains on the tendon, and it can be palpated like a guitar string on stretch. Failure to correctly align the lateral advancement flap with the lateral conjunctiva and upper lid results in rounding of the lateral canthus. Good cosmesis is achieved with the Tenzel curvilinear incision; however, the results with a straight lateral skin incision are acceptable (see Figure 3–5). Spinelli and Jelks noted that canthal abnormalities were responsible for over 50 percent of the major complications in their series of patients who had lid reconstruction after removal of a lid tumor.[32]

Tarsoconjunctival Pedicle Flap (Hewes-Beard Procedure)

Either a Hughes or a Hewes-Beard procedure can be used for simple reconstruction of the entire lower lid.[29,30] The goal of surgery is to create a relatively rigid mucous membrane–lined posterior lamella and to cover it with either a free or an advancement skin graft. If the lid defect involves more than 60 percent of the lower lid (unless it is predominantly the medial portion of the lid), and if the lateral canthus is not involved, a Hewes-Beard procedure can be used (Figure 3–7A). The author prefers the tarsoconjunctival pedicle flap to the Hughes procedure because the former does not require temporary closure of the involved eye. If the Hughes procedure is used, the eye must be occluded for 2 to 6 weeks after surgery. Either of these procedures is preferable to other lower lid reconstructions, such as a Mustardé procedure, for two major reasons: (1) these are simpler procedures for an ophthalmic surgeon to perform; and (2), in our experience, the results are excellent.

In the Hewes-Beard procedure, a tarsoconjunctival pedicle flap is created. The upper lid is everted over a Desmares retractor (Figure 3–7B). The medial remnant of the lower lid is grasped and pulled laterally, and its relative horizontal position is identified by a vertical scratch incision in the upper tarsus. If only a small remnant of the lateral lower lid remains, we usually sacrifice it. A No. 67 Beaver blade is used to make an incision in the upper lid tarsus and conjunctiva. Horizontal incisions are made to create a 4-mm wide tarsoconjunctival flap. The tarsal incision closest to the lash margin is approximately 4 mm away from it, while the superior horizontal tarsal incision is made approximately at the upper margin of the tarsus. The length of the tarsoconjunctival pedicle is predicated on the amount of surgical lid defect remaining after the lid remnants are grasped with forceps and pulled together. The tarsal flap should fit this defect; too large a pedicle uniformly results in lower lid ectropion. The tarsoconjunctival flap is then mobilized using toothed forceps and sharp scissors. We attempt to minimize cauterization of bleeding from the flap, especially at its lateral aspect, to lessen damage to its vascular supply. While the author is uncertain whether there is a good blood supply to the entire length of the flap, Beard feels strongly that it has at least some circulation (personal communication).

The tarsoconjunctival pedicle flap is mobilized at the lateral aspect of the lid and rotated so that the conjunctival side of the flap faces the inferior bulbar conjunctiva (see Figure 3–7B). The distal ends of the tarsoconjunctival pedicle flap are sutured with two interrupted 5-0 chromic sutures to the tarsus of the medial remnant of the lower lid (Figure 3–7C). An interrupted 5-0 chromic suture is used to anchor the inferolateral aspect of this pedicle to the remnant of the inferior canthal tendon. A running 6-0 plain gut suture anastomoses the conjunctiva on the inferior edge of the pedicle flap to the remnant of conjunctiva in the lower lid defect.

A number of options exist for creating an anterior lid lamella, the best of which is an advancement myocutaneous or "bucket handle" flap from below. A free skin graft can be placed on top of the pedicle flap, but its chances for survival may not be as good. In order of preference, the graft should be taken from the upper lid, retroauricular skin, or, least desirably, the supraclavicular fossa. If the last area of skin is used as a donor site, we usually create an advancement bridge flap from the lower cheek to cover the margin of the reconstructed lower lid; we then place the supraclavicular skin in the inferior defect. Regardless of the donor site, the skin graft should be approximately 25 percent larger than the defect to be filled to allow for shrinkage. All donor skin should be turned over and the subcutaneous tissues removed prior to transplantation.

After 6-0 cardinal sutures are placed at the superior, inferior, lateral, and medial edges of the skin graft, the superior edge of the graft is sutured to the superior edge of the tarsoconjunctival pedicle flap, using a continuous 6-0 plain gut suture. We attempt to have the edge of the tarsoconjunctival pedicle graft slightly higher than the skin to avoid abrading the cornea (Figure 3–7D). A number of small, linear cuts are made in the graft with a scalpel to avoid post-transplantation exudation. The eye and orbit are pressure-patched with an antibiotic ointment for 24 hours and pressure-patched again for an additional 24 hours after the surgical site is dressed again. In some large cutaneous grafts, the ends of the sutures are tied over cotton bolsters to put additional pressure on the graft.

A number of complications are associated with the tarsoconjunctival pedicle flap reconstruction of the lower lid defect. First, if the tarsal pedicle flap is too long, an ectropion invariably occurs (Figure 3–8). In order to avoid this problem, it is imperative that the tarsoconjunctival flap be short enough to create reasonable tension along the lower lid. This necessitates measuring the horizontal length of the flap with the medial lid remnant stretched laterally with a forceps. Second, with any form of lower lid reconstruction, there is loss of eyelashes. In the author's experience, lash grafts have been uniformly disappointing in correcting this relatively minor cosmetic defect. Third, in some patients, the pedicle is

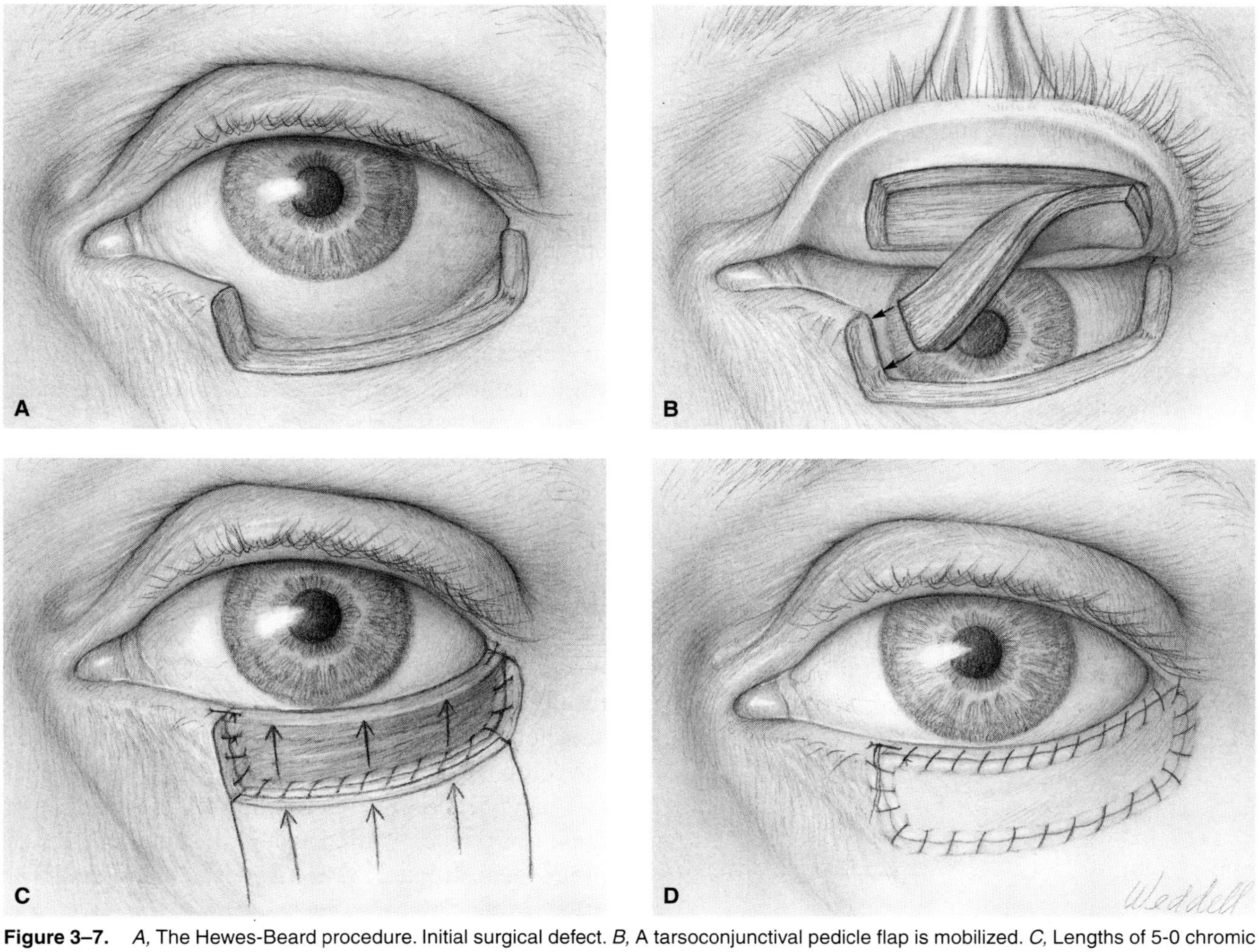

Figure 3–7. *A,* The Hewes-Beard procedure. Initial surgical defect. *B,* A tarsoconjunctival pedicle flap is mobilized. *C,* Lengths of 5-0 chromic and 6-0 plain gut sutures are used to create the posterior lamella. *D,* A free skin graft from the contralateral upper lid is used to create the anterior lid lamella.

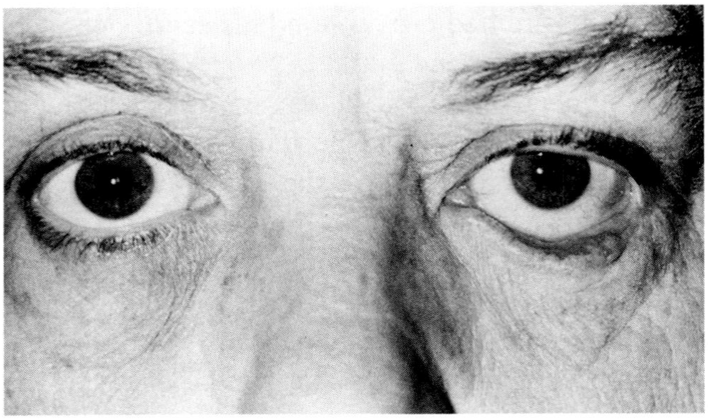

Figure 3–8. Ectropion caused by a tarsoconjunctival pedicle graft that was too long.

left in situ, which yields a rounded lateral canthus (Figure 3–9). In most patients, approximately 6 weeks after surgery, 2 percent lidocaine (Xylocaine) and 1:100,000 epinephrine are injected into the pedicle in the lateral intrapalpebral fissure, and then it is incised in the office.

The two major contraindictions to the Hewes-Beard procedure are tumors involving the entire lower lid, canthus, and lateral upper lid region, and malignancies involving only the medial lower lid.

Tarsoconjunctival Advancement Flap (Hughes Procedure)

The Hughes procedure was an early approach to correcting a 50 to 100 percent lower lid defect.[30] The author has not used this approach for the last 10 years because the tarsoconjunctival pedicle flap is equally effective and does not require eye closure during the recuperative period. Performance of a Hughes procedure is relatively straightforward. Instead of a pedicle flap, the inner lamella of the lower lid defect is reconstructed, using an advancement flap of tarsus and conjunctiva from the upper lid.

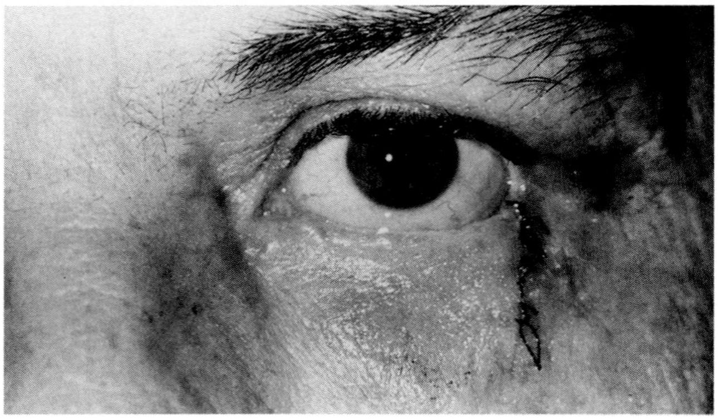

Figure 3–9. Rounded lateral canthus after a tarsoconjunctival pedicle graft.

As shown in Figure 3–10, a tarsoconjunctival advancement from the upper lid is brought down to fill the lower lid defect. After the upper lid is everted on a Desmares retractor, a scalpel is used to mark the tarsal extent of donor tissue (Figure 3–10A). As with a tarsoconjunctival pedicle flap, the remnants of the lateral and medial lower lid defects should be positioned as close together as possible to minimize the amount of upper lid material needed to cover the defect. The incision should be approximately 4 mm from the lash margin to prevent upper lid instability. Blunt dissection of the tarsus and conjunctiva from the more superficial layers of the upper lid is performed. Care should be taken to avoid damage to Müller's muscle and the flap's vascular supply. The tarsoconjunctival advancement flap is sutured to the respective conjunctival and tarsal surfaces of the lower lid defect using interrupted 5-0 chromic sutures for the tarsus and running 6-0 plain gut for the conjunctiva (Figure 3–10B). A free skin graft or an advancement bridge flap is then sutured in the defect to recreate the anterior lamella of the lower lid (Figure 3–10C). The skin graft should be approximately 25 percent larger than the defect. The surgical technique of graft placement is described under the Hewes-Beard procedure.

Approximately 1 to 6 weeks after initial surgery, the tissue of the upper lid is incised just above the reconstructed lower lid edge (see Figure 3–10C), using a convex superior curved incision. By angling the scissors anteriorly and making a convex incision, retraction and scarring leave an even tissue surface with a slight excess of conjunctiva; this method also results in a lower incidence of secondary corneal abrasions. Other authors have recommended cutting the conjunctiva flush with the skin. They believe that this modification results in improved cosmesis.[33] If there is too much conjunctiva in the anterior surface of the reconstructed lower lid, it can either keratinize or be cauterized.

A number of complications have been reported in association with the Hughes procedure. If too lit-

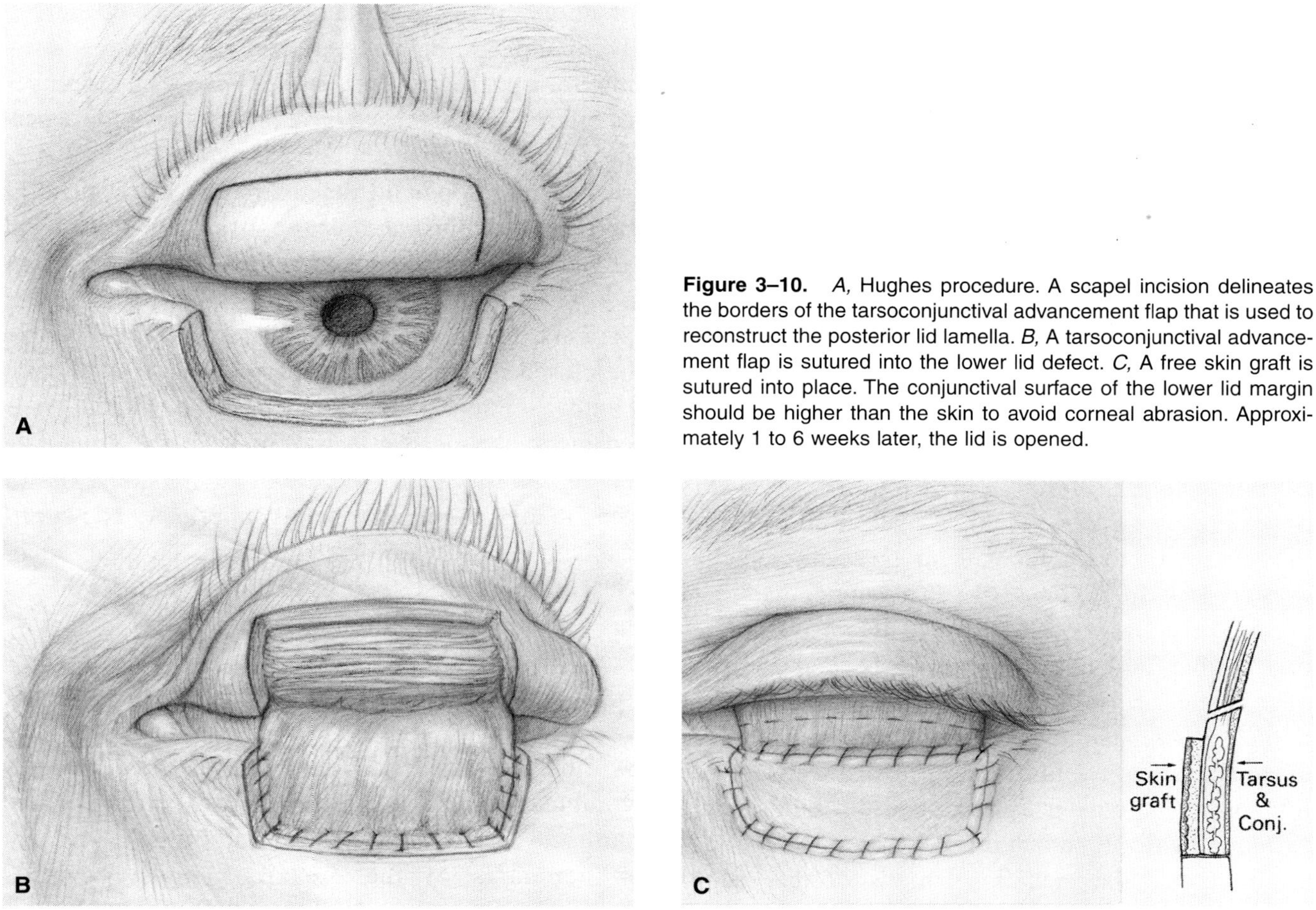

Figure 3–10. *A,* Hughes procedure. A scapel incision delineates the borders of the tarsoconjunctival advancement flap that is used to reconstruct the posterior lid lamella. *B,* A tarsoconjunctival advancement flap is sutured into the lower lid defect. *C,* A free skin graft is sutured into place. The conjunctival surface of the lower lid margin should be higher than the skin to avoid corneal abrasion. Approximately 1 to 6 weeks later, the lid is opened.

tle upper lid tarsus remains, an upper lid entropion with trichiasis can result. Similarly, secondary retraction of the upper lid can occur if the conjunctiva superior to the tarsus in the upper fornix is not dissected free from Müller's muscle when the advancement flap is created from the posterior lamella of the upper lid. As with the tarsoconjunctival pedicle flap, if too large a donor graft is placed in the lower lid defect, the occurrence of a lower lid ectropion is likely; if the graft is too small, entropion can occur. If insufficient conjunctiva is left on the anterior edge of the lower lid, fine residual hairs can abrade the cornea. The reconstructed lower lid is less mobile than normal. Some authors have suggested using an orbicularis muscle advancement as a modification of this procedure to increase mobility.[34,35] Less commonly used lower lid procedures (glabellar flap, Mustardé, laissez faire) and the Gorney procedure are discussed at the end of the chapter.

Posterior Free Tarsal Graft

Recently, many surgeons are using more free grafts to replace the posterior lamellae of the lower eyelid. The two most used donor sites are either ipsilateral

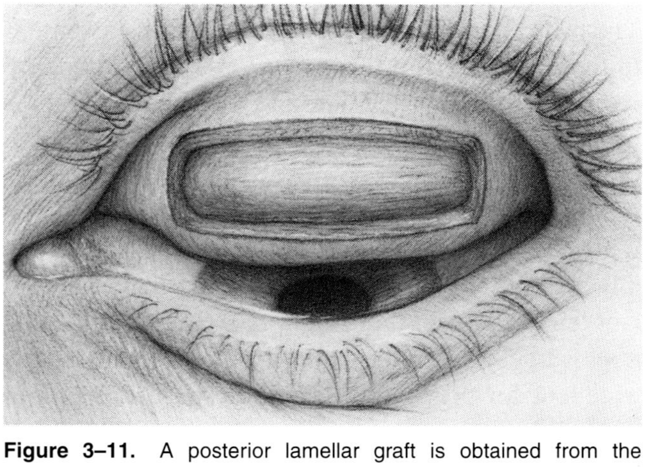

Figure 3–11. A posterior lamellar graft is obtained from the everted upper eyelid.

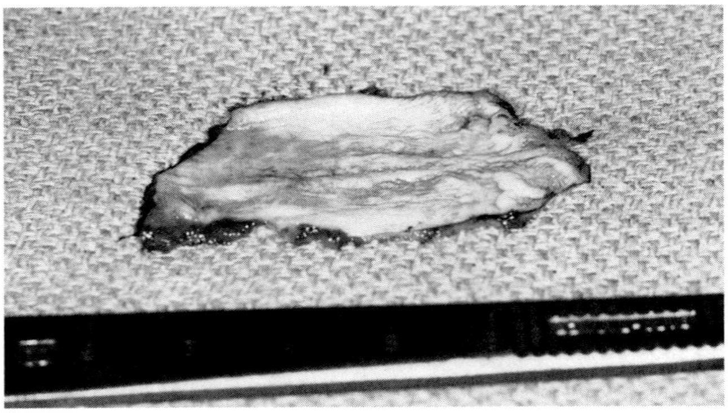

Figure 3–12. A large hard palate graft harvested. Care is taken to avoid both the midline and the soft palate.

or contralateral posterior upper eyelid (Figure 3–11) or hard palate (Figure 3–12).[36–40] The author prefers the variant of the composite or posterior lamellar graft shown in Figure 3–11. The upper eyelid is everted on a Desmares retractor with a 4-0 silk traction suture. The length of the tarsus needed (with the edge of the surgical defect relatively tightly apposed to measure this length) is marked with a scalpel. We take care to leave 2 to 3 mm of tarsus near the lash line. Sutures are used, as described for the previous two procedures, to attach this conjunctival tarsal tissue to create the posterior lamella of the reconstructed lower lid. The anterior lamella is reconstructed with a sliding or bridge flap. Hard palate grafts (see Figure 3–12) for lower eyelid defects also work well, but it is more difficult for the ophthalmologist who performs this type of procedure only rarely to obtain such tissue.

UPPER LID RECONSTRUCTION

The principles of upper lid reconstruction are similar to those of lower lid repair but with three important caveats. First, since the normal Bell's phenomenon is usually preserved, the placement of buried knots in the central portion of an upper lid reconstruction is crucial to avoid corneal abrasions and pain. Even with correct closure of upper lid defects, occasionally we find it necessary to use a soft bandage contact lens to protect the cornea in the first few weeks after surgery. Second, while the upper lid tarsus is excellent for providing a stable posterior lamella in lower lid reconstructions, the much smaller and less stable lower lid tarsus does not provide equal support or utility for reconstruction of an upper lid defect. Third, the hard palate is probably not a good substitute for upper eyelid tarsus. We have seen a number of referred patients who have had this procedure performed with significant corneal damage.

In small upper lid defects (usually less than 33 percent of the lid), a direct apposition of the medial and lateral remnants is performed in the same manner as primary closure of the lower lid. In older patients, a defect as large as 60 percent of the lid can be closed by cutting the superior crus of the lateral canthal tendon. To close an upper lid defect, it is cosmetically more effective to have the convexity curved inferiorly, instead of having the convexity of the lateral skin incision point superiorly. The surgical techniques to perform these procedures are identical to those described in the lower lid and do not need further description.

Lateral Cantholysis and Sliding Tarsal Flap

A moderate-sized lid defect can be closed with a combination of a lateral cantholysis sliding procedure and a transposition tarsal flap from the remnant or remnants of the medial, lateral, or upper tarsi.[34,41,42] This approach is shown in Figure 3–13.

In this procedure, after maximum sliding is obtained with lateral cantholysis, a full-thickness tarsal incision is made from the superior edge of the tarsus to within 1 mm of the inferior border and 2 to 3 mm from the cut tarsal edge (Figure 3–13A). This tarsal strip is rotated to create a posterior lamella in the upper lid defect. The superior conjunctiva is mobilized and brought down as an advancement flap and sutured with 6-0 plain gut to the upper edge of the transposed tarsus, and a free skin graft is placed over the entire defect, as shown in Figures 3–13B and C. Figure 3–14 shows a slight modification of this technique in a 40-year-old man with sebaceous gland carcinoma. In this case, the tarsal transposition flap from the medial lid remnant was sutured to a raised strip of orbital periosteum.[43] Schematically, this procedure utilizes a rotated tarsal strip attached to the raised piece of periosteum of the lateral orbital rim. This procedure is schematically shown in Figure 3–15.

In patients with a carcinoma that only involves the distal 2 to 5 mm of the eyelid near the eyelashes,

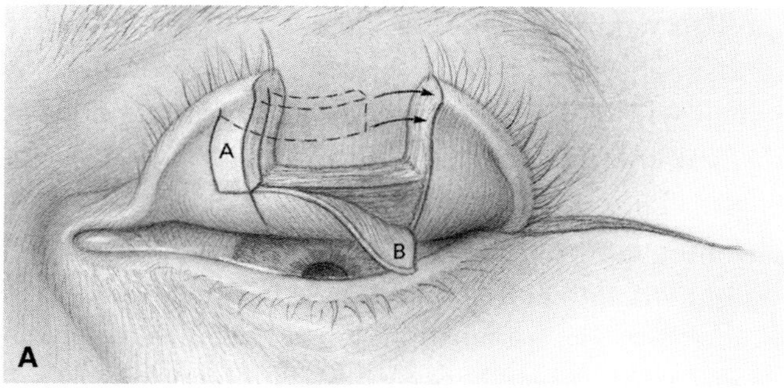

Figure 3–13. *A,* A tarsoconjunctival transpositional flap is used to create the posterior lamella of the upper lid. *B,* Conjunctiva from the superior fornix is advanced to the tarsal flap. *C,* A free skin graft or myocutaneous advancement is placed over the rotated tarsal flap to reconstruct the upper lid defect.

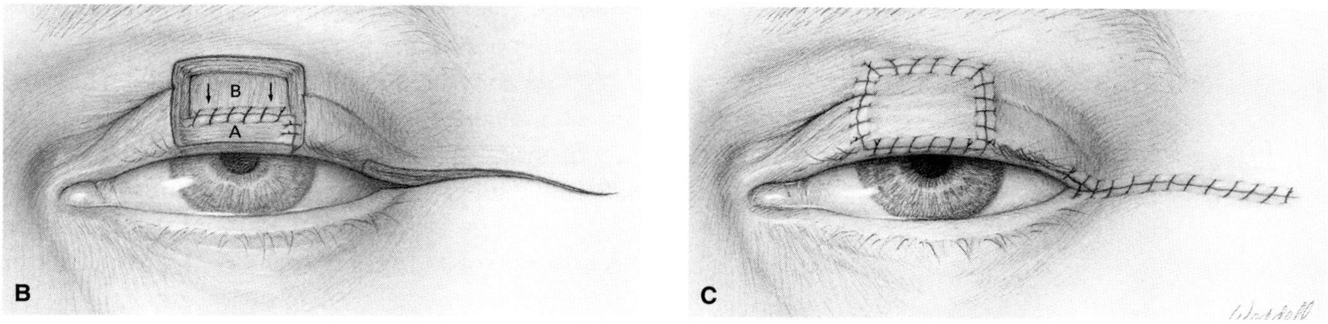

another approach to closure is shown in Figure 3–16. The remaining tarsus is brought down to fill the posterior defect and a free skin graft is placed anteriorly. It has not been necessary to alter the normal levator aponeurosis-tarsal relationship with this small advancement.[44] We have not had a problem with eyelid retraction postoperatively.

Cutler-Beard Procedure

The reconstruction of a defect involving more than 60 percent of the upper lid is best accomplished using a Cutler-Beard procedure.[45] The surgery is straightforward, but the technique requires some functional levator aponeurosis as well as a two-stage repair. The surgical upper lid defect is trimmed to rectangular shape, and a full-thickness lower lid donor flap is fashioned approximately 4 to 5 mm inferior to the lower lid margin (Figure 3–17A). The length of the horizontal lower lid incision should parallel the amount of defect present in the upper lid. As discussed above under "Lower Lid Reconstruction," this upper lid defect should be minimized by creating moderate traction with forceps on both the lateral and medial lid remnants. A flat ribbon retractor is placed in the inferior cul-de-sac, and a No. 15 Bard-

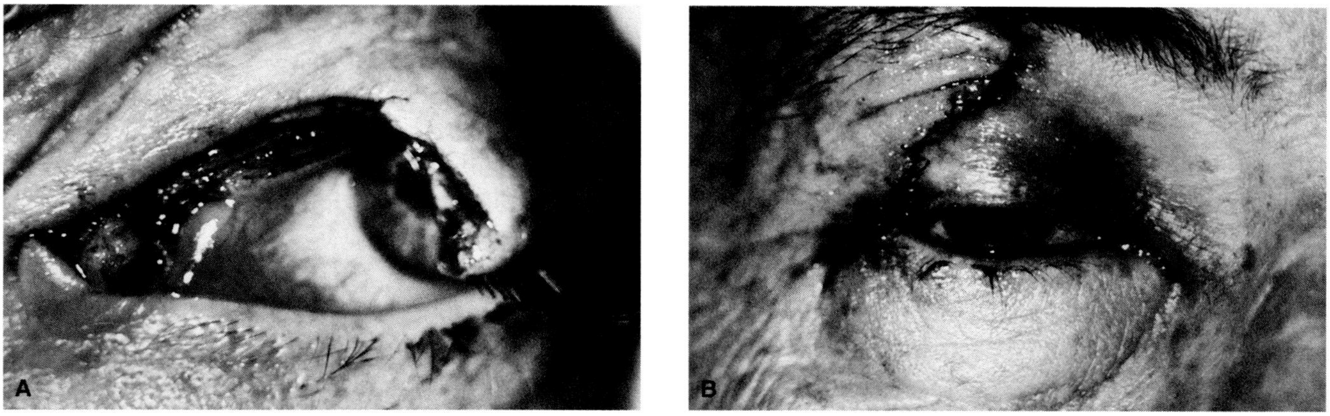

Figure 3–14. *A,* Intraoperative view of a large upper lid defect after resection of a sebaceous gland carcinoma. *B,* The defect is closed by rotating an upper lid tarsal flap and suturing it to lateral orbital periosteum. The mycutaneous layer is closed with an advancement flap.

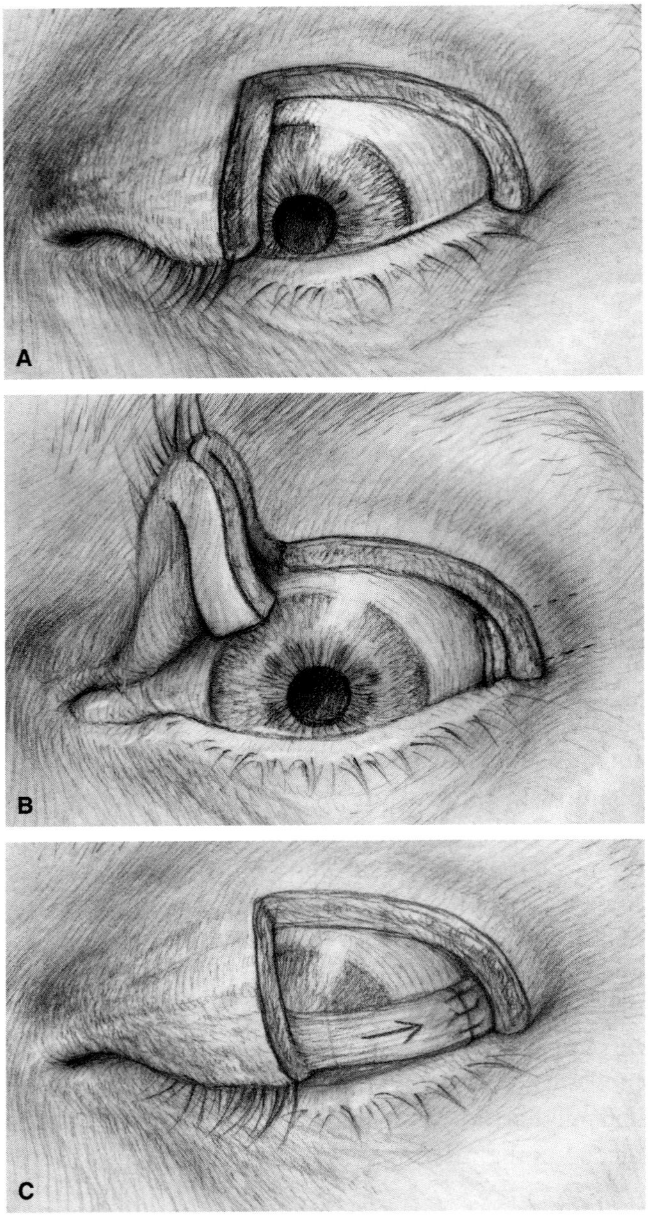

Figure 3–15. *A*, Schematic approach to closure of a upper lid lateral defect with a rotational tarsus graft. *B*, A tarsal graft is mobilized as discussed previously. It is sutured to the raised strip of periosteum from the lateral orbital rim. *C*, This tarsal-periosteal anastomosis is used as a reconstruction point for the posterior lamellae of the upper lid.

Parker blade is used to make the horizontal incision through the entire lower lid onto the anterior surface of the retractor. The medial and lateral edges of the lower lid advancement flap are incised with sharp scissors, and the full-thickness flap is passed under the bridge of the margin of the lower lid (Figure 3–17B). A three-layer closure of conjunctival, then subcutaneous, and finally skin tissues is used to unite the flap with the tissues at the edges of the upper lid defect. The corners of the conjunctiva are approximated with 6-0 interrupted gut, and the remainder of the conjunctiva is closed with a running 7-0 plain gut suture. The subcutaneous tissues are closed with 5-0 chromic gut suture, and the skin is approximated with interrupted and continuous 7-0 silk sutures (see Figure 3–17B). Some surgeons believe that insertion of eye bank sclera between the conjunctiva and the myocutaneous layers produces a more stable reconstructed upper lid margin.[46]

While some authors have advocated closing the open remnant of the lower lid bridge, we usually do not; instead, we place an eye pad, cut in half, on each side of the lower lid margin, put antibiotic on its surface, and pressure-patch the entire area. There have been rare, isolated reports of necrosis of the lower lid bridge, but we have never observed this.

The eye must remain closed for between 4 and 12 weeks after surgery to allow stretching of the advancement flap and re-establishment of vascular as well as lymphatic supply. It is not rare to have transient lymphedema in the advancement flap (Figure 3–18B).

The second stage of the reconstructive procedure is done under local anesthesia, using 2 percent lidocaine and 1:100,000 epinephrine. Two muscle hooks are used to elevate the lid away from the bulbar conjunctiva, and an inferiorly pointing convex incision is made with angled scissors to leave the conjunctiva slightly longer than the skin of the upper lid (see Figure 3–17C). An incision is made approximately 2 mm below the intended upper lid margin to allow for normal shrinkage. If the incision is cut straight across, retraction results in an unsightly scar and possible exposure. The slight increase in conjunctiva length to overlap the shorter skin edge decreases the likelihood of corneal abrasion (see Figure 3–17C). The upper lid margin is closed with a 6-0 plain gut suture. The inferior aspect of the marginal lower lid remnant is freshened with either a scalpel or scissors, and the severed lower lid bridge flap is resutured in three layers using a 6-0 plain gut to appose conjunctiva, 5-0 chromic interrupted suture for the subcutaneous layer, and 7-0 silk for the skin. Figures 3–18A to C show the use of a Cutler-Beard procedure to reconstruct an 85 percent defect in the upper lid after resection of a melanoma. Figure 3–18D

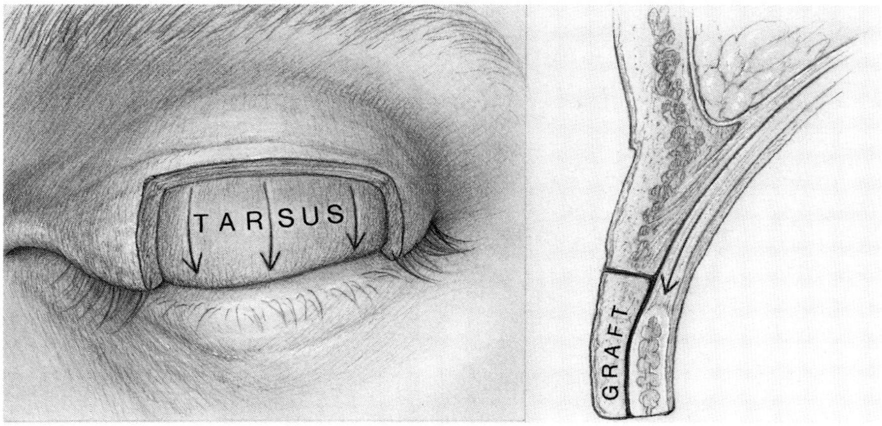

Figure 3–16. For a small defect involving just the lash, the margin of the upper lid tarsus can be brought down to fill the posterior gap. A free graft can be placed anteriorly.

demonstrates the final result of a squamous cell carcinoma defect in a 50-year-old man who had lid repair with a Cutler-Beard procedure.

In our experience, the major complication associated with the Cutler-Beard lower lid advancement technique has been the loss of lashes. Retraction of both the upper lid and lower lid scars can occur, but it is unlikely. Rarely, delicate hairs on the advanced lower lid skin can abrade the cornea. A number of modifications of the Cutler-Beard procedure have

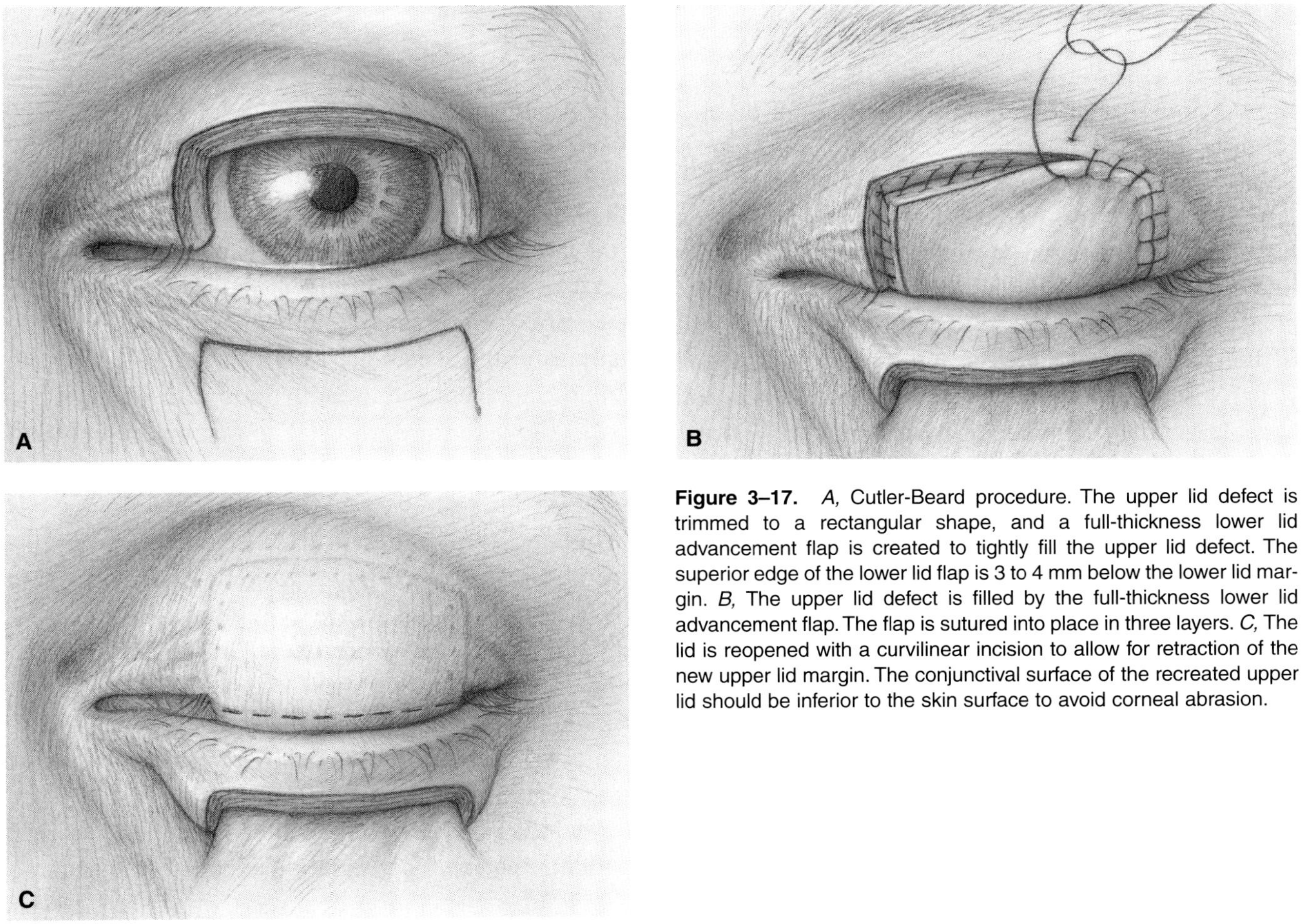

Figure 3–17. *A,* Cutler-Beard procedure. The upper lid defect is trimmed to a rectangular shape, and a full-thickness lower lid advancement flap is created to tightly fill the upper lid defect. The superior edge of the lower lid flap is 3 to 4 mm below the lower lid margin. *B,* The upper lid defect is filled by the full-thickness lower lid advancement flap. The flap is sutured into place in three layers. *C,* The lid is reopened with a curvilinear incision to allow for retraction of the new upper lid margin. The conjunctival surface of the recreated upper lid should be inferior to the skin surface to avoid corneal abrasion.

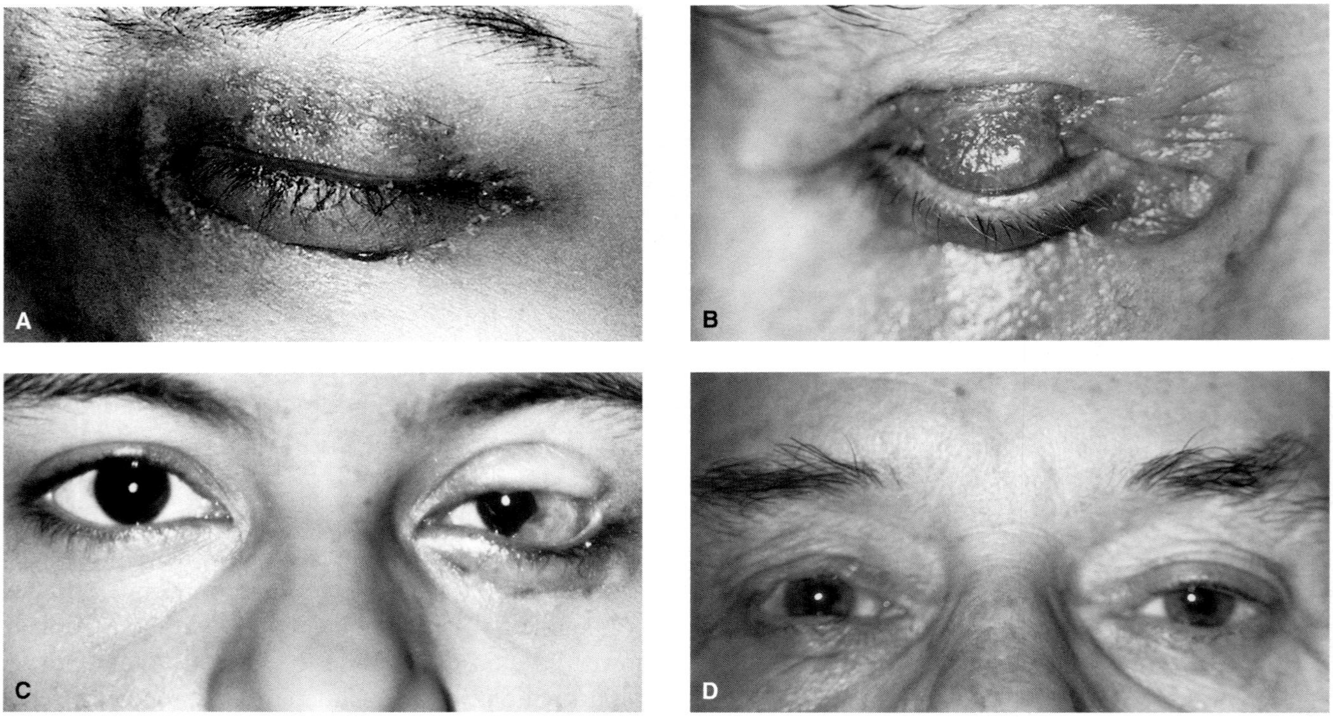

Figure 3–18. *A,* Clinical photographs of the Cutler-Beard procedure. Closure of an 85 percent upper lid defect. *B,* Transient edema is not uncommon. *C,* Postoperative view 1 week after second stage of the procedure shown in Figure 3–17A. *D,* Postoperative view 3 months after the repair shown in Figure 3–17B.

been proposed, but the author has not used them.[47] Entropion also has been reported after this procedure,[48] but the author has not had this problem.

The author has not used the Mustardé technique for the upper lid reconstruction, in which the lower lid is rotated to replace the upper lid and the defect created inferiorly is replaced with a posterior graft of the nasal septal mucosa and a rotational cheek flap. This procedure, while effective in Mustardé's capable hands, seems much more complex without any obvious advantages.[49] Similarly, a variant of the reverse Mustardé—using the upper eyelid to close a lower eyelid defect—seems a less optimal procedure than the others described above.[50]

OTHER PROCEDURES

As mentioned at the outset of this chapter, the discussion has been limited to the procedures found most useful for the repair of surgically created lid defects by an ophthalmologist. The procedures listed below are less commonly useful in managing either canthal lesions or isolated lid tumors.

Composite grafts taken from the contralateral lid have been used for over 35 years to repair lid defects.[51,52] The initial composite grafts were of full thickness and involved both the posterior and anterior lamellae of the lid; necrosis of a portion of the graft was not an infrequent complication. More recently, Putterman and others have suggested using only a posterior lamella from the opposite lid with an advancement flap of skin and muscular tissue to cover the anterior defect.[53] The maximum length of a full-thickness composite graft is approximately 8 mm. We have rarely used this procedure since it has a greater risk of necrosis than the other options listed. In a one-eyed patient with a tumor involving the upper lid of the seeing eye, a posterior composite graft from the contralateral lid in combination with lateral cantholysis may be used to avoid closing the lid. As discussed above, we usually elect to use either a modification with a free tarsal conjunctival graft or a rotational tarsal flap.

A larger complete upper lid defect in a one-eyed patient may be one situation where the Mustardé lower lid transposition operation would be another reasonable alternative. In a large upper eyelid defect where the cancer does not reach more than 10 to 12 mm above the eyelid margin, a variation of this option has been used by the author in a few cases. A free tarsal graft from the contralateral upper eyelid is sewn in place, and the skin from below the brow is brought down in a modified "bucket-handle" approach. A series of these cases will be published from other centers.

If upper lid tarsus is not available for the reconstruction of a lower lid defect, or if an attempt at repair of a large upper lid defect is made without a Cutler-Beard procedure, a free tarsal graft and a nasal septum mucosa free graft to create a posterior lid lamella are other options.[54,55] Free chondrodermal auricular cartilage or eye bank sclera grafts have also been used in selected cases.[56–58] The technique to obtain a nasal-septal graft is discussed under the Mustardé procedure.

Procedure for Closing Medial Canthal Defects

Large medial defects involving both the upper and lower lids can be repaired with a free skin graft, a glabellar transposition flap, or a laissez-faire approach.[59–61] Figure 3–19 shows a case in which a malignant adnexal tumor was superficial and deep canthal structures were clear of tumor. A free skin graft from the supraclavicular area was used to close the defect. Usually, an upper lid tarsal transposition flap, a free posterior composite graft, or a nasal-septal graft is used to create the posterior lamellae, and a sliding skin flap is used to form the anterior lid structure. If the canthal tendon is sacrificed during tumor resection, the posterior grafts or flaps are sutured to a raised periosteum. As discussed above, under "Lateral Cantholysis" and "Sliding Tarsal Flap," the posterior lamellae must be anchored toward the posterior lacrimal crest area to maintain proper lid-eye position. In cases with a medial canthal fistula, more extensive surgery is required, and this is nicely summarized elsewhere.[61]

The laissez faire technique for repair of lid defects was first described in the 18th century.[62] We have used this approach in patients who have had multiple tumors, such as in basal cell nevus syndrome or xeroderma pigmentosum syndrome, and in those who have experienced local recurrence after many surgeries and extensive cryotherapy and radiation treatment.[22,63–65] The size of the medial defect is reduced by cutting the lateral canthal tendon and mobilizing both the upper and lower lids medially. The remnants of the upper and lower lids are individually sutured to the remains of the medial canthal tendon or orbital periosteum with a 4-0 nonabsorbable suture (Figure 3–20). The wound is cleaned and allowed to granulate. The cosmetic appearance is adequate, but not excellent (Figure 3–21). In smaller defects, laissez faire cosmesis can be quite good.

Usually, the lacrimal drainage system must be repaired if an extensive medial canthal tumor is removed. If any of the canalicular system is present, silicone tubes can be used to reconstruct the drainage system.[66] We intubate the remaining portion of the system and tie the tubes in the nose in the usual manner. A posterior notch in the reconstructed lid is used to reconstruct the punctum, and the tubes are secured in those positions. If there is no canalicular system left when the tumor is resected, a Jones tube can be placed secondarily. We usually wait until

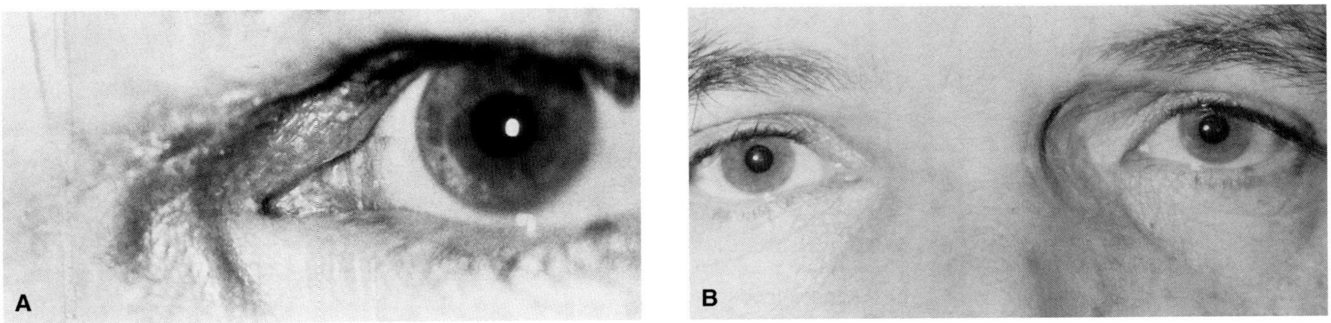

Figure 3–19. *A,* Superficial medial canthal maligant adnexal tumor. *B,* Free skin graft to repair the superficial defect after removal of the tumor.

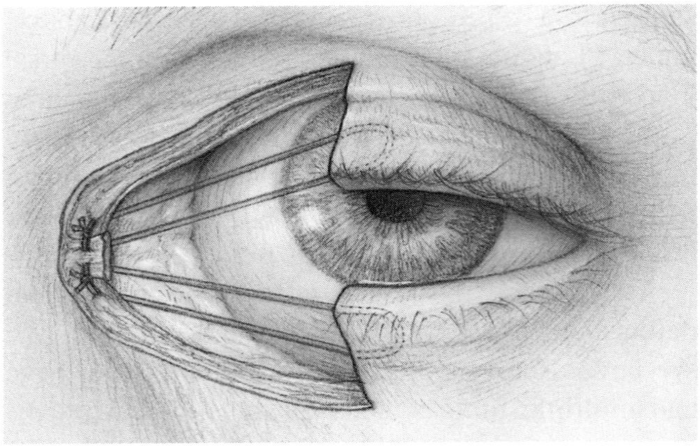

Figure 3–20. Laissez-faire approach. The lateral canthal tendons are severed, and the medial lid remnants are sutured to the orbital periosteum. Healing occurs by granulation.

healing of the reconstructed lid has been accomplished before doing this latter procedure.

Ancillary Surgical Procedures

The glabellar forehead flap is not among our frequently used approaches for lid repair. We only use it to reconstruct a medial canthal tumor, if we are unable to obtain skin from lower lid or adjacent sites. Extensive undermining has to be performed, and the length of the flap should be not more than five times its width.

We have tried not to use Mustardé's lower lid reconstruction technique for several reasons:[49] (1) it is a technically more difficult procedure for the ophthalmic surgeon and no more effective than other techniques; (2) it usually results in a long scar line; (3) there is a necessity for excising a large triangle of normal cheek skin, since the medial vertical lid incision must be 1.5 to 2 times the length of the horizontal defect to be closed; (4) the lid is less mobile than we are able to produce with other types of lower lid repair; and (5) with time, most of these reconstructed lower eyelids sag. The Mustardé procedure is shown schematically in Figure 3–22A. Usually the posterior lamella of the lid is recreated with a nasal-septal graft or hard palate (Figure 3–22B). Prior to obtaining the nasal-septal graft, the nose is packed with 4 percent lidocaine and 1:100,000 epinephrine. At least 1 cm of nasal cartilage must be left in situ anterior to the graft donor site to support the nasal bridge. A submucosal injection of 1:100,000 epinephrine in 2 percent lidocaine is given to strip the mucosa from the contralateral cartilage. In some cases, the nasal opening is too small to be separated effectively, and a lateral rhinotomy in the nasal fold can be made to provide easier access to the nasal septum. The rhinotomy is closed in two layers, after the graft is obtained. A scalpel is used to create the nasal-septal flap. The flap is stripped from the opposite mucosa using a periosteal elevator to avoid a through-and-through septal defect (see Figure 3–22B). If the contralateral mucosa is surgically invaded, it should be either sutured or packed. Scissors are then used to complete the resection. This material is used in a manner analogous to a tarsoconjunctival free graft (Figure 3–22C). A very large myocutaneous flap must be created with the superior edge of the flap at the top of the tragus and brought down vertically just in front of the ear. The semicircle's height, at least to the level of the brow, tends to counteract lower lid sagging (Figure 3–22D). The amount of medial triangle that must be excised varies with the size of the rotation flap. As mentioned above, usually, the medial vertical cut is 1.5 to 2 times the length of the horizontal defect. We have used the Mustardé procedure if there is diffuse involvement of the canthus, if the lid cancer extends down from the lower lid onto the cheek, or if a patient is referred with a large recurrence or incomplete resection of a tumor previously repaired with a Hughes or a Hewes-Beard procedure. The closure of skin should begin with reconstruction of the canthal angle and proceed from there (see Figure 3–22D). Figure 3–23 shows a case in which we used a Mustardé reconstruction. The patient had a malignant melanoma that had been

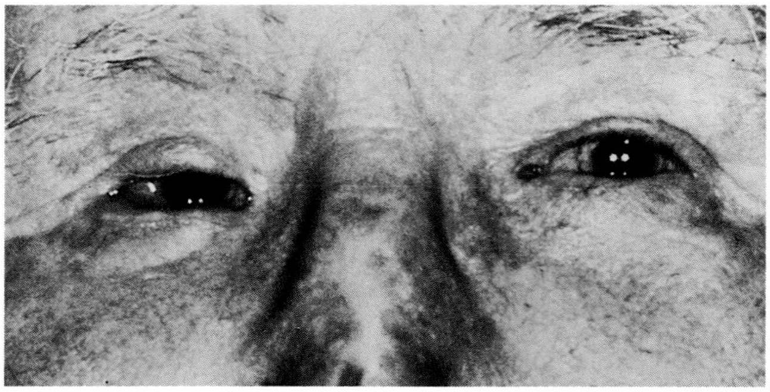

Figure 3–21. Laissez-faire healing of a large tumor in xeroderma pigmentosum patient; the tumor involved over 50 percent of both upper and lower lids.

described by an outside pathologist as clear on frozen sections. The ophthalmic surgeon repaired the lower lid defect with a Hughes procedure, but he found on perusal of the final selections that all three margins were involved by melanoma.

The Gorney procedure (Figure 3–24) for medial lower lid reconstruction was originally described to repair either medial or lateral lower lid defects, but in our unit, we have used it mainly as an alternative to reconstruct lesions confined to the medial one-half or two-thirds of the lower lid.[67] Reconstruction is performed using a full-thickness pedicle flap from the upper lid skin, muscle, tarsus, and conjunctiva.

After obtaining clear tumor margins, the length of donor skin tissue needed to fill the defect is marked, and an incision is made in the upper lid just inferior to the lid crease and carried down

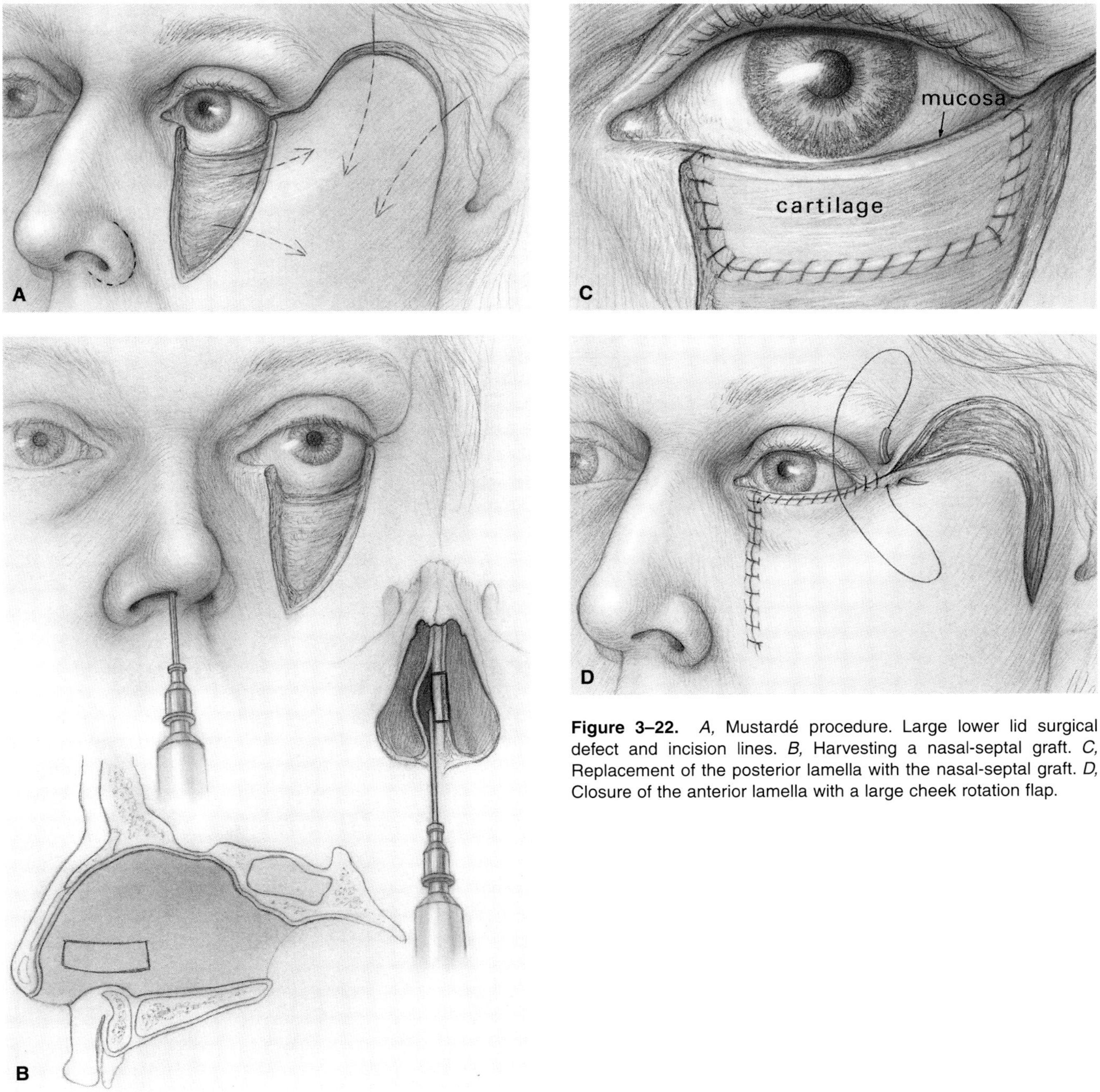

Figure 3–22. *A,* Mustardé procedure. Large lower lid surgical defect and incision lines. *B,* Harvesting a nasal-septal graft. *C,* Replacement of the posterior lamella with the nasal-septal graft. *D,* Closure of the anterior lamella with a large cheek rotation flap.

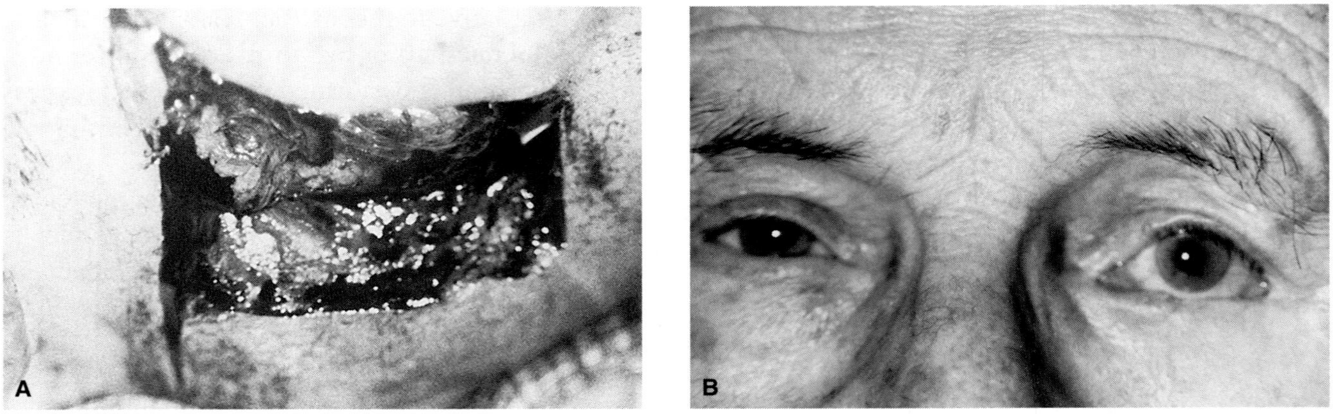

Figure 3–23. *A,* A large lower lid defect resulting from a Mustardé resection of a cutaneous malignant melanoma. *B,* Postoperative view 2 weeks after the procedure.

through the orbicularis. The upper lid is then everted on a Desmares retractor. The amount of tarsus needed to fill the lower lid tarsal defect is measured, and this is incised using a scalpel and sharp scissors (see Figure 3–24A). The entire flap consisting of skin, muscle, tarsus, and conjunctiva is rotated into the lower lid defect and closed in three layers (see Figures 3–24B and C). Similar to the Hewes-Beard procedure, the closure should be taut to avoid late development of ectropion. Some additional procedures have been used that are not discussed in this chapter. A number of authors have described the use of island rotational pedicle grafts for reconstruction. This is nicely outlined in another publication.[68] In some cases where we have had to remove the benign lid tumors, especially

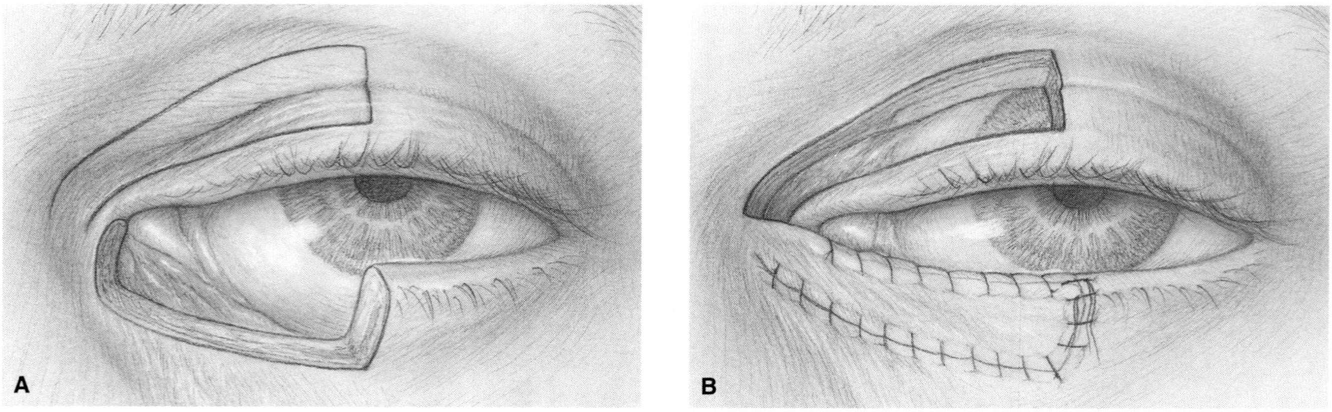

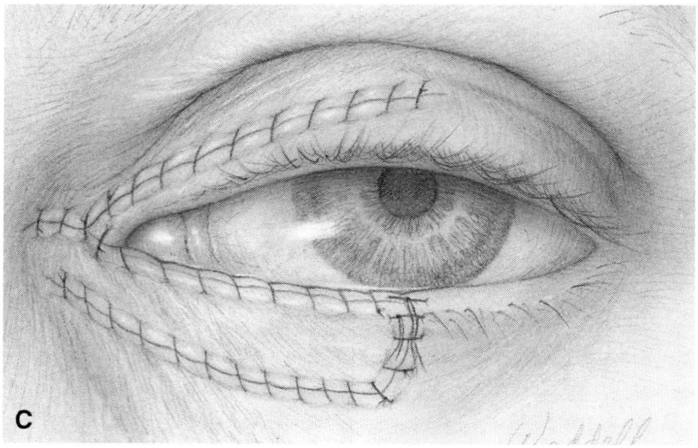

Figure 3–24. An upper lid cutaneous flap is used and shown in A–C to close the anterior lamella of the lower lid medial defect.

with neurofibromatosis, the use of a lid expander has been quite helpful, and this is described well in a separate publication.[69]

REFERENCES

1. Beard C. Observations on the treatment of basal cell carcinoma of the eyelids. The Wendell L. Hughes Lecture. Trans Am Acad Ophthalmol Otolaryngol 1975;79:664–70.
2. Einaugler RB, Henkind P. Basal cell epithelioma of the eyelid: apparent incomplete removal. Am J Ophthalmol 1969;67:413–7.
3. Aurora AL, Blodi FC. Reappraisal of basal cell carcinoma of the eyelids. Am J Ophthalmol 1970;70: 329–36.
4. Rakofsky SI. The adequacy of the surgical excision of basal cell carcinoma. Ann Ophthalmol 1973;5: 596–600.
5. Chalfin J, Putterman AM. Frozen section control in the surgery of basal cell carcinoma of the eyelid. Am J Ophthalmol 1979;87:802–9.
6. Doxanas MT, Green WR, Iliff CE. Factors in the successful surgical management of basal cell carcinoma of the eyelids. Am J Ophthalmol 1981;91:726–36.
7. Gooding CA, White G, Yatsuhashi M. Significance of marginal extension in excised basal cell carcinoma. N Engl J Med 1965;273:923–4.
8. Frank WJ. Frozen section control of excision of eyelid basal cell carcinomas: 8 1/2 years' experience. Br J Ophthalmol 1989;73:328–32.
9. Older JJ, Quickert MH, Beard C. Surgical removal of basal cell carcinoma of the eyelids utilizing frozen section control. Trans Am Acad Ophthalmol Otolaryngol 1975;79:658–63.
10. Wolfe JT III, Yeatts RP, Wick MR, et al. Sebaceous carcinoma of the eyelid. Errors in clinical and pathologic diagnosis. Am J Surg Pathol 1984;8:597–606.
11. Landthaler M, Braun-Falco O, Leitl A, et al. Excisional biopsy as the first therapeutic procedure versus primary wide excision of malignant melanoma. Cancer 1989;64:1612–6.
12. Mohs FE. Chemosurgery; microscopically controlled method of cancer excision. Arch Surg 1941;42: 279–95.
13. Mohs FE. Chemosurgical treatment of cancer of the eyelid; microscopically controlled method of excision. Arch Ophthalmol 1948;39:43–59.
14. Mohs FE. The chemosurgical method for microscopically controlled excision of external cancer with reference to cancer of the eyelids. Trans Am Acad Ophthalmol Otolaryngol 1958;62:335–6.
15. Mohs FE. Microscopically controlled surgery for periorbital melanoma: fixed-tissue and fresh-tissue techniques. J Dermatol Surg Oncol 1985;11:284–91.
16. Mohs FE. Micrographic surgery for the microscopically controlled excision of eyelid cancers. Arch Ophthalmol 1986;104:901–9.
17. Callahan M, Monheit GD, Callahan A. Mohs histologically controlled excision for management of orbital invasion of eyelid carcinomas. Acta Int Congress Ophthalmol 1982;2:998–1001.
18. Mohs FE. Microscopically controlled excision of medial canthal carcinomas. Ann Plast Surg 1981;7: 308–11.
19. Grove AS Jr. Staged excision and reconstruction of extensive facial-orbital tumors. Ophthalmic Surg 1977;8:91–109.
20. Anderson RL, Ceilley RI. A multispecialty approach to the excision and reconstruction of eyelid tumors. Ophthalmology 1978;85:1150–63.
21. Robins P, Henkind P, Menn H. Chemosurgery in treatment of cancer of the periorbital area. Trans Am Acad Ophthalmol Otolaryngol 1971;75:1228–35.
22. Harrington JN. Reconstruction of the medial canthus by spontaneous granulation. (Laissez-Faire): a review. Ann Ophthalmol 1982;14:956–60.
23. Leib ML, Johnson DA, Eliezri YD. Mohs histographic surgery and ophthalmic plastic reconstruction. Ophthal Plast Reconst Surg 1992;8:262–70.
24. Bieley HC, Kirsner RS, Reyes BA, Garland LD. The use of Mohs micrographic surgery for determination of residual tumor and incompletely excised basal cell carcinoma. J Am Acad Dermatol 1992;26:754–6.
25. Stephenson C. Reconstruction of the eyelid using a myocutaneous island flap. Ophthalmology 1983;90: 1060–5.
26. Reese AB. Epithelial tumors of the lid, conjunctiva, cornea, and lacrimal sac. In: Reese AB, editor. Tumors of the eye, 3rd ed. New York, NY: Harper and Row; p. 50.
27. Tenzel RR. Reconstruction of the central one half of an eyelid. Arch Ophthalmol 1975;93:125–6.
28. Tenzel RR, Stewart WB. Eyelid reconstruction by the semicircle flap technique. Ophthalmology 1978;85: 1164–9.
29. Hewes EH, Sullivan JH, Beard C. Lower eyelid reconstruction by tarsal transposition. Am J Ophthalmol 1976;81:512–4.
30. Hughes WL. New method for rebuilding a lower lid; report of a case. Arch Ophthalmol 1937;17:1008–17.
31. Levine MR, Buckman G. Semicircular flap revisited. Arch Ophthalmol 1986;104:915–7.
32. Spinelli HM, Jelks GW. Periocular reconstruction: a systematic approach. Plast Reconstruct Surg 1993; 91:1017–24.
33. Bartley GB, Putterman AM. A minor modification of Hughes' operation for lower eyelid reconstruction. Am J Ophthalmol 1995;119:96–7.
34. Doxanas MT. Orbicularis muscle mobilization in eyelid reconstruction. Arch Ophthalmol 1986;104:910–4.

35. Cies WA, Bartlett RE. Modification of the Mustardé and Hughes methods of reconstructing the lower lid. Ann Ophthalmol 1975;7:1497–1502.
36. Holds JB, Anderson RL. Medial canthotomy and cantholysis in eye-lid reconstruction. Am J Ophthalmol 1993;116:218–23.
37. Werner MS, Olson JJ, Putterman AM. Composite grafting for eyelid reconstruction. Am J Ophthalmol 1993;116:11–6.
38. Bartley GB, Kay PP. Posterior lamellar eyelid reconstruction with a hard palate mucosal graft. Am J Ophthalmol 1989;107:609–12.
39. Jordan DR, McDonald H, Anderson RL. Irradiated homologous aorta in eyelid reconstruction. Part II. Human data. Ophthal Plast Reconstruct Surg 1994; 10:227–33.
40. Cohen MS, Shorr N. Eyelid reconstruction with hard palate muscosa grafts. Ophthal Plast Reconstr Surg 1992;8:183–95.
41. Beard C. Surgery of lid tumors. In: Fox SA, editor. International ophthalmology clinics, Vol. 4, Number 1. Boston, MA: Little, Brown; 1964.
42. Kersten RC, Anderson RL, Tse DT, Weinstein GL. Tarsal rotational flap for upper eyelid reconstruction. Arch Ophthalmol 1986;104:918–22.
43. Weinstein GS, Anderson RL, Tse DT, Kersten RC. The use of a periosteal strip for upper eyelid reconstruction. Arch Ophthalmol 1985;103:357–9.
44. Jordan DR, Anderson RL, Nowinski TS. Tarsoconjunctival flap for upper eyelid reconstruction. Arch Ophthalmol 1989;107:599–603.
45. Cutler NL, Beard C. A method for partial and total upper lid reconstruction. Am J Ophthalmol 1955;39:1–7.
46. Wesley RE, McCord CD Jr. Transplantation of eyebank sclera in the Cutler-Beard method of upper eyelid reconstruction. Ophthalmology 1980;87:1022–8.
47. Hecht SD. An upside-down Cutler-Beard bridge flap. Arch Ophthalmol 1970;84:760–4.
48. Carroll RP. Entropion following the Cutler-Beard procedure. Ophthalmology 1983;90:1052–5.
49. Mustardé JC. Repair and reconstruction in the orbital region. New York, NY: Churchill Livingstone Inc.; 1971.
50. Papp C, Maurer H, Geroldinger E. Lower eyelid reconstruction with the upper eyelid rotational flap. Plast Reconstruct Surg 1990;86:563–5.
51. Callahan A. Free composite lid graft. Arch Ophthalmol 1951;45:539–45.
52. Fox SA. Autogenous free full-thickness eyelid grafts. Am J Ophthalmol 1969;67:941–5.
53. Putterman AM. Viable composite grafting in eyelid reconstruction. Am J Ophthalmol 1978;85:237–41.
54. Stephenson CM, Brown BZ. The use of tarsus as a free autogenous graft in eyelid surgery. Ophthal Plast Reconstr Surg 1985;1:43–50.
55. Brown BZ. The use of homologous tarsus as a donor graft in lid surgery. Ophthal Plast Reconstr Surg 1985;1:91–5.
56. Robbins TH. Chondrodermal graft reconstruction of the lower eyelid. Br J Plast Surg 1981;34:140–1.
57. Beyer CK, Albert DM. The use and fate of fascia lata and sclera in ophthalmic plastic and reconstructive surgery. (The Wendel Hughes Lecture 1980). Ophthalmology 1981;88:869–86.
58. Baylis HI, Rosen N, Neuhaus RW. Obtaining auricular cartilage for reconstructive surgery. Am J Ophthalmol 1982;93:709–12.
59. Leone CR Jr, Hand SI Jr. Reconstruction of the medial eyelid. Am J Ophthalmol 1979;87:797–801.
60. Mehta HK. Simultaneous, spontaneous, and primary surgical repair of eyelids. Br J Ophthalmol 1989;73: 488–93.
61. Putterman AM. Reconstruction of nasal fistulas of the medial canthus. Am J Ophthalmol 1989;108:68–74.
62. Marmelzat W. "Noli me tangere" circa 1754; Jacques Daniel's forgotten contribution to skin cancer. Arch Dermatol 1964;90:280–3.
63. Fox SA, Beard C. Spontaneous lid repair. Am J Ophthalmol 1964;58:947–52.
64. Fier RH, Older JJ. Spontaneous repair of the medial canthus after removal of basal cell carcinoma. Ophthal Surg 1982;13:737–40.
65. Mehta HK. Spontaneous reformation of lower eyelid. Br J Ophthalmol 1981;65:202–8.
66. Quickert MH, Dryden RM. Probes for intubation in lacrimal drainage. Trans Am Acad Ophthalmol Otolaryngol 1970;74:431–3.
67. Gorney M, Falces E, Jones H, Manis JR. One-stage reconstruction of substantial lower eyelid margin defects. Plast Reconstr Surg 1969;44:592–6.
68. Beyer-Machule CK, Grewers H, Kestember E. Island rotational pedicle graft for reconstruction. Orbit 1994;13:183–6.
69. Tse DT, McCafferty LR. Controlled tissue expansion in periocular reconstructive surgery. Ophthalmology 1993;100:260–8.

4

Conjunctival Malignancies

The pathogenesis and pathophysiology of squamous cell carcinoma, melanoma, sebaceous cell carcinoma, and Kaposi's sarcoma (KS) are covered in the chapters on lid tumors. The oncogenesis and progression of melanomas are discussed in the chapters on eyelid and uveal melanomas, and the mechanism of lymphoid tumor development is discussed in the section on the orbit.

Five malignancies often involve the conjunctiva: squamous cell carcinoma, melanoma, lymphoid tumors, KS, and sebaceous cell carcinoma, secondarily from contiguous lid involvement. Squamous cell carcinoma is the most common malignant lesion of the conjunctiva. Melanomas occur less frequently, followed by lymphoid lesions, sebaceous gland carcinoma, and KS. Sebaceous gland carcinoma is discussed in Chapters 1 and 3. Although basal cell carcinoma of the conjunctiva has been reported, the estimated ratio of squamous cell conjunctival carcinoma to basal cell conjunctival carcinoma is greater than 20:1.[1–3] In one large series of conjunctival malignancies, the 6 patients with basal cell carcinoma all had a history of an identical neoplasm involving the eyelid.[4] There are some epidemiologic data on squamous cell carcinoma of the conjunctiva. Newton and co-workers studied the geographic distribution of this malignancy in relation to ambient solar ultraviolet (UV) radiation. They noted that the incidence of squamous cell carcinoma declined by approximately 49 percent for each 10-degree increase in latitude. In Uganda, there are 12 cases per million per year in contrast to 0.2 cases per million per year in the United Kingdom.[5] In a study from the United States, Sun and co-workers noted that the incidence was 0.3 per million per year, with the rate being fivefold higher in Caucasian males. They also noted a very strong UV-B exposure and both conjunctival melanoma as well as squamous cell carcinoma of the conjunctiva.[6]

Unlike both cutaneous and uveal melanomas, where several cytogenetic abnormalities have been documented, there is a paucity of data on conjunctival melanoma. McCarthy and colleagues noted a translocation in chromosome 1 and 14 in a patient with dysplastic nevus syndrome.[7] Dahlenfors and colleagues have noted a small abnormality in a few cells, but it appears that conjunctival melanomas probably have a different genomic alteration than uveal melanomas.[8,9]

BENIGN CONJUNCTIVAL TUMORS

A number of benign lesions can occur in the conjunctiva and simulate malignancy. The most common simulating lesions include pterygium, viral papilloma (Figure 4–1), amelanotic nevus, dermolipoma (Figure 4–2), pyogenic granuloma (Figures 4–3A and B), and corneal pannus. In most cases, these lesions do not require biopsy, but in uncommon presentations, incisional biopsy or cytopathologic evaluation of surface scrapings is necessary.

Viral papillomas are one of the more frequent simulating conjunctival lesions (see Figure 4–1).[1–4,10] They most commonly occur in young children than in adults, often in multiple areas.[11] Recently, workers have demonstrated that some benign conjunctival papillomas appear to be caused by the human papillomavirus (HPV). Management of these lesions is often quite difficult.[12] Surgery, topical chemotherapy, cimetidine, and cryotherapy have been effective

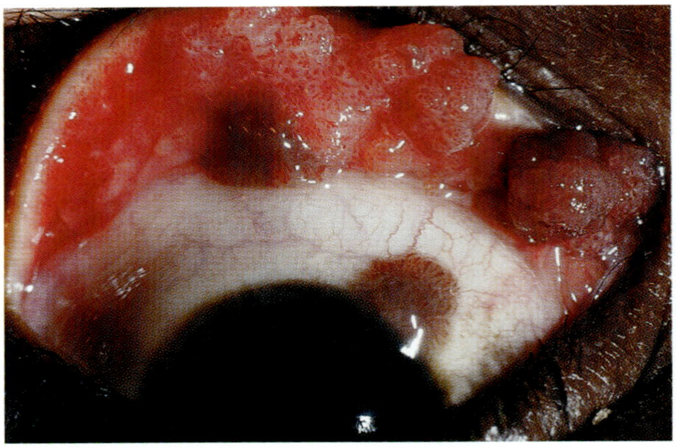

Figure 4–1. Nonmalignant viral conjunctival papilloma.

in some patients.[13–15] As discussed below, viruses also may be important in the pathophysiology of squamous cell carcinomas of the conjunctiva.[16–19]

A number of less common benign conjunctival lesions can simulate a malignancy; many can only be correctly diagnosed on histologic evaluation. As an example, we have seen a discoid lupus of the eyelid and conjunctiva simulate a malignancy.[20]

Ectopic lacrimal gland tissue has been described at the corneal limbus.[21] Similarly, respiratory epithelium has been reported to produce a limbal cystic choristoma in a neonate.[22] Localized amyloid deposits can occur on the bulbar conjunctiva, although this process more commonly involves either the palpebral or forniceal conjunctiva or the lid (Figure 4–4).[23] Unlike a carcinoma that is initially epithelial in origin, often amyloid appears as a subepithelial mass, usually without intrinsic vasculature. Pyogenic granulomas can simulate a malignancy. They usually occur in young patients after strabismus or ptosis surgery (see Figure 4–3B) and in older patients following chronic infection or trauma.[24] In older patients, a biopsy is usually necessary to differentiate a pyogenic granuloma at the corneal limbus from the squamous cell carcinoma it mimics.[25]

Dermoids and osseous choristomas can involve the conjunctival limbus (see Figure 4–2). Usually, these lesions do not grow and are not difficult to differentiate from malignancies, since they appear in a younger age group.[26–28] They can be confused, however, with fibromas, lipomas, or nonpigmented nevi.[26–29] As Crawford has emphasized, excision of these benign pediatric lesions, especially if they involve the lateral fornices, has been associated with significant ocular morbidity. Similarly, limbal dermoids, when excised too deeply, can result in a filtering wound, staphyloma, or corneal ulcer.[30–32] As discussed in the section on anterior uveal tumors, high-frequency ultrasonography has sufficient reso-

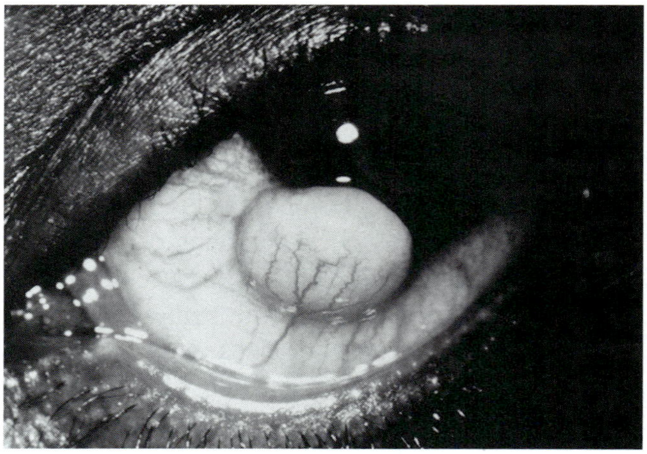

Figure 4–2. Conjunctival limbal dermoid.

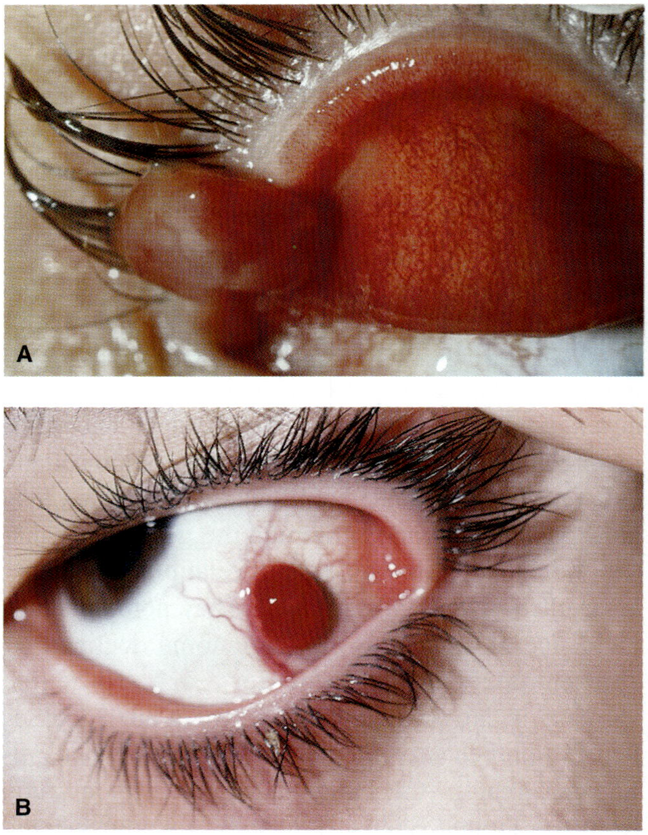

Figure 4–3. *A,* Pyogenic granuloma of the conjunctiva after ptosis. *B,* Pyogenic granuloma of the conjunctiva after strabismus surgery.

lution to delineate the intracorneal borders of such lesions. In a study by Elsas and Green, < 1.5 percent of pediatric conjunctival tumors that were biopsied were malignant.[33] Several clinicians have reported "teddy bear" granulomas of the conjunctiva that can simulate a tumor. These granulomas are caused by the synthetic fibers of the toy.[34] Rarely, a meningoencephalocele can simulate a conjunctival mass in an infant.[35] Occasionally, a conjunctival dermoid cyst can produce a chronic red eye.[27]

Fibrous histiocytomas can sometimes simulate a lymphoid lesion. However, they are more tan and yellow in color, whereas lymphoid tumors are salmon-pink. Unlike malignant processes, these lesions generally do not have intrinsic tumor vessels or episcleral vessels feeding the tumor.[36–39] An isolated episcleral neurofibroma can also have a yellowish-white appearance and, if incompletely excised, has a tendency to recur.[39–41] These tumors have been associated with both neurofibromatosis types 1 and 2 (*NF1*, *NF2*).[42] Only 13 cases of benign myxoma involving the conjunctiva have been reported. In appearance, myxomas are smooth, fleshy, or gelatinous, and they are often pink in color. Unlike their behavior in other locations, myxomas of the conjunctiva usually do not regrow after they are excised.[43,44] Nodular fasciitis can rarely involve the conjunctiva; this author has usually seen it in the orbit.[45] Usually, the diagnosis of lymphangiomas of the conjunctiva in the orbit is straightforward; rarely, in an older patient, because of hemorrhage, they can simulate a malignancy.[46]

Neurilemmomas and trans-scleral leiomyomas can also rarely simulate a conjunctival mass; usually, these appear to be vascularized.[47–49] In contrast, while the orbital hemangioperiocytoma is vascularized, the rare conjunctival manifestations of the tumor often are not, although there is usually dilated overlying vasculature.

There are several benign variants of systemic lymphoid lesions and other simulating tumors that can mimic a conjunctival lymphoid lesion.[50,51] Rarely, a conjunctival salmon-patch mass may be the first manifestation of a recurrence of systemic acute leukemia.[52] Other rare simulating lesions include dacryoadenoma, sinus histocytosis, and, rarely, infectious mononucleosis.[53–56]

Several indeterminate squamous cell lesions of the conjunctiva have been described. As has been described in the cutaneous literature, the spectrum between keratoacanthoma and squamous cell carcinoma, inverted papillomas, and recurrent papillomas in adults is poorly delineated. The paucity of these possibly benign squamous cell proliferations and their limited follow-up make it difficult to draw conclusions about their management.[57–60] In the few that the author has, on the basis of very little data, the tendency has been to manage them as if they were squamous cell carcinomas.

SQUAMOUS CELL CARCINOMA

The nomenclature of conjunctival epithelial neoplasia is confusing. McGavic coined the term "Bowen's disease" for this condition, since in situ conjunctival dysplasias have bizarre cells, often with giant nuclei or multinucleated configurations.[61] Unfortunately, this has proven to be a misnomer. Bowen's disease was initially thought to be a skin cancer associated with visceral malignancy, but more recent studies have cast doubts on that association.[62,63]

Most clinicians now use the term "conjunctival intraepithelial neoplasia" (CIN) for what was previously referred to as Bowen's disease, conjunctival dysplasia, or conjunctival epithelioma.[64–67] CIN usually connotes partial- to full-thickness intraepithelial neoplasia, whereas carcinoma has full-thickness involvement with invasion. Neither CIN nor invasive conjunctival squamous cell carcinoma is associated with visceral malignancies.[63,68] Several workers

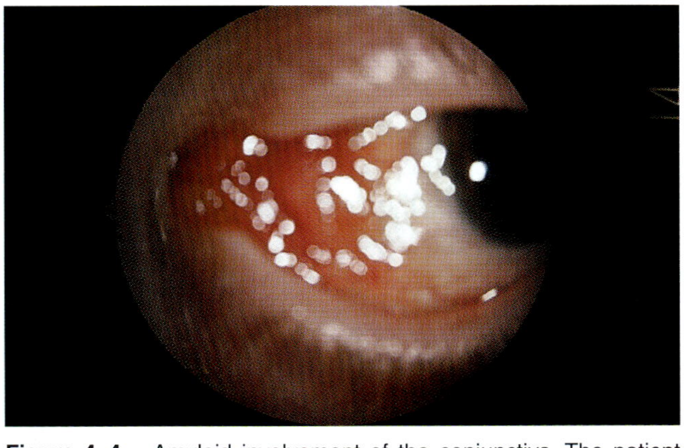

Figure 4–4. Amyloid involvement of the conjunctiva. The patient had no systemic abnormalities

have shown that proliferation rates appear to affect the chance of malignant progression.[69]

The incidence of CIN lesions in an equatorial sunny climate was noted to be approximately 1 to 2.8 per 100,000 people per year.[70,71] The strongest risk factor for squamous cell carcinoma of the conjunctiva is past history of cutaneous malignancy. As above, the role of UV radiation has been demonstrated.[63,72]

Several reports and studies have emphasized that in a patient under 50 years old who presents with a conjunctival squamous cell carcinoma the possibility of human immunodeficiency virus (HIV) infection should be considered.[73] It is estimated there is an 8- to 13-fold increased incidence of conjunctival carcinoma in this setting. In addition, immunosuppressed transplantation patients may also have an increased risk of this neoplasm.[74]

Diagnosis

The pathogenesis and pathophysiology of squamous cell carcinoma is uncertain. As discussed in Chapter 1, UV radiation can produce "signature" mutations in *p53*, a tumor suppressor gene, that is probably important in the pathophysiology of these neoplasms. Recent work in a transgenic mouse model of cutaneous squamous cell carcinoma has illustrated the importance of the *p53* suppressor gene in this tumor.[75]

In cervical carcinoma, several groups have observed human papillomavirus (HPV) types 16 and 18.[76] McDonnell and colleagues noted that 88 percent of 37 CIN lesions had HPV-16, as demonstrated with polymerase chain reaction (PCR) on paraffin-embedded tissue.[6,17] The HPV oncogenes inactivate both the *p53* and *Rb* proteins and some experimental treatments are being studied in an attempt to alter this process.[77,78] Since many of these patients also had evidence of the virus in the contralateral, uninvolved eye, they postulated that HPV was only one of a number of factors important in the initiation and progression of CIN lesions. Other reports have described bilateral conjunctival carcinomas that were positive for this virus.[79] There have now been approximately 15 reports, with variable rates of detection of HPV in squamous cell carcinoma.[74] What becomes problematic are studies of nonmalignant conjunctival lesions associated with excess solar exposure, where there are alterations of either *p53* or HPV. Tan and associates found that 3 of 8 pterygia specimens were positive for abnormal *p53* staining.[80]

A conjunctival squamous cell carcinoma appears to occur more commonly in equatorial regions, and older men with high solar exposure appear to have a higher risk of developing it.[65,81] This epidemiology would be consistent with the *p53* data shown with squamous cell carcinomas involving the skin. Some studies have shown that the E6 and E7 viral proteins interact with *p53* and *Rb* proteins and can form complexes that then inactivate these proteins.[82] Several studies have questioned whether HPV is, in fact, a main driving force or a passenger in the development of squamous cell carcinomas.[83] Karcioglu and Issa noted that HPV was present in 20 percent of climatic droplet keratopathy patients, 35 percent in scarred corneas, and in 30 percent of conjunctiva biopsies from otherwise normal cataract patients in Saudi Arabia.[84]

In most series, approximately three-quarters of conjunctival carcinoma cases have occurred in male patients. While children as young as 4 years have been reported with squamous cell carcinoma, the usual age of onset is in the mid-60s.[84,85] In the series from the Mayo Clinic, patients with invasive squamous cell carcinoma had a mean age 7.6 years older than those with CIN.[65]

Most CIN lesions developed at the limbus in the interpalpebral fissure (Figure 4–5) and are amelanotic. The presence of a neoplastic conjunctival lesion distant from the limbus suggests the possibility of a sebaceous gland carcinoma or another tumor.[85]

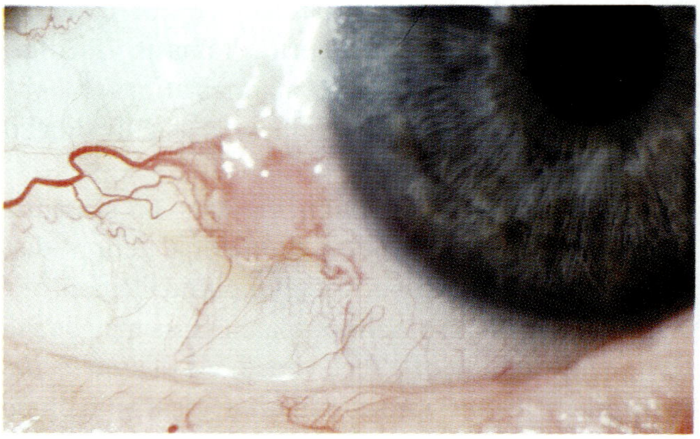

Figure 4–5. Conjunctival intraepithelial neoplasm (CIN) usually develops in the epithelium at the limbus.

Occasionally, squamous cell tumors can be pigmented, and nevi can sometimes simulate these lesions.[86] In one histologic report, a malignant nerve sheath tumor simulated a conjunctival squamous cell carcinoma.[87] We recently managed a patient who had both primary acquired melanosis and CIN in the same biopsy specimen (personal observation).

Whereas CIN lesions usually develop at the limbus and more commonly involve the bulbar conjunctiva, a more subtle CIN lesion may occur in the cornea. Waring and co-workers described a gray limbal intraepithelial plaque in the interpalpebral fissure (Figure 4–6). Often, this sheet of tissue had a characteristic fimbriated margin with isolated clusters of gray spots (Figure 4–7). None of the 17 reported cases of these very early lesions progressed to invasive carcinoma, on serial evaluation.[66]

Invasive squamous carcinomas have four common clinical presentations: (1) a gelatinous lesion with intrinsic vessels (Figure 4–8), (2) a leukoplakia lesion (Figure 4–9), (3) a vascular papilloma-like lesion (Figures 4–10 and 4–11), or (4) pagetoid spread onto the cornea (Figures 4–12 and 4–13). Most commonly, if a mass is present (in contrast to a pagetoid flat

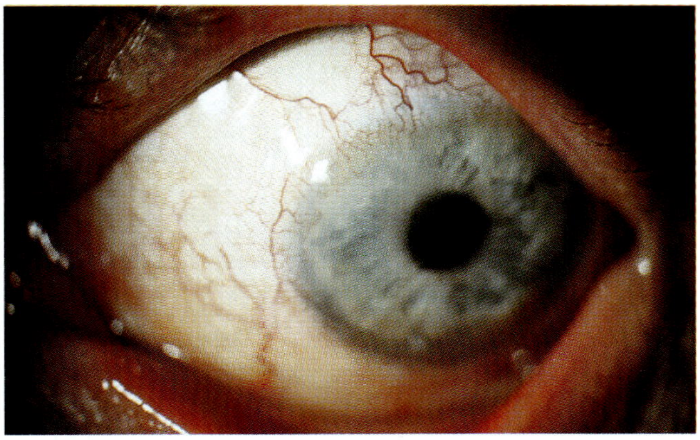

Figure 4–6. Small, early CIN lesion with an intraepithelial plaque.

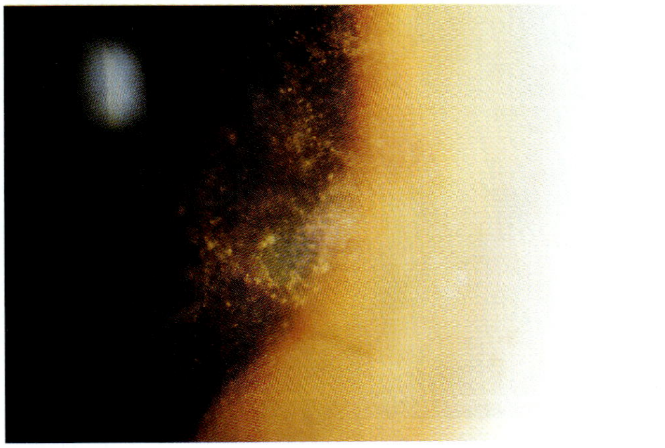

Figure 4–7. Small early CIN lesion with some intrinsic pigmentation.

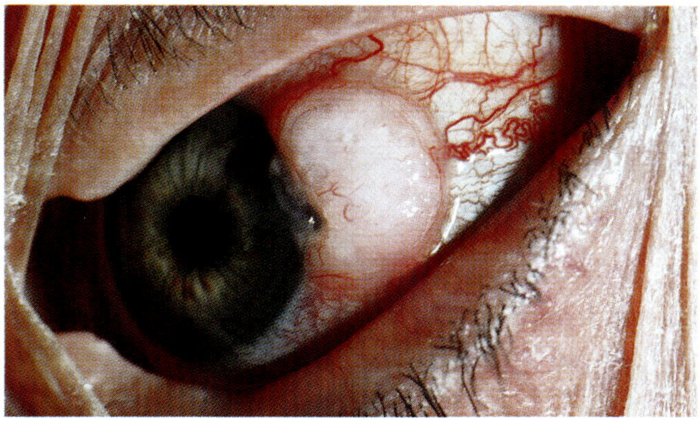

Figure 4–8. Gelatinous conjunctival squamous cell carcinoma with intrinsic vessels.

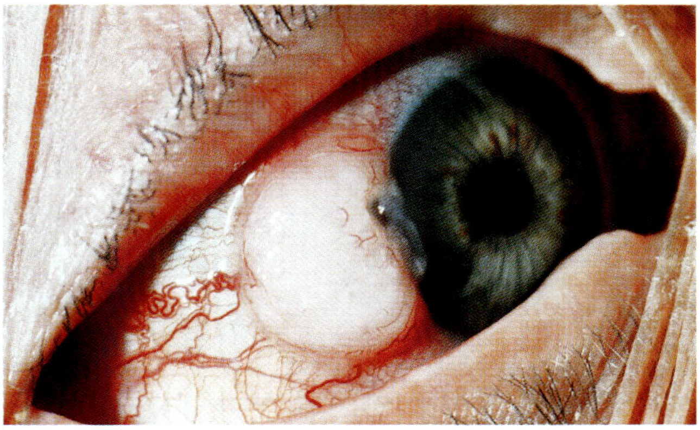

Figure 4–9. Leukoplakic presentation of invasive conjunctival squamous cell carcinoma.

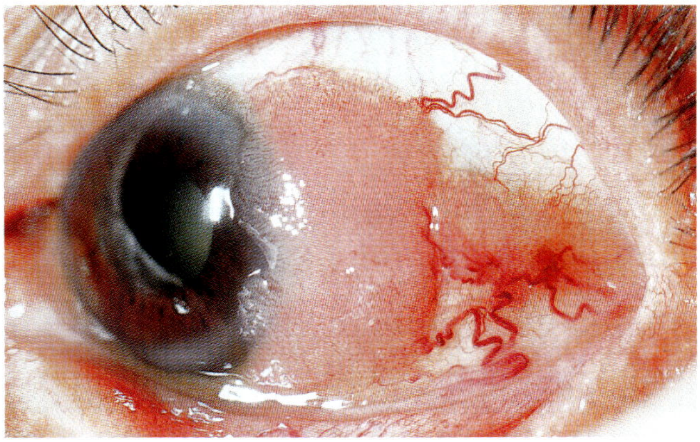

Figure 4–10. Vascular papillomatous presentation of squamous cell carcinoma.

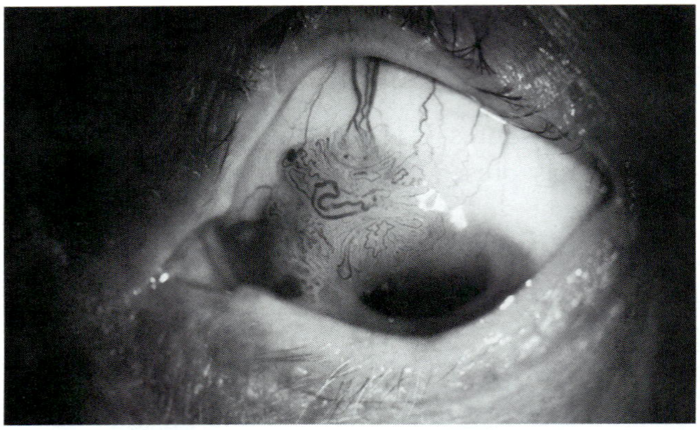

Figure 4–11. Papillomatous vascular appearance of a biopsy-proven conjunctival carcinoma.

lesion), it has intrinsic vasculature, as shown in Figure 4–5. Occasionally, CIN or invasive carcinoma can simulate a pterygium (Figure 4–14). Most often, the pseudopterygium is either not in the palpebral fissure, or if it is, it is in the temporal location instead of in the more common nasal location. Rarely, the vascular pattern is atypical and may simulate a peripheral corneal degeneration as shown in Figure 4–15. Occasionally, only the cornea appears to be involved by this neoplasm.[66–67]

Advanced invasive squamous cell carcinoma of the conjunctiva is often misdiagnosed as a chronic unilateral conjunctivitis (Figure 4–16). Consequently, any older patient with a refractory unilateral conjunctivitis should have a biopsy.[88–90] Exfoliative cytology is helpful in establishing a diagnosis in patients suspected of having a conjunctival malignancy. As shown in Figure 4–17, a stained specimen scraped from the surface of the lesion may demonstrate typical neoplastic cells with an abnormal

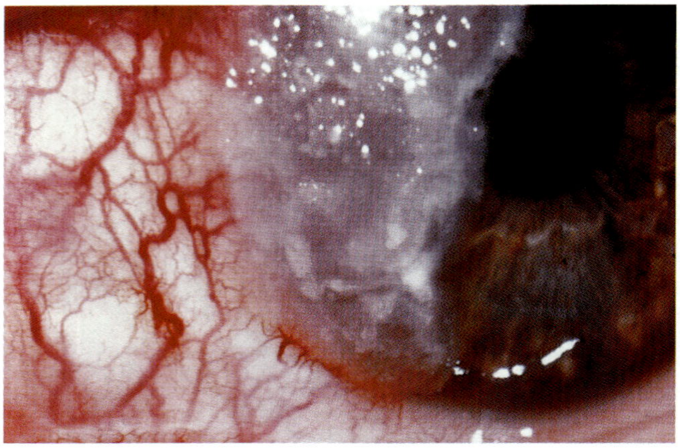

Figure 4–12. Pagetoid spread of a conjunctival carcinoma onto the cornea.

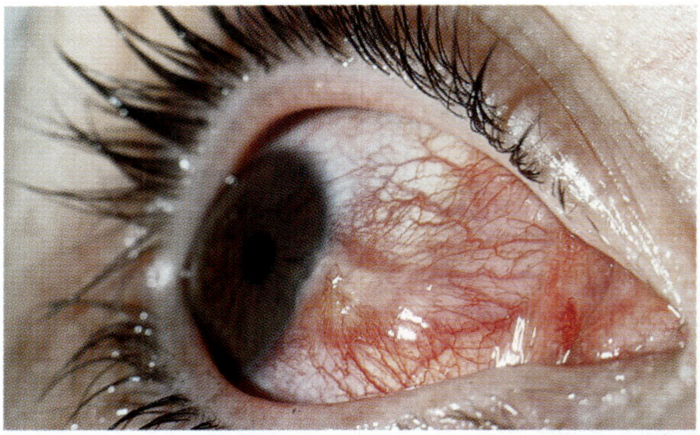

Figure 4–14. Invasive conjunctival carcinoma simulating a pyterigium. Unlike pterygia, which usually occur in the nasal intrapalpebral fissure, the carcinoma can involve any area of the limbus.

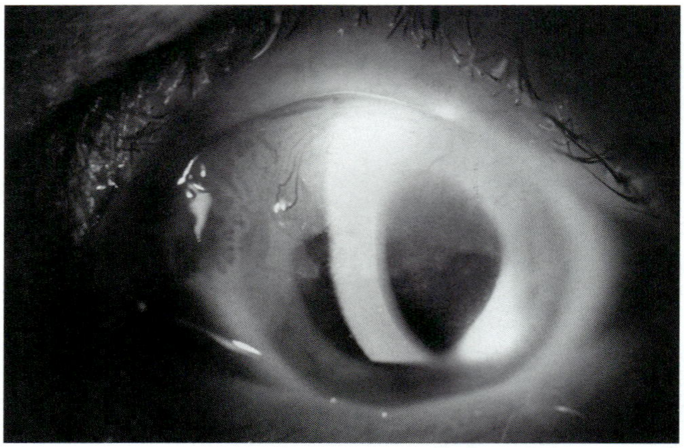

Figure 4–13. Corneal involvement of squamous carcinoma is usually anterior to Bowman's membrane. The advancing edge of the neoplasm is irregular.

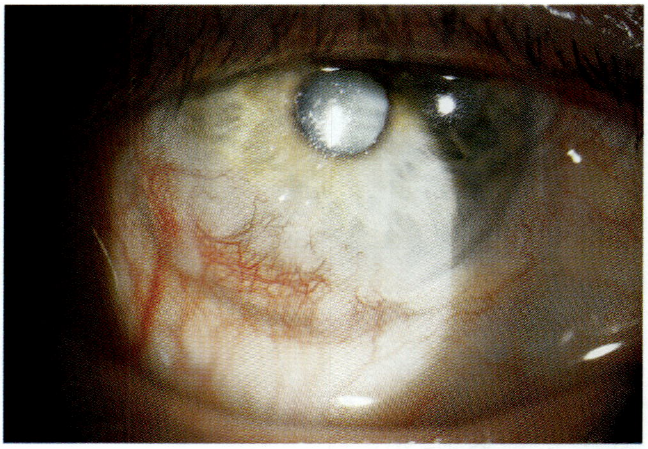

Figure 4–15. Carcinoma simulating a marginal corneal degeneration.

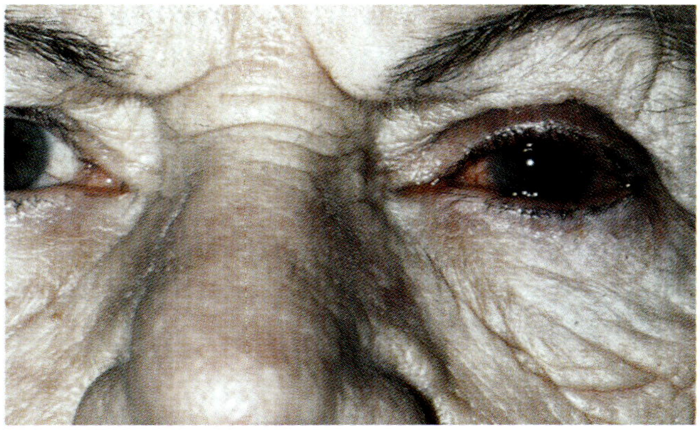

Figure 4–16. Diffuse squamous cell carcinoma of the bulbar and palpebral conjunctiva simulates "chronic unilateral conjunctivitis."

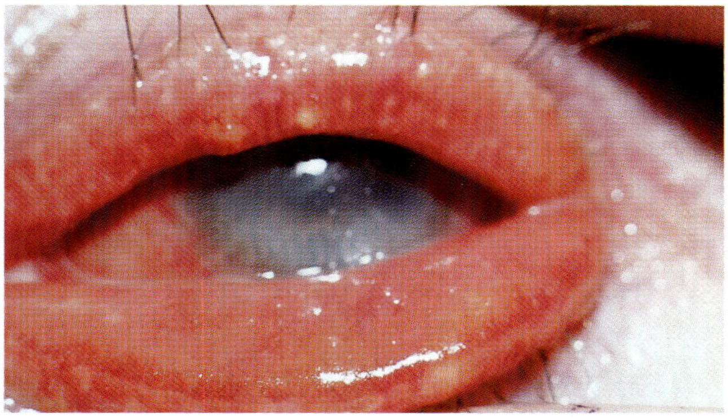

Figure 4–18. Sebaceous gland carcinoma of the lid presenting as a conjunctival tumor. An epithelial malignancy of the conjunctiva that arises away from the limbus should suggest this diagnosis.

nuclear- cytoplasm ratio, coarse nuclear, and chromatin.[91,92] In a recent small report from an experienced center, cytology had 100 percent accuracy.[93] Some authors have suggested using rose bengal to label dead or degenerative epithelial cells and to delineate the margins of this tumor.[94] We have not found this technique sufficiently accurate to be useful. Sebaceous gland carcinoma of the lid can present with mainly conjunctival involvement (Figure 4–18).

CIN may progress to invasive squamous cell carcinoma, although a few have been reported to have undergone spontaneous regression.[95] Many CIN lesions do not progress to invasive squamous cell carcinoma.[65] Fully developed conjunctival carcinomas often have a pathognomonic appearance of a mulberry gelatinous tumor with fronds of superficial vessels (see Figure 4–8). The histologic features of CIN lesions may appear quite malignant, but the

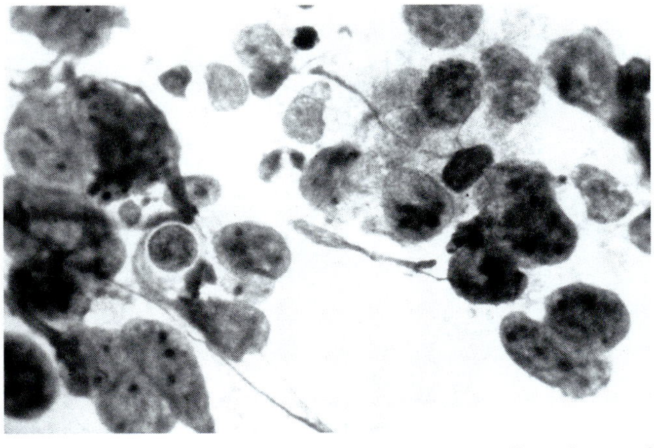

Figure 4–17. Exfoliative cytology of a squamous cell carcinoma of the conjunctiva. Large malignant nuclei are seen.

risk of metastatic disease is almost zero.[1,10,96,97] The recurrence rate of both CIN and invasive squamous cell carcinoma is mainly a function of the completeness of tumor resection. Previous series, often with incomplete tumor removal, have reported recurrence rates ranging from 10 to 64 percent.[98] In some studies, the correlation between clear microscopic margins and survival were not as good as in others.[99] In the author's experience, as discussed below, surgical margins have been quite accurate as a means to prevent recurrence.[100] The low historic figure of a 10 percent recurrence rate is from a series in which over half the cases had either no follow-up or follow-up for less than 1 year, and most older series had a short-term recurrence rate of approximately 40 percent.[85,92,94] Fifty-three percent of incompletely excised CIN lesions recurred versus < 5 percent of lesions that were completely resected.[65] In the cases that did recur, the mean interval between excision and recurrence was approximately 22 months.

Usually, recurrences develop at the limbus (Figure 4–19) and spread superficially onto the cornea rather than toward the cul-de-sac. Alternatively, there can be intraconjunctival metastatic lesions. As discussed in Chapter 1, for basal cell carcinomas of the eyelid and probably by analogy germane for these conjunctival neoplasms, these patients are also at risk for new as well as recurrent squamous cell carcinoma of the conjunctiva, although the former hypothesis has not been proven. Rarely, there can be intraocular extension of a squamous cell carcinoma.[101–108] Invasion into the globe has been very difficult to diagnose. The author has personally had

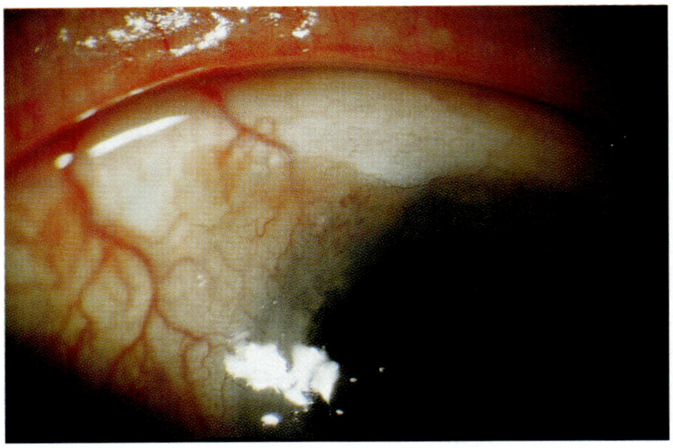

Figure 4–19. Recurrent conjunctival carcinoma in the interpalpebral fissure at the limbus.

experience with 6 such cases. In 3, gonioscopic examination showed broad-based synechiae and a "velvety appearing" tumor in the anterior segment. In 1, there appeared to be just anterior segment inflammation, as others have noted.[104] Occasionally, cytologic examination of an anterior chamber paracentesis may be diagnostic.[103] The fifth case that the author managed presented with a flat anterior chamber after the referring physician had attempted to perform a conjunctival scraping for cytopathologic diagnosis (Figure 4–20). The intraocular penetration was secondary to tumor erosion through the cornea. Another case of focal intraocular recurrence after multiple treatments is shown in Figure 4–21. In the latter case, we were able to resect the tumor with an 18-mm en-bloc scleral-iridocyclochoroidectomy. Five years later, the patient was tumor free, with a visual acuity of 20/25 in the involved eye.[109] The spindle cell variant of squamous cell carcinoma has a higher incidence of intraocular invasion.[110,111] In one reported case, this tumor resulted in the patient's death within 14 months of the initial incision.[112] Unfortunately, the appearance of a spindle cell tumor is not diagnostic (Figure 4–22). Rarely, squamous cell carcinoma can be bilateral (Figure 4–23).

Management

Surgery

As discussed under "Conjunctival Surgery" (see below), the mainstay of treatment of conjunctival epithelial tumors is excisional biopsy with frozen section control. In the author's personal experience with approximately 100 CINs and invasive conjunctival epithelial carcinomas, < 5 percent recur when frozen sections are used to evaluate margins.[100] There are two problems with this technique: (1) it is imperative that accurate orientation be given to the pathologist. We have a life-sized, sterilized ocular pathology form (see Figure 3–1), and all specimens are submitted on it; and (2) while it is relatively straightforward to establish whether the margins distal to the limbus are clear of tumor, the corneal edge usually cannot be accurately sampled, and similarly, the deep scleral surface of the tumor is often not precisely surveyed with standard frozen section control.

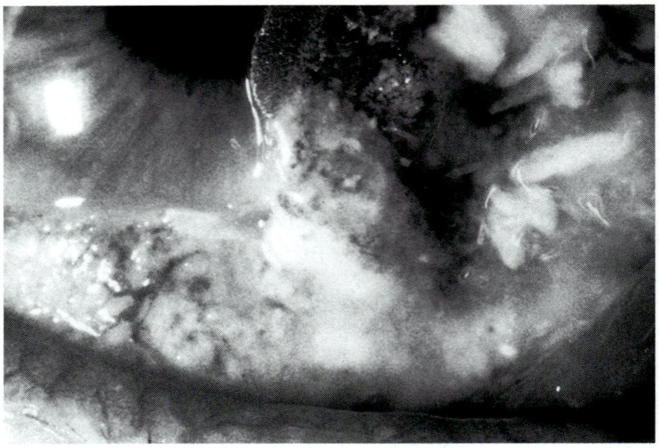

Figure 4–20. Intraocular invasion of a conjunctival carcinoma. Intraocular penetration (and subsequent gluing) occurred when the referring physician attempted diagnostic scraping.

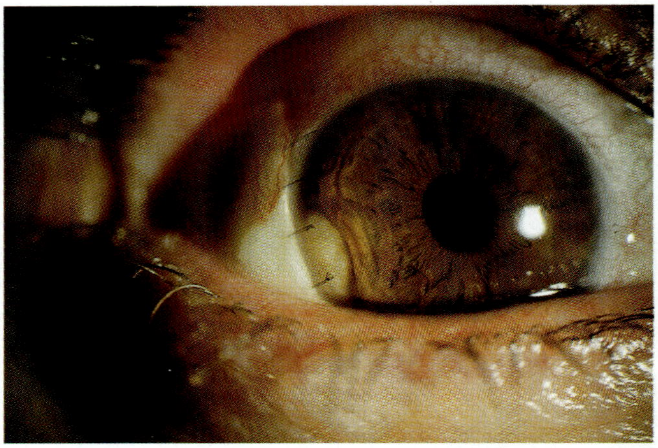

Figure 4–21. A case referred for a focal intraocular recurrence after multiple treatments. The tumor was removed with a large iridocyclectomy and a free graft.

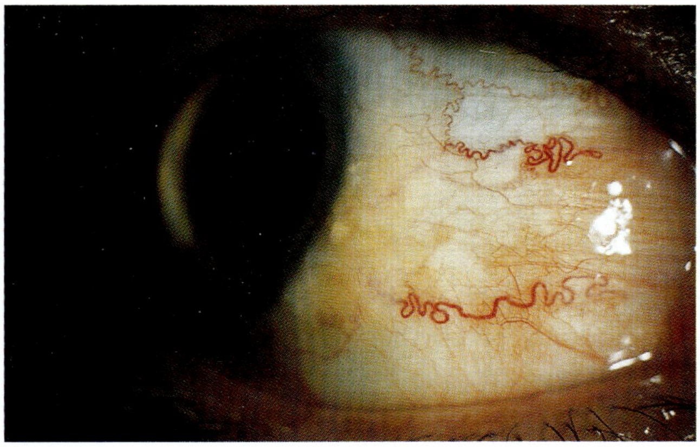

Figure 4–22. The clinical appearance of the spindle cell variant of squamous cell carcinoma is not diagnostic. These tumors are more aggressive.

Usually, Bowman's membrane offers considerable resistance to deep invasion; however, occasionally a lamellar keratectomy is required to completely excise a tumor.[55,65,86]

We routinely use adjunctive cryosurgery with a double freeze-thaw technique (see Chapter 2) at the scleral base of the tumor as well as on presumably "tumor-free" conjunctival margins. Fraunfelder and Wingfield reviewed 36 patients with squamous cell carcinoma of the conjunctiva who were treated and followed up for more than 3 years. Two of six who were only excised had recurrences, as did 3 of 9 who were treated with only freezing. Excision plus cryotherapy had a recurrence rate of approximately 9 percent.[113] Other workers, including ourselves, have had a similar experience.[114–116] Rarely, after cryosurgery, a Wesseley ring can occur, last for several months, and produce decreased vision; however, the author has never seen this complication.[117]

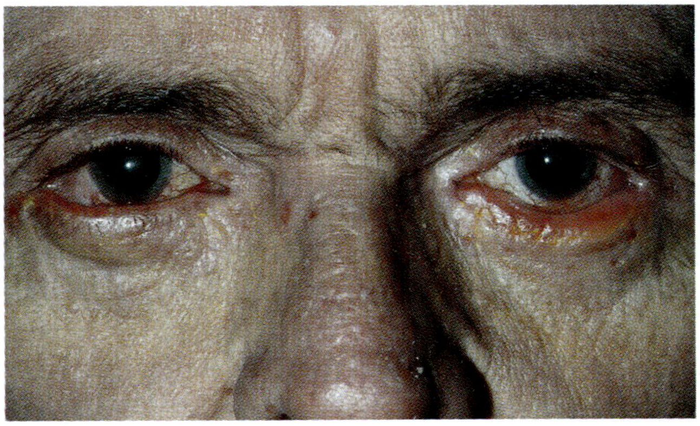

Figure 4–23. Bilateral conjunctival squamous cell carcinoma.

Often with a small carcinoma, the tumor area that has been treated with resection and cryotherapy can be closed primarily. If too large a defect has been created, we cover the muscles with either an autologous conjunctival membrane or a buccal mucous membrane graft, since symblepharon or fibrosis with secondary strabismus can occur, if these areas treated by freezing are not covered with mucosal epithelium.[118]

A major problem with tumors that involve more than 40 percent of the corneal surface has been post-treatment morbidity and resultant decreased visual acuity. On the basis of the work by Thoft and colleagues, we have treated such patients with limbal grafts after superficial resection and cryotherapy.[119,120] A 3 × 5 mm limbal graft is harvested from the contralateral eye and sutured into place at the limbus with four interrupted No. 10-0 nylon sutures. Figure 4–24 shows fluorescein staining 36 hours after removal of a tumor involving most of the corneal surface, cryotherapy, and placement of limbal grafts. Note that > 85 percent of the cornea has been re-epithelialized as a result of the limbal graft. Figures 4–25A and B show a lesion prior to and after resection, cryotherapy, and placement of limbal grafts. Visual acuity improved from 20/100 to 20/20. An alternative approach to reconstruction is the use of amniotic membrane transplantation; however, the long-term experience for this approach for tumors is extremely limited.[121] An additional surgical option that has been tried in only a few patients is the use of excimer laser keratectomy to resect the corneal portion of the tumor.[122] The problems with this

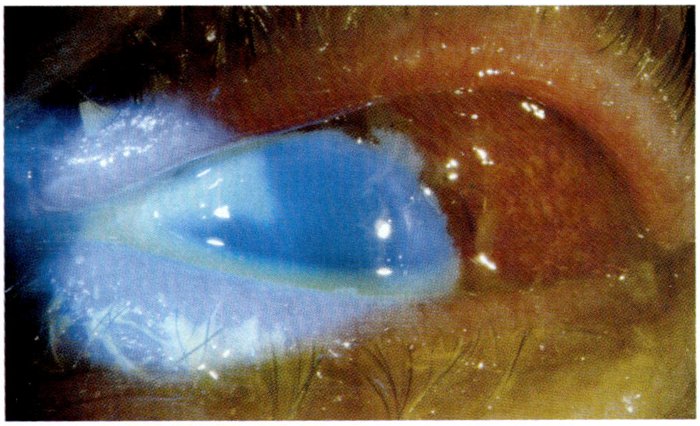

Figure 4–24. Fluorescein staining 36 hours after complete removal of involved epithelium, cryotherapy and placement of limbal grafts. This figure shows that > 80 percent of the corneal surface had become re-epithelialized by that time.

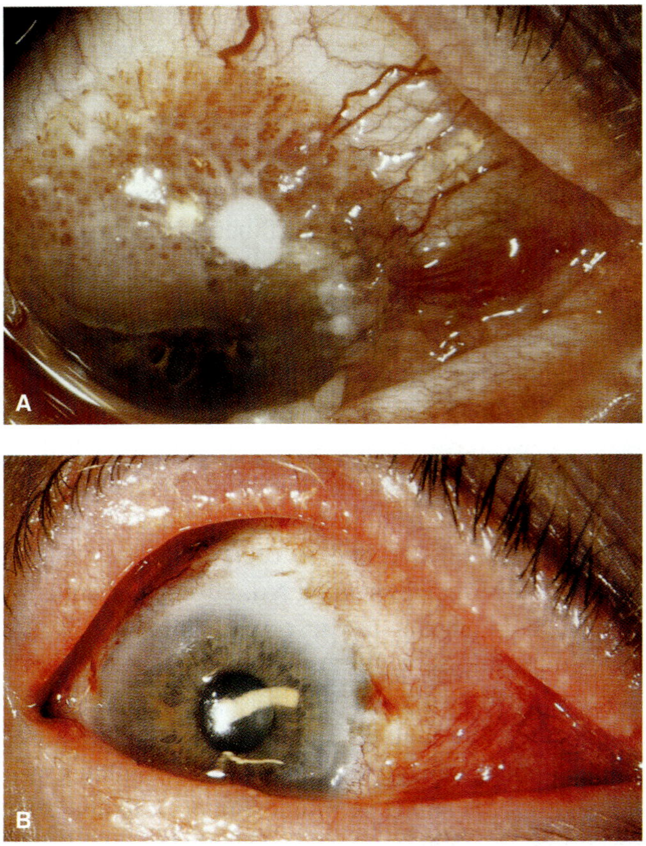

Figure 4–25. *A,* A large conjunctival—corneal squamous cell carcinoma. *B,* Removal of the tumor, cryotherapy, and placement of autologous limbal grafts resulted in a good visual outcome.

approach are at least threefold. The major issue is that since it vaporizes tissue, there is no material available for histologic evaluation of the margins or of the lesion itself. A second less important issue is that since these tumors do not grow in a symmetric fashion, sculpting an area with the laser would be somewhat difficult. Third, there is a paucity of data.

Recently, the group in Miami has reported excellent results using only Mohs' technique (see Chapter 3) under a local anesthesia without cryotherapy. None of 19 patients developed a recurrence with a follow-up between 6 and 60 months.[123] In 4 of the 19 patients, however, a second procedure was required, since the initial surgical margins were positive.

We have had one intraocular occurrence that was present at the time of initial surgery, though we failed to recognize it. The patient, who had had her first surgical procedure in a developing country, appeared to have a rough scleral surface as a result of a partial-thickness sclerectomy. Three months after we removed one tumor with clear margins and treated the resected tumor base with triple freeze-thaw cryotherapy to –30° C, intraocular invasion was documented.

Radiation

Some, generally diffuse carcinomas have been treated with brachytherapy or teletherapy. Lommatzsch reported treating 15 patients with beta irradiation for localized tumors, with excellent results. In 6 patients followed up over 5 years, no recurrences were noted. One patient developed a cataract, but it was bilateral, and 1 developed a partial symblepharon. Two patients developed glaucoma, and 1 case of corneal degeneration also occurred.[124]

Several other groups have reported radiation therapy results with different forms of brachytherapy (ruthenium-106 [^{106}Ru], iridium-125 [^{125}I], strontium-90 [^{90}Sr]) in small number of cases.[125–129] Radiation doses have varied from 30 to over 100 gray (Gy) in single or fractionated treatments. Cataract occurred in some of these patients and recurrences were reported in 4 of 27 cases in one series.[125] ^{90}Sr has been used as an adjunctive therapy after surgical resection of conjunctival squamous cell carcinoma. In 131 evaluable cases, approximately 6 percent developed recurrences. Cataract and scleral damage were noted in $<$ 5 percent of cases.[130] Scleral damage at lower radiation doses after pterygium repair has been previously reported.[131] Possibly, if radiation-induced scleral necrosis occurs, hyperbaric oxygen can be used, although the author's inclination would be to biopsy the area to ensure there is no recurrent tumor, and then graft the site.[132]

Topical Therapy

Several evolving experimental therapies are being investigated for CIN and invasive squamous cell carcinoma. Maskin reported a single case of a CIN lesion treated with topical interferon.[133] Dausch and colleagues reported a single case with a 26-month follow-up of a patient who had a CIN lesion removed by phototherapeutic keratectomy.[134] Frucht-Pery and Rozenman reported 3 patients treated with topical mitomycin-C for between 10 and 22 days. After 4 to

12 months of follow-up, none of the 3 had recurrences.[135] While they noted no major complications, others have seen severe vision problems when this medicine has been used after pterygium surgery.[136]

There have been several small series reported with the use of topical mitomycin-C, mainly for intraepithelial disease. A few patients have been treated with 5-fluorouracil with short-term good results.[137] A number of authors have reported under 10 patients each, using various concentrations of mytomycin-C, usually either 0.02 percent or 0.04 percent four times a day for either 7 or 14 days. In a follow-up paper by Frucht-Pery and associates, 17 patients with CIN were treated. After one course of therapy, the tumors were eradicated in 10 cases, but in 6 regrowth occurred. In 5 of the 6 cases where there were CIN lesions (the latter was an invasive carcinoma), they were able to eradicate the tumor.[138] Wilson and colleagues treated 7 eyes with 0.04 percent mitomycin-C four times a day for 7 days in alternate-week cycles, and 2 of 7 required a resection.[139–141] Vann and Karp have treated 6 patients with biopsy proven lesions using 3 megaunits of interferon 2-beta and achieving complete resolution, with a mean follow-up of 7.2 months.[142]

Management of Widespread Conjunctival or Orbital Invasion by Squamous Cell Carcinoma

Unfortunately, a number of invasive conjunctival squamous cell carcinoma patients are initially misdiagnosed as having chronic unilateral conjunctivitis when they actually have a diffuse conjunctival carcinoma involving both the palpebral and bulbar conjunctiva (Figure 4–26). In this group of patients, it is very difficult to retain a functional eye. In one or two heroic cases, we resected the entire conjunctival area and used extensive grafts. We have been able to control the tumors with 50 Gy of radiation; however, as a result of damage to the goblet cells and lacrimal ductules, none of these eyes has retained useful vision, and most required anterior exenteration after they became painful and nonfunctional.[143]

Orbital or intraocular invasion in these patients is often an indication for anterior exenteration (see Figure 4–20). We have had to perform total orbital exenteration in only a few cases, as orbital involvement is almost always limited to the anterior portion of the orbit. (See Chapter 8 for a discussion of exenteration techniques). In an anterior exenteration, we make incisions distal to the lashes and elevate a myocutaneous flap as shown in Figure 8–71. The entire conjunctiva and globe are removed en bloc, but the muscles posterior to their insertions as well as other orbital structures are left in situ. Hemostasis is achieved with both pressure and cautery. The orbital tissues are closed with 4-0 chromic gut suture. A small Penrose drain is left in place, and the skin is sutured with interrupted 6-0 silk. The orbit is pressure-patched for 48 hours, and re-dressed with another 48-hour pressure-patch after the first dressing change. Thereafter, the bandage is changed daily. Figure 4–27 shows a patient 1 week after an anterior exenteration.

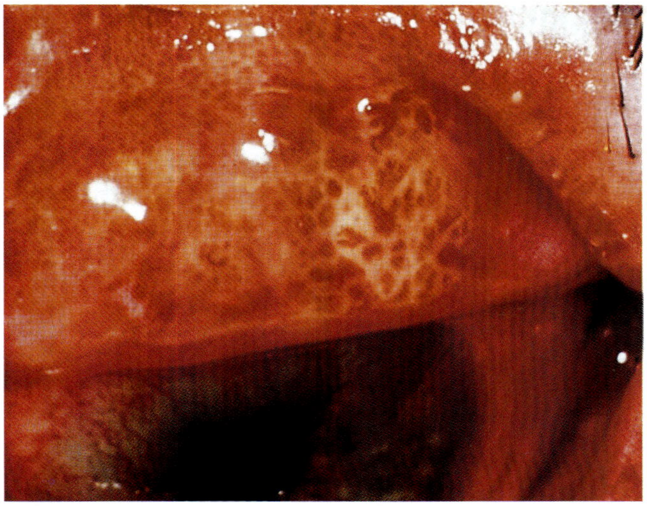

Figure 4–26. Diffuse involvement of both palpebral and bulbar conjunctiva by squamous cell carcinoma.

Metastases from squamous cell carcinoma of the conjunctiva are quite rare; only 3 tumor deaths have been reported in the United States, and only 1 of these was documented with postmortem examination.[5,62,63] In the world's literature, there have been approximately 10 cases of tumor-related mortality associated with conjunctival squamous cell carcinoma.[3,144]

Variants of Conjunctival Squamous Cell Carcinoma

Some variants of conjunctival squamous cell carcinoma that have a greater tendency to behave aggres-

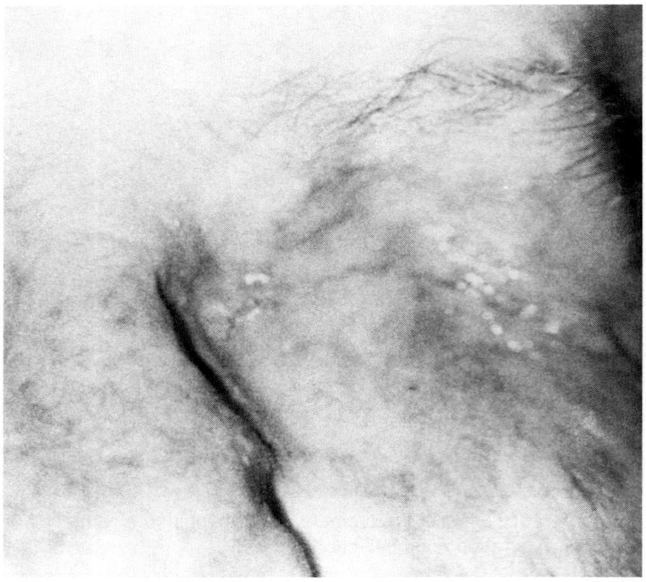

Figure 4–27. One week after anterior exenteration for intraocular invasion of a diffuse squamous cell carcinoma.

sively have been reported. Margo and Groden described a case of a CIN lesion with mucoepidermoid differentiation.[145] There have been approximately 15 cases of mucoepidermoid carcinomas of the conjunctiva described. There is a high tendency for these spindle cell variants to invade the globe and the orbit, and local excision has been of limited efficacy (see Figure 4–22).[110,111,146] In 2 of 6 spindle cell carcinomas of the conjunctiva, reported by Huntington and colleagues, intraocular extension developed.[147]

Campanella and colleagues report two cases of conjunctival carcinoma in enucleated sockets and hypothesize that the prosthesis may have caused sufficient irritation to promote tumor development.[148] The author personally has never seen such a case.

CONJUNCTIVAL MELANOMA

Conjunctival melanoma is an uncommon ocular tumor that accounts for 2 percent of all eye malignancies.[149,150] In Sweden, the annual incidence of this tumor is approximately 0.024 per 100,000.[151] In an American study of 4,836 cases of melanomas at all sites, 5.2 percent involved ocular structures, and of the ocular structures, 85 percent were uveal and 4.8 percent involved the conjunctiva.[152] The estimated incidence of melanoma in the uvea is between 20 and 40 times that in the conjunctiva.[149–152]

Pathogenesis

The pathogenesis of conjunctival melanomas is controversial. They can arise de novo, from nevi, or from malignant degeneration of acquired melanosis.[153–155] Reese believed that most conjunctival melanomas arise from an area of acquired melanosis.[156] Although some oncologists continue to believe that conjunctival melanomas arise de novo in approximately 50 percent of cases, most oncologists no longer do.[157] Folberg and colleagues reviewed 131 cases of conjunctival melanoma and concluded that 98 (75%) arose from primary acquired melanosis, while 33 were either new tumors or tumors arising from nevi.[158] Other workers believe that only 50 to 60 percent of conjunctival melanomas arise from acquired melanosis.

The importance of environmental factors in the etiology of conjunctival melanomas is uncertain. In cutaneous melanomas, sun exposure plays an important role, and melanomas occur more frequently in patients living closer to the equator. Similar, but smaller, data sets are available for both uveal and conjunctival melanoma.[63,159,160] Because of the paucity of tissue, there have been few molecular biologic investigations on conjunctival melanoma. In some work in the author's laboratory several years ago, we did not find increased *p53* abnormalities, and others have found similar results.[161,162]

Diagnosis

Establishing the correct diagnosis in a patient suspected of having a conjunctival melanoma can be difficult. Three general principles are helpful: (1) the patient's age is a factor; melanomas rarely occur in teenagers and younger children; most occur in middle-aged or older individuals. Fewer than 10 cases of conjunctival melanoma have been reported in children;[163–166] (2) conjunctival melanoma is an epithelial lesion. Many of the pigmented simulating lesions, such as melanosis oculi (Figure 4–28), oculodermal melanosis (nevus of Ota), and blue nevi are in the sclera; and (3) conjunctival nevi will often have cystic inclusions visible on slit-lamp examination (Figure 4–29); cystic inclusions are almost never found in melanomas.

The patient's ocular history is important in differentiating simulating lesions from melanomas. A

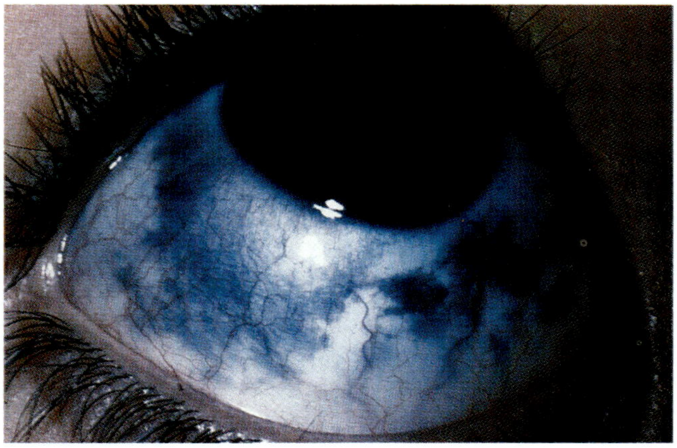

Figure 4–28. Melanosis oculi.

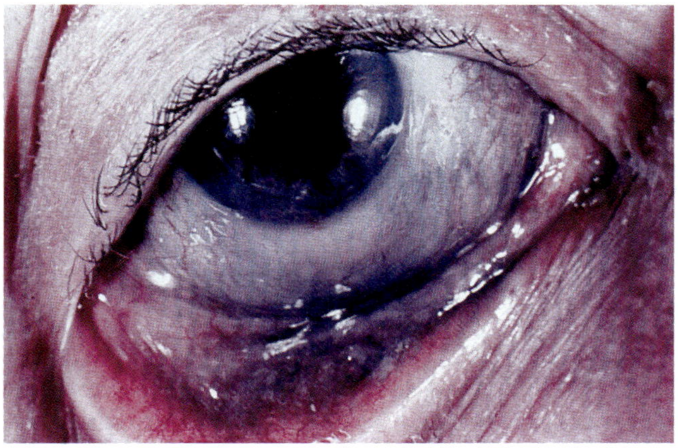

Figure 4–30. Argyrosis.

history of previous conjunctival inflammation, such as trachoma, the use of certain eyedrops (argyrosis or adrenochrome staining) (Figures 4–30 and 4–31), exposure to radiation or arsenic, and certain systemic conditions, such as pregnancy or Addison's disease, can produce benign superficial pigmentation.[167,168] In Carney's complex, an autosomal dominant disorder characterized by cardiac myxomas, endocrine disease, and spotty pigmentation, conjunctival pigmentation has been described.[169]

Simulating Lesions

Lesions that can simulate conjunctival melanomas include nevi (see Figure 4–29), staphylomas, subconjunctival hematomas, foreign bodies (Figure 4–32), and extraocular extensions of uveal melanomas (Figure 4–33). While previously thought to be uncommon, we have noted that combined nevi are not rare and can closely mimic melanomas.[170]

Conjunctival melanomas are rare in dark-skinned races.[171,172] As is the case with uveal melanomas, African Americans are much less commonly affected by this process. Approximately 5 to 10 percent of Caucasians have limbal conjunctival epithelial pigmentation.[173] In contrast, approximately 50 percent of Oriental and Hispanic patients have limbal pigmentation, and it is present in almost 95 percent of black patients.[172] Some clinicians have used an overly inclusive definition of primary acquired melanosis (PAM). Gloor and Alexandrakis thought it was present in 36 percent of outpatient examinations in one center.[174]

Conjunctival nevi may be difficult to differentiate either clinically or histologically from melanomas. Jay reported 43 conjunctival nevi that had previously been histologically classified as melanomas.[175] He

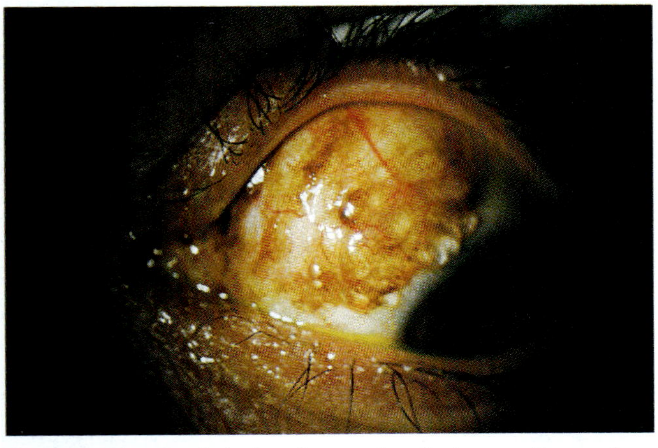

Figure 4–29. Cystic lesions in a conjunctival nevus; these microcysts are never clinically observed in conjunctival melanomas.

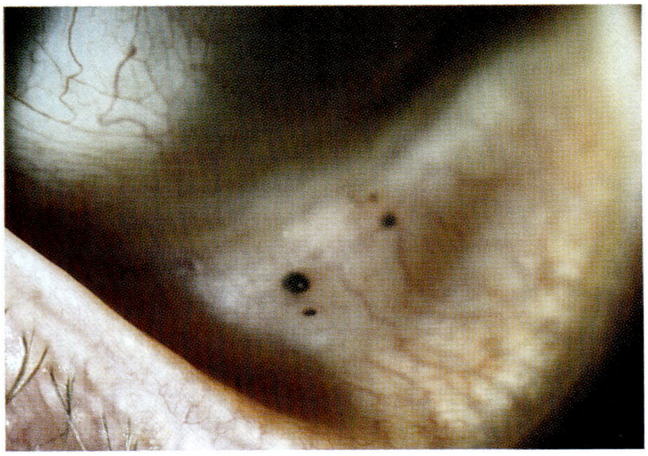

Figure 4–31. Adenochrome staining of the conjunctiva

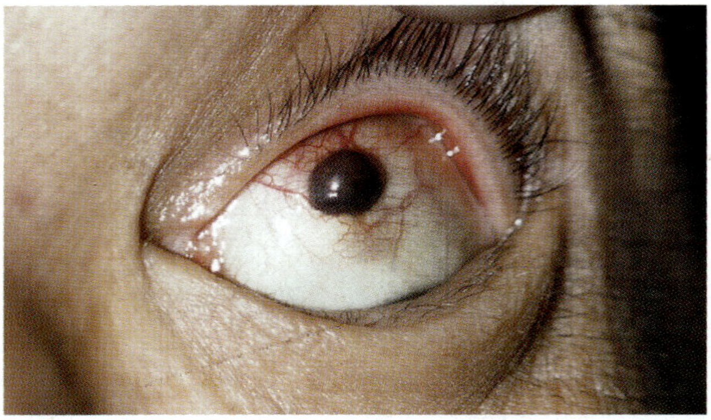

Figure 4–32. Conjunctival foreign bodies simulating melanoma.

noted that it is often difficult to correctly diagnose a conjunctival melanoma, since the cells can have bizarre shapes and there can be marked inflammation surrounding the lesion. Others have queried whether some presumed conjunctival nevi that later appear to undergo malignant degeneration may actually be undiagnosed melanomas in the radial growth phase.[176] Using several markers, such as S-100, HMB-45, NKI/C3, there is not good enough differentiation to delineate benign and malignant pigmented conjunctival lesions. Preliminary work using an antibody toward MAGE-3, Mab57b, showed reasonable specificity between benign and malignant pigmented lesions but only 44 percent of sensitivity.[177] More recent studies have shown that even in expert centers, there is diagnostic uncertainty in these indeterminant cases.[178]

The clinical as well as the histologic differentiation of nevi from melanomas may be confusing. Most commonly, conjunctival nevi are present at birth and arise at the limbus.[179] Often, nevi appear to grow at puberty as a result of the increased pigmentation of the nevus cells. Conjunctival nevi and melanomas can be amelanotic (Figure 4–34A and 4–34B). Alternatively, nevi can occasionally be red. Kantelip and colleagues reported a Spitz nevus in a 15-year-old boy that was at the limbus, red and 6 mm in size.[180]

If the clinical diagnosis of a conjunctival pigmented lesion is not definitive, a biopsy should be performed. Incisional biopsy followed by definitive therapy does not alter the patient's prognosis.[181] Some authors have also advocated tear cytology.[182] In atypical cases of either a possible amelanotic melanoma or melanoma versus a nonpigmented lesion, HMB-45, a monoclonal antibody that is positive for both benign and malignant melanocytic processes, can be useful.[183,184]

Acquired melanosis of the conjunctiva, an entity first defined by Reese, can be difficult to differentiate from melanoma.[163] Some authors have suggested that "primary epithelial melanosis" might be a better term, but it has not had wide acceptance. Usually, the onset of acquired melanosis of the conjunctival epithelium occurs in early middle age. Patients who develop malignant degeneration are, on average, slightly older than those with benign acquired melanosis.[181]

Patients initially develop patchy brown areas of conjunctival epithelial pigmentation (Figure 4–35); occasionally, the lesion can secondarily involve the cornea or lid (Figure 4–36A). The clinical course of acquired melanosis is varied.[173] New areas of con-

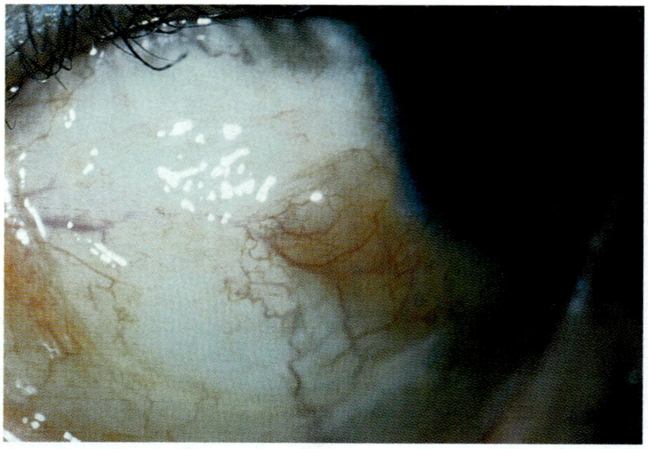

Figure 4–33. Extraocular extension of a uveal melanoma; unlike a conjunctival melanoma, the lesion is subepithelial.

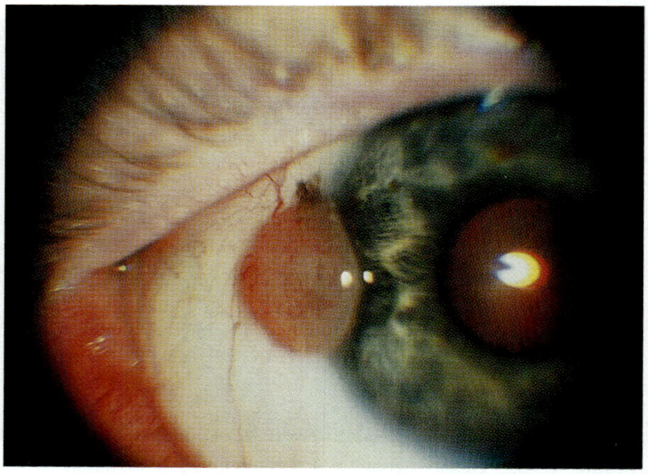

Figure 4–34. Amelanotic melanoma of the conjunctiva.

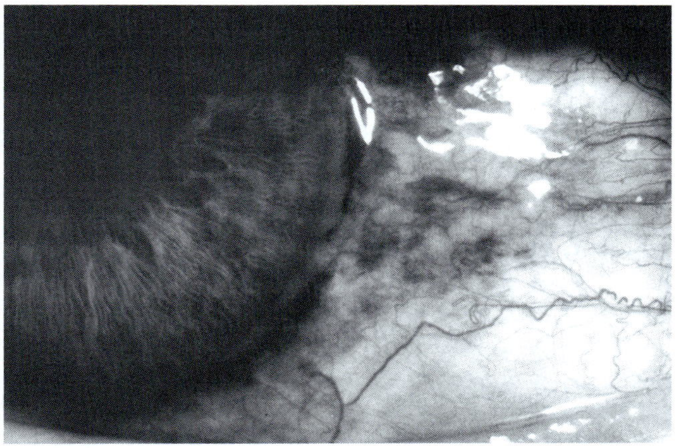

Figure 4–35. Limbal conjunctival acquired melanosis.

junctival involvement may develop as other sites lose pigmentation. Total spontaneous regression occasionally occurs, whereas other patients develop malignant degeneration. Approximately 17 percent of the patients followed up by Reese developed areas of malignant degeneration.[173] Figure 4–36B illustrates malignant degeneration of the case shown in Figure 4–36A. Figures 4–37A and B demonstrate another case of malignant progression in a patient with primary acquired melanosis. Histologically, the progression of acquired melanosis to invasive melanoma has been well delineated.[184,185]

Zimmermann classified acquired melanosis into four stages. In stage I, there is minimal junctional activity. In stage Ib, there is marked junctional activity, with nesting of the nevus cells. Stage II can be divided into cancerous melanosis with minimal invasion (IIa) or marked invasion (IIb). The histologic changes noted on biopsy are important prognostically, even if no malignancy is noted.[184] Folberg and colleagues demonstrated that approximately 50 percent of primary acquired melanosis cases with basal atypical cells later developed into invasive melanoma.[156,185] A particularly difficult form of primary acquired melanosis to diagnose is a tumor that arises out of a primary melanosis sine pigmento.[186] Most cases of corneal melanomas probably arise from either the limbus or from an unsuspected primary melanosis sine pigmento.[172,186,187]

Unfavorable prognostic signs in conjunctival melanoma include tumor thickness, location, (involvement of caruncle, palpebral conjunctiva, or fornix), diffuse melanomas, multifocality, more malignant cell type, lymphocytic infiltration, the presence of marked cytologic atypia, cell proliferation, pigmentation of the lid margin, and pagetoid spread (Table 4–1).[158,175,188–193] In a Danish retrospective study of 55 cases with a minimum follow-up of 10 years, the 5- and 10- year survival rates were 86 percent and 73 percent, respectively. The local recurrence rate at 5 years was 5 percent, and at 10 years 42 percent.[194] In a French series, in 49 of 56 patients who had surgery plus external beam radiation, the overall survival was 77 percent at 5 and 64 percent at 10 years. Tumors that arose de novo had a worse prognosis.[195] In another series of 61 patients reported from Yugoslavia, tumor thickness was the most important predictor of survival in multivariant analysis. Other important factors were mitosis, pigmentation, and inflammation.[195] Most series have shown that tumors > 1.8 mm thick have a poor prognosis, but some have not.[175,180,189,192] In some cases, melanomas that arose from the nevi had a better prognosis than those that

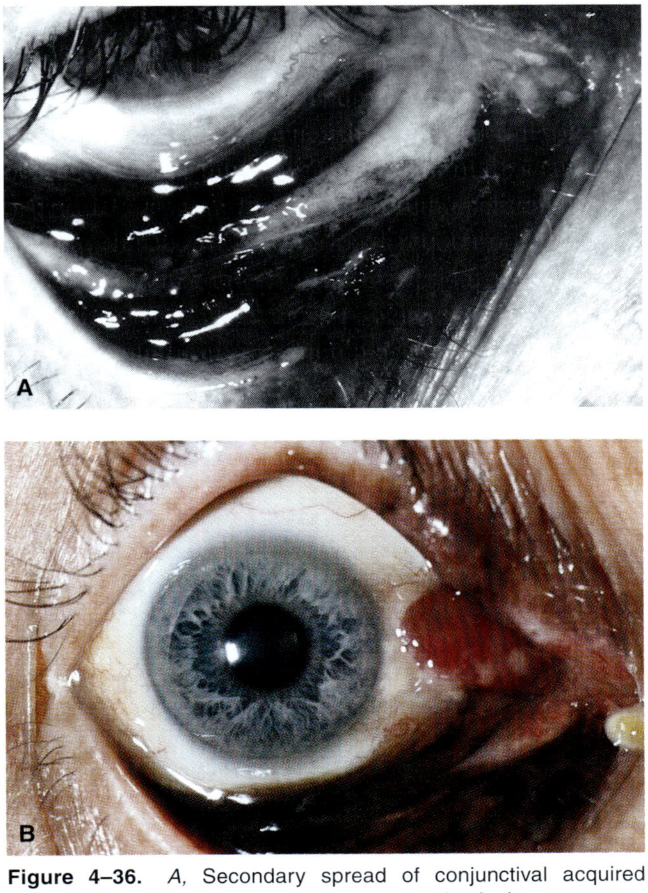

Figure 4–36. *A,* Secondary spread of conjunctival acquired melanosis onto the lid. *B,* Malignant degeneration in the same case, with vertical growth phase in bulbar melanoma.

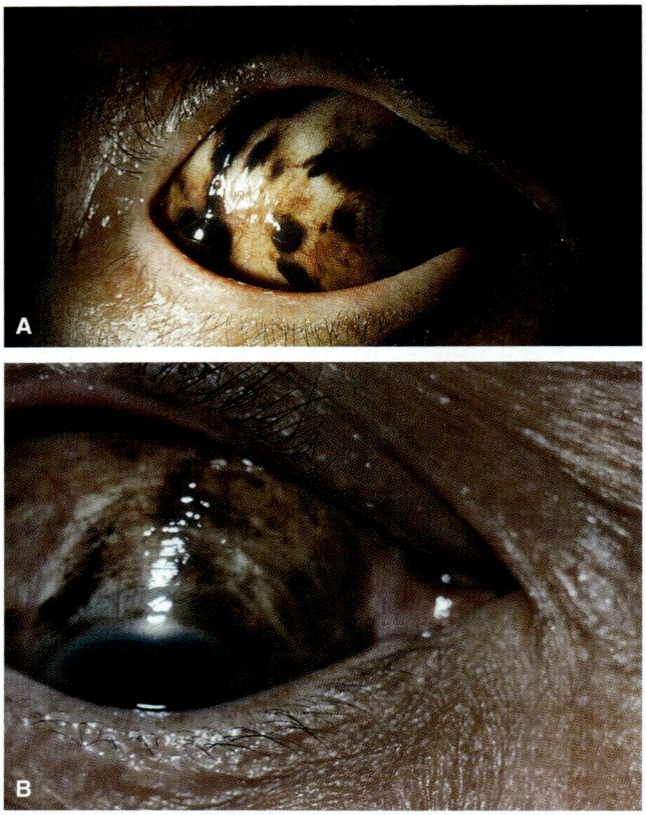

Figure 4–37. *A* and *B,* Malignant progression in multiple areas in a patient with PAM.

arose de novo or from acquired melanosis, but this is not evident in other series.[158,196]

Almost 20 percent of patients with acquired melanosis develop malignant transformation. If the patient has a relatively small area of PAM that is easily resected at the limbus, it is probably prudent to do so in a young person. In patients with diffuse involvement, an incisional biopsy in the thickest area or one with inflammation should be performed along with careful serial examinations. The presence of new vessels, discrete tumor thickening, inflammation, or spread of diffuse disconnected pigment suggests malignant degeneration.

Management

Optimal management of acquired melanosis is uncertain. There are no randomized prospective clinical trial data on which to base management decisions, and there have been no statistically significant data demonstrating the superiority of any therapeutic modality in the management of conjunctival melanoma. In general, patients with relatively thin melanomas that are localized on the bulbar conjunctiva do quite well (see Table 4–1). We excise suspicious conjunctival lesions in the office and send the specimens for pathologic examination. If the clinical appearance of the lesion suggests a melanoma, given its thickness, lack of cysts, and epithelial origin, we remove it under frozen section control in the operating room. If the margins are free of tumor, even if there is no clinical evidence of scleral extension, the base and resection margins are treated with double freeze-thaw cryotherapy. The techniques used in conjunctival surgery are discussed at the end of the chapter.

Some authors have advocated various forms of radiation therapy.[197–201] Radiation is relatively effec-

Table 4–1. CONJUNCTIVAL MELANOMA: PROGNOSTIC PARAMETERS FOR TUMOR-RELATED MORTALITY*

	Fornix/Caruncular Involvement	Diffuse Involvement	Bulbar Involvement Only	Tumor Thickness < 1.95 mm	Tumor Thickness > 1.8 mm
Silvers, et al.[157]	8/10	10/15	1/9	0/16	12/12
Jeffrey, et al.[189]	7/10	2/6	1/21	2/18	8/16†
Liesegang, et al.[196]	2/8		2/20	6/6†	
Crawford.[31]	4/4		3/10	4/5	
Folberg, et al.[158]	8/25	9/63‡	36/94‡		
Jay[155]					
Paridaens, et al.[220]	Favorable location (see text) cell type, advanced age, lymphocytic infiltration and multifocality.		Unfavorable location (hazards ratio 2.18), thickness > 4mm versus < 1mm		

*Data presented as number of patients who died of tumor over number with prognostic sign.
† Tumor thickness > 2.0 mm
‡ Tumor thickness > 1.6 mm

tive in controlling local disease; however, its effect on conjunctival melanoma metastases is unclear.[202] We use radiation to treat diffuse conjunctival melanomas arising from acquired melanosis when they cannot be surgically resected and the patients refuse exenteration. In a few such cases, we have saved the eye; however, most had enough ocular damage from wide-field irradiation so that only a limited function was achieved (Figure 4–38). Slightly better results have been described by Zografos and colleagues with protons, cobalt, and cryotherapy.[203] Other investigators have used approximately 100 Gy of beta radiation to treat more localized melanomas, with good results. Lommatzsch noted that 31 of 45 conjunctival melanomas could be controlled with ^{90}Sr beta applicators.[199] As is the case with uveal melanomas, tumor shrinkage is often delayed for 2 to 4 years, and complications including cataract, conjunctival telangiectasia, keratitis, anterior uveitis, neovascular glaucoma, and loss of the eye can occur. Approximately, 12 percent of conjunctival melanomas treated with radiation develop a significant ocular complication, including loss of the eye.[198] In Lommatzsch's series, 11 of 65 patients died, 4 with proven metastases.[199]

Contraindications for radiation therapy include bulky tumors in the fornix, tumor involvement of the palpebral conjunctiva and lid, and recurrent melanoma previously treated with radiation.

Cryotherapy is usually used as an adjunct in the management of conjunctival melanomas. Not much data are available on this technique, even though it has been used in ophthalmic oncology since the late 1960s.[13,204] Limited data indicate that in conjunction with surgery for local disease, cryotherapy is as effective as ionizing radiation and is associated with fewer complications. Cryotherapy can have significant complications, including trichiasis, ptosis, loss of lashes, symblepharon, and paresis of the recti muscles.[205,206] The use of this modality for benign acquired melanosis is uncertain. Jakobiec and coworkers have reported results in 5 such patients with acquired melanosis without malignant degeneration.[207] Severe corneal changes and cataract occurred in 1 patient. While cryotherapy can destroy nevoid as well as melanoma cells, it does have significant complications, and the value of intervention in patients with benign disease is uncertain.[206] Cryotherapy in an area of acquired melanosis usually destroys all pigmentation. The technique may be effective even when melanoma has superficially involved the sclera.[207,208] It has been the author's experience that if the tumor is limited to the conjunctival epithelium, it is useful to elevate this layer with a 30-gauge needle using topical anesthesia before freezing the tumor. The author believes that this technique decreases the morbidity to both Tenon's capsule and the eye that otherwise might occur with this therapy. The author also places a symblepharon conformer for 5 to 7 days if a wide area of conjunctiva has been treated with cryotherapy to prevent adhesions.

Experimental treatments with heat have been reported, but sufficient data are not available to determine their utility.[209] Several reports using mitomycin-C, analogous in dose and schedule with that used for conjunctival squamous cell carcinoma have been reported with melanoma.[210–213] Frucht-Pery and Pe'er treated a patient with PAM with atypia, without progression over 7 months. Starting in 1995, Lomatzsch and colleagues treated 14 patients, 9 with melanoma and 5 with PAM. With local excision, they received 0.02 percent mitomycin-C for 4 to 6 weeks.[214] Two cases developed progression. Finger and colleagues reported 10 cases treated at 0.04 percent qid. Six of the 10 had been treated after the excision in cryotherapy, and all developed transient conjunctivitis, with 1 developing epithelial defect. Those tumors which had a

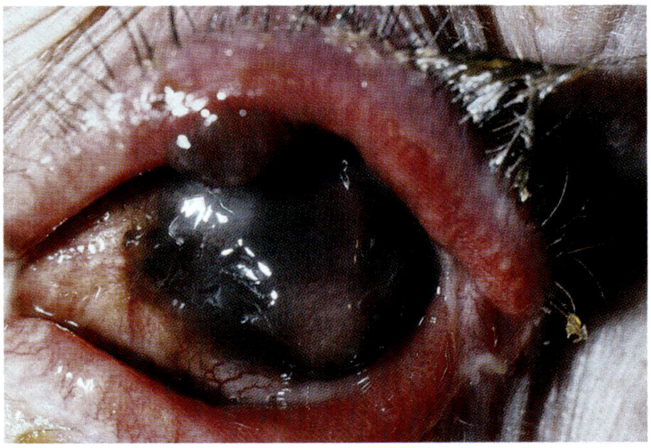

Figure 4–38. Diffuse conjunctival melanoma treated with wide-field radiation. Loss of goblet cells and secondary xerophthalmia has resulted in loss of visual function.

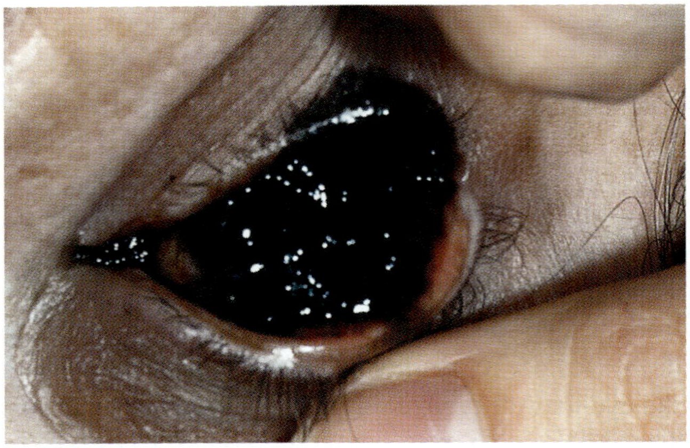

Figure 4–39. Bulky, diffuse conjunctival and eyelid melanomas.

nodular component were resistant to treatment, and 4 which were treated with topical mitomycin-C all recurred. Exenteration is necessary for some conjunctival melanomas that have intraocular or orbital extension, diffuse, bulky fornix involvement (Figure 4–39), or recurrence after irradiation.[215] The intraocular pattern of conjunctival melanoma invasion is not pathognomonic; often, it appears as a flat, diffuse choroidal tumor (Figure 4–40) or as a pupillary irregularity (Figure 4–41).

Prior to exenteration, a complete metastatic evaluation should be performed. In addition, as several authors have pointed out, inspection of the nasal sinuses with the endoscope to detect possible extension down the nasal lacrimal duct should be performed. This includes a general physical examination, serum liver function tests, and chest and abdominal computed tomography (CT) or magnetic resonance imaging (MRI) evaluation.

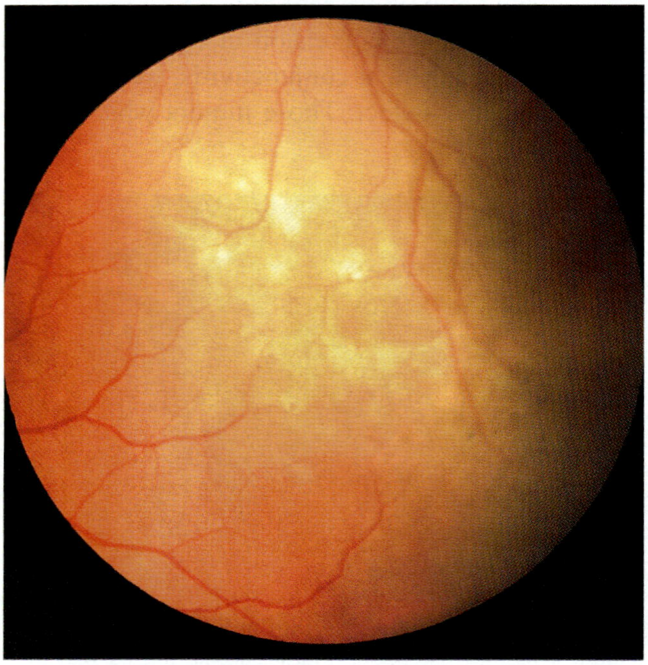

Figure 4–40. Histologically confirmed diffuse choroidal infiltration from intraocular penetration of conjunctival melanoma.

The effect of exenteration on the natural history of conjunctival melanoma is unclear.[216] The surgical techniques for exenteration are shown in Chapter 8.

Conjunctival melanomas can metastasize to the conjunctiva, sinus mucosa, local cervical nodes, submandibular or preauricular nodes, intra-abdominal nodes, subcutaneous tissues, liver, bone, parotid gland, and brain.[2,197,216,219] In a large series Paridaens and co-workers noted that 27 percent of treated patients had recurrences in the previous site, lymph node involvement developed in 11 percent, 5 percent had orbital recurrence, and 3 percent developed sinus involvement.[220] Tumor-related mortality from conjunctival melanomas is affected by the extent, location, cell type, lymphocytic invasion, mitotic rate, and thickness of the tumor (see Table 4–1). There is a slight tendency for women to have a better prognosis than men, but this is not statistically significant.[175,221] Larger, more diffuse, and thicker tumors have a worse prognosis. Patients with diffuse malignant degeneration of acquired melanosis probably have a worse prognosis than those with localized tumors.[155,175] In the largest series of 256 consecutive invasive primary conjunctival melanomas, Paridaens and co-workers studied prognostic factors with multivariate analyses. Tumors in unfavorable

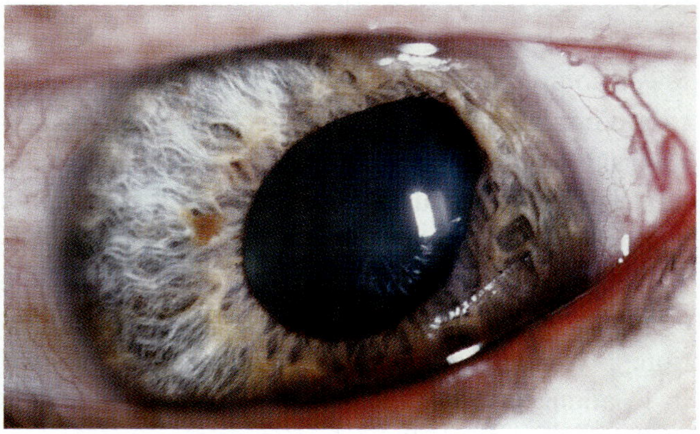

Figure 4–41. Iris invasion from conjunctival melanoma presenting as a pupillary abnormality.

locations, which they defined as palpebral conjunctiva, fornices, caruncle, and lid margins, had over twofold higher mortality, compared with those melanomas on the globe.[220] Similarly, patients with mixed tumors had three times higher mortality than those with pure spindle melanomas, and lymphocytic invasion was associated with a fourfold increased death rate. Multifocal tumors on the surface of the eye were associated with a fivefold increase in mortality. Unlike other smaller series, Paridaens and colleagues employed Cox modeling to adjust for effects of multiple parameters on survival.[220] They noted that some factors that appeared to be important in univariate analysis lost their significance when multivariate analysis was performed. As an example, when all tumors were considered, melanomas arising from PAM had a worse prognosis; however, this effect was lost when location and cell type were considered. Tumor location, lymphocytic invasion, and cell type were important prognostic parameters when all melanomas were considered together. In tumors in favorable locations, cell type, lymphocytic invasion, multifocality, and advanced age were also prognostically significant. In tumors in unfavorable locations, only thickness > 4mm, compared with < 1 mm, added to prognostic risk.[220]

Fuchs and others have also found that tumor location is important for survival.[222] As previously noted, Folberg and colleagues have found that the pagetoid spread in PAM-derived melanomas is also an important prognostic indicator for the development of metastases.[223] In this series, gender, age, and whether the tumor arose from an area of PAM, de novo, or from a nevus was not prognostically significant.[220] This group did not find evidence of nucleolar organizer regions associated with prognosis.[224] In a combination of several large series, the 5-year tumor-related mortality with conjunctival melanomas has been approximately 17 percent, and the 10-year mortality has been approximately 30 percent.[151,154,158,175,189,193,194,220,225]

There is controversy regarding the use of systemic adjunctive treatment in high-risk cutaneous melanoma. In some studies, the use of interferon alpha-2b has increased the relapse time and overall survival, while in other studies, this has not been demonstrated.[225] There is significant morbidity with this agent, and its efficacy in either conjunctival or uveal melanoma has not been demonstrated.

CONJUNCTIVAL KAPOSI'S SARCOMA

KS of the conjunctiva has become a common tumor in patients with acquired immunodeficiency syndrome (AIDS).[226] This neoplasm was first described in 1872 and has most commonly occurred in the lids or conjunctiva of elderly Italian or Jewish men. Before 1980, there were approximately 30 reported cases.[227,228] In Africa, the prevalence of this tumor paralleled the prevalence of malaria with its immunosuppression. The tumor also occurs in other immunosuppressed populations.[229] As discussed in the section on lid tumor pathogenesis, human herpes virus-8 (HHV-8) is important in the etiology of this tumor.[230] The role of the herpes virus in the etiology of this tumor would fit with the epidemiology of the disease.[230] The clinical presentation with a reddish or bluish, relatively diffuse, vascular conjunctival lesion is almost pathognomonic in a patient with AIDS.[2331–232] Approximately 75 percent of patients with ocular involvement exhibit oral lesions.[233] The author has never seen a patient with conjunctival KS who does not have the diagnosis or symptoms of AIDS. Three publications cite rare cases of patients with AIDS in whom KS was the first manifestation of the disease.[234] A typical example is shown in Figure 4–42. Occasionally, these tumors present as a focal mass (Figure 4–43). This vascular malignancy is very different in appearance from a benign conjunctival vascular malformation (Figure 4–44).

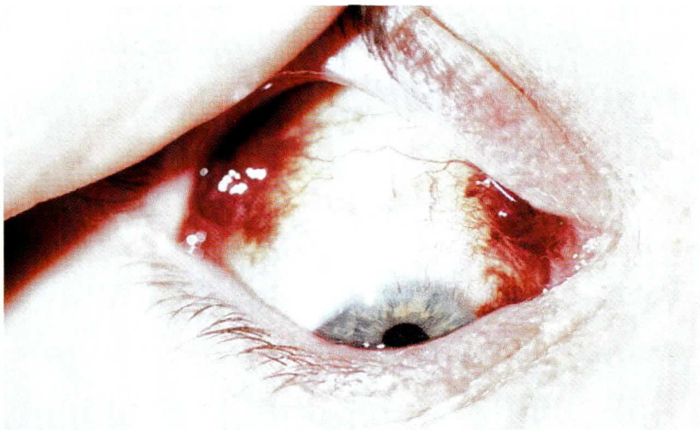

Figure 4–42. Typically, Kaposi's sarcoma in the conjunctiva are multifocal, diffuse, and reddish lesions.

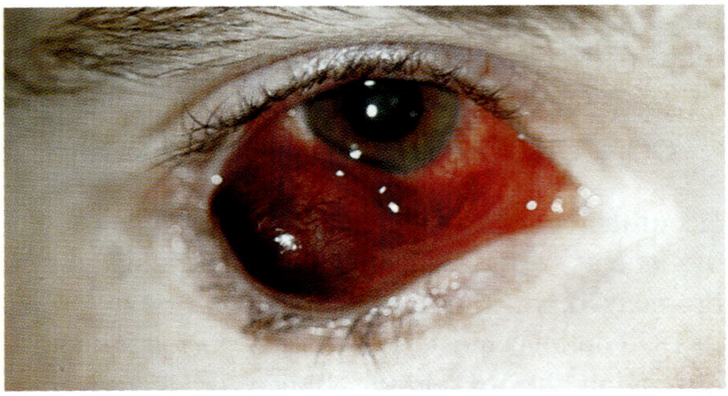

Figure 4–43. Solitary conjunctival Kaposi's sarcoma in an AIDS patient.

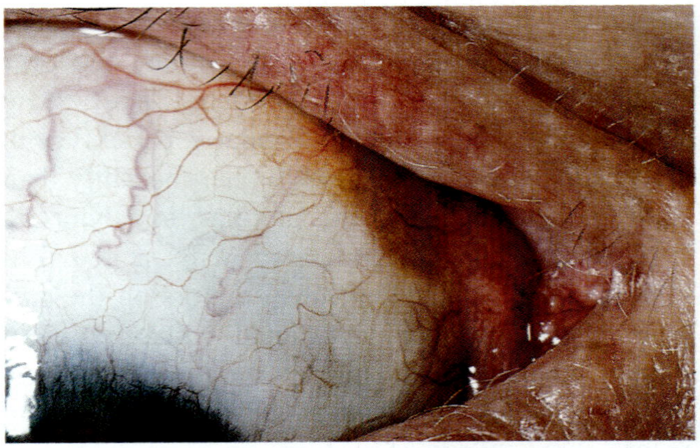

Figure 4–45. Lesion shown in Figure 4-42 after low-dose superficial electron irradiation.

Fortunately, with the use of multiple protease inhibitors, the incidence of KS lesions of both the lid and conjunctiva has markedly diminished. KS lesions respond rapidly to a number of therapeutic modalities, including cryotherapy, surgery, irradiation, and chemotherapy with vinblastine.[233–238] The patient shown in Figure 4–43 received 6 megavoltage (MeV) electrons with excellent results (Figure 4–45). In our experience, equivalent results are obtained with a single fraction of photon irradiation with less morbidity than using cryotherapy, intralesional chemotherapy, or surgery.[233]

CONJUNCTIVAL LYMPHOID LESIONS

The conjunctiva can be involved by a number of benign or malignant lymphoid lesions, including lymphoid hyperplasia, pseudotumor, leukemia, and various types of lymphoma. It is estimated that conjunctival lymphoid tumors account for between 0.2 and 1 percent of all ocular tumors. Lymphoid lesions characteristically present as a salmon-colored, subconjunctival infiltrate (Figure 4–46). Occasionally, diagnosis of a lymphoma can be difficult, and these can simulate a conjunctivitis or a scleritis.[239,240] While usually lymphoid lesions involve the bulbar conjunctiva, occasionally they will present with involvement mainly with the palpebral conjunctiva.[241] Differentiating between benign and malignant lymphoid infiltrates can be exceedingly difficult; one large series with a 5-year follow-up showed that it is often not possible to distinguish between the two.[242] Scarring of the overlying conjunctival epithelium is more common with benign processes (Figure 4–47); it is not usually seen in malignant lymphomas (Figure 4–48).

Less common lesions that have involved the conjunctiva include plasmacytoma, acute monocytic leukemia, Hodgkin's disease, Burkitt's lymphoma, T-cell lymphoma, mycosis fungoides, and large cell lymphomas.[243–251]

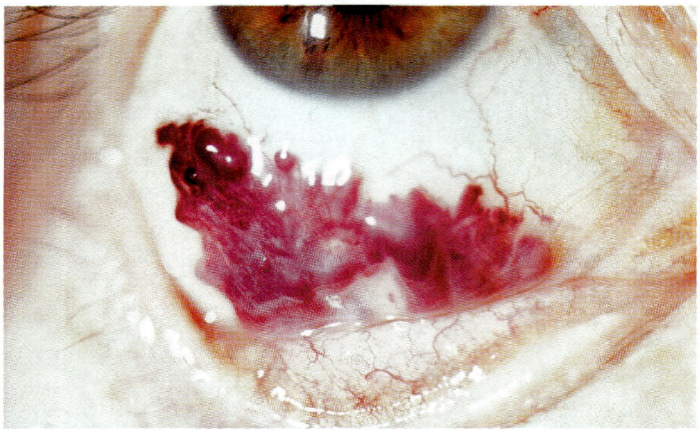

Figure 4–44. Benign conjunctival vascular malformation.

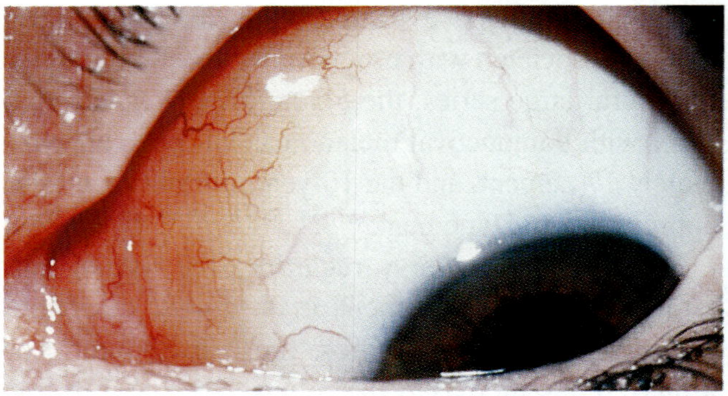

Figure 4–46. Typical salmon-colored lymphoid lesion. It is usually impossible to predict benign or malignant histology on the basis of the clinical appearance.

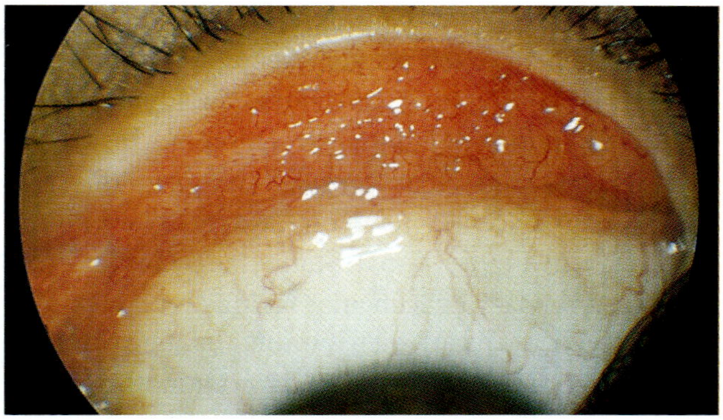

Figure 4–47. Scarring over a benign lymphoid process.

The laboratory diagnosis of lymphoid lesions is by standard histology, immunohistologic marker studies, and, in some cases, Southern blot or polymerase chain reaction (PCR) technique. These newer diagnostic modalities are discussed in Chapter 26.

Localized lesions can be excised (Figure 4–49). Fraunfelder and colleagues reported the use of cryotherapy in a diffuse mixture of lymphoid lesions. Thirty-nine out of 42 responded with two treatments, and 41 of 42 with a third treatment.[252] Diffuse malignant lesions isolated to the ocular adnexa are treated with 30 to 40 Gy of irradiation. If the lesion involves only the conjunctiva, after being biopsied, it is irradiated using either orthovoltage (approximately 250 lev) or electrons with appropriate shielding (see Chapter 2) (Figure 4–50A and B). If orbital involvement is present, megavoltage photon irradiation is used (see Chapter 26). Isolated conjunctival small cell lymphomas respond rapidly to irradiation, and in our experience and that of most others, less than 10 percent develop widespread disease on long-term follow-up.[253] In the study by Coupland and co-workers, however, they noted no difference in the incidence or development of systemic lymphoma between conjunctival or orbital lymphomas.[254] As discussed in the chapter on orbital lymphoma, orbital tumors generally have a higher likelihood of developing widespread disease; in another series, this was not been observed.[254] In the more poorly differentiated lesions, the risk of systemic disease is substantially higher.[255,256] Pre-existing systemic lymphoma was present in approximately 10 percent of our cases, but it was not always diagnosed.

All patients with conjunctival lymphomas should have a thorough evaluation, including complete blood count (CBC), plasma protein electrophoresis, body scans, and bone marrow biopsies. In benign lymphoid lesions that are symptomatic and involve a diffuse area, low-dose irradiation with 10 to 20 Gy is used, with shielding of the cornea and lens. A case of conjunctival–anterior orbital pseudotumor (diagnosed with Southern blot and monoclonal antibodies) is shown before and after low-dose irradiation (Figures 4–51A, B, and C). In rare circumstances, other therapies have been employed. Cellini and colleagues reported an HIV-positive patient with conjunctival lymphoma who responded to a short course of interferon.[257]

CARUNCLE LESIONS

Most lesions of the caruncle are benign. In two large series, < 10 percent of these tumors were malignant.

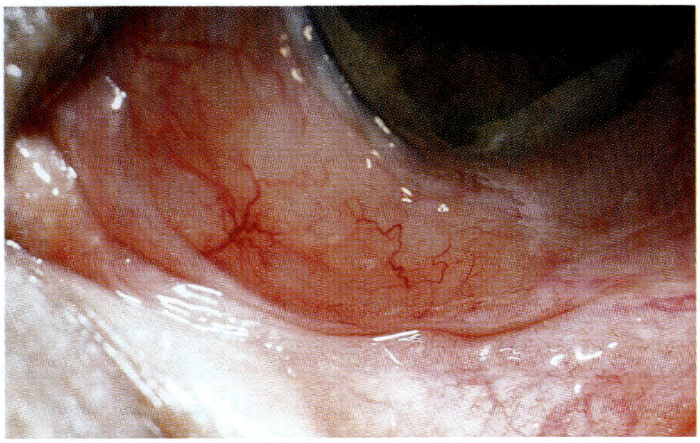

Figure 4–48. Absence of scarring with malignant lymphoma or leukemia.

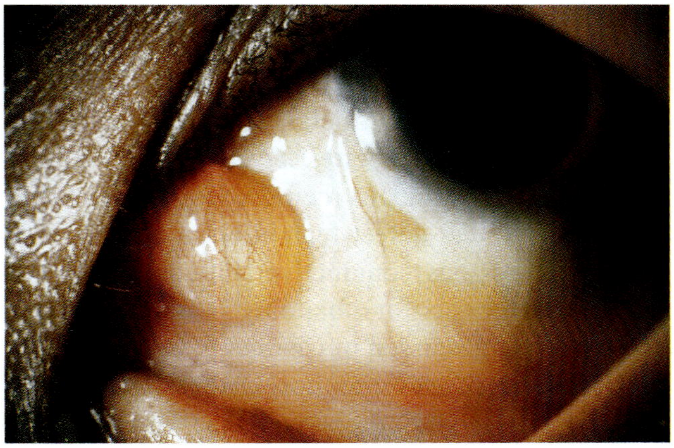

Figure 4–49. Localized lymphoid conjunctival lesion.

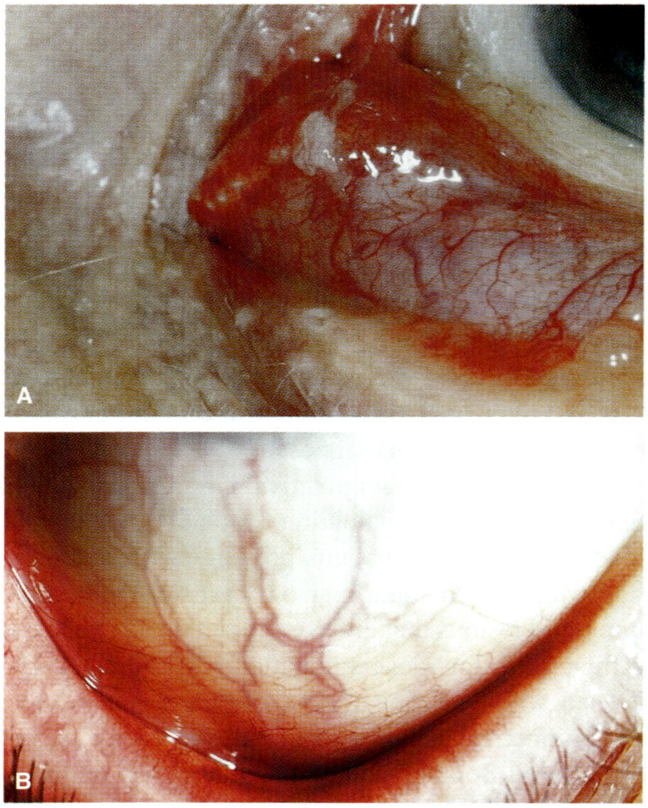

Figure 4–50. *A,* Conjunctival lymphoma involving the superior conjunctiva and anterior orbit before radiation. *B,* Appearance after receiving 40 Gy of photon irradiation.

In a series from the Wilmer Institute, nevi accounted for 43 percent of caruncle lesions, followed by papilloma (13%), sebaceous gland hyperplasia (8%), and nonspecific inflammation (4.5%). The most common malignancies were squamous cell carcinoma of the conjunctiva, sebaceous gland carcinoma of the lid, and conjunctival melanoma.[258] There have been four cases reported of primary basal carcinomas of the caruncle.[259] Other rare lesions include a mucoepidermoid carcinoma of the caruncle.[260] These lesions are managed like conjunctival squamous cell carcinoma or melanoma, with one exception. We find that better cosmetic results are obtained when a mucous membrane graft is used to cover the surgical defect than either a primary closure or autologous conjunctiva (Figure 4–52). The surgical technique for obtaining a mucous membrane graft is discussed in Chapter 3.

A number of less common lesions may involve the caruncle, including oncocytoma, which characteristically is a striking cherry red, and, rarely, adenocarcinoma.[261–264] A caruncular nevus is shown in Figure 4–53, a sebaceous gland carcinoma in Figure 4–54, a squamous cell carcinoma in Figure 4–55, and a melanotic melanoma in Figure 4–56. In the last case, despite clear surgical margins, this had orbital recurrence as shown on the axial T_1-weighted MRI scan in Figure 4–57. Santos and Gomez-Leal have described 113 caruncular lesions with a similar histologic patterns of distribution. In their referral base series, only 114 out of 2,624 conjunctival biopsies involved the caruncle.[265]

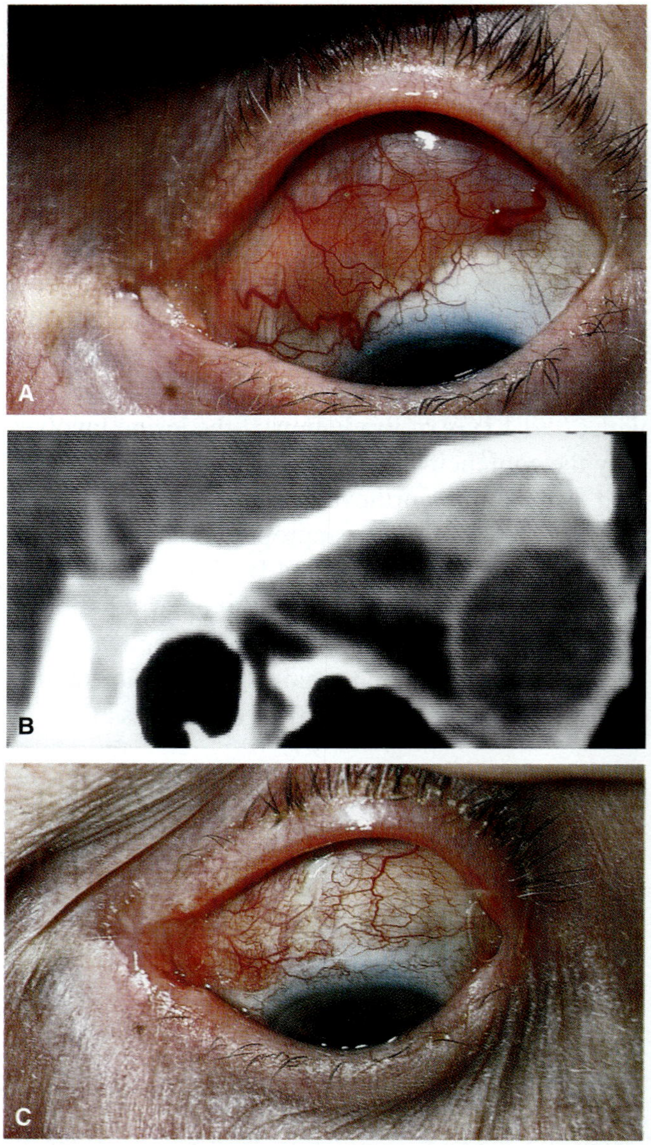

Figure 4–51. *A,* Conjunctival-anterior orbital pseudotumor diagnosed with monoclonal antibodies and Southern blot technique prior to treatment. *B,* Post resection with tumor regression. *C,* Appearance after receiving 20 Gy of photon irradiation.

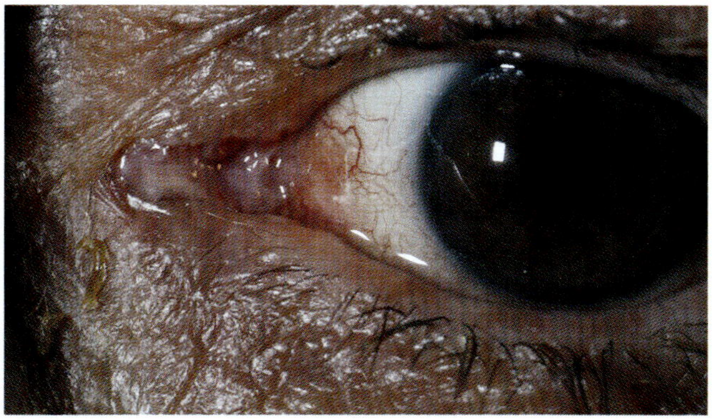

Figure 4–52. Mucous membrane graft used to cover caruncular defect after excision of sebaceous carcinoma.

RARE CONJUNCTIVAL MALIGNANCIES

Rare types of conjunctival malignancies are so uncommon that definitive statements about management cannot be made. Several case reports have included descriptions of primary tumors such as leiomyosarcoma, malignant fibrous histiocytoma, and metastatic carcinoid.[266–270] In addition, a paraneoplastic syndrome involving the conjunctiva and producing pemphigus has been described.[271,272] Rare conjunctival malignancies include mucoepidermoid carcinoma of the conjunctiva and spindle cell carcinoma of the conjunctiva.[151,153] Metastases to the conjunctiva rarely occur, and they have been described with a number of tumors, including melanoma, metastatic rhabdomyosarcoma, lung cancer, larynx, and uveal melanoma.[272–277]

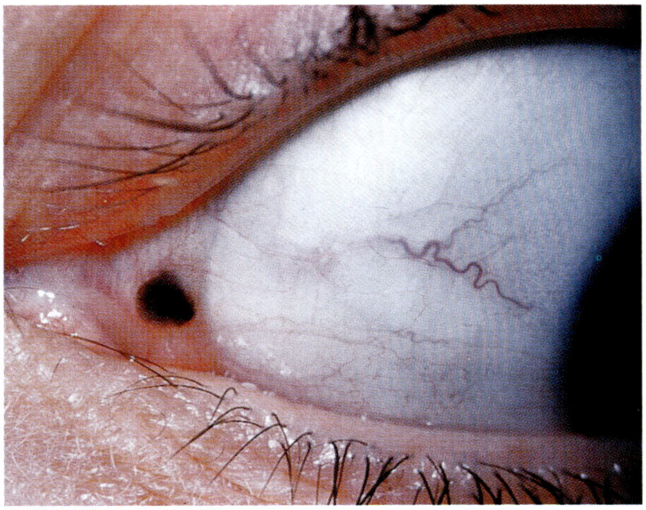

Figure 4–53. Caruncular nevus.

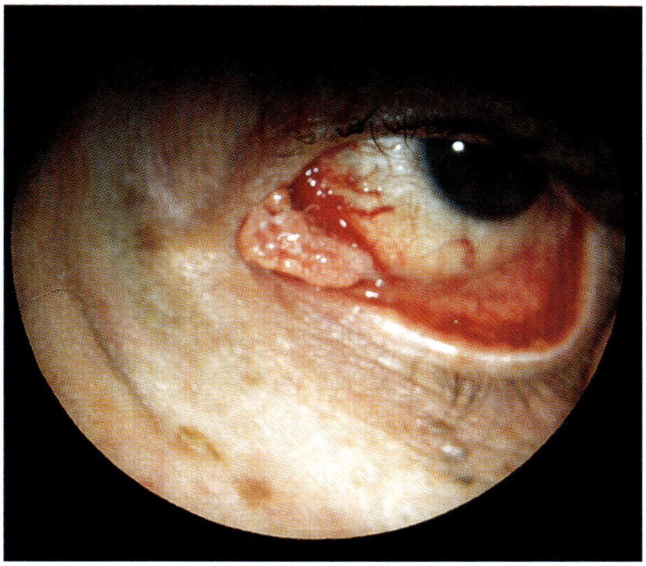

Figure 4–54. Sebaceous gland carcinoma of the caruncle.

CONJUNCTIVAL SURGERY

The control of tumor margins in the surgical resection of conjunctival malignancies is difficult owing to the limited amount of tumor tissue available for frozen section analysis, problems of accurate orientation, and difficulty in assessing the deep, scleral surface or the corneal margin. Adjunctive double freeze-thaw cryotherapy is routinely used by us in all our conjunctival melanomas and carcinomas because of these inherent limitations regarding accurate histologic sampling of margins, especially the deep surface if some tissue is used for horizontal margin assessment.

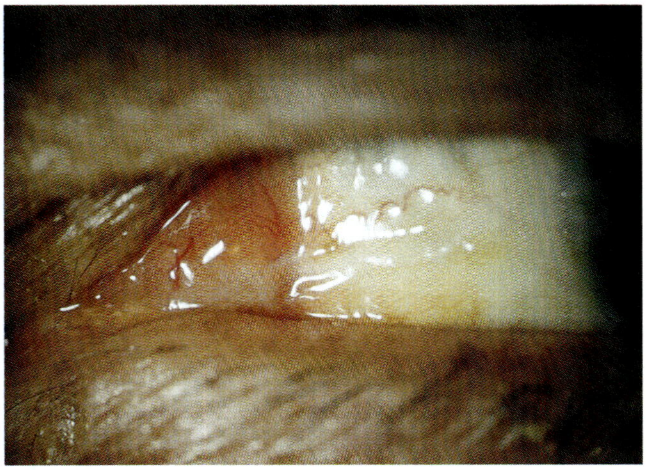

Figure 4–55. Caruncular squamous cell carcinoma.

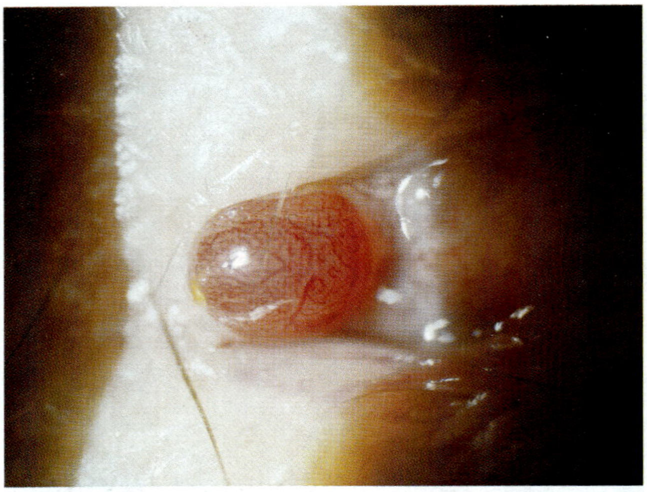

Figure 4–56. Caruncular amelanotic malignant melanoma.

Tissue orientation is crucial. For accurate histologic evaluation, it is vital to relate the neoplasm to normal structures and ensure that the specimen is not folded into itself. We always place conjunctival samples on a sterile ocular map (see Figure 3–1) and label the superior edge of the specimen with a long 4-0 silk suture and the inferior edge with a short 4-0 silk suture. In lesions that extend into the superficial cornea, we have not found frozen section control of that margin to be useful, since usually only tissue anterior to stroma is removed, often in a piecemeal manner. The bulk of the tumor is removed and the underlying corneal stroma is treated with double freeze-thaw cryotherapy.

In general, surgery is not effective management for diffuse conjunctival malignancies that extensively involve both bulbar and palpebral conjunctiva (see Figure 4–26). In tumors that superficially involve the corneal epithelium but not stroma, a Took knife is useful to perform a lamellar scleral and corneal dissection (Figure 4–58).

A number of unique problems are associated with resection of large areas of conjunctiva for either diffuse conjunctival squamous cell carcinoma or melanoma. Tumors that involve a large enough area so that loss of goblet cells results in inadequate tear film, tumors that completely surround the cornea, tumors that involve both bulbar and palpebral conjunctiva, and tumors in the area of the lacrimal ductules are difficult to manage surgically with long-term retention of a useful eye. Although in one heroic case at our institution, the entire conjunctiva was removed and replaced with vaginal mucosa, usually eyes with diffuse tumors that involve both palpebral and bulbar conjunctiva eventually are lost. Some of the surgical techniques discussed below are shown on the CD-ROM accompanying this book.

In some diffuse neoplasms, we combine surgery with irradiation. The perilimbal and corneal tumor is resected so that the cornea and lens can be shielded with a lead contact lens; ionizing radiation is delivered to the remainder of the conjunctival malignancy. Unfortunately, the amount of radiation necessary to sterilize a diffuse tumor usually results in a dry, painful eye that eventually needs anterior exenteration.

In diffuse acquired melanosis with focal areas of malignant degeneration, the melanoma is resected with frozen section control and adjunctive double

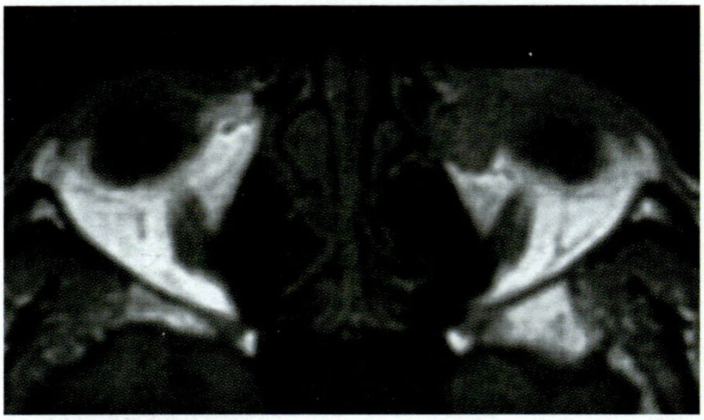

Figure 4–57. A T_1-weighted MRI image showing orbital invasion 2 years after resection, with clear margins, of the lesion shown in Figure 4-56. This was demonstrated to be a melanoma recurrence on fine-needle aspiration biopsy and was locally resected with good margins.

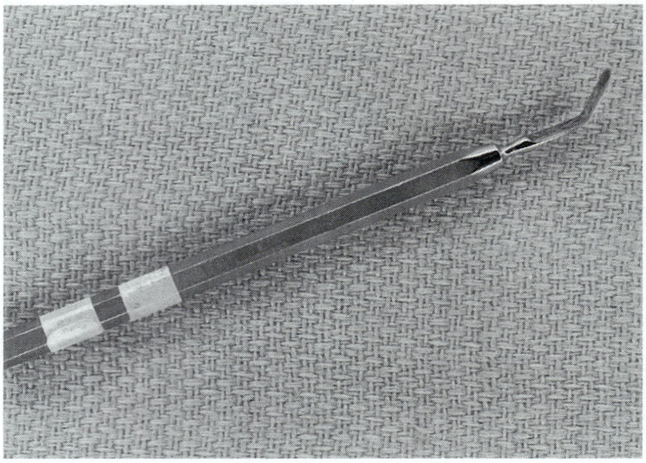

Figure 4–58. Took knife for lamellar disection.

freeze-thaw cryotherapy. In the operating room, we use either liquid nitrogen spray, or a hammerhead probe (Figure 4–59) without a thermocouple. The temperature on the control console is brought to –40° C, the tissue is allowed to thaw, then it is frozen to –40° C again. For larger areas, we use a liquid nitrogen spray. As mentioned previously, these areas of malignant transformation can usually be identified by their increased thickness, vascularity, inflammation, or new spread of pigment. If there is malignant melanoma in association with diffuse acquired melanosis after the malignancy is excised, flat areas of pigmentation are treated with double freeze-thaw cryotherapy after the epithelium is elevated from underlying tissue using a 30-gauge needle and local anesthesia.

Five methods can be used to restore ocular integrity after tumor removal. These are primary closure, bare sclera, advancement conjunctival flaps, free autologous conjunctival grafts, and free buccal mucosa grafts. As previously discussed, when over 40 percent of the cornea is involved, we use a free limbal graft from the opposite eye.

In diffuse perilimbal tumors, if the defect cannot be closed primarily, a bare sclera approach is adequate. It is less satisfactory to leave the bare sclera if tumor resection extends < 5 mm from the limbus. While strabismologists routinely have left even larger areas of extraocular muscles denuded of conjunctival epithelium, it has been our experience that if adjunctive cryotherapy has been used (with its associated inflammation), significant complications occur. In small defects, the conjunctiva can be undermined, mobilized, and closed primarily. In larger defects, we obtain a free conjunctival graft, either from the superior nasal quadrant of that eye (if that area is uninvolved) or from the contralateral superior nasal quadrant. If the conjunctiva is harvested correctly, there should be neither postoperative discomfort nor scarring.

Topical anesthesia is applied to the donor area of the conjunctiva, and a 30-gauge needle is placed directly under the conjunctival epithelium. A conjunctival intraepithelial bleb is created with either balanced salt solution (if the patient is under general anesthesia) or 2 percent lidocaine with 1:100,000 epinephrine. The objective is to obtain only epithelium, without disturbing the underlying Tenon's capsule. The conjunctival graft should be approximately 25 percent larger than is needed to fill the defect. The donor area of the graft is removed with Steven's scissors and forceps. It is often difficult to differentiate the epithelial surface from the subepithelial surface, and care is taken to orient the conjunctival epithelium on a wet tongue depressor with the superficial surface away from the board.

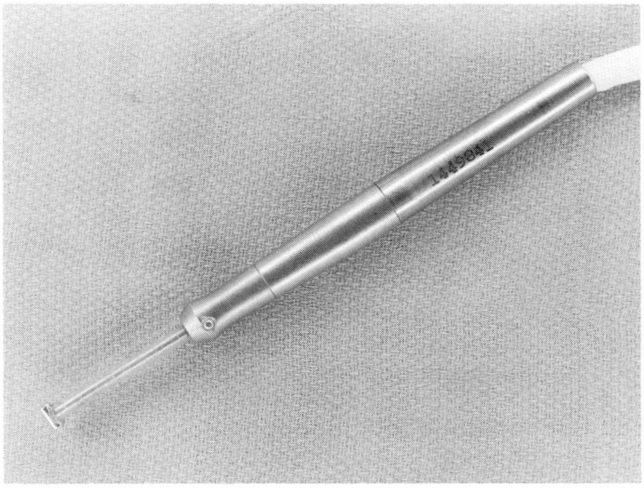

Figure 4–59. Hammerhead cryotherapy probe. Alternatively, a liquid nitrogen applicator or spray can be used.

The conjunctival graft is sutured into the area of tumor resection, using 8-0 vicryl cardinal sutures and running 10-0 nylon suture. Figure 4–60A and B demonstrates a conjunctival melanoma before and after resection with a free autologous conjunctival graft.

If a defect > 15 mm is present, buccal mucosa is obtained from the inner surface of the lip. If an extensive conjunctival resection with buccal mucosal graft is anticipated, the operation is usually performed under general anesthesia. Two towel clips are placed just below the vermilion border at the nasal and lateral aspects of the lower lip (Figure 4–61). The lip is everted over a rolled sponge. Two percent lidocaine with 1:100,000 epinephrine is used to infiltrate just under the epithelial surface of the buccal mucosa (Figure 4–62). Either a Davol dermatome (Figure 4–63) or a free buccal mucosal graft is obtained. The author prefers this method, since harvesting a graft with scissors and forceps is slower and the tissue is both thicker and uneven. The

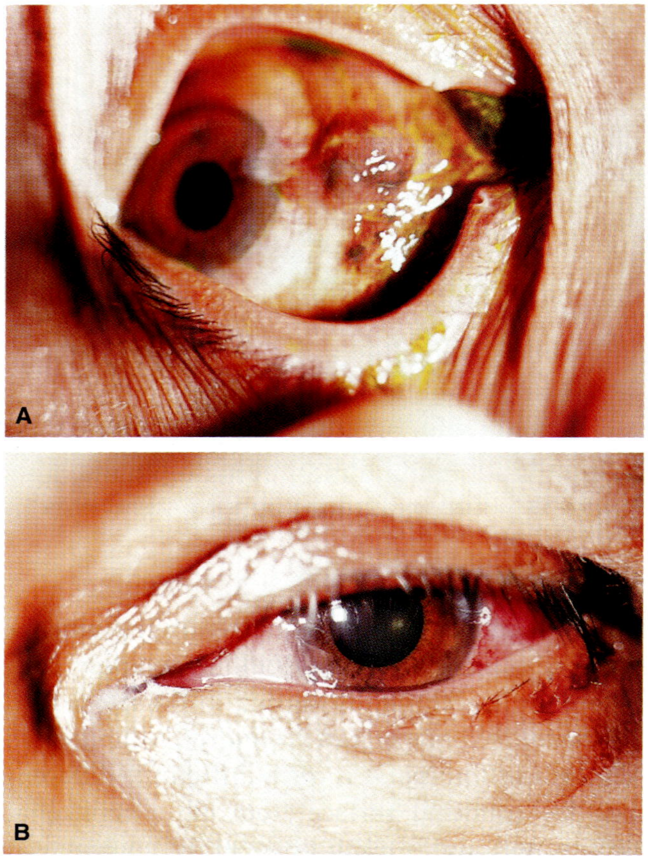

Figure 4–60. *A,* Conjunctival melanoma treated with resection under frozen section control, double freeze-thaw cryotherapy and a free, conjunctival graft. *B,* One week postoperative appearance.

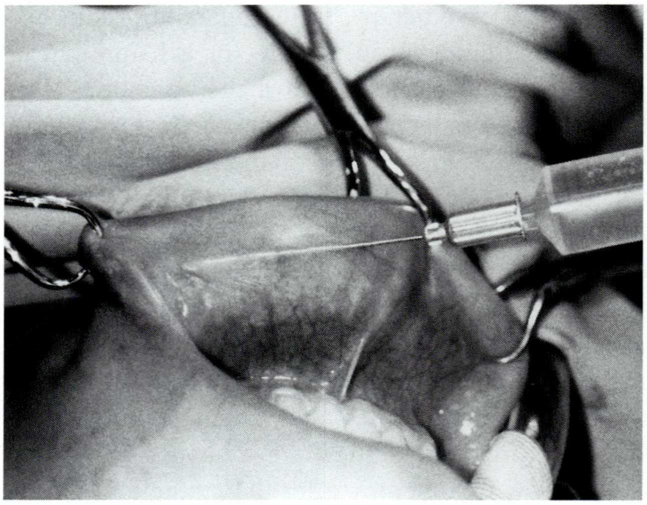

Figure 4–62. Subepithelial infiltration prior to obtaining graft.

towel clips are removed, and a thrombin-soaked sponge is placed between the front surface of the lower teeth and the posterior aspect of the lip. The buccal defect is not closed and results in surprisingly little postoperative discomfort or complications.[278] If the conjunctival defect extends into the fornix, deep mattress 5-0 chromic gut sutures are used to construct the fornix; at the end of the procedure, a vault conformer (also known as a symblepharon

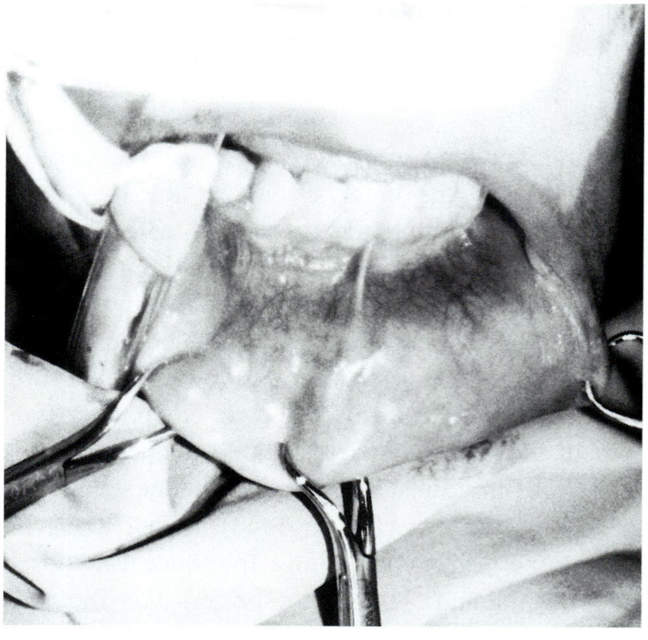

Figure 4–61. Placement of towel clips to evert lower lip in preparation for obtaining buccal mucous membrane graft.

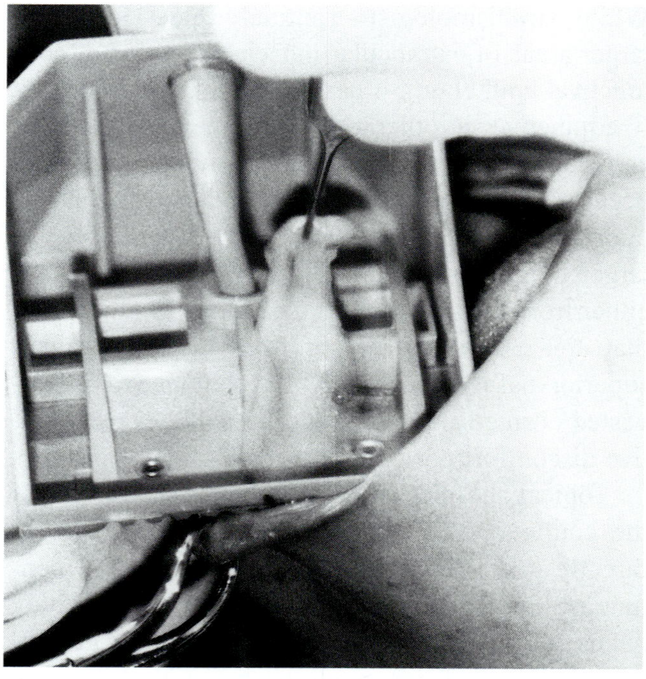

Figure 4–63. The use of Davol dermatome to obtain a buccal mucous membrane graft.

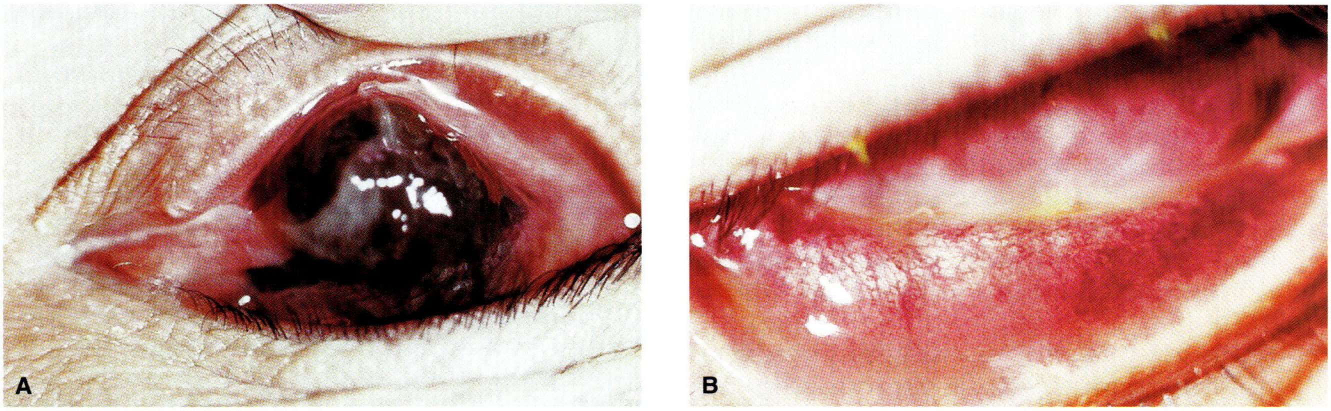

Figure 4–64. *A,* Large fornix-palpebral conjunctival melanoma. *B,* Five years after frozen section-controlled resection, cryotherapy and placement of a large, autologous mucous membrane graft.

conformer) is placed in the space, and a Frost or reverse Frost suture of 4-0 silk is placed in the lid to tightly close the eye for 48 hours. We have found that if this is not done when the fornix is reconstructed, symblepharon is almost inevitable.

In Figures 4–64 A and B, a case of a large fornix palpebral conjunctival melanoma in a patient who refused exenteration is shown prior to surgery and 5 years after resection, cryotherapy, and placement of a large mucous membrane graft.

REFERENCES

1. Ash JE. Epibulbar tumors. Am J Ophthalmol 1950;33:1203–19.
2. Reese AB. Tumors of the eye, 3rd ed. Hagerstown, MD: Harper and Row; 1976. p. 257.
3. Quillen DA, Goldberg SH, Rosenwasser GO, Sassani JW. Basal cell carcinoma of the conjunctiva. Am J Ophthalmol 1993;116:244–5.
4. Grosssniklaus HE, Green WR, Luckenbach M, Chan CC. Conjunctival lesions in adults. A clinical and histopathologic review. Cornea 1987;6:78–116.
5. Newton R. A review of the etiology of squamous cell carcinoma of the conjunctiva. Br J Cancer 1996;74:1511–3.
6. Sun EC, Fears TR, Goedert JJ. Epidemiology of squamous cell conjunctival cancer. Cancer Epidemiol Biomarkers Prev 1997;6:73–7.
7. McCarthy JN, Rootman J, Horseman D, White BA. Conjunctival and uveal melanoma in dysplastic nevus syndrome. Surv Ophthalmol 1993;37:377–86.
8. Dahlenfors R, Tornquist GU, Wettrell K, Mark J. Cytogenetic observations in nine ophthalmic malignant melanomas. Anticancer Res 1993;13:415–20.
9. Aubert C, Rouge F, Reilaudou M, Metge P. Establishment and characterization of human ocular melanoma cell lines. Int J Cancer 1993;54:784–92.
10. Ash JE, Wilder HC. Epithelial tumors of the limbus. Am J Ophthalmol 1942;25:926–32.
11. Noojin RO. Multiple ophthalmic verrucae. Arch Dermatol 1968;97:176–7.
12. Petrelli R, Cotlier E, Robins S, Stoessel K. Dinitrochlorobenzene immunotherapy of recurrent squamous papilloma of the conjunctiva. Ophthalmology 1981;88:1221–5.
13. Harkey ME, Metz HS. Cryotherapy of conjunctival papillomata. Am J Ophthalmol 1968;66:872–4.
14. Burns RP, Wankum G, Giangiacoma J, Anderson PC. Dinitrochlorobenzene and debulking therapy of conjunctival papilloma. J Pediatr Ophthalmol Strabismus 1983;20:221–6.
15. Shields CL, Lally MR, Singh AD, et al. Oral cimetidine (Tagamet) for recalcitrant, diffuse conjunctival papillomatosis. Am J Ophthalmol 1999;128:362–4.
16. Lass JH, Grove AS, Papale JJ, et al. Detection of human papillomavirus DNA sequences in conjunctival papilloma. Am J Ophthalmol 1983;96:670–4.
17. McDonnell JM, McDonnell PJ, Mounts P, et al. Demonstration of papillomavirus capsid antigen in human conjunctival neoplasia. Arch Ophthalmol 1986;104:1801–5.
18. Odrich MG, Jakobiec FA, Lancaster WD, et al. A spectrum of bilateral squamous conjunctival tumors associated with human papillomavirus type 16. Ophthalmology 1991;98:628–35.
19. McDonnell JM, McDonnell PJ, Sun YY. Human papillomavirus DNA in tissues and ocular surface swabs of patients with conjunctival epithelial neoplasia. Invest Ophthalmol Vis Sci 1992;33:184–9.
20. Uy HS, Pineda R, Shore JW, et al. Hypertropic discoid lupus erythematosis of the conjunctiva. Am J Ophthalmol 1999;127:604–5.

21. Kessing SV. Ectopic lacrimal gland tissue at the corneal limbus (glands of Manz?). Acta Ophthalmol 1966; 46:398–403.
22. Young TL, Buchi ER, Kaufman LM, et al. Respiratory epithelium in a cystic choristoma of the limbus. Arch Ophthalmol 1990;108:1736–9.
23. Blodi FC, Apple DJ. Localized conjunctival amyloidosis. Am J Ophthalmol 1979;88:346–50.
24. Boockvar W, Wessely Z, Ballen P. Recurrent granuloma pyogenicum of limbus. Arch Ophthalmol 1974;91: 42–4.
25. Minckler D. Pyogenic granuloma of the cornea simulating squamous cell carcinoma. Arch Ophthalmol 1979;97:516–7.
26. Ortiz JM, Yanoff M. Epipalpebral conjunctival osseous choristoma. Br J Ophthalmol 1979;63:173–6.
27. Martinez LM, Cohen KL. Conjunctival dermoid cyst seen on examination as a chronically red eye. Arch Ophthalmol 1998;116:1109–11.
28. Mansour AM, Barber JC, Reinecke RD, Wang FM. Ocular choristomas. Surv Ophthalmol 1989;33:339–58.
29. Jakobiec FA, Bonanno P, Sigelman J. Conjunctival adnexal cysts and dermoids. Arch Ophthalmol 1978; 96:1404–9.
30. Emamy H, Ahmadian H. Limbal dermoid with ectopic brain tissue. Report of a case and review of the literature. Arch Ophthalmol 1977;95:2201–2.
31. Crawford JS. Benign tumors of the eyelid and adjacent structures: should they be removed? J Pediatr Ophthalmol Strabismus 1979;16:246–50.
32. Frucht-Pery J, Sugar J, Baum J, et al. Mitomycin C treatment for conjunctival-cornea intraepithelial neoplasia. Ophthalmology 1997;104:2085–93.
33. Elsas FJ, Green WR. Epibulbar tumors in childhood. Am J Ophthalmol 1975;79:1001–7.
34. Ferry AP. Synthetic fiber granuloma. 'Teddy Bear' granuloma of the conjunctiva. Arch Ophthalmol 1994;112:1339–41.
35. Terry A, Patrinely JR, Anderson RL, Smithwick W IV. Orbital meningioencephalocele manifesting as a conjunctival mass. Am J Ophthalmol 1993;115:46–9.
36. Iwamoto T, Jakobiec FA, Darrell RW. Fibrous histiocytoma of the corneoscleral limbus: the ultrastructure of a distinctive inclusion. Ophthalmology 1981;88: 1260–8.
37. Jakobiec FA. Fibrous histiocytoma of the corneoscleral limbus. Am J Ophthalmol 1974;78:700–6.
38. Faludi JE, Kenyon K, Green WR. Fibrous histiocytoma of the corneoscleral limbus. Am J Ophthalmol 1975; 80:619–24.
39. Litricin O. Fibrous histiocytoma of the corneosclera. Arch Ophthalmol 1983;101:426–8.
40. Perry HD. Isolated episcleral neurofibroma. Ophthalmology 1982;89:1095–8.
41. Dabezies OH Jr, Penner R. Neurofibroma or neurilemmoma of the bulbar conjunctiva. Arch Ophthalmol 1961;66:73–5.
42. Kalina PH, Bartley GB, Campbell RJ, Buettner H. Isolated neurofibromas of the conjunctiva. Am J Ophthalmol 1991;111:694–8.
43. Pe'er J, Ilsar M, Hidayat A. Conjunctival myxoma: a case report. Br J Ophthalmol 1984;68:618–22.
44. Patrinely JR, Green WR. Conjunctival myxoma. Arch Ophthalmol 1983;101:1416–20.
45. Ferry AP, Sherman FE. Nodular fasciitis of the conjunctiva apparently originating in the fascia bulbi (Tenon's capsule). Am J Ophthalmol 1974;78: 514–7.
46. Rohrbach JM, Wohlrab TM, Kuper K. Lymphangioma of the conjunctiva. Klin Monatsbl Augenheilkd 1997;311:211–2.
47. Graham CM, McCartney ACE, Buckley RJ. Intrascleral neurilemmoma. Br J Ophthalmol 1989;73:378–81.
48. Shields CL, Shields JA, Varenhorst P. Transscleral leiomyoma. Ophthalmology 1991;98:84–7.
49. Charles NC, Fox DM, Avendano JA, et al. Conjunctival neurilemmoma. Arch Ophthalmol 1997;115:547–9.
50. Charles NC, Fox DM, Glasberg SS, Swicki J. Epibulbar granular cell tumor. Ophthalmology 1997;104: 1444–56.
51. McLeod SD, Edward DP. Benign lymphoid hyperplasia of the conjunctiva in children. Arch Ophthalmol 1999;117:832–5.
52. Cook BE Fr, Bartley GB. Acute lymphoblastic leukemia manifesting in an adult as a conjunctival mass. Am J Ophthalmol 1997;124:104–5.
53. Jakobiec FA, Perry HD, Harrison W, Krebs W. Dacryoadenoma. A unique tumor of the conjunctiva epithelium. Ophthalmology 1989;96:1014–20.
54. Allaire GS, Hidayat AA, Zimmerman LE, Minardi L. Reticulohistiocytoma of limbus and cornea. A clinicopathologic study of two cases. Ophthalmology 1990;97:1018–22.
55. Urbak SF. Infectious mononucleosis presenting as a unilateral conjunctival tumour. Acta Ophthalmologica 1993;71:133–5.
56. Stopak SS, Dreizen NG, Zimmerman LE, O'Neill JF. Sinus histiocytosis presenting as an epibulbar mass. A clinicopathologic case report. Arch Ophthalmol 1988;106:1426–8.
57. Migliori ME, Putterman AM. Recurrent conjunctival papilloma causing nasolacrimal duct obstruction. Am J Ophthalmol 1990;110:17–22.
58. Streeten BW, Carrillo R, Jamison R, et al. Inverted papilloma of the conjunctiva. Am J Ophthalmol 1979;88:1062–6.
59. Grossniklaus HE, Martin DF, Solomon AR. Invasive conjunctival tumor with keratoacanthoma features. Am J Ophthalmol 1990;109:736–8.
60. Munro S, Brownstein S, Liddy B. Conjunctival keratoacanthoma. Am J Ophthalmol 1993;116:654–5.

61. McGavic JS. Intraepithelial epithelioma of the cornea and conjunctiva (Bowen's disease). Am J Ophthalmol 1942;25:167–76.
62. Arbesman H, Ransohoff DF. Is Bowen's disease a predictor for the development of internal malignancy? A methodological critique of the literature. JAMA 1987;257:516–8.
63. Sun EC, Fears TR, Goedert JJ. Epidemiology of squamous cell conjunctival cancer. Cancer Epidemiol Biomarkers Prev 1997;6:73–7.
64. Pizzarello LD, Jakobiec FA. Bowen's disease of the conjunctiva: a misnomer. In: Jakobiec FA, editor. Ocular and adnexal tumors. Birmingham, AL: Aesculapius; 1978. p. 553–71.
65. Erie JC, Campbell RJ, Liesegang TJ. Conjunctival and corneal intraepithelial and invasive neoplasia. Ophthalmology 1986;93;176–83.
66. Waring GO III, Roth AM, Ekins MB. Clinical and pathologic description of 17 cases of corneal intraepithelial neoplasia. Am J Ophthalmol 1984;97:547–59.
67. Zimmerman LE. Squamous cell carcinoma and related lesions of the bulbar conjunctiva. In: Boniuk M, editor. Ocular and adnexal tumors, St Louis, MO: CV Mosby Co; 1964. p 49–74.
68. Char DH. The management of lid and conjunctival malignancies. Surv Ophthalmol 1980;24:679–89.
69. Boone CW, Kelloff GJ, Steele VE. Natural history of intraepithelial neoplasia in humans with implications for cancer chemoprevention strategy. Cancer Res 1992;52:1651–9.
70. Lee GA, Hirst LW. Incidence of ocular surface epithelial dysplasia in metropolitan Brisbane. Arch Ophthalmol 1992;110:525–7.
71. Newton R, Ferlay J, Reeves G, et al. Effects of ambient solar ultraviolet radiation on incidence of squamous-cell carcinoma of the eye. Lancet 1996;347:1450–1.
72. Newton R. A review of the etiology of squamous cell carcinoma of the conjunctiva. Br J Cancer 1996;74: 1511–3.
73. Marc'hadour FL, Romanet JP, Fdilia A, et al. Schwannoma of the bulbar conjunctiva. Arch Ophthalmol 1996;114:1258–60.
74. Macarez R, Bossis S, Robinet A, et al. Conjunctival epithelial neoplasias in organ transplant patients receiving cyclosporine therapy. Cornea 1999;18: 495–7.
75. Li G, Ho VC, Berean K, Tron VA. Ultraviolet radiation induction of squamous cell carcinomas in p53 transgenic mice. Cancer Res 1995;55:2070–4.
76. Jha PK, Beral V, Hack S, et al. Antibodies to human papillomavirus and to other genital infectious agents and invasive cervical cancer risk. Lancet 1993;341: 1116–8.
77. Liang J, Mei Q, Da-Zhi C, et al. Indole-3-carbinol prevents cervical cancer in human papilloma virus type 16 (HPV16) transgenic mice. Cancer Res 1999;59: 3991–7.
78. Sauter ER, Nesbit M, Litwin S, et al. Antisense cyclin D1 induces apoptosis and tumor shrinkage in human squamous carcinomas. Cancer Res 1999;59: 4876–81.
79. Tabandeh H, Gopal S, Teimory M, et al. Conjunctival involvement in malignancy-associated acanthosis nigricans. Eye 1993;7:648–51.
80. Tan DTH, Lim ASM, Goh H-S, Smith DR. Abnormal expression of the p53 tumor suppressor gene in the conjunctiva of patients with pterygium. Am J Ophthalmol 1997;123:404–5.
81. Clear AS, Chirambo MC, Hutt MS. Solar keratosis, pterygium, and squamous cell carcinoma of the conjunctiva in Malawi. Br J Ophthalmol 1979;63:102–9.
82. Alani RM, Munger K. Human papillomaviruses and associated malignancies. J Clin Oncol 1998;330–7.
83. Koss LG. Human papillomavirus—passenger, driver, or both? Hum Pathol 1998;29;309–10.
84. Karcioglu ZA, Issa TM. Human papilloma virus in neoplastic and non-neoplastic conditions of the external eye. Br J Ophthalmol 1997;81:595–8.
85. Iliff WJ, Marback R, Green WR. Invasive squamous cell carcinoma of the conjunctiva. Arch Ophthalmol 1975;93:119–22.
86. Jauregui HO, Klintworth GK. Pigmented squamous cell carcinoma of cornea and conjunctiva: a light microscopic, histochemical, and ultrastructural study. Cancer 1976;38:778–88.
87. Verderber L, Wesley RE, Glick AD. Malignant peripheral nerve sheath tumor presenting at the limbal conjunctiva. Orbit 1995;14:81–6.
88. Cameron JA, Hidayat AA. Squamous cell carcinoma of the cornea. Am J Ophthalmol 1991;111:571–4.
89. Steinhorst U, von Domarus D. Carcinoma in situ of the cornea. Ophthalmologica 1990;200:107–10.
90. Daxecker F, Philipp W, Mikuz G. Corneal carcinoma. Ophthalmologica 1989;198:163–5.
91. Spinak M, Friedman AH. Squamous cell carcinoma of the conjunctiva. Value of exfoliative cytology and diagnosis. Surv Ophthalmol 1977;21:351–5.
92. Tsubota K, Kajiwara K, Ugajin S, Hasegawa T. Conjunctival brush cytology. Acta Cytologica 1990; 34:233–5.
93. Nadjari B, Kersten A, Ross B, et al. Cytologic and DNA cytometric diagnosis and therapy monitoring of squamous cell carcinoma in situ and malignant melanoma of the cornea and conjunctiva. Anal Quant Cytol Histol 21:387-96, 1999.
94. Wilson FM II. Rose bengal staining of epibulbar squamous neoplasms. Ophthalmic Surg 1976;7:21–3.
95. Morsman CD. Spontaneous regression of a conjunctival intraepithelial neoplastic tumor. Arch Ophthalmol 1989;107:1490–1.

96. Irvine AR Jr. Dyskeratotic epibulbar tumors. Trans Am Ophthalmol Soc 1963;61:243–73.
97. Carroll JM, Kuwabara T. A classification of limbal epitheliomas. Arch Ophthalmol 1965;73:545–51.
98. Seitz B, Fischar M, Holbach LM, Naumann GOH. Differential diagnosis and progress of 122 excised epibulbar epithelial neoplasias. Klin Monatsvl Augenheilkd 1995;207:239–46.
99. Tabin G, Lewvin S, Snibson G, et al. Late recurrences and the necessity for long-term follow-up in corneal and conjunctival intraepithelial neoplasia. Ophthalmology 1997;104:485–92.
100. Spraul CW, Lang GK. Oncocytoma of the conjunctiva. Klin Monatsbl Augenheildkd 1996;209:176–7.
101. Sanders N, Bedotto C. Recurrent carcinoma in situ of the conjunctiva and cornea (Bowen's disease). Am J Ophthalmol 1972;74:688–93.
102. Stokes JJ. Intraocular extension of epibulbar squamous cell carcinoma of limbus. Tr Acad Ophthalmol 1955;59:143–6.
103. Nicholson DH, Herschler J. Intraocular extension of squamous cell carcinoma of the conjunctiva. Arch Ophthalmol 1977;95:843–6.
104. Li WW, Pettit TH, Zakka KA. Intraocular invasion by papillary squamous cell carcinoma of the conjunctiva. Am J Ophthalmol 1980;90:697–701.
105. Wexler SA, Wallow IH. Squamous cell carcinoma of the conjunctiva presenting with intraocular extension. Arch Ophthalmol 1985;103:1175–7.
106. Blodi FC. Squamous cell carcinoma of the conjunctiva. Doc Ophthalmol 1973;34:93–108.
107. Shields JA, Shields CL, Gunduz K, Eagle RC. Intraocular invasion of conjunctival squamous cell carcinoma in five patients. Ophthal Plast Reconstr Surg 1999;15:153–60.
108. Lindenmuth KA, Sugar A, Kincaid MC, et al. Invasive squamous cell carcinoma of the conjunctiva presenting as necrotizing scleral perforation and uveal prolapse. Surv Ophthalmol 1998;33:50–4.
109. Char DH, Crawford JB, Howes EL Jr, Weinstein AJ. Resection of intraocular squamous cell carcinoma. Br J Ophthalmol 1992;76:123–5.
110. Brownstein S. Mucoepidermoid carcinoma of the conjunctiva with intraocular invasion. Ophthalmology 1981;88:1226–30.
111. Cohen BH, Green WR, Iliff NT, et al. Spindle cell carcinoma of the conjunctiva. Arch Ophthalmol 1980;98:1809–13.
112. Seregard S, Kock E. Squamous spindle cell carcinoma of the conjunctiva. Fatal outcome of a pterygium-like lesion. Acta Ophthalmol Scand 1995;73:464–6.
113. Fraunfelder FT, Wingfield D. Management of intraepithelial conjunctival tumors and squamous cell carcinomas. Am J Ophthalmol 1983;95:359–63.
114. Dutton JJ, Anderson RL, Tse DT. Combined surgery and cryotherapy for scleral invasion of epithelial malignancies. Ophthalmic Surg 1984;15:289–94.
115. Divine RD, Anderson RL. Nitrous oxide cryotherapy for intraepithelial epithelioma of the conjunctiva. Arch Ophthalmol 1983;101:782–6.
116. Peksayar G, Soyturk MK, Demiryont M. Long-term results of cryotherapy on malignant epithelial tumors of the conjunctiva. Am J Ophthalmol 1989; 107:337–40.
117. Fraunfelder FT, Wingfield D. Therapy of intraepithelial epitheliomas and squamous cell carcinoma of the limbus. Trans Am Ophthalmol Soc 1980;78: 290–300.
118. Kenyon KR, Wagoner MD, Hettinger ME. Conjunctival autograft transplantation for advanced and recurrent pterygium. Ophthalmology 1985;92:1461–70.
119. Turgeon PW, Nauheim RC, Roat MI, et al. Indications for keratoepithelioplasty. Arch Ophthalmol 1990; 108:233–6.
120. Copeland RA Jr, Char DH. Limbal autograft reconstruction after conjunctival squamous cell carcinoma. Am J Ophthalmol 1990;110:412–5.
121. Tseng SC, Prabhasawat P, Lee SH. Amniotic membrane transplantation for conjunctival surface reconstruction. Am J Ophthalmol 1997;124:765–74.
122. Maloney RK, Thompson V, Ghiselli G, et al. A prospective multicenter trial of excimer laser phototherapeutic keratectomy for corneal visual loss. Am J Ophthalmol 1996;122:149–60.
123. Buus DR, Tse DT, Folberg R. Microscopically controlled excision of conjunctival squamous cell carcinoma. Am J Ophthalmol 1994;117:97–102.
124. Lommatzsch P. Beta-ray treatment of malignant epithelial tumors of the conjunctiva. Am J Ophthalmol 1976;81:198–206.
125. Cerezo L, Otero J, Aragon G, et al. Conjunctival intraepithelial and invasive squamous cell carcinomas treated with strontium-90. Radiother Oncol 1990;17:191–7.
126. Behrendt S, Bernsmeier H, Randzio G. Fractionated beta-irradiation of a conjunctival lymphangioma. Ophthalmologica 1991;203:161–3.
127. Jones DB, Wilhelmus KR, Font RL. Beta radiation of recurrent corneal intraepithelial neoplasia. Trans Am Ophthal Soc 1991;89:285–91.
128. Zehetmayer M, Menapace R, Kulnig W. Combined local excision and brachytherapy with ruthenium-106 in the treatment of epibulbar malignancies. Ophthalmologica 1993;207:133–9.
129. Ullman S, Augsburger JJ, Brady LW. Fractionated epibulbar I-125 plaque radiotherapy for recurrent mucoepidermoid carcinoma of the bulbar conjunctiva. Am J Ophthalmol 1995;119:102–3.
130. Kearsley JH, Fitchew RS, Taylor RG. Adjunctive radiotherapy with strontium-90 in the treatment of con-

junctival squamous cell carcinoma. Int J Radiat Oncol Biol Phys 1988;14:435–43.
131. Moriarty AP, Crawford GJ, McAllister IL, Constable IJ. Severe cornealscleral infection: a complication of beta irradiation scleral necrosis following pterygium excision. Arch Ophthalmol 1993;111:947–51.
132. Green MO, Brannen AL. Hyperbaric oxygen therapy for beta- irradiation-induced scleral necrosis. Ophthalmology 1995;102:1038–41.
133. Maskin SL. Regression of limbal epithelial dysplasia with topical interferon. Arch Ophthalmol 1994;112: 1145–6.
134. Dausch D, Landesz M, Schroder E. Phototherapeutic keratectomy in recurrent corneal intraepithelial dysplasia. Arch Ophthalmol 1994;112:22–3.
135. Frucht-Pery J, Rozenman Y. Mitomycin C therapy for corneal intraepithelial neoplasia. Am J Ophthalmol 1994;117:164–8.
136. Rubinfeld RS, Pfister RR, Stein RM, et al. Serious complications of topical mitomycin-C after pterygium surgery. Ophthalmology 1992;99:1647–54.
137. Midena E, Boccato P, Degli Angeli DC. Conjunctival squamous cell carcinoma treated with topical 5-fluorouracil. Arch Ophthalmol 1997;115:1600–1.
138. Frucht-Perry J, Assil K, Ziegler E, et al. Fibrin-enmeshed tobramycin liposomes: single application topical therapy of Pseudomonas keratitis. Cornea 1992;11:393–7.
139. Wilson MW, Hungerford JL, George SM, Madraperla SA. Topical mitomycin C for the treatment of conjunctival and corneal epithelial dysplasia and neoplasia. Am J Ophthalmol 1997;124:303–11.
140. Grossniklaus HE, Aaberg TM. Mitomycin C treatment of conjunctival intra-epithelial neoplasia. Am J Ophthalmol 1997;124:381–3.
141. Heigle TJ, Stulting RD, Palay DA. Treatment of recurrent conjunctival epithelial neoplasia with topical mitomycin C. Am J Ophthalmol 1997;124:397–401.
142. Vann RR, Karp CL. Lesional perilesional entopical interferon alpha-B for conjunctival and corneal neoplasia. Ophthalmology 1999;106:91–7.
143. Wolter JR, Bromley WC. Intraepithelial sebaceous epithelioma of lids, conjunctiva, and cornea treated with minimal orbital exenteration. Ophthal Surg 1991;22:341–4.
144. Johnson TE, Tabbara KF, Weatherhead RG, et al. Secondary squamous cell carcinoma of the orbit. Arch Ophthalmol 1997;115:75–8.
145. Margo CE, Groden LR. Intraepithelial neoplasia of the conjunctiva with mucoepidermoid differentiation. Am J Ophthalmol 1989;108:600–1.
146. Carrau RL, Stillman E, Canaan RE. Mucoepidermoid carcinoma of the conjunctiva. Ophthal Plast Reconst Surg 1994;10:163–8
147. Huntington AC, Langloss JM, Hidayat AA. Spindle cell carcinoma of the conjunctiva. An immunohistochemical and ultrastructural study of six cases. Ophthalmology 1990;97:711–7.
148. Campanella PC, Goldberg SH, Erlichman K, Abendroth C. Squamous cell tumors and ocular prostheses. Ophthalmol Plast Reconstr Surg 1998;14:45–9.
149. Keller AZ. Histology, survivorship and related factors in the epidemiology of eye cancers. Am J Epidemiol 1973;97:386–93.
150. Scotto J, Fraumeni JF Jr, Lee JA. Melanomas of the eye and other noncutaneous sites: epidemiologic aspects. J Natl Cancer Inst 1976;56:489–91.
151. Seregard S, Kock E. Conjunctival malignant melanoma in Sweden 1969–1991. Acta Ophthalmol 1992;70: 289–96.
152. Chang AE, Karnell LH, Menck HR. The national cancer data base report on cutaneous and noncutaneous melanoma: a summary of 84,836 cases from the past decade. Cancer 1998;83:1664–78.
153. Verhoeff FH, Loring RG. A case of primary epibulbar sarcoma with secondary growths in limbus and sclera, and invasion of the choroid, ciliary body, and iris. Arch Ophthalmol 1903;32:97–102.
154. Stefani FH. A prognostic index for patients for malignant melanoma of the conjunctiva. Graefe's Arch Clin Exp Ophthalmol 1986;224:580–2.
155. Jay B. A follow-up study of limbal melanomata. Proc R Soc Med 1964;57:497–500.
156. Reese AB. Precancerous and cancerous melanosis of conjunctiva. Am J Ophthalmol 1955;39:96–100.
157. Silvers DN, Jakobiec FA, Freeman TR, et al. Melanoma of the conjunctiva: a clinical pathologic study. In: Jakobiec, editor. Ocular and adnexal tumors, Birmingham, AL: Aesculapius; 1978. p. 585–99.
158. Folberg R, McLean IW, Zimmerman LE. Malignant melanoma of the conjunctiva. Hum Pathol 1985;16: 136–43.
159. Tucker MA, Shields JA, Hartge P, et al. Sunlight exposure as risk factor for intraocular malignant melanoma. N Engl J Med 1985;313:789–92.
160. Swerdlow AJ. Epidemiology of eye cancer in adults in England and Wales, 1962-1977. Am J Epidemiol 1983;118:294–300.
161. Jay V, Ho M, Hunter W, et al. Expression of p53 in conjunctival melanocytic nevi. An immunohistochemical study. Arch Pathol Lab Med 1996;120:378–9.
162. Seregard S. Cell growth and p53 expression in primary acquired melanosis and conjunctival melanoma. J Clin Pathol 1996;49:338–42.
163. McDonnell JM, Carpenter JD, Jacobs P, et al. Conjunctival melanocytic lesions in children. Ophthalmology 1989;96:986–93.
164. Margo CE, Roper DL, Hidayat AA. Borderline melanocytic tumor of the conjunctiva: diagnostic and theraputic considerations. J Pediatr Ophthalmol Strabismus 1991;28:268–70.

165. Strempel I, Kroll P. Conjunctival malignant melanoma in children. Ophthalmology 1999;213:129–32.
166. Hitzer S, Bialasiewica AA, Richard G. Immunohistochemical markers for cytoplasmic antigens in acquired melanosis, malignant melanomas, and nevi of the conjunctiva. Klin Monatsbl Augenheilkd 1998;213:230–7.
167. Soong HK, McKeeney MJ, Wolter JR. Adrenochrome staining of senile plaque resembling malignant melanoma. Am J Ophthalmol 1986;101:380.
168. Bartley GB, Buller CR, Campbell RJ, Bullock JD. Pigmented episcleral mass from argyrosis following strabismus surgery. Arch Ophthalmol 1991;109:775–6.
169. Kennedy RH, Flanagan JC, Eagle RC Jr, Carney JA. The Carney complex with ocular signs suggestive of cardiac myxoma. Am J Ophthalmol 1991;111:699–702.
170. Crawford JB, Howes EL Jr, Char DH. Combined nevi of the conjunctiva. Arch Ophthalmol 1999;117: 1121–7.
171. Charles NC, Stenson S, Taterka HB. Epibulbar malignant melanoma in a black patient. Arch Ophthalmol 1979;97:316–8.
172. Welsh NH, Jhavery Y. Malignant melanoma of the cornea in an African patient. Am J Ophthalmol 1971;72:796–800.
173. Reese AB. Precancerous and cancerous melanosis. Am J Ophthalmol 1966;61:1272–7.
174. Gloor P, Alexandrakis G. Characteristics of primary choroidal melanosis. Invest Ophthalmol Basic Sci 1995;36:721–9.
175. Jay B. Naevi in melanomata of the conjunctiva. Br J Ophthalmol 1965;49:169–204.
176. Jakobiec FA. Conjunctival melanoma. Arch Ophthalmol 1980;98:1378–84.
177. Hofbauer GF, Schaefer C, Noppen C, et al. MAGE-3 immunoreactivity in formalin-fixed, paraffin-embedded primary and metastatic melanoma: frequency and distribution. Am J Pathol 1997;151: 1549–53.
178. Grossniklaus HE, Margo CE, Solomon AR. Indeterminate melanocytic proliferations of the conjunctiva. Arch Ophthalmol 1999;117:1131–6.
179. Folberg R, Jakobiec FA, Bernardino VB, Iwamoto T. Benign conjunctival melanocytic lesions. Clinicopathologic features. Ophthalmology 1989;96:436–61.
180. Kantelip B, Boccard R, Nores JM, Bacin F. A case of conjunctival spitz nevus: review of literature and comparison with cutaneous locations. Ann Ophthalmol 1989;21:176–9.
181. Weiss JS, Perusse P, Reale F. Tear cytology in conjunctival melanoma. Am J Ophthalmol 1991;111:648–49.
182. Glasgow BJ, McCall LC, Foos RY. HMB-45 antibody reactivity in pigmented lesions of the conjunctiva. Am J Ophthalmol 1990;109:696–700.
183. McDonnell JM, Sun YY, Wagner D. HMB-45 immunohistochemical staining of conjunctival melanocytic lesions. Ophthalmology 1991;98:453–8.
184. Zimmerman FA. Criteria for management of melanosis. Arch Ophthalmol 1966;76:307–8.
185. Jakobiec FA, Folberg R, Iwamoto T. Clinicopathologic characteristics of premalignant and malignant melanocytic lesions of the conjunctiva. Ophthalmology 1989;96:147–66.
186. Jay V, Font RL. Conjunctival amelanotic malignant melanoma rising in the primary melanosis sine pigmento. Ophthalmol 1998;105:91–4.
187. Clune JP. Primary malignant melanoma of the cornea. Am J Ophthalmol 1963;55:147–50.
188. Guillen FJ, Albert DM, Mihm MC Jr. Pigmented melanocytic lesions of the conjunctiva — a new approach to their classification. Pathology 1985;17: 275–80.
189. Jeffrey IJ, Lucas DR, McEwan C, Lee WR. Malignant melanoma of the conjunctiva. Histopathology 1986;10:363–78.
190. Crawford JB. Conjunctival melanomas: prognostic factors. A review and an analysis of a series. Trans Am Ophthalmol Soc 1980;78:467–502.
191. Seregard S. Cell proliferation as a prognostic indicator in conjunctival malignant melanoma. Am J Ophthalmol 1993;116:93–7.
192. Lommatzsch PK, Lommatzsch RE, Kirsch I, Fuhrmann P. Therapeutic outcome of patients suffering from malignant melanomas of the conjunctiva. Br J Ophthalmol 1990;74:615–9.
193. Seregard S. Conjunctival melanoma. Surv Ophthalmol 1998;42:321–50.
194. Norregaard JC, Gerner N, Jensen OA, Prause JU. Malignant melanoma of the conjunctiva: Reoccurrence and survival following surgery and radiotherapy in a Danish population. Graefes Arch Clin Exp Ophthalmol 1996;234:569–72.
195. Desjardins L, Poncet P, Levy C, et al. Prognostic factors in malignant melanoma of the conjunctiva. An anatomo-clinical study of 56 patients. J Fr Ophtalmol 1999;22:315–21.
196. Liesegang TJ, Campbell RJ. Mayo Clinic experience with conjunctival melanomas. Arch Ophthalmol 1980;98:1385–9.
197. Lederman M. Radiotherapy of malignant melanomata of the eye. Br J Radiol 1961;34:21–42.
198. Lederman M. Discussion of pigmented tumors of the conjunctiva. In: Boniuk M, editor. Ocular and adnexal tumors. St Louis, MO: CV Mosby; 1964. p. 24–48.
199. Lommatzsch PK. Beta-ray treatment of malignant epibulbar melanoma. Albrecht Von Graefes Arch Klin Exp Ophthalmol 1978;209:111–24.
200. Napel JA. Conjunctival melanoma, a retrospective study. Doc Ophthalmol 1977;42:321–8.

201. Lederman M, Wybar K, Busby E. Malignant epibulbar melanoma: natural history and treatment by radiotherapy. Br J Ophthalmol 1984;68:605–17.
202. Kreusel KM, Wiegel T, Bechrakis NE, et al. Treatment of advanced conjunctival melanoma by external beam irradiation. Front Radiat Ther Oncol 1997; 30:150–3.
203. Zografos L, Uffer S, Bercher L, Gailloud C. Chirurgie, cryocoagulation et radiotherapie combinee pour le traitmement des melanomes de la conjonctive. Klin Monatsbl Augenheilkd 1994;204:385–90.
204. Matthaus W, Lange G, Roitzsch E. Cryotherapy of eyelid and conjunctival tumors. Ophthalmologica 1976;173:53–62.
205. Jakobiec FA, Brownstein S, Wilkinson RD, et al. Combined surgery and cryotherapy for diffuse malignant melanoma of the conjunctiva. Arch Ophthalmol 1980;98:1390–6.
206. Jakobiec FA, Brownstein S, Albert W, et al. The role of cryotherapy in the management of conjunctival melanoma. Ophthalmology 1982;89:502–15.
207. Brownstein S, Jakobiec FA, Wilkinson RD, et al. Cryotherapy for precancerous melanosis (atypical melanocytic hyperplasia) of the conjunctiva. Arch Ophthalmol 1981;99:1224–31.
208. Freedman J, Rohm G. Surgical management and histopathology of invasive tumours of the cornea. Br J Ophthalmol 1979;63:632–5.
209. Engin K, Leeper DB, Tupchong L, Waterman FM. Thermoradiotherapy in the management of superficial malignant tumors. Clin Cancer Res 1995;1:139–45.
210. Akpek EK, Ertoy D, Kalayci D, Hasiripi H. Postoperative topical mitomycin C in conjunctival squamous cell neoplasia. Cornea 1999;18:59–62.
211. Frucht-Pery J, Pe'er J. Use of mitomycin C in the treatment of conjunctival primary acquired melanosis with atypia. Arch Ophthalmol 1996;114:1261–4.
212. Werschnik C, Lommatzsch PK. Mitomycin C in treatment of conjunctival melanoma and primary acquired melanosis. Klin Monatsbl Augenheilkd 1998;212:465–8.
213. Finger PT, Cxechonska G, Liarikos S. Topical mitomycin C chemotherapy for conjunctival melanoma and PAM with atypia. Br J Ophthalmol 1998;82:476–9.
214. Gow JA, Spencer WH. Intraocular extension of an epibulbar malignant melanoma. Arch Ophthalmol 1993;90:57–9.
215. Werschnik C, Lommatzsch PK. Mitomycin C in treatment of conjunctival melanoma and primary acquired melanosis. Klin Monatsbl Augenheilkd 1998;212:465–8.
216. Travis LW, Rice DH, McClatchey KD, Wallace SW. Malignant melanoma of the conjunctiva metastatic to parotid gland. Reports of cases and discussion of surgical management. Laryngoscope 1977;87:2000–7.
217. Robertson DM, Hungerford JL, McCartney A. Pigmentation of the eyelid margin accompanying conjunctival melanoma. Am J Ophthalmol 1989;108:435–9.
218. Jakobiec FR, Buckman G, Zimmerman LE, et al. Metastatic melanoma within and to the conjunctiva. Ophthalmology 1989;96:999–1005.
219. Robertson DM, Hungerford JL, McCartney AL. Malignant melanomas of the conjunctiva, nasal cavity, and paranasal sinuses. Am J Ophthalmol 1989; 108:440–2.
220. Paridaens AD, Minassian DC, McCartney AC, Hungerford JL. Prognostic factors in primary malignant melanoma of the conjunctiva: a clinicopathologic study of 256 cases. Br J Ophthalmol 1994;78:252–9.
221. Birns JW, Jenkins HA. Melanoma of the conjunctiva — a rational approach to management. Head Neck Surg 1979;2:99–106.
222. Fuchs U, Kivela T, Leisto K, Tarkkanen A. Prognosis of conjunctival melanoma in relation to histopathologic features. Br J Cancer 1989;59:261–7.
223. Folberg R, McLean IW, Zimmerman LE. Primary acquired melanosis of the conjunctiva. Hum Pathol 1985;16:129–35.
224. Paridaens AD, Seregard S, Minassian D, et al. AgNOR counts in conjunctival malignant melanoma lack prognostic value. Br J Ophthalmol 1992;76:621–3.
225. Kirkwood JM. Systematic adjuvant treatment of high-risk melanoma: the role of interferon alfa-2b and other immunotherapies. Eur J Cancer 1998;34:S12–7.
226. Holland GN, Pepose JS, Pettit TH, et al. Acquired immune deficiency syndrome. Ocular manifestations. Ophthalmology 1983;90:859–73.
227. Kalinske M, Leone CR Jr. Kaposi's sarcoma involving eyelid and conjunctiva. Ann Ophthalmol 1982;14: 497–9.
228. Lieberman PH, Llovera IN. Kaposi's sarcoma of the bulbar conjunctiva. Arch Ophthalmol 1972;88:44–5.
229. Bedrick JJ, Savino PJ, Schatz NJ. Conjunctival Kaposi's sarcoma in a patient with myasthenia gravis. Arch Ophthalmol 1981;99:1607–9.
230. Chang Y, Cesarman E, Pessin MS, et al. Identification of Herpes virus-like DNA sequences in AIDS-associated Kaposi's sarcoma. Science 1994;266:1865–9.
231. Macher AM, Palestine A, Masur H, et al. Multicentric Kaposi's sarcoma of the conjunctiva in a male homosexual with the acquired immunodeficiency syndrome. Ophthalmology 1983;90:879–84.
232. Weiter JJ, Jakobiec FA, Iwamoto T. The clinical and morphologic characteristics of Kaposi's sarcomas of the conjunctiva. Am J Ophthalmol 1980;89:546–52.
233. Ghabrial R, Quivey JM, Dunn JP Jr, Char DH. Radiation therapy of acquired immunodeficiency syndrome related Kaposi's sarcoma of the eyelids and conjunctiva. Arch Ophthalmol 1992;110:1423–6.
234. Kurumety UR, Lustbader JM. Kaposi's sarcoma of the

bulbar conjunctiva as an initial clinical manifestation of acquired immunodeficiency syndrome. Arch Ophthalmol 1995;113:978.

235. Shuler JD, Holland GN, Miles SA, et al. Kaposi sarcoma of the conjunctiva and eyelids associated with the acquired immunodeficiency syndrome. Arch Ophthalmol 1989;107:858–62.
236. Dugel PU, Gill PS, Frangieh GT, Rao NA. Ocular adnexal Kaposi's sarcoma in acquired immunodeficiency syndrome. Am J Ophthalmol 1990;110:500–3.
237. Cooper JS, Steinfeld AD, Lerch I. Intentions and outcomes in the radiotherapeutic management of epidemic Kaposi's sarcoma. Int J Radiat Oncol Biol Phys 1991;20:419–22.
238. Dugel PU, Gill PS, Frangieh GT, Rao NA. Treatment of ocular adnexal Kaposi's sarcoma in acquired immune deficiency syndrome. Ophthalmology 1992;99:1127–32.
239. Akpek EK, Polcharoen W, Ferry JA, Foster CS. Conjunctival lymphoma masquerading as chronic conjunctivitis. Ophthalmology 1999;106:757–60.
240. Yanoff M, Sharaby ML. Multiple endocrine neoplasia type IIB. Arch Ophthalmol 1996;114:228–9.
241. Kuper KD, Rohrbach JM. Atypical non-Hodgkin's lymphoma of the conjunctiva as an incidental finding in lower lid entropion. Klin Monatsbl Augenheilkd 1998;212:125–6.
242. Morgan G, Harry J. Lymphocytic tumours of indeterminate nature: a 5-year follow-up of 98 conjunctival and orbital lesions. Br J Ophthalmol 1978;62:381–3.
243. Franklin RM, Kenyon KR, Green WR, et al. Epibulbar IgA plasmacytoma occurring in multiple myeloma. Arch Ophthalmol 1982;100:451–6.
244. Seddon JM, Corwin JM, Weiter JJ, et al. Solitary extramedullary plasmacytoma of the palpebral conjunctiva. Br J Ophthalmol 1982;66:450–4.
245. Font RL, Mackay B, Tang R. Acute monocytic leukemia recurring as bilateral perilimbal infiltrates: immunohistochemical and ultrastructural confirmation. Ophthalmology 1985;92:1681–5.
246. Wolter JR, Leenhouts TM, Hendrix RC. Corneal involvement in mycosis fungoides. Am J Ophthalmol 1963;55:317–22.
247. Kremer I, Loven D, Mor C, Lurie H. A solitary conjunctival relapse of Hodgkin's disease treated by radiotherapy. Ophthal Surg 1989;20:494–6.
248. Petrella T, Bron A, Foulet A, et al. Report of a primary lymphoma of the conjunctiva. A lymphoma of MALT origin? Pathol Res Pract 1991;187:78–84.
249. Hardman-Lea S, Kerr-Muir M, Wotherspoon AC, et al. Mucosal-associated lymphoid tissue lymphoma of the conjunctiva. Arch Ophthalmol 1994;112:1207–12.
250. Weisenthal RW, Streeten BW, Dubansky AS, et al. Burkitt lymphoma presenting as a conjunctival mass. Ophthalmology 1995;102:129–30.
251. Friedman B, Borrelli FJ, Geleris I. Lymphosarcoma of bulbar conjunctiva: report of a case. Arch Ophthalmol 1955;54:381–5.
252. Eichler MD, Fraunfelder FT. Cryotherapy for conjunctival lymphoid tumors. Am J Ophthalmol 1994;118: 463–7.
253. Jakobiec FA, Iwamoto T, Patell M, Knowles DM II. Ocular adnexal monoclonal lymphoid tumors with a favorable prognosis. Ophthalmology 1986;93: 1547–57.
254. Coupland SE, Kraus L, Delecluse HJ, et al. Lymphoproliferative lesions of the ocular adnexa: analysis of 112 cases. Ophthalmology 1998;105:430–9.
255. Dunbar SF, Linggood RM, Doppke KP, et al. Conjunctival lymphoma: results and treatment with a single anterior electron field. A lens sparing approach. Int J Radiat Oncol Biol Phys 1990;19:249–57.
256. Letschert JGJ, Gonzalez DG, Oskam J, et al. Results of radiotherapy in patients with stage I orbital non-Hodgkin's lymphoma. Radiother Oncol 1991;22: 36–44.
257. Cellini M, Possati GL, Poddu P, Caramazza C. Interferon alpha in the therapy of conjunctival lymphoma in an HIV+ patient. Eur J Ophthalmol 1996; 6:475–7.
258. Luthra CL, Dozanas MT, Green WR. Lesions of the caruncle: clinicohistopathologic study. Surv Ophthalmol 1978;23:183–95.
259. Poon A, Sloan B, McKelvie P, Davies R. Primary basal cell carcinoma of the caruncle. Arch Ophthalmol 1997;115:1585–7.
260. Rodman RC, Frueh BR, Elner BM. Mucoepidermoid carcinoma of the caruncle. Am J Ophthalmol 1997; 123:564–5.
261. Shields CL, Shields JA, Arbizo V, Augsburger JJ. Oncogenes of the caruncle. Am J Ophthalmol 1986; 102:315–9.
262. Biggs SL, Font RL. Oncocytic lesions of the caruncle and other ocular adnexa. Arch Ophthalmol 1977; 95:474–8.
263. Lamping KA, Albert DM, Ni C, Fournier G. Oxyphil cell adenomas. Three case reports. Arch Ophthalmol 1984;102:263–5.
264. Meythaler H, Koniszewski G. Light and electron microscopic finding of an adenocarcinoma of the caruncle. Albrecht Von Graefes Arch Klin Exp Ophthalmol 1980;213:49–58.
265. Santos A, Gomez-Leal A. Lesions of the lacrimal caruncle. Ophthalmology 1994;101:943–9.
266. Margo CE, Horton MB. Malignant fibrous histiocytoma of the conjunctiva with metastasis. Am J Ophthalmol 1989;107:433–4.
267. White VA, Damji KF, Richards JS, Rootman J. Leiomyosarcoma of the conjunctiva. Ophthalmology 1991;98:1560–4.

268. Gritz DC, Rao NA. Metastatic carcinoid tumor diagnosis from a caruncular mass. Am J Ophthalmol 1991; 112:470–2.
269. Allaire GS, Corriveau C, Teboul N. Malignant fibrous histiocytoma of the conjunctiva. Arch Ophthalmol 1999;117:685–7.
270. Heuring AH, Hutz WW, Eckhardt HB, Bohle RM. Inverted transitional cell papilloma of the conjunctiva with peripheral carcinomatous transformation. Klin Monatsbl Augenheilkd 1998;212:61–3.
271. Lam S, Stone MS, Goeken JA, et al. Paraneoplastic pemphigus, cicactricial conjunctivitis, and in acanthosis nigricans with pachydermatoglyphy in a patient with bronchogenic squamous cell carcinoma. Ophthalmology 1992;99:108–13.
272. Blumenthal EZ, Arzozi H, Bahir J, Pe'er J. Multiple conjunctival metastases as the initial sign of metastatic uveal melanoma. Ophthalmol 1997;124: 549–50.
273. Kiratli H, Shields CL, Shields JA, DePortter P. Metastatic tumours of the conjunctiva: report of 10 cases. Br J Ophthalmol 1996;80:5–8.
274. Shields JA, Gunduz K, Shields CL, et al. Conjunctival metastases as initial manifestation of lung cancer. Am J Ophthalmol 1997;124:399–400.
275. Kwapiszeski BR, Savitt ML. Conjunctival metastases midcutaneous melanoma as initial sign of dissemination. Am J Ophthalmol 1997;123:266–8.
276. Sekundo W, Roggenkamper P, Fischer HP, et al. Primary conjunctival rhabdomyosarcoma: 2.5 years' follow-up after combined chemotherapy and brachytherapy. Graefes Arch Clin Exp Ophthalmol 1998;236:873–5.
277. Wood C. Metastases to the conjunctiva. Br J Ophthalmol 1996;80:1.
278. Neuhaus RW, Baylis HI, Shorr M. Complications at mucous membrane donor sites. Am J Ophthalmol 1982;93:643–46.

5

Posterior Uveal Tumors

Several benign and malignant tumors have a predilection for the posterior uvea. An organized approach is important to establish a differential diagnosis, select the most useful diagnostic studies, and optimally treat these lesions. Since choroidal tumors are a central component of ocular oncology, the chapters on uveal tumors are dense. This chapter introduces choroidal melanoma, its etiology, and its diagnosis. Chapter 6 discusses nevi, retinal pigment epithelium lesions, metastases, hemangiomas, and disciform and other lesions that may be misdiagnosed as melanoma. Chapter 7 overviews the management of melanomas and "nevomas." Lastly, Chapter 8 discusses in depth the management of uveal tumors.

CHOROIDAL MELANOMA

Choroidal malignant melanoma is the most common primary intraocular tumor of adults; its incidence is approximately 5 to 7 per million per year in the United States and Western Europe.[1,2] In the United States, approximately 1,200 to 1,500 new cases are diagnosed each year. In comparison, about 47,700 cutaneous melanomas are diagnosed in this country each year.[3] Uveal melanomas occur most commonly in middle-aged and older Caucasian patients, rarely in dark-skinned populations.[4] In a relatively small Florida study, Caucasian males had a 72-fold increased risk for uveal melanoma, compared with black males.[5] Epidemiologic studies have shown a slightly increased incidence of uveal melanomas in populations with more sun exposure.[6] This malignancy is also more prevalent in Caucasian patients with ocular or oculodermal melanosis (nevus of Ota) (Figure 5–1).[7,8] In a study of 56 Caucasians with oculodermal melanocytosis, the authors estimates that about 1 out of 400 will develop a uveal melanoma. While uveal nevi are more frequent in patients with the dysplastic nevus syndrome, the frequency of uveal melanoma in that population does not appear to be above the baseline.[9–12] It has been stated that neurofibromatosis type-1 (NF1) is associated with choridal melanomas, although there have been fewer than 20 cases reported.[13] In contrast to cutaneous melanoma, which has shown a fivefold to sixfold increase in incidence over the last several decades, the frequency of uveal melanoma appears not to have changed.[14] Approximately 12 percent of all melanomas arise in the uveal tract. Eighty percent of uveal melanomas occur in the choroid; 5 to 8 percent are iris lesions; and 10 to 15 percent of tumors involve the ciliary body.[15]

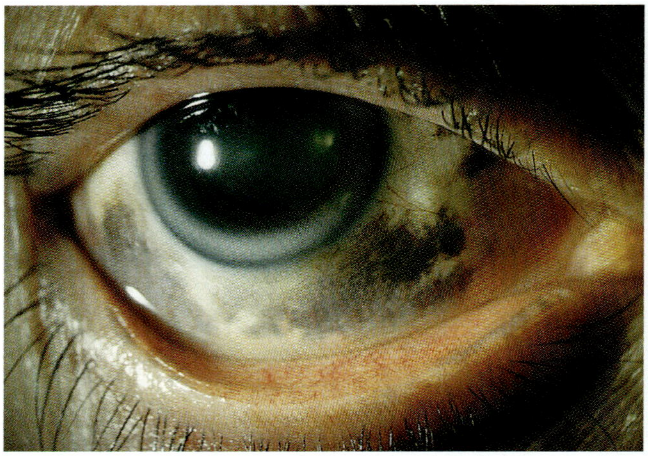

Figure 5–1. Melanosis oculi with increased scleral pigmentation. In Caucasians, this problem is associated with an increased risk of uveal melanoma, as seen in this patient.

ETIOLOGY

The etiology of uveal melanoma remains an enigma. Epidemiologic data have shown that sunlight may be important; similarly, we have also noted an association with arc welding.[7,16] Approximately 20 families have been reported with uveal melanomas in more than one generation since the initial description in 1892.[17–20] While some viral-associated models of uveal melanomas have been reported, viral oncogenes have not been reproducibly demonstrated in human intraocular melanoma.[21,22] Occupational correlations with uveal melanoma development are unclear.[17]

In cutaneous melanoma, a number of molecular alterations have been described during the development and progression of that neoplasm that are disparate from uveal melanoma.[13,23–26] The most common chromosomal alterations in cutaneous melanoma are in chromosome 1, 6q, 7, 9, 10, and 11.[27] Tumor suppressor loci are present on 6q and 9p, and loss or rearrangement in the latter area is found in about 50 percent of cutaneous melanomas.[13, 24–28] The alteration on 9p, which appears to code for p16 (CDKN2A), an inhibitor of cyclin-dependent kinase 4, had not been found to be altered in uveal melanoma.[17,18, 27,29,30]

Several groups, including ours, have described reproducible genomic changes in uveal melanomas.[31–35] The most consistent finding in uveal melanoma has been loss of chromosome 3 and increased copy number of 8q.[32–40] Alterations have been described on several other chromosomes including 6p and 6q.[31,33,35]

Loss of chromosome 3 (monosomy of 3) and increase in chromosome 8 have been associated with an adverse prognosis.[33,36] Prescher and colleagues in a study of 54 patients with enucleated uveal melanoma found that the closest correlation with tumor mortality was monosomy of chromosome 3.[35] In that series, ciliary body involvement was also highly associated with loss of chromosome 3, although in other series that latter association has not been noted.[37] White and co-workers assessed the effect of the genomic uveal melanoma changes and prognosis in 54 patients with enucleated uveal melanoma. They noted that when both abnormalities on chromosomes 3 and 8 were present together, there was a relative increased risk of metastases.[38] In that study, an alteration of chromosome 6 had a slightly protective effect, and the alterations were independent of tumor location. A recent investigation has demonstrated p16 inactivation in approximately 27 percent of uveal melanomas.[39] The alterations in chromosome 8 were only observed in patients who had either a monosomy of chromosome 3 or alteration of chromosome 6p. Thus, 8q alterations probably occur relatively late in tumor development.[36] Workers had previously thought that chromosome 3 changes might occur earlier, but data for that were equivocal.[36,40]

In cutaneous melanoma, several different cytokine arrays have been demonstrated to be altered during tumor progression.[41] A number of these are vasogenic cytokines and probably are important in both tumor growth as well as the side effects that occur when these eyes with uveal melanoma are irradiated.[42] Different genes have been proposed that might relate to metastases; however, their importance in uveal melanoma is uncertain.[43,44] We and others have done a number of studies with both parafin-fixed and fresh tissue to look at clonal changes in uveal melanoma progression. The results of these studies are quite preliminary.[45,46]

Controversy exists regarding whether alterations of another tumor suppressor gene, *p53*, are important in uveal melanomas.[19,47] In familial uveal melanomas, an alteration of *p53* has been described with most mutations documented at codons 238 and 253.[18,48] Unfortunately, work from our laboratory and others (personal communication, Ian McLean) has failed to find *p53* alterations in the vast majority of uveal melanomas using the same methodology.[50] Recently Coupland and associates reported cyclin D1 and *p53* positivity had an adverse association with prognosis, with cyclin D1 being an independent prognostic factor using a multiple regression model.[49]

Immunologic investigations of uveal melanoma have continued, but progress remains slow. Alteration of HLA expression on uveal melanomas has been associated with prognosis.[48] The expression of epidermal growth factor receptor in animal models appear to correlate with prognosis.[48]

A number of other proteins are present on the uveal melanoma cell surface that might be candidates for immunotherapy.[51,52] These antigens include

MART-1, tyrosinase, and the MAGE family of proteins.[52] Ksander and colleagues have begun studies of tumor-infiltrating lymphocytes, which have been cultured with a lymphocyte stimulating factor (interleukin-2) and have noted a different pattern of response with cutaneous melanomas.[53] This group believes that it may be possible to develop effective immune therapy, but that is yet to be demonstrated.[54]

Several other etiologic avenues have been explored for uveal melanoma development. As with cutaneous melanoma, pregnancy does not appear to affect either the development or the prognosis in this tumor.[55–58] We and others have rarely noted uveal melanomas arising in an area of a chorioretinal scar.[59,60] The importance of trauma in tumor development would appear to be minimal. The author can recall only 3 such cases in approximately 3,000 uveal melanomas that have been examined.

DIAGNOSIS

Making the correct diagnosis of a posterior uveal tumor can be difficult.[61,62] History and presentation vary; approximately 33 percent of patients with uveal melanoma are asymptomatic when they are first diagnosed. Patients may complain of flashing lights or a scotoma. If there is a large uveal melanoma, symptoms may develop as a result of exudative retinal detachment. Patients with tumors in or near the macula may present with metamorphopsia. In anterior uveal tumors that involve the ciliary body, sentinel vessels (Figure 5–2) are often present, and the patient may seek medical evaluation for a red eye.

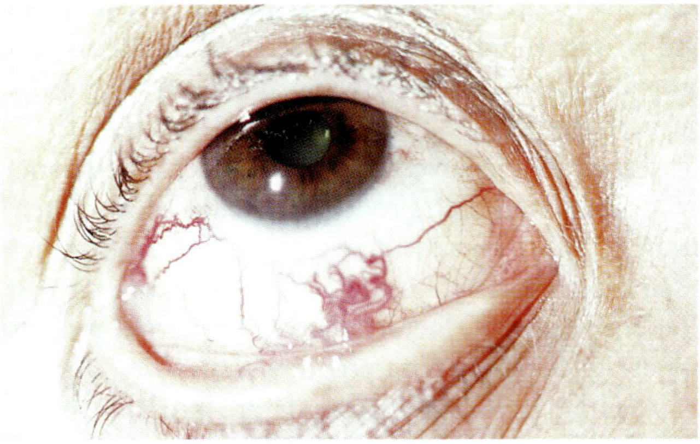

Figure 5–2. Episcleral sentinel vessels in association with an anterior uveal melanoma.

Some of these latter patients first present with visual distortion due to astigmatism caused by a growing ciliary body melanoma pressing against the lens.

Subjective findings are more helpful in identifying a simulating lesion than in diagnosing a uveal melanoma. Atypical findings for a choroidal melanoma include severe eye pain, which is uncommon unless a uveal tumor has destroyed vision, inflamed the eye, caused glaucoma, or produced extraocular extension. Patients who have systemic hypertension, recent intraocular surgery, or collagen vascular disease are more likely to have some simulating lesions, such as ruptured arterial microaneurysms, localized hemorrhagic choroidal detachments, macular disciform lesions, and scleritis. A history of systemic malignancy should be sought, since especially with gastrointestinal, renal, and lung carcinoma, the eye findings often predate the discovery of the primary neoplasm.

Melanoma very rarely presents in patients < 20 years old. In a series reported by Barr and coworkers, only 100 of 6,350 uveal melanomas occurred in that group.[63,64] Congenital melanomas in all body sites have been reported in fewer than 30 patients.[65]

An intraocular malignancy should be included in the differential diagnosis of any patient with a unilateral cataract or opaque media.[66] Figure 5–3 shows a patient who was referred with a unilateral advanced cataract due to an undiagnosed necrotic melanoma.

The lesions that most commonly simulate uveal melanoma are listed in Table 5–1. They include uveal nevi, choroidal hemangiomas, choroidal metastases, rhegmatogenous retinal detachments, and disciform lesions. Other less common lesions that may also be confused with uveal melanomas include retinal pigment epithelial (RPE) tumors, RPE hypertrophy, RPE hyperplasia, melanocytoma, choroidal detachment (especially after cataract surgery), retinal cysts, choroidal osteoma, neurilemmoma, sclerochoroidal calcification, inflammatory disease (such as tuberculomas), uveal effusion syndrome, lymphoid lesions, and intraocular foreign bodies.[67–85]

The appearance of fundus lesions on indirect ophthalmoscopy is often diagnostic. A 20-diopter Nikon indirect lens can be used to estimate the diameter of posterior choroidal lesions.[86] The diam-

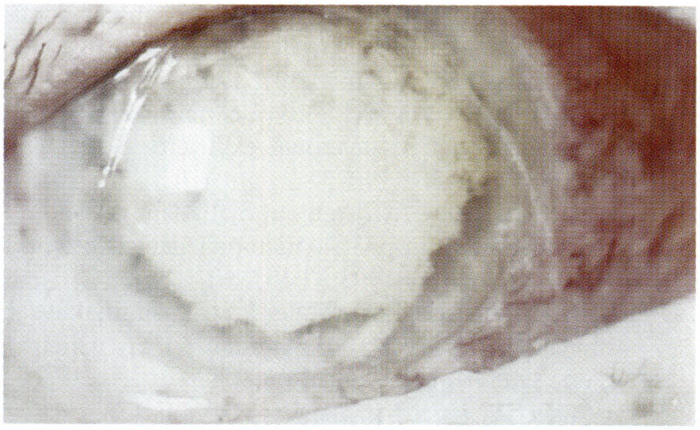

Figure 5–3. Necrotic uveal melanoma presenting as a unilateral cataract.

eter of the retinal field viewed through the lens is approximately 12 mm, so the tumor diameter can be inferred; for example, a lesion that fills one half the lens diameter is 6 mm in diameter, and one that fills three-fourths of the field is 9 mm.

The major goals in the evaluation of posterior uveal tumors are to determine whether an intraocular malignancy is present and if intervention is necessary. As discussed below, if a lesion is > 4 mm in thickness and the media are clear, the diagnosis can usually be made with indirect ophthalmoscopy alone. Similarly, the evaluation and management of flat tumors is straightforward. An asymptomatic, small, (< 6 mm in diameter) flat lesion without subretinal fluid is usually not serious and requires little further evaluation other than a fundus drawing. If a flat lesion is > 6 mm in diameter, fundus photographs should be obtained, and the lesion monitored. Ultrasonography is not helpful for lesions < 1 to 2 mm in thickness but may be useful as a baseline for serial evaluation.

As discussed in Chapter 8, rarely a peripapillary uveal melanoma can have its major growth outside the eye and present as an orbital tumor.[13] It is hypothesized that tumors progress from a less malignant state to a more malignant one, and multiple, serial genomic changes occur during that process.[87,88] In colon carcinoma, the progression of these genetic changes has become clearer.[25,36] In uveal melanomas, the timing and relative importance of these genetic changes are uncertain. In cutaneous melanomas, changes on 6q appear early, while alterations on 9p appear to be a later event.[89] In an immunohistochemical study, p16 (CDKN2), coded for on 9p, was found on early melanocytic lesions but was lost in many later tumors and those that developed metastases.[90] As shown in the first figure, in the introduction, the p16 protein is part of a cell cycle control loop involving the *Rb1* gene. Probably, in uveal melanoma, monosomy of chromosome 3 occurs relatively early, but the sequence of events is unclear.

One of the most challenging diagnostic groups of lesions is pigmented uveal tumors 1 to 3 mm thick. It is very difficult, sometimes impossible, to differentiate a small melanoma from an atypical, large nevus. A combination of noninvasive diagnostic tests that usually include indirect ophthalmoscopy, visual field testing, slit-lamp biomicroscopy with contact lens, fundus photography, fluorescein angiography, and ultrasonography are used to evaluate elevated posterior uveal masses. An invasive diagnostic test such as fine-needle aspiration biopsy is indicated only if therapeutic intervention is planned. These approaches are discussed under alternative therapy. In Chapter 6, a

Table 5–1. LESIONS THAT SIMULATE CHOROIDAL MELANOMA

Choroidal Neoplasms
- Choroidal nevus
- Choroidal metastasis
- Choroidal hemangioma
- Choroidal osteoma
- Choroidal neurilemmoma
- Choroidal neurofibroma
- Peripheral melanocytoma
- Benign lymphoid tumor
- Choroidal hemangiopericytoma
- Choroidal leiomyoma

Hemorrhagic Processes
- Involutional macular degeneration
- Extramacular disciform lesion
- Ruptured arteriolar macroaneurysm
- Localized choroidal detachment/hemorrhage

Retinal Pigment Epithelial Processes
- Retinal pigment epithelial hyperplasia
- Retinal pigment epithelial hypertrophy
- Retinal pigment epithelial adenocarcinoma

Inflammatory Processes
- Posterior scleritis
- Posterior uveitis

Miscellaneous
- Hemorrhagic retinal detachment
- Retinoschisis with hemorrhage
- Staphyloma
- Intraocular foreign body granuloma
- Massive retinal gliosis
- Acquired retinal hemangioma
- Retinal glioma

brief review of various lesions in the differential diagnosis of posterior uveal melanomas demonstrates the role of the different diagnostic techniques as well as their limitations.

REFERENCES

1. Scotto J, Fraumeni JF Jr, Lee JA. Melanomas of the eye and other noncutaneous sites: epidemiologic aspects. J Natl Cancer Inst 1976;56:489–91.
2. Keller AZ. Histology, survivorship and related factors in the epidemiology of eye cancers. Am J Epidemiol 1973;97:386–93.
3. Grin-Jorgensen C, Berke A, Grin M. Ocular melanoma. Dermatol Clin 1992;10:663–8.
4. Margo CE, McLean IW. Malignant melanoma of the choroid and ciliary body in black patients. Arch Ophthalmol 1984;102:77–9.
5. Margo CE, Mulla Z, Billiris K. Incidence of surgically treated uveal melanoma by race and ethnicity. Ophthalmology 1998;105:1087–90.
6. Tucker MA, Shields JA, Hartge P, et al. Sunlight exposure as risk factor for intraocular malignant melanoma. N Engl J Med 1985;313:789–92.
7. Gonder JR, Shields JA, Albert DM, et al. Uveal malignant melanoma associated with ocular and oculodermal melanocytosis. Ophthalmology 1982;89:953–60.
8. Dutton JJ, Anderson RL, Schelper RL, et al. Orbital malignant melanoma and oculodermal melanocytosis: report of two cases and review of the literature. Ophthalmology 1984;91:497–507.
9. Rodriguez-Sains RS. Ocular findings in patients with dysplastic nevus syndrome. Ophthalmology 1986; 93:661–5.
10. Albert DM, Chang MA, Lamping K, et al. The dysplastic nevus syndrome. A pedigree with primary malignant melanomas of the choroid and skin. Ophthalmology 1985;92:1728–34.
11. Greene MH, Sanders RJ, Chu FC, et al. The familial occurrence of cutaneous melanoma, intraocular melanoma, and the dysplastic nevus sydrome. Am J Ophthalmol 1983;96:238–45.
12. McCarthy JM, Rootman J, Horsman D, White VA. Conjunctival and uveal melanoma in the dysplastic nevus syndrome. Surv Ophthalmol 1993;37:377–86.
13. Friedman SM, Margo CE. Choroidal melanoma and neurofibromatosis type 1. Arch Ophthalmol 1998; 116:694–5.
14. Osterlind A. Trends in incidence of ocular malignant melanoma in Denmark 1943-1982. Int J Cancer 1987;40:161–4.
15. Hogan MJ, Zimmerman LE. Ophthalmic pathology: an atlas and textbook, 2nd ed. Philadelphia, PA: WB Saunders; 1962.
16. Holly EA, Aston DA, Char DH, et al. Uveal melanoma in relation to ultraviolet light exposure and host factors. Cancer Res 1990;50:5773–7.
17. Lutz JM, Cree I, Foss AJ. Risk factors for intraocular melanoma and occupational exposure. Br J Ophthalmol 1999;83:1190–3.
18. Jay M, McCartney AC. Familial malignant melanoma of the uveal and p53: a Victorian detective story. Surv Ophthalmol 1993;37:457–62.
19. Singh AD, Shields CL, De Potter P, et al. Familial uveal melanoma. Clinical observations on 56 patients. Arch Ophthalmol 1996;114:392–9.
20. van Hees CL, Jager MJ, Bleeker JC, et al. Occurrence of cutaneous and uveal melanoma in patients with uveal melanoma and their first degree relatives. Melanoma Res 1998;8:175–80.
21. Mintz B, Silvers WK. Transgenic mouse model of malignant skin melanoma. Proc Natl Acad Sci USA 1993;90:8817–21.
22. Mooy CM, Van der Helm MJ, Van der Kwast TH, et al. No N-ras mutations in human uveal melanoma: the role of ultraviolet light revisited. Br J Cancer 1991; 64:411–7.
23. Rivers JK, Ho VC. Malignant melanoma. Who shall live and who shall die? Arch Dermatol 1992;128:537–42.
24. Cannon-Albright LA, Goldgar DE, Meyer LJ, et al. Assignment of a locus for familial melanoma, MLM to chromosome 9p13-p22. Science 1992;258:1148–52.
25. Yamanishi DT, Meyskens FL Jr. Alterations in gene expression and signal transductions in human melanocytes and melanoma cells. Crit Rev Oncogenesis 1994;5:429–50.
26. Zhang J, Glattfelter AA, Taetle R, Trent JM. Frequent alterations of evolutionarily conserved regions of chromosome 1 in human malignant melanoma. Cancer Genet Cytogenet 1999;111:119–23.
27. Nelson MA, Thompson FH, Emerson J, et al. Clinical implications of cytogenetic abnormalities in melanoma. Surg Clin North Am 76:1257–71.
28. Trent JM, Thompson FH, Meyskens FL Jr. Identification of a recurring translocation site involving chromosome 6 in human malignant melanoma. Cancer Res 1989;49:420–3.
29. Ohta M, Nagai H, Shimizu M, et al. Rarity of somatic and germline mutations of the cyclin-dependent kinase 4 inhibitor gene, CDK41, in melanoma. Cancer Res 1994;54:5269–70.
30. Fountain DW, Karayyoirgou M, Ernstoff MS, et al. Homozyogous deletions within human chromosomes band 9p21 in melanoma. Proc Natl Acad Sci USA 1992;89:10557–61.
31. Wiltshire RN, Elner VM, Dennis T, et al. Cytogenetic analysis of posterior uveal melanoma. Cancer Genet Cytogenet 1993;66:47–53.
32. Sisley K, Cottam DW, Rennie IG, et al. Non-random abnormalities with chromosome 3,6, and 8 associ-

ated with posterior uveal melanoma. Genet Chrom Cancer 1992;5:197–200.
33. Prescher G, Bornfeld N, Horsthemke B, Becher R. Chromosomal aberrations defining uveal melanoma of poor prognosis. Lancet 1992;339:691–2.
34. Dehlenfors R, Tornqvist G, Wettrell K, Mark J. Cytogenetical observations in nine ocular malignant melanomas. Anticancer Res 1993;13:1415–20.
35. Prescher G, Bornfield N, Hirche H, et al. Prognostic implications of monosomy 3 in uveal melanoma. Lancet 1996;347:1222–5.
36. Parrella P, Sidransky D, Merbs SL. Allelotype of posterior uveal melanoma: implications for a bifurcated tumor progression pathway. Cancer Res 1999;59: 3032–7.
37. Prescher G, Bornfeld N, Becher R. Two subclones in a case of uveal melanoma. Cancer Genet Cytogenet 1994;77:144–6.
38. White VA, Chambers JD, Courtright PD, et al. Correlation of cytogenetic abnormalities with the outcome of patients with uveal melanoma. Cancer 1998;83: 354–9.
39. Merbs SL, Sidransky D. Analysis of p16(CDKN2/MTS-1/INK4A) alterations in primary sporadic uveal melanoma. Invest Ophthalmol Vis Sci 1999; 40:779–83.
40. Gordon KB, Thompson CT, Char DH, et al. Comparative genomic hybridization in the detection of DNA copy number abnormalities in uveal melanoma. Cancer Res 1994;54:4764–8.
41. Bishop JAN. Molecular pathology of melanoma. Cancer Metastasis Rev 1997;16:141–54.
42. Casey R, Li WW. Perspective: factors controlling ocular angiogenesis. Am J Ophthalmol 1997;124:521–9.
43. Lee JH, Miele ME, Hicks DJ, et al. KiSS-1, a novel human malignant melanoma metastasis-suppressor gene. J Natl Cancer Inst 1996;88:1731–7.
44. Greco IM, Calvisi G, Ventura L, Cerrito F. An immunohistochemical analysis of nm23 gene product expression in uveal malanoma. Melanoma Res 1997; 3:231–6.
45. Larouche N, Larouche K, Beliveau A, et al. Transcriptional regulation of the alpha 4 integrin subunit gene in the metastatic spread of uveal melanoma. Anticancer Res 1998;18:3539–47.
46. Ghazvini S, Char DH, Kroll S, et al. Comparative genomic hybridization analysis of archival formalin-fixed paraffin-embedded uveal melanomas. Cancer Genet Cytogenet 1996;90:95–101.
47. Tobal K, Warren W, Cooper CS, et al. Increased expression and mutation of p53 in choroidal melanoma. Br J Cancer 1992;66:900–4.
48. Blom D Jr, Lyten GPM, Mooy C, et al. Human leucocyte antigen class I expression: marker of poor prognosis in uveal melanoma. Invest Ophthalmol Vis Sci 1997;38:1865–72.
49. Coupland SE, Antastassiou G, Stang A, et al. The prognostic value of D-1, p53 and mom_2 protein expression in uveal melanoma. J Pathol 2000;191:120–6.
50. Kishore K, Ghazvini S, Char DH, et al. Accumulation of nuclear p53 protein correlates with high cell cycling in uveal melanoma. Am J Ophthalmol 1996; 121:561–7.
51. De Vries TJ, Tancikova D, Ruiter DJ, van Muihen GNP. High expression of immunotherapy candidate proteins gp 100, MART-100, tyrosinase and TRP-1 in uveal melanoma. Br J Cancer 1998;78:1156–61.
52. Mucalhy KA, Rimoldi D, Brasseur F, et al. Infrequent expression of the MAGE family in uveal melanomas. Int J Cancer 1996;66:738–42.
53. Verbik DJ, Murray TG, Tran JM, Ksander BR. Melanomas that develop within the eye inhibit lymphocyte proliferation. Int J Cancer 1997;73:470–8.
54. Ksander BR, Geer DC, Chen PW, et al. Uveal melanomas contain antigenically specific and nonspecific infiltrating lymphocytes. Curr Eye Res 1998;17:165–73.
55. Colbourn DS, Nathanson L, Belilos E. Pregnancy and malignant melanoma. Semin Oncol 1989;16:377–87.
56. Hannaford PC, Billard-Mackintosh L, Vessey MP, Kay CR. Oral contraceptives and malignant melanoma. Br J Cancer 1991;63:430–3.
57. Kjems E, Krag C. Melanoma in pregnancy. A review. Acta Oncologica 1993;32:371–8.
58. Shields CL, Shields JA, Eagle RC Jr, et al. Uveal melanoma and pregnancy. A report of 16 cases. Ophthalmology 1991;98:1667–73.
59. Zografos L. Occurrence of uveal melanoma in contact with a chorioretinal cryocoagulation scar. Ophthalmologica 1990;201:213–5.
60. Vicary D. Malignant melanoma at the site of penetrating ocular trauma. Arch Ophthalmol 1986;104:1130.
61. Ferry AP. Lesions mistaken for malignant melanoma of the posterior uvea: a clinical pathologic analysis of 100 cases with ophthalmoscopically visible lesions. Arch Ophthalmol 1964;72:463–9.
62. Shields JA. Lesions simulating malignant melanoma of the posterior uvea. Arch Ophthlamol 1973;89: 466–71.
63. Barr CC, McLean IW, Zimmerman LE. Uveal melanoma in children and adolescents. Arch Ophthalmol 1981;99:2133–6.
64. Shields CL, Shields JA, Milite J, et al. Uveal melanoma in teenagers and children. A report of 40 cases. Ophthalmology 1991;98:1662–6.
65. Broadway D, Lang S, Harper J, et al. Congenital malignant melanoma of the eye. Cancer 1991;67:2642–52.
66. Makley TA Jr, Teed RW. Unsuspected intraocular malignant melanomas. Arch Ophthalmol 1958;60: 475–8.
67. Schachat AP, Robertson DM, Mieler WF, et al. Sclerochoroidal calcification. Arch Ophthalmol 1992; 110:196–9.

68. Kindermann WR, Shields JA, Eiferman RA, et al. Metastatic renal cell carcinoma to the eye and adnexae; a report of three cases and review of the literature. Ophthalmology 1981;88:1347–50.
69. Packard RB, Harry J. Choroidal neurilemmoma — an unusual clinical misdiagnosis. Br J Ophthalmol 1981;65:189–91.
70. Buettner H. Congential hypertrophy of the retinal pigment epithelium. Am J Ophthalmol 1975;79:177–89.
71. Ryan SJ, Zimmerman LE, King FM. Reactive lymphoid hyperplasia. An unusual form of intraocular pseudotumor. Trans Am Acad Ophthalmol Otolaryngol Soc 1972;76:652–71.
72. Cibis GW, Fratkin J. Hemorrhage into retinoschisis diagnosed as malignant melanoma. Am J Ophthalmol 1979;87:96–7.
73. Laqua H, Wessing A. Congenital retino-pigment epithelial malformation, previously described as hamartoma. Am J Ophthalmol 1979;87:34–42.
74. Howard GM, Forrest AW. Incidence and location of melanocytomas. Arch Ophthalmol 1967;77:61–6.
75. Tso MO, Albert DM. Pathological condition of the retinal pigment epithelium. Neoplasms and nodular non-neoplastic lesions. Arch Ophthalmol 1972;88:27–38.
76. Kannan KA. Lymphomatous pseudo-tumor of the choroid with secondary retinal detachment. Ind J Ophthalmol 1976;23:28–31.
77. Campo RV, Aaberg TM. Choroidal granuloma in sarcoidosis. Am J Ophthalmol 1984;97:419–27.
78. Cunha SL. Osseous choristoma of the choroid. A familial disease. Arch Ophthalmol 1984;102:1052–4.
79. Jakobiec FA, Witschel H, Zimmerman LE. Choroidal leimyoma of vascular origin. Am J Ophthalmol 1976;82:205–12.
80. Papale JJ, Frederick AR, Albert DM. Intraocular hemangiopericytoma. Arch Ophthalmol 1983;101:1409–11.
81. Jabbour NM, Faris B, Trempe CL. A case of pulmonary tuberculosis presenting with a choroidal tuberculoma. Ophthalmology 1985;92:834–7.
82. Perry HD, Zimerman LE, Benson WE. Hemorrhage from isolated aneurysm of a retinal artery: report of two cases simulating malignant melanoma. Arch Ophthalmol 1977;95:281–3.
83. Minckler D, Allen AW Jr. Adenocarcinoma of the retinal pigment epithelium. Arch Ophthalmol 1978;96:2252–4.
84. Lipper S, Eifrig DE, Peiffer RL, Bagnell CR. Chorioretinal foreign body simulating malignant melanoma. Am J Ophthalmol 1981;92:202–5.
85. Bellows AR, Chylack LT Jr, Hutchinson BT. Choroidal detachment. Clinical manifestation, therapy and mechanism of formation. Ophthalmology 1981;88:1107–15.
86. Char DH, Stone RD, Irvine AR, et al. Diagnostic modalities in choroidal melanoma. Am J Ophthalmol 1980;89:223–30.
87. Fearon ER, Vogelstein B. A genetic model for colorectal tumorigenesis. Cell 1990;61:759–67.
88. Usmani BA. Genomic instability and metastatic progression. Pathobiology 1993;61:109–16.
89. Walker GJ, Palmer JM, Walters MK, Hayward NK. A genetic model of melanoma tumorigenesis based on allelic losses. Genes Chromosomes Cancer 1995;12:134–41.
90. Reed JA, Loganzo F Jr, Shea CR, et al. Loss of expression of p16/cyclin-dependent kinase inhibitor 2 tumor suppressor gene in melanocytic lesions correlates with invasive stage of tumor progression. Cancer Res 1995;55:2713–8.

6

Choroidal Simulating Lesions

A number of uveal lesions can simulate a choroidal melanoma. The most common simulating lesions are nevi, metastases to the uvea, hemangiomas, hemorrhagic processes, inflammatory lesions, and detachments. The clinical patterns of these processes are described in this chapter.

CHOROIDAL NEVI

Choroidal nevi are usually flat, or minimally elevated, slate gray lesions, almost always < 6 mm in diameter (Figure 6–1). Most are asymptomatic; rarely, they may produce subretinal neovascularization or overlying retinal changes that cause visual distortion. Visual field tests usually demonstrate either no scotoma or a relative defect.[1] Characteristic flat, asymptomatic choroidal nevi are documented on the first visit with either photography or a fundus drawing, then serially examined every 2 years without ancillary tests.

Uveal nevi may have overlying light yellow or white drusen that are either isolated or confluent (Figures 6–1 and 6–2). Less frequently nevi can be blond (Figure 6–3), have associated subretinal neovascularization (Figure 6–4), a hypopigmented surround (Figure 6–5), or changes in the overlying retinal pigment epithelium (RPE). Unlike metastatic lesions that may mimic them, blond nevi do not have associated subretinal fluid, and they do not have a predilection for the posterior pole. Subretinal neovascularization is a sign of chronicity. Some of the lesions with surrounding RPE hyperplasia probably had subretinal fluid which resorbed.

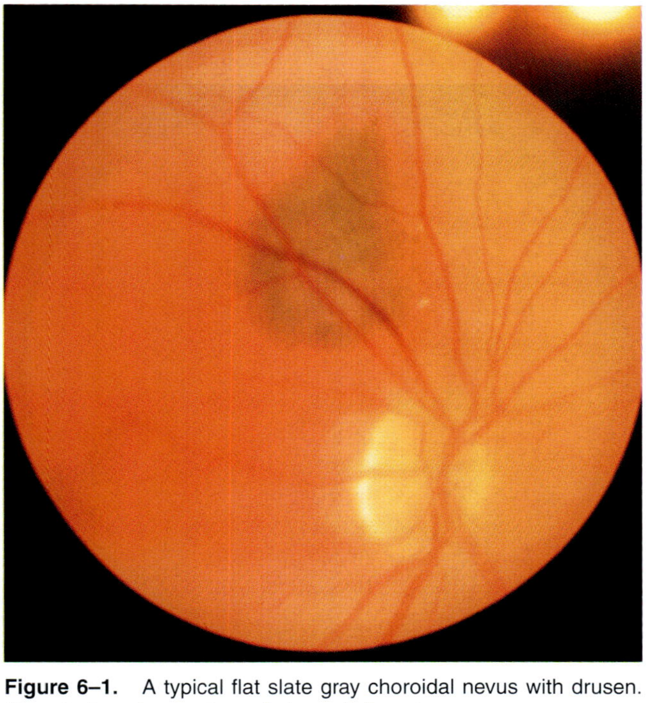

Figure 6–1. A typical flat slate gray choroidal nevus with drusen. Almost all nevi are < 6 mm in largest diameter.

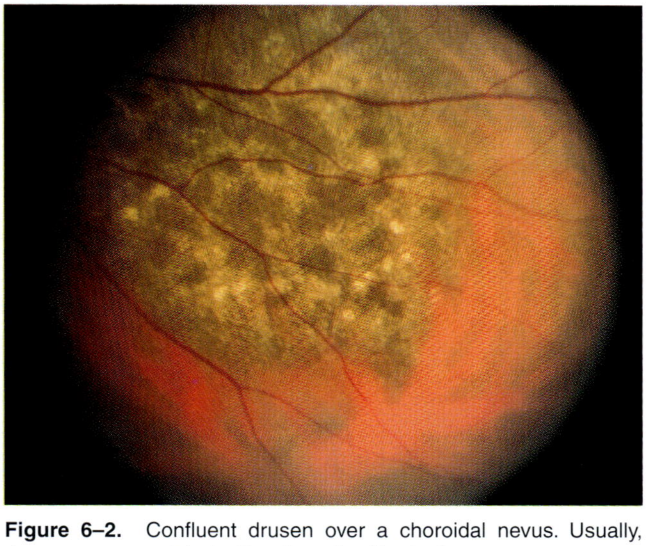

Figure 6–2. Confluent drusen over a choroidal nevus. Usually, drusen are associated with a longstanding lesion.

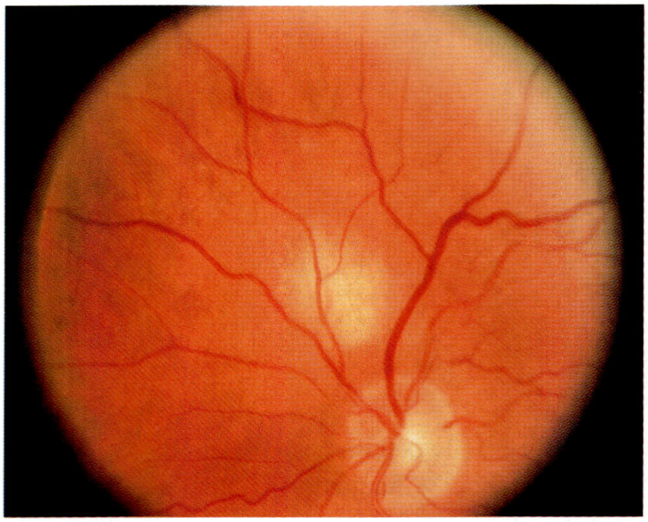

Figure 6–3. A blond nevus. Such nevi can simulate metastatic tumor.

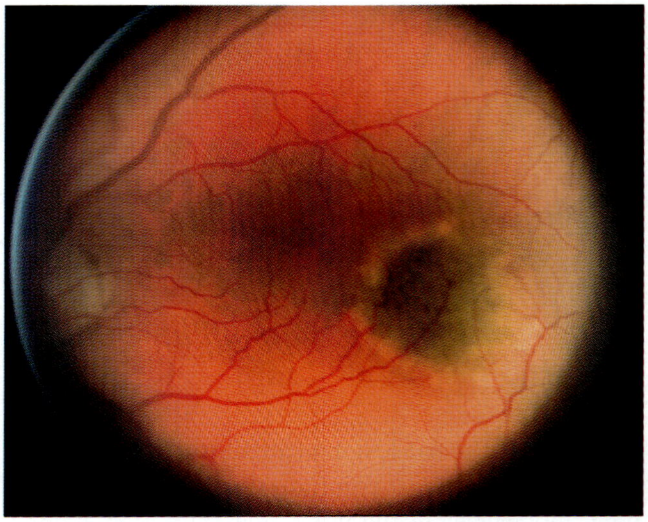

Figure 6–5. A hypopigmented area surrounding a choroidal nevus. This finding usually indicates a chronic, stable lesion.

Less common causes of flat choroidal pigmentation include multiple choroidal nevi, which occur as a normal variant, or proliferations of uveal melanocytes that are rarely observed as a form of a paraneoplastic syndrome in patients with widespread metastases.[2,3] In the latter syndrome of bilateral diffuse melanocytic proliferations in association with carcinoma, most patients develop ocular symptoms prior to the detection of the primary neoplasms.[2–5] Exudative detachments and cataracts develop rapidly in this paraneoplastic process.

Finally, as discussed under choroidal melanocytomas, diffuse, benign, flat choroidal pigmented lesions can occur. More extensive evaluation of presumptive nevi is indicated if any of the following is present:

1. Visual symptoms, such as decreased acuity or an absolute scotoma
2. An elevated lesion (Figure 6–6), or one with a diameter > 6 mm
3. Overlying orange pigmentation (Figure 6–7)

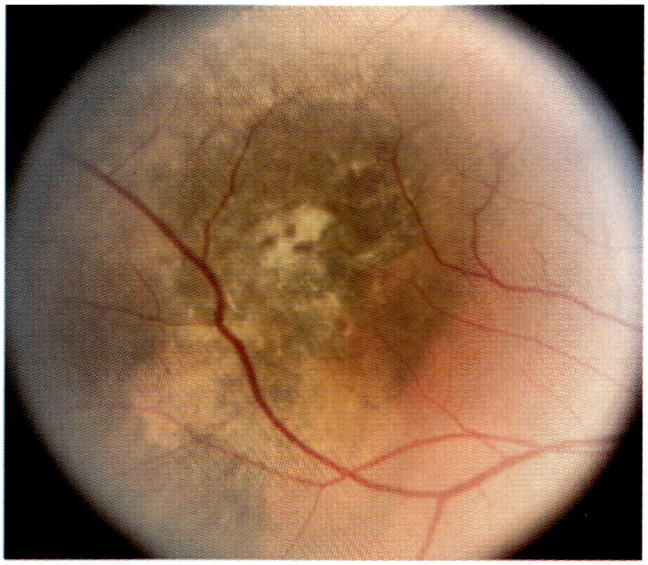

Figure 6–4. Subretinal neovascularization in association with a choroidal nevus. Like drusen, subretinal neovascularization is a sign of chronicity.

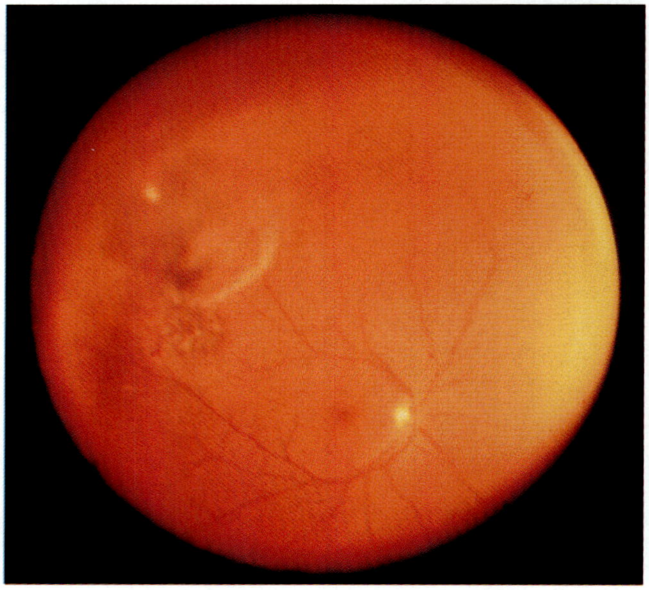

Figure 6–6. An elevated presumed choroidal nevus with no evidence of growth during over 5 years of serial observation.

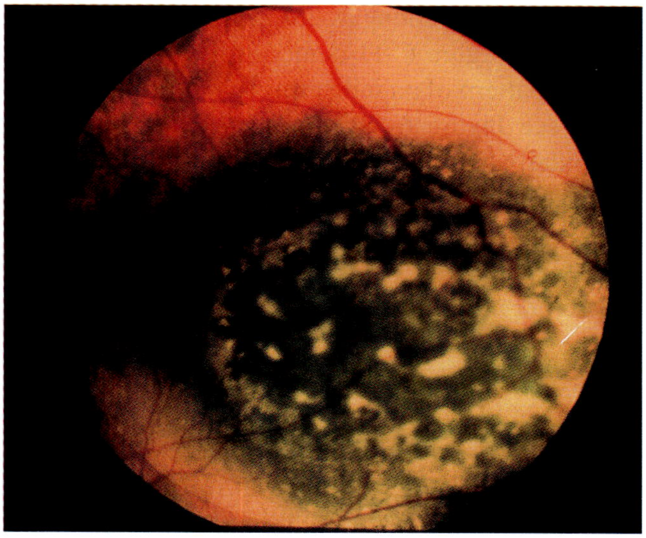

Figure 6–7. Orange pigmentation over a nevus, which has been monitored for over 10 years, with a change.

4. Overlying subretinal fluid. (Figure 6–8)

Orange pigmentation, visible because of the contrast between lipofuscin and melanin, is most commonly observed over melanomas.[6] Nevi with orange pigment are more likely to progress to melanomas; however, the patient with the lesion in Figure 6–7 has been followed up for over 20 years without change. As previously mentioned, it is almost impossible to differentiate atypical nevi from small melanomas of this size. The majority of small pigmented tumors that sometimes progress into small uveal melanomas (< 3 mm thick and < 10 mm in diameter), are initially asymptomatic, do not have subretinal fluid, and can be safely watched until growth is documented (see Chapter 7).[7] Fluorescein angiography is usually not useful in differentiating small melanomas from nevi; in a study we performed several years ago, the overall accuracy of fluorescein angiography in all sizes of uveal melanoma was approximately 50 percent.[8,9]

Fluorescein angiography may be helpful in diagnosing a few conditions including choroidal hemangiomas and subretinal hemorrhages, disciform degenerations, and arterial macroaneurysms.[9] Figure 6–9 shows an arterial macroaneurysm with secondary hemorrhage, a condition that clinically simulates a small uveal melanoma. The corresponding fluorescein angiogram nicely delineates the correct diagnosis with closure of the vessel, hemorrhage obscuring underlying detail, and exudate (Figure 6–10).

Indocyanine green angiography data have been reported in various tumors. The author has not been impressed that it has been a useful diagnostic adjuvant.[10,11] As discussed under uveal melanoma prognosis, it is possible that confocal indocyanine green laser scanning ophthalmoscopy may be useful, if it can reliably demonstrate the uveal melanoma microvascular

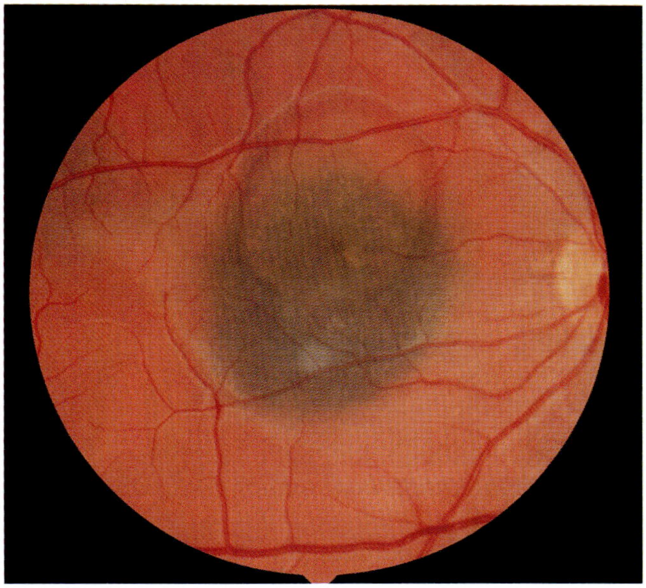

Figure 6–8. A nevus with secondary exudative detachment. On quantitative echography, the lesion measured < 1.5 mm thick.

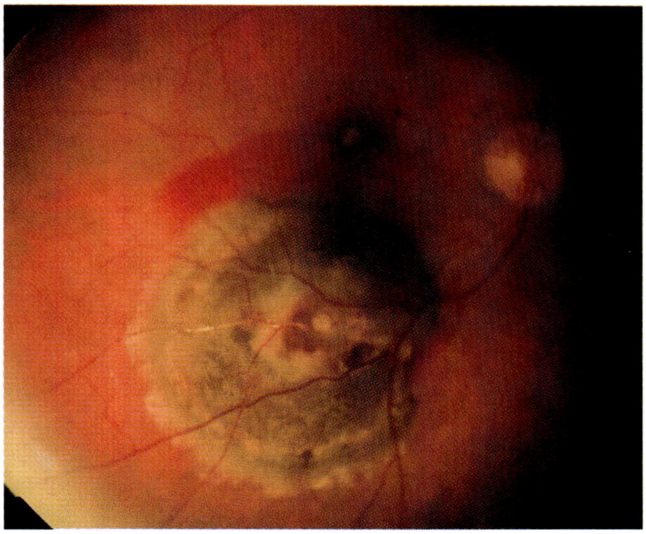

Figure 6–9. An arterial macroaneurysm clinically simulating a uveal melanoma, with what appears to be overlying orange pigment. Closer examination shows subretinal hemorrhage around the base of the lesion and an occluded arteriole distal to the macroaneurysm.

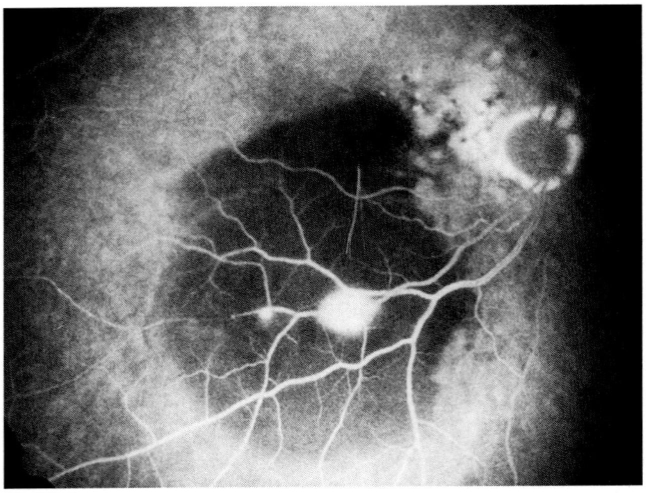

Figure 6–10. Fluorescein angiogram of an arterial macroaneurysm with hemorrhage obscuring underlying detail.

patterns.[12,13] At present the use of optical coherence tomography is of limited value in choroidal tumor diagnosis.[14]

The accuracy of ultrasonography in the differentiation of atypical uveal nevi from melanoma is unclear. I have not been willing to diagnose a melanoma on the basis of ultrasonographic criteria alone unless it is > 3 mm in thickness. We have serially examined some of these indeterminate pigmented lesions, that have many A- and B-scan melanoma characteristics (see section on choroidal melanoma), for as long as 20 years without evidence of growth. Figure 6–11 demonstrates the ultrasonographic pattern of an indeterminate pigmented uveal mass (see Figure 6–7). On B-scan, there is some choroidal excavation (Figure 6–11A). The absence of orbital shadowing and an acoustic quiet zone (findings characteristic of larger uveal melanomas) probably does not represent a significant difference in internal architecture from larger melanomas but, rather, reflects the fact that the mass is too thin for these ultrasound features to have developed. Similarly, the A-scan pattern is not classic for a melanoma; the area of low-medium reflectivity is minimal, and the lesion often has medium to high reflectivity (Figure 6–11B). We recently examined a patient we had diagnosed as a nonpigmented nevoma (indeterminant pigmented lesion) approximately 10 years ago. The patient had 20/20 vision and no symptoms until recently. The correct nature of the enlarged lesion could now be ascertained both clinically and on ultrasonography. It was an obvious hemangioma; however, neither the initial clinical ultrasound pattern nor the fluorescein angiogram was diagnostic when it was 2.0 mm thick.

There have been a few modifications in the ultrasound technique that may be helpful in monitoring in unusual settings. Several investigators have attempted to use new ultrasound contrast agents to differentiate

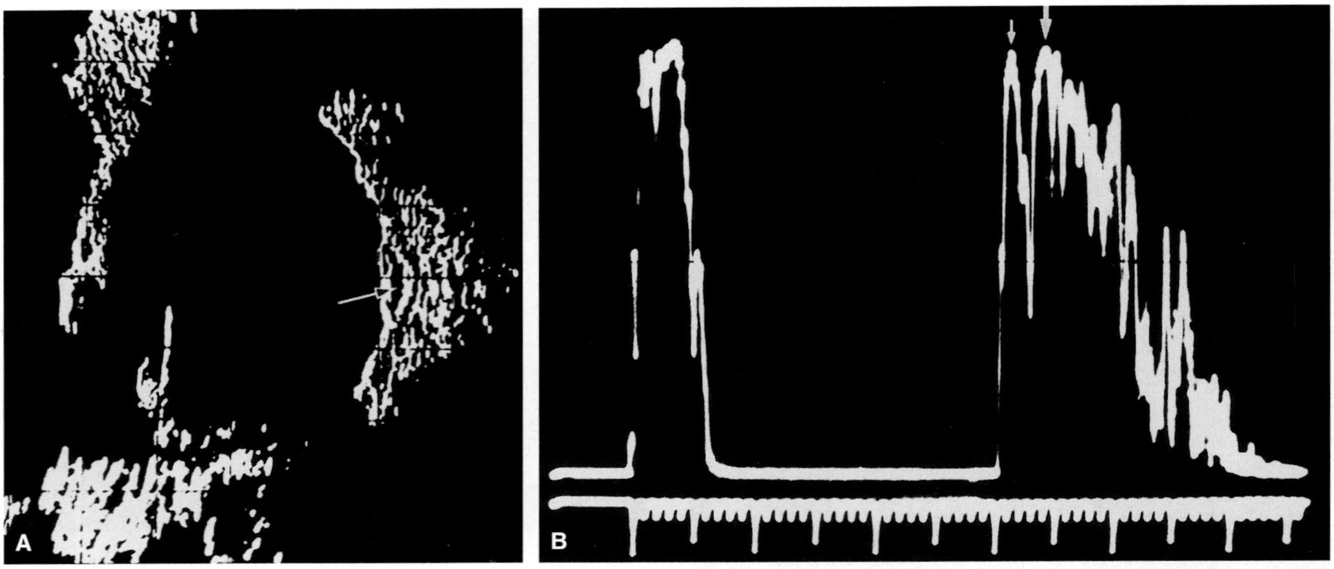

Figure 6–11. *A,* The B-scan appearance of a "nevoma", an indeterminate, elevated, pigmented choroidal lesion. On B-scan, there is an area of choroidal excavation (*arrow*). *B,* The quantitative A-scan appearance of the lesion shown in Figure 6–11A. The mass is noted with intermediate reflectivity between the anterior retinal (*small arrow*) and posterior scleral (*large arrow*) spikes.

lesions of varying vascular nature. While not helpful diagnostically, three-dimentional ultrasonography may be useful for the post-treatment serial evaluation of tumors.[15,16]

Positron emission tomography (PET) scanning can be used to visualize some larger uveal melanomas.[17] Our experience, and that of most investigators, has been that choroidal tumors < 7 mm in diameter and 5 mm thick are poorly evaluated with this technique, and yet that is the size in which many diagnostic difficulties occur (unpublished observations). Use of magnetic resonance imaging (MRI) is discussed in Chapter 7. It is an expensive technique, and does not appear to increase intraocular diagnostic accuracy; MRI is mainly used to detect localized extrascleral extension of a uveal melanoma.[18–20]

In indeterminate pigmented choroidal lesions, there are a few signs that suggest a melanoma. Obviously, growth, while not an absolute criterion of a small melanoma, is such a finding. Other factors suggesting malignancy are visual symptoms, orange pigmentation, and subretinal fluid. As discussed under management, we do not treat most patients with asymptomatic, indeterminate pigmented lesions, since no diagnostic modality accurately differentiates these nevomas into nevi and melanomas, and we have observed no tumor related-mortality in lesions that have not grown. As discussed in Chapter 8, we have been able to accurately delineate those nevomas at very high risk for growth; we intervene especially in those cases with tumors distant from the nerve and fovea.

RETINAL PIGMENT EPITHELIAL LESIONS

RPE lesions can occasionally be confused with melanomas. Most RPE proliferations are almost always flat. Congenital RPE hypertrophies often have a halo, scalloped margins, and lacunae and usually have areas that are much more darkly pigmented than either melanomas or nevi (Figures 6–12 and 6–13).[21–23] Occasionally, as patients age, these lesions may become entirely amelanotic. The RPE hypertrophy lesions that are associated with Gardner's syndrome (familial polyposis) are much smaller in area than lesions that could be confused with an uveal melanoma.[24] The pattern of these small RPE proliferations generally at the posterior pole is helpful, especially to identify family members at risk for Gardner's syndrome.[25,26]

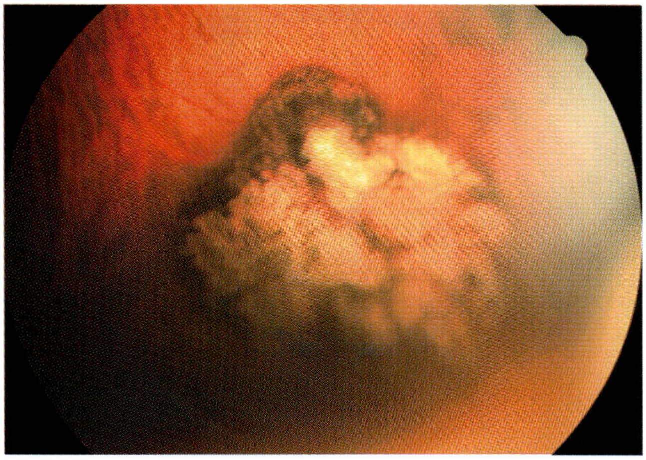

Figure 6–12. Retinal pigment hypertrophy with characteristic scalloped margins and lacunae.

RPE hyperplasia is a reactive process that occurs as a result of infection, trauma, or uveitis; these lesions are typified by flat, black pigmentation with ragged margins (Figure 6–14).[27] Occasionally, these lesions can have an atypical appearance.[28]

Occasionally, RPE proliferations can be very difficult to diagnose correctly. In the case of lesions in the periphery, it is often difficult to determine tumor

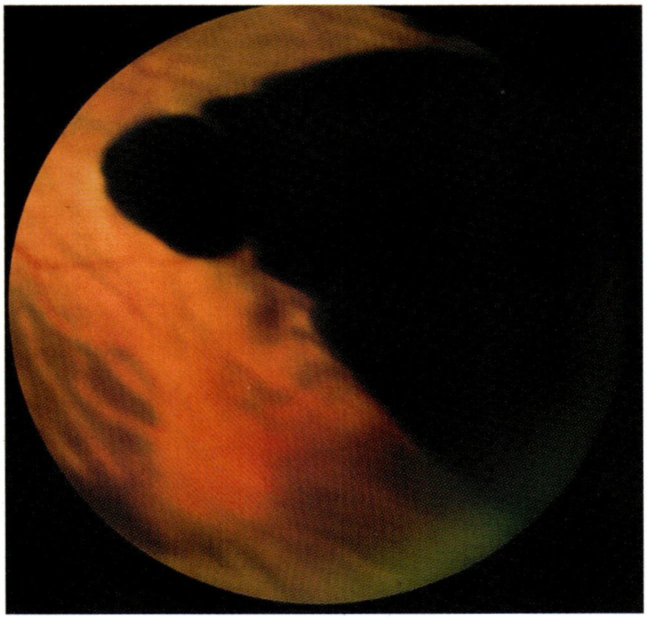

Figure 6–13. Grouped pigmentation, a forme fruste of RPE hypertrophy.

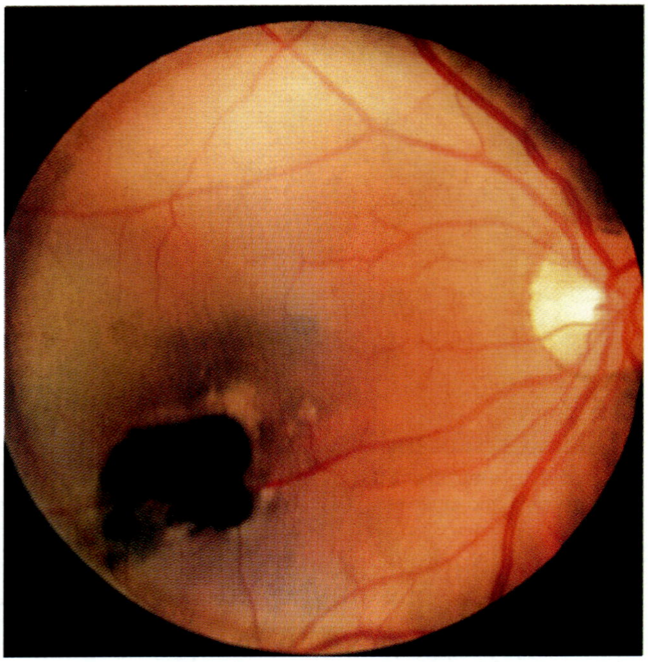

Figure 6–14. Retinal pigment epithelial hyperplasia with typically ragged margins. The nature of the margins and absence of lacunae help differentiate this acquired lesion from congenital RPE hypertrophy.

thickness. The patient shown in Figure 6–15 was referred for a melanoma because the flat nature of this RPE hypertrophy was not appreciated. In one case, even with a fine-needle aspiration biopsy (FNAB), the diagnosis was not established until after enucleation.[29]

Shields and colleagues, on the basis of some cases in which histologic data became available, have noted a typical feature of a prominant feeder vessel in elevated RPE adenomas. Figures 6–16 and 6–17 demonstrate such cases that we have followed up for many years, with lesions that almost look like small, black, mini-collar buttons with a feeder vessel.[30–32] These tumors are, presumably, RPE adenomas.

Adenocarcinomas of the RPE have been described, although they are quite rare and, fortunately, do not metastasize. An ultrasound may have a pattern different from a uveal melanoma.[32,33]

CHOROIDAL METASTASES

Differentiation of a uveal metastasis from a primary uveal melanoma can be difficult. Approximately 6 to 10 percent of patients with documented uveal melanomas have had another systemic malignancy treated previously.[34,35] We have not found an excess of systemic malignancies in uveal melanoma patients.[36] The finding of a past history of systemic malignancy on review of systems in a patient with a uveal tumor can present problems. We have managed several patients with uveal melanoma who were initially treated elsewhere with insufficient radiation because of their past medical history and an incorrect diagnosis of a presumed metastatic choroidal mass prior to

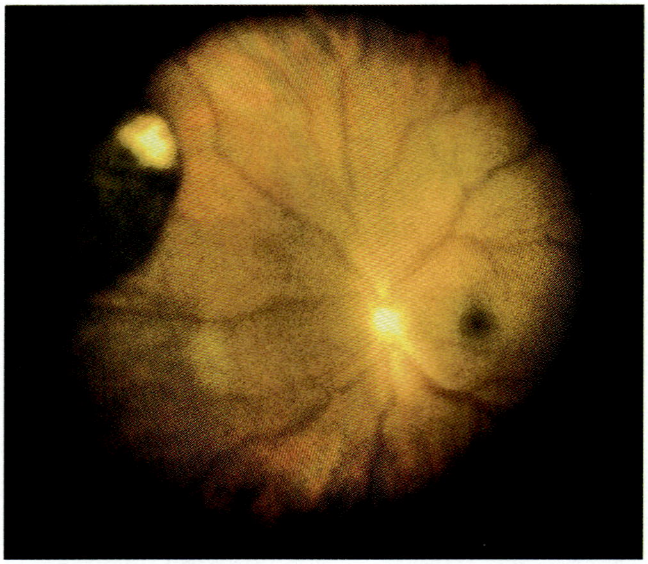

Figure 6–15. RPE proliferation in the periphery can appear to be elevated, when in reality, it is flat. In the former setting, it can simulate a uveal melanoma.

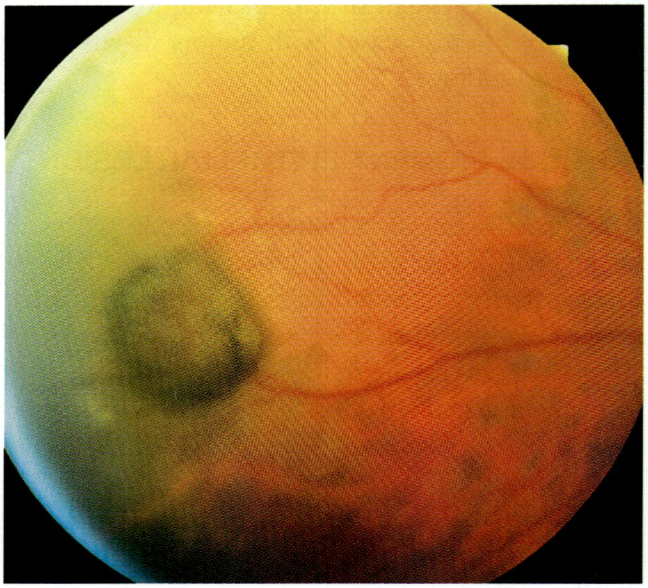

Figure 6–16. RPE adenoma with typical pseudo-collar button and feeder vessels.

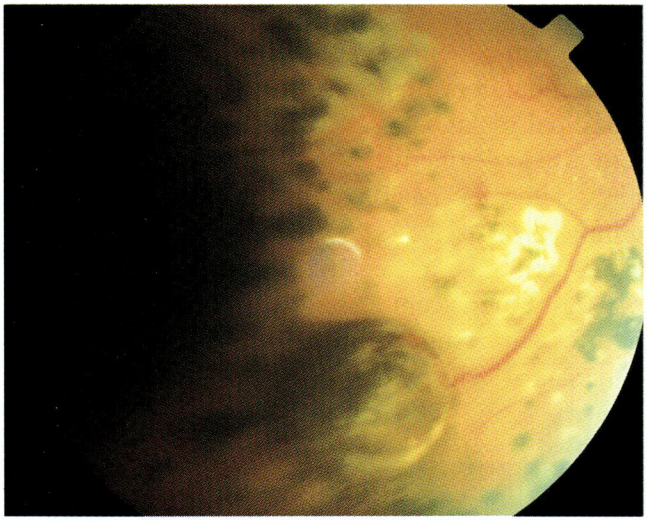

Figure 6–17. Another RPE adenoma similar to one shown in Figure 6–16.

their referral. In one patient with a history of localized breast carcinoma, 50 gray (Gy) of photon radiation plus combination chemotherapy was given for a choroidal nevus (Figure 6–18). Conversely, some patients have been treated for uveal melanomas but who have had obvious metastatic choroidal tumors.

Metastatic deposits in the uveal tract may be the first sign of a systemic malignancy in as many as 50 percent of patients.[37] The most common primary tumors that secondarily involve the choroid are breast, lung, kidney, gastrointestinal tract, and genitourinary tumors. In over 80 percent of patients with lung and renal tumor metastases, the eye lesion is the first manifestation of malignancy. In contrast, over 90 percent of patients with breast metastases to the uvea have a history of primary tumor treatment. In different series, the incidence of primary sites has varied.[38]

Metastatic choroidal tumors are amelanotic, usually involve the posterior pole, especially the macula, and are associated with subretinal fluid. In approximately one-fourth of cases, metastases to the uveal tract are bilateral and/or multifocal (Figure 6–19). Metastatic deposits are much less frequent in the optic nerve, retina, iris, ciliary body, or vitreous.[39,40] In a recent report from Philadelphia, the iris was involved in 9 percent, the ciliary body in 2 percent, and the choroid in 88 percent of uveal metastases.[41]

The mushroom shape or collar-button configuration associated with a uveal melanoma is almost never associated with a metastatic choroidal tumor. In one such case with a mini-collar button, the patient was diagnosed elsewhere with a presumed choroidal metastasis on the basis of a known primary. This patient was referred to the author after she failed to respond to 40 Gy of photon radiation. Cytology confirmed that the correct diagnosis was a uveal melanoma. There is no intrinsic tumor pigmentation in uveal metastases; however, overlying RPE alteration may produce hyperplastic RPE pigmentation. The clinical pattern of different histologic types of metastatic tumors is not diagnostic. Breast carcinomas metastatic to the uveal tract often have a peau d'orange pattern of pigmentary alteration (Figure 6–20). Metastatic foci can be quite large, as the tumor shown in Figure 6–21 demonstrates.

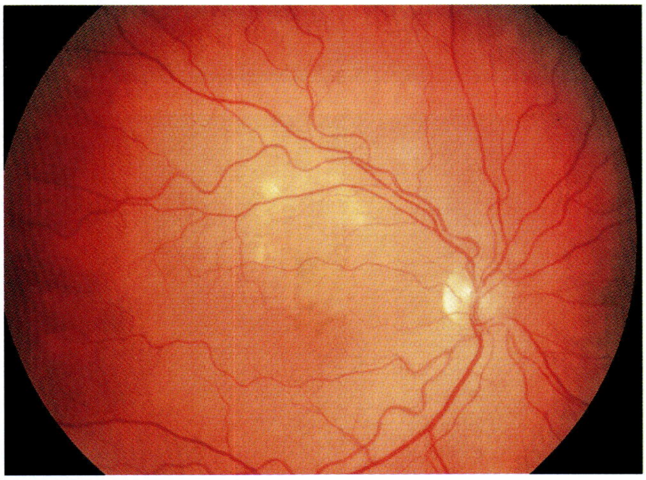

Figure 6–18. A history of treated breast carcinoma led to radiation and chemotherapy for a presumed choroidal nevus.

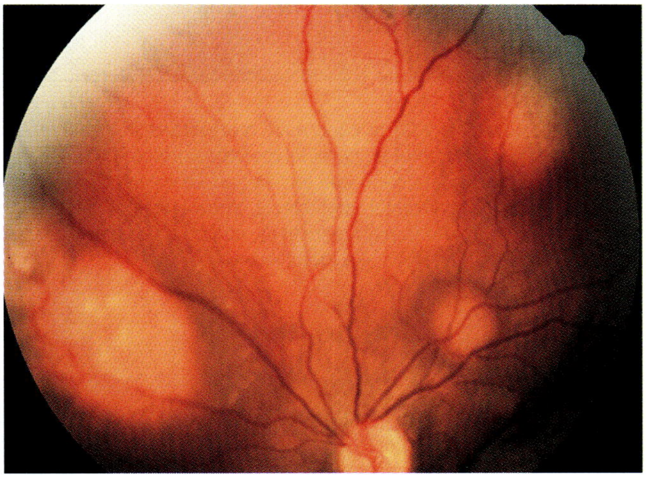

Figure 6–19. Multiple amelanotic tumors in a patient with bilateral uveal metastases.

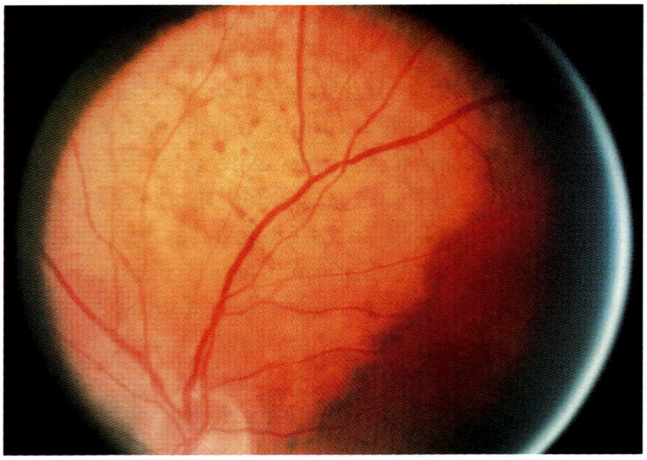

Figure 6–20. A breast carcinoma with a typical peau d'orange pattern.

The metastasis pattern on both B-scan and quantitative echography is often distinctive and differs from that of a uveal melanoma.[42] Figure 6–21B is an immersion B-scan of the pancreatic metastasis shown in Figure 6–21A. There is a solid choroidal tumor without an acoustic quiet zone, choroidal excavation, or orbital shadowing usually observed in choroidal melanomas. The quantitative A-scan pattern is also distinctive. The reflectivity is medium to high; often the back portion of the tumor pattern climbs towards the sclera (arrow), a finding sometimes termed "a negative-angle kappa" (Figure 6–21C). Fluorescein angiography is not particularly helpful in establishing a diagnosis in these patients.[43,44] The plasma carcinoembryonic antigen

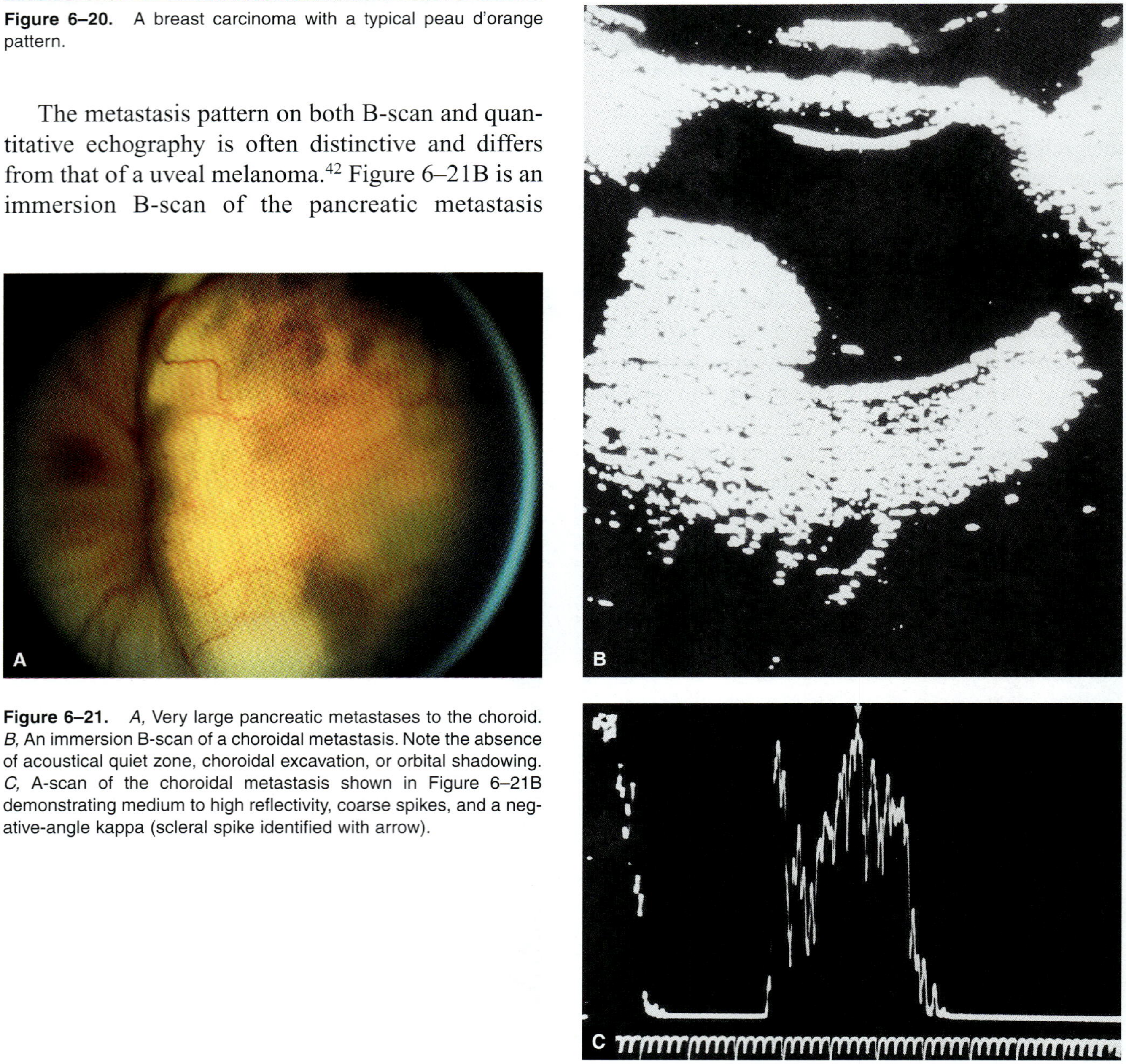

Figure 6–21. *A,* Very large pancreatic metastases to the choroid. *B,* An immersion B-scan of a choroidal metastasis. Note the absence of acoustical quiet zone, choroidal excavation, or orbital shadowing. *C,* A-scan of the choroidal metastasis shown in Figure 6–21B demonstrating medium to high reflectivity, coarse spikes, and a negative-angle kappa (scleral spike identified with arrow).

(CEA) level is elevated above 10 ng/mL in approximately 50 percent of these cases versus almost no uveal melanoma patients.[45]

In some cases, the clinical and ultrasonographic pattern in metastatic uveal tumors is not clear cut (Figures 6–22A to C).[46,47] As described below, FNAB has been a very important adjunct in cases with atypical choroidal metastases.[39,48–52]

The reason for the relative incidence of choroidal metastases as compared with other ocular sites is uncertain. The choroid has, perhaps, the highest blood flow of any body site.[53] In approximately, 3 to 4 percent of metastatic carcinoma patients, a primary malignancy is not identifiable; in referral centers, this incidence is approximately 10 percent.[54]

Rarely, metastases to the choroid can occur many years after the primary tumor has been treated or removed.[55] This can be especially true with carcinoid tumors and renal cell carcinoma, and in one case, ocular metastases were discovered 9 years after resection of the primary lesion.[56] The pattern of metastases is partially predicated on the vascular endothelial differences as well as surface antigens of the tumors.[57] The treatment of metastatic choroidal tumors is discussed in Chapter 8. Depending on the systemic status of the patient, this can include chemotherapy, conventional teletherapy, laser, or brachytherapy.

CHOROIDAL HEMANGIOMA

Choroidal hemangiomas may occur as solitary, focal lesions or as a diffuse process, often in association with Sturge-Weber syndrome.[58–60] The focal lesions have a typical clinical pattern; they are moderately elevated (2 to 5 mm) pinkish-orange lesions, often with overlying subretinal fluid (Figure 6–23). The fluorescein angiographic pattern is believed by some to be diagnostic; however, we have seen two patients with typical patterns, in whom we histologically confirmed the diagnosis of a melanoma.[59,60] On fluorescein angiography, the lesion is usually characterized by early lobular filling of the choroidal ves-

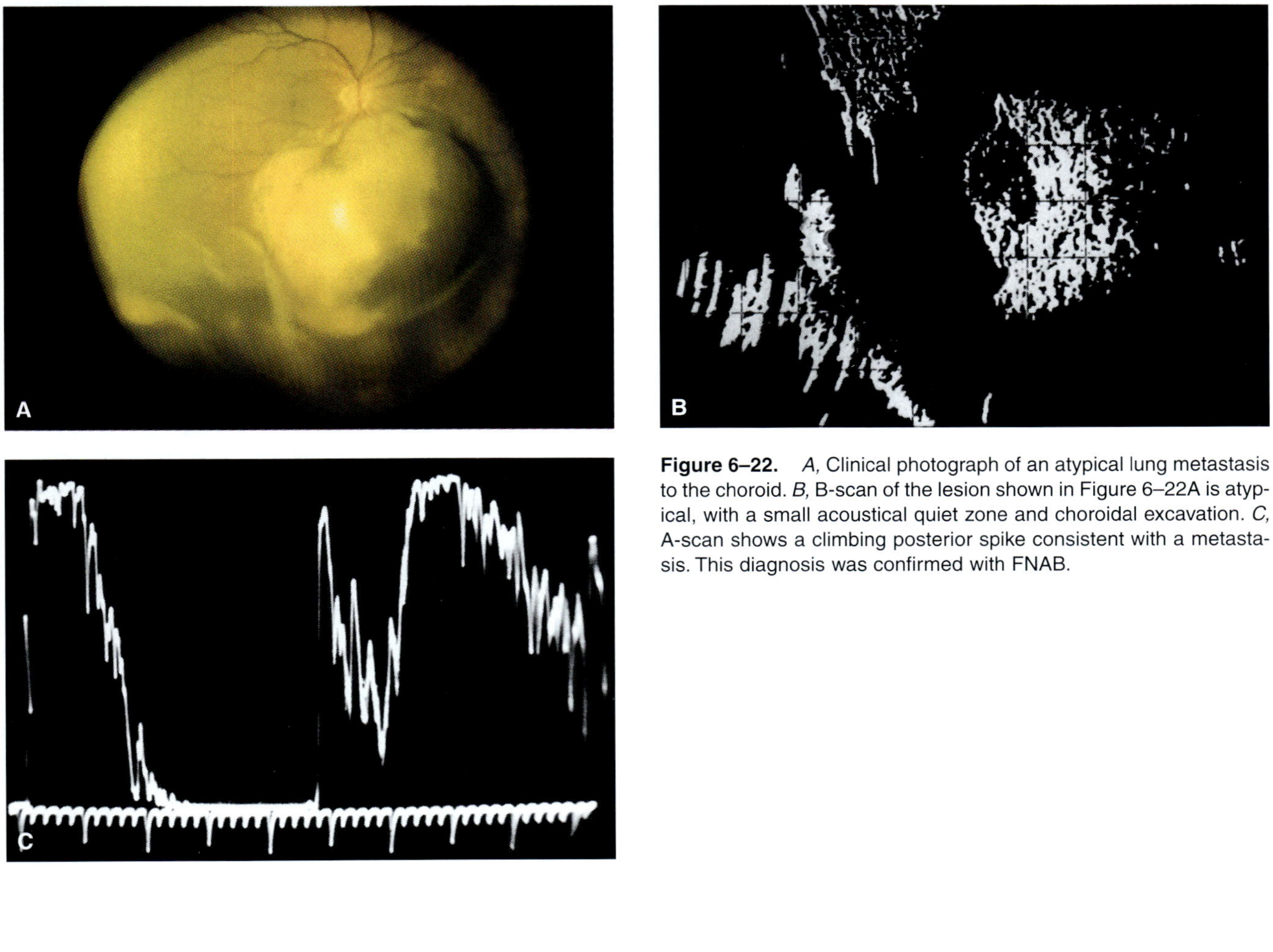

Figure 6–22. *A,* Clinical photograph of an atypical lung metastasis to the choroid. *B,* B-scan of the lesion shown in Figure 6–22A is atypical, with a small acoustical quiet zone and choroidal excavation. *C,* A-scan shows a climbing posterior spike consistent with a metastasis. This diagnosis was confirmed with FNAB.

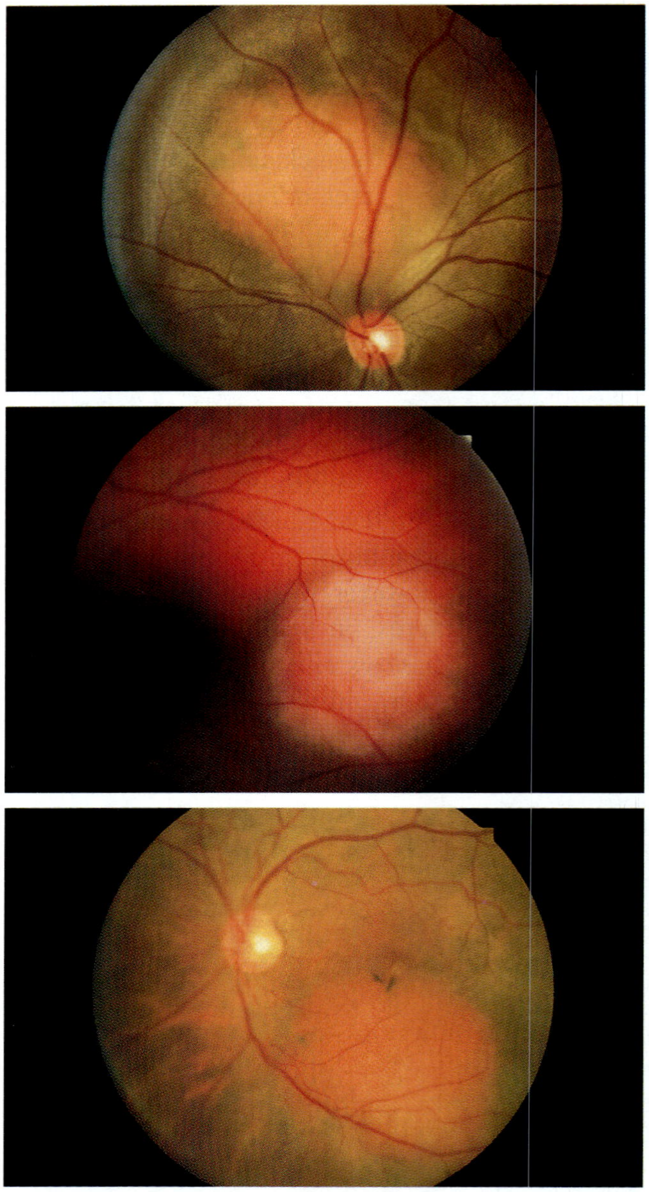

Figure 6–23. Solitary choroidal hemangiomas.

sels in the area of the tumor prior to filling of the retinal vessels (Figures 6–24A and B). The ultrasonographic pattern is diagnostic. The B-scan appearance is similar in some respects to a metastasis; a choroidal hemangioma appears solid without choroidal excavation, acoustic quiet zone, or orbital shadowing (Figure 6–25A). On A-scan, the lesion has uniform high reflectivity (Figure 6–25B).

These tumors have rarely been demonstrated to grow. In one report, Medlock and colleagues noted 5 patients who showed an enlargement, with a mean interval of 52 months.[61] We have recently examined a patient who was intially seen with 20/20 vision with a small macular lesion, who demonstrated growth over an interval of 10 years (Figures 6–26A and B). These tumors can also produce choroidal neovascularization.[62] Rarely, these have been documented to spontaneously resolve and produce a chorioretinal scar.[62] In diffuse choroidal hemangiomas, usually associated with Sturge-Weber syndrome, diagnosis is often straightforward. Patients have distinct facial features, and the entire posterior pole of the affected eye is usually involved (Figures 6–27A to C).[46] The managment of choroidal hemangiomas is covered in Chapter 8.

MACULAR AND EXTRAMACULAR DISCIFORM LESIONS

Involutional macular disciform lesions (AMD) can simulate a melanoma, especially if the patient has

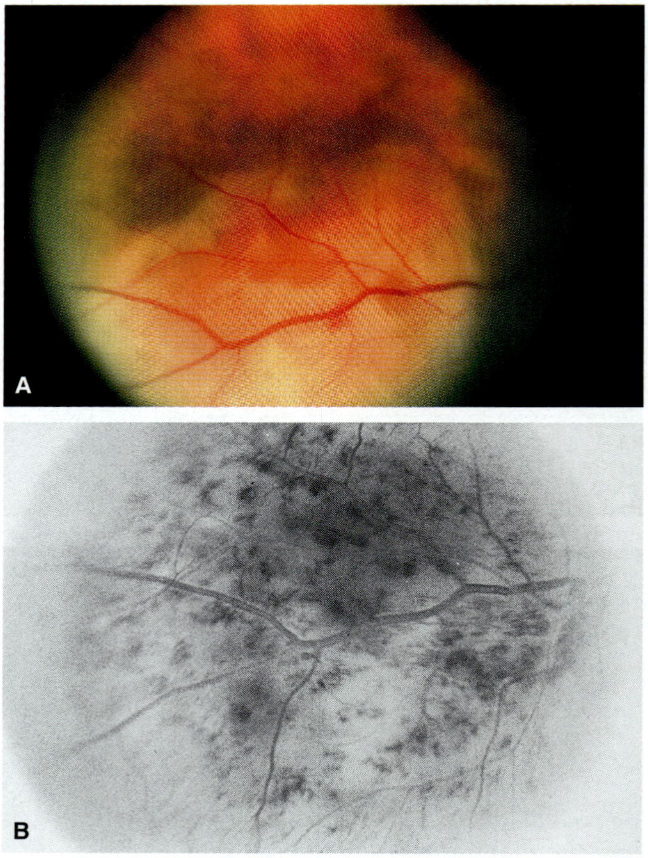

Figure 6–24. *A,* Clinical photograph of a choroidal hemangioma with a typical orangish-pink coloration. *B,* Early lobular fluorescence prior to the filling of retinal vessels, typical for a choroidal hemangioma. (Fluorescein angiogram of Figure 6–24A: early lobular fluorescence).

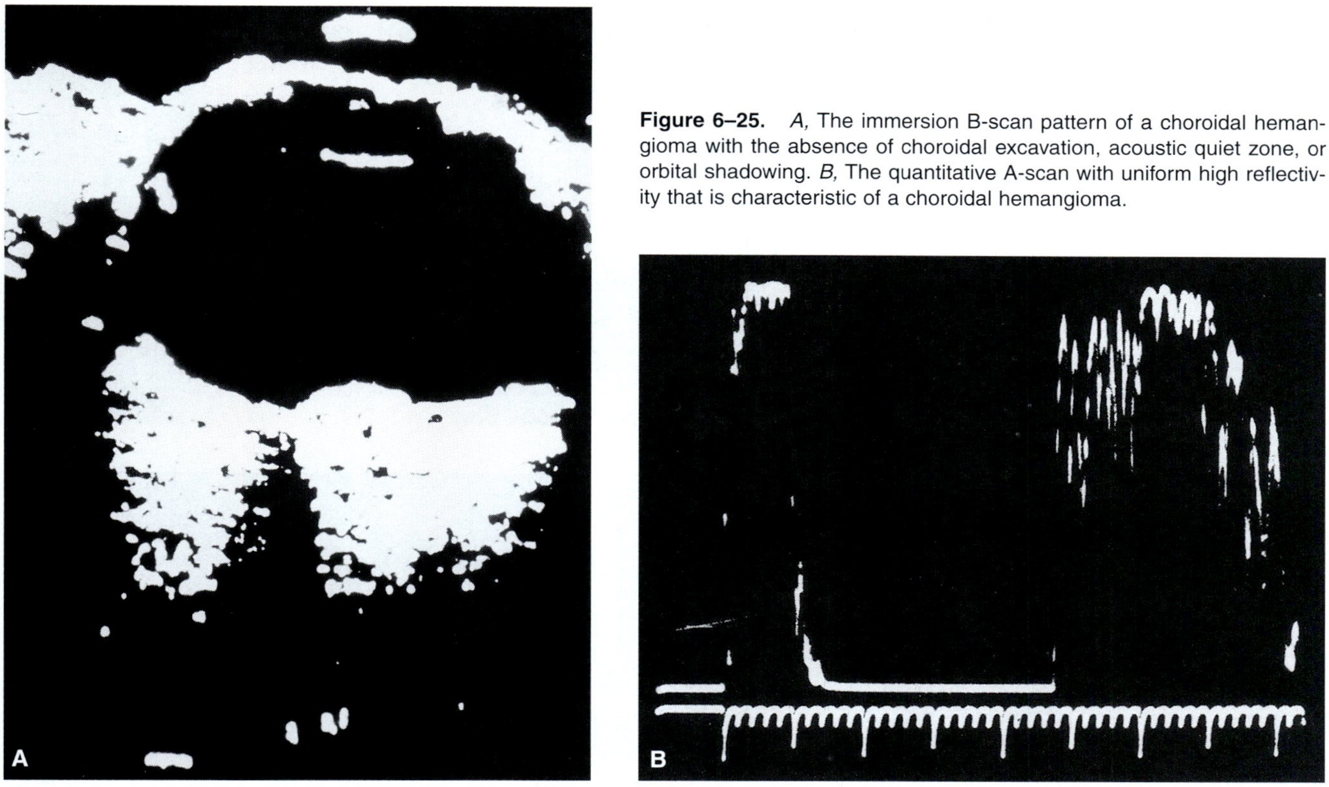

Figure 6–25. *A,* The immersion B-scan pattern of a choroidal hemangioma with the absence of choroidal excavation, acoustic quiet zone, or orbital shadowing. *B,* The quantitative A-scan with uniform high reflectivity that is characteristic of a choroidal hemangioma.

markedly asymmetric disease, or if the lesion occurs outside the anatomic macula (Figures 6–28 and 6–29). It is important to evaluate the contralateral macula in any patient suspected of harboring a foveal uveal melanoma, since the finding of macular degeneration in the contralateral eye helps to determine the true nature of the lesion (Figures 6–30A and B). Hemorrhage, as seen in Figures 6–28 and 6–29, would be very unusual in a uveal melanoma this thin; melanomas generally only produce a vitreous hemorrhage when an overlying retinal vessel is torn as the tumor breaks through Bruch's membrane. Lipid exudation is also common in a disciform process but relatively rare in an untreated melanoma. The ultra-

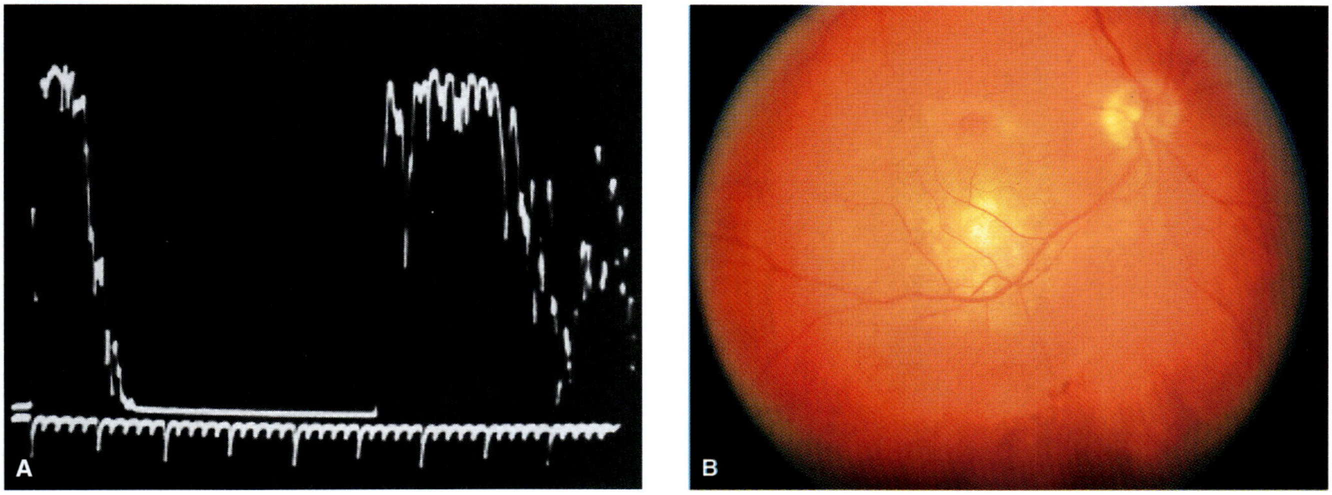

Figure 6–26. *A,* Nondiagnostic A-scan demonstrating a lesion of approximately 2.3 mm thickness. *B,* A scan 10 years later showing lesion grown to 3.4 mm thickness and has a typical pattern of a choroidal hemangioma.

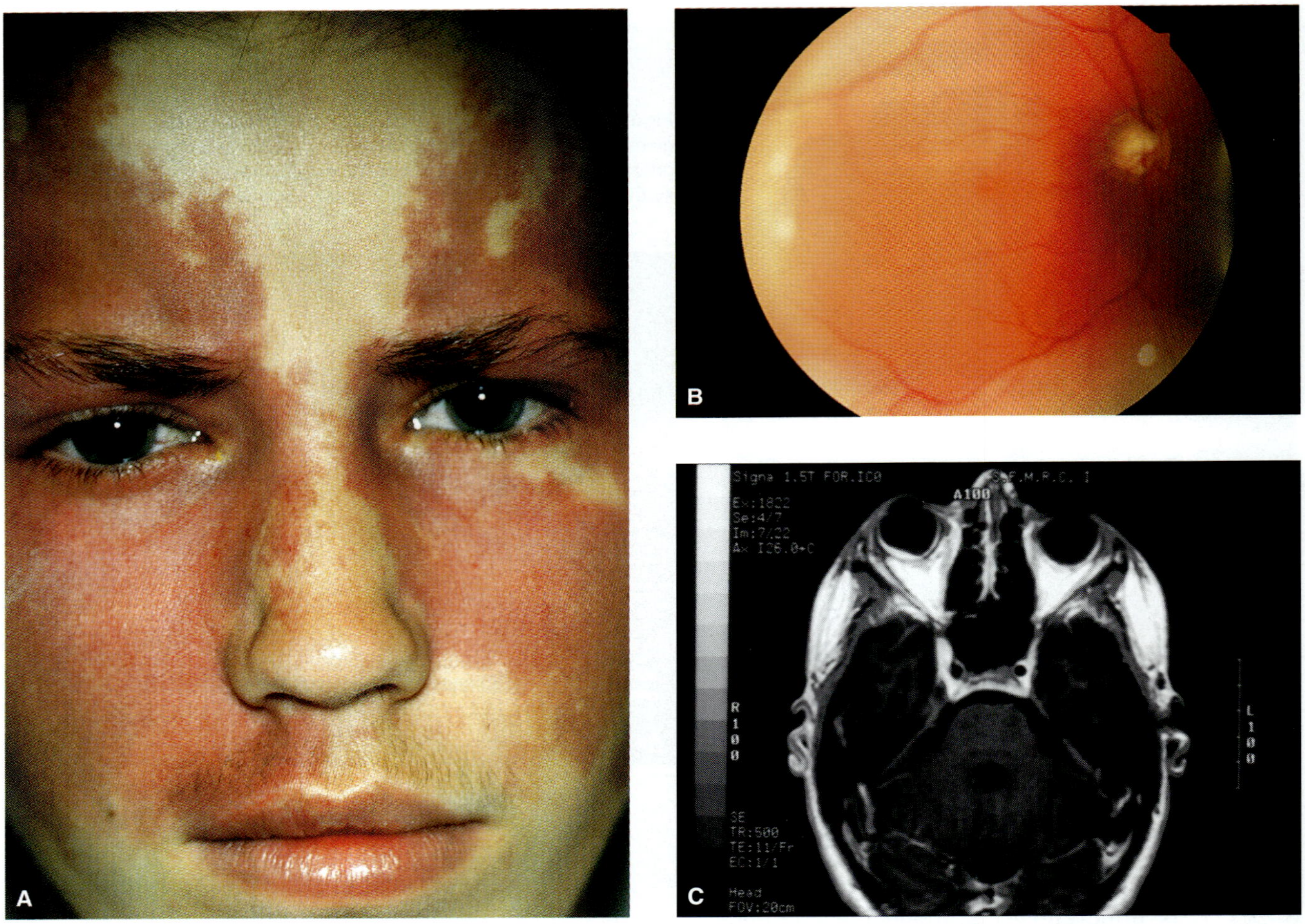

Figure 6–27. *A,* Patients with diffuse hemangiomas often have distinct facial features. *B,* The entire posterior pole is involved; a shallow exudative detachment has decreased visual acuity. *C,* T_1-weighted axial MRI shows the diffuse nature of this hemangioma.

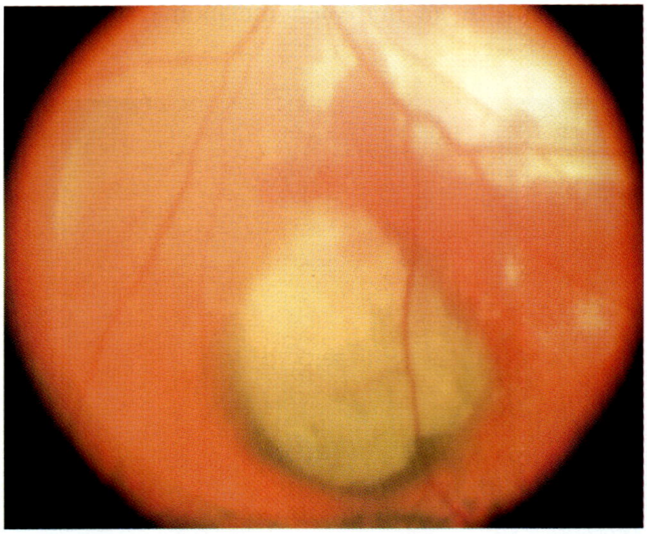

Figure 6–28. Clinical photograph of an extramacular disciform lesion simulating a uveal melanoma. Hemorrhage is very uncommon with a choroidal melanoma, unless it is thick enough to have broken through Bruch's membrane.

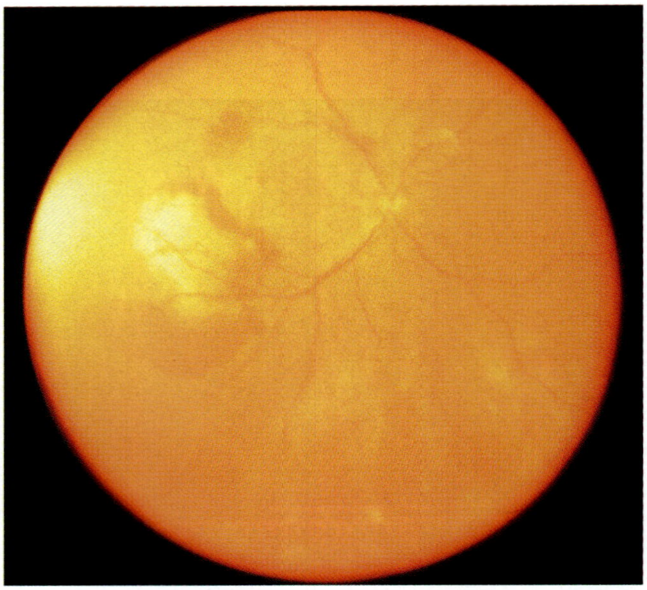

Figure 6–29. Example of an extramacular disciform lesion with exudate and hemorrhage.

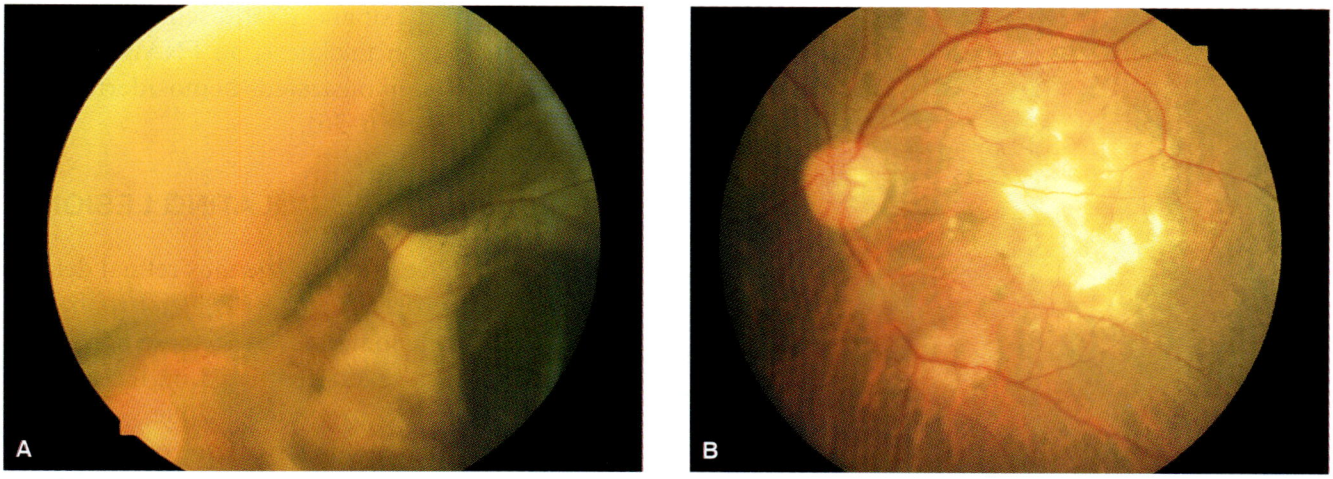

Figure 6–30. *A,* Large tumor with exudate superior. The clinical features of the mass are most consistent with old blood. *B,* The contralateral fundus shows age-related macular degeneration.

sonographic pattern of subretinal hemorrhage on both A-scan and B-scan can simulate a melanoma; however, often the acoustic quiet zone is not as homogeneous on B-scan, and on A-scan, there are no vascular pulsations and higher internal reflectivity (Figures 6–31A and B). The fluorescein angiogram in these patients with AMD and extramacular disciform (EMD) lesions is sometimes useful; there is no intrinsic tumor vasculature, and the underlying choroidal vasculature is obscured by hemorrhage (Figure 6–32). In patients referred to an oncology unit because of a diffuse vitreous hemorrhage, it is more likely caused by an extraocular disciform lesion than by a uveal melanoma, particularly if the lesion is < 5 mm in elevation. While MRI may be useful, given that on acute hemorrhage has a pattern different from that of a melanoma, we have observed a number of errors where MRI scans had been used to attempt to establish the diagnosis. The patient shown in Figure 6–33 had an MRI pattern consistent with a melanoma. As seen in Figure 6–34, a serial observation demonstrated shrinkage of this EMD lesion. These lesions can also sometimes simulate an RPE rip.[62] Rarely, we have observed these lesions to enlarge transiently. Figures 6–35A and B demonstrate such a case in which the patient was followed

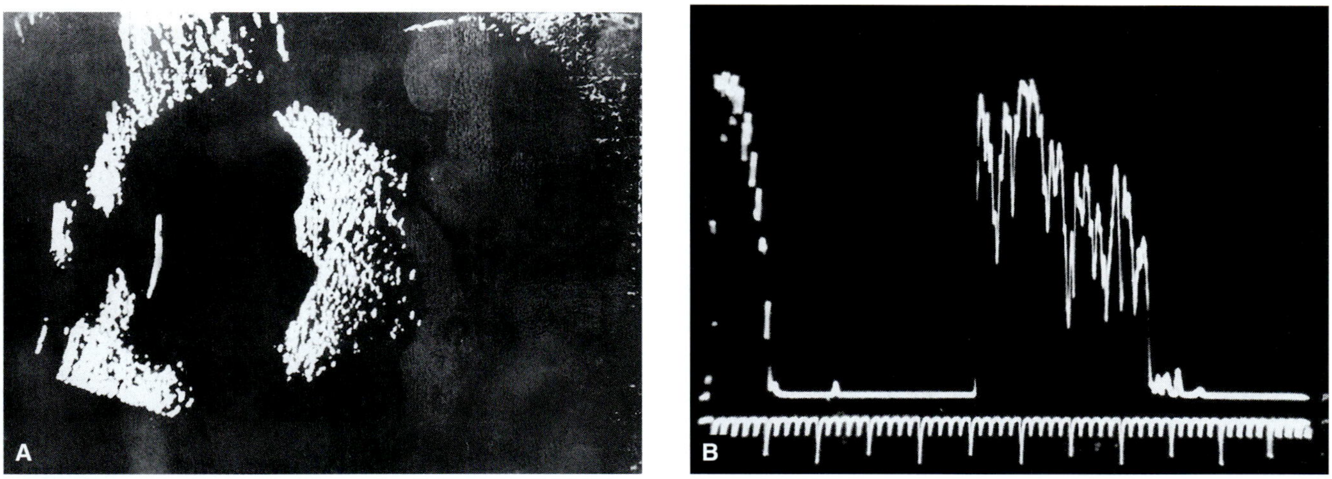

Figure 6–31. *A,* An immersion B-scan pattern of a subretinal hemorrhage that clinically simulated a choroidal melanoma. These sometimes can have an acoustical quiet zone (not present) and choroidal excavation (not seen). *B,* The A-scan pattern of a subretinal hemorrhage shown in Figure 6–31A. While this case has a diagnostic ultrasound, in some hemorrhagic processes, we have noted almost perfect simulation of a melanoma, except for the absence of vascular pulsations.

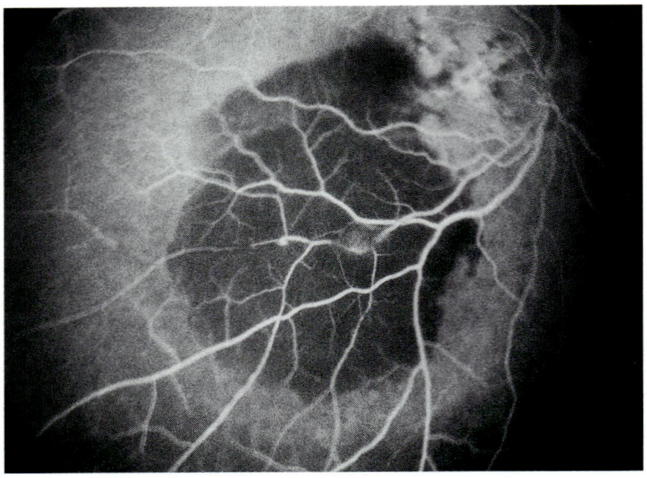

Figure 6–32. A fluorescein angiogram of a subretinal hemorrhage showing no intrinsic vasculature and blockage.

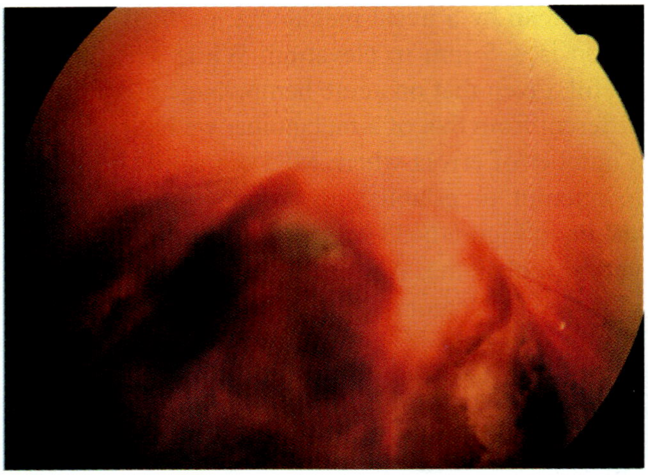

Figure 6–33. A clinical photograph of extramacular disciform with MRI features of uveal melanoma.

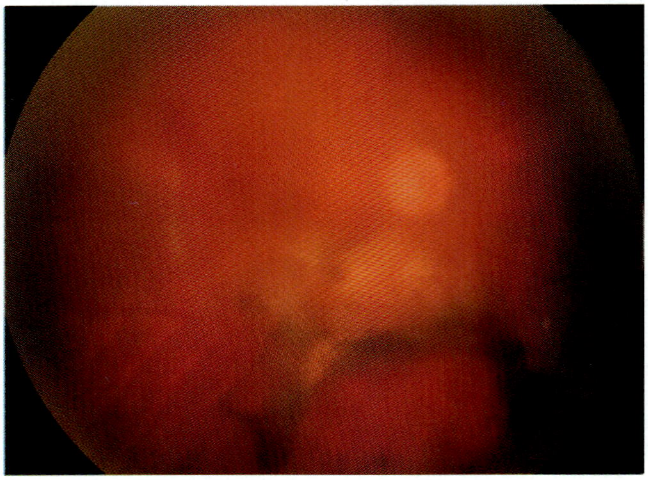

Figure 6–34. Serial follow-up shows involution of the lesion shown in Figure 6–33.

up for a presumed extramacullar disciform. When it enlarged > 2 mm in thickness, an FNAB was performed, which demonstrated hemosiderin-laden macrophages (Figure 6–36).

MISCELLANEOUS SIMULATING LESIONS

As discussed above, rhegmatogenous retinal detachment, RPE hyperplasia, and RPE hypertrophy can all simulate a melanoma; however, these conditions can almost always be differentiated on the basis of indirect ophthalmoscopy findings alone.

A melanocytoma not involving the optic disc can be difficult to diagnose; a uniform jet black color is more consistent with a diagnosis of melanocytoma than one of uveal melanoma.[62,63] Rarely, melanocytomas present in children and diffusely involve the

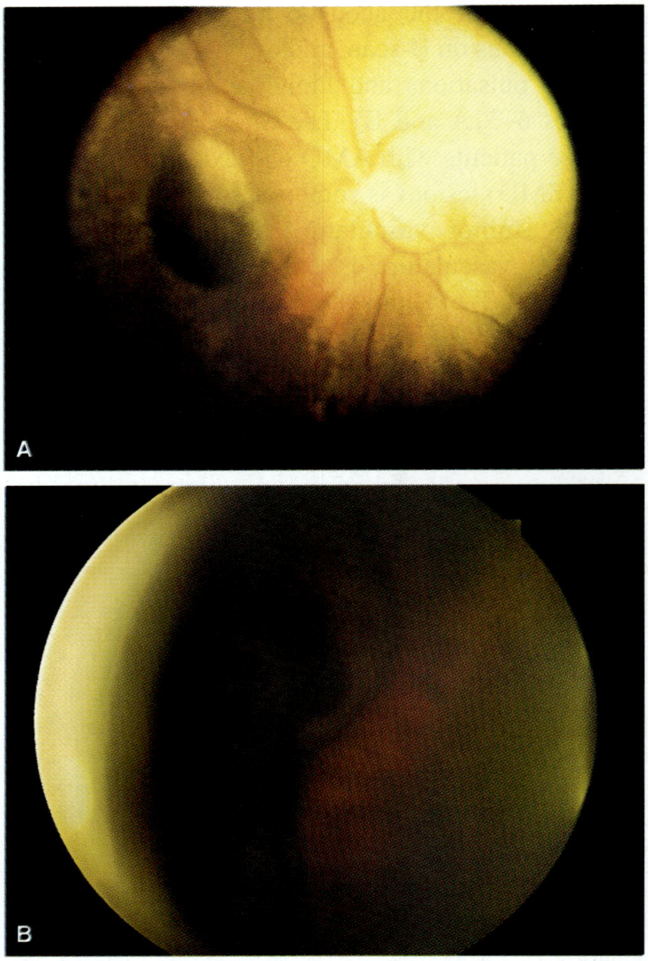

Figure 6–35. *A*, Extramacular disciform lesion prior to growth. *B*, Same patient 6 months later, demonstrating a 2-mm enlargement of the lesion without any obvious hemorrhage.

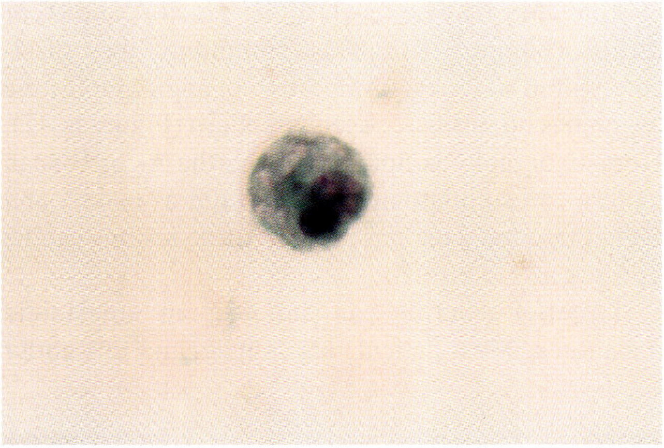

Figure 6–36. Fine-needle biopsy of the lesion shown in Figure 6–35 with hemosiderin-laden macrophages. This lesion shrank over the next year.

choroid.[63] We have monitored the lesion shown in Figure 6–37, a presumed peripheral uveal melanocytoma, for 20 years and observed no change. Melanocytomas can undergo necrosis, and in one report, 10 of 23 had that feature. Figure 6–38 shows an FNAB- confirmed melanocytoma approximately 8 mm thick. Six years after biopsy, the lesion remained stable, and vision was still 20/20. As discussed previously, melanocytoma can perfectly simulate the MRI or ultrasound pattern of a melanoma, as was noted in this case. Occasionally, they can also undergo malignant degeneration.[64,65]

A choroidal osteoma can appear similar to a metastatic tumor, sclerochoroidal calcification, or an amelanotic melanoma on ophthalmoscopic examination.[66–71] Clinically, choroidal osteomas are amelanotic and relatively flat with an irregular surface and may grow. A typical lesion is shown in Figure 6–39A. On fluorescein angiography, there is often an area of capillary tufting circumferentially (Figure 6–39B). Intralesional calcium is visible by ultrasonography or computed tomography (CT) (Figures 6–39C and D). While intralesional calcium is classic for an osteoma, we as well as others have seen that only rarely in choroidal melanomas.[72] Usually, osteomas are more common in women in their 20s and 30s, and approximately 75 percent are unilateral.[73]

Approximately 70 choroidal osteomas have been reported. They usually occur near the optic nerve. Rarely, they have been reported to have developed in later life; two siblings were noted to have normal fundi at an earlier age and then developed this process.[74] Occasionally, patients develop these lesions in an area of previous uveitis, and one-quarter of cases have been bilateral. In young children, these lesions can occasionally be diagnosed when there is rapid enlargement.[75] In other familial reports, bilateral disease has been documented.[76] While initially most patients have had good vision, almost one-half eventually develop poor vision due to retinal atrophy

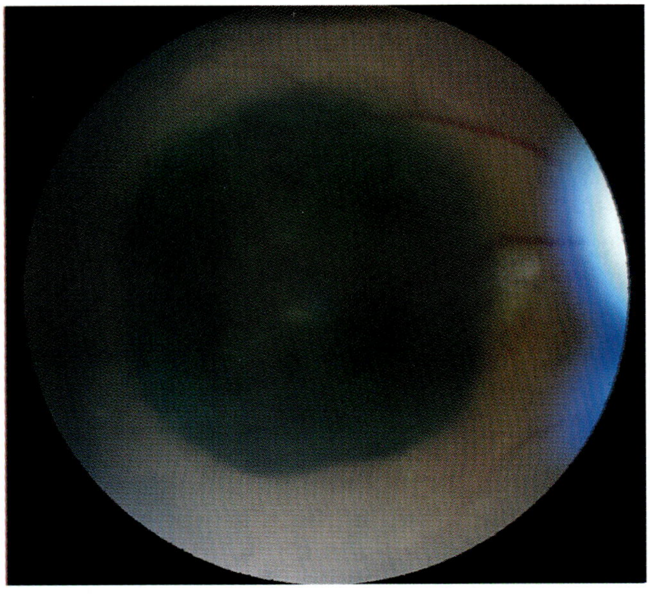

Figure 6–37. A uveal melanocytoma, which has been followed up for 15 years, without change.

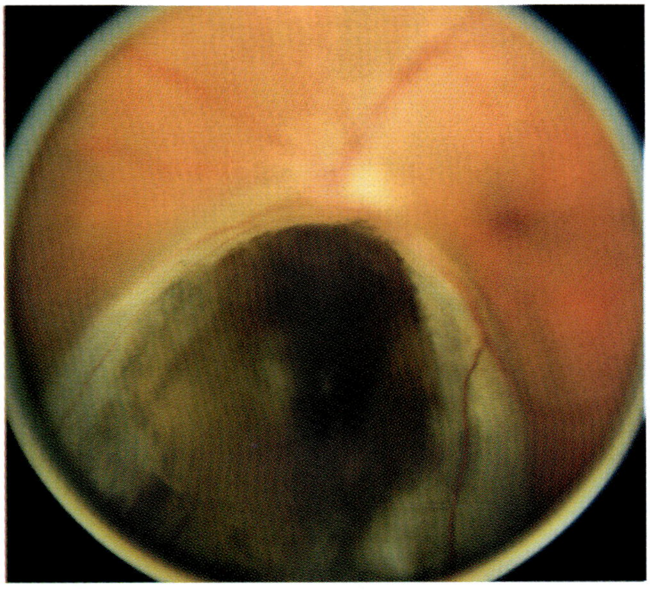

Figure 6–38. An 8-mm thick melanocytoma with good vision 6 years after FNAB-confirmed diagnosis.

or subretinal neovascularization. In a series from the Bascom Palmer Institute, with a mean follow-up of 10 years, growth was observed in 9 of the 36 patients studied and visual loss to ≤ 20/200 was noted in 58 percent of the cases, mainly from choroidal vascularization.[77]

Choroidal detachments, especially those after cataract surgery, can also be mistaken for melanoma.[78] While these usually occur after prolonged hypotony and involve a large area of the choroid, they may be focal (Figures 6–40A and B) or diffuse (Figure 6–41). Most commonly, they dissipate within 6 weeks; on fluorescein angiography, the lesion has no intrinsic vascular pattern (Figure 6–42). Ultrasonography is not diagnostic; the A- or B-scan pattern can simulate melanoma (Figures 6–43A and B) in these focal lesions. Rarely, these lesions can be as thick as 5.5 mm.[79]

Posterior scleritis can simulate an amelanotic melanoma. Most patients are female, and this entity

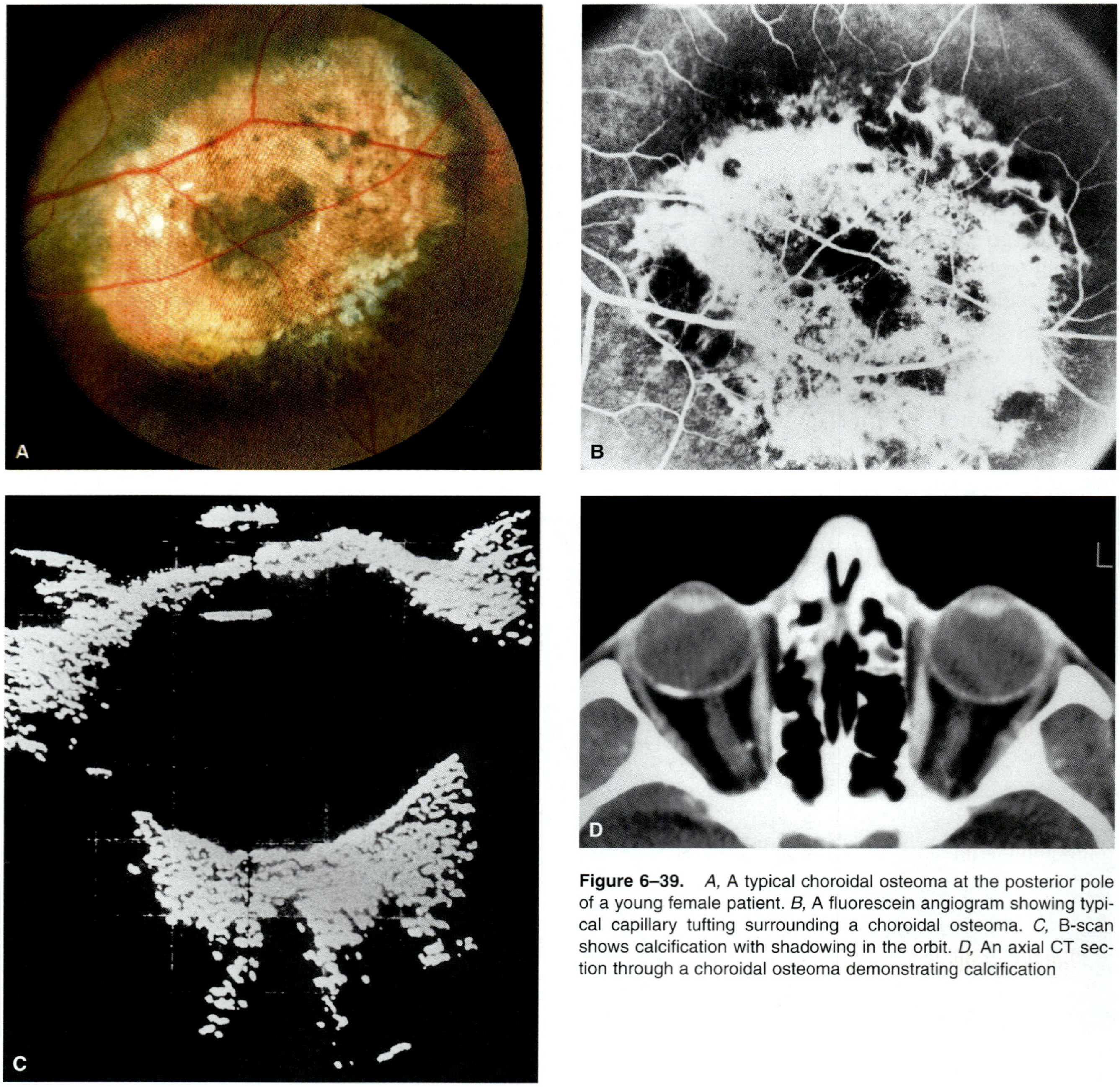

Figure 6–39. *A,* A typical choroidal osteoma at the posterior pole of a young female patient. *B,* A fluorescein angiogram showing typical capillary tufting surrounding a choroidal osteoma. *C,* B-scan shows calcification with shadowing in the orbit. *D,* An axial CT section through a choroidal osteoma demonstrating calcification

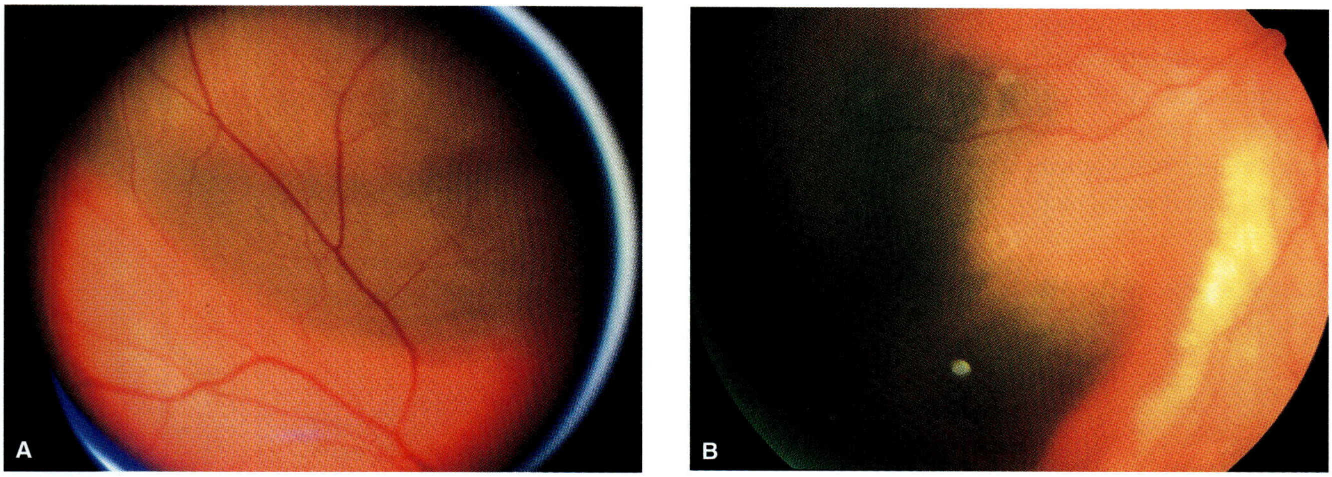

Figure 6–40. *A,* A focal choroidal detachment occurring after cataract surgery; 6 weeks later, the lesion had entirely dissipated. *B,* A focal hemorrhage after cataract extraction.

often occurs in association with rheumatoid disease.[80] Patients often present with a deep boring pain, especially during ocular versions. The ultrasonographic pattern (Figure 6–44), often with fluid in Tenon's space, is typical; the CT pattern, as shown in Figure 6–45, is also characteristic. Clinically, there may be an associated exudative detachment over an amelanotic lesion, with associated choroidal folds. Occasionally, anterior extension of the scleritis is noted. Rarely, a metastatic focus can simulate this entity, as in the testicular uveal metastasis shown in Figure 6–46. Rarely, a plaque-like melanoma can simulate scleritis and even partially respond to corticosteroids.[81,82]

There are a myriad of other lesions that can simulate uveal melanoma.[83] As an example, in the patient shown in Figures 6–47A and B, there was a longstanding rheumatoid arthritis and probably an old inactive scleritis. Alternatively, this lesion could have been a herniation of the vortex vein wall, but the author thinks that is less likely. On the patient looking up, a small tumor was noted (see Figure 6–47A). When the patient looked down, the tumor disappeared.

Rarely, lymphoid lesions can simulate uveal melanoma. Many of these tumors will have a classic fleshy pink subconjunctival change in association with diffuse choroidal thickening. Often, on ultrasonography, these lesions have vascularity noted.[83–85]

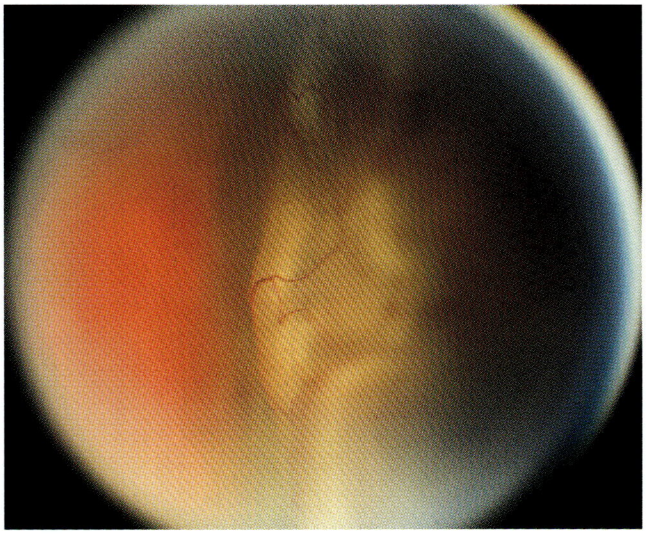

Figure 6–41. A diffuse choroidal detachment.

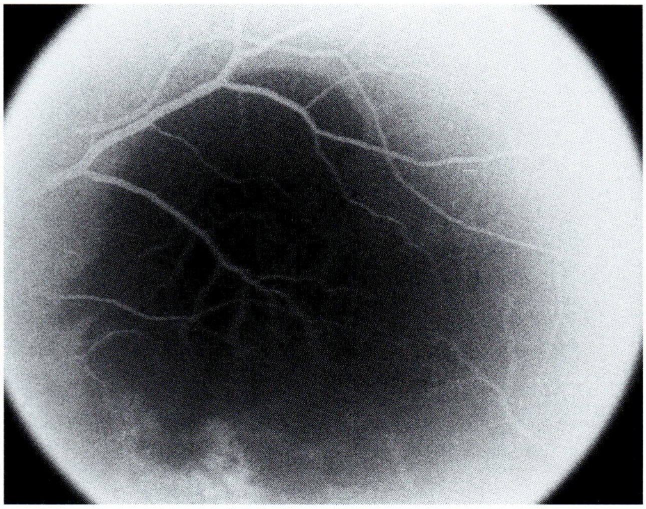

Figure 6–42. A fluorescein angiogram of a focal choroidal detachment with no evidence of intrinsic vasculature.

As many case reports have documented, most rare simulating tumefactions have had clinical, fluorescein, or ultrasound characteristics of melanoma, and the correct diagnosis only became apparent when the eye was studied histologically.[86–92] In many such cases, growth was documented prior to enucleation. Unfor-

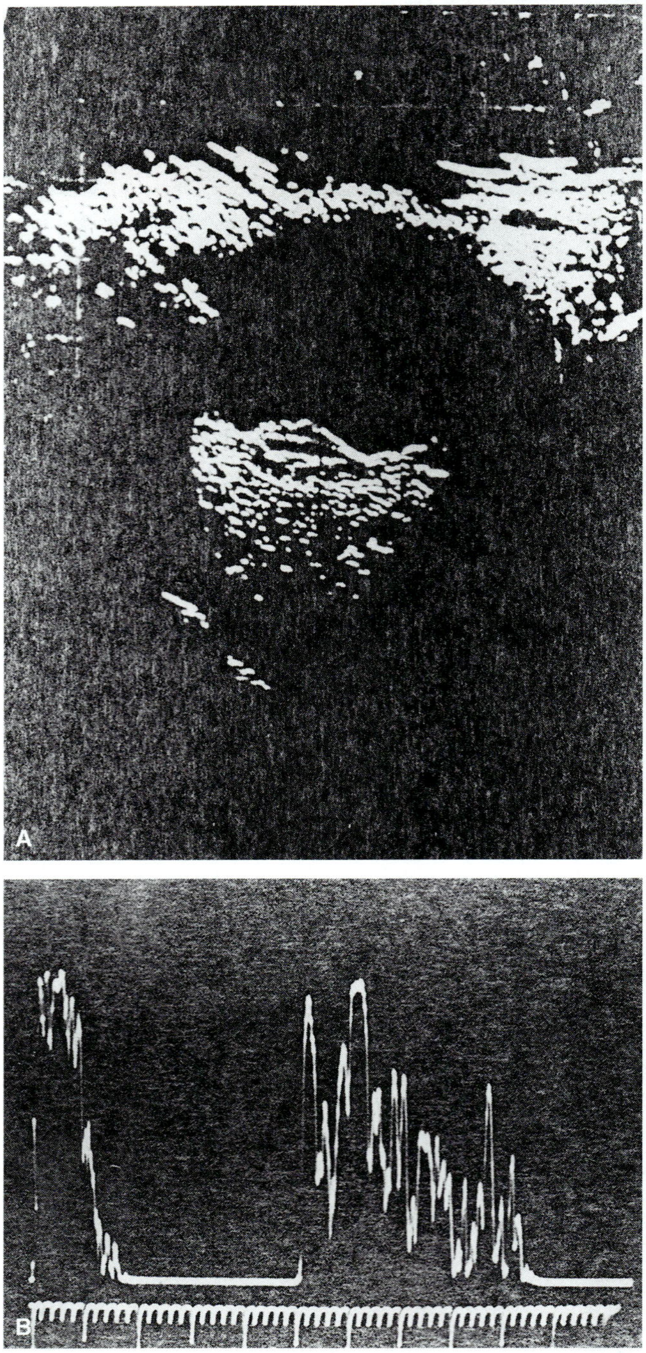

Figure 6–43. *A,* An immersion B-scan of a focal choroidal detachment after cataract surgery which disappeared within 3 months. *B,* A-scan pattern of the choroidal detachment.

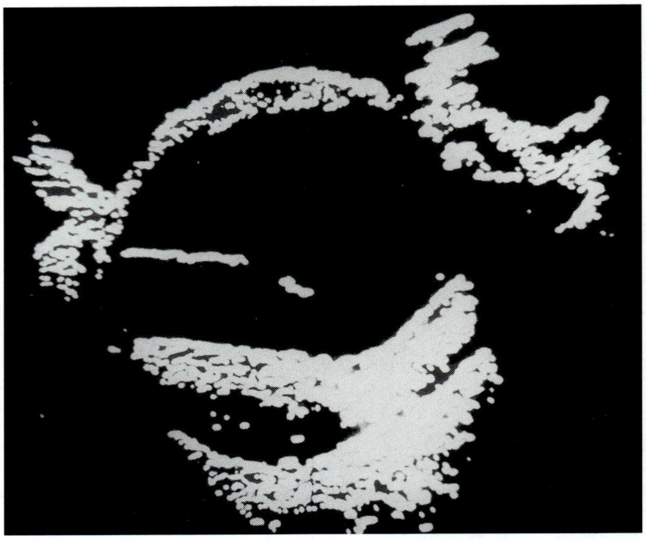

Figure 6–44. An ultrasound pattern showing typical fluid in Tenon's space and an edematous sclera in posterior scleritis.

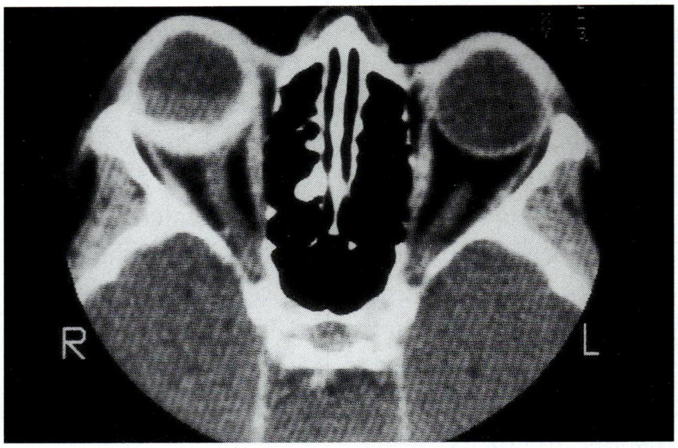

Figure 6–45. A brawny sclera on a CT study of a posterior scleritis.

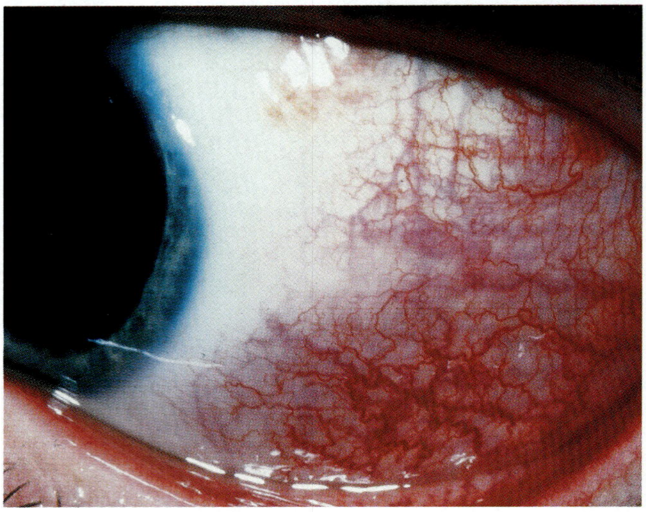

Figure 6–46. Simulating scleritis. A uveal testicular metastasis.

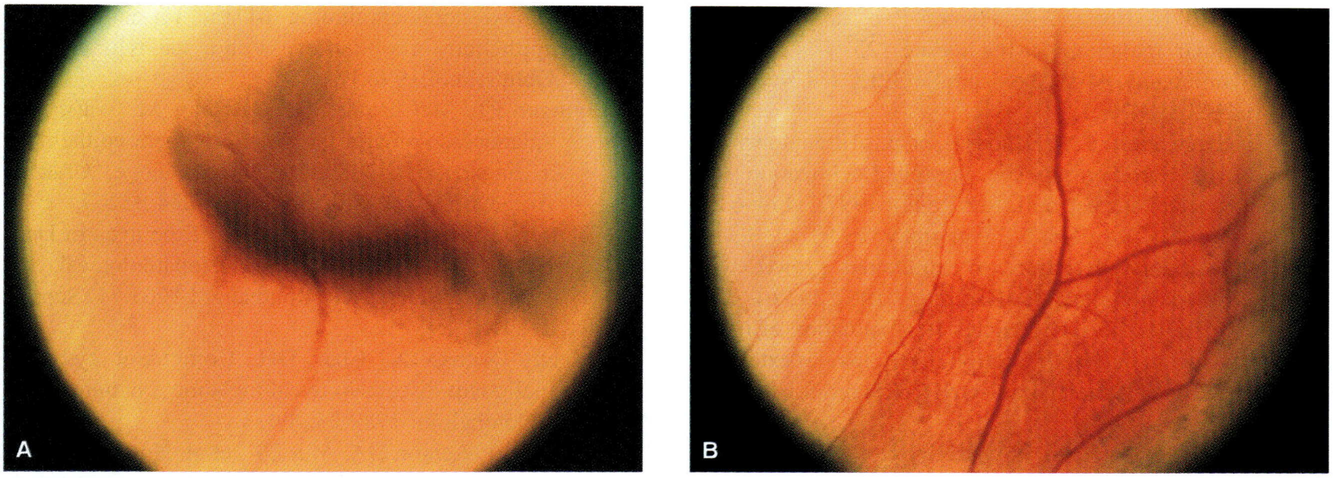

Figure 6–47. *A,* Rheumatoid arthritis patient with presumed inactive scleritis. In upgaze, there is a small tumor. *B,* On downgaze, the tumor shown in Figure 6–47A has disappeared.

tunately, many of these unusual simulating lesions cannot be correctly diagnosed with noninvasive techniques. As discussed in a later chapter, FNAB may decrease enucleation of these very atypical simulating lesions. There are insufficient data to determine the diagnostic accuracy and sensitivity of that technique with atypical pseudomelanomas. In one report, however, FNAB data altered the therapeutic plan in 48 percent of the patients who had this procedure.[93] In our experience, as discussed in Chapter 8, it has altered the management in about 10 percent of cases.

REFERENCES

1. Flindall RJ, Drance SM. Visual field studies of benign choroidal melanomata. Arch Ophthalmol 1969; 81:41–4.
2. Gass JD, Gieser RG, Wilkinson CP, et al. Bilateral diffuse uveal melanocytic proliferation in patients with occult carcinoma. Arch Ophthalmol 1990;108:527–33.
3. Leys AM, Dierick HG, Sciot RM. Early lesions of bilateral diffuse melanocytic proliferation. Arch Ophthalmol 1991;109:1590–4.
4. Murphy MA, Hart WM Jr, Olk RJ. Bilateral diffuse uveal melanocytic prolifeation simulating an arteriovenous fistula. J Neuroophthalmol 1997;17:166–9.
5. De Potter P. Ocular manifestations of cancer. Curr Opin Ophthalmol 1998;9:100–4.
6. Smith LT, Irvine AR. Diagnostic significance of orange pigment accumulation over choroidal tumors. Am J Ophthalmol 1973;76:212–6.
7. Char DH. The management of small choroidal melanomas. Surv Ophthalmol 1978;22:377–86.
8. Rodriguez-Sains RS. Ocular findings in patients with dysplastic nevus syndrome. Ophthalmology 1986; 93:661–5.
9. Hogeweg M, Bos PJ, Greve EL. Malignant melanomas of the choroid that on fluorescein angiography and perimetry gave the impression of naevi. Doc Ophthalmol 1976;40:30118.
10. Schalenbour A, Zografos L, Chamot L, et al. Interert de l'angiographic numerisee au vert d'indocyanine dans le diagnostic differentiel des tumeurs non pigmentees de la choroide. Klin Monatsbl Augenheilkd 1996;208:330–2.
11. Romani A, Baldeschi L, Genovesi-Ebert F, et al. Sensitivity and specificity of ultrasonography, fluorescein videoangiography, indocyanine green videoangiography, magnetic resonance and radioimmunoscintigraphy in the diagnosis of primary choroidal malignant melanoma. Ophthalmologica 1998;212: 44–6.
12. Mueller AJ, Bartsch DU, Folberg R, et al. Imaging the microvasculature of choroidal melanomas with confocal indocyanine green scanning laser ophthalmoscopy. Arch Ophthalmol 1998;116:31–9.
13. Ghazvini S, Char DH, Kroll S, et al. Comparative genomic hybridization analysis of archival formalin-fixed paraffin-embedded uveal melanomas. Cancer Genet Cytogenet 1996;90:95–101.
14. Schaudig U, Hassenstein A, Bernd A, et al. Limitations of imaging choroidal tumors in vivo by optical coherence tomography. Graefes Arch Clin Exp Ophthalmol 1998;236:588–92.
15. Finger PT, Romero JM, Rosen RB, et al. Three-dimensional ultrasonography of choroidal melanoma. Arch Ophthalmol 1998;116:305–12.
16. Cusumano A, Coleman DJ, Silverman RH, et al. Three-dimensional ultrasound imaging: clinical applications. Ophthalmology 1998;105:300–6.

17. Everaert H, Bossuyt A, Flamen P, et al. Visualizing ocular melanoma using iodine-123-N- (2-Deithylaminoethyl) 4-iodobenzamide SPECT. J Nucl Med 1997;38:870–3.
18. Hosten N, Lemke AJ, Sander B, et al. MR anatomy and small lesions of the eye: improved delineation with a special surface coil. Eur Radiol 1997;7:459–63.
19. Hosten N, Bornfeld N, Wassmuty R, et al. Uveal melanoma: detection of extraocular growth with MR imaging and US. Radiology 1997;202:61–7.
20. Scott IU, Murray TG, Hughes JR. Evaluation of imaging techniques for detection of extraocular extension of choroidal melanoma. Arch Ophthalmol 1998;116: 879–9.
21. Buettner H. Congenital hypertrophy of the retinal pigment epithelium. Am J Ophthalmol 1975;79:177–89.
22. Ryan SJ, Zimmerman LE, King FM. Reactive lymphoid hyperplasia. An unusual form of intraocular pseudotumor. Trans Am Acad Ophthalmol Otolaryngol Soc 1972;76:652–71.
23. Lloyd WC III, Eagle RC Jr, Shields JA, et al. Congenital hypertrophy of the retinal pigment epithelium. Electron microscopic and morphometric observations. Ophthalmology 1990;97:1052–60.
24. Shields JA, Shields CL, Shah PG, et al. Lack of association among typical congenital hypertrophy of the retinal pigment epithelium, adenomatous polyposis, and Gardner syndrome. Ophthalmology 1992;99: 1709–13.
25. Ruhswurm I, Zehetmayer M, Dejaco C, et al. Ophthalmic and genetic screening in pedigrees with familial adenomatous polyposis. Am J Ophthalmol 1998;125:680–6.
26. Reck AC, Bunyan D, Eccles D, Humphry R. The presence of congenital hypertrophy of the retinal pigment epithelium in a subgroup of patients with adenomatous polyposis coli mutations. Eye 1997;11: 298–300.
27. Howard GM, Forrest AW. Incidence and location of melanocytomas. Arch Ophthalmol 1967;77:61–6.
28. Olsen TW, Frayer WC, Meyers FL, et al. Idiopathic reactive hyperplasia of the retinal pigment epithelium. Arch Ophtholmol 1999;117:50–4.
29. Shields JA, Eagle RC Jr, Barr CC, et al. Adenocarcinoma of retinal pigment epithelium arising from a juxtapapillary histoplasmosis scar. Arch Ophthalmol 1994;112:650–3.
30. Shields JA, Shields CL, Gunduz K, Eagle RC Jr. Neoplasms of the retinal pigment epithelium: the 1998 Albert Ruedemann Sr memorial lecture, Part 2. Arch Ophthalmol 1999;117:601–8.
31. Loose IA, Jampol LM, O'Grady R. Human adenoma making a juxtapapillary melanoma. Arch Ophthalmol 1999;117:120–2.
32. Edelstein C, Shields CL, Shields JA, Eagle RC Jr. Presumed adenocarcinoma of the retinal pigment epithelium in a blind eye with a staphyloma. Arch Ophthalmol 1998;116:525–8.
33. Finger PT, McCormic SA, Davidian M, Walsh JB. Adenocarcinoma of the retinal pigment epithelium: a diagnostic and therapeutic challenge. Graefe's Arch Clin Exp Ophthalmol 1996;234:S22–7.
34. Jensen OA. Malignant melanomas of the uvea in Denmark 1943-1952. A clinical, histopathological, and prognostic study. Acta Ophthalmol 1963;75 (Suppl): 1–220.
35. Kindy-Degnan N, Char DH. Coincident systemic malignant disease in uveal melanoma patients. Can J Ophthalmol 1989;24:204–6.
36. Holly EA, Ashton DA, Ahn DK, et al. No excess prior cancer in patients with uveal melanoma. Ophthalmology 1991;98:608–11.
37. Ferry AP, Font RL. Carcinoma metastatic to the eye and orbit. I. A clinicopathologic study of 227 cases. Arch Ophthalmol 1974;92:276–86.
38. De Potter P, Shields CL, Shields JA, Tardio DJ. Uveal metastasis from prostate carcinoma. Cancer 1993; 71:2791–6.
39. Char DH, Schwartz AS, Miller TR, Abele JS. Ocular metastases from systemic melanoma. Am J Ophthalmol 1980;90:702–7.
40. Bowman CB, Guber D, Brown CH III, Curtin VT. Cutaneous malignant melanoma with diffuse intraocular metastases. Arch Ophthalmol 1994;112:1213–6.
41. Shields CL, Shields JA, Gross NE, et al. Survey of 520 eyes with uveal metastases. Ophthalmol 1997;104: 1265–76.
42. Sobattka B, Schlote T, Krumpaszky HG, Kreissig I. Choroidal metastases and choroidal melanomas: comparison of ultrasonographic findings. Br J Ophthalmol 1998;82:159–61.
43. Davis DL, Robertson DM. Fluorescein angiography of metastatic choroidal tumors. Arch Ophthalmol 1973; 89:97–9.
44. Harner RE, Smith JL, Reynolds DH. Fluorescein fundus study of metastatic breast carcinoma following cryohypophysectomy. Arch Ophthalmol 1967;78: 300–5.
45. Michelson JB, Felberg NT, Shields JA. Evaluation of metastatic cancer to the eye. Carcinoembryonic antigen and gamma glutamyl transpeptidase. Arch Ophthalmol 1977;95:692–4.
46. Perri P, Chiarelli M, Monari P, et al. Choroidal metastases. Echographic experience from 42 patients. Acta Ophthalmologica 1992;204 (Suppl):96–8.
47. Verbeek AM, Thijssen JM, Cuypers MH, et al. Echographic classification of intraocular tumours. A 15-year retrospective analysis. Acta Ophthalmologica 1994;72:416–22.
48. Augsburger JJ. Fine needle aspiration biopsy of sus-

pected metastatic cancer to the posterior uvea. Trans Am Ophthal Soc 1988;86:500–60.
49. Leff SR, Yarian DL, Shields JA, et al. Tumor-associated retinal pigment epithelial proliferation simulating retinal pigment epithelial tear. Retina 1989;9: 267–9.
50. Char DH, Miller TR, Ljung BM, et al. Fine needle aspiration biopsy in uveal melanoma. Acta Cytologica 1989;33:599–605.
51. Shields JA, Shields CL, Ehya H, et al. Fine needle aspiration biopsy of suspected intraocular tumors. Ophthalmology 1993;100:1677–84.
52. Davila RM, Miranda MC, Smith ME. Role of cytopathology in the diagnosis of ocular malignancies. Acta Cytol 1998;42:362–6.
53. Weiss L. Analysis of the incidence of intraocular metastasis. Br J Ophthalmol 1993;77:149–51.
54. Greenberg BR, Lawrence HJ. Metastatic cancer with unknown primary. Med Clin North Am 1988;72: 1055–65.
55. Haimovici R, Gragoudas ES, Gregor Z, et al. Choroidal metastases from renal cell carcinoma. Ophthalmology 1997;104:1152–8.
56. Holbach LM, Chevez P, Snyder WB, Font RL. Unsuspected renal cell carcinoma metastatic to the choroid nine years after nephrectomy. Am J Ophthalmol 1990;110:441–3.
57. Auerbach R. Patterns of tumor metastasis: organ specificity and the spread of cancer cells. Lab Invest 1988;58:361–4.
58. Witschel H, Font RL. Hemangioma of the choroid. A clinicopathologic study of 71 cases and a review of the literature. Surv Ophthalmol 1976;20:415–31.
59. Augsburger JJ, Shields JA, Moffat KP. Circumscribed choroidal hemangiomas: long-term visual prognosis. Retina 1981;1:56–61.
60. Hayreh SS. Choroidal tumors: role of fluorescein fundus angiography in their diagnosis. Curr Concepts Ophthalmol 1974;4:168.
61. Medlock RD, Augsburger JJ, Wilkinson CP, et al. Enlargement of circumscribed choroidal hemangiomas. Retina 1991;11:385–8.
62. Shields JA, Font RL. Melanocytoma of the choroid clinically simulating a malignant melanoma. Arch Ophthalmol 1972;87:396–400.
63. Haas BD, Jakobiec FA, Iwamoto T, et al. Diffuse choroidal melanocytoma in a child. A lesion extending the spectrum of melanocytic hamartomas. Ophthalmology 1986;93:1632–8.
64. el Baba F, Hagler WS, De la Cruz A, Green WR. Choroidal melanoma with pigment dispersion in vitreous and melanomalytic glaucoma. Ophthalmology 1988;95:370–7.
65. Shields JA, Shields CL, Eagle RC Jr, et al. Malignant melanoma associated with melanocytoma of the optic disc. Ophthalmology 1990;97:225–30.
66. Cunha SL. Osseous choristoma of the choroid. A familial disease. Arch Ophthalmol 1984;102:1052–4.
67. Buettner H. Spontaneous involution of a choroidal osteoma. Arch Ophthalmol 1990;108:1517–8.
68. Char DH, Stone RD, Irvine AR, et al. Diagnostic modalities in choroidal melanoma. Am J Ophthalmol 1980;89:223–30.
69. Gass JD, Guerry RK, Jack RL, Harris G. Choroidal osteoma. Arch Ophthalmol 1978;96:428–35.
70. Gass JD. New observations concerning choroidal osteomas. Int Ophthalmol 1979;1:71–84.
71. Coston TO, Wilkinson CP. Choroidal osteoma. Am J Ophthalmol 1978;86:368–72.
72. Chan TKJ, Atta HR, Scott GB. Ossification in choroidal melanoma. Br J Opthalmol 1995;79:705–6.
73. Shields CL, Shields JA, Augsburger JJ. Choroidal osteoma. Surv Ophthalmol 1988;33:17–27.
74. Eting E, Savir H. An atypical fulminant course of choroidal osteoma in two siblings. Am J Ophthalmol 1992;113:52–5.
75. Mizota A, Tanabe R, Adachi-Usami E. Rapid enlargement of choroidal osteoma in a three year old girl. Arch Ophthalmol 1998;116:1128–9.
76. Noble KG. Bilateral choroidal osteoma in three siblings. Am J Ophthalmol 1990;109:656–60.
77. Aylward GW, Chang TS, Paulter SE, Gass JD. A long-term follow-up of choroidal osteoma. Arch Ophthalmol 1998;116:1337–41.
78. Bellows AR, Chylack LT Jr, Hutchinson BT. Choroidal detachment. Clinical manifestation, therapy, and mechanism of formation. Ophthalmology 1981;88: 1107–15.
79. Augsburger JJ, Coats TD, Lauritzen K. Localized suprachoroidal hematomas. Ophthalmoscopic features, fluorescein angiography, and clinical care. Arch Ophthalmol 1990;108:968–72.
80. Feldon SE, Sigelman J, Albert DM, Smith TR. Clinical manifestations of brawny scleritis. Am J Ophthalmol 1978;85:781–7.
81. Yap EY, Robertson DM, Buettner H. Scleritis as an initial manifestation of choroidal malignant melanoma. Ophthalmology 1992;99:1693–7.
82. Janknecht P, Mittelviefhaus H, Loffler KU. Sclerochoroidal granuloma in Wegener's granulomatosis simulating a uveal melanoma. Retina 2000 [In press].
83. Oh KT, Polk TD, Boldt HC, Turner JF Jr. Systemic small noncleaved cell lymphoma presenting as a posterior choroidal mass. Am J Ophthalmol 1998; 125:560–2.
84. Chang TS, Byrne SR, Gass JDM, et al. Echographic findings in benign reactive lymphoid hyperplasia of the choroid. Arch Ophthalmol 1996;114:669–75.

85. Grossniklaus HE, Martin DF, Avery R, et al. Uveal lymphoid infiltration report of four cases and clinicopathologic review. Ophthalmology 1998;105: 1265–73.
86. Strempel I. Rare choroidal tumor simulating a malignant melanoma. Ophthalmologica 1991;202:110–14.
87. Shields JA, Font RL, Eagle RC, et al. Melanotic schwannoma of the choroid. Immunohistochemistry and electron microscopic observations. Ophthalmology 1994;101:843–9.
88. Ben-Ezra D, Sahel JA, Harris NL, et al. Uveal lymphoid infiltrates: immunohistochemical evidence for a lymphoid neoplasia. Br J Ophthalmol 1989;73: 846–51.
89. Fan JT, Robertson DM, Campbell RJ. Clinicopathologic correlation of a case of adenocarcinoma of the retinal pigment epithelium. Am J Ophthalmol 1995; 119:243–5.
90. Fredrick DR, Char DH, Ljeung BM, Brinton DA. Solitary intraocular lymphoma as an initial presentation of widespread disease. Arch Ophthalmol 1989;107: 395–7.
91. Jurgens I, Roca G, Sedo S, et al. Presumed melanocytoma of the macula. Arch Ophthalmol 1994;112: 305–6.
92. Barondes MJ, Sponsel WE, Stevens TS, Plotnik RD. Tuberculous choroiditis diagnosed by chorioretinal endobiopsy. Am J Ophthalmol 1991;112:460–61.
93. Eide N, Syrdalen P, Walaas L, Hagmar B. Fine needle aspiration biopsy in selecting treatment for inconclusive intraocular disease. Acta Ophthalmol Scand 1999;77:448–52.

7

Choroidal Nevomas and Melanomas

Making the correct diagnosis in suspected uveal melanomas is a function of observer experience, media clarity, and tumor size. In most ocular oncology practices, over 99 percent of tumors that require therapeutic intervention can be correctly diagnosed.[1–6] The diagnostic accuracy reported in various series is partially predicated on the criteria used. In a recent study, we noted that 9 of 100 small to medium uveal tumors that were scheduled for radiation therapy on a basis of a noninvasive test diagnosis of uveal melanoma did not have that diagnosis confirmed with fine-needle aspiration biopsy (FNAB).[7] In another series, findings from a fine-needle biopsy altered the therapeutic plan in 48 percent of the cases.[2] In our experience with uveal melanomas that have required enucleation, there has been < 1 percent diagnostic error rate.[1] A recent publication from the Collaborative Ocular Melanoma Study (COMS) cited an even lower diagnostic error rate; however, the difficult diagnostic cases, such as those with opaque media, were excluded from that analysis since the COMS inclusion criteria included a readily diagnosable melanoma to be part of that study.[8] In small centers, the diagnostic accuracy is less. In 5 of 53 eyes enucleated with the diagnosis of a uveal melanoma by community ophthalmologists in Florida, another diagnosis was noted on histologic examination.[9]

It is almost impossible to differentiate a small melanoma from a large, atypical nevus; patients with such small, indeterminate lesions 1 to 3 mm thick are usually monitored. Very few physical findings are pathognomonic for the diagnosis or exclusion of a small uveal melanoma. Pragmatically, we often classify indeterminate pigmented lesions < 10 mm in diameter and < 3 mm thick as "nevomas." Clinically, it is difficult to distinguish tumors that will grow from those that will remain stable for many years. The fluorescein pattern is not diagnostic, and on ultrasonography, while homogeneity is most often associated with a potentially active small melanoma, it is not pathognomonic.[10] Gass and others have stressed that certain clinical features, such as subretinal neovascularization, drusen, and a hypopigmented surround, are signs of chronicity; however, the author has observed indeterminant pigmented choroidal lesions with each of these features which demonstrated growth.[6] Therefore, even when factors associated with chronicity are noted, the lesions are still closely monitored.

Uveal melanoma pigmentation is variable; there is usually some intrinsic tumor pigmentation, although 25 percent of cases are amelanotic. Most melanomas are light to medium gray in color; a moderately elevated (< 4 mm) black lesion is more likely to be either a melanocytoma or an extramacular disciform lesion, especially if there is significant vitreous hemorrhage.[11,12] Some clinicians have used transillumination to differentiate melanomas with intrinsic pigmentation from other simulating lesions. I do not use transillumination diagnostically for posterior tumors. I have seen histologically documented uveal melanomas that do not block transillumination and nonmelanoma lesions that do. As previously mentioned, orange pigmentation over melanomas is quite common.[6,13] A typical pattern is shown in Figure 7–1 in a small

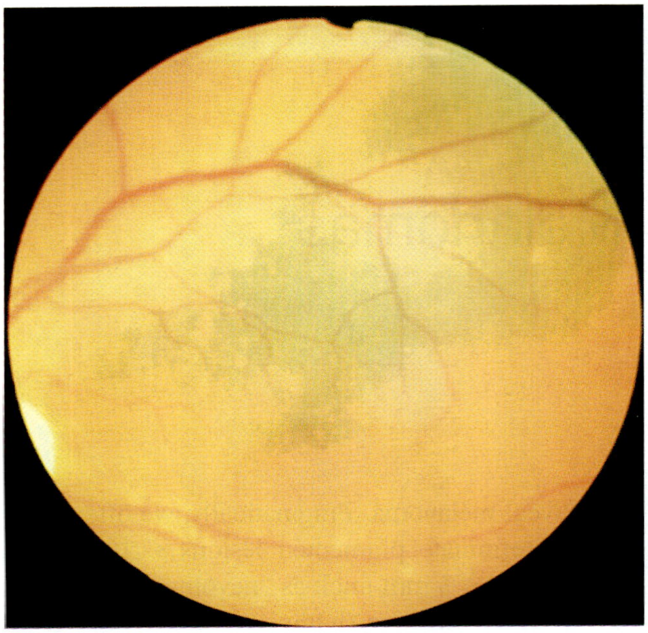

Figure 7–1. Orange pigmentation (lipofusin) over a uveal melanoma.

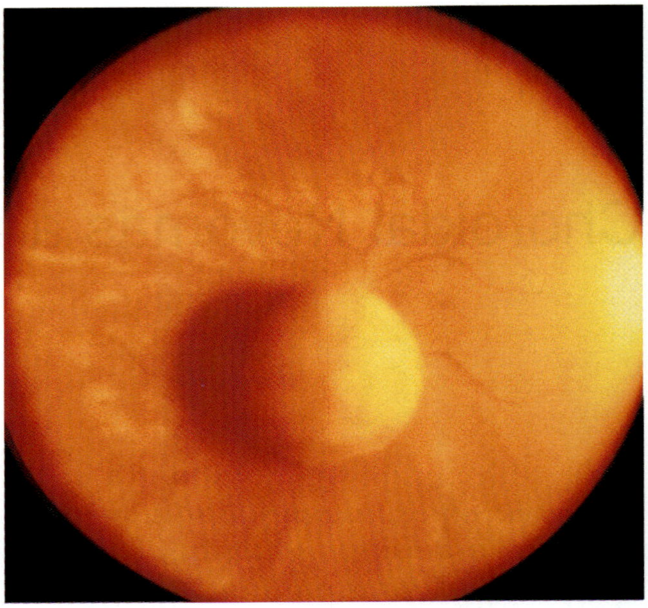

Figure 7–2. A large uveal melanoma with a typical "mushroom shaped" collar button lesion.

lesion that eventually grew and was treated. The orange pigmentation may be discrete or confluent and may vary in its intensity.

There are a number of typical clinical, ultrasonographic, and photographic features for medium (10 to 15 mm diameter and 3 to 5 mm thick) and large uveal melanomas (> 15 mm in diameter or > 5 mm in thickness). Interestingly, there are different definitions now in use for small, medium, and large tumors. The COMS considers a small tumor < 16 mm in diameter, and < 3 mm thickness. A large tumor is > 16 mm diameter or > 10 mm thick.[14] Figure 7–2 demonstrates a large uveal melanoma with the typical collar button ("mushroom shaped") appearance that occurs when the tumor breaks through Bruch's membrane. This topography is almost pathognomonic for a uveal melanoma. Retinal invasion is often associated with a collar button configuration; on ophthalmoscopic examination, the melanoma surface appears velvety brown atop the collar button (Figure 7–3). Uncommonly, a dense vitreous hemorrhage occurs secondary to a uveal melanoma that has broken through Bruch's membrane (Figure 7–4).[8] If a mass is < 5 mm thick, a Bruch's membrane rupture is unlikely; a dense vitreous hemorrhage in such cases is more suggestive of an extramacular or macular disciform process, although a melanoma must be ruled out.[15] Figure 7–5 demonstrates a histologically benign lesion simulating this process.

Usually, eyes with large choroidal melanomas have an associated exudative retinal detachment. Occasionally, an area of choroidal detachment is also present.[15] Figure 7–6 shows a large, relatively amelanotic melanoma, with almost 30 percent of the retina secondarily detached. It is sometimes difficult to differentiate a rhegmatogenous from an exudative

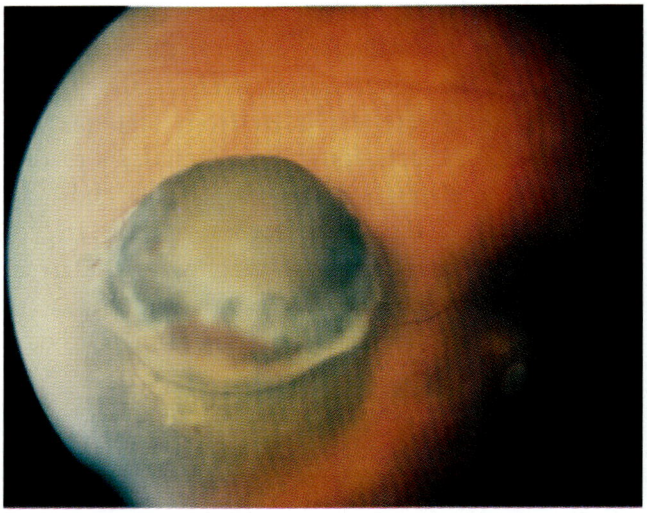

Figure 7–3. Retinal invasion in an area in which the melanoma has broken through Bruch's membrane. Clinically, retinal invasion has a typical velvety surface texture.

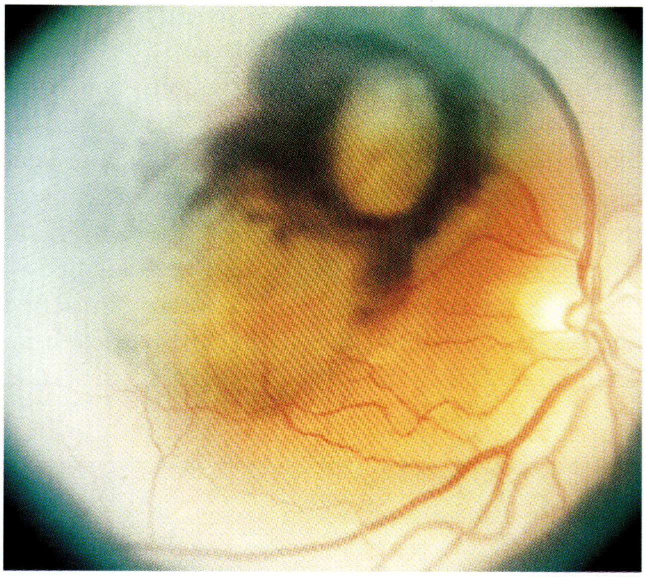

Figure 7–4. A small vitreous hemorrhage at the crest of a collar-button-shaped uveal melanoma secondary to damage of the retinal vessels when the tumor broke through Bruch's membrane.

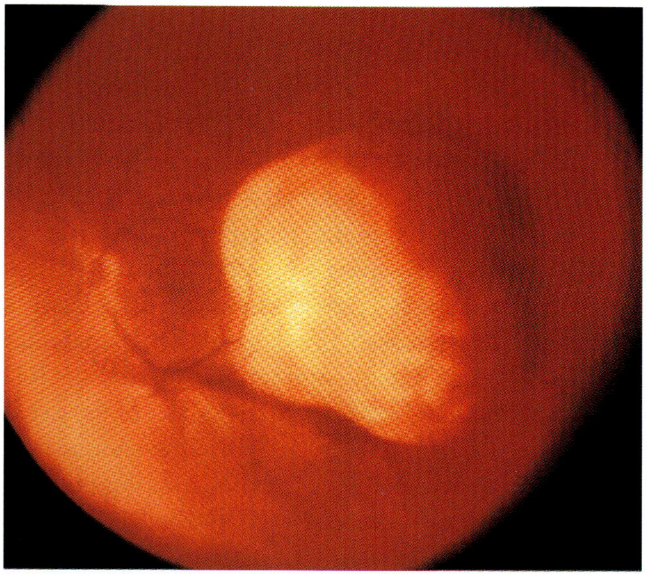

Figure 7–6. Wide-angle fundus photograph demonstrating subretinal fluid in association with a uveal melanoma.

retinal detachment. Four features are helpful in differentiating these conditions: (1) retrolental detachments (Figure 7–7), (with the exception of those associated with proliferative vitreo-retinopathy), are almost never rhegmatogenous; if the retina is easily visible on routine slit-lamp biomicroscopy, the detachment is almost always secondary to tumor or inflammation; (2) exudative detachments have shifting subretinal fluid margins; the fluid pools inferiorly when the patient is upright and superiorly if the patient is placed with his head down; (3) subretinal fluid associated with a melanoma is usually quite clear and the retinal marking distinct. Often, these exudative detachments can be either missed or mistaken for retinoschisis by an inexperienced observer; this clarity of retinal detail is also observed in some long-standing rhegmatogenous detachments. It is quite common for smaller melanomas to have subretinal fluid, either just over the tumor or visible only in the

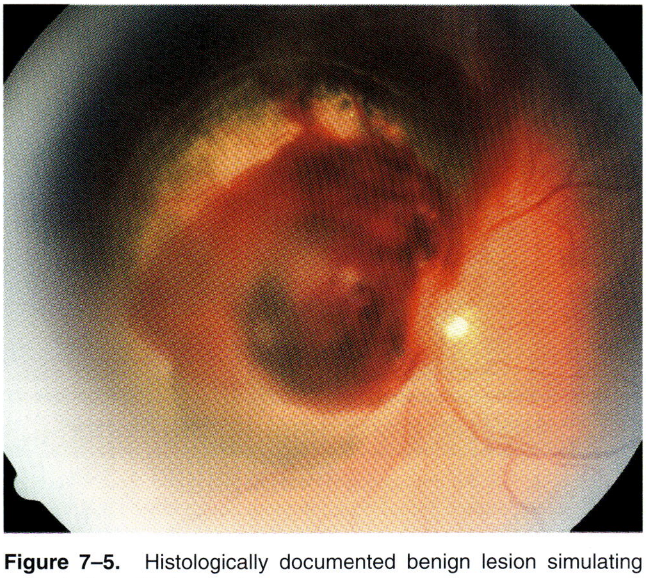

Figure 7–5. Histologically documented benign lesion simulating collar button with hemorrhage.

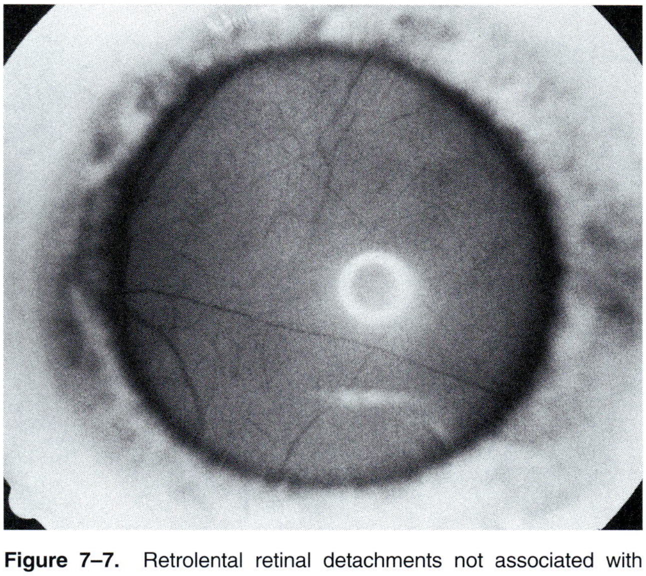

Figure 7–7. Retrolental retinal detachments not associated with proliferative vitreoretinopathies are almost always exudative in nature.

inferior fundus; this is most easily detected by indirect ophthalmoscopic examination to identify elevated retinal vessels; and (4) patients with exudative detachment do not have retinal holes, although a careful fundus examination will detect retinal breaks in as many as 6 percent of uveal melanoma patients, an incidence comparable with that in the general population.

A variant of the more common globular-shaped choroidal melanoma is the diffuse uveal melanoma which has an increased predilection for extraocular extension.[16] The most common definition of this lesion is that it involves at least 25 percent of the uveal tract and is < 5 mm thick.[17] A diffuse melanoma simulating a large atypical nevus is shown in Figure 7–8.

Ultrasound evaluation is the most useful diagnostic test in the evaluation of patients with elevated uveal mass lesions, especially those > 3 mm in thickness. A complete description of ultrasound technique and analysis is beyond the scope of this book; a number of excellent reviews have been written.[18–20] We have found that a combination of both immersion B-scan and Kretz A-scan (quantitative echography) are most reliable. Their performance and interpretation are acquired skills; for the novice, pattern recognition is a good first step in differentiating choroidal lesions. Figure 7–9A shows an immersion B-scan of a uveal melanoma. On quantitative echography (Figure 7–9B), the reflectivity of the tumor is medium to low. Vascular pulsations can often be observed during the actual performance of this test. Figure 7–10 shows extrascleral extension of uveal melanoma.

In some centers, duplex sonography and color Doppler ultrasonography have also been used. No blood flow has been noted in choroidal nevi or age-related macular degenerations, in contrast to uveal melanomas.[20,21] This technique may also be useful to detect vascular changes that occur after radiation of the uveal melanomas.[22–24] Several other ultrasound approaches for volume measurement have also been reported.[25–28]

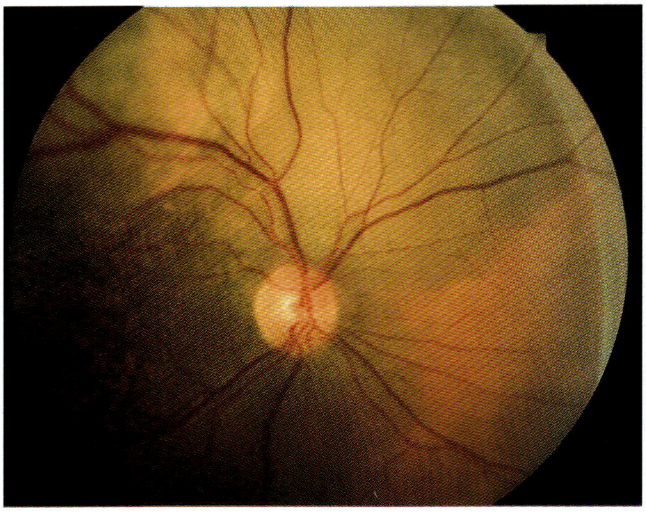

Figure 7–8. A diffuse uveal melanoma (< 5 mm in thickness and involving at least 25 percent of the uveal tract).

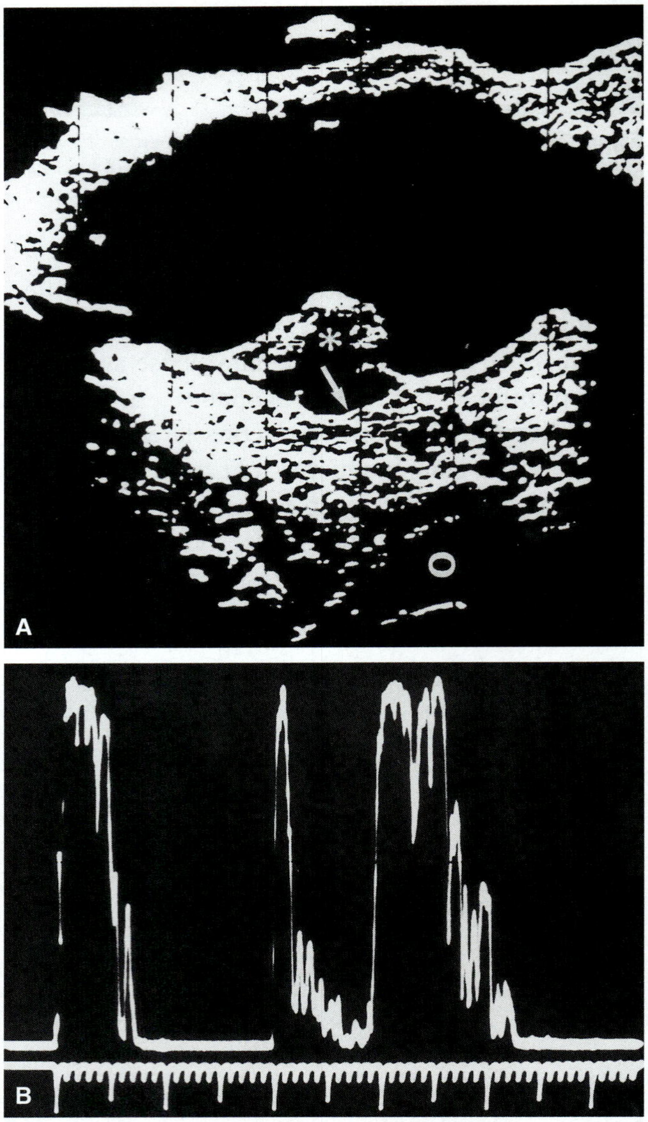

Figure 7–9. *A,* An immersion B-scan showing the typical findings of a uveal melanoma including an acoustic quiet zone (*), choroidal excavation (*arrow*), and orbital shadowing (o). *B,* A quantitative A-scan demonstrating medium to low reflectivity which is characteristic of a uveal melanoma.

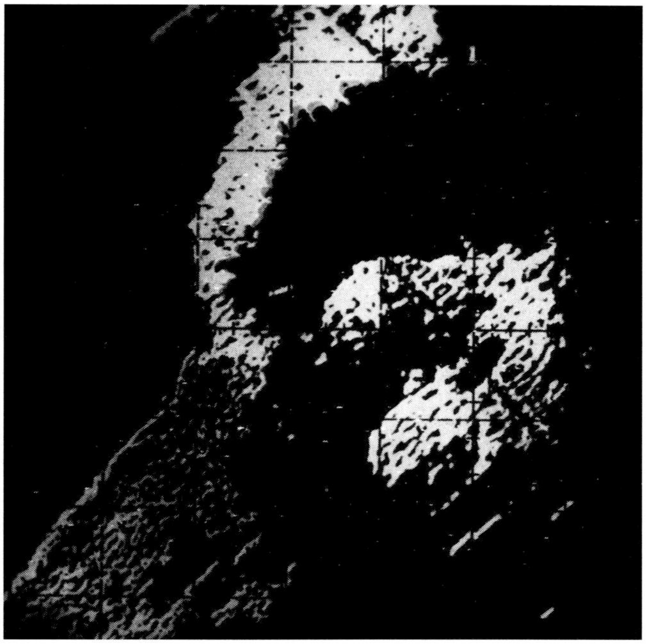

Figure 7–10. Immersion B-scan shows a uveal melanoma with localized extrascleral extension.

It is important to emphasize that in an eye with opaque media, ultrasonic biometry to establish IOL power cannot be used to exclude a uveal melanoma. We have examined a number of patients, including one in whom we removed a 12 mm thick ciliary body choroidal tumor with a cyclochoroidectomy, that had "normal" ultrasound biometry results. Others have noted similar problems with that technique.[29,30]

As mentioned previously, the diagnostic accuracy of fluorescein angiography in uveal melanoma diagnosis is less than 50 percent.[1] Fluorescein angiographic findings suggestive of a choroidal melanoma are an intrinsic vasculature (Figure 7–11), "hot spots," which are initially point-source leakage that became diffuse over time (Figure 7–12), vascular leakage, and blockage of fluorescence by orange pigment. Often, there are prominent tumor vessels in the collar-button portion of a melanoma (Figure 7–13). As mentioned in Chapter 6, confocal indocyanine green scanning laser ophthalmoscopy may allow evaluation of other prognostic factors that are currently not available in eyes in which histology has not been attained.[31]

Computed tomography (CT) (Figure 7–14) and magnetic resonance imaging (MRI) (Figure 7–15) both generate images of uveal melanomas and simulating lesions. In some cases, CT can detect extraocular extension of a choroidal melanoma (Figure 7–16); however, we have not noted significantly better sensitivity with either CT or MRI, compared with ultrasonography. Other workers have found that MRI is more sensitive for the detection of extraocular extension of a tumor, although the relative sensitivity of these techniques has not been proven.[32] On MRI, the T_1 and T_2 parameters of uveal melanoma may be characteristic due to the melanin free radical. The typical appearance of a uveal melanoma on an MRI scan is hyperintense, in comparison with the

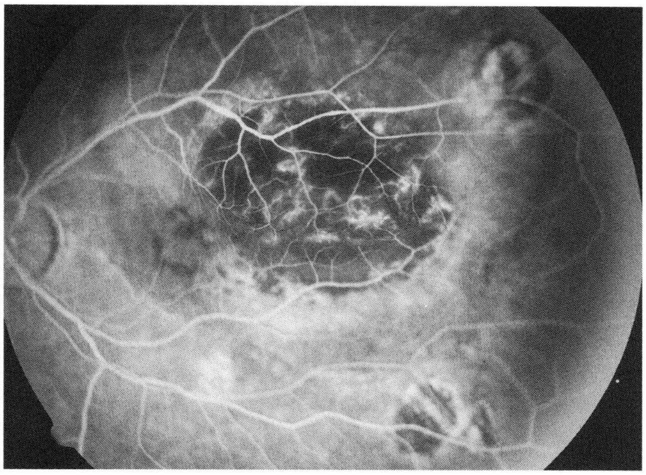

Figure 7–11. Fluorescein angiogram demonstrating an intrinsic vasculature ("double circulation") in a large melanoma.

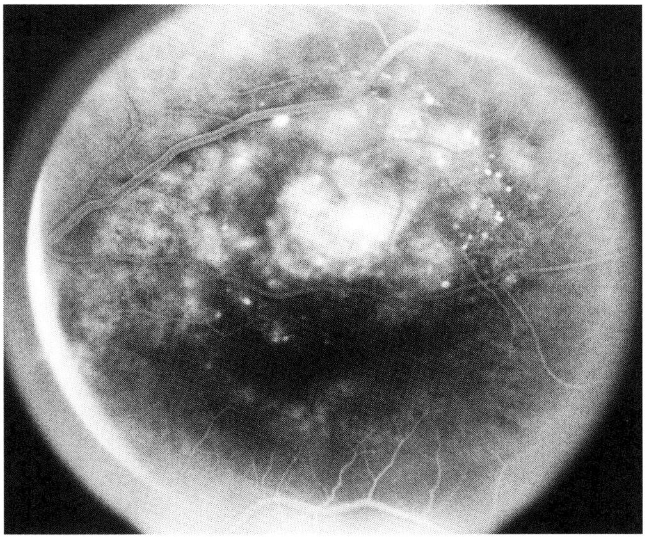

Figure 7–12. Fluorescein angiogram demonstrating "hot spots," which initially are point- source leakage, not window defects, which gradually show enlargement during the course of the study.

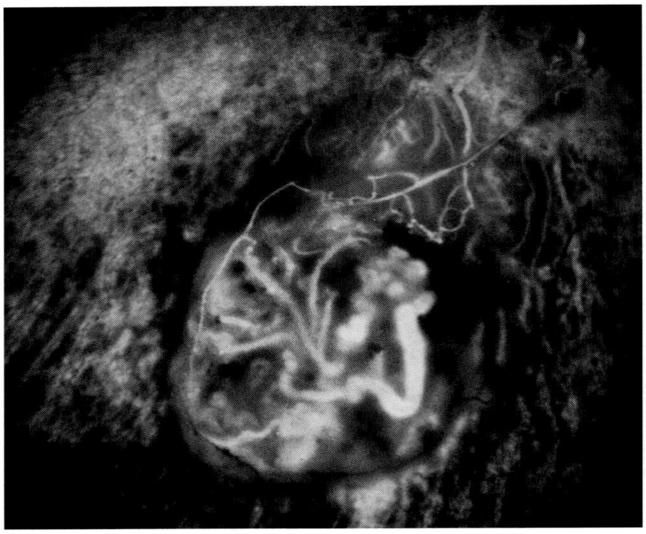

Figure 7–13. Fluorescein angiogram shows a prominent intrinsic tumor vessels in the collar-button portion of the tumor.

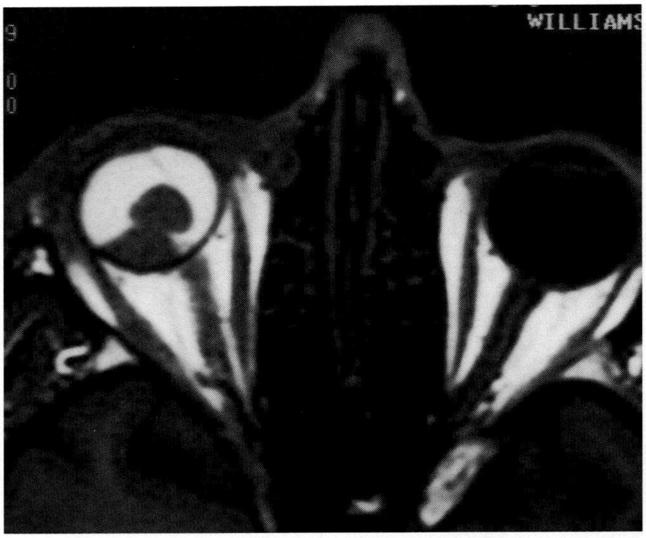

Figure 7–15. Axial T_1-weighted MRI scan showing a collar-buttoned shaped choroidal melanoma.

vitreous on T_1–weighted and a hypointense image on T_2–weighted scan (Figures 7–17A and B).[33] Unfortunately, the pattern of a melanocytoma on MRI is identical to a melanoma.[34–40]

Subsequent studies reported different T_1 and T_2 patterns of uveal melanomas on MRI.[35–40] As an example, a typical MRI pattern of a uveal melanoma has been reported in 7 to 93 percent of cases.[37] Clearly, some of these differences are due to equipment or imaging strategies; however, MRI is much less cost effective than ultrasonography and does not offer more information for the diagnosis of most uveal melanomas.[37–43] We initially thought that this technique might be very useful in differentiating a choroidal hemorrhage or an extramacular disciform from a uveal melanoma. Unfortunately, it is not always diagnostic. Figures 7–18A and B show the MRI pattern in an elderly patient who had multiple repeat dense hemorrhages. MRI was nondiagnostic, as was ultrasonography. The patient had a FNAB, which was also negative. The author felt the recurrent hemorrhage was due to the tumor and therefore removed the eye since it was not functional. On examination of the enucleated specimen, this was a

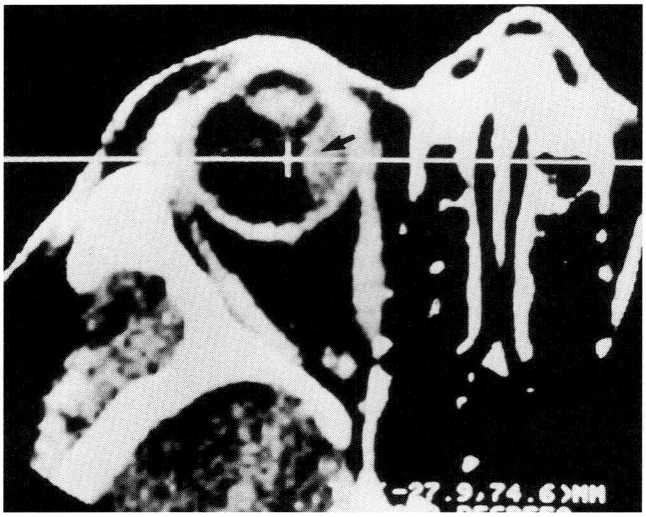

Figure 7–14. Axial CT scan demonstrates a choroidal melanoma (*arrow*).

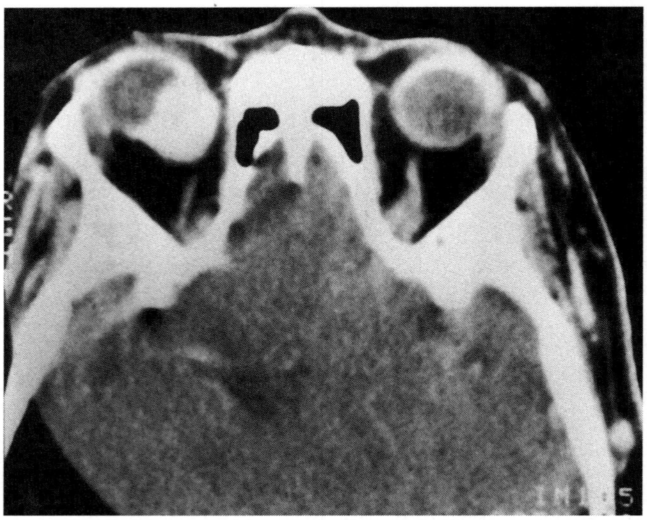

Figure 7–16. CT scan documents extrascleral extension of a uveal melanoma.

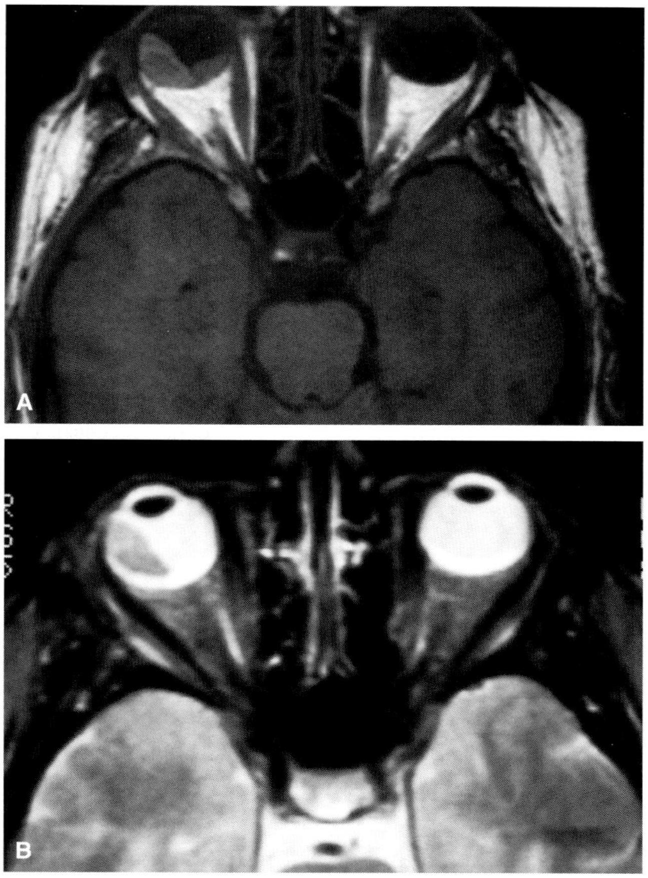

Figure 7–17. *A* and *B,* On T_1-weighted MRI, the uveal melanoma is hyperintense to brain, while on T_2-weighted scan it is hypointense.

necrotic melanoma with only a few viable cells in the midvitreous.[41]

Magnetic resonance spectroscopy has been described in uveal melanomas by several groups including ours. Currently, that technique, positron emission tomography (PET) scans, and immunoscintography with monoclonal antibodies directed toward melanoma-associated antigens are research tools.[44–49] As discussed in Chapter 6, the data supporting the use of these imaging techniques in tumors < 7 mm in diameter and 5 mm thickness are tenuous.[50,51]

We use CT or MRI to confirm the extraocular extension noted on ultrasonography.[47] An example of a melanoma in which the main tumor mass was extrascleral is shown in Figure 7–16. In our experience, small areas of extrascleral tumor extensions can produce false-negative ultrasound, CT, and MRI data.[33]

It is possible that a Doppler ultrasonography, PET, and ^{31}P spectroscopy may improve our ability to accurately predict prognosis and enhance the monitoring of melanomas after alternative therapy, although currently this is only supposition.[52–54] ^{31}P MRS can be used to determine the metabolism, pH, membrane transport, and oxygenation of a tumor. The ^{31}P MRS pattern of uveal melanoma is distinctive; there are unusually high concentrations of a phospholipid metabolite and two phosphodiesters.[55,56] After hyperthermia in experimental models, the MRS pattern demonstrated significant changes, which quite accurately reflected an early tumor response. Unfortunately, our experience with MRS after a combination of hyperthermia and radiation or radiation alone does not show as much promise.[33,57]

Despite newer diagnostic modalities, errors still occur. The two most common settings in which we have seen errors made even by excellent clinicians have been either when subjective data (either history

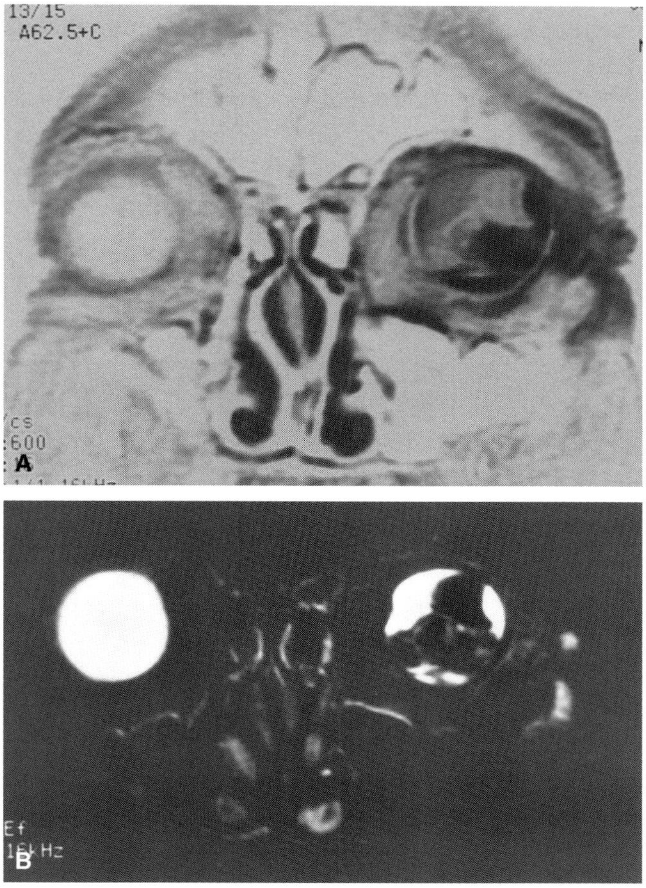

Figure 7–18. *A,* MRI T_1-weighted coronal scan shows a hyperintense uveal lesion in relation to brain. *B,* MRI T_2-weighted coronal scan shows both hype- and hypointensity consistent with either a hemorrhage or a melanoma and intratumor hemorrhage.

or review of systems) are confusing or when a patient is referred for a second opinion after an intraocular surgery with a presumed hemorrhage, and the true nature of the intraocular pathology was not correctly established. Figures 7–19 and 7–20 demonstrate one of these difficult diagnostic settings. In both cases, the patient was referred to superb retinal surgeons with presumed vitreous hemorrhages that had occurred after glaucoma or cataract surgery. Extraocular extension of both uveal melanomas had occurred after the surgeries.

METASTATIC EVALUATION

Approximately 1 percent of patients with uveal melanoma simultaneously present with both ocular and systemic disease.[58,59] It is likely that many more patients have microscopic disease, but we are unable to detect it with current imaging and blood studies. The author has not seen a patient with a small- or medium-sized melanoma present with simultaneous metastases.

Microscopic tumor that has undergone only 10 to 15 doublings and is < 1 mm^3 in size will be missed with current diagnostic modalities (ophthalmoloscopy, ultrasound, FNAB). If one assumes that the tumor starts as one malignant cell and that it takes approximately 40 doublings to kill a host, until a tumor is "middle aged" and has gone through 20 doublings, it is not detectable.[59]

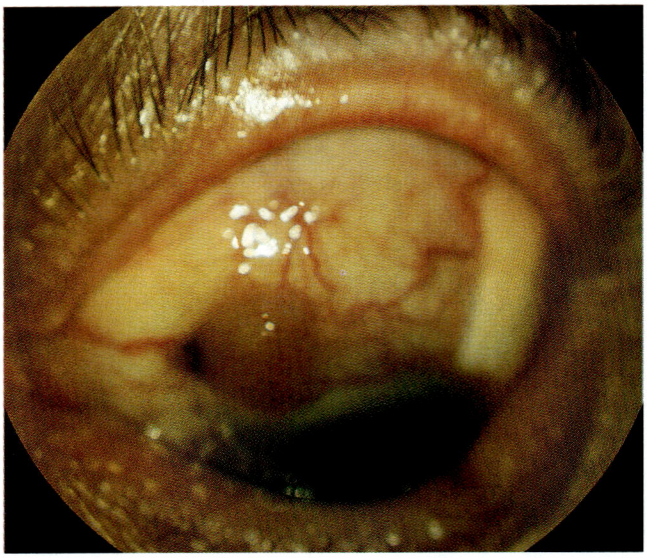

Figure 7–19. Patient was referred for retinal evaluation because of vitreous hemorrhage following glaucoma seton surgery. The melanoma was not detected until extrascleral extension was noted.

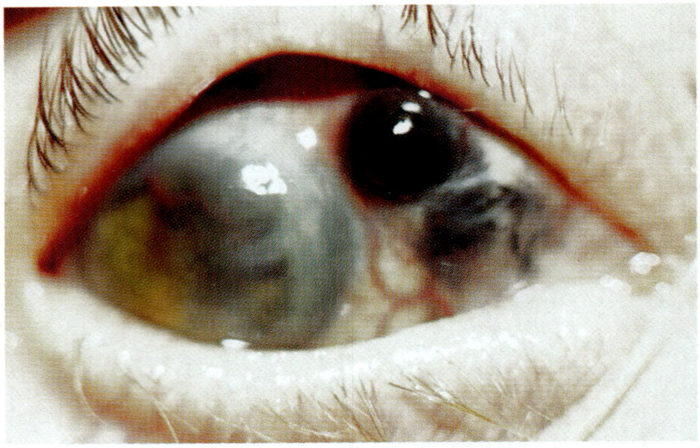

Figure 7–20. Patient was referred for retinal evaluation because of vitreous hemorrhage following cataract surgery. Similar to the case in Figure 7–19, there was no underlying melanoma detected until extrascleral extension was noted.

The rate of uveal melanoma tumor growth is uncertain, and probably it varies during the natural history of the tumor. We and others have used clinical and cell cycling studies to demonstrate that melanomas are relatively slow growing.[60,61] Manschot speculated that it takes up to 7 years to develop metastases from an active uveal melanoma; however, that hypothesis assumes a constant doubling time.[62] Folkman and colleagues have demonstrated that micrometastases are probably not initially vascularized, but while the cells are rapidly dividing, they are in "in equalibrium" with apoptosis.[63]

We studied the initial site of metastatic disease in enucleated uveal melanoma patients who developed clinically detectable metastases. The initial site of metastasis from primary uveal melanoma is shown schematically in Figure 7–21. The most common initial presentation for metastases is in the liver; approximately 60 to 70 percent of patients first develop liver metastases. Usually, these patients have right upper quadrant pain, fullness, tenderness, nausea, vomiting, and weight loss.[58] Other less common presentations of metastatic uveal melanoma include subcutaneous nodules, lung disease, bone involvement, and central nervous system disease. In a subsequent study by Gragoudas and colleagues, 94 percent of patients with metastatic disease had liver involvement.[64] In another study of 24 metastatic uveal melanoma patients, 87 percent had liver involvement, 46 percent had lung lesions, 29 percent had bone lesions, and 17 percent had subcutaneous metastases.[65]

The sensitivity of radiologic imaging tests versus serum studies to detect metastases is unclear.[66–68] A number of investigations have demonstrated that the serum lactic dehydrogenase (LDH) or glutamyl transpeptidase (GTP) have a false-negative rate of approximately 3 percent.[69] In a study by Hicks and colleagues, the sensitivity of GTP was 21 percent with the specificity of 92 percent. In contrast, the sensitivity of ultrasonography was 14 percent. The relative sensitivity of serum tests versus chest-abdominal MRI or CT is unclear. All patients evaluated by the author receive standard chest radiography, liver function tests (alkaline phosphatase, LDH, GGP), and a general physical examination. If these preliminary studies are negative, we do not order other metastatic investigations. If the chest radiograph is positive, we obtain chest CT; if the liver function tests are positive (and there is a false-positive rate of up to 40 percent), we obtain body abdominal CT and use a FNAB if a lesion is noted. A study from Finland has disagreed with our approach. This was a retrospective cohort study. Interestingly, they diagnosed 74 percent of the metastases by screening; 26 percent were symptomatic. In that study, liver ultrasonography was diagnostic 78 percent of the time, while liver function tests were only abnormal in 70 percent of cases. More importantly, the false-negative rate was 33 percent with the serum liver function test versus 4 percent with ultrasonography. They also found that the use of chest radiography, given the relatively low pick-up, was not very cost effective.[67] Typical liver metastases on liver CT is shown in Figures 7–22A and B. Rarely, other patterns of metastases can occur. We have managed a few patients with metastatic tumors of the opposite orbit. Figures 7–23A and B show a primary uveal melanoma that was irradiated. Two years later, the patient presented with a FNAB-diagnosed metastasis to the other eye as the initial manifestation of widespread disease (Figure 7–23A).

SERIAL OBSERVATION WITHOUT INTERVENTION FOR NEVOMAS

The effect of intervention on uveal melanoma mortality has been controversial for over 100 years.[70–74] There have been a few patients who refused enucleation for large, growing melanomas yet lived many years without the development of metastatic disease, although historically almost all untreated patients died of widespread disease.[75,76]

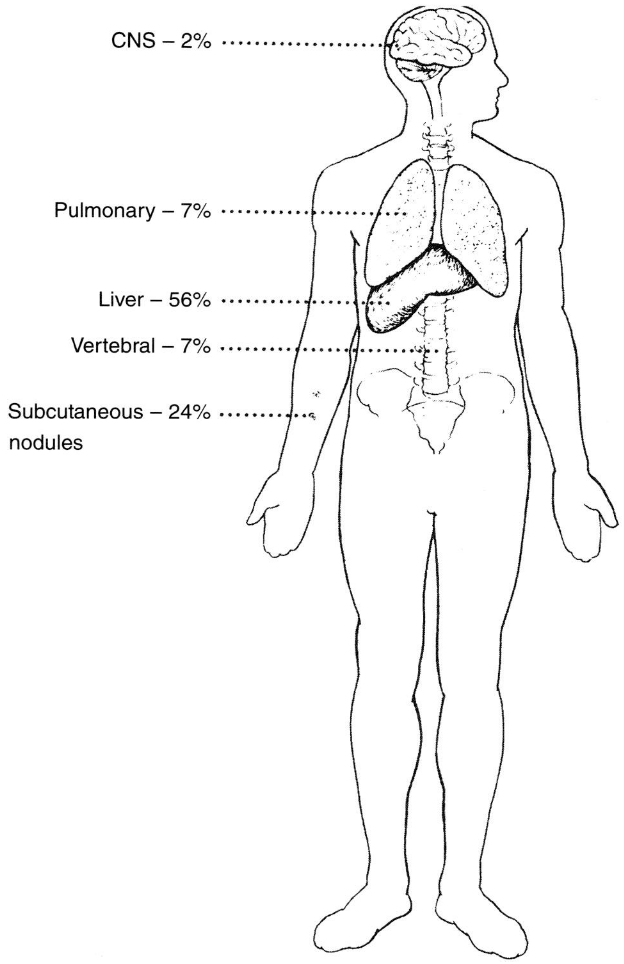

Figure 7–21. The initial site of uveal melanoma metastasis (Reprinted from Char DH. Metastatic choroidal melanoma. Am J Ophthalmol 1978;86:76–80).

There is a reasonable amount of retrospective data that suggest that patients with small uveal melanomas or indeterminate pigmented tumors < 3 mm in thickness and < 10 mm in diameter can be safely monitored without therapeutic intervention until growth is documented.[74] Figures 7–24A and B document a 10-year follow-up, without apparent growth of a pigmented tumor that remained 3.5 mm thick on quantitative echographic measurement. Figure 7–25 shows a similar lesion followed up for 10 years, until the patient died of a myocardial infarct. Histologic examination of the choroidal mass showed only benign pigmented cells.

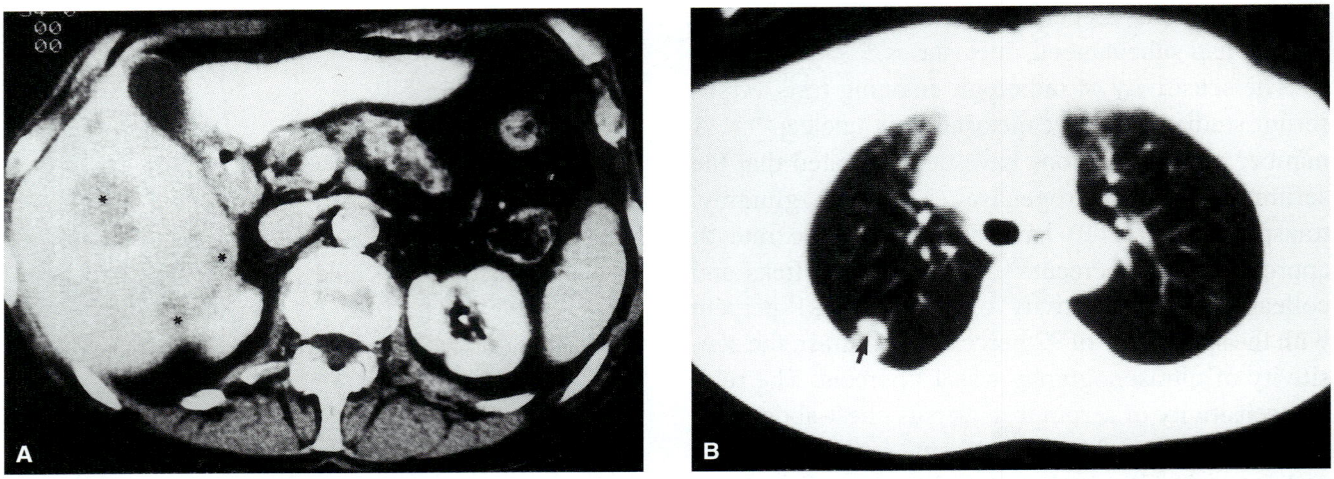

Figure 7–22. *A,* Abdominal CT scan demonstrating liver metastases (*arrows*). *B,* Chest CT with fine needle in a uveal melanoma metastatic to the lung (*arrow*)

We monitor many small, indeterminate pigmented choroidal tumors for three reasons: (1) as mentioned above, it is usually not possible to determine (with the exceptions noted below) which tumors will remain stationary and which will grow; (2) in over 500 cases we have followed up, without signs of growth, many for as long as 10 years, no mortality has occurred. In those lesions that eventually grew, the tumor-related mortality has been < 5 percent, 5 years after treatment.[77] In the later group of patients who were followed until growth was documented, there is no evidence to suggest that delaying therapeutic intervention increases mortality rates, compared with rates in patients who have been treated elsewhere with immediate intervention;[78,79] and (3) there is a morbidity associated with any form of treatment. Two subsequent large trials have found relatively similar results. As part of the collaborative ocular melanoma study, there was a significantly higher death rate from other causes than tumor, and in their analysis (with slightly different size inclusion criteria) the 8-year melanoma mortality was 3.7 percent. Similarly, a study by Shields and colleagues that included some

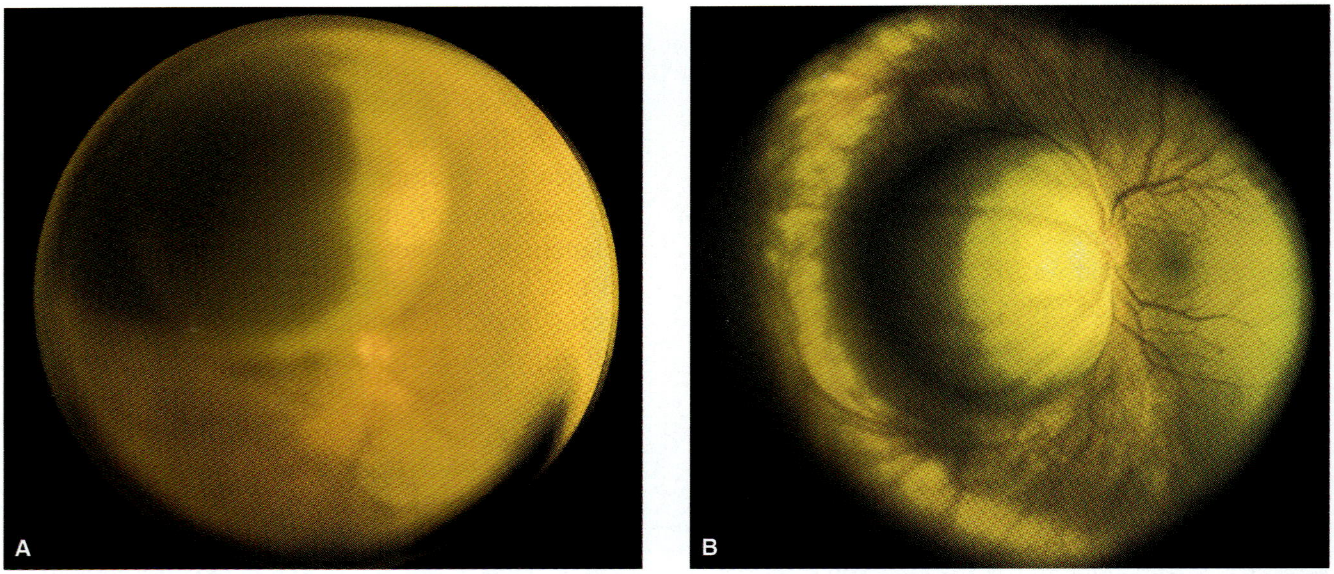

Figure 7–23. *A,* Primary uveal melanoma. *B,* Opposite fundus 2 years later when the patient presented with choroidal metastases (FNAB confirmed) as initial manifestation of widespread disease.

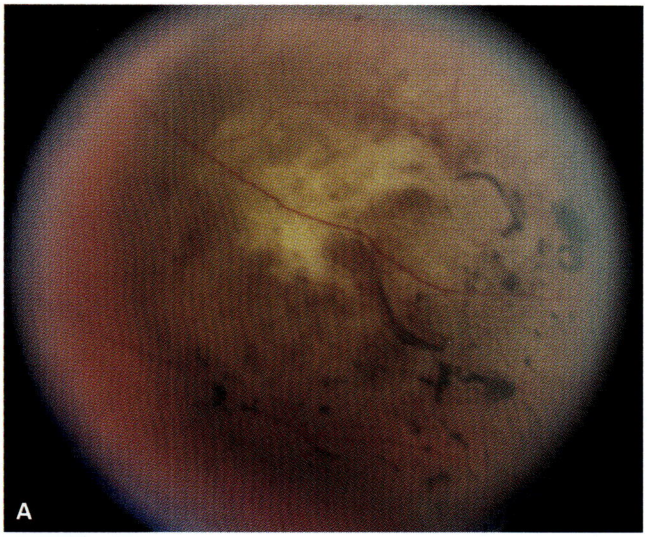

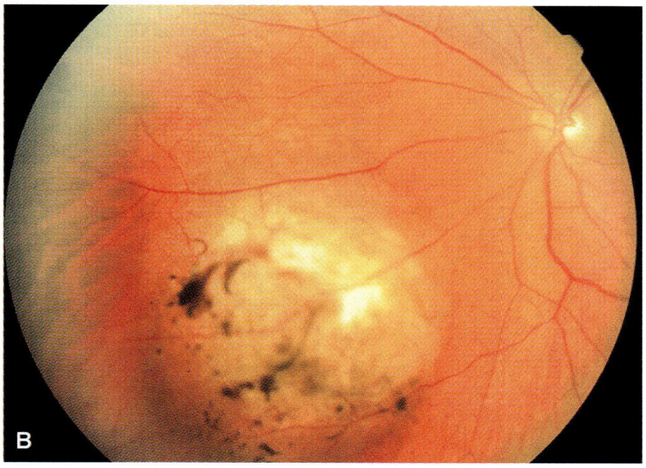

Figure 7–24. *A,* An indeterminant uveal pigmented mass lesion in 1974. *B,* The same lesion 11 years later demonstrating no growth.

small active melanoma on first visit also had similar tumor-related mortality. [80]

Many tumors, especially with extensive drusen, retinal pigment epithelium (RPE) hyperplastic changes, hypopigmented surround, or subretinal neovascularization, remain stationary for many years, and it seems reasonable to not intervene.[77] Figures 7–26 and 7–27 document an exception to a rule, a tumor in which growth occurred in the presence of extensive, overlying drusen. Similarly, other exceptions to rules can occur, such as small melanomas that were treated and the patient died with metastases, or those with extraocular extension noted at enucleation.[81–83] Fortunately, such cases are rare.

It is very difficult to differentiate a small melanoma (< 10 mm in diameter and < 3 mm thick) from an atypical nevus, and we have therefore labeled these lesions, with a neologism, termed "nevomas." There are five inclusion criteria for patients to be serially examined without therapy:

1. tumor size (< 10 mm diameter and < 3 mm thickness),
2. the presence of good vision,
3. absent or minimal subretinal fluid,
4. informed consent, and
5. willingness to have frequent serial examinations, including fundus photography and ultrasonography.

A small amount of subretinal fluid just over a tumor can come and go; however, our experience has been that most tumors with dependent fluid are active and should be treated. Figure 7–28 shows typical RPE changes inferior to a tumor due to resorbed subretinal fluid. Signs that suggest tumor activity are extensive orange pigmentation or an area of the tumor apparently entering a vertical growth phase (Figure 7–29). Figures 7–30A and B show a similar case followed up with 20/20 vision until growth occurred. At that juncture, the tumor was irradiated.

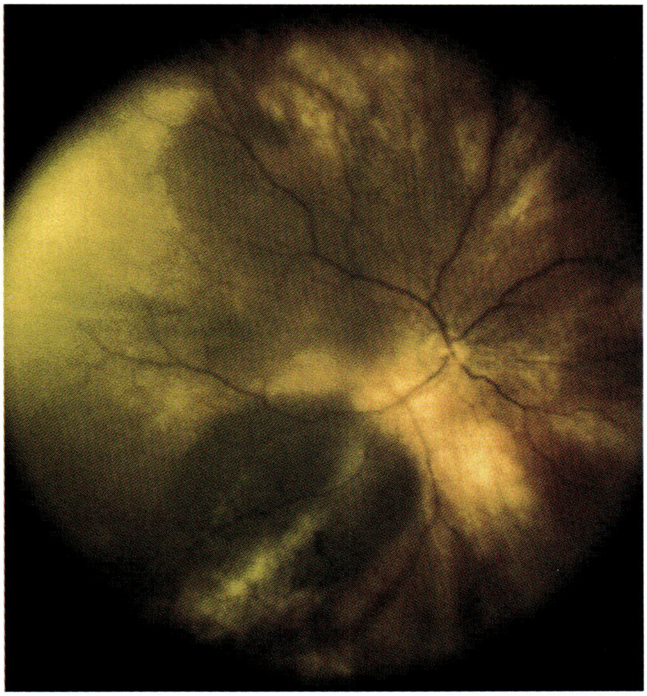

Figure 7–25. A 10-year follow-up without change in this 7.5 x 7.5 x 2.6 mm lesion. At autopsy, this lesion consisted of benign nevoid cells.

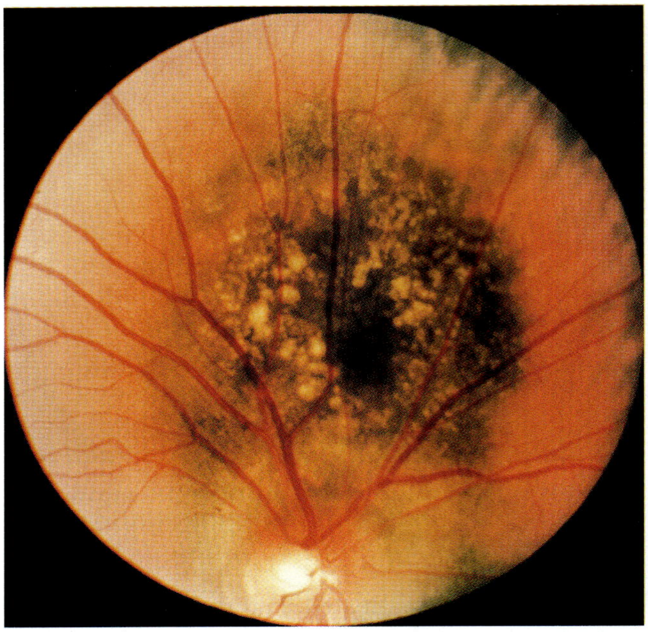

Figure 7–26. A small indeterminate uveal pigmented lesion with extensive drusen; these findings would suggest chronicity and a low potential for growth.

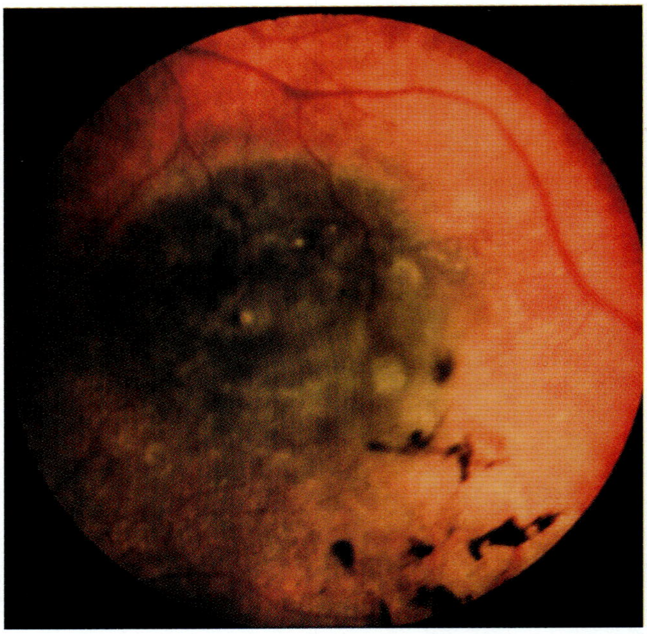

Figure 7–28. Retinal pigment epithelial changes in an area of resorbed subretinal fluid inferior to a mass.

As discussed above, almost all patients with presumed nevomas versus small uveal melanomas are initially monitored clinically (indirect ophthalmoscopic fundus drawing and visual field) and have both photography and ultrasonography performed. The first two visits are usually spaced approximately 3 months apart. During the first year, if no growth is documented horizontally by photography or vertically by ultrasonography, patients are examined every 3 months. After the first year, the interval between return visits is gradually increased.

It is difficult, even with quantitative echography and serial fundus photographs, to be certain whether a very small amount of growth has occurred. Usually, when definite growth occurs, it is readily apparent on clinical observation as well as with ancillary tests (Figure 7–31). The accuracy of ultrasonographic measurements depends on equipment, operator skill, tumor topography, and melanoma loca-

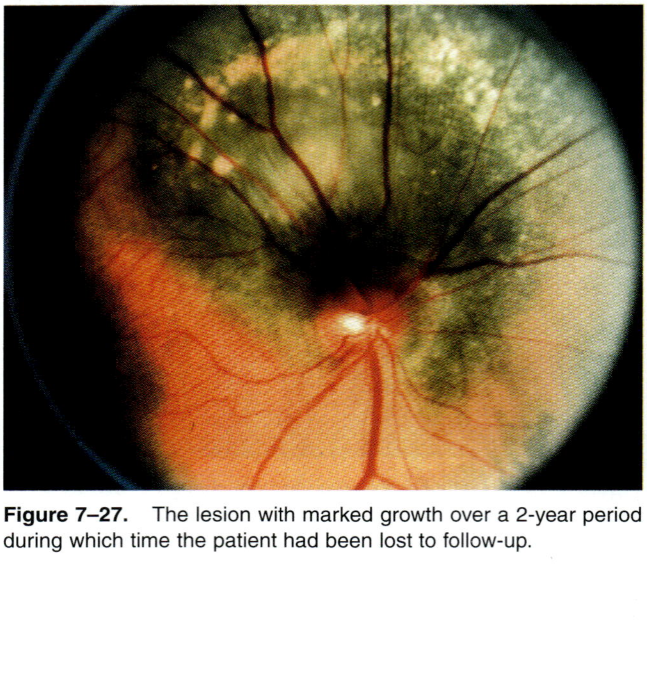

Figure 7–27. The lesion with marked growth over a 2-year period during which time the patient had been lost to follow-up.

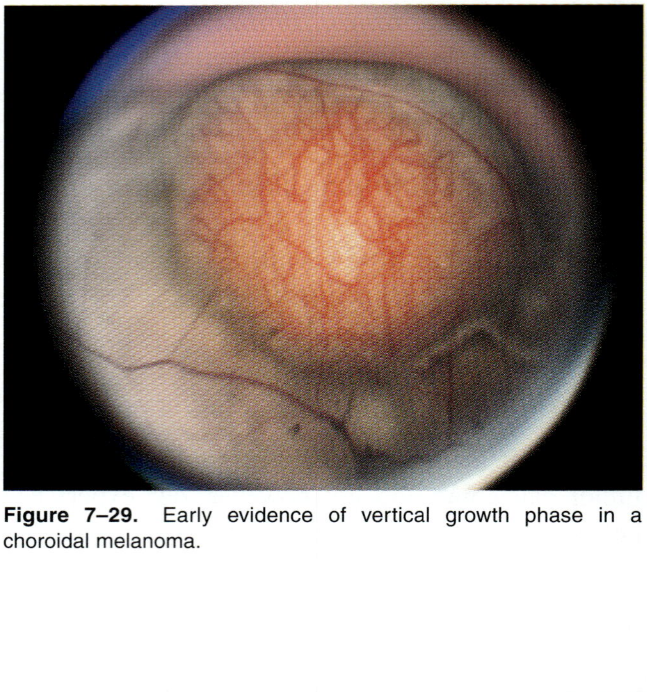

Figure 7–29. Early evidence of vertical growth phase in a choroidal melanoma.

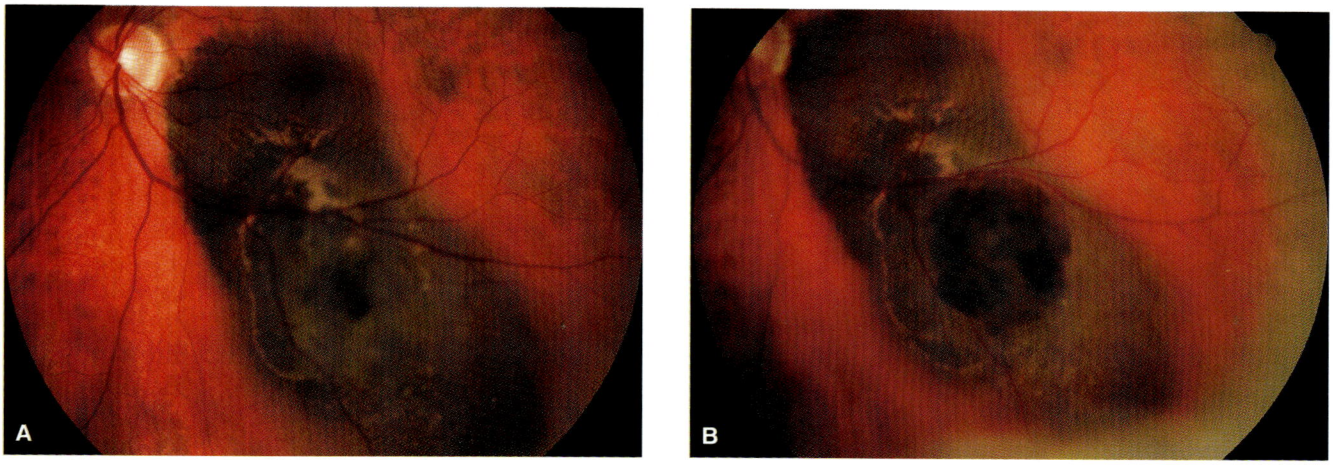

Figure 7–30. *A,* Peripapillary nevoma with orange pigment and 20/20 vision. *B,* One year later, growth occurred, and the eye was irradiated.

tion.[84,85] In regularly shaped posterior pole lesions, a quantitative A-scan increase of 0.5 mm is probably significant. In anterior lesions or in those with an irregular surface contour, ultrasound differences of < 1 mm have to be interpreted cautiously. Similarly, differences in the film, lighting, and camera technique mandate caution, unless the change on serial photographs is unequivocal.

We retrospectively reviewed approximately 300 nevoma patients.[77] In approximately two-thirds of patients, the tumor did not grow over a 5-year observation. We developed a five parameter model to predict growth (Figure 7–32). Each of the factors was given 1 point, except for tumor height, for which 1 point was given for each millimeter of tumor thickness. Symptoms, tumor thickness, presence of orange pigment, hot spots on fluorescein angiography, and homogeneity on ultrasonography were measured. A score of 1 to 2 was associated with < 10 percent chance of tumor growth versus over 90 percent likelihood if a score of 5 or more was established. In approximately 100 cases where the melanoma grew, there were 5 tumor deaths. In 3 of these, the patients delayed therapy despite recommendations for intervention. In one case, the tumor was initially seen when it was 1mm thick; the patient refused enucleation until the tumor filled the eye and became painful. In patients who allowed prompt intervention when growth was detected, the 5-year tumor-related mortality was < 3 percent.[73]

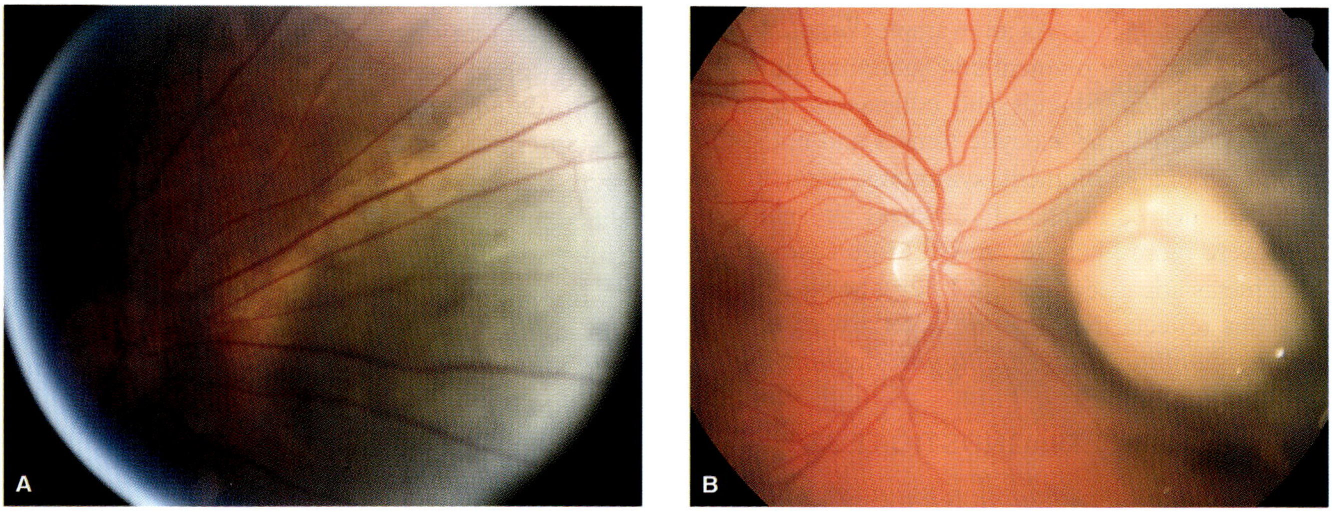

Figure 7–31. *A,* A small uveal melanoma versus a nevoma with good vision. *B,* The lesion shown in Figure 7-31A 9 months later. At this junction the tumor was treated. Five years after combined laser (posterior portion), and helium ion (vertical growth portion), vision is 20/25.

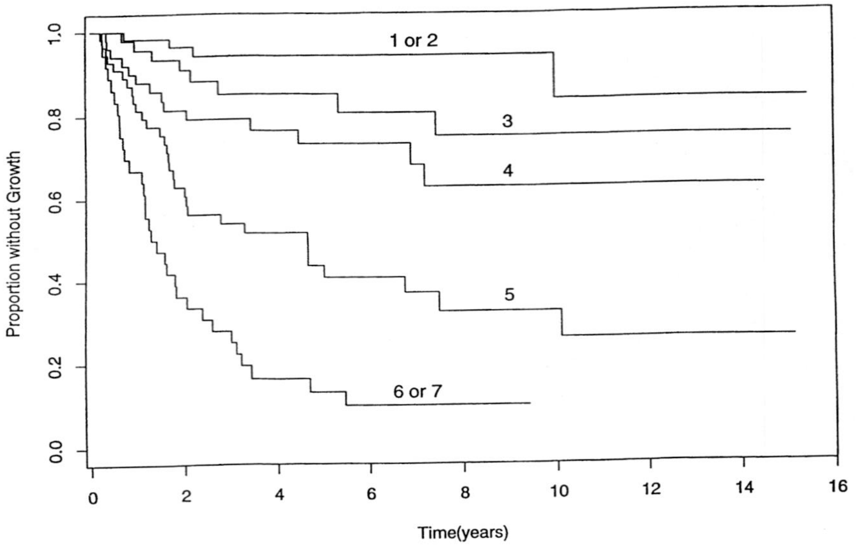

Figure 7–32. Five- parameter model to estimate growth risk in patients with indeterminate pigmented choroidal masses ("nevomas" versus small melanomas).

On the basis of our data and these studies, we no longer monitor all nevomas; if they have a score of 4 or more on our risk table, especially if they are distant from the optic nerve or fovea, we promptly treat them.[77]

Augsburger reviewed the literature on small melanocytic lesions, and noted that between 12 and 44 percent had growth documented; lesions classified as "dormant melanomas" had a 50 percent rate of enlargement.[86] Other investigators have published slightly discrepant results, compared with our nevoma data, probably due to differences in case selection.[68,80] In our analysis, we only included small, indeterminate lesions. As an example, a melanocytic tumor with orange pigment and subretinal fluid was promptly treated. Shields and colleagues reviewed over 1,000 small melanocytic tumors and noted that those with orange pigment, symptoms, contiguity to the optic nerve, increased thickness or subretinal fluid were more likely to grow.[87] More cases developed metastatic disease (35 of 1,329); however, probably this reflects the selection criteria used and the percentage of metastatic events was similarly low.

INVASIVE DIAGNOSTIC TESTS

The use of invasive diagnostic tests is appropriate when therapeutic intervention is indicated and when noninvasive test results are unclear. For example, in a patient with a growing lesion, with nondiagnostic clinical, ultrasound, and fluorescein angiographic findings, additional tests are indicated.

The radioactive phosphorus uptake test is no longer used because of its limited sensitivity and specificity in diagnostically difficult cases. It was routinely positive in large uveal melanomas that were easy to diagnose clinically or with ultrasonography. Its accuracy in atypical simulating lesions including atypical nevi, hemangioma, and metastases was limited.[88,89]

In difficult cases, in which therapeutic intervention is necessary but the diagnosis cannot be established with noninvasive tests, FNAB is the most useful diagnostic assay. There have been over 100,000 fine needle biopsies reported in the systemic cancer literature with no increased tumor-related mortality.[90] A complete discussion of the history and principles of FNAB is found in Chapter 15. In a recent study, we retrospectively reviewed, with the use of Cox multi-variate analysis, the effects of FNAB on melanoma-related mortality and found no adverse effect.[91]

A few case reports of tumor spread with large-bore needle biopsies for solid intraocular tumors were published in the early 20th century through the 1950s.[92–101] Since the late 1970s, a number of authors have reported FNAB diagnosis of uveal melanomas.[102–110]

FNABs are especially useful in patients with opaque media or atypical lesions that require intervention because of their size but cannot be definitively diagnosed with other tests.[7,109] We use a 25-gauge needle, via the transvitreal or trans-scleral route, with minimal morbidity. Surprisingly, when we have used the transvitreal route and entered the tumor by piercing the retina, we have not produced a rhegmatogenous retinal detachment in those eyes that have subsequently undergone alternative therapy. When we use a trans-scleral approach directly over the tumor, we carefully isolate and dry that area and, as we remove the needle, close the minipuncture sites with a drop of histoacryl tissue adhesive.

We have not had any false-positive FNABs. In a few large necrotic melanomas, a false-negative diagnosis was obtained. In 5 small growing tumors, we did not establish a cytopathologic diagnosis. In a few atypical simulating lesions, we have been able to correctly differentiate a benign tumefaction from melanomas.[7,108] We have established an FNAB diagnosis on growing adenomas of the ciliary epithelium, melanocytomas, uveal lymphoid tumors, various metastases, and a probable choroidal neurilemmoma. As a general rule, a positive FNAB result is useful, but a negative one, especially if there is an inadequate sample (too few cells), is not helpful. Other investigators have noted some false-positive and false-negative results.[103,109,111]

The most important expertise in a FNAB is that of a superb cytopathologist. We have examined a number of specimens that were incorrectly diagnosed in other hospitals; if cytologic expertise is not available, this approach should not be used. It is invaluable to have a cytopathologist in the operating room. We immediately perform a quick stain on all aspirates. There are two reasons for this procedure: (1) we can establish the cytologic diagnosis in the operating room in over 98 percent of cases; and (2) if an inadequate specimen is obtained, a second biopsy can be performed. The attendance of a cytopathologist has resulted in a much lower false-negative rate than has been observed in other series.[103,111]

A number of adjuvant studies can be performed on cells obtained with FNAB techniques, including laboratory studies to assess DNA content, cell cycling, flow cytometry, ultrastructure, special stains, and fluorescent in situ hybridization (FISH) analysis. In a study of FNABs performed in eyes treated with either brachytherapy or charged particles, the cytopathologic determination of cell type was strongly correlated with prognosis.[112] It is also possible to perform cell cycling studies on FNAB specimens.[113] In one histologic study of irradiated eyes, positive cycling, as measured with a PC-10 antibody, was associated with ineffective radiation.[112] In addi-

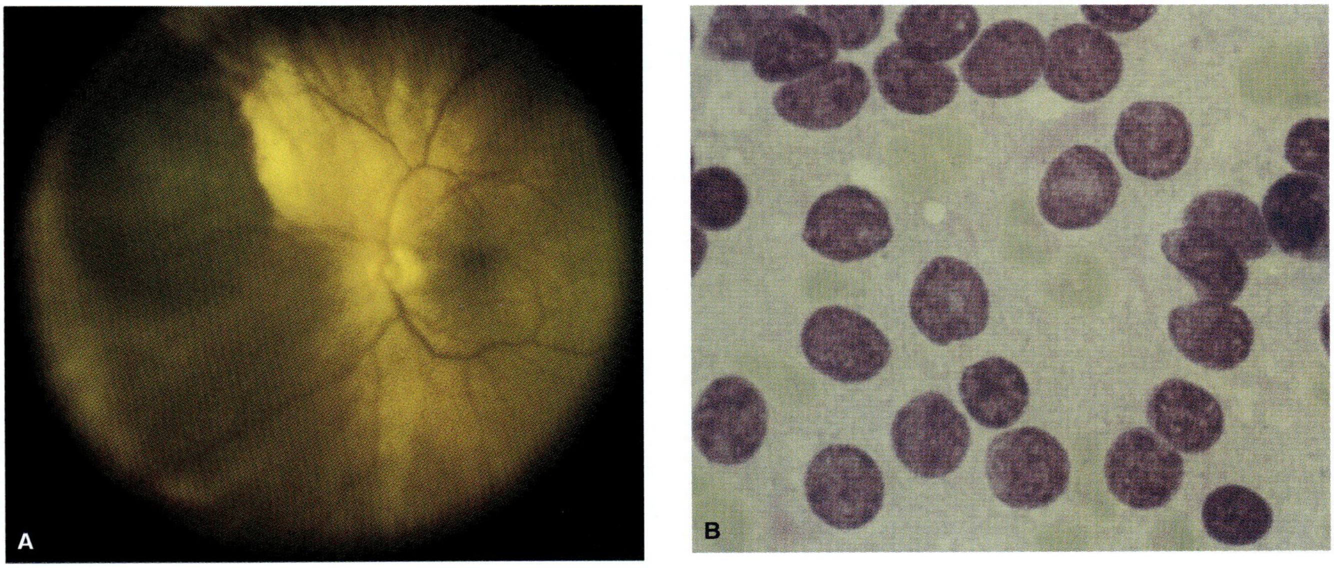

Figure 7–33. *A,* A typical carcinoid with FA and US pattern of a melanoma. A FNAB was positive for carcinoid. *B,* Carcinoid uveal tumor.

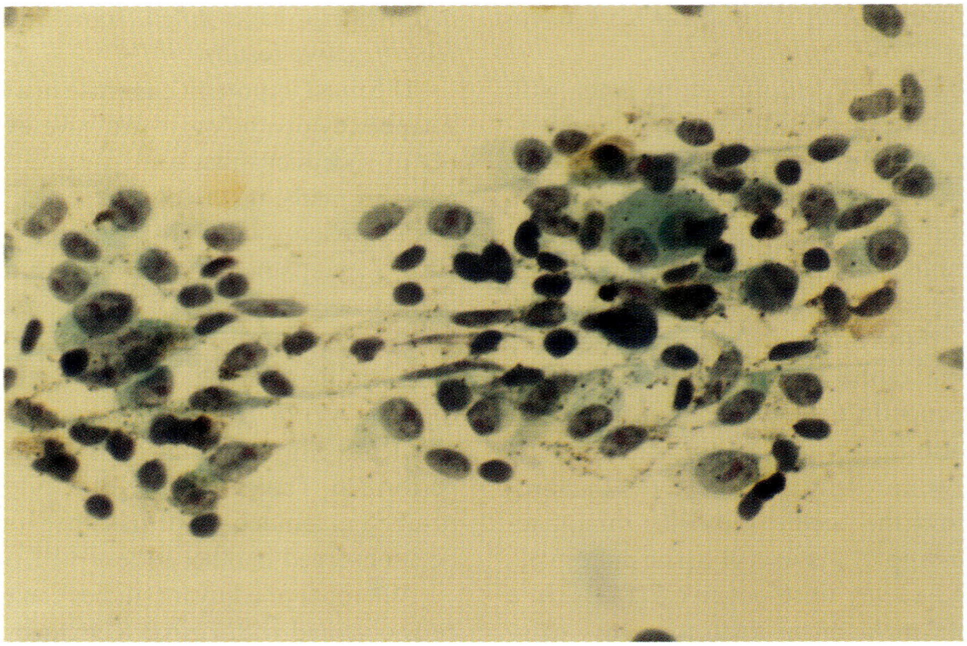

Figure 7–34. Cytopathology of a mixed cell melanoma.

tion, we have recently shown using multivariate anaylsis that data from FNABs add important prognostic information in addition to other paramenters in nonenucleated eyes.[91]

There has been no evidence of spread of a nonocular malignancy caused by FNAB when a 23-gauge or smaller needle was used. Even when extremely malignant, noncohesive animal tumors in syngeneic hosts are studied, no adverse effects on tumor-related mortality as a result of FNAB have been reported. While tumor cells can be observed in the needle track of such animals or in some human sites,

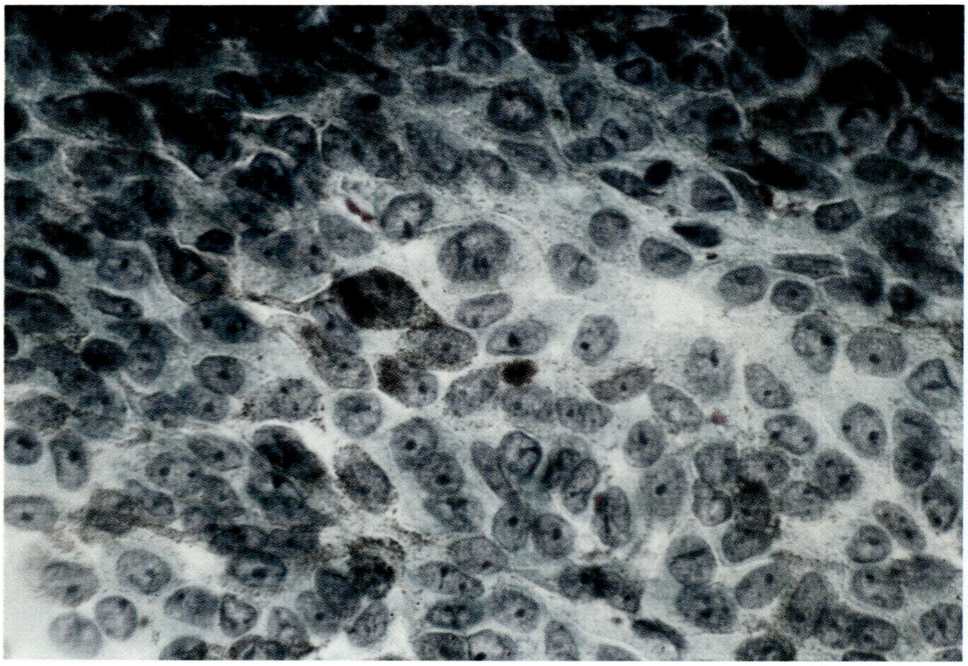

Figure 7–35. Cytopathology of an epithelioid melanoma.

too few cells are present to either develop a successful implant or spread elsewhere.[114]

Figure 7–33A shows an example of an atypical carcinoid tumor; FNAB correctly categorized the lesion (Figure 7–33B), and it completely regressed with a much lower radiation dose and no morbidity. If this tumor had been treated with standard radiation for a melanoma, significant ocular morbidity would probably have occurred. In our experience, we have been able to differentiate spindle, mixed, and epithelioid melanomas on cytopathology. Figure 7–34 shows a mixed melanoma (note both the spindle and epithelioid cells), while Figure 7–35 is a epithelioid melanoma.

REFERENCES

1. Flindall RJ, Drance SM. Visual field studies of benign choroidal melanomata. Arch Ophthalmol 1969;81: 41–4.
2. Eide N, Syrdalen P, Walaas L, Hagmar B. Fine-needle aspiration biopsy in selecting treatment for inconclusive intraocular disease. Acta Ophthalmol Scand 1999;77:448–52.
3. Shields JA, McDonald PR. Improvements in the diagnosis of posterior uveal melanomas. Arch Ophthalmol 1974;91:259–64.
4. Robertson DM, Campbell RJ. Errors in the diagnosis of malignant melanoma of the choroid. Am J Ophthalmol 1979;87:269–75.
5. Davidorf FH, Letson AD, Weiss ET, Levine E. Incidence of misdiagnosed and unsuspected choroidal melanomas. A 50-year experience. Arch Ophthalmol 1983;101:410–2.
6. Gass JD. Problems in the differential diagnosis of choroidal nevi and malignant melanoma. XXXIII Edward Jackson Memorial lecture. Trans Am Acad Ophthalmol Otolaryngol 1977;83:19–48.
7. Char DH, Miller T. Accuracy of presumed melanoma diagnosis prior to alternative therapy. Br J Ophthalmol 1995;79:692–6.
8. Collaborative Ocular Melanoma Study Group. Accuracy of diagnosis of choroidal melanomas in the Collaborative Ocular Melanoma Study. COMS Report No. 1. Arch Ophthalmol 1990;108:1268–73.
9. Margo CE. The accuracy of diagnosis of posterior uveal melanoma. Arch Ophthalmol 1997;115:432–3.
10. Butler P, Char DH, Zarbin M, Kroll S. Natural history of indeterminant pigmented choroidal tumors. Ophthalmology 1994;101:710–7.
11. Kielar RA. Choroidal melanoma appearing as vitreous hemorrhage. Ann Ophthalmol 1982;4:461–4.
12. Bardenstein DS, Char DH, Irvine AR, Stone RD. Extramacular disciform lesions simulating uveal tumors. Ophthalmology 1992;99:944–51.
13. Smith LT, Irvine AR. Diagnostic significance of orange pigment accumulation over choroidal tumors. Am J Ophthalmol 1973;76:212–6.
14. Mortality in patients with small choroidal melanoma. COMS Report No. 4: The collaborative ocular melanoma study group. Arch Ophthalmol 1997; 115:886–93.
15. Sneed SR, Byrne SF, Mieler WF, et al. Choroidal detachment associated with malignant choroidal tumors. Ophthalmology 1991;98:963–70.
16. Char DH, Stone RD, Crawford JB, et al. Diffuse melanoma of the choroid. Br J Ophthalmol 1980; 64:178–80.
17. Font RL, Spaulding AG, Zimmerman LE. Diffuse malignant melanoma of the uveal tract: a clinicopathologic report of 54 cases. Am Acad Ophthalmol Otolaryngol Trans 1968;72:877–95.
18. Ossoinig K. Echography of the eye, orbit, and periorbital region. In: Arger PH, editor. Orbit roentgenology. New York, NY: John Wiley & Sons; 1977. p. 224–69.
19. Coleman DJ, Lizzi FL, Jack RL. Ultrasonography of the eye and orbit. Philadelphia, PA: Lea & Febiger; 1977.
20. Byrne SF, Green RL. Ultrasound of the eye and orbit. St. Louis, MO: Mosby-Year Book; 1992.
21. Wolff-Kormann PG, Kormann BA, Hasenfratz GC, Spengel FA. Duplex and color Doppler ultrasound in the differential diagnosis of choroidal tumors. Acta Ophthalmologica 1992;204 (Suppl):66–70.
22. Guthoff RF, Berger RW, Winkler P, et al. Doppler ultrasonography of malignant melanomas of the uvea. Arch Ophthalmol 1991;109:537–41.
23. Abramson DH, Servodidio CA, McCormick B, et al. Changes in height of choroidal melanomas after plaque therapy. Br J Ophthalmol 1990;74:359–62.
24. Wolff-Kormann PG, Kormann BA, Riedel KG, et al. Quantitative color doppler imaging in untreated and irradiated choroidal melanoma. Invest Ophthalmol Vis Sci 1992;33:1928–33.
25. Gosbell AD, Barry WR, Favilla I, Burgess F. Volume measurement of intraocular tumors by cross-sectional ultrasonographic scans. Austr NZ J Ophthalmol 1991;19:327–33.
26. Jensen PK, Hansen MK. Ultrasonographic, three-dimensional scanning for determination of intraocular tumor volume. Acta Ophthalmol 1991;69:178–86.
27. Finger PT, Romero JM, Rosen RB, et al. Three-dimensional ultrasonography of choroidal melanoma. Arch Ophthalmol 1998;116:305–12.
28. Cusumano A, Coleman DJ, Silverman RH, et al. Three-dimensional ultrasound imaging: Clinical applications. Ophthalmol 1998;105:300–6.

29. O'Leary SW, Ramsey MS. Unsuspected uveal melanoma diagnosed after cataract extraction. Can J Ophthalmol 1990;25:333–5.
30. Aldard WLM, Byrne SF, Hughes JR, Hodapp EA. Dislocated lens nuclei simulating choroidal melanomas. Arch Ophthalmol 1989;107:1463–4.
31. Mueller A, Bartsch D-U, Folberg R, et al. Imaging the microvasculature of choroidal melanomas with confocal indocyanine green scanning laser ophthalmoscopy. Arch Ophthalmol 1998;116:31–9.
32. Scott IU, Murray TG, Hughes JR. Evaluation of imaging techniques for detection of extraocular extension of choroidal melanoma. Arch Ophthalmol 1998;116:897–9.
33. Raymond WR, Char DH, Norman D, Protzko EE. Magnetic resonance imaging evaluation of uveal tumors. Am J Ophthalmol 1991;111:633–41.
34. Jurgens I, Roca G, Sedo S, et al. Presumed melanocytoma of the macula [letter]. Arch Ophthalmol 1994;112(3):305–6.
35. Schilling A, Seiler T, Bender T, Wollensak J. Amelanotisches Melanom und Kernspintomographie—Kasuistik. Fortschr Ophthalmol 1989;86:472–3.
36. Zimmerman RA, Bilaniuk LT. Ocular MR imaging. Radiology 1988;168:875–6.
37. Ferris JD, Bloom PA, Goddard PR, Collins C. Quantification of melanin and iron content in uveal malignant melanomas and correlation with magnetic resonance image. Br J Ophthalmol 1993;77:297–301.
38. Mihara F, Gupta KL, Murayama S, et al. MR imaging of malignant uveal melanoma: role of pulse sequence and contrast agent. Am J Nucl Radiol 1991; 12:991–6.
39. De Potter T, Flanders AE, Shields JA, et al. The role of fat-suppression technique and gadopentetate dimeglumine in magnetic resonance imaging evaluation of intraocular tumors and simulating lesions. Arch Ophthalmol 1994;112:340–8.
40. Bloom PA, Ferris JD, Laidlaw DAH, Goddard PR. Magnetic resonance imaging. Diverse appearances of uveal malignant melanomas. Arch Ophthalmol 1992;110:1105–11.
41. Peyster RG, Augsburger JJ, Shields JA, et al. Choroidal melanoma: comparison of CT, fundoscopy, and US. Radiology 1985;156:675–80.
42. deKeizer RJ, Vielvoye GJ, deWolff-Rouendaal D. Nuclear magnetic resonance imaging of intraocular tumors. Am J Ophthalmol 1986;102:438–41.
43. Jones H, Manners R, Elkington AR, Weller RO. Complete infarction of the eye complicating a choroidal malignant melanoma. Br J Ophthalmol 1991;75: 471–2.
44. Brancato R, Lucignani G, Modorati G, et al. Metabolic imaging of uveal melanoma using positron emission tomography. Arch Ophthalmol 1990;108:326–7.
45. Pascal SG, Liggett PE, Chen CP, et al. Immunoscintigraphy of primary metastatic uveal melanoma with technetium-99M labeled monoclonal antibody. Ophthalmology 2000 [In press].
46. Karczmar GS, Meyerhoff DJ, Boska MD, et al. P-31 spectroscopy study of response to superficial human tumors to therapy. Radiology 1991;179:149–53.
47. Modorati G, Brancato R, Paganelli G, et al. Immunoscintigraphy with three step monoclonal pretargeting technique in diagnosis of uveal melanoma: preliminary results. Br J Ophthalmol 1994;78:19–23.
48. De Potter P, Von Weymarn C, Zografos L. In vivo phosphorus-31 magnetic resonance spectroscopy of human uveal melanomas and other intraocular tumors. Am J Ophthalmol 1991;111:276–88.
49. Rennie I. Imaging posterior uveal melanomas. Br J Ophthalmol 1994;78:241.
50. Yakobson EA, Zlotogorski A, Shafir R, et al. Screening for tumour suppressor p16 (CDKN2A) germline mutations in Israeli melanoma families. Clin Chem Lab Med 1998;36:645–7.
51. Char D, Caputo G, Miller T. Orbital fibrous histiocytomas. Orbit; 2000 [In press].
52. Grimson BS, Cohen KL, McCartney WH. Concomitant ocular and orbital neoplasms. J Comput Assist Tomogr 1982;6:617–9.
53. Lashkari K, Lee KY, Cheng HM, et al. Gadolinium-enhanced magnetic resonance imaging of melanomas treated with iodine plaque and laser coagulation. Ophthalmology, 2000 [In press].
54. Cousins JP. Clinical MR spectroscopy: fundamentals, current applications, and future potential. AJR Am J Roentgenol 1995;164:1337–47.
55. Kolodny NH, Albert DM, Epstein J, et al. Characterization of human uveal melanoma cells by phosphorous 31 nuclear magenetic resonance spectroscopy. Am J Ophthalmol 1985;100:38–44.
56. Gomori JM, Grossman RI, Shields JA, et al. Choroidal melanomas: correlation of NMR spectroscopy and MR imaging. Radiology 1986;158:443–5.
57. Kurhanewicz J, Char DH, Stauffer P, et al. ^{31}P magnetic resonance spectroscopy after combined hyperthermia and radiation. Current Eye Res 1993;13: 151–6.
58. Char DH, Metastatic choroidal melanoma. Am J Ophthalmol 1978;86:76–80.
59. Char DH, Heilbron DC, Juster RP, Stone RD. Choroidal melanoma growth patterns. Br J Ophthalmol 1983;67:575–8.
60. Bardenstein DS, Char DH, Kaleta-Michaels S, Kroll SM. Ki-67 and bromodeoxyuridine labeling of human choroidal melanoma cells. Current Eye Res 1991;10:479–84.

61. Kroll S, Char DH, Kaleta-Michaels S. A stochastic model for dual label experiments: an analysis of the heterogeneity of S-phase duration. Cell Proliferation 1995;28:545–67.
62. Manschot WA, Van Strik R. Uveal melanoma: therapeutic consequences of doubling times and irradiation results: a review. Intl Ophthalmol 1992;16:91–9.
63. Holmgren L, O'Reilley MS, Folkman J. Dormancy of micrometastases: balance, proliferation, and apoptosis in the presence of angiogenesis suppression. Nature Med 1995;1:149–50.
64. Gragoudas ES, Egan KM, Seddon JM, et al. Survival of patients with metastases from uveal melanoma. Ophthalmology 1991;98:383–9.
65. Kath R, Hayungs J, Bornfeld N, et al. Prognosis and treatment of disseminated uveal melanoma. Cancer 1993;72:2219–23.
66. Inouye SK, Sox HC Jr. Standard and computed tomography in the evaluation of neoplasms of the chest. A comparative efficacy assessment. Ann Intern Med 1986;105:906–24.
67. Eskelin S, Pyrhonen S, Summanen P, et al. Screening for metastatic malignant melanoma of the uvea revisited. Cancer 1999;85:1151–9.
68. Hicks C, Foss AJE, Hungerford JL. Predictive power of screening tests for metastasis in uveal melanoma. Eye 1998;2:945–8.
69. Albert DM, Niffenegger AS, Willson JK. Treatment of metastatic uveal melanoma: review and recommendations. Surv Ophthalmol 1992;36:429–38.
70. Lawford JB, Collins ET. Sarcoma of the uveal tract, with notes of one hundred and three cases. London Ophthal Hosp Rep 1891;13:104–65.
71. von Hippel E. Zur Prognose der Uvealsarkome. Arch Ophthalmol 1930;124:206–20.
72. Westerveld-Brandon ER, Zeeman WP. The prognosis of melanoblastomata of the choroid. Ophthalmologica 1957;134:20–9.
73. Char DH. History of ocular oncology. Ophthalmology 1996;103:S90–101.
74. Albert DM. The ocular melanoma story. LII Edward Jackson Memorial Lecture. Am J Ophthalmol 1997; 123:729–41.
75. Dunphy EB. Management of intraocular malignancy: the Gifford Memorial Lecture. Am J Ophthalmol 1957;44:313–22.
76. Koenig IJ. Malignant melanoma of the iris and ciliary body of a one-eyed patient: case observed for 20 years. Arch Ophthalmol 1954;51:656–62.
77. Butler P, Char DH, Zarbin M, Kroll S. Natural history of indeterminant pigmented choroidal tumors. Ophthalmology 1994;101:710–7.
78. Shields JA, McDonald PR. Improvements in the diagnosis of posterior uveal melanomas. Arch Ophthalmol 1974;87:259–64.
79. Diener-West M, Hawkins BS, Markowitz JA, Schachat AP. A review of mortality from choroidal melanoma. II. A meta-analysis of 5-year mortality rates following enucleation. Arch Ophthalmol 1992;110:245–50.
80. Shields CL, Shields JA, Kiratli H, et al. Risk factors for growth and metastasis of small choroidal melanocytic lesions. Trans Am Ophthalmol Soc 1995;93:259–75.
81. Raivio I. Uveal melanoma in Finland. An epidemiological, clinical, histological and prognostic study. Acta Ophthalmol Suppl 1977;133:1–64.
82. Ruiz RS. Early treatment in malignant melanomas of the choroid. In: Brockhurst RJ, Boruchoff SA, Hutchinson BT, Lessell S, editors. Controversy in ophthalmology. Philadelphia, PA: WB Saunders; 1977. p. 604–10.
83. Davidorf FH, Pajka JT, Makley TA Jr, Kartha MK. Radiotherapy for choroidal melanoma. An 18-year experience with radon. Arch Ophthalmol 1987; 105:352–5.
84. Char DH, Stone RD, Irvine AR, et al. Diagnostic modalities in choroidal melanoma. Am J Ophthalmol 1980;89:223–30.
85. Verbeek AM. Differential diagnosis of intraocular neoplasms with ultrasonography. Ultrasound Med Biol 1985;11:163–70.
86. Augsburger JJ. Is observation really appropriate for small choroidal melanomas. Trans Am Ophthalmol Soc 1993;91:147–75.
87. Shields CL, Shields JA, Kirali H, et al. Risk factors for metastasis of small choroidal melanocytic lesions. Are we waiting too long? Ophthalmology 1995; 102:1351–61.
88. Zakov ZN, Smith TR, Albert DM. False-positive 32P uptake tests. Arch Ophthalmol 1978;96:2240–3.
89. Shammas HF, Burton TC, Weingeist TA. False-positive results with the radioactive phosphorus test. Arch Ophthalmol 1977;95:2190–2.
90. Tao LC, Pearson FG, Delarue NC, et al. Percutaneous fine-needle aspiration biopsy. I. Its value to clinical practice. Cancer 1980;45:1480–5.
91. Char DH, Kroll SM, Miller T, et al. Irradiated uveal melanomas: cytopathologic correlation with prognosis. Am J Ophthalmol 1996;122:509–13.
92. Esser F. Zur Diagnose des Aderhaut-Sarkoms. Klin Monatsbl Augenheilk 1924;73:192–4.
93. Meisner W. Zur Diagnose des Aderhautsarkoms. Klin Monatsbl Augenheilk 1923;70:722–32.
94. Velhagen K. Uber die diagnostische Punktion bei Verdacht auf Srakom der Aderhaut. Klin Monatsbl Augenheilk 1941;107:354–61.
95. Popovic JM. Zur Diagnose des Aderhautsarkoms: Modifikation der Meisnerschen Punktion zwechs mikroskopischer Feststellung des Aderhautsarkoms. Klin Monatsbl Augenheilk 1931;86:816–9.
96. Kauffman ML. Aspiration biopsy of malignant

melanoma of choroid. Arch Ophthalmol 1952;47: 541–2.
97. Veasey CA Jr. Intraocular biopsy. Am J Ophthalmol 1951;34:432–4.
98. Long JC, Black WC, Danielson RW. Aspiration biopsy in intraocular tumors. Arch Ophthalmol 1953;50: 303–10.
99. Gonzales VF, Pateyro P, Grosso O. Cytologic diagnosis of melanoma of the choroid. Arch Soc Ophthalmol Hispano Am 1950;10:579.
100. Sanders TE, Smith ME. Biopsy of intraocular tumors: a re-evaluation. Int Ophthalmol Clin 1972;12:163–76.
101. Makley TA Jr. Biopsy of intraocular lesions. Am J Ophthalmol 1967;64:591–9.
102. Prescher G, Bornfeld N, Horsthemke B, Becher R. Chromosomal aberrations defining uveal melanoma of poor prognosis. Lancet 1992;339:691–2.
103. Shields JA, Shields CL, Ehya H, et al. Fine-needle aspiration biopsy of suspected intraocular tumors. Ophthalmology 1993;100:1677–84.
104. Jakobiec FA, Coleman DJ, Chattock A, Smith M. Ultrasonographically guided needle biopsy and cytologic diagnosis of solid intraocular tumors. Ophthalmology 1979;86:1662–81.
105. Czerniak B, Woyke S, Domagala W, Krzysztolik Z. Fine-needle aspiration cytology of intraocular malignant melanoma. Acta Cytologica 1983;27:157–65.
106. Augsburger JJ, Shields JA, Folberg R, et al. Fine-needle aspiration biopsy in the diagnosis of intraocular cancer. Cytologic-histologic correlations. Ophthalmology 1985;92:39–49.
107. Palma D, Canall N, Scaroni P, Torri AM. Fine needle aspiration biopsy: its use in the management of orbital and intraocular tumors. Tumor 1989;75: 598–603.
108. Char DH, Miller TR, Crawford JB. Cytopathologic diagnosis of benign lesions simulating choroidal melanomas. Am J Ophthalmol 1991;112:70–5.
109. Davila RM, Miranda MC, Smith ME. Role of cytopathology in the diagnosis of ocular malignanices. Acta Cytol 1998;42:362–6.
110. Char DH, Kroll SM, Stoloff A, et al. Cytomorphometry of uveal melanoma. Comparison of fine needle aspiration biopsy samples with histologic sections. Analytical Quantitative Cytol Histol 1991;13:293–9.
111. Shields JA, Eagle RC Jr, Barr CC, et al. Adenocarcinoma of retinal pigment epithelium arising from a juxtapapillary histoplasmosis scar. Arch Ophthalmol 1994;112:650–3.
112. Pe'er J, Gnessin H, Shargal Y, Livni N. PC-10 immunostaining of proliferating cell nuclear antigen in posterior uveal melanoma. Enucleation versus enucleation postirradiation groups. Ophthalmology 1994;101:56–60.
113. Char DH, Kroll SM, Stoloff A, et al. Cytomorphometry of uveal melanomas: fine-needle aspiration biopsy versus standard histology. Trans Am Ophthalmol Soc 1989;87:197–212.
114. Glasgow BJ, Brown HH, Zargoza AM, Foos RY. Quantitation of tumor seeding from fine needle aspiration of ocular melanomas. Am J Ophthalmol 1988;105:538–46.

8

Management of Posterior Uveal Tumors

The management of both nevomas (indeterminate pigmented choroidal neoplasms) and uveal melanomas is controversial. A number of unresolved issues make it difficult to make definitive statements about the effect of various therapies on vision and on tumor-related mortality.[1–3] The two most important clinical questions are: at what stage in the natural history of a uveal melanoma does it develop the capacity to metastasize, and at what stage must ocular intervention occur to avoid the development of widespread disease? In other words, what is the most effective form of treatment for a given uveal melanoma? The third paramount question is: what treatment, for a given tumor, will produce local control with the least ocular morbidity?

A number of clinical uveal melanoma parameters correlate with prognosis. Increased tumor diameter, increased age, extraocular extension, and involvement of the ciliary body and anterior choroid all adversely affect prognosis.[4] Lighter iris color was correlated with higher tumor-related mortality.[5] In women, a history of childbearing was associated with improved survival (relative risk 1.23).[6] Several studies have shown no adverse effect of pregnancy on survival of melanoma patients.[7]

A number of histologic parameters correlate with prognosis. These parameters include cell type (worse with mixed or epithelioid tumors), measures of increased nucleolar area (mean area of largest nucleoli is easier to compute than the inverse of the standard deviation), increased DNA content (aneuploidy), increased cell cycling (increased bromodeoxyuridine uptake, increased mitoses, Ki67 and proliferating cell nuclear antigen [PCNA]), complex microvascular patterns (see below), and the presence of tumor-infiltrating lymphocytes (TIL).[8–16] The relative prognostic importance of each parameter, and their inter-relationship is uncertain. Different investigators using retrospective data sets have discrepant conclusions.[17–23] There are a few other parameters which have been studied and have shown promise, including the pattern of tumor infiltration by peripheral blood lymphocytes as well as the level of various antigens (ICAM) on the tumor cell surface; however, these data have not been replicated in other studies.[24,25] Gamel, McLean, and colleagues have shown that tumor diameter, mean nucleolar area, and cell type all affect prognosis and probably are pertubated by other different tumor parameters.[9–13,26] Folberg and associates noted that vascular loops, vascular networks, parallel vessels with crosslinks, and arcs were associated with more malignant cell types.[11] In their multivariate analysis, vascular pattern and largest tumor diameter were the most important prognostic parameters, although increased mitoses were also associated with worse outcome.[27] In my laboratory using a smaller data set, we noted that measures of cell cycling (increased mitoses or bromodeoxyuridine uptake) correlated better with survival than did vascular patterns.[28] Pe'er and coworkers found that nucleolar area did not contribute in a prognostic model when vascular patterns had already been entered into it; other investigators have disagreed with that assessment.[27–29]

The presence of tumor-infiltrating lymphocytes was associated with worse prognosis. Whelcher and colleagues found that both T-cell and B-cell infiltration in uveal melanomas were associated more with tumor-related mortality.[30] At 18 years the mortality was 73 percent when lymphocytes were present and only 32 percent when there were only a few of these infiltrating cells. In our experience, only a small number of uveal melanomas have over 5 percent tumor-infiltrating lymphocytes.[31] Several other experimental assays are under investigation. As an example, the presence of gelatinolytic metalloproteinase has correlated with increased metastatic risk.[32]

McLean and co-workers have used histologic parameters to ascertain factors that affect survival times, compared with cure rates, in uveal melanomas. In their analysis, cell type was associated with survival time but not with cure rate. Increasing age markedly affected mean survival time but did not affect cure.[19,33]

INTERVENTION OPTIONS

The different treatment options for uveal melanomas include various forms of brachytherapy (radioactive plaques), charged particle beams (helium ions and protons), gamma knife, intensity-modulated conformal teletherapy, xenon photocoagulation, krypton laser, tunable dye laser, laser-induced hyperthermia (transpupillary thermotherapy [TTT]), adjunct hyperthermia, various approaches to resect the tumor with eye retention, and enucleation with or without adjunct radiation. There is minimal randomized prospective treatment data for any of these modalities, except pre-enucleation radiation and comparison of plaques and charged particles. A large body of retrospective treatment data and some prospective studies can be used as a basis for rational therapy.

Our indications for therapy with the intent to preserve the globe are nevomas with > 80 percent chance of growth, small melanomas with dependent subretinal fluid into the fovea decreasing vision, small uveal melanomas with documented growth, and most medium- and many large-sized uveal melanomas. The author is unaware of any data that show better survival with enucleation than with other therapies. The relative merits of a Collaborative Ocular Melanoma Study (COMS) are discussed later. Several American ocular oncologists did not participate in this trial for four reasons:[34] (1) as discussed below, the tumor-related mortality rate in the patient cohort that the study initially randomized to enucleation versus iodine-125 (^{125}I) brachytherapy was only 10 percent at 5 years after helium ion radiation.[34] Several investigators felt that this tumor-related mortality was too low to detect a difference between radiation versus enucleation if one existed; (2) in the patients who would be randomized to enucleation, several leading ocular oncologists believed that many of these patients would retain excellent vision and did not think it was ethical to randomize them, since there were no data suggesting better survival with enucleation;[35] (3) the trial did not include some of the newer therapies, such as charged particle (proton) radiation; and (4) in a subset of patients with even larger melanomas who were randomized to pre-enucleation radiation versus enucleation alone, we and others, as discussed below, had shown that there was no advantage in that adjunctive treatment. The COMS trial of pre-enucleation radiation has similarly shown no significant advantage.[35,36]

We do not recommend alternative therapy to patients who, when confronted with the fact that they have a malignant tumor, wish to have the eye removed and to those with melanomas that involve > 40 percent of the ocular volume, melanomas in blind eyes, tumors in eyes with iris neovascularization, or most melanomas in eyes with significant localized extrascleral extension.

Xenon Photocoagulation and Laser Treatment

Conventional photocoagulation and laser treatment have only limited value in uveal melanoma therapy; < 5 percent of melanomas meet the criteria for this form of treatment.[37] This technique was used in small growing melanomas < 3.0 mm thick located between 1 and 3 mm from the optic nerve or fovea. The use of any radiation modality in these areas is very likely to produce visually destructive radiation vasculopathy. We have also used older and newer forms of laser or photocoagulation in growing small melanomas farther from the nerve or fovea, but behind the equator. In addition to the thickness limit, in our experience, of < 3.5 mm, we have restricted the use of this modality to tumors < 10 mm in diameter. Vogel and colleagues have listed a number of criteria for photocoagulation treatment.[38] That probably remains germane for newer approaches, such as TTT. The pupil must be easily dilated and the media clear. Tumors > 10 mm in diameter or > 4.0 mm thick are poor candidates for laser or photocoagulation treatment, as are lesions with extensive overlying detachment.

We have had poor results with conventional laser treatment of patients with growing foveal melanomas; < 40 percent of the melanomas were successfully destroyed (unpublished observations). These data demonstrated that tumors at the fovea are not good candidates for conventional laser treatment. Amelanotic tumors have also been relatively resistant. We, as well as others, have found argon laser therapy less effective than either krypton or xenon.[39] The author has not used a tunable dye laser for melanomas.

A number of different photocoagulation protocols have been published.[40,41] Retrobulbar anesthesia with an equal combination of 4 percent lidocaine (Xylocaine) and 0.75 percent bupivacaine (Marcaine) is given for both older and newer photocoagulation and laser therapies. Xenon arc photocoagulation was done with a 6° aperture and a setting of green I or II. The tumor was surrounded with at least two confluent rows of photocoagulation; their purpose was fourfold: (1) in subsequent treatment sessions, the overlying retina was destroyed; unless a barrier was created between the treatment area and the normal retina, an iatrogenic retinal break could cross into normal retina and produce a detachment; (2) approximately 10 percent of patients treated with photocoagulation had late tumor recurrence (Figure 8–1); a wide area of surrounding retinal ablation decreased the likelihood of a marginal miss; (3) before extensive destruction occurred, it was easier to establish a safe distance between the edge of treatment and the fovea or optic nerve; and (4) destruction of the surrounding retinal and choroidal vessels diminished the vascular supply to the melanoma.

After surrounding the tumor, moderately heavy treatment was delivered to the entire tumor. Examples of a tumor before and after four treatments are shown in Figure 8–2. We waited between 6 and 8 weeks for repigmentation before commencing the second treatment session. Either xenon arc photocoagulation (green I-IV) or krypton laser (500 micron spot size, 0.2-second duration, and 500 to 1,200 mW power) was used. The tumor was treated relatively heavily, but care was taken to try not to destroy the overlying Bruch's membrane. Subsequent treatment sessions were similarly spaced. Usually, during the third or fourth treatment sessions, audible "pigment pops" were heard as Bruch's membrane was destroyed. Often an overlying, poorly pigmented scar developed, and it had to be destroyed with heavier treatment.

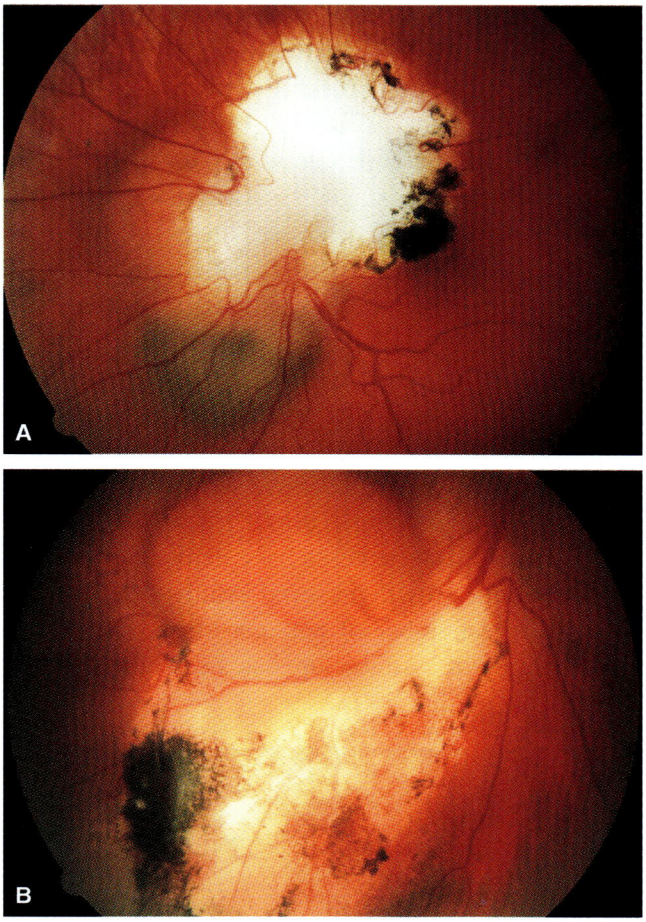

Figures 8–1. *A* and *B*, Recurrent melanomas treated with photocoagulation several years earlier at another center.

Other workers have used different time, power, and fractionation protocols. Some investigators have used very low powers for extremely long durations (up to 1 minute) to treat these tumors. Retrospectively, those investigators were probably heating the tumor, although that was not considered a major mechanism of tumor cytoxicity at the time.

The author has seen a few patients treated up to 18 times and referred with active, growing melanomas. Usually, with either laser or photocoagulation, tumor control is achieved in four to six treatments. The author has not treated any patient more than eight times with this modality.

It is difficult to determine when a melanoma has been destroyed after either laser or photocoagulation.[42] Usually, a successfully treated melanoma appears as an area of scleral show surrounding a brown to black pigment area with interspersed areas of bare sclera; this stage is shown in Figure 8–2. Often, it takes up to 2 years for the entire tumor to dissipate; as mentioned above, patients need ongoing follow-up, since there is late recurrence in up to 10 percent of cases (see Figure 8–1).[43–45]

We have treated a few indeterminate, elevated, pigmented choroidal lesions with photocoagulation or laser to eradicate vision-reducing subretinal fluid. All these cases have had diffuse serous leakage, and treatment with moderate burns has not been successful; most of these cases have demonstrated subsequent tumor growth on serial evaluation.[46]

In a large number of patients treated with TTT, unfortunately, the follow-up has been too short to draw definitive conclusions.[47] Probably, the concept on which this was based was predated by Brockhurst, who suggested using very low-energy, long-duration treatments with argon many years ago (personal communications). The current approach uses a very large spot size (generally 2,000 or 3,000 microns), long duration (1 minute), relatively low intensity (generally in the range of 400- 1,000 mW) overlapping treatments. The commercial unit is made by Iris Medical and is shown in Figure 8–3. A good example prior to and following this form of therapy is shown in Figures 8–4 to 8–7. The Dutch group has had the longest experience with this approach.[48] In histologic studies, they demonstrated depth of tumor penetration up to 3.9 mm. However, in those histologic studies, 4 out of the 11 enucleated eyes had minimal tumor damage.[49] Most of the patients initially treated with this regime were managed with a combination of brachytherapy and this laser modality.[50] The Dutch group was concerned about the use of only this laser approach, since in one histologic specimen, there was a viable cluster of cells deep in the sclera.[51]

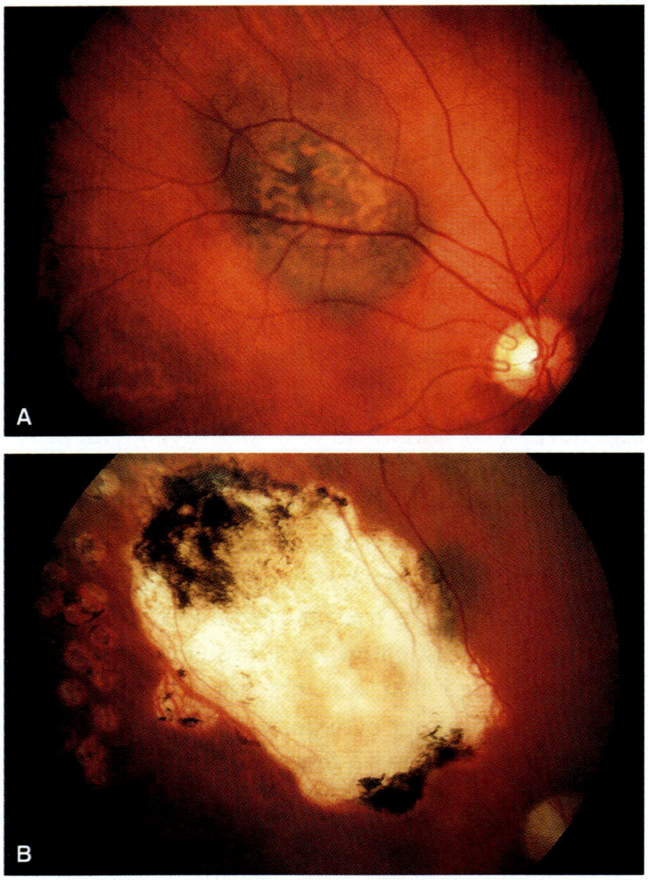

Figure 8–2. *A,* Prior to photocoagulation for a growing tumor. *B,* After photocoagulation for growing tumor shown in Figure 8–2A. Lesion appears to be destroyed and vision remains good.

Several investigators in the United States have used a slight modification of this approach, as primary treatment for nevomas or small uveal melanomas. The author's results have not been published because the long-term efficacy is not known. In one paper, 100 consecutive cases of tumors with a mean diameter of 7.1 mm and a mean thickness of 2.8 mm were treated. After an average of three treatment sessions, the tumor thickness had markedly diminished, and only 6 percent of the eyes had failed, with relatively short follow-up. As many of the tumors were under the macula, there was a 42 percent incidence of decreased vision, as expected.[52] A recent small study by Robertson and colleagues demonstrates that many small tumors probably only require a single therapy session and long follow-up. They treated a group of generally smaller tumors with a mean height of approximately 2 mm with one session of laser and found with follow-up that almost all of them had regressed.[53] As we have also noted, it can sometimes take over a year to see the onset of response after this form of therapy, and regression can continue without additional treatment for 2 to 3 more years.

Godfrey and colleagues reported 14 patients treated with TTT with a mean tumor thickness of

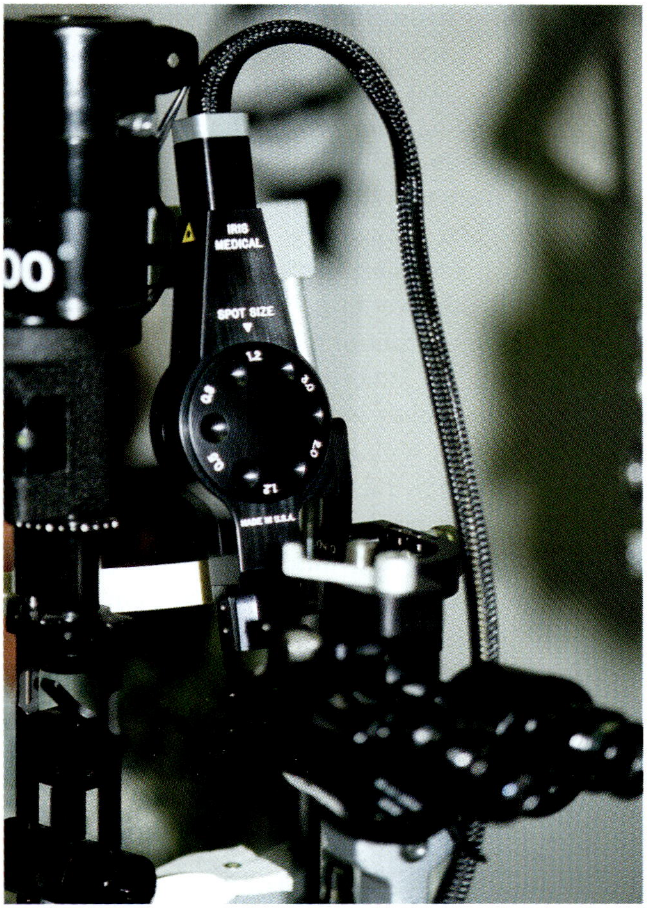

Figure 8–3. A slit-lamp laser delivery system used to deliver presumed laser-induced hyperthermia, also termed "transpupillary thermal therapy."

1.8 mm. Three of 14 required re-treatment, and one eye had to be enucleated. Complications included hemorrhage, vessel occlusion, retinal traction, and pain.[54,55]

Seven major complications are associated with either photocoagulation or laser treatment of uveal melanomas: (1) excessive treatment can produce a retinal break and detachment, especially if there is an insufficient barrier between the tumor and the normal retina; (2) during the third or fourth treatment session, the melanoma may bleed (Figure 8–8). Rarely, this can produce a vitreous hemorrhage, usually stopped by gentle digital pressure; (3) in tumors that are < 1 mm from the fovea, structural alteration of the macula and diminished vision have almost always been unavoidable; (4) a major late complication has been choroidal-retinal-vitreal neovascularization at the edge of treatment.[56] An example of this

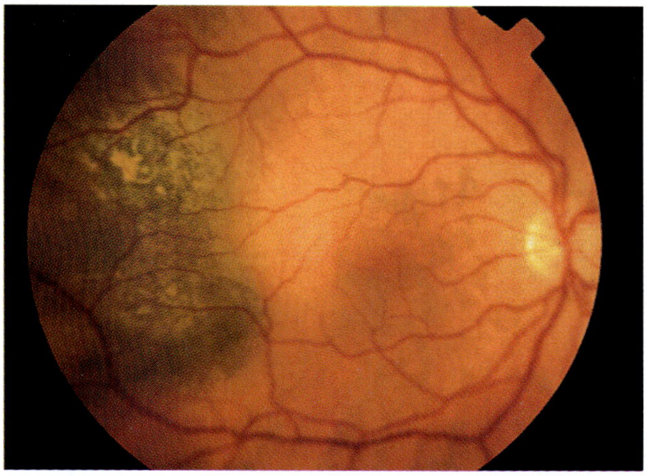

Figure 8–4. A patient before treatment with laser-induced hyperthermia

complication is shown in Figure 8–9. This neovascularization is extremely difficult to manage. Some patients have had 20/20 vision after tumor destruction, only to present 4 to 12 months later with a total detachment and diffuse vitreous hemorrhage from late neovascularization. Scatter photocoagulation peripheral to the tumor in the area of major vessels may diminish peripheral retinal ischemia and prevent this complication from occurring; (5) a few patients have developed visual loss from treatment-induced branch vessel occlusion with secondary macular edema; (6) especially with thick tumors or lesions inside the vascular arcade, incomplete tumor control has necessitated other therapy; and (7) when xenon arc photocoagulation is used, corneal damage

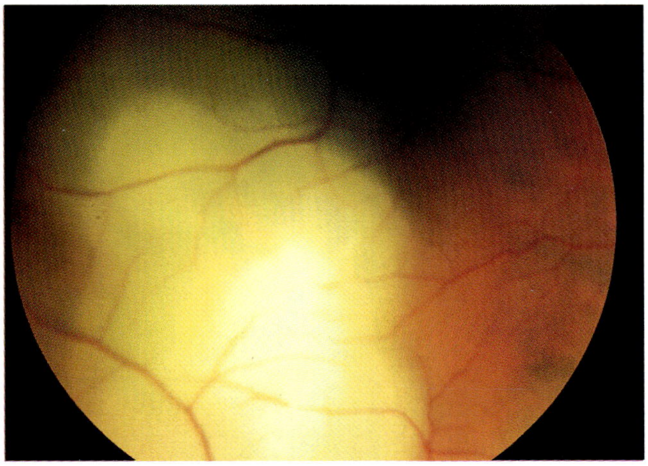

Figure 8–5. Lesion shown in 8–4 immediately following laser-induced hyperthermia.

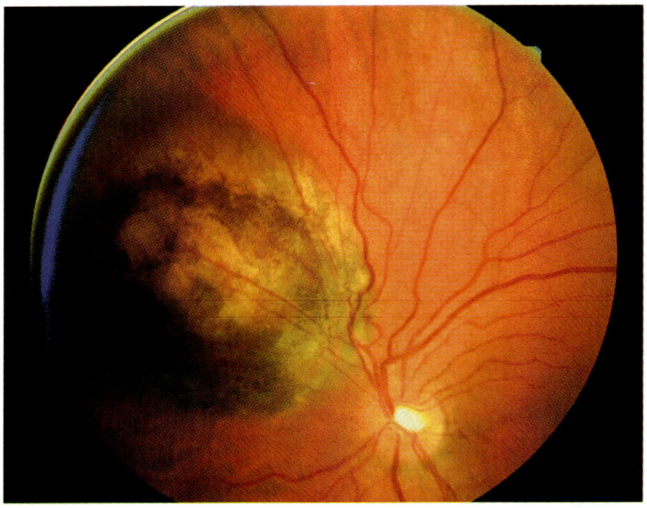

Figure 8–6. A patient with a small growing tumor prior to laser-induced hyperthermia.

can occur; this complication can be avoided by using artificial tears instead of balanced salt solution, to maintain corneal hydration. We also avoid using a lid speculum for the same reason.

Less common and, in some cases, avoidable complications include damage to the iris (atrophy or synechiae) due to treatment in an inadequately dilated eye, lens opacification, pigment migration into the vitreous, and development of acute angle-closure glaucoma or neovascular glaucoma.[57]

A similar set of complications has been noted after TTT. Especially in children with retinoblastoma, but also in patients with uveal melanoma, if the iris is not adequately dilated and in the field, an area of iris atrophy and cataract can occur, as shown in Figure 8–10. A number of other complications have also been observed, including damage to the overlying or surrounding retina, retinal traction, and retinal vascular occlusions (Figure 8–11). In the Philadelphia series, there was significant retinal traction in 10 percent, vascular occlusion in 5 percent, disc edema in 12 percent, and ocular ischemia in 1 percent.[52] As mentioned above, we do not know the incidence of incomplete tumor control with this modality.

A number of other experimental laser-based treatment approaches have been used. A combination of treatment with a photoactivated dye preferentially taken up by the tumor and treatment using a tunable dye laser has been employed in several animal models and a few human uveal melanomas.[58] Most of the work has been performed using several generations of hematoporphyrin dye derivatives (HPD); its major mechanism of action appears to be vascular closure rather than tumor cytotoxicity. While theoretically this approach holds promise, a number of histologic studies have demonstrated only partial tumor destruction, thus limiting its applicability.[59,60]

Several newer compounds have been used in models, including chloroaluminum sulfonated phthalocyanine, rose bengal, metaporphyrin, lipoprotein-delivered benzoporphyrin, benzoporphyrin derivative, and mono-L-aspartyl chlorine.[61–66] Kim and co-workers have used a different formula for a light-activating compound therapy in

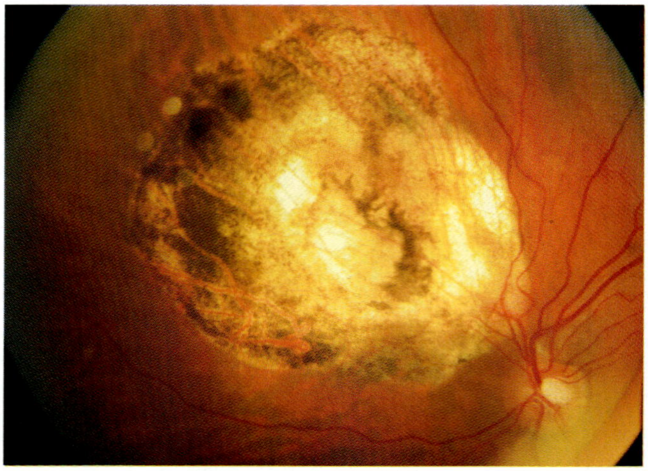

Figure 8–7. The same patient shown in Figure 8–6 after transpupillary thermal therapy.

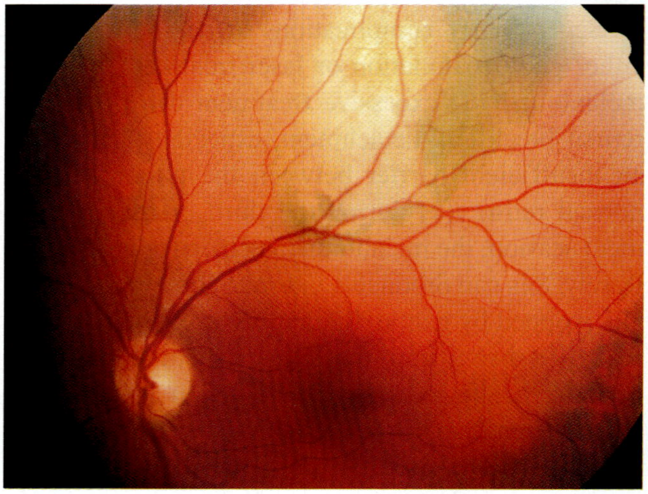

Figure 8–8. Small growing uveal melanoma.

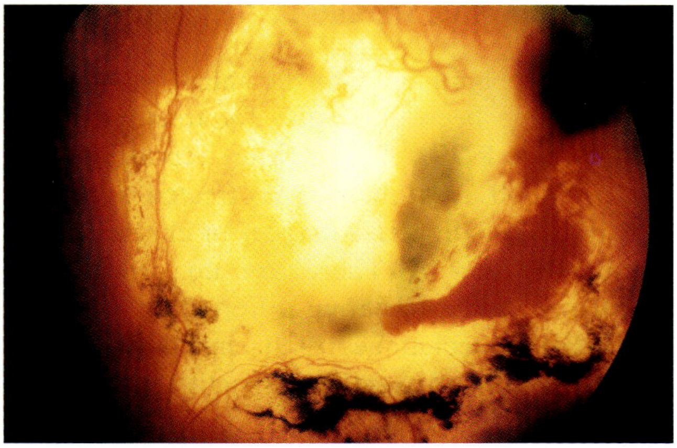

Figure 8–9. Tumor shown in Figure 8–8 was destroyed after four photocoagulation treatments. Note choroidal-retinal-vitreal neovascularization at treatment edge.

an animal model, with significantly more cytotoxicity oberserved.[54]

Favilla and colleagues treated 19 patients with HPD (5 to 7.5 mg/kg) and a 620 to 630-nm laser. Six of 19 had a complete remission; however, follow-up was < 3 years.[67] The presumed mechanism of action utilized in this approach is a photochemical absorption of light to cause excited singlet and triplet states with subsequent damage. Several other investigators have used endogenously created procompounds, morphrins, and photodynamic therapies, with positive results in nonophthalmic systems. The applicability of this to uveal melanoma and other intraocular tumors remains to be shown.[16,68]

Choroidectomy and Eye Wall Resection

Most reported uveal resections have been for anterior melanomas (see Chapter 9). A smaller number of patients have been reported to have local resections for posterior uveal melanomas. The technique is similar, with slight variations, for tumors in either location. We have arbitrarily discussed the technique and results in Chapter 9. Figures 8–12 to 8–16 show several choroidal melanomas that we have treated with eye wall resection. Routinely, we encircle and support the vitreous base with a 42 or similar band.

The role of posterior uveal resections is uncertain. The author has mainly used this approach in tumors > 8 mm in thickness. As discussed below, the rationale for this is straightforward. In irradiated uveal melanomas, independent of tumor location in relation to the optic nerve or fovea, increased tumor thickness is associated with both higher incidence of eye loss and poor visual outcome. As an example, an eye with a tumor 8 mm thick is roughly 8 to 10 times more likely to have a poor outcome than one with a tumor 5 mm thick. Given the much larger incidence of complications in irradiated eyes with thick tumors, we have treated many of these using eye wall resection. One of the major problems in eye wall resection, discussed in Chapter 9, is a lack of predictability. As a general rule, relatively small-diameter tumors (< 12 mm) and those associated with a retinal overlying detachment not involving the ciliary body

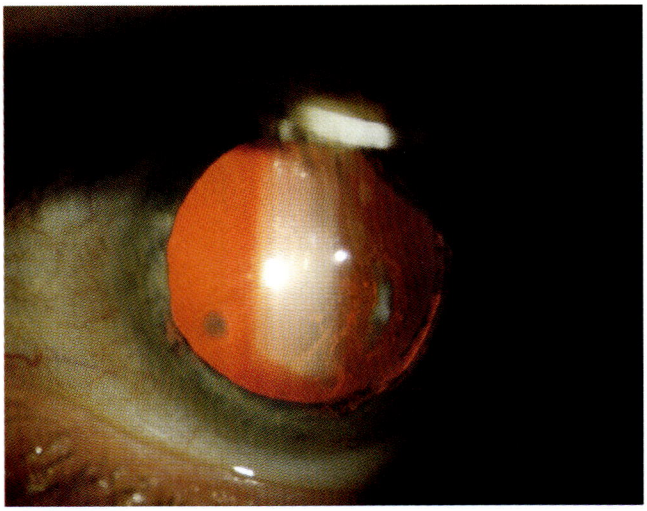

Figure 8–10. Localized lens opacity developed after laser-induced thermal therapy due to inadvertent heating when the pupil constricted.

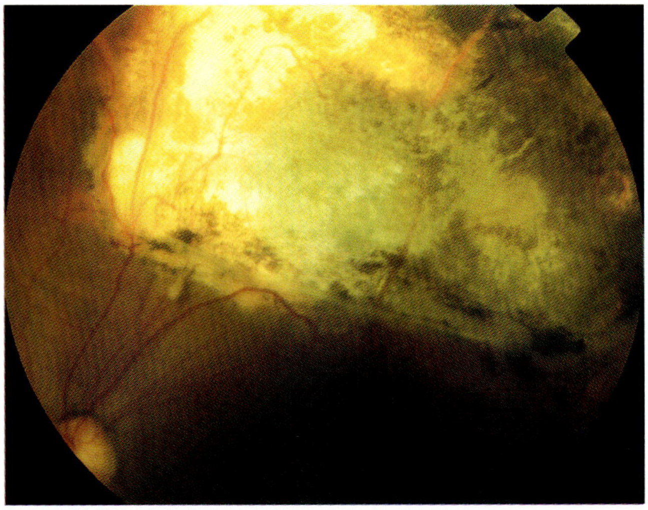

Figure 8–11. Retinal vascular occlusion after laser-induced hyperthermia.

have the best outcome.[69,70] Larger-diameter tumors, > 16 mm in size, and those that have broken through Bruch's membrane and invaded the retina have a much higher failure.[71,72] In addition, since surgery is optimally performed under hypointensive anesthesia, older hypertensive patients are not good candidates for this procedure.

Several authors have noted a relatively high incidence of intrascleral invasion in thick melanomas. Partially this reason, as well as the inability to accurately obtain clear surgical margins, has led most of us to add adjunctive radiation, either with a plaque or particles to the bed of the resected tumors. Damato and colleagues noted that the risk of both metastasis and local recurrence was significantly higher in eyes that did not receive postoperative radiation.[71,72] Interestingly, in the large series from Glasgow, death due to metastasis was not associated with an incomplete tumor excision, especially if later occurrence was adequately dealt with.[71–73]

One group has advocated an internal approach for posterior tumors where the tumor is removed piecemeal using vitrectomy instrumentation.[74] The author has not tried this technique, nor is it considered optimal. It is conceivable that doing incisional biopsies and piecemeal resection through vitrectomy ports may very well spread tumor, not only inside, but outside the eye, and there is little advantage and only major potential disadvantages of this approach, compared with other surgical options. A central tenet of cancer surgery is to avoid piecemeal resection of a malignancy, and this procedure violates that concept.[75]

Alternative Radiation Techniques

Radiation techniques with the intent to preserve the eye have been an option for treating ocular tumors since 1929.[76] The literature reports approximately 7,700 uveal melanomas treated with various forms of radioactive plaques or charged particle irradiation.[77–91] There are no randomized prospective data comparing different eye-preserving radiation techniques with enucleation; however, there is sufficient retrospective material to draw a number of conclusions regarding indications, contraindications, efficacy, and complications of radiation therapy. A COMS group is prospectively investigating the relative efficacy of enucleation versus ^{125}I brachytherapy, but after more than 10 years, no data have yet been published on this aspect of their investigation.

The major goal of radiation therapy is to destroy the tumor cell's reproductive capacity. Detectable tumor shrinkage after any form of radiation therapy is delayed. In our experience, usually the first sign of tumor response is the loss of subretinal fluid. This occurs approximately 6 to 12 months after treatment. Usually, tumor shrinkage is not detected for approximately 1 year after treatment; however, in as many as 30 percent of the cases, the tumor just stabilizes and does not show growth for as long as 15 years after radiation. Radiation complications may have a long latency. The first eye change as a result of radiation was noted in 1897.[92] Stallard's data, going back to the 1930's, demonstrates that

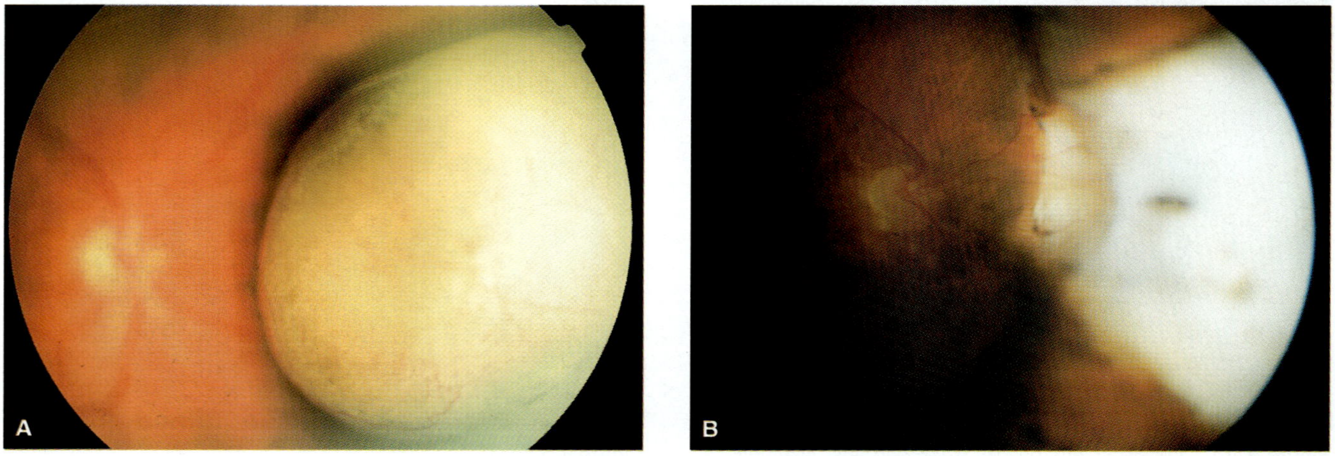

Figure 8–12. *A,* Uveal melanoma prior to choroidectomy. *B,* After choroidectomy, 5 years later, the visual acuity was 20/40.

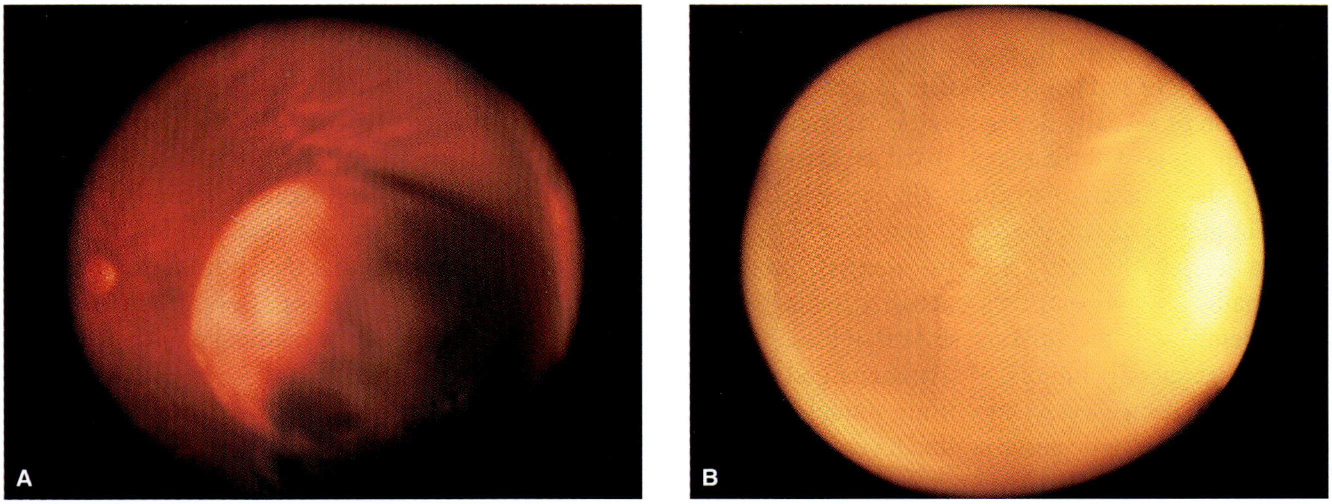

Figure 8–13. *A* and *B,* Choroidal melanoma, 11-mm thick, prior to and after resection with clear margins.

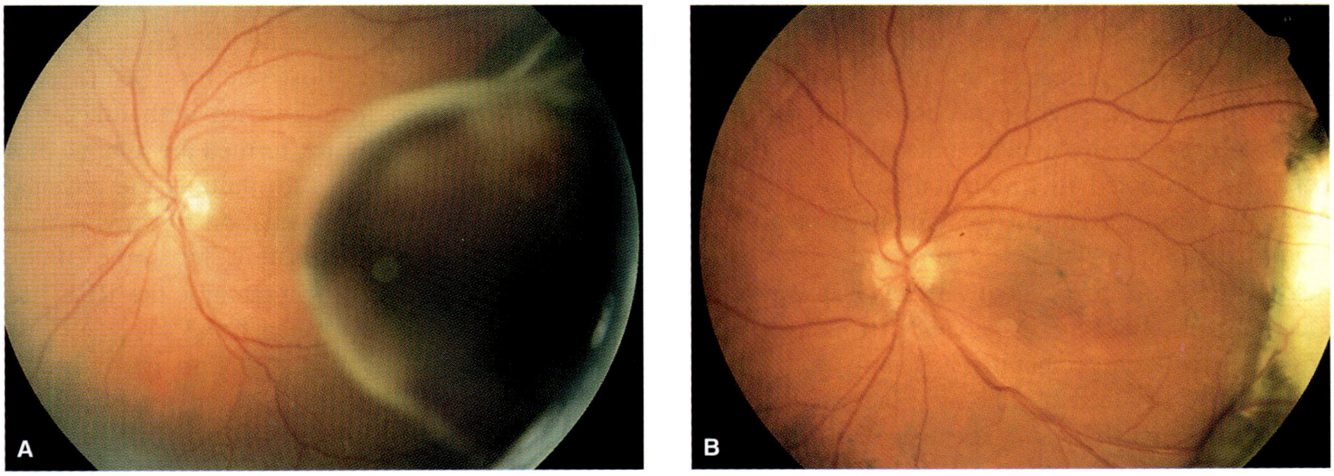

Figure 8–14. *A* and *B,* Very large choroidal melanoma. Six months after surgery, vision was 20/200 due to cystoid macular edema.

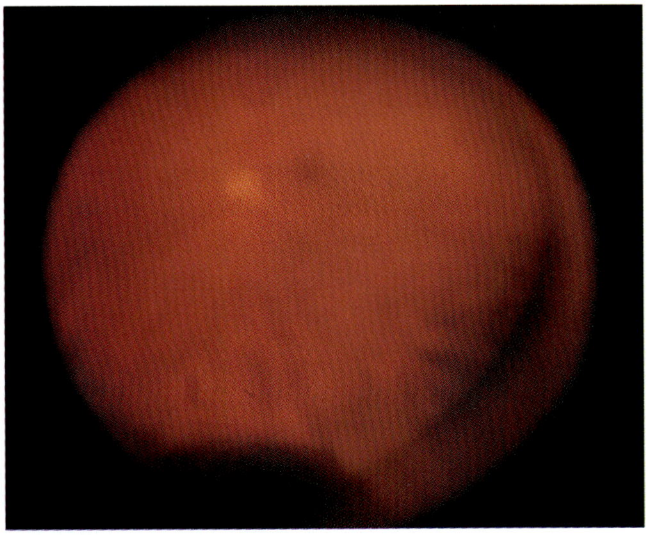

Figure 8–15. Large uveal melanoma prior to resection.

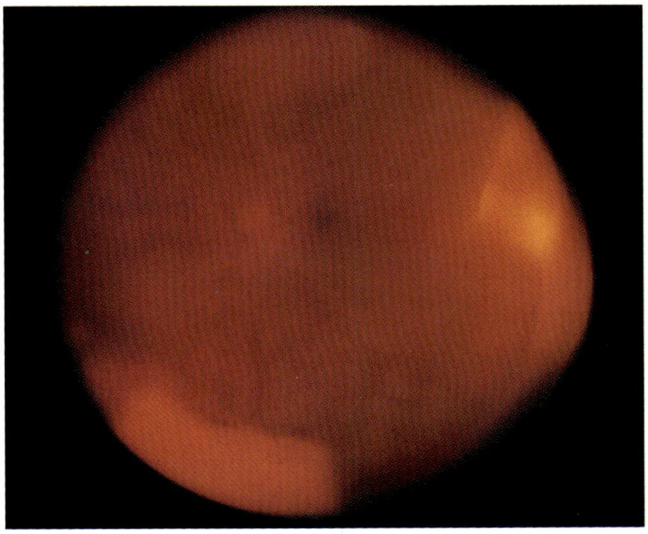

Figure 8–16. Photograph of the patient after tumor was removed.

radiation vasculopathy associated with cobalt plaques can develop 20 years after treatment.[79]

The roles of radiation versus tumor effects in the production of visually destructive ocular morbidity is uncertain. Eyes with untreated uveal melanomas can develop disc neovascularization (Figure 8–17), neovascular glaucoma (Figure 8–18), and cystoid macular edema (Figure 8–19). In proliferative diabetic retinopathy, a number of vasoactive cytokines have been identified in the vitreous; several of these factors are also secreted by tumors.[93,94] After charged particle irradiation, decreased vision from retinal damage, when neither the optic nerve nor the fovea has received significant radiation, has been noted.[95,96] It is probable that both a uveal melanoma and the host's response to it (cytokines and lymphocytic infiltration) produce significant ocular morbidity, independent of damage from either irradiation or other therapeutic modalities. This is discussed further below. If this hypothesis is correct, then it limits the potential of adjunct treatments to decrease eye damage after radiation. Ocular complications noted after radiation therapy are multifactorial in etiology. Patient age, tumor size (especially increased tumor thickness > 7 mm) and proximity to disc and fovea all independently affect visual outcome. Overall, approximately 85 percent of irradiated eyes are retained after treatment in many large centers, with patient survival affected by the same factors associated with primary uveal melanoma enucleation.[88,90,95,97]

Brachytherapy

Choice of Isotope

A number of different isotopes including cobalt-60 (^{60}Co), iodine-125 (^{125}I), iridium-192 (^{192}Ir), ruthenium-106 (^{106}Ru), gold-198 (^{198}Au), palladium-103 (^{103}Pd), strontium-90 (^{90}Sr), and radom-222 (^{222}Ra) have been used in radioactive plaques (brachytherapy) for uveal melanoma treatment.[79–93,95,98–101] All forms of ocular brachytherapy share several features. First, the maximum radiation dose is delivered to the area contiguous to the plaque; the radiation exposure decreases exponentially over distance. Therefore, thicker tumors require exponentially more irradiation of the tumor base in order to deliver a tumoricidal dose to the apex of a melanoma. Second, unless shielding is possible (see below), treatment of thicker tumors results in increased lateral radiation spread, placing more of the contiguous retina and optic nerve at risk for radiation vasculopathy. Third, with any form of radioactive plaque therapy, the dose for each melanoma must be calculated by a radiation physicist, and the plaque must be correctly positioned so that the entire tumor receives a therapeutic radiation dose. Several publications cite technical details of the medical physics involved in brachytherapy planning.[102–105]

There are a number of uncertainties in ocular brachytherapy. We do not know the ideal therapeutic dose that destroys a melanoma and minimizes radiation vascular complications. Most uveal melanomas have been treated with a total apical dose of between 70 and 100 gray (Gy) (7,000 and 10,000 rad) although doses between 50 and 120 Gy have been reported. The inaccuracy dose rate for ^{106}Ru is probably about 30 percent and varies with other isotopes.[106] A numerical figure, termed the relative biologic effect (RBE), is used to multiply the physical gray of different types of radiation to provide biologic equivalence. Unfortunately, for some of the istopes used in ocular brachytherapy, the RBE has been widely estimated between 1 and 4.

As reviewed elsewhere, radiation morbidity is mainly a function of total dose, volume treated, radiation characteristics, and dose fractionation. As discussed below, there are definite advantages (in terms of both tumor destruction and ocular morbidity) to some isotopes and charged particle irradiation. As examples, in a randomized prospective dynamically balanced study, we noted significantly better local tumor control with helium ions as compared with ^{125}I brachytherapy. There is similarly a higher failure rate with ^{106}Ru, compared with protons; the efficacy with ^{125}I is strongly affected by dose rate.[106] In contrast, while there are certain theoretic advantages to ^{125}I over ^{60}Co, as discussed below, the scleral dose to tumors approximately 5 mm thick is similar.[107]

The molecular mechanisms of both radiation cytotoxity and apoptosis in both uveal melanoma and retinoblastoma is unclear; direct tumor damage and indirect compromise of the vascular supply both play a role in radiation therapy's effect.[108] Most likely, the former is of greater importance, since we

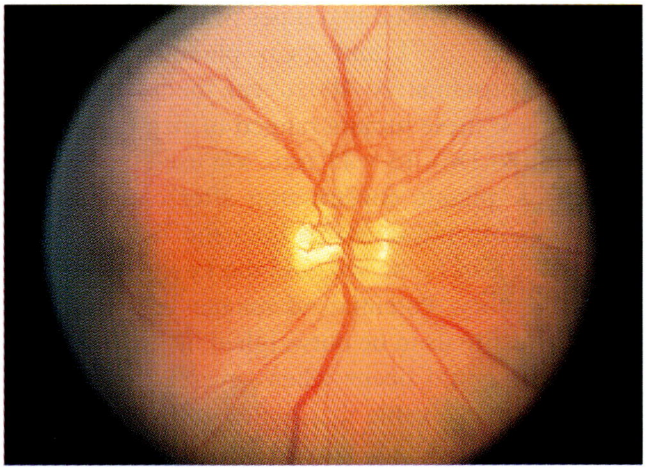

Figure 8–17. Disc neovascularization in a melanoma-containing eye prior to therapy.

have observed a number of tumors with almost complete regression prior to development of radiation vascular changes.

The effect of brachytherapy versus enucleation on uveal melanoma–related mortality is uncertain. The majority of patients who have been treated with brachytherapy have had smaller tumors than those treated with enucleation.[109] Retrospective studies have demonstrated no survival advantage with either radiation or enucleation.[109–114]

Historically, in most cases of uveal melanoma, brachytherapy was performed with either ^{60}Co or ^{106}Ru plaques.[79–83,86] ^{106}Ru does not produce sufficiently penetrant radiation to be useful for very thick tumors. Perhaps because some larger lesions have been treated with this isotope, there has been a relatively high failure rate.[106,114,115] In one series of 100 cases, with a mean follow-up of 3.3 years, there was a 5-year local control rate of 59 percent.[116] Eighteen metastases were reported in that series, and 7 occurred in the 19 patients who had local relapses. In another ^{106}Ru series, 9 of 49 patients had local failures.[117] In smaller tumors, up to 85 percent of eyes are retained at 5 years.[118] Probably because of the problems with ^{106}Ru in the case of thick tumors, adjuctive treatment with other modalities has often been used.[114,119] Seregard recently reported in meta-analysis over 1,000 patients treated with ^{106}Ru.[120] Unfortunately, the problems with meta-analysis, in general, have shown up to a 35 percent inaccuracy in some studies, compared with randomized control data.[121] In reports with ^{106}Ru brachytherapy, there appears to be a slightly lower incidence of optic neuropathy than in some series, although selection criteria are probably different. In one report, the incidence of optic neuropathy was 10 percent.[122,123] Over 2,500 cases of ^{106}Ru radiation have been reported.[114,120] Usually, the pattern of regression is the same as described for ^{125}I; however, in 3 cases, calcification of the lesion did occur.[87]

As has been reported with helium ion, protons, and cobalt, faster shrinkage after plaque therapy is associated with the worse survival.[95,97,114] This observation may appear to be counterintuitive; however, it is logical. More malignant, rapidly cycling tumors grow faster and respond to the DNA-induced radiation damage with rapid shrinkage; these cases have high tumor-related mortality.

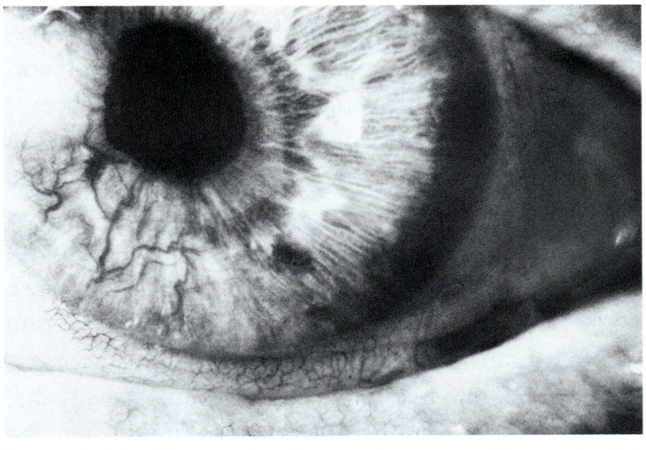

Figure 8–18. Neovascular glaucoma in an eye with an untreated melanoma.

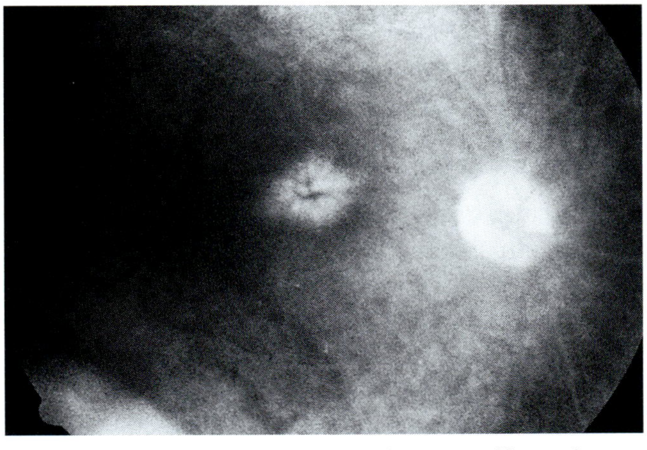

Figure 8–19. Cystoid macular edema in an eye with a melanoma prior to treatment.

Several studies have been reported with long-term follow-up ^{60}Co plaques.[79–117,124–127] The local control rate with ^{60}Co plaques has been approximately 70 to 80 percent. There is a significantly higher metastatic rate in those which have a local relapse.[124,127] There is a higher incidence of failure in larger-diameter, thinner tumors, especially those located near the optic nerve.[124,128] Local recurrences develop contiguous to the original tumor, although rarely, they can occur in another part of the eye. Figure 8–20 shows a marginal recurrence next to an area of presumed complete tumor destruction with chorioretinal atrophy. Figure 8–21 shows a recurrence inferior to a melanoma that had been treated elsewhere with ^{60}Co radioactive plaque. In the latter instance and in the literature, 3 of 4 such cases developed metastatic disease.[129] We reported metastatic risk as a correlate of postradiation recurrence patterns after ^{125}I brachytherapy. Diffusely enlarging tumors were at significantly increased risk, but even those that had a small, relatively flat marginal recurrence also had a higher death rate.[130] Of a reported 116 uveal melanomas treated with brachytherapy between 1968 and 1987, 20 had local recurrences; significant cataracts occurred with 32. The percentage of patients who retained 20/200 or better vision declined by 10 percent per year.[127] Brady estimated that 58 percent of patients treated with cobalt plaques retained useful vision 5 years after treatment.[126]

Several different techniques have been used to monitor brachytherapy in addition to standard modalities, such as ultrasonography, clinical examination, and photography. These modalities may include different types of ultrasonography, magnetic resonance imaging (MRI), gadolinium-DTPA, and histologic measures of cell cycling.[131–134] Doppler ultrasonography has been used to monitor radiation response; loss of tumor vascularity has been associated with effective radiation in a small number of ^{106}Ru-treated cases.[93–95]

In a retrospective analysis of lens opacities after ^{60}Co plaque brachytherapy, Kleineidam and colleagues noted that 22 percent developed cataract within 5 years; factors important in cataract production are tumor thickness, location of the anterior margin relative to the ora, and the diameter of the plaque.[135]

We have only used two types of uveal melanoma brachytherapy: ^{125}I and ^{60}Co plaques. We have treated approximately 400 uveal melanomas with ^{125}I plaques; these tumors ranged in size from $6 \times 6 \times 2.3$ mm to $18 \times 15 \times 11$ mm. We used only ^{125}I in radioactive plaque construction after consultations with radiation physicists at both the University of California, San Francisco, and the Lawrence Berkeley Laboratory. Potential advantages of other isotopes appear to us to be outweighed by possible confusion that could occur when several isotopes are used. It is conceivable that higher risk of treatment planning errors could ensue. There are a number of potential advantages and disadvantages with ^{125}I, compared with other isotope radioactive plaques. We do not use beta-emitting isotopes, since they have much less penetration and cannot be optimally used with tumors 3 to 5 mm thick.[86]

Although we prefer to use ^{125}I plaques, there are four potential advantages of ^{60}Co plaque therapy over ^{125}I brachytherapy: (1) a ^{60}Co plaque has a long (5.26 year) half -life and can be reused for at least 5 years without recharging which decreases patient cost; (2) the radiophysics calculations associated with a long half -life, highly penetrant, high-energy isotope like ^{60}Co are easier than those associated with ^{125}I plaque construction. With ^{60}Co, essentially the same treatment plan can be used on a number of patients over a several-month period because the slow radioactive decay results in little change in the isodose lines. At an institution with limited radiophysics expertise, errors are probably less likely with ^{60}Co plaques. There are also higher failure and complication rates in less experienced centers;[136] (3) cobalt plaques deliver a wider field of radiation for a given apical dose than does ^{125}I plaque therapy; if localizing a tumor correctly is difficult, there may be a lower incidence of marginal misses with cobalt plaques; and (4) cobalt plaques may have a smaller radiation gradient between the tumor base and the apex in progressively thicker tumors. Fortunately, in our experience, this fourth potential limitation of ^{125}I brachytherapy has not been borne out. We have treated tumors as thick as 11 mm without significant scleral necrosis. Scleral necrosis is probably not due to direct radiation, but is usually due to the release of inflammatory cytokines when the conjunctiva is not closed well over a lesion, and a

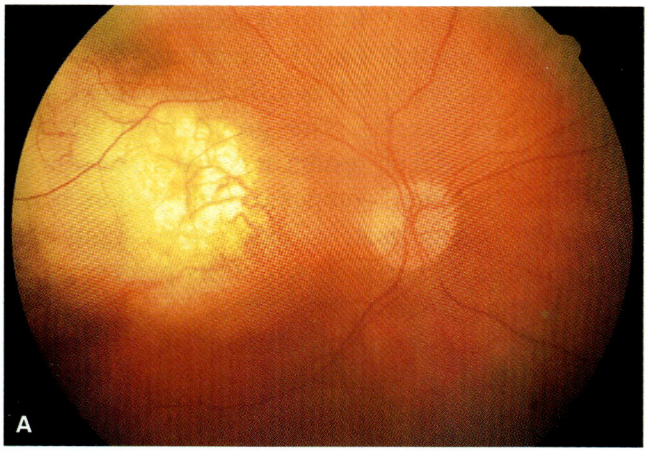

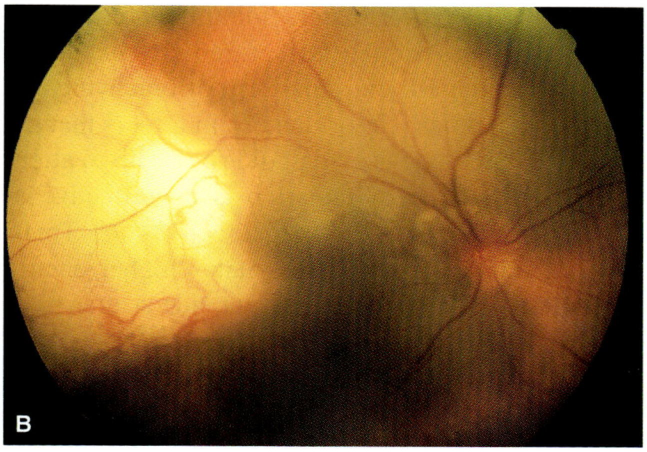

Figure 8–20. *A,* Shows almost complete destruction of tumor. *B,* Demonstrates marginal recurrence of the lesion shown in Figure 8-20A.

localized area of inflammation or infection ensues. Figure 8–22 shows scleral melt that occurred in a patient who had conjunctival retraction after removal of a plaque and suturing of the conjunctiva.

There are a number of potential advantages of ^{125}I over ^{60}Co plaques. ^{125}I can be easily shielded with as little as 0.3 mm of gold; this thickness produces less than one part per million transmission.[98,100,137] In contrast, ^{60}Co plaques cannot be adequately shielded to protect noninvolved ophthalmic structures or the surgical team. More than one foot thickness of lead is needed to give equivalent ^{60}Co shielding versus 0.3 mm thickness of gold for ^{125}I. The ability to shield ^{125}I plaques has a number of clinical ramifications. First, there is significantly less radiation exposure for the operative team, especially if a large number of cases are treated. Second, there may be fewer radiation induced vascular complications in both the eye and in contiguous orbital structures; however, no conclusive data support this hypothesis. With a very thick anteriorly located tumor, ^{125}I can produce cataract, eyelash loss, and, if the tumor is in a superior temporal location, significant dryness. ^{60}Co plaque therapy of a superior temporal melanoma usually results in a dry eye due to lacrimal gland radiation damage; this can usually be avoided with a conventionally shielded ^{125}I plaque, unless a very thick, broad-based tumor in this location is being treated. Similarly, in an anterior nasal tumor, sufficient ^{60}Co plaque radiation is delivered to the lacrimal excretory system to produce closure of the puncta and resultant epiphora; this complication can usually be avoided with ^{125}I use. The lower penetration and softer gamma emission of ^{125}I, compared with ^{60}Co, results in lesser radiation spread. Various shapes and sizes of ^{125}I plaque carriers have been constructed as shown in Figure 8–23. Cut-outs are used for tumors next to the optic nerve or sometimes when the isodose array is appropriately arranged so that the plaque carrier can be placed with the cut-out around the insertion of an extraocular muscle that is contiguous to the tumor and thus avoid the necessity of temporarily removing that muscle. The ability to attenuate ^{125}I with a thin layer of gold has also allowed the production of rimmed

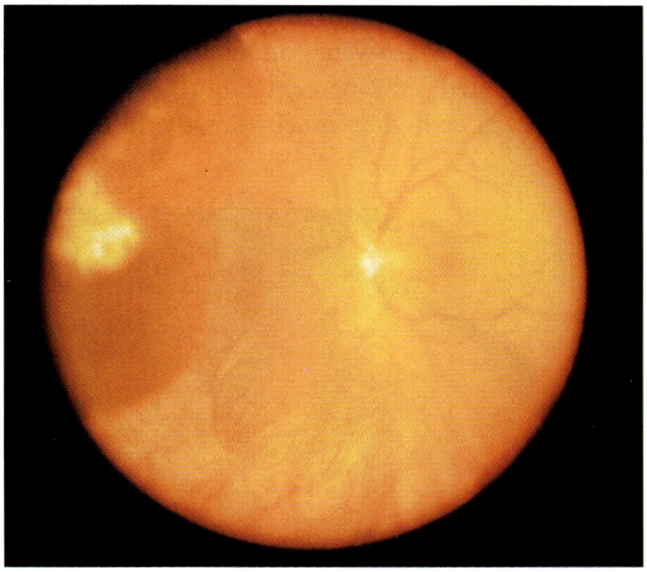

Figure 8–21. Recurrent tumor inferior to a melanoma treated in another center with ^{60}Co radioactive plaque.

plaques. Many investigators initially thought that rimmed plaques might further reduce the lateral spread of radiation with this form of brachytherapy in thin melanomas. Unfortunately, in tumors that are > 4.8 mm thick, the use of a gold rim or lip to attenuate lateral spread of radiation is not effective to decrease ocular morbidity (Figure 8–24).[138] Treatment of thicker tumors necessitates higher energy seeds and the lip does not prevent side scatter from the seeds that are well away from it. In retrospective analysis of our ^{125}I brachytherapy data, we did not observe a significant difference in visual outcome 3 years after treatment between those who did and those who did not receive rimmed or unrimmed ^{125}I plaques (unpublished data).

There are no randomized prospective data comparing various isotopes used in uveal melanoma brachytherapy. As thicker tumors are treated, the complications associated with therapy increase, regardless of the isotope utilized. In our experience with over 400 ^{125}I brachytherapy cases, we have a long-term ocular retention rate of approximately 85 percent.[139,140] As reported with ^{60}Co plaques, we noted a higher local failure rate when tumors were relatively thin and near the optic nerve.

The initial use of ^{125}I brachytherapy was for small tumors.[98,99] Two groups reported a 12 to 14 percent local failure rate in 140 patients with a mean follow-up of under 4 years[141,142] Garretson and colleagues noted a lower local failure rate in 26 patients, with a similar duration of follow-up.[143] In a small series with a 6-year follow-up, Hill and collaborators noted a 29 percent failure rate.[144] Lean has observed a higher brachytherapy failure rate with larger tumors.[145] In our experience with larger tumors, local control was 91 percent at 3 years and 83 percent at 5 years.[146] It is difficult to compare the nonrandomized series. The group from London recently reported their results in patients treated with radioactive plaques, compared with proton beam irradiation. Unfortunately, there were significant differences in tumor size as well as percentage of tumors in the posterior pole in the different treatment arms, thus making it difficult to demonstrate meaningful differences. In that series, ^{106}Ru had a higher failure rate than either ^{125}I or proton radiation; however, these results must be interpreted cautiously.[147] Similarly, it will be difficult to compare the COMS plaque data with many older series. We and others have noted higher plaque failure rates in tumors that are thin and come to the edge of the optic nerve. Such cases were excluded in the COMS, hence it should increase their local control rate.

In a randomized prospective study comparing ^{125}I brachytherapy with helium ion–charged particle irradiation, we did not note, for the entire group of cases, a significant difference in visual outcome.[139] As discussed above, in a retrospective analysis, we did not find the use of a rimmed plaque carrier more effective in improving visual outcome; however, surprisingly, we also did not find that this type of carrier increased our rate of marginal recurrences.

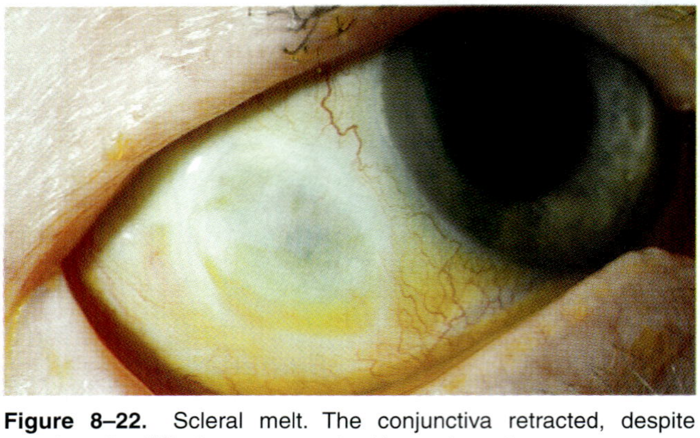

Figure 8–22. Scleral melt. The conjunctiva retracted, despite suturing after ^{125}I plaque removal, with resultant damage.

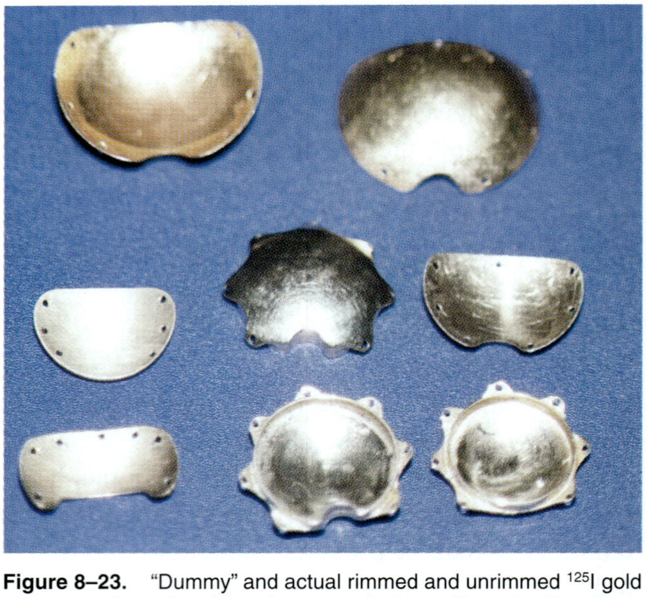

Figure 8–23. "Dummy" and actual rimmed and unrimmed ^{125}I gold plaque carriers of various shapes and sizes with and without cutouts for the optic nerve and extraocular muscle insertions.

There are approximately 136 centers in the United States that have used ^{125}I brachytherapy for various malignancies.[148] The COMS is currently enrolling patients in a prospective, randomized trial to compare the tumor-related mortality of patients with tumors > 2 mm from the optic nerve that are < 16 mm in largest diameter and 2.5 to 10 mm in thickness. The two experimental groups receive either ^{125}I brachytherapy or enucleation. The author's scepticism that this trial will show any difference is based on three objections: (1) there have never been any data to suggest better survival with enucleation than with radiation. In a study with a 5-year follow-up rate of 100 percent after helium ion radiation, we noted only a 10 percent tumor-related mortality in patients with tumors of the size the COMS originally chose to randomize in this trial.[95] If those less-experienced centers attain a similar tumor control rate, it is very doubtful that radiation will do worse than enucleation; (2) given the control rates demonstrated with particles and plaques, it seems that for most patients, there are strong advantages to retain an eye rather than undergoing enucleation. The latter point is especially germane in a subset of patients of whom almost 70 percent have long-term visual acuities of ≥ 20/40; these patients have melanomas < 5 mm thick that are > 4 mm from the optic nerve and fovea;[149] and (3) the pragmatic objection is to the design of the brachytherapy portion of that trial. For smaller tumors, "one size fits all" radiation dosimetry to a constant depth is being used. While undoubtedly it may allow a lower failure rate in thin tumors, this excess radiation will increase the morbidity.

There are a number of potential disadvantages with ^{125}I brachytherapy. Figure 8–25 shows the limitations of a rimmed plaque for tumors contiguous with the optic nerve. The exterior diameter of the optic nerve is approximately 1 mm wider than it is inside the eye. A rimmed plaque cannot be used for a tumor in close proximity to the optic nerve, or a marginal miss (insufficient radiation to the posterior edge of the tumor) will occur. This issue undoubtably led the COMS participants not to treat tumors within 2 mm of the disc as part of the trial; and this should result in a better tumor control rate than we reported when tumors contiguous with the disc were treated. In tumors that are treated next to the disc, some other

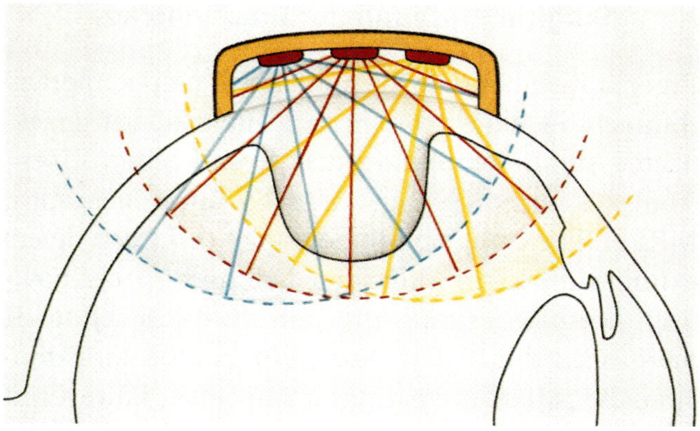

Figure 8–24. In tumors > 5 mm in height (tumor + sclera ≥ 6 mm) the required ^{125}I seed strength to treat the apex is such that a rim does sufficiently attenuate lateral radiation spread to decrease ocular morbidity.

approaches to suturing plaques may be advantageous.[150] There is a higher incidence of secondary strabismus and vitreous hemorrhage after brachytherapy.[139,151] In a few centers, patients with longstanding exudative detachments after brachytherapy have been treated with good results.[152]

^{125}I plaques are more expensive to construct and have a shorter half-life than ^{60}Co sources. Treatment planning is more complex, and since the ^{125}I plaques are created with multiple radioactive seeds, irregular radiation isodose curves do occur.[102,103,137,153]

Some investigators have used a different isotope, ^{103}Pd, that is a softer gamma emitter than ^{125}I.[100,154] We have chosen not to use this isotope for three reasons: (1) the basic radiobiology regarding its relative biologic effect is still uncertain;[133,155,156] (2) as has been queried for thicker tumors when ^{125}I is compared with ^{60}Co, it is doubtful that the softer energy distribution of ^{103}Pd will decrease ocular morbidity in the majority of the melanomas treated; and (3) as discussed above, we believe that unless there are substantial advantages in the use of an additional isotope, the risk of errors in calculations when more than one type of radiation source is used negates potential advantages. As discussed previously with ^{106}Ru, it is difficult to compare patient groups, but a review of a recent paper on ^{103}Pd demonstrates that many of these lesions were extrordinarily small, and probably in a significant minority, we would have opted for observation over treatment.[155] The excellent survival and low failure rates are partially predicated on patient selection.

Surgical Procedure for Brachytherapy

Preoperative consent for radioactive plaque therapy routinely includes consent for enucleation if unsuspected significant extraocular scleral tumor extension is found at surgery. Usually ultrasonography, MRI and/or computed tomography (CT) can detect extraocular tumor extension before surgery; however, these techniques are not always accurate. If there is a small, flat, focal area of extraocular extension, the patient is treated with a plaque; however, if a larger or diffuse extension is present, enucleation is usually, but not always, performed instead (Figures 8–26A and B).[157]

Radioactive plaque therapy requires accurate tumor localization. We routinely perform a 360° limbal peritomy and sling all four rectus muscles using 2-0 silk sutures. The tumor is localized with two separate techniques. An O'Malley light pipe with a corneal transilluminator is placed on the cornea (Figure 8–27A); the tumor casts a scleral shadow which is demarcated with diathermy marks to outline the borders of the lesion. In very elevated tumors, corneal transillumination alone produces an inaccurately large posterior shadow. This problem can be overcome in two ways: (1) we place a transilluminator 180° away from the tumor; and (2) we routinely localize posterior uveal tumors, using indirect ophthalmoscopy and a fiberoptic light pipe incorporated into a diathermy unit (Figures 8–27 and 8–28).

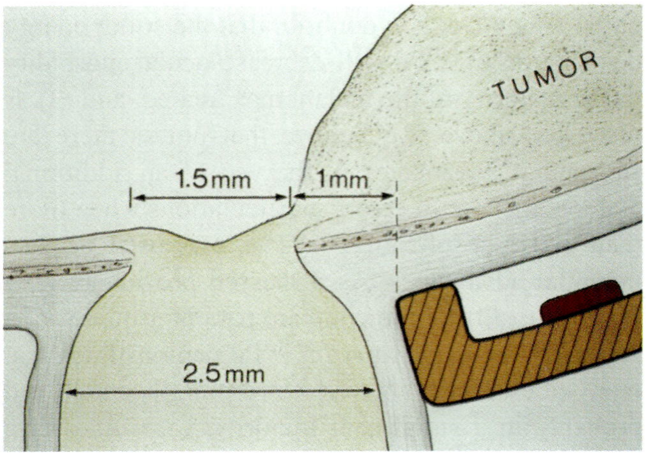

Figure 8–25. Rimmed plaques cannot be used next to the optic disc since the larger exterior diameter of the nerve, vis-a-vis the rim, delivers insufficient radiation for a tumor that is contiguous to the optic nerve.

Sutures of 5-0 dacron are used to attach an identical carrier ("dummy" plaque) without the radioactive isotope to the scleral area overlying the tumor. The carrier location is reconfirmed with point-source transillumination and indirect ophthalmoscopy; this allows sutures to be placed which will hold the actual plaque in situ, while minimizing radiation exposure to the surgical team (Figure 8–28).

The location of the radioactive plaque itself may not be an accurate guideline to the radiation delivery. The calculated radiation isodose lines necessary to encompass a given field with the appropriate radiation and their location, vis-a-vis both the plaque margins and tumor, are necessary to correctly situate the plaque. In many centers ^{125}I plaques are individually fabricated; the tumor must be in the exact center of some plaques, and other plaques are constructed so that tumoricidal radiation is delivered up to 5 mm lateral to the plaque edge. Similarly, some plaques are constructed such that the radiation isodose lines are quite asymmetric; the plaque cannot be haphazardly placed over a tumor. We routinely have a radiation physicist with the isodose curves in the operating room at the time of surgery. We have found the above-mentioned plaque localization method acceptable. In a series of eyes enucleated for late complications after helium ion radiation, the location of the tantalum marker rings were within 0.5 mm of where they had been supposedly placed in all cases.[158] We have, therefore, not routinely used ultrasonographic localization of radioactive plaques, since they are easier to localize than placing tantalum marker rings for particle radiation. We always suture a plaque with sutures that are at least 180° apart to avoid possible displacement of a plaque or tilting of its surface, overlying the sclera surface. Other investigators have used this technique, as shown in Figure 8–29. One can visualize the plaque correctly positioned under a uveal melanoma.

After placing a plaque, the eye is irrigated with antibiotic solution and the conjunctiva closed with a 6-0 gut suture. We are currently using a 70-GyE apical dose radiation to treat uveal melanomas; plaques usually remain in situ for 3 to 4 days to deliver this dose. We chose this dose arbitrarily to compare in a randomized prospective trial (see below) with 70 GyE of helium ion irradiation. Quivey and colleagues noted

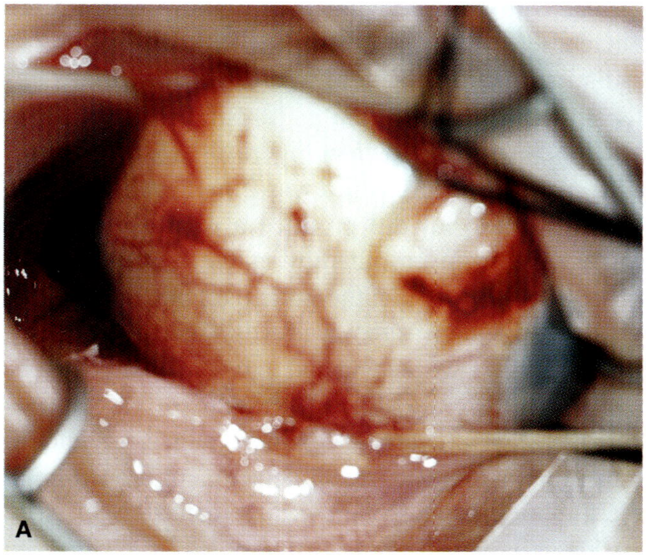

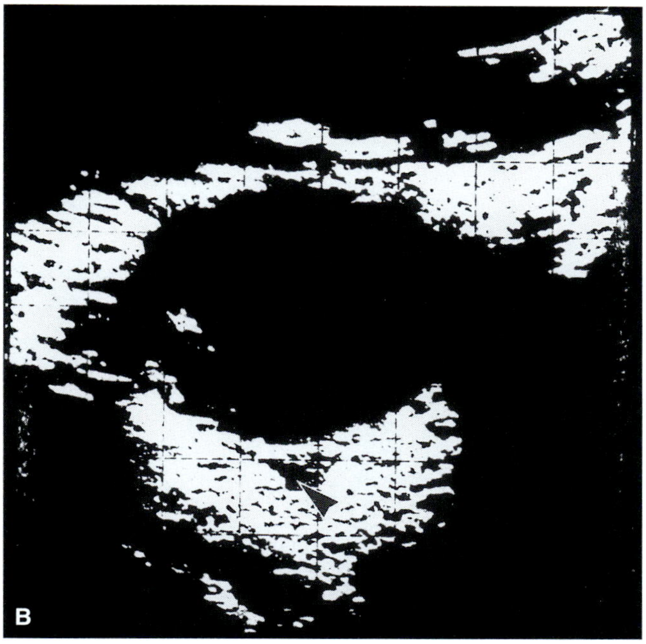

Figure 8–26. *A,* Extraocular extension of a uveal melanoma. *B,* Ultrasound of case in Figure 8–26A; arrow shows extraocular extension.

that the lower dose rate delivered with ^{125}I plaques was a significant correlate of tumor failure, as was a location of the tumor close to the optic disc.[159] The clinically observed radiation response with both plaques and charged particles is similar, and it is discussed under the section on charged particle radiation.

There are some problems specific to radioactive plaques. First, occasionally, a tumor's location requires temporary disinsertion of an extraocular muscle to deliver adequate irradiation. Even when a muscle does not have to be detached, the placement of the plaque under a muscle causes stretching. This results in a greater incidence of transient diplopia than is seen after charged particle irradiation; however, we have rarely had to surgically correct strabismus. Second, there is a small increased risk that an untoward event could occur during the second operation necessary to remove a plaque; obviously a second procedure is not necessary with charged particle irradiation.

Figures 8–30 and 8–31 demonstrate successful brachytherapy of a small growing and a large (16 mm diameter and 8 mm thick) choroidal melanoma. In both these cases, long-term control was achieved with an excellent visual outcome. As discussed below, since both radiation shrinkage and complications are usually delayed, often by more than 1 year,

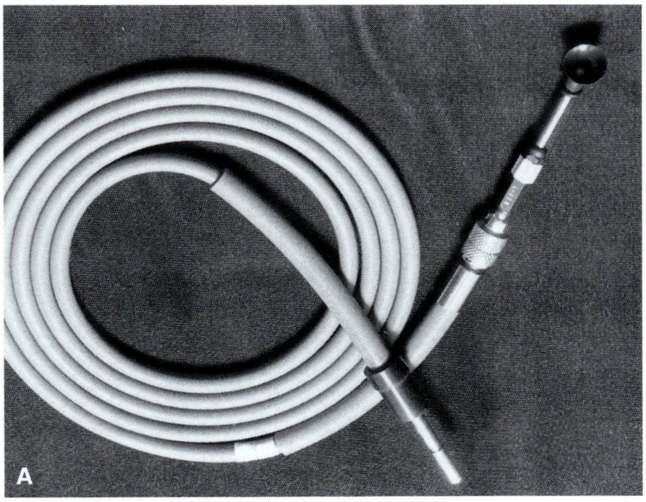

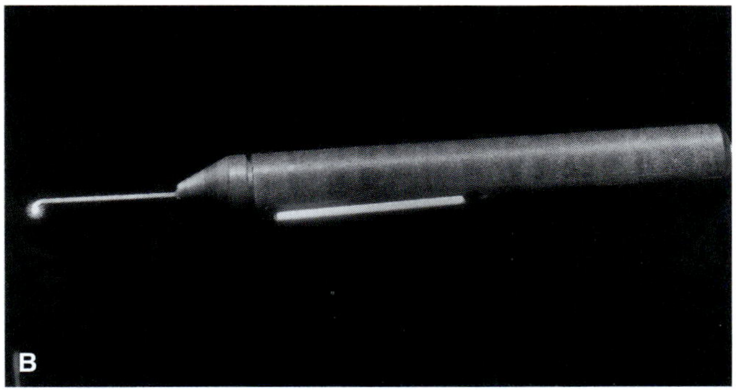

Figure 8–27. *A* and *B,* Corneal transilluminator and a diathermy with an integrated fiber optic light source are used for tumor localization.

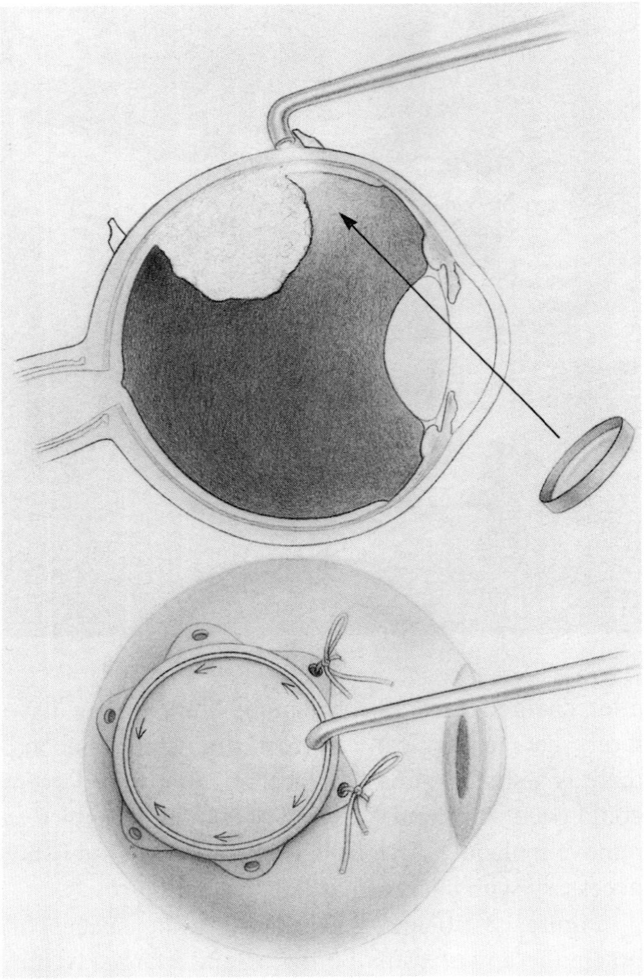

Figure 8–28. Indirect ophthalmoscopy and point-source transillumination to delineate the margins of the tumor and the relationship to the edges of a rimmed radioactive plaque carrier.

long-term follow-up is necessary to ascertain the relative merits of newer radiation treatment modalities. Figure 8–32 illustrates a late marginal recurrence, after ^{125}I brachytherapy. The tumor appeared to shrink after radiation, with exudate along the posterior aspect of the melanoma (Figures 8–32B). The tumor then developed some marginal "creep" toward the macula (Figure 8–32C), and this was successfully treated with laser (Figure 8–32D). While it would be expected that a tumor this close to the optic disc would have a poor visual outcome, acuity remains 20/50 approximately 10 years after laser.

A number of immediate and late complications can occur after radiation. Surgical complications include damage to the extraocular muscles, vitreous hemorrhage (especially with thick tumors that have broken through Bruch's membrane), and retinal detachment due to either an exudative response to radiation or an inadvertent suture. We caused this latter surgical complication in 2 out of about 1,000 patients. The case shown in Figure 8–33 is instructive. The easier, anterior, suture was 2 mm away from the tumor margin but did produce a retinal break. We treated this with cryotherapy at the time of plaque placement, but while the retina remained attached when the plaque was removed 4 days later, it detached in the next few weeks and had to be re-repaired. Probably, the radiation delivered to the tumor base and its surroundings prevented adequate adhesion, and in retrospect, perhaps a retinal detachment procedure at the time of plaque explant was indicated.

Several issues remain unresolved regarding the use of brachytherapy. Dose rate has been empiric, yet some preliminary data suggest that a relatively high dose delivery over 4 days results in better control than when plaques have been left in situ for as long as 10 to 14 days.[159] The utility of adjuvant treatment with brachytherapy remains uncertain. Hyperthermia is discussed both under photocoagulation and after charged particles. Photocoagulation and, more recently, laser-induced hyperthermia (see section on laser) after plaque therapy have been used by several investigators.[160,161] Augsburger and colleagues have noted that there is faster tumor regres-

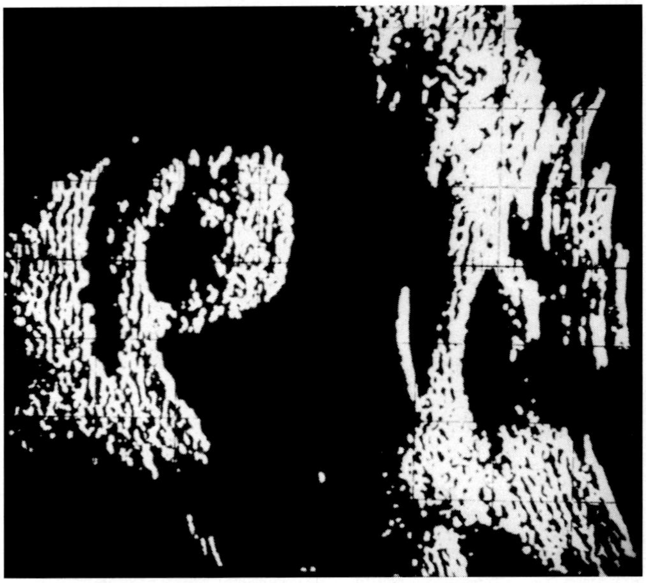

Figure 8–29. B-scan ultrasound demonstrates radioactive plaque correctly positioned on the sclera surface of a melanoma.

sion but worse short-term visual outcome when sequential brachytherapy and laser are used.[161] Finally, as mentioned previously, the results of the prospective trial of ^{125}I brachytherapy and enucleation are awaited. Approximately 80 percent of patients treated with alternative brachytherapy and teletherapy irradiation have had their tumors successfully controlled without the need of enucleation.[79–88,98–100,117,122–132,139–141,142,162–164]

Charged Particle Irradiation

Two different charged particles (proton and helium ion) have been used to treat uveal melanomas. Centers in Boston, San Francisco, Switzerland, France, England, Japan, Southern California, and Russia, have used proton-charged particle irradiation. Our center in San Francisco initially used helium ion radiation; more recently, because of cost constraints, we have switched to protons. Approximately 7,000 patients have been treated with these techniques.[77,78,89–91,95,111,116,139,165,166] Charged particle irradiation has four potential advantages over brachytherapy for uveal melanoma therapy:[167] (1) charged particle irradiation can be more precisely focused than any form of radioactive plaque. The lateral spread of helium ion irradiation decreases from 100 to 10 percent in 2.3 mm. Figure 8–34 compares lateral radiation spread with helium ions versus ^{125}I radioactive plaques; (2) a uniform radiation dose is delivered to the entire tumor with charged particles; there is no gradient between the base and the apex of the lesion; (3) in some experimental tumors, the high linear energy transfer (LET) associated with some heavier particles makes them more tumoricidal than

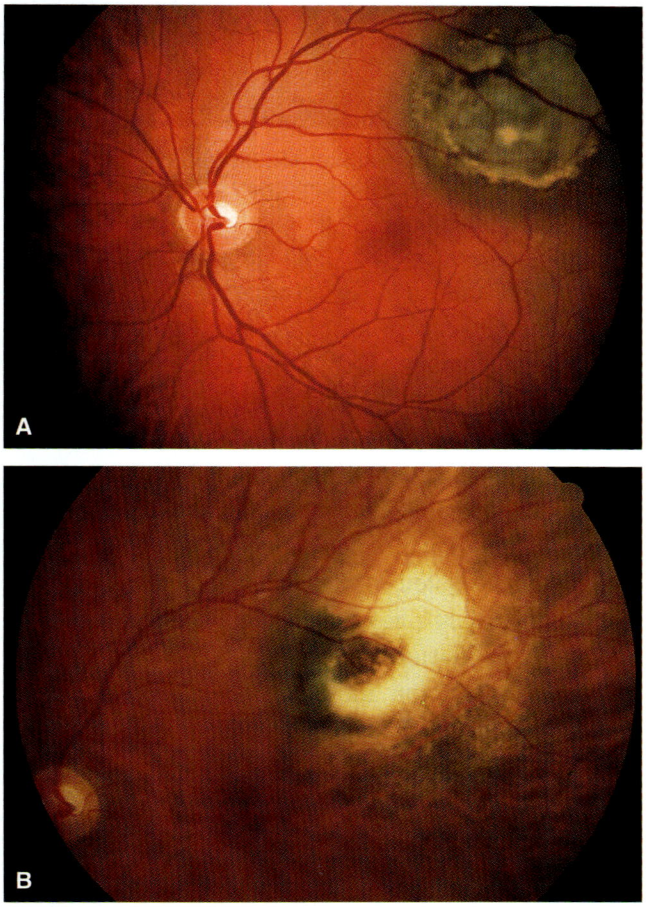

Figure 8–30. *A,* Small growing choroidal melanoma near the fovea. *B,* Five years later, vision remains good and the tumor has shrunk.

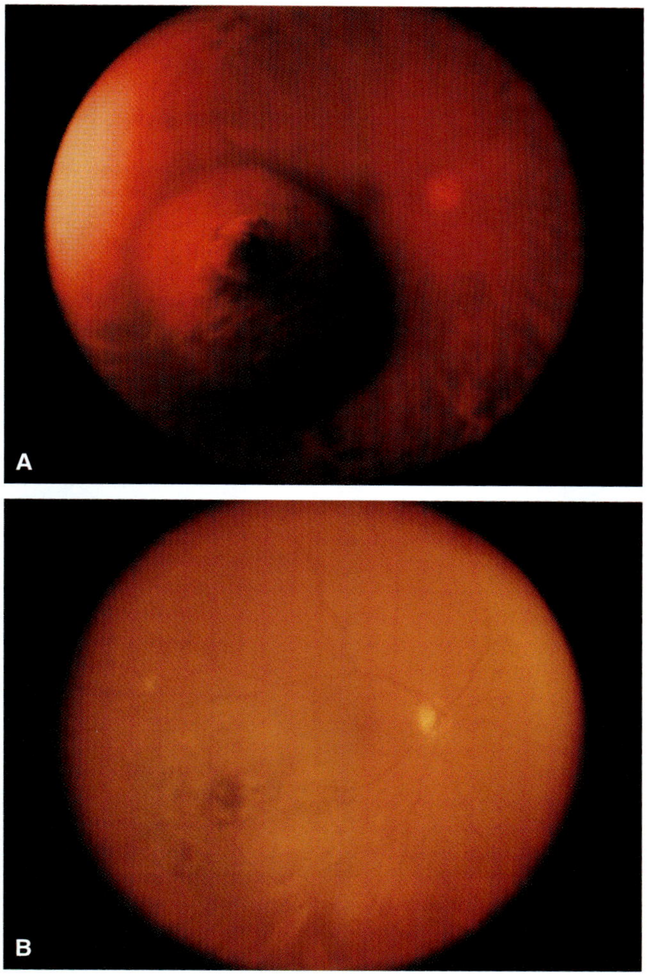

Figure 8–31. *A,* Larger (16 mm largest diameter and 8 mm thickness) choroidal melanoma. *B,* Tumor shown in Figure 8–31A with marked regression. Eye retained excellent vision.

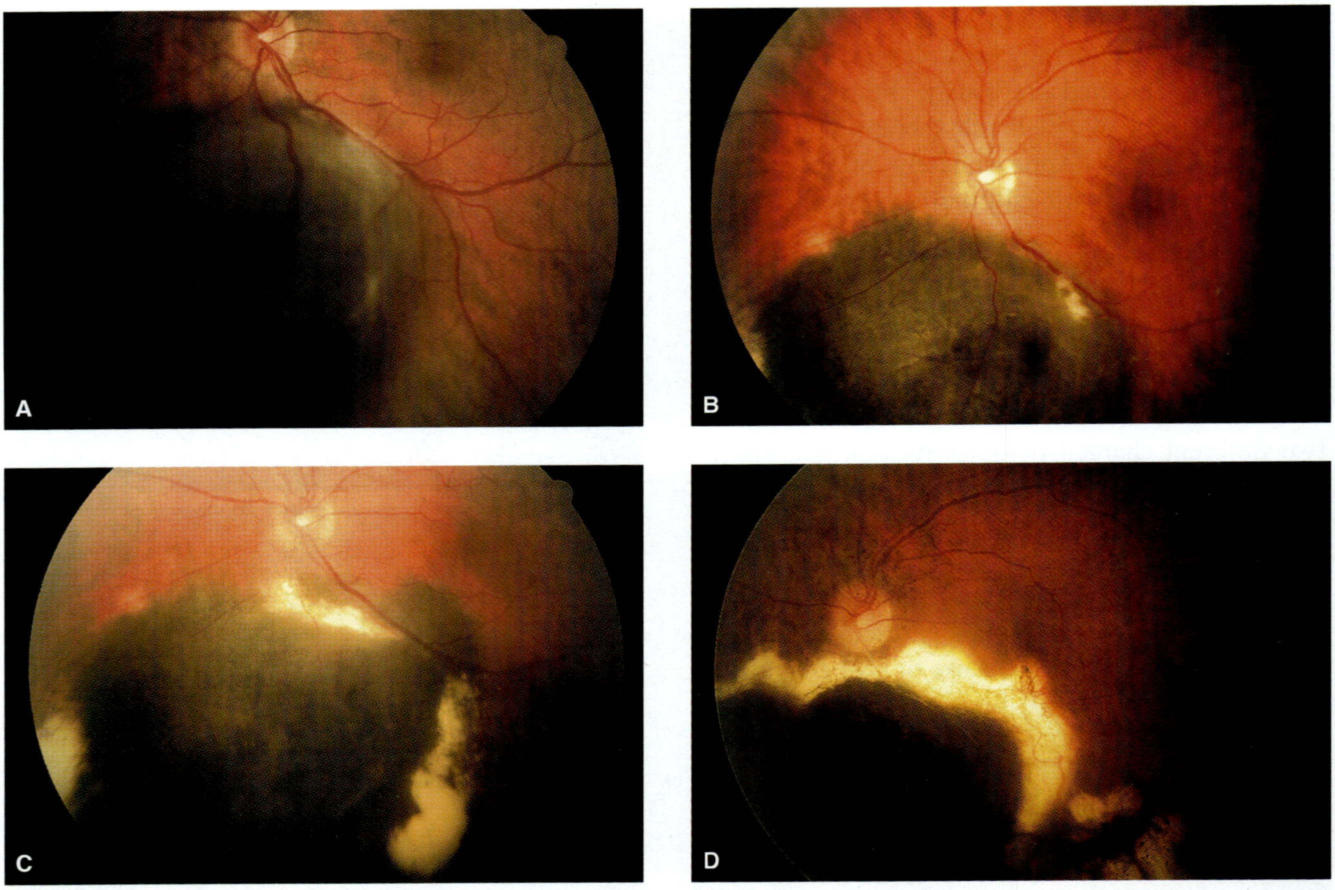

Figure 8–32. *A,* After ^{125}I brachytherapy for a peripapillary melanoma. *B,* Early regression with some intratumor radiation vasculopathy manifested by exudate. *C,* Marginal recurrence toward the macula. *D,* Five years after laser, with good tumor control and surprisingly good vision (20/50).

conventional forms of radiation; and (4) particles can effectively treat larger tumors than can brachytherapy. Definitive trial data supporting the first three potential advantages have not been published.

There are a number of potential disadvantages to charged particle beam therapy. First, these techniques are only available in a few centers. The facilities are costly to build and maintain and they require a technically sophisticated support staff. Second, the external complications, as a result of the radiation beam passing through normal tissue on its path towards the tumor, are greater than similar adnexal complications associated with plaques; some of these complications, such as lash loss or transient epitheliitis (Figure 8–35), are usually minor. Cataract and neovascular glaucoma are more frequent with particles, although, as discussed below, the latter problem has been markedly diminished using multiple treatment beams.[168] Treatment of superior temporal or anterior nasal melanomas with particles can produce lacrimal gland damage in the first instance or lacrimal drainage system damage in the latter as the external radiation beam passes through and damages adnexal structures contiguous with the ocular tumor.[169]

Over 85 percent of eyes treated with either protons or helium ions have been retained.[139,166,168,170,171] The 5-year tumor-related mortality appears to be approximately 20 percent; almost all metastatic events have occurred in patients with large or very large tumors.[139,171] Seddon and colleagues analyzed tumor mortality after enucleation versus proton irradiation in a group of patients treated by two different groups of physicians at Harvard University.[112] These retrospective data demonstrated that survival after proton beam irradiation was not worse than after enucleation, even though the proton-treated melanomas appeared to be slightly larger than those treated with

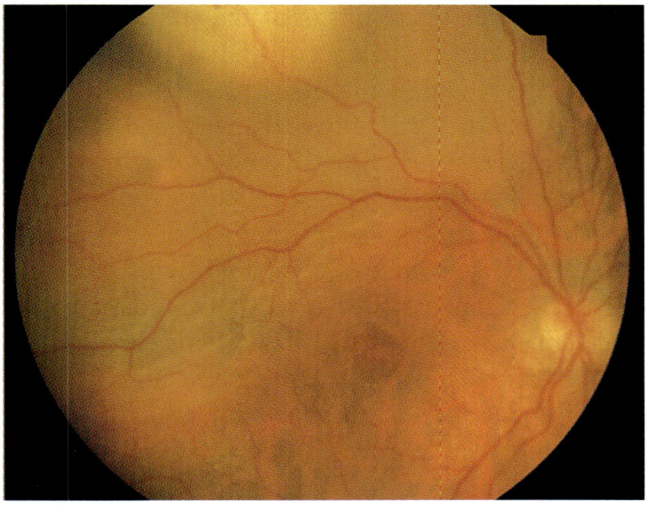

Figure 8–33. Rhegmatogenous retinal detachment after ^{125}I brachytherapy. Detachment was repaired with good visual outcome.

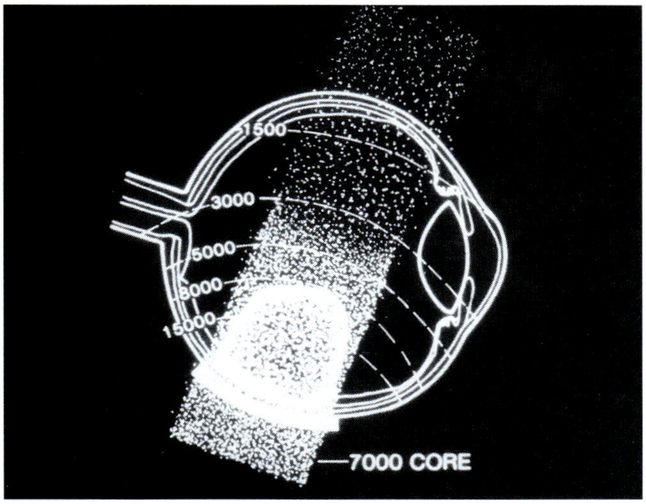

Figure 8–34. A schematic comparison of lateral radiation spread with helium ions versus a radioactive ^{125}Iplaque.

enucleation; other known risk factors were similar in the two groups.

The indications and contraindications for charged particle irradiation of uveal melanomas are still in flux. We have been able to control over 97 percent of treated tumors (with control defined as either stability or shrinkage of the intraocular tumor); however, some melanomas have a very high incidence of treatment complications that result in the eventual loss of the eye.[139,171]

The treatment of uveal melanomas with charged particle irradiation entails tumor localization with 2.5 mm tantalum marker rings for treatment planning, and radiation. The tumor and a 2-mm normal surround of uvea and retina are included in the high dose radiation field. The tumor is localized with both diffuse corneal transillumination and point-source transillumination with indirect ophthalmoscopy. The marker rings are usually placed on the sclera approximately 2 mm away from the tumor borders. A computer program—utilizing the clinical drawing, wide-angle fundus photograph, and plain orthogonal radiographs of the tantalum marker rings—is used to develop the treatment field.[172,173] As shown in Figure 8–36, the relationship of the visual structures, especially the optic nerve, fovea, and lens, to the radiation field is determined. Both the angle of gaze and the radiation beam are aligned to irradiate the tumor and minimize the dose to visually vital structures. In Figure 8–36A the melanoma and the optic nerve and fovea would be in the treatment field; Figure 8–36B demonstrates that alteration in beam and gaze angle decreases dose to the optic nerve and fovea, while the tumor receives the full radiation scheduled.

Most serious treatment complications have occurred in eyes with large and very large tumors. One approach to decrease complications has been to lower the radiation dose. This foveal melanoma shown in Figure 8–37 was successfully controlled with 50 GyE; however, visually destructive radiation vasculopathy developed. In a phase I/II study, we found no difference in control, enucleation, or survival rate in cases that were treated with 50, 60, 70, or 80 GyE irradiation.[174] In a prospective study

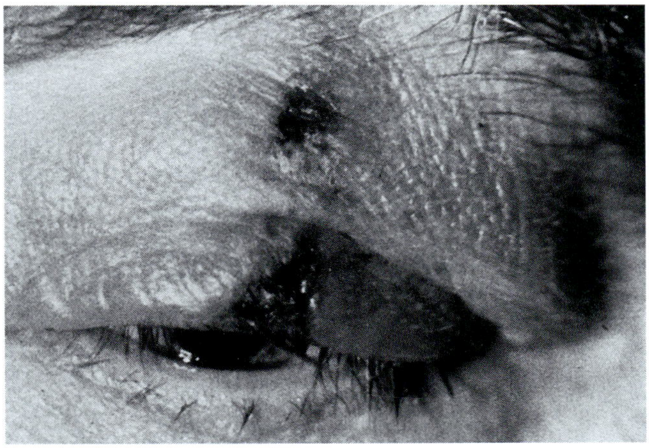

Figure 8–35. Lid complications. Severe lash loss and epitheliitis after helium ion irradiation. Usually, if the eyelid can be moved out of the entrance beam, the changes are less severe.

using between 50 and 70 cGy, Gragoudas and colleagues found similar results.[175]

In both the Boston and San Francisco experiences, an independent risk factor for visual outcome was tumor size. Initially, it was thought that tumors that were at least 3 mm from the nerve or the fovea could be treated without radiation damage to these structures and therefore with retention of good vision. We have observed, with longer follow-up, that increasingly large tumors, especially those > 8 mm thick, have significantly poorer visual outcome, regardless of location.[139] As discussed elsewhere, the marked increase in eye damage observed after irradiation of tumors > 8 mm thick has led us to attempt to resect especially tumors that are not > 12 mm in diameter and use adjunct radiation.

We have not been able to save functional eyes when the melanoma involves more than 40 percent of the ocular volume. Anterior tumors that involve more than 180° of the ocular circumference also have a grim prognosis for retention of an useful eye. Many of these tumors have been sterilized, but most of these eyes were eventually lost due to radiation complications, such as neovascular glaucoma, scleral or corneal melt, or intractable pain.[139,176] The advantage of retaining an eye with minimal vision is uncertain. Ross has pointed out that patients with some light perception probably have less sleep disturbances and less depression.[177]

We reported the results of a randomized, prospective, dynamically balanced trial comparing ^{125}I brachytherapy and helium ion irradiation in primary uveal melanomas < 15 mm in diameter and < 10 mm thick.[139] Several pertinent findings from that study influence our management of patients. As mentioned previously, there was a significantly greater local failure rate with plaques, compared with particles ($p < .001$). Comparison with most other non-randomized series have shown that this discrepancy in local failure rates with particles compared with plaques is real. The causation is multifactorial. One, the tumor shape and position affected this parameter; thinner, posterior tumors near the optic nerve had a much higher failure rate in our and other series.[125,128,139] In addition, either the higher dose delivery rate with particles (in most centers four or five 1-minute fractions over 1 week) or the relative biologic effect of charged particles, compared with plaques, probably contributes to the better local tumor control.

In both treatment arms, if tumors were > 3 mm from the disc and fovea and < 6 mm thick, most had vision ≥ 20/50 at 3 years.[139] The incidence of metastases was slightly higher in the brachytherapy group, although this has not yet reached statistical significance.

There were more external complications after treatment with particles, including lash loss,

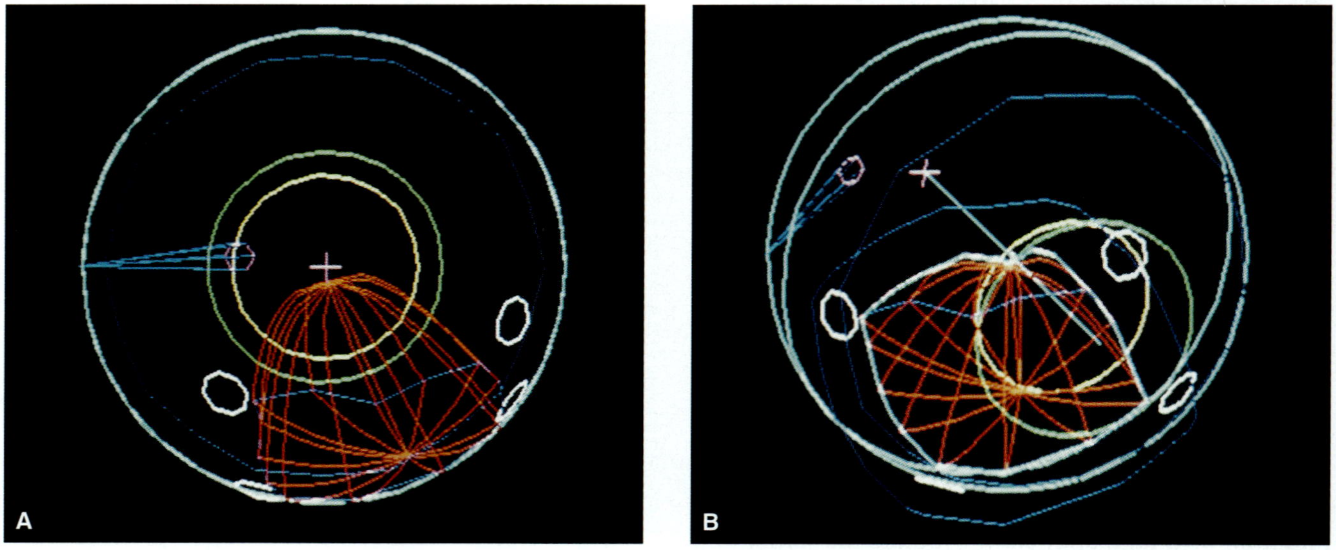

Figure 8–36. *A* and *B,* Computer treatment planning of charged particle ion irradiation. The tumor, if treated in the position shown *(A)*, would result in radiation to the melanoma as well as the fovea. Computer treatment plan demonstrates that movement of position of gaze and beam angle *(B)* allows radiation of tumor without inclusion of the optic nerve or the fovea in the high radiation dose.

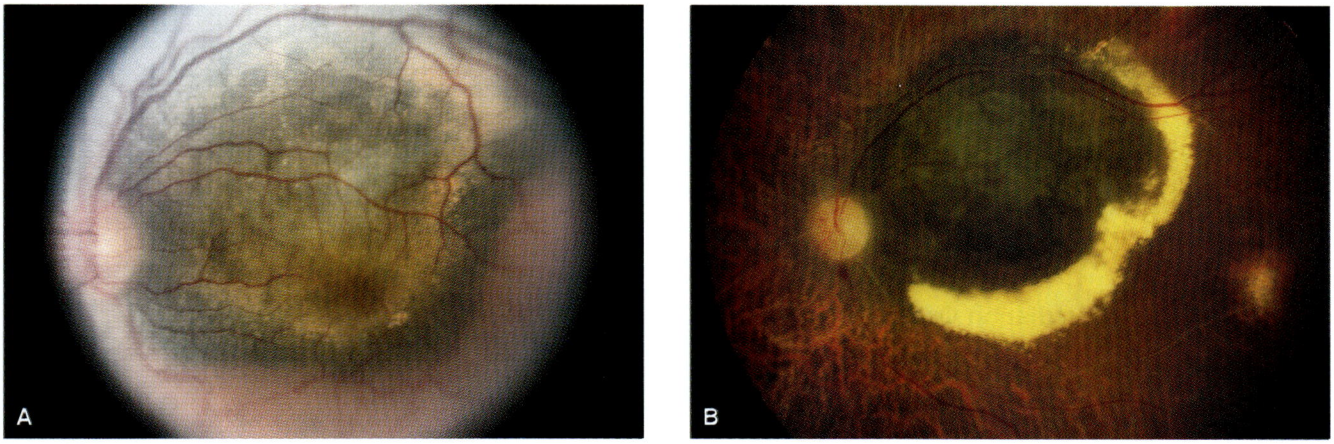

Figure 8–37. Radiation retinopathy in an eye treated with 50 GyE of helium ion radiation. *A*, Prior to radiation therapy. *B*, Four years after radiation therapy.

cataract, and neovascular glaucoma. Most of these anterior segment complications were the result of including a large percentage of these structures in the entrance beam.[176] Most neovascular glaucoma developed in the first 2 years after treatment, while cataract continued to develop at 7 percent per year with an overall incidence of 44 percent (Figure 8–38). Currently, we are using two field techniques in difficult larger tumors (Figure 8–39A, B, and C) to minimize anterior segment radiation. This newer approach with avoidance of the anterior segment in the entrance beam has diminished the incidence of neovascular glaucoma in our experience to less than 7 percent. Our current rate of neovascular glaucoma development is similar between particles and plaques.[141,168]

We attempted to further lower the radiation dose for uveal melanoma, using protons. Unfortunately, when we dropped below 40 Gy we had two failures. Given that there is an increased incidence of metastatic disease associated with local failure, we considered further dose diminution unwarranted.[130,178]

Several issues remain unresolved regarding the role of particle beams in uveal melanoma treatment. There is little question that particle beams provide better local control, and that there is less discrepancy in control rates if small, thin posterior tumors are excluded from brachytherapy. There is also no question that there is greater anterior segment complications with these proton beams, although the most serious anterior complication, neovascular glaucoma, has been reduced with multiple treatment fields. Currently, we use particles extensively in three situations: (1) small, thin tumors near the disc; in these cases there is better local control; (2) in tumors < 6 mm thick, and 3 to 6 mm from the optic nerve and fovea; in this group, we believe the visual results are slightly better than with brachytherapy; and (3) in very large tumors. In contrast, we prefer to use plaques in three other settings: (1) in relatively thick tumors near or involving the fovea, where with either technique, there will be radiation induced severe visual loss, but with a plaque there will not be as great anterior segment complications; (2) in tumors < 6 mm thick located anterior to the superior temporal equator where ^{125}I brachytherapy is less likely to produce lacrimal gland damage; and (3) in patients who have lesions that could be treated by either approach, but find the logistics of particle treatment more onerous. There is little data on new approaches to decrease tumor-related mortality after particle irradiation. Glynn and colleagues noted that several different factors influence early as compared with late metastatic disease.[179] Local failure, as would be expected, is associated with a worse prognosis, although in our experience, there is not as strong an association if the eye can be salvaged.[180,181]

Gragoudas and colleagues have noted that about 50 percent of patients who had cataract extraction after particles had > 20/100 vision.[182] The reason many of these patients do not have better vision is that cataract is associated with larger tumors, and larger tumors also have more complications. In our experience, unfortunately, many of the patients who developed cataracts had very large tumors and also developed neovascular glaucoma with poor visual outcome.

The Boston group has shown that enucleation for late radiation complications does not negatively impact a patient's survival.[166] We have also analysed our data and have noted the same results (unpublished data).

Other Radiation Options

Other radiation approaches are being investigated. The gamma knife, which has been evolving since the 1970s, became a more useful delivery device when it was linked to a computer so that dose delivery with the multiple cobalt sources could be more precisely controlled (Figure 8–40). While a gamma knife does not produce as sharp a dose gradient as can be obtained with a proton beam, it is significantly better than most forms of brachytherapy for small volume (< 10 mm^3) tumors. There is only phase I/II data available with this modality.[183–185] The optimum dose in a single fraction to control the uveal melanoma and not produce excess morbidity is unknown.[183–185] In approximately 200 reported patients, short-term local control has been good, but complications have been noted in single-fraction doses between 45 and 60 Gy.[186–188] The issue of single-fraction doses is paramount for both tumor control (where single fraction gives more tumor destruction) and for ocular complications, where single fractions would have a higher chance of damage. As an example, in the treatment of age-related maculopathy, a single 7-Gy fraction is equivalent to approximately 16 Gy given in four fractions over a week.[189]

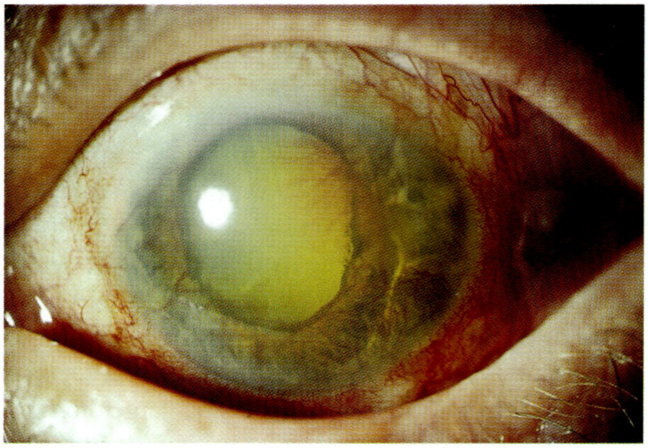

Figure 8–38. Neovascularization of the iris anterior lens capsule and cataract after helium ion radiation.

Another approach is to use fractionated teletherapy either with a gamma knife or other approaches, such as intensity-modulated conformal therapy.[190] There is a paucity of data available with this latter approach, although in other sites (see chapter on orbital sinus tumors) it has produced a good tumor destruction with markedly reduced complications.

In some centers, another means to deliver radiation, boron neutron capture, is also being investigated.[191,192] There is insufficient human uveal melanoma data with this technique to allow meaningful analyses.

Effects of Radiation Therapy and Follow-Up Guidelines

The major effect of ocular irradiation is to destroy the reproductive integrity of the tumor; tumors rarely regress completely. In large series from many centers, following successful treatment, tumors regress to approximately 40 percent of their pretreatment volume; only 10 percent of tumors entirely disappear on long-term follow-up. Direct radiation tumor damage primarily and indirect damage as a result of radiation vasculopathy that decreases tumor perfusion destroy the neoplastic proliferation capacity. While there are some immediate radiation effects on a tumor, most evidence of radiation tumor damage is delayed. DNA errors are induced in the cell at the time of treatment. These errors are manifested as tumor destruction when the cells enter mitosis; since the intermitotic phase of melanomas is variable and often prolonged, evidence of tumor shrinkage is usually delayed 3 to 18 months.[139,193] In addition, as discussed previously, apoptotic pathways are activated by radiation and radiation alters the cytokine expression in tumor cells. Also, tumors that have rapid growth are more likely to regress more rapidly but have a poorer prognosis.[139]

After any form of alternative uveal melanoma irradiation, five features indicate tumor response. The most frequent early finding is resorption of subretinal fluid. Figures 8–41A and B demonstrate a uveal melanoma with an inferior exudative hemidetachment of the retina prior to helium ion therapy and the same tumor approximately 3 months later.

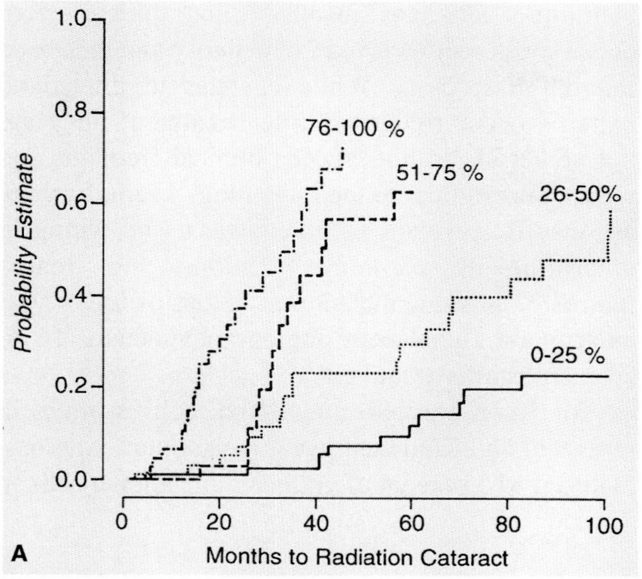

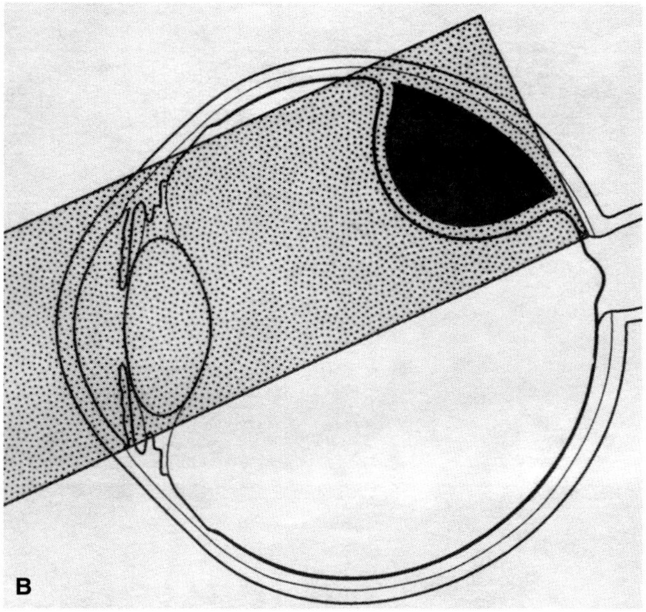

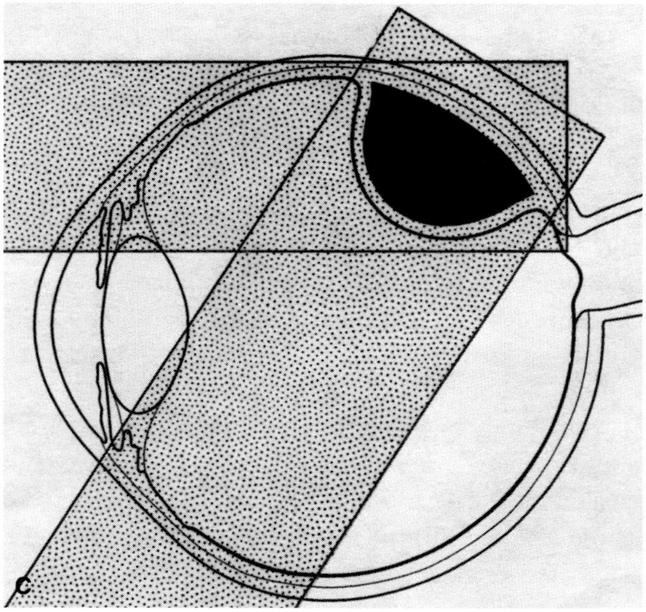

Figure 8–39. *A,* In retrospective analysis, percentage of the anterior segment in the charged particle entrance beam was associated with both neovascular glaucoma and cataracts. *B,* A schematic single field approach. The anterior segment received approximately 70% of the tumor dose. *C,* Two-field technique delivers identical tumor dose but decreases radiation to the anterior segment.

Usually, subretinal fluid is resorbed in 6 to 9 months. Loss of subretinal fluid usually occurs after treatment; however, in 10 percent of cases, there has been a transient increase in subretinal fluid, not associated with continued tumor activity. We hypothesize that some regressing tumors produce vasoactive and inflammatory humoral factors that result in transient, increased fluid. In those treated melanomas that have a transient increase in subretinal fluid and later show a decrease in tumor size, the fluid is resorbed in the first 12 to 15 months after treatment. Unfortunately, while transient macular detachments associated with exudative detachment in uveitis have a good prognosis for visual recovery, longstanding exudative macular detachments associated with tumors result in permanent central visual loss. We have treated some irradiated melanomas that had increased subretinal fluid after radiation with large spot size (3,000 micra) 810 mm long-duration confluent laser treatments and we noted marked diminution of the retinal detachment (unpublished observation).

The second clinical sign of radiation response is diminution of tumor thickness. There is a tendency

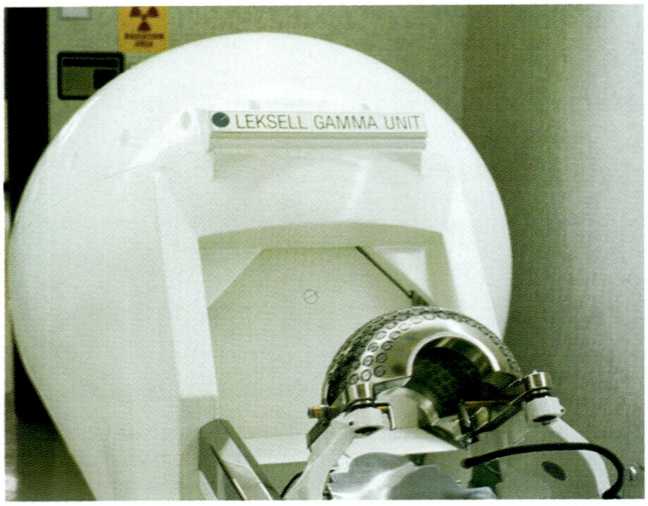

Figure 8–40. Gamma Knife is a computer-controlled multiport cobalt device.

for continued tumor shrinkage to be most marked in the first 2 to 4 years after treatment, but it continues as long as 10 years. Figures 8–42A and B demonstrate a tumor prior to and after helium ion irradiation, showing regression from approximately 10 mm to 2.5 mm in thickness in 6 years. Figures 8–43A and B represent another case with marked regression, with the tumor regressing to approximately 20 percent of its pretreatment volume. Sometimes, the collar-button portion of the lesion will shrink less rapidly, although this is variable.[194]

Some tumors appear to either not shrink or shrink very slowly over a 5- to 10-year period. We have enucleated several eyes, with good tumor control (defined as the absence of growth or actual tumor shrinkage), but there were late complications that produced blindness and painful eyes. In none of those eyes were tumor cells cycling.[195] In one case, we noted that while the tumor did not change after irradiation, it was entirely necrotic on histologic examination (Figure 8–44).[196] As mentioned previously, enucleation of such eyes does not adversely affect survival.

As discussed under brachytherapy, several newer approaches including magnetic resonance spectroscopy (MRS), MRI, Doppler ultrasonography, and three-dimensional ultrasonography have been used to monitor melanomas after radiation. Quantitative A-scan is the most accurate method to demonstrate changes in tumor height; as previously discussed, however, there are limitations in the accuracy of this technique. Changes in the echographic pattern occur, most notably loss of vascularity and increased internal reflectivity. While changes in ultrasound patterns occur frequently after treatment, they are not universal, do not precede clinical findings, and we are uncertain as to their meaning. Similarly, there are insufficient data with acoustic tissue typing to determine its accuracy in monitoring treated tumors.[197] In some melanomas, a loss of tumor vascularity on fluorescein angiography occurs 12 to 24 months after treatment.

We have studied melanoma cell cycling in untreated and irradiated uveal melanomas. Approximately 1 to 5 percent of untreated melanoma cells in

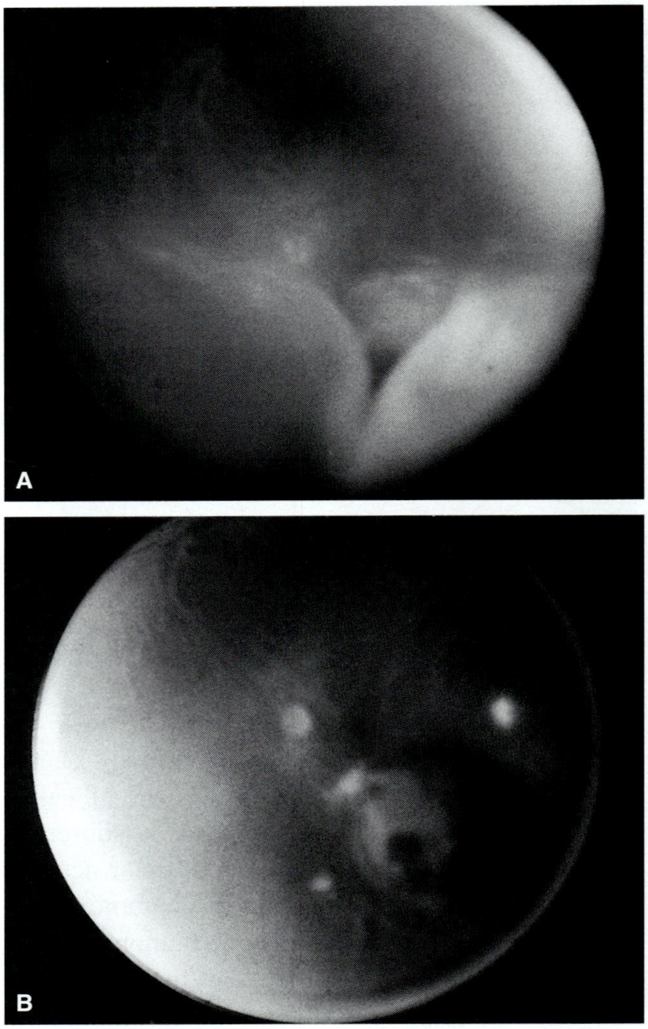

Figure 8–41. *A,* A large uveal melanoma with a secondary exudative detachment of the inferior fundus. *B,* The same melanoma 3 months after helium ion irradiation; the white areas are diathermy marks outlining the tantalum marker rings. Note the absence of subretinal fluid.

untreated tumors incorporate bromodeoxyuridine and are in the DNA synthesis phase of the cell cycle. In contrast, no cells are actively cycling after successful irradiation. We have incorporated DNA cell cycling studies into fine-needle aspiration biopsy (FNAB) techniques in a few patients. One patient with a uveal melanoma in his only eye that had been treated with a ^{60}Co plaque was referred because of presumed tumor growth. FNAB and cell cycling studies were negative, and the patient has been followed up for 7 years since that time, and there has been no evidence of enlargement. In another one-eyed patient who had been treated at another institution with 60 Gy of photon radiation for his melanoma, FNAB and cell cycling studies demonstrated that the tumor was still active, and the eye was removed. Histologically, this tumor demonstrated numerous mitoses. The use of FNAB and DNA studies in the serial evaluation of irradiated patients with uveal melanomas remains experimental with very limited indications.

Finally, the clinical appearance of a successfully radiated melanoma is characteristic. These lesions develop a surface charcoal-like appearance (Figure 8–45). Usually, there is loss of normal retinal and choroidal vasculature in the area along with change in the retinal pigment epithelium (RPE), and decreased tumor thickness.[198]

It is not uncommon to have minimal or even no evidence of tumor shrinkage after radiation. Unless definite enlargement (at least 1 to 2 mm) is present on sequential ultrasound examinations or serial fundus photographs, we do not consider the treatment a failure. The dilemma is predicated on the observation that occasionally, immediately after surgery or radiation, there is some hemorrhage or edema. Further, in some cases, intratumor radiation vasculopathy can produce hemorrhagic enlargement of the mass. The destruction and removal of tumor cells and debris after irradiation is inefficient. We have examined a number of eyes, either at autopsy or after enucleation (because of radiation complications and pain), in which the tumor was entirely necrotic, yet a significant mass remained.[196,197]

The follow-up visit after any form of alternative radiation therapy is empiric; we chose these intervals because they seem reasonable. A post-treatment baseline is established 3 months after treatment, since hemorrhage and edema can occur after surgery and irradiation. Patients are then examined every 4 months for the first year, using clinical and ultrasound evaluation, and then at progressively longer intervals. After the first year, we obtain fluorescein angiograms every 6 months to determine if radiation vasculopathy is present.

Most recurrences develop within 3 years of treatment. We have, however, seen rare recurrences as long as 10 years after plaque and 5 years after particle therapy (Figure 8–46).[139,181] Three patterns of recurrence can typically develop: (1) a marginal recurrence, more common with a plaque, in which there is a small flat area of lateral extension from a side of the irradiated tumor. In a small minority of

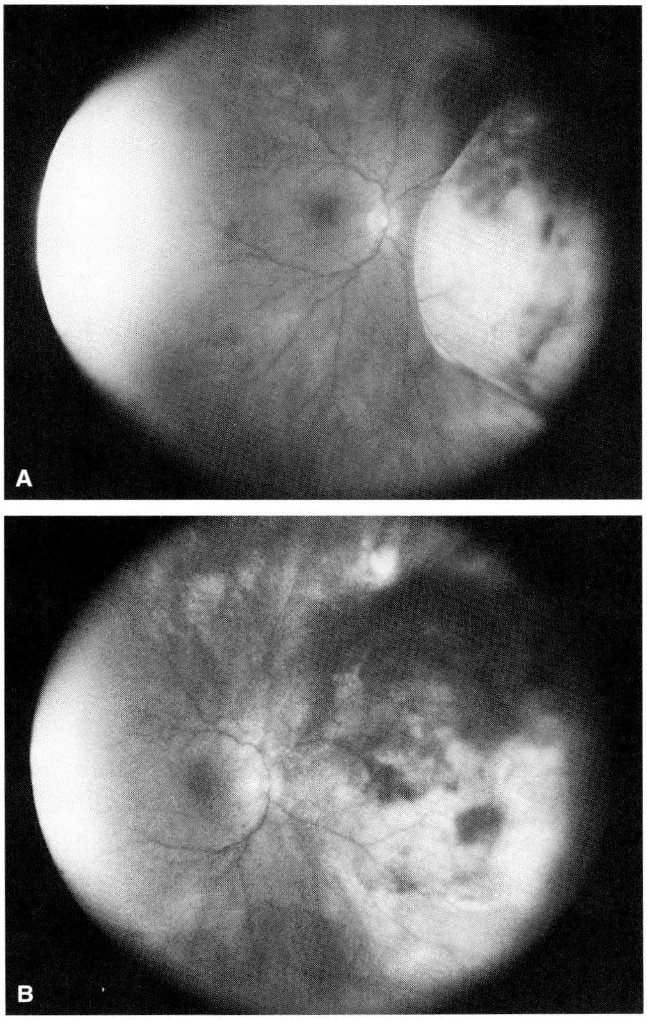

Figure 8–42. *A*, A large uveal melanoma prior to treatment. *B*, The tumor shown approximately 6 years after helium ion irradiation.

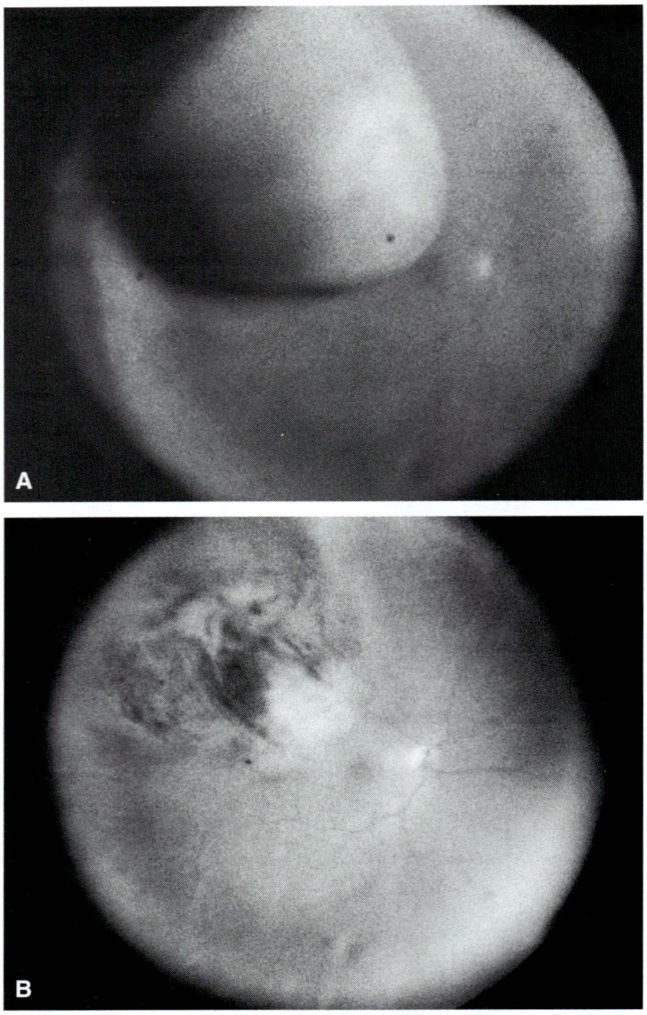

Figure 8–43. *A,* A large melanoma prior to treatment. *B,* One year after helium ion irradiation, the tumor is markedly reduced in size.

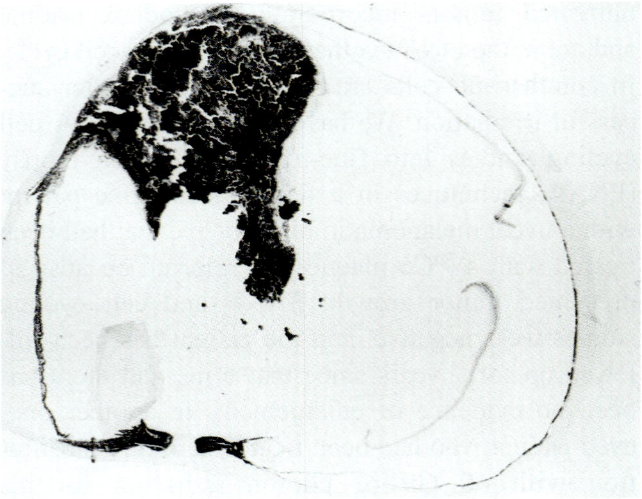

Figure 8–44. A histologic section of an 11-mm thick tumor 1 year after irradiation, which had not demonstrated regression clinically nor on ultrasound. On histology the tumor consisted almost entirely of necrotic cells.

cases, retrospective replanning of radiation shows an inadequate dose was delivered to that area of the neoplasm; (2) a generalized marked enlargement of the tumor, usually associated with increased thickness and diameter and recurrent subretinal fluid; and (3) a distant or ring (diffuse, 360°) recurrence.

The delineation of tumor enlargement resulting from radiation vasculopathy, as distinguished from neoplastic cell proliferation, can be more difficult. Usually, the time course and appearance are helpful in distinguishing these two etiologies of melanoma enlargement. If a tumor has no hemorrhagic changes around it or any intratumor hemorrhage and is enlarging rapidly within the first 2 years after treatement, it is most likely due to continued neoplastic proliferation. In contrast, if the tumor was treated more than 5 years ago and had regressed considerably but now is enlarged with other significant signs of radiation vasculopathy, possible hemorrhagic enlargement is more likely the diagnosis. Other signs of radiation vasculopathy should be present, and significant hemorrhage should be visible in and around the tumor. The time course is often helpful to differentiate the etiology of a post-treatment tumor enlargement, since radiation vasculopathy as an etiology of tumor enlargement usually occurs later than does recurrent tumor cell proliferation. As discussed previously, tumor recurrence after radiation is associated with increased melanoma-associated mortality.

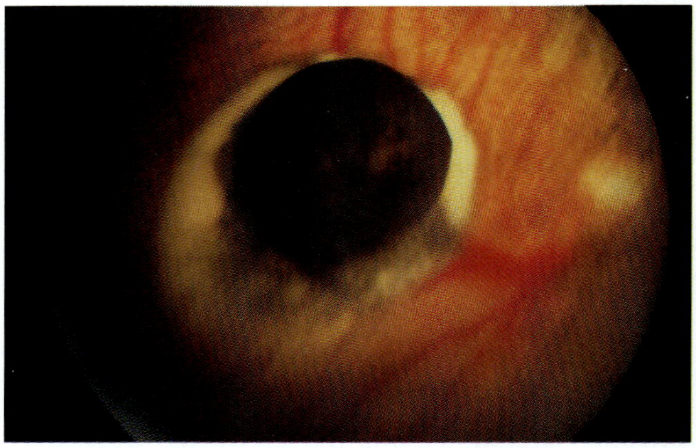

Figure 8–45. A clinical "charcoal" appearance associated with a necrotic melanoma following irradiation treatment.

Post-treatment Complications

A number of radiation complications destructive to vision are associated with 50 GyE or more of brachytherapy or charged particle irradiation. We have treated smaller melanomas with as little as 42 GyE of helium ion irradiation and still encountered radiation retinopathy.

Intraocular radiation vasculopathy after any form of irradiation occurs within approximately 6 to 36 months.[199] Retinopathy is usually characterized by areas of capillary nonperfusion, cottonwool spots, hemorrhages, microaneurysms, and exudates (Figures 8–47 to 8–49). Optic neuropathy has a typical appearance as shown in Figures 8–50 and 8–51; early changes are the presence of flame hemorrhages and edema of the nerve head; later atrophy with loss of normal disc microvasculature occurs.

Radiation retinopathy occurs slightly earlier with charged particle irradiation than it does with radioactive plaques; however, the incidence of posterior pole complications with plaques appears to be higher than with charged particles in our randomized intra-institutional study.[139] The tumor plus 2 mm of normal surround are routinely treated with high-dose charged particle radiation to avoid the possibility of either a marginal miss secondary to clinically inapparent tumor or movement of the patient during treatment. Thus, if the tumor is within 3 mm of the fovea or nerve, (2 mm of normal surround plus lateral radiation beam fall-off), it is likely that these visually vital structures will receive sufficient irradiation to develop clinically significant irradiation vasculopathy.

The pattern and time course of radiation vascular complications vary. Lash loss and both conjunctival and lid erythema become evident within the first 6 weeks after charged particle irradiation (Figure 8–52). To avoid epiphora secondary to radiation stenosis of the lacrimal drainage system, silicone tubes are placed prior to irradiation of uveal melanomas in the nasal portion of the eye.[169] In approximately 10 percent of patients with large anterior uveal melanomas, keratopathy develops because a significant portion of the cornea is in the high-dose radiation field. Radiation cataracts develop within 6 to 12 months, if the majority of the lens is included in the high-dose region of the treatment beam or in the high-dose region for brachytherapy. In a series of 558 patients treated in Boston for posterior tumors that were within 6 mm of the optic disc, it was noted that the 5-year rates were 64 percent for maculopathy, 35 percent for radiation optic neuropathy, and 68 percent for vision loss.[200] As we had previously described, diabetes was also noted to be an increased risk factor for vision loss in this latter series. The authors noted that the safe radiation dose to the optic nerve was about 30 Gy.[201] Similar studies of eyes treated with brachytherapy have been done.[202]

We have previously studied the accuracy of charged particle radiation delivery; if the treated tumor is > 4 mm from the fovea or the nerve, these structures seldom receive significant radiation.[200] We initially hypothesized that the focusability of charged particle beams would decrease the incidence of post-treatment visual loss; however, we had been overly optimistic. Retrospective evalua-

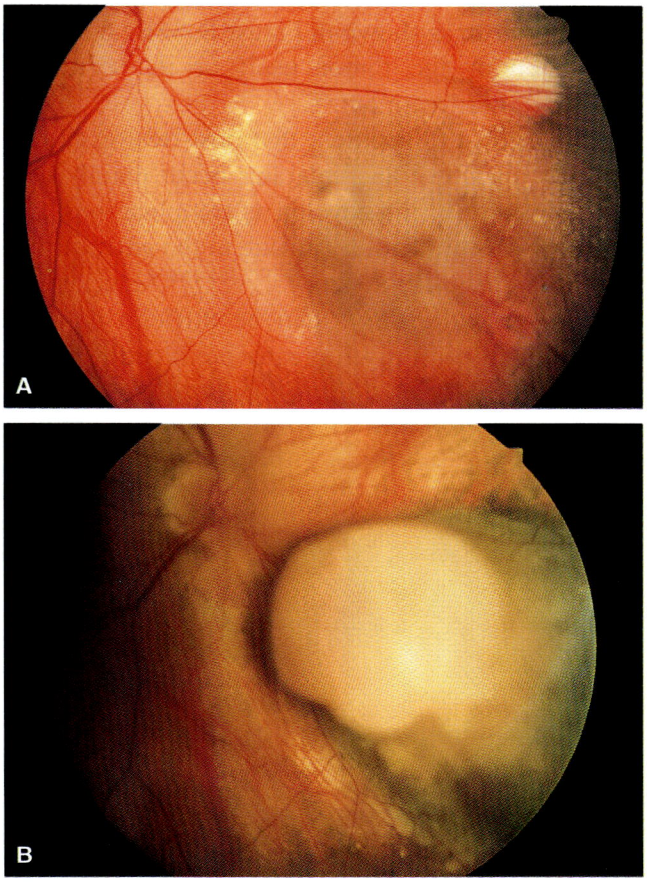

Figure 8–46. *A* and *B*, Melanoma has been nicely flattened by ^{125}I radioactive plaque. The new area of vertical growth occurred about 10 years after radiation.

tion of patients treated with either protons or helium ions has demonstrated ocular complications both inside and outside the radiation field. Uveal melanoma patients whose tumors are distant from the fovea and the nerve can still develop loss of vision after charged particle therapy. The data from both Boston and San Francisco demonstrate that tumor thickness is a major factor in determining whether patients will or will not have good post-treatment vision, independent of the tumor's location and the radiation field dose to the nerve or the fovea. Figure 8–53A demonstrates a case of a peripheral uveal melanoma treated with helium ion irradiation, where neither the optic nerve nor the fovea received any significant radiation. Unfortunately, 8 months later, the visual acuity was permanently diminished, secondary to an exudative detachment into the fovea. Since untreated large melanomas may produce rubeosis iridis, cystoid macular edema, and other visually destructive complications, it is unclear whether the post-radiation distant effects, as shown in Figure 8–53B, are due to irradiation or the tumor itself or its regression response after treatment.[203]

Similarly, it is apparent that post-treatment neovascular glaucoma and cataracts occur mainly with large melanomas and develop as complications, as a result of direct radiation damage to the anterior segment as well as tumor size.[168,177,204–206] Anterior segment neovascularization can be difficult to diagnose, since it has a much greater predilection for the chamber angle rather than the anterior iris surface. All patients with elevated intraocular pressures should have gonioscopy. The glaucoma in many of these cases can be controlled with steroids, glaucoma medications, and retinal ablation (panretinal photocoagulation or cryotherapy) procedures.

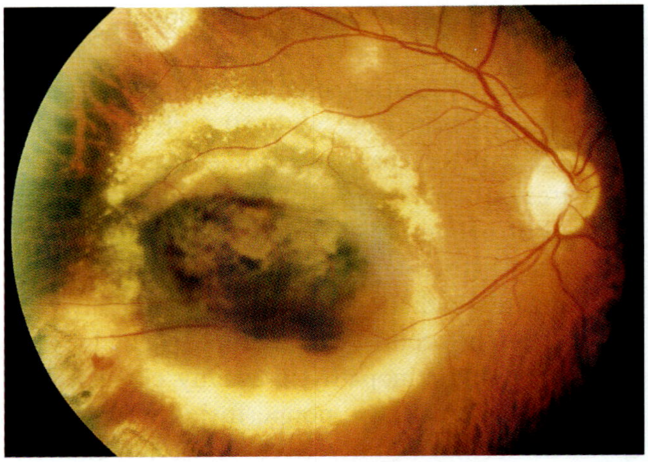

Figure 8–48. Radiation-induced exudates.

Radiation: Conclusion

Our experience of both particle and plaque therapies demonstrates some advantages and disadvantages of these techniques. Larger melanomas are more advantageously treated with proton therapy than with any form of radioactive plaque. If melanomas > 18 mm in diameter and > 10 mm thick are not removed, they should be managed with charged particle irradiation.

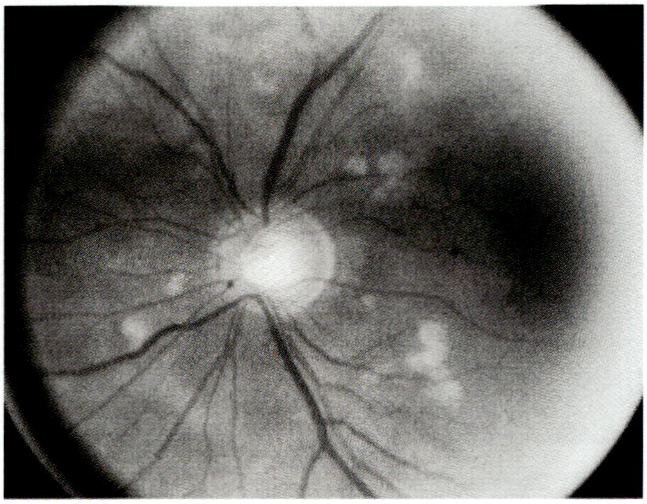

Figure 8–47. Radiation retinopathy with cotton wool spots.

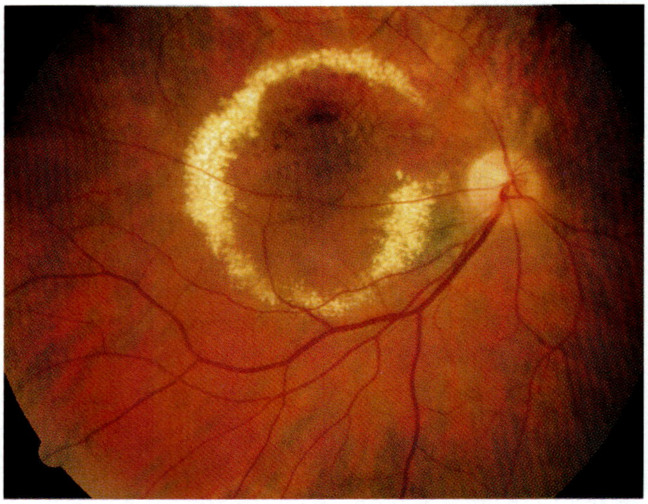

Figure 8–49. Radiation-induced maculopathy.

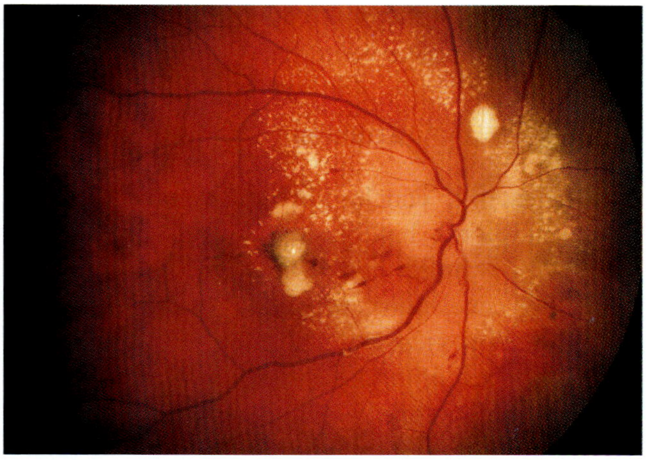

Figure 8–50. Acute radiation optic neuropathy.

Unfortunately, < 15 percent of irradiated eyes with tumors of that thickness retained 20/200 or better vision, and approximately 25 percent of such eyes are eventually enucleated from late complications.

There is usually less external eye damage if thick posterior uveal melanomas are treated with radioactive plaques. Shielding the ^{125}I plaque with a gold carrier minimizes damage to the adnexal structures, which, depending on tumor position, include the lacrimal gland, puncta, and eye lashes. There may be more intraocular radiation damage, such as radiation retinopathy, with plaques. Lesions contiguous to the optic nerve head are more difficult to treat with plaques than with particles. Radiation complication rates associated with the treatment of larger anterior melanomas are high.[207]

Several molecular biologic approaches are being studied to attempt to decrease radiation ocular morbidity. However, there is a paucity of even phase I ophthalmic data. In vitro, alteration of the manganese superoxide dismutase gene alters relative damage to the tumor, compared with normal cells.[208] Similarly, alterations of the *Egr-1* gene appear to alter the relative effect on normal versus tumor cells.[209,210] Several studies have addressed the mechanisms of radiation-induced vascular compromise; however, clinical trials are just being initiated.[211,212] Vascular central nervous system (CNS) injuries have shown some response to anticoagulation, but the effectiveness of this approach in radiation-induced injury is uncertain.[213,214]

Adjunctive Hyperthermia

Hyperthermia, which has been known to have anticancer properties since the 19th century, has a synergistic effect with radiation.[215–217] A number of investigators have used hyperthermia to treat animal models of intraocular melanoma, and a few patients have been treated. Laboratory data have also demonstrated that heat can alter the antigenic array on uveal melanoma in vitro.[218] Initial long-term results reported by Finger and colleagues looked promising;[219] however, patients in that series were derived from highly selected cases, with approximately two-thirds having good prognosis both for vision and life, and the results should

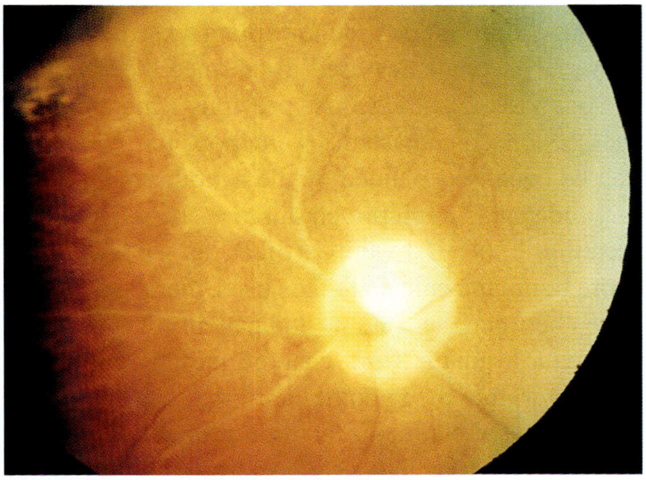

Figure 8–51. Radiation optic atrophy with vascular closure after cobalt plaque therapy.

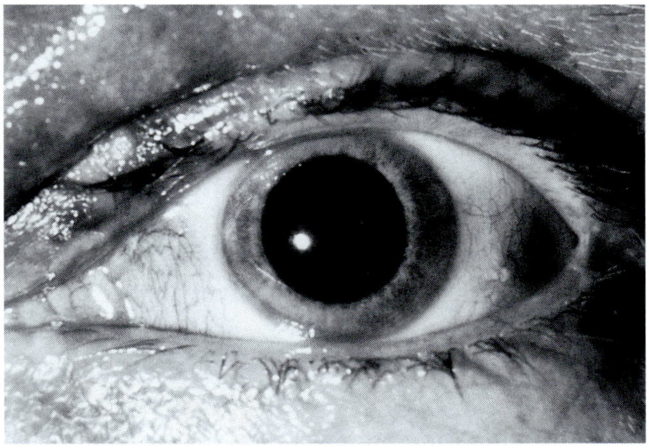

Figure 8–52. Lash loss and both conjunctival and lid erythema occur within the first 6 weeks after charged paticle irradiation, when the lids are included in the treatment field.

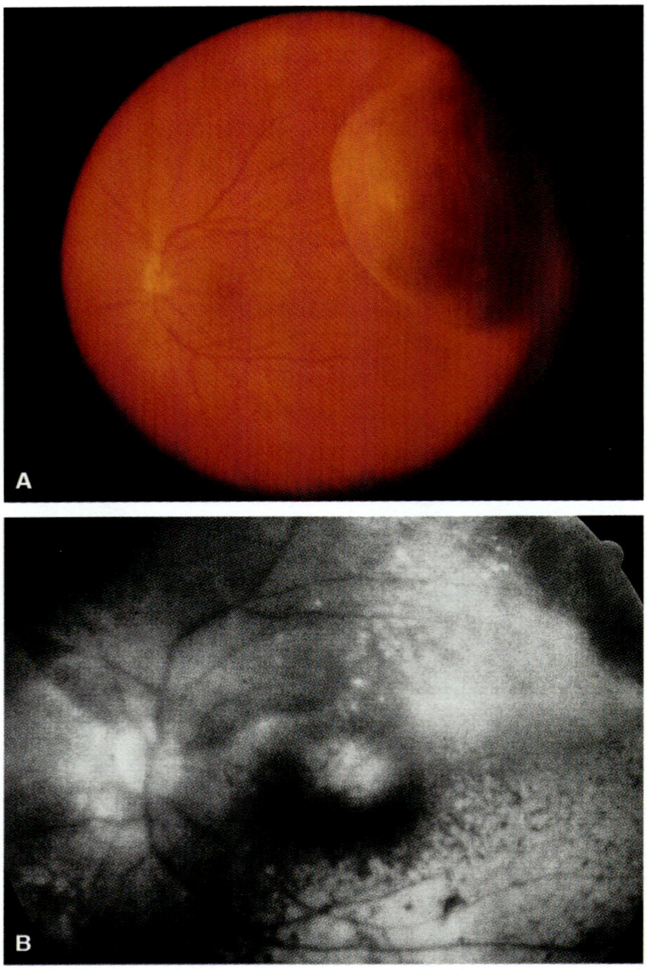

Figure 8–53. *A,* Large peripheral melanoma treated with helium ion radiation. *B,* Exudative changes in the macula 8 months after treatment of the above peripheral uveal melanoma. Both the fovea and the optic nerve were outside the radiation treatment field.

therefore have been excellent.[219] There is little evidence to suggest that this approach has been demonstrated to increase the control rate or decrease the morbidity, compared with radiation alone. It is also uncertain whether it will be better to use ultrasound, microwave, laser, or ferromagnetic seed-induced hyperthermia to treat ocular tumors, if this modality is used. In a collaborative European systemic hyperthermia study, technical problems with therapeutic delivery were noted; only 14 percent of cases received optimal heating.[220] Several groups, including ours, have shown in animals that there is at least a two-fold enhancement of radiation effect with heating.[221,222] Therefore, it is likely that if there will be a role for hyperthermia, a markedly reduced radiation dose will have to be given in order to avoid the complications that previously have been noted.

Enucleation

The efficacy of enucleation in the management of uveal melanoma has been controversial for many years. Early workers noted widely discrepant survival rates after enucleation; between 20 to 96 percent of patients died as a result of the tumor.[223,224] Some investigators believed that early enucleation decreased tumor-related mortality, while others did not.[224–226]

Zimmerman and colleagues suggested a potentially deleterious effect of enucleation on tumor-related mortality.[227,228] There are a number of data that demonstrate that enucleation does not adversely affect prognosis.[229,230]

Zimmerman and his colleagues hypothesized that pressure on the eye during enucleation could seed tumor cells into the circulation and increase the risk of metastases. In one hamster model, there were data consistent with this viewpoint, but not in another animal model.[231,232] Retrospective clinical pathologic data from the Armed Forces Institute of Pathology (AFIP) demonstrated that the peak incidence of metastases occurred during the first 2 years after enucleation, and the researchers inferred that the increased risk of metastases during this time period could be due to surgical manipulation.

There are a number of data that do not support that hypothesis. (1) Several other malignancies treated with nonsurgical techniques have a similar tumor-related mortality curve; an adverse effect from surgical trauma cannot be used to explain these data.[233] (2) Some of the statistics used to advance the argument are open to question. (3) As previously mentioned in the section on metastatic evaluation, the AFIP data can be equally explained by the hypothesis that there are undetectable micrometastases at the time of enucleation.[230] (4) If myelin artifact, as evidence of a more traumatic enucleation, is used, there is no correlation between that finding and patient survival.[231] (5) The data available from charged particle irradiation partially refute the hypothesis. If pressure at the time of surgery were a major factor in promoting metastasis, it is likely that those patients treated with charged particle beams, in whom tantalum marker rings are often sutured at the posterior of the globe, would be at greater risk for metastases than those patients who underwent enucleation. Retrospective matched studies comparing enucleation and proton beam irradiation have shown that the latter technique appears to have a lower incidence of metastases.[112] (6) Animal studies have demonstrated that pressure alone at the time of enucleation is not enough to increase tumor-related mortality.[112]

Prior to considering a patient as a candidate for enucleation, we perform a metastasis evaluation. If a patient has uveal melanoma metastases, the mean survival is < 1 year, and enucleation should not be performed, unless the eye is painful.

It is important to establish a correct diagnosis before enucleation is considered. As previously discussed, using modern diagnostic techniques, false-positive enucleation for suspected melanomas should occur in < 1 percent of cases. In the last 10 years, we have not enucleated any eyes in which the diagnosis of uveal melanoma was not confirmed on histopathologic examination.

In an eye with a suspected large melanoma with opaque media or in other very atypical cases, we perform either trans-scleral or transvitreal FNAB with a 25-gauge needle. As the needle is withdrawn from the sclera, the area is sealed with histoacryl glue. The cytologist in the operating room can usually make the diagnosis immediately (Figure 8–54); if the biopsy is positive for melanoma, the eye is enucleated.

Enucleation is the recommended therapy for a number of uveal melanomas. It should be used in patients who, after informed consent, request removal of the eye. It is also best in patients whose melanoma involves over 40 percent of ocular volume or over 50 percent of the ocular circumference. Our experience has demonstrated that while such tumors can be destroyed with charged particle irradiation, visual function is lost.[139] If the melanoma is associated with significant neovascularization or is in a blind eye, the eye should be enucleated.

Surgical Procedure

There are a number of enucleation techniques. We usually perform a standard enucleation with minimal pressure on the eye. We have not used a cryoenucleation technique. It is unwieldy; if one were a strong advocate of this procedure, it would be necessary to perform a lateral orbitotomy to insert the cryo-apparatus against the tumor area of the eye with minimal trauma.[232] We do not use a paracentesis to decrease intraocular pressure during eye removal.[233]

A 360° limbal peritomy is performed (Figure 8–55). The quadrants are gently opened, using a Bishop Harman forceps and Steven's scissors, to separate Tenon's capsule from the globe and isolate the muscles (Figure 8–56). If there is a previously undetected area of extraocular extension, we routinely isolate the Tenon's capsule in that quadrant and extirpate it, along with contiguous extraocular muscle, and the globe en bloc.[234] In this situation, since some of these cases are treated with adjunct radiation, 50 Gy can result in loss of the implant and some cosmetic defect.

In routine enucleation, the four recti muscles are isolated and detached. We routinely use scleral-wrapped hydroxyapatite (HA) integrated implants, and the muscles are imbricated with 5-0 vicryl (Figure 8–57).[235] If an older approach with only a sphere is used, the muscles are severed from the globe. Regardless of technique, we leave 2 mm stumps of the medial and lateral recti muscles on their insertions. After the recti and oblique muscles are severed from the globe, the two stumps are used to grasp the globe, using either 4-0 silk sutures or mosquito forceps (Figure 8–58). We usually use forceps instead of sutures in a resident teaching institution, since we are concerned about the possibility of penetrating a tumor-filled eye with a suture needle. A Steven's or curved enucleation scissors is placed into the medial orbit after the optic nerve is located using a Steven's muscle hook. The blades of the scissors are placed around the optic nerve, and it is severed (Figure 8–59). A test tube filled with warm water is placed in the orbit; a 4 × 4 sponge is used to create pressure for approximately 7 minutes. It is not necessary to use an optic nerve snare for hemostasis, and not using it avoids some myelin artifacts on histologic sections.

After enucleation, the eye should be carefully examined in the operating room. If there is a significant area of extraocular extension which had not been noted during the enucleation procedure, the orbit is explored using Sewell retractors. If a small area of extraocular extension was transsected

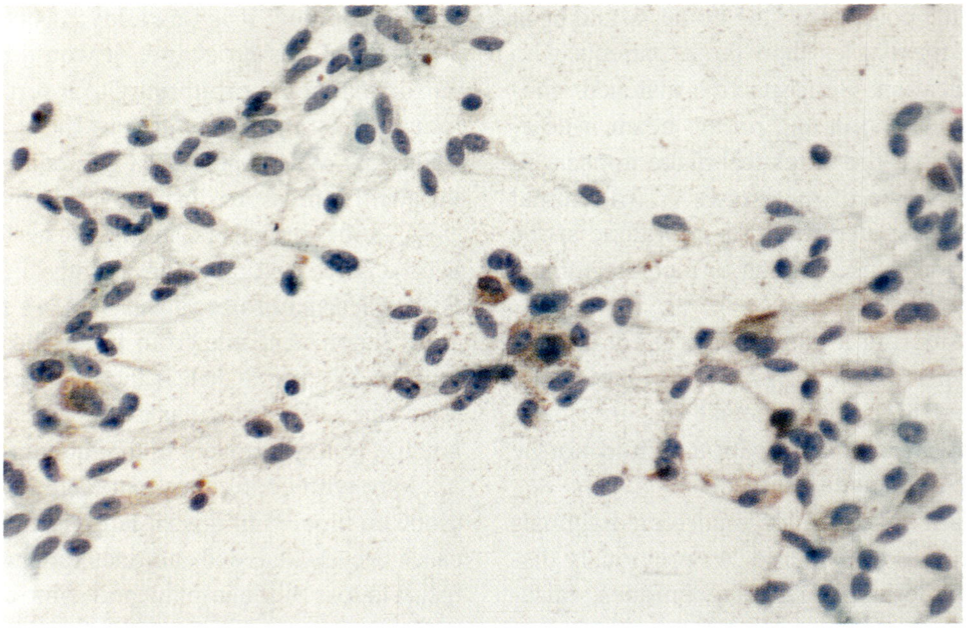

Figure 8–54. Cytologic appearance of FNAB of a spindle cell uveal melanoma.

at the time of enucleation, the gross residual tumor should be removed and no implant inserted into the orbital space.

In adults, we generally use a 20-mm HA implant soaked in antibiotic solution and 0.5 percent bupivacaine (Marcaine). An allogenic scleral shell from which the cornea has been harvested is sutured with 5-0 dacron so that the corneal space is facing posteriorly. Windows, approximately 3 × 5 mm in size, are cut through the sclera at the equator (Figure 8–60).

When hemostasis is achieved, the implant is placed in the orbit. If a scleral-wrapped HA implant is used, the ends of the horizontal and vertical muscles are imbricated into the respective anterior lip of each scleral window, as shown in Figure 8–61.

If an older implant is used, the largest size compatible with the patient's orbital anatomy is selected; in adults, a 20- or 22-mm sphere or a large Moore or Ellis implant is inserted (Figure 8–62). In infants or children, implant size varies between 14 and 20 mm.

If an older modified Ellis or Moore implant is used instead of a sphere, the horizontal muscles are imbricated together and the vertical muscles are imbricated together over the surface of the implant (Figure 8–63). This should not be done with a plain sphere, since it will cause implant migration. Tenon's capsule is closed in three layers. A 4-0 chromic suture or 4-0 vicryl is used in a "purse-string" manner (Figure 8–64A). Two rows of interrupted 4-0 chromic suture are used to close the remaining gaps in Tenon's capsule (Figures 8–64B and C). The conjunctiva is closed with a running 6-0 plain gut suture (Figure 8–64D).

A conformer is placed into the orbit, approximately 2 mL of 0.75 percent bupivacaine is then injected into the orbital quadrants, and the orbit is

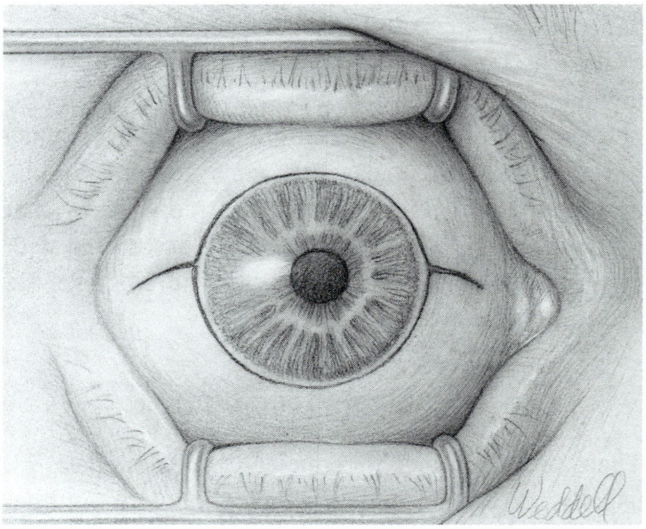

Figure 8–55. A 360° peritomy with relaxing incisions.

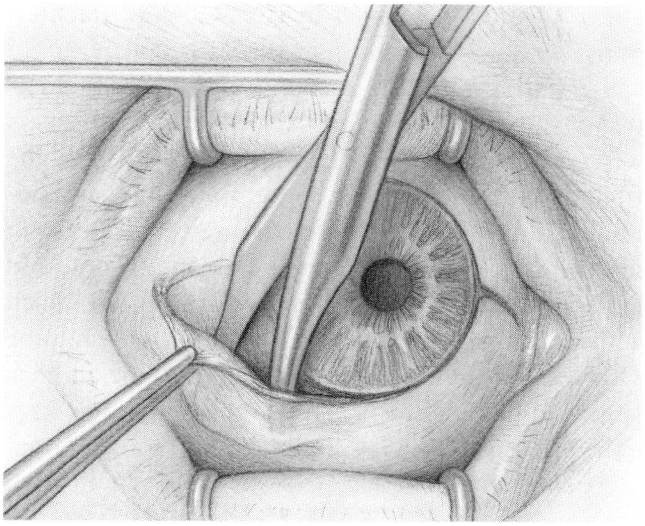

Figure 8–56. A Stevens scissors is used to open Tenon's capsule between the rectus muscles.

firmly pressure-patched for approximately 48 hours. The use of an injectable long-acting anesthetic markedly reduces postoperative pain, and many patients leave the hospital either the same day or the morning after surgery. The patch is removed at 48 hours, and the patient is then repatched for an additional 48-hour period. After that time, the orbital dressing is changed daily by the patient.

We have not used a dermis-fat graft as a primary procedure after enucleation for two reasons: (1) We do not believe that it markedly enhances cosmesis; and (2) there is continual remodeling, and in tumors where there might be a question of local recurrence, this has led to confusion in a number of cases.[236,237]

The patient is examined by an ocularist within 2 weeks after enucleation so that the painting of the orbital prosthesis can be begun. The fitting of the orbital prosthesis generally occurs between 4 and 8 weeks after surgery.

While HA implants are now in vogue, their ultimate role in enucleated sockets is uncertain.[238–240] These are expensive, can rarely become exposed, and do not always produce better cosmesis than a much less expensive plastic or silicone sphere.[241] Several newer synthetic implants that may be less expensive and equally effective have become available.[242] Some of the results with these approaches have been less effective.[243] An advantage of the HA implant is that it is easy to shape in the operating room, if contour alteration or size reduction is required.[244] Several complications have been reported with HA implants, especially when they are pegged for better motility. The discussion of that cosmetic approach is outside the scope of this book. In the author's experience, less than one-half of the patients require pegging to obtain excellent motility.[245–253] After either enucleation or, more often, exeneration, placement of an orbital epidermal catheter may be useful to control discomfort.[254]

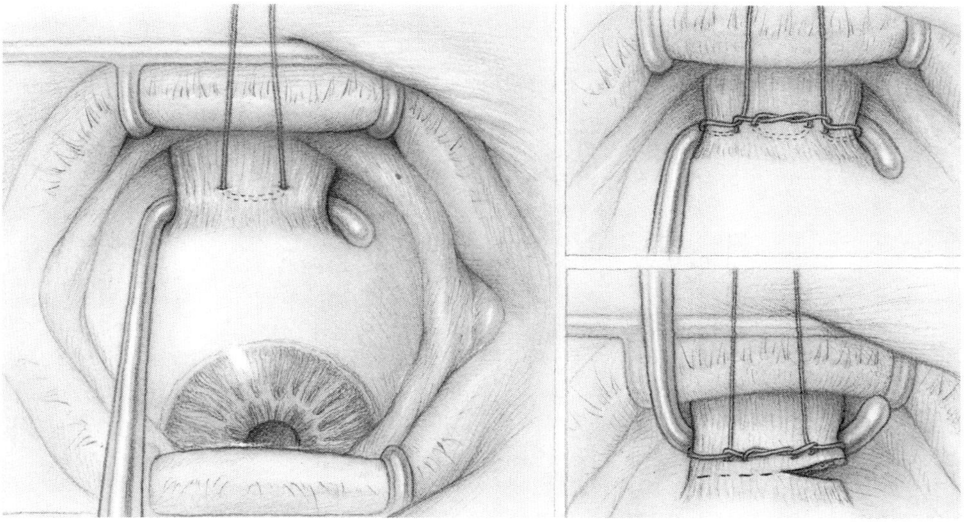

Figure 8–57. If an integrated implant is used, the rectus muscles are individually imbricated with 5-0 vicryl sutures and disinserted from the globe.

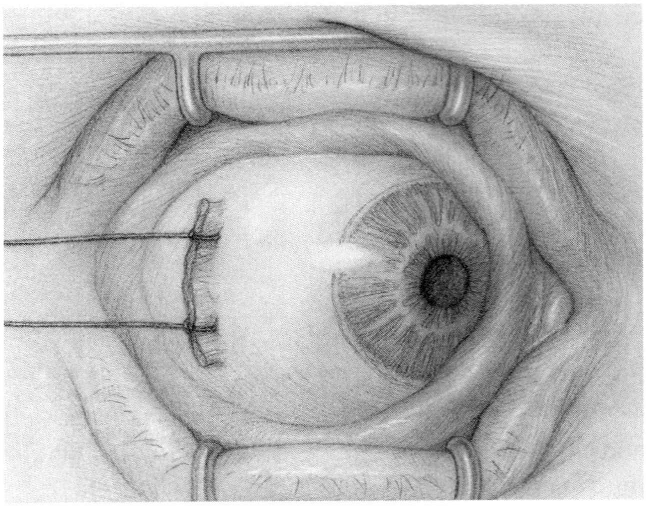

Figure 8–58. The stumps of the medial and lateral rectus muscles can either be grasped with mosquito forceps or, as shown, imbricated with 5-0 silk traction sutures.

Adjunctive Pre-enucleation Radiation

While several groups were questioning the usefulness of pre-enucleation radiation, we initiated a phase I/II trial, whose design was the basis for a portion of the COMS in 1977. In patients with large uveal melanomas scheduled for enucleation, 20 Gy of photon irradiation was given in five 400-cGy fractions over 1 week.[245,246] In some systemic malignancies, the use of perioperative irradiation has decreased tumor-related mortality. Anterior lateral wedge pair ports were used, as shown in Figure 8–65. Either on the final day of irradiation or on the following day, enucleation was performed. We observed no significant untoward effects with this fractionation schedule and radiation dose.[246] The theoretical advantages of such an irradiation dose were (1) it has been shown to be effective in other malignancies; (2) melanomas appear to be more responsive to relatively high fraction sizes (400 cGy) rather than conventional (200 cGy) fractionation; (3) 20 Gy given in high fraction sizes is probably as effective as 30 Gy given with conventional size fractions; (4) this dose and fractionation schedule could be delivered in a short period, whereas increasing radiation to 40 Gy would entail 6 weeks of radiation; and (5) this dose and fractionation were safe and entailed little risk to the uninvolved contiguous structures.

There are a number of potential limitations to this approach. (1) If micrometastases have already occurred at the time of diagnosis, it is unlikely that ocular irradiation will decrease tumor-related mor-

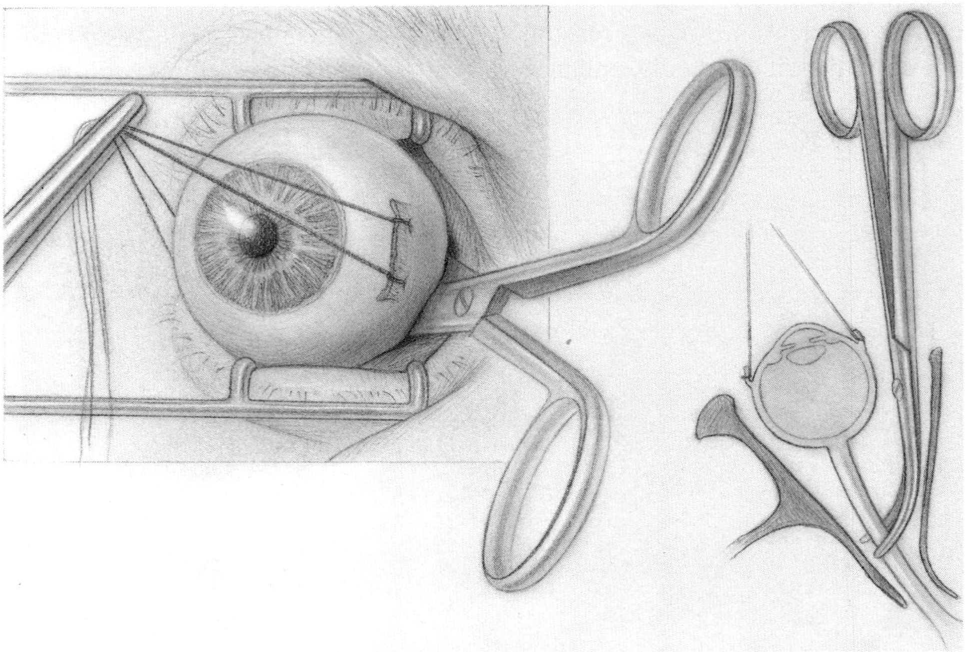

Figure 8–59. The globe is enucleated by exerting traction on the stumps of the medial and lateral rectus muscles and placing enucleation scissors medially into the posterior orbit to obtain a long section of optic nerve.

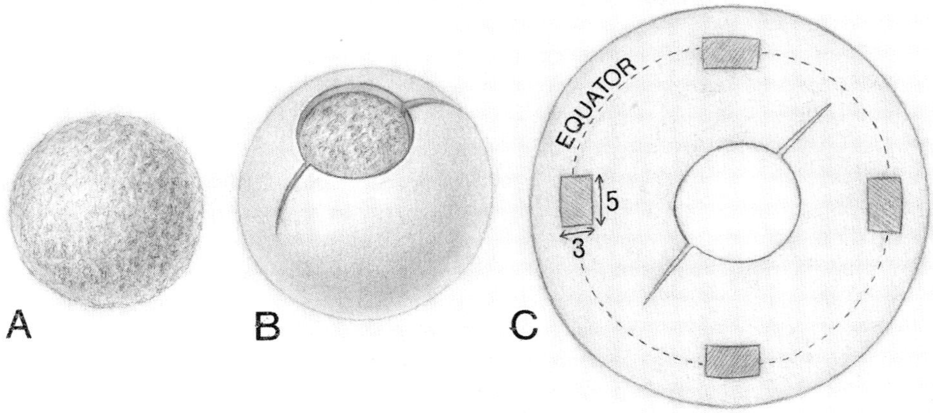

Figure 8–60. Hydroxyapatite implant has a scleral shell sutured around it with 5.0 dacron sutures. Four 3 x 5 mm windows are cut at the equator.

tality. (2) The dose and fractionation schedule chosen, while reasonable, may be inadequate to destroy the tumor. (3) Perioperative irradiation has been most effective in tumors in which there has been either local or lymph node recurrence; this is not the pattern for uveal melanoma spread.

Unfortunately, although the rationale for this study seemed reasonable, the approach proved to be ineffective in our experience. We used Cox model analysis to compare the survival of 42 patients treated with this protocol with 33 patients with similar tumors enucleated by the same surgeon.[247] Tumor size, cell type, and use of pre-enucleation irradiation were all significant parameters associated with worse prognosis. The data indicate that pre-enucleation irradiation did not improve survival. The failure of this technique does not appear to be

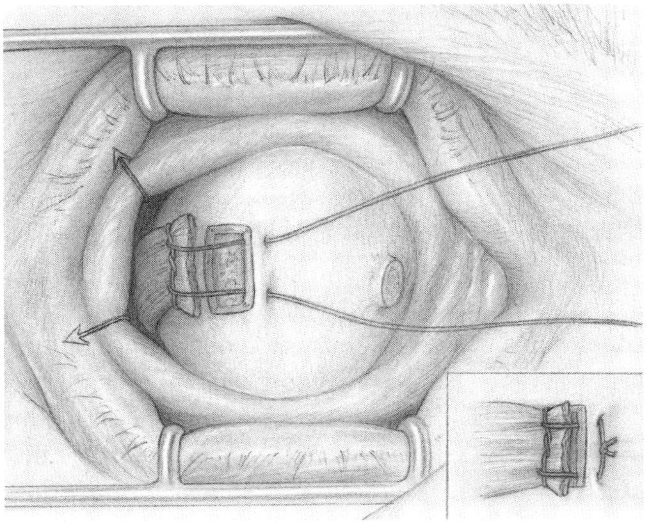

Figure 8–61. Muscles attached to the anterior lips with the scleral windows.

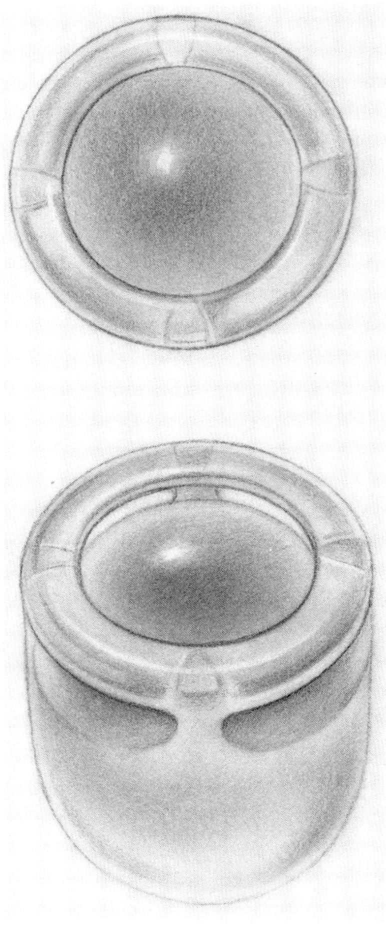

Figure 8–62. A Moore implant, one of a number of different integrated implants.

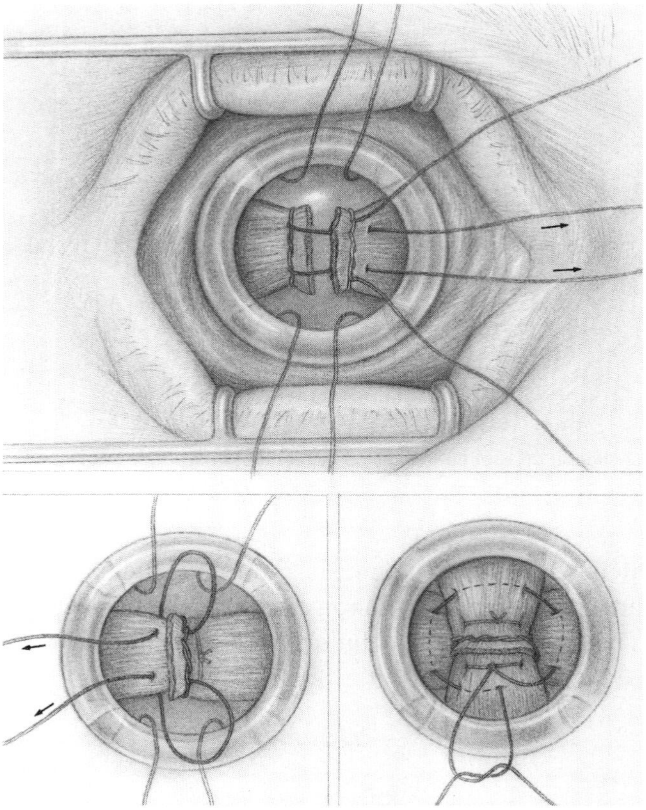

Figure 8–63. If an integrated implant is used, the medial and rectus muscles are tied together, as are the superior and inferior rectus muscles. The four rectus muscles are then imbricated together in a circular fashion to avoid slippage. If a sphere is used and the muscles are not tied over the implant, migration is inevitable.

due to inadequate radiation dose, since irradiated tumor cells had significantly less tumor culture growth or cell cycling than had cells from nonirradiated melanomas. On the basis of these data, we have abandoned this modality.

Luyten and colleagues used two 400-cGy fractions in 145 cases and used Cox model analysis to compare them with a historic control group; no improvement in survival was noted.[248] Similarly, four other trials found no beneficial effect with pre-enucleation radiation.[249,255–257]

The COMS reported its results in a prospective randomized trial of enucleation versus pre-enucleation radiation followed by enucleation in 1,003 patients (pre-encleation radiation of 497 and enucleation alone in 506 patients). They found no statistically significant difference in the 5-year survival in the two groups. While there was slightly better survival in the group that received radiation, the difference and balances in the baseline covariates may have accounted for this. A few were biopsied for recurrence in the eyes that received pre-enucleation radiation versus enucleation alone (0 versus 5), and surprisingly, the patients who received radiation had a slightly lower incidence of ptosis. However the author thinks that the latter finding was probably spurious.[258]

Exenteration

There are very few indications for exenteration in uveal melanoma, even when there is focal, extraocular extension.[259] If there is diffuse extraocular extension, then exenteration is indicated to remove the tumor, provided there are no metastases (Figure 8–66). Often, these patients have metastases. The patient shown in Figure 8–67 was referred for exenteration of an orbital recurrence; however, metastatic evaluation revealed widespread disease. Prior to exenteration, a complete metastatic evaluation is performed. Exenteration can be performed either with lid-sparing or non–lid sparing techniques (Figures 8–68 to 8–79). I prefer to remove the lids at the time of exenteration in uveal melanoma cases. We have managed a few patients with local recurrences that, after exenteration, were controlled because they were detected very early, since the only volume in the orbit was a split-thickness skin graft. If we had elected to do surgery and had chosen to spare the lids, allow self-granulation, or place a temporalis flap, the tumor would have grown beyond local control by the time it was noted.

Surgical Procedure

Exenteration techniques, for both sparing and removing of the lids, are shown (see Figures 8–68 to 8–79). If the eyelids are to be retained, a skin incision is made with a No. 15 blade scalpel in the upper and lower lids, approximately 2 mm from the eyelash margin. The skin is mobilized, and a myocutaneous flap elevated to the area of the orbital rim in all directions (see Figures 8–68 and 8–71). If the lids are to be sacrificed, then an incision is made just inside the orbital rim with a scalpel (see Figures 8–69 and 8–72). Using a cutting Bovie, the incision

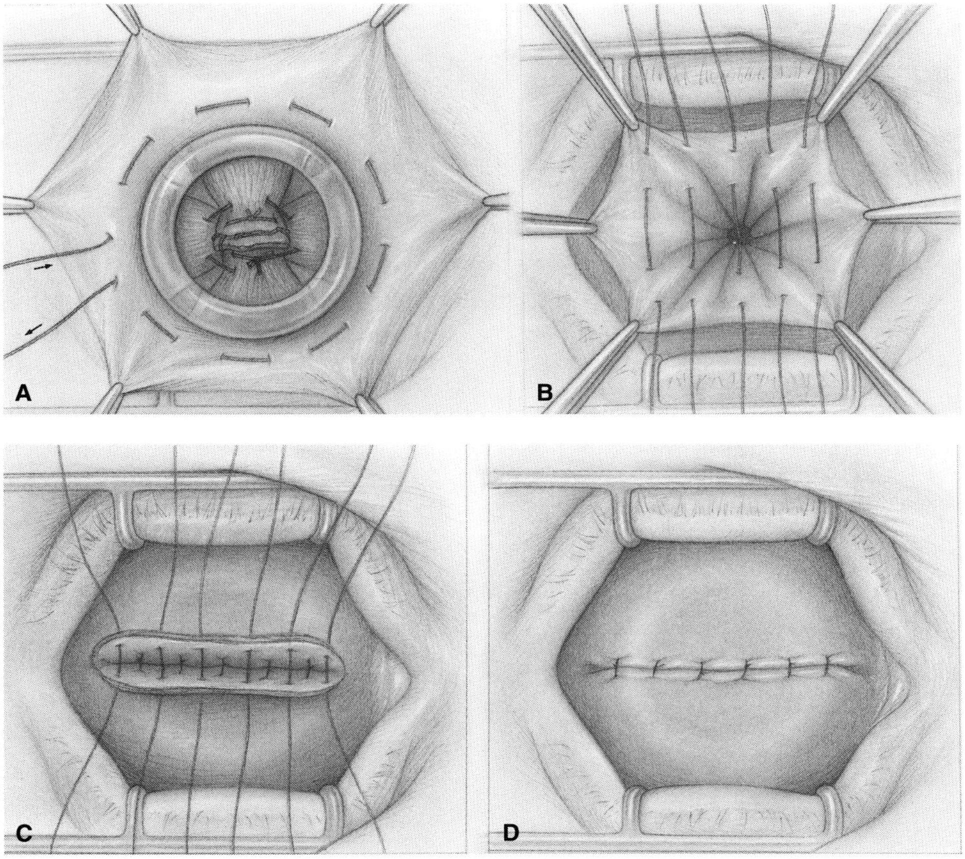

Figure 8–64. *A* to *C,* In any enucleation procedure, whether a sphere or an integrated implant is used, Tenon's capsule should be closed in three layers. As shown on the left, the first layer is a "pursestring" 4-0 chromic suture. Two additional layers of 4-0 interrupted chromic sutures are used to close the remaining gaps. *D,* The conjunctiva is closed with either a running or interrupted 6-0 plain gut suture.

is carried down to the orbital rim for 360°. A Bovie cautery along with mosquito clamps is used to achieve hemostasis. The orbital rim is incised with a scalpel; Freer elevators are used to undermine the periosteum for 360° (Figure 8–73). Scissors are used to cut the medial and lateral canthal tendons. The periosteum is elevated to the orbital apex, and the orbital contents are cut and removed, using curved scissors. Hemostasis is achieved with Bovie cautery, by obliterating flow in the ophthalmic artery and temporary packing. It is important to remove the lacrimal sac and avoid, if possible, creating defects in the adjacent sinuses.

If the lids have been removed, we obtain a split-thickness skin graft from the lateral aspect of the upper thigh. A Brown dermatome (or similar instrument) is used to harvest the graft, which is sutured with interrupted and running 6-0 silk around the outer aspect of the orbit to the remaining periorbital skin (see Figure 8–77). The graft is then placed against the orbital walls and sutured to itself. A pressure dressing of Xeroform gauze packing is left in situ for 7 days. We change the dressing three times in the first month, each time leaving the dressing in place for 7 days, and then gradually decrease the pack over the next 2 weeks. This ensures the survival of the split-thickness graft, as shown in Figure 8–78**.** Since the split-thickness skin is not against any pressure-bearing surfaces, normal desquamation does not occur. The orbit should be cleaned by the patient, a family member, or a nurse every week, with a dilute solution of hydrogen peroxide and cotton tip applicators.

If the lid skin is left at the time of exenteration, we suture it together and put pressure against the skin to force it into contact with the walls of the orbit. We then pressure-pack with gauze and antibiotic ointment for approximately 7 days, and then gradually decrease the pressure and the pack.

The cosmesis achieved with any form of orbital implant after exenteration is limited. While the patient in Figure 8–79 appears to have reasonable cosmesis, the lids do not blink and the eye does not move. Most patients have not been willing to wear a prosthesis over extended lengths of time.

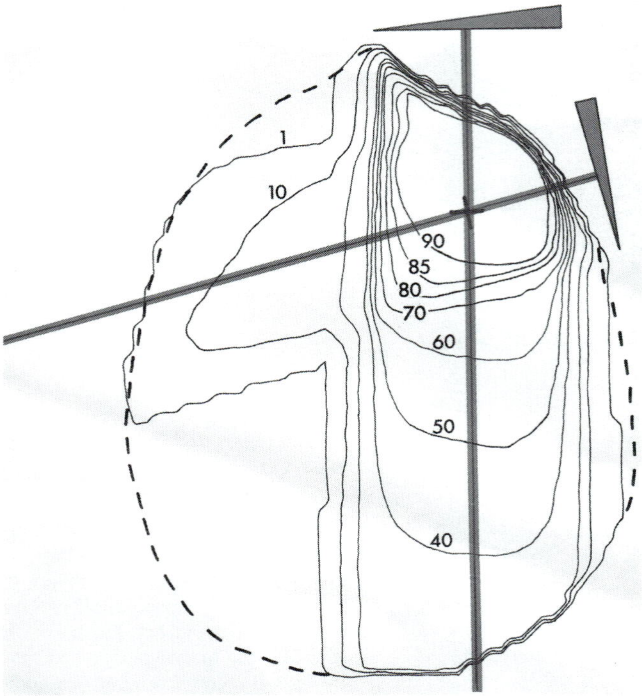

Figure 8–65. Anterior lateral wedge pair ports used to deliver five 400 cGy fractions to a total dose of 20 Gy of photon irradiation, for poor-risk uveal melanomas.

Follow-up after Enucleation and Exenteration and Treatment of Metastatic Uveal Melanoma

Metastatic evaluations are performed every 6 months after enucleation or exenteration. This includes screening liver function tests, physical examination, and chest radiography. The use of abdominal ultrasonography has been shown in

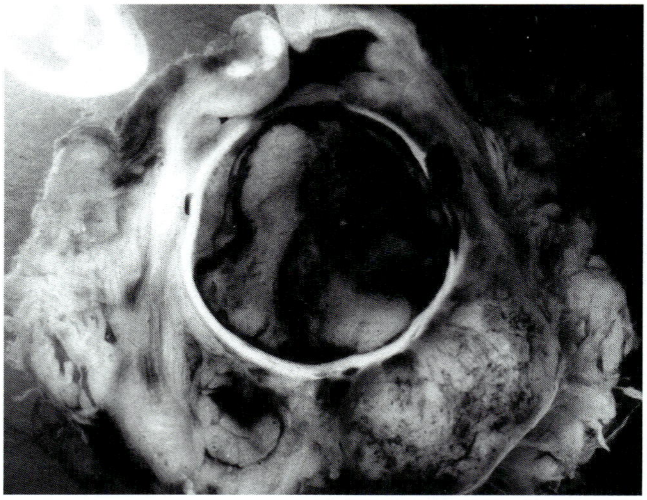

Figure 8–66. Diffuse orbital extension.

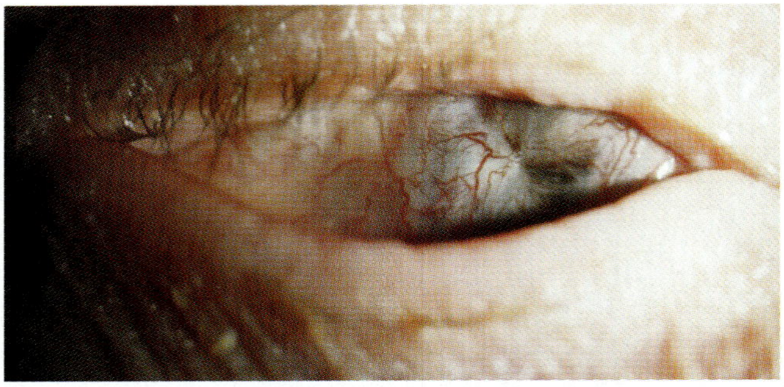

Figure 8–67. Recurrent orbital melanoma 5 years after enucleation. On metastatic evaluation, widespread tumor was noted.

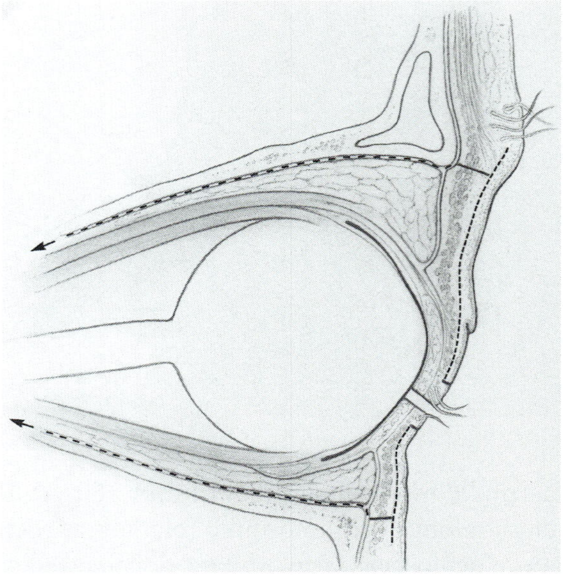

Figure 8–68. Sagittal schematic for a lid-sparing exenteration.

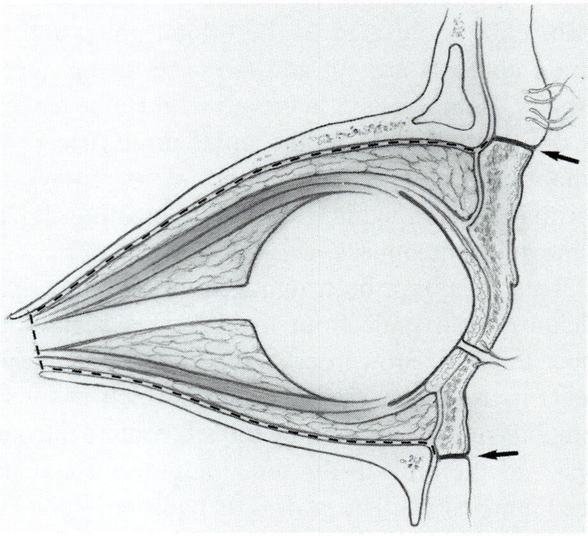

Figure 8–69. Sagittal schematic for an extenteration including the eyelids and entire orbit.

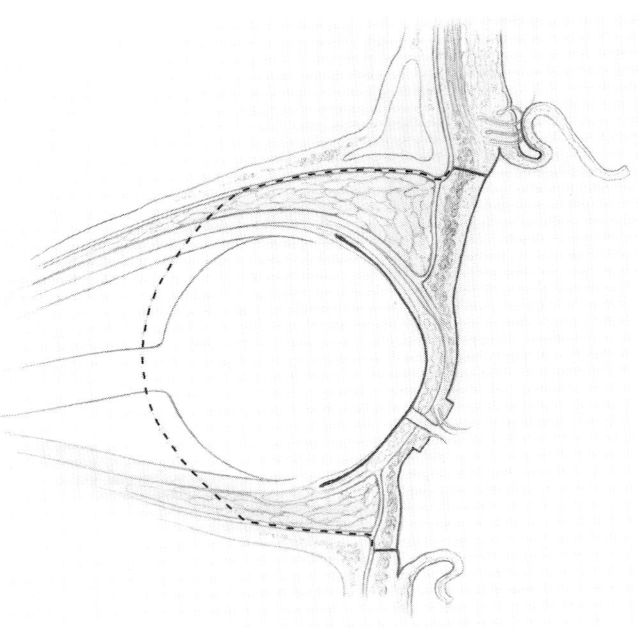

Figure 8–70. Sagittal schematic of an anterior exenteration that is used for invasive conjunctival carcinoma.

some studies to be more sensitive than serum liver function tests, but not in others.[260] While initally having some theoretical promise, the use of PCR technology to detect tyrosinase messenger RNA (mRNA) have not been effective to detect early metastases. In our experience, PCR for tyrosinase mRNA has not been effective in detecting early metastases (unpublished data).[261,262]

Metastases of uveal melanomas are usually first found in the liver. The peak incidence of metastasis is within the first 24 to 36 months after treatment.[263–265] Unfortunately, uveal melanoma, unlike breast carcinoma, can metastasize as late as 50 years after treatment, and therefore, all patients have to be followed up throughout their lives.[266–268] In melanomas from all body sites that metastasized more than 10 years after initial therapy, 12 of 168 were from the eye and the longest intervals (45 and

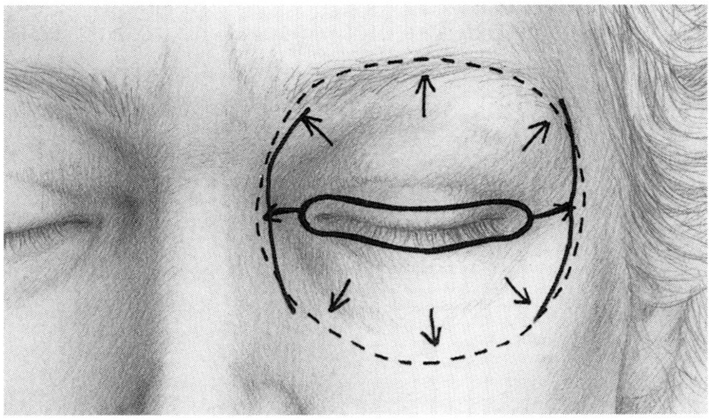

Figure 8–71. Lid approach for a lid-sparing exenteration. An incision is made 2 mm distal to the lash margins. Myocutaneous flaps are mobilized past the bony orbital rim.

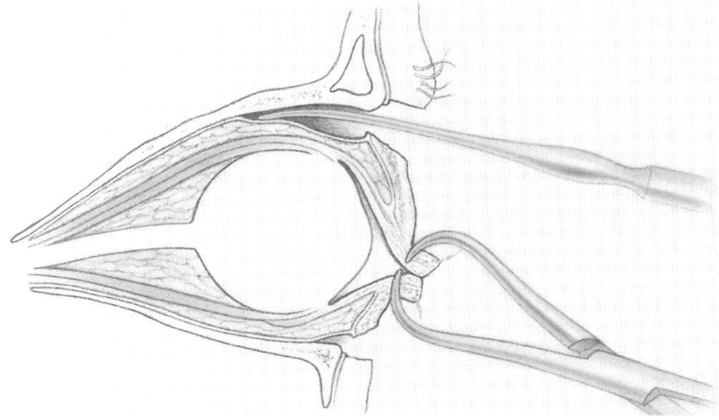

Figure 8–73. Whether the lids are spared or (as shown) sacrificed, the area of the lashes and lid margins is grasped with a towel clip for traction after an incision is made through the periosteum at the orbital rim to free orbital contents from the orbital bones.

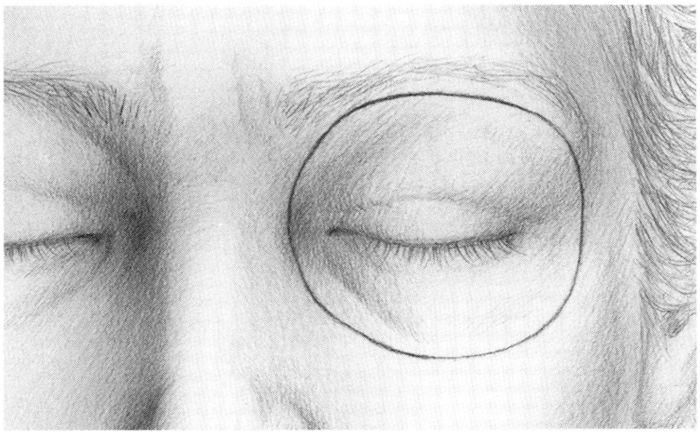

Figure 8–72. Outline of the skin incision for a non–lid-sparing exenteration.

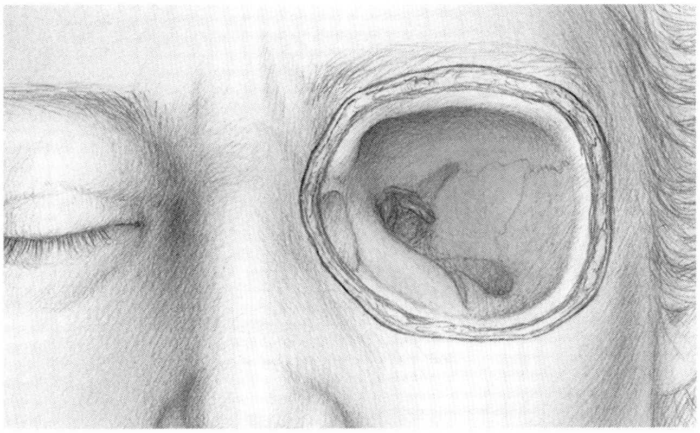

Figure 8–74. Appearance of orbital bones after removal of the orbital contents.

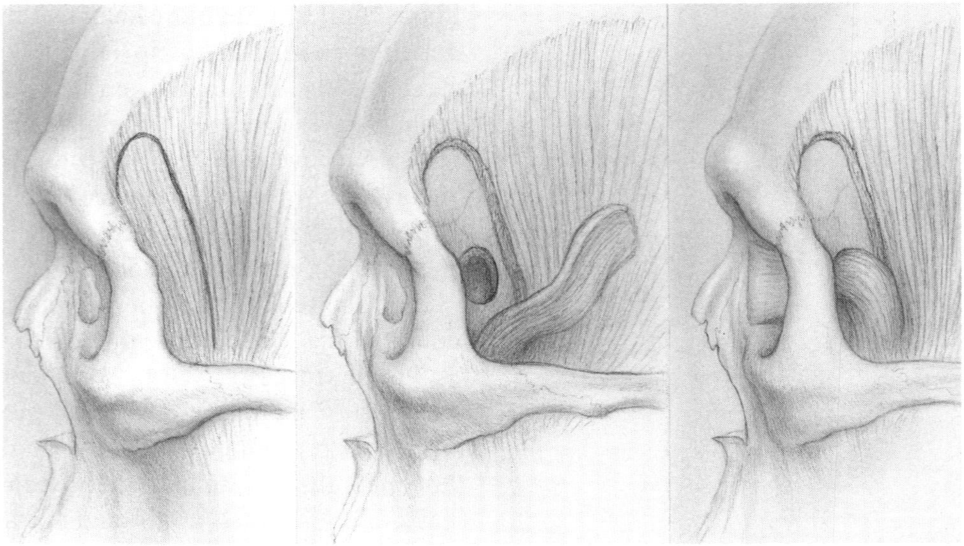

Figure 8–75. If a temporalis flap is to be made, a skin incision is taken laterally from the lateral canthus posteriorly. The anterior edge of the temporalis muscle is mobilized, and, as shown, a circular defect in the lateral orbital bone is produced with a dental burr.

47 years) were from the ocular, compared with the cutaneous, cases.[269]

The mean survival with live involvement of metastatic melanoma is approximately 7 months.[270,271] Single or combined forms of chemotherapy have had rather dismal results in controlling visceral metastatic melanoma.[272–278] In our experience, both single-drug chemotherapy with DTIC or methyl-CCNU and chemotherapy with as many as five agents produce only a partial response in up to 20 percent of patients with visceral metastases. The results with current chemotherapy are so poor and have sufficient toxicity that we do not believe it is indicated as adjunctive therapy in patients who do not have symptomatic metastases.[279,280] Bedikian and colleagues reported 201 patients with a response rate of < 1 percent. Various other drug regimes have produced incomplete responses in 36 percent of

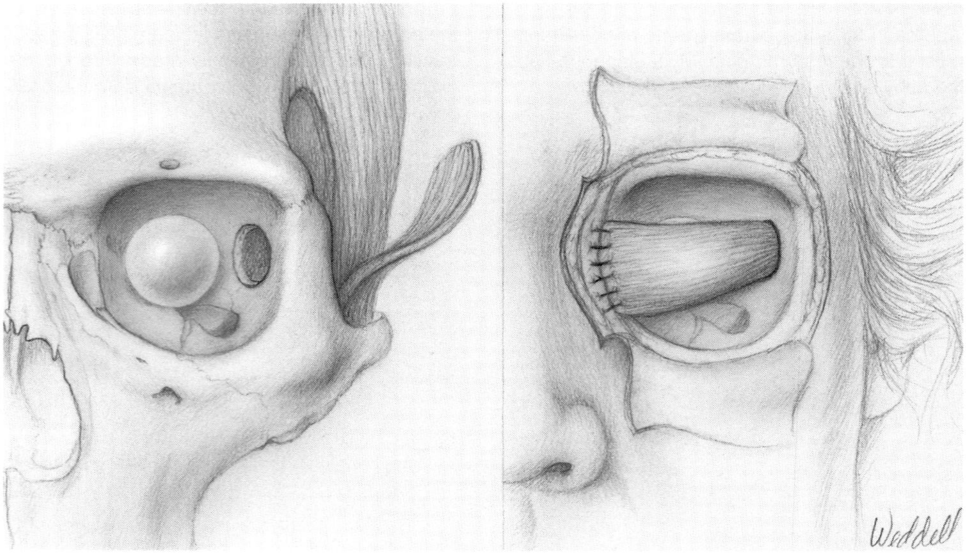

Figure 8–76. An 18-mm HA implant is placed behind the temporalis muscle flap, and this muscle is sutured to a remnant of the medial periorbita.

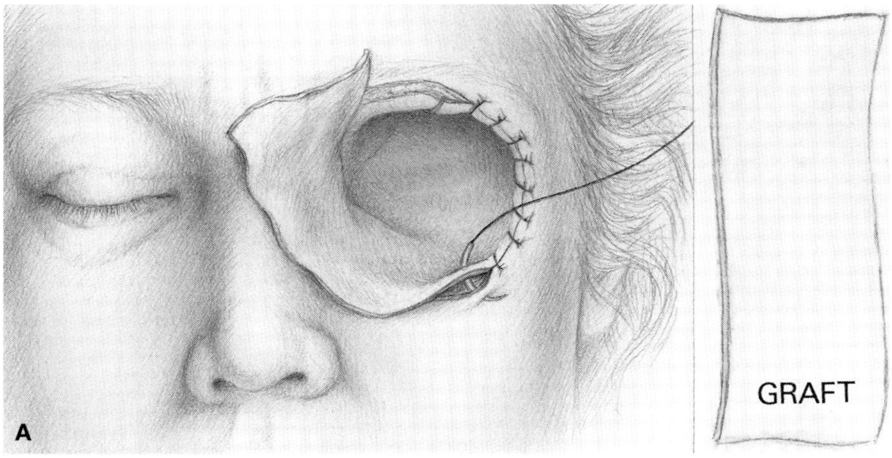

Figure 8–77. *A* to *C,* A partial-thickness skin graft is obtained using a Brown dermatome from the buttock or lateral thigh. This is sutured to the cut edge of skin with interrupted and running 6-0 plain gut sutures. It is placed into the orbital apex and pressure-packed with Xeroform gauze. The pressure-packing is changed weekly.

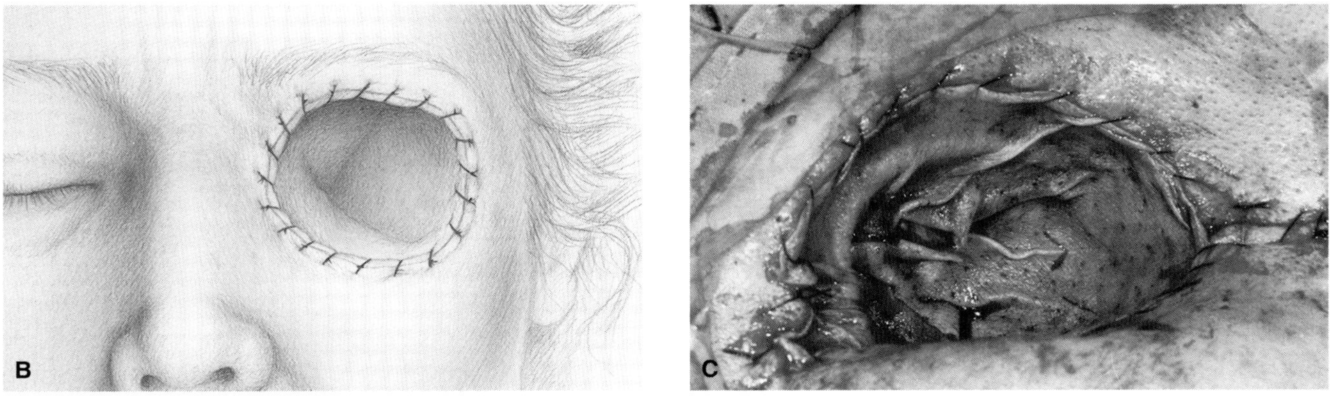

patients with metastatic melanoma[279–281] Leyvraz and his colleagues in Switzerland have treated asymptomatic uveal melanoma patients, whose metastases were found on routine ultrasonography, with a third-generation nitrourea, fotemustin, and found that they had objective responses in 12 of 30 patients, with a median duration of 11 months.[282] Unfortunately, in that later study, the treatment of asymptomatic patients probably did not obtain an increase in life span above and beyond what one might have noted if they had been treated after they developed symptoms. In some centers, the combination of hepatic resection of metastases with intra-arterial chemotherapy appeared to prolong survival; however, most patients could not have the entire tumor removed, and the mean survival was not significantly different from historic controls.[283–288] Several patients with solitary metastatic disease to the liver have had resection.[289]

While there has been some early promise with interferon-alpha (IFN-α) and interleukin-2 (IL-2) as adjuvant therapy, it has not shown benefit in metastatic melanoma.[290–292] Other groups have been working on either in vitro or in vivo studies with immune modulation and uveal melanoma, but those approaches have similarly been relatively disappointing.[293–296]

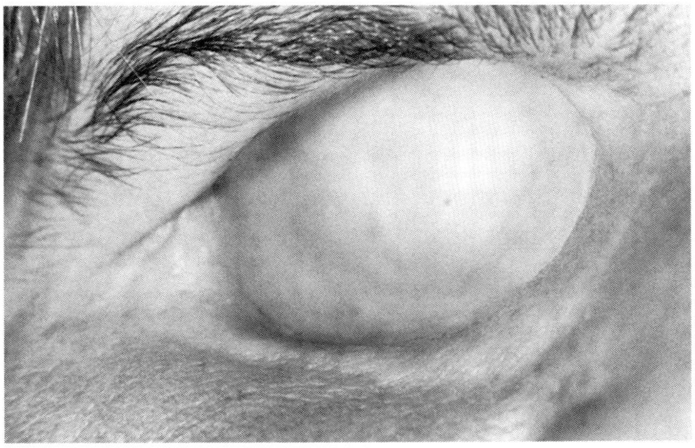

Figure 8–78. Appearance of an exenterated socket covered by a split thickness skin graft.

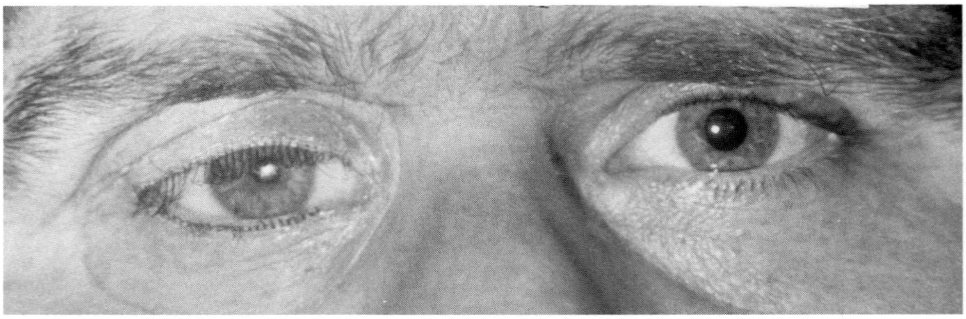

Figure 8–79. Clinical photograph of a prosthesis in situ. Most patients are not satisfied with the cosmetic appearance of an exenteration prosthesis because it does not move or blink.

UVEAL MELANOMA MANAGEMENT: CONCLUSION

Significant progress has been made in uveal melanoma management. Inaccurate diagnoses in ocular oncology units have virtually been eliminated. In our experience, over 80 percent of the melanoma-containing eyes that we examine can be salvaged. The two major goals over the next decade will be to decrease ocular morbidity in eyes that are retained, and to decrease metastases, especially in larger tumors that are not amenable to alternative therapies. Several problems will make the attainment of those goals difficult. (1) While we are able to retain many eyes with current techniques, it is uncertain if funding of research will allow the same degree of advances we have observed until now. (2) Especially for metastatic melanoma, there has been very little advancement in our ability to treat this problem effectively, regardless of the site of the primary tumor. Several groups, including our own, have noted tumor-infiltrating lymphocytes in uveal melanomas, and these may be exploitable for therapy in the future.[30,31,288,297–299] Further, while most immunomodulatory approaches for primary uveal melanoma have not shown promise, in one case report, a melanoma-derived vaccine appeared to decrease tumor size.[300,301]

UVEAL METASTASES

The management of choroidal metastases is dependent on the patient's general health, the presence or absence of CNS spread, and chemotherapy status. Therapeutic decisions must be made in conjunction with the patient's medical oncologist, after a complete metastatic evaluation, including brain MRI with contrast performed when ocular metastases are diagnosed. In most cases, the presence of choroidal metastatic disease is a very poor prognostic sign; most patients die within 1 year of diagnosis.[302] In a series of 32 ocular metastases, of which 18 involved the choroid, the mean interval between diagnosis and death was 7 months. Patients with choroidal metastases had slightly longer survival than those with orbital disease.[303] In that study, 10 of 32 patients developed CNS metastases. Some patients have isolated choroidal metastases and live for a number of years after diagnosis. There are five treatment options for most forms of choroidal metastases: observation, chemotherapy, radiation, laser, and enucleation.[302–312] Only when an eye with metastatic disease has intractable pain is enucleation indicated. Choroidal metastatic foci are as responsive as other body sites to systemic chemotherapy. Especially when the primary cancer is a breast carcinoma, chemotherapy is probably the first choice for treatment of choroidal metastases (Figures 8–80A and B). We have seen some metastatic breast tumors respond to just tamoxifen. As has been known for many years, tamoxifen can produce intraretinal crystals, although this side effect usually occurs after long-term administration.[313] There is usually some residual tumor after effective treatment, and often there are overlying RPE changes.

When multiple uveal metastases are present and they are not overly amenable to chemotherapy or various drugs have been tried without success, and both the choroidal and systemic tumors are progressive, either external beam photon radiation for multiple ocular lesions or an ^{125}I plaque for a solitary focus is indicated.[306,309,312,314]

Prior to radiation therapy, brain imaging studies are indicated. If the patient has some chance of a long survival, it is important to minimize radiation complications. We have seen a few tragic cases in which brain MRI with contrast and a lumbar puncture for cerebrospinal fluid cytology were not performed, and a second course of radiation for an initially unsuspected frontal lobe tumor delivered a visually destructive additional radiation dose to the eye. In terminally ill patients who are visually symptomatic and require ocular palliation, we radiate with large fraction sizes up to approximately 35 Gy. While this approach has a lower cure rate and a higher incidence of late complications, treatment can be performed over a shorter time, with little chance of problems developing during the patient's limited life span. However, if the patients have only choroidal metastases and are otherwise functional, they are treated with 200 cGy fractions over a 3-week period for a total dose of 35 to 40 Gy of photon irradiation (Figures 8–81 and 8–82). In rare patients with solitary choroidal metastases, it is sometimes more efficient to treat these to 40 Gy using a ^{125}I plaque (Figures 8–83A and B).

Often patients have either multiple or diffuse choroidal metastases, and so there is no added value over external beam photon irradiation with localized, invasive radiation techniques, using either radioactive plaques or charged particle therapy. For the same reason, it is rare that either xenon arc photocoagulation or laser therapy is used. Figures 8–84A and B show a lesion lateral to the fovea (A) treated with laser (B). When the patient developed widespread disease, the area just posterior and inferior to the laser therapy reactivated (B). The patient died 2 weeks later.

The overall success rate in terms of local ocular control and retention of vision with choroidal metastases is approximately 75 percent. Vision is usually maintained if it is better than 20/200 at the outset; lesions producing a retrolental detachment or diffuse tumors surrounding the disc have a poor visual prognosis. In another study of choroidal metastases, complete response of the ocular lesion was noted in 53 percent, with slightly better results when photon

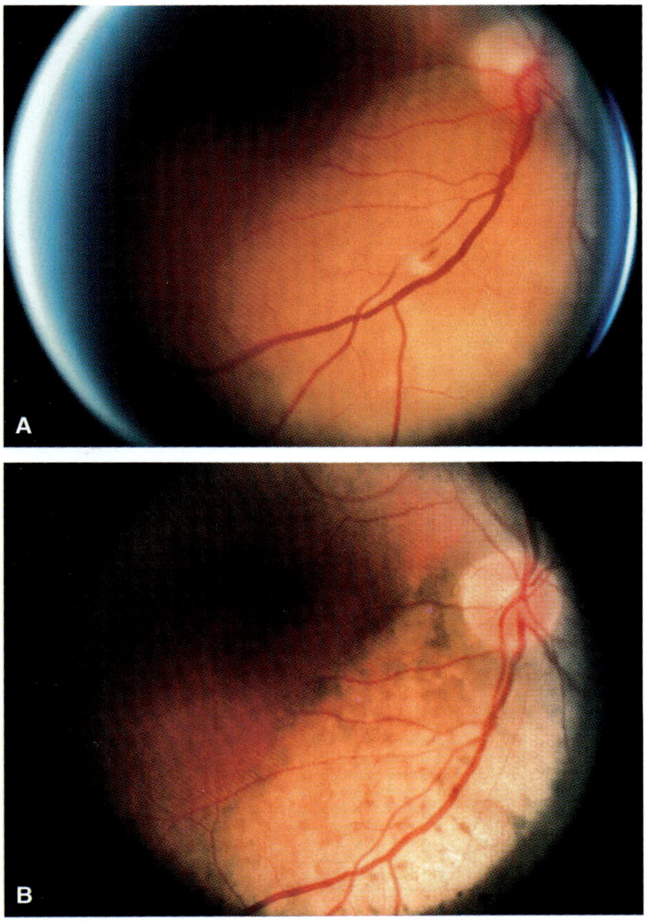

Figure 8–80. *A,* Uveal metastasis of breast cancer prior to chemotherapy. *B,* After chemotherapy. The tumor is flatter, and there are changes in the overlying retinal pigment epithelium.

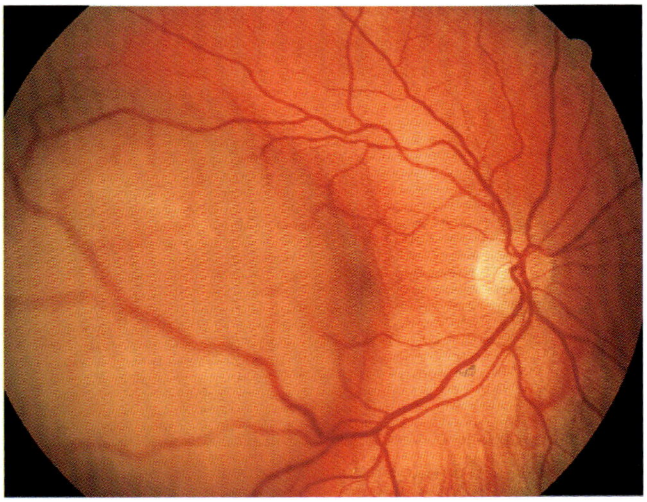

Figure 8–81. Bilateral uveal metastases of breast cancer.

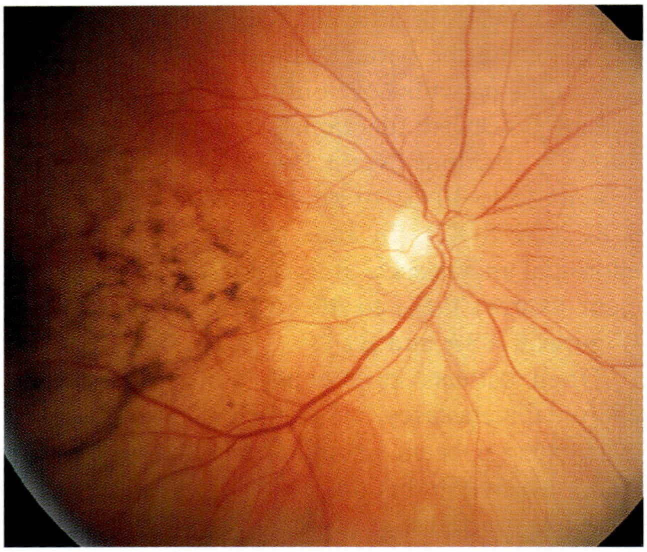

Figure 8–82. Lesion shown in Figure 8–81 after 40 Gy of photon irradiation.

therapy was given above 35.5 Gy. Overall, in that study, 62 percent had improved vision.[212]

CHOROIDAL HEMANGIOMA

Historically, difuse lesions have been difficult to treat, and focal lesions were treated with laser. It often took up to three laser sessions to heavily scar the tumor surface and dry up the subretinal fluid. Usually, a tumor was not destroyed, but the subretinal fluid would be resorbed with this techniuque (Figure 8–85).

Unfortunately, while we could often obliterate the exudative detachment, the long-term visual results were not excellent. In one study, less than one-third of patients had better than 20/200 acuity 10 years later.[303] Visual loss can be due to subretinal

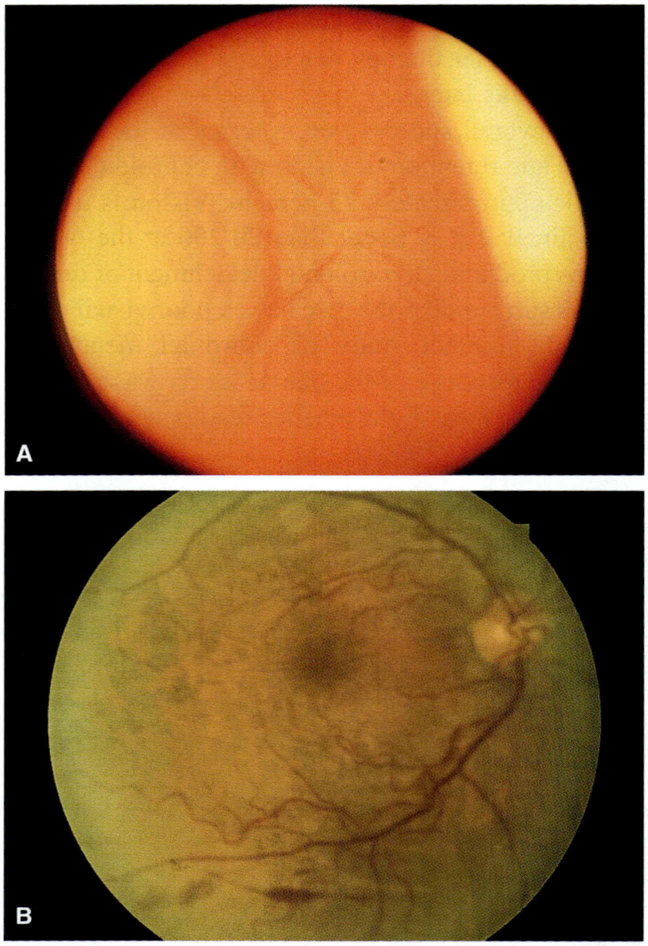

Figure 8–83. *A,* Solitary metastasis involving only a discrete area of choroid. FNAB was positive for estrogen receptor breast carcinoma. *B,* Case in Figure 8–83A after 40 Gy of ^{125}I brachytherapy.

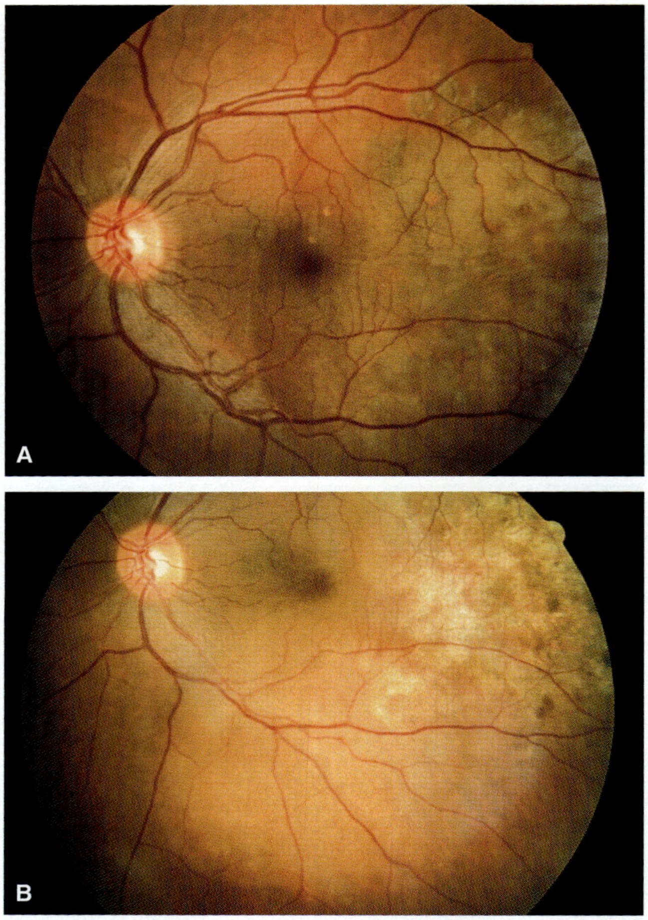

Figure 8–84. *A,* Breast cancer metastasis lateral to the fovea. *B,* Lesion shown above was controlled with laser; however, the patient developed widespread metastases and 2 weeks prior to death, activation along the posterior-inferior edge was noted.

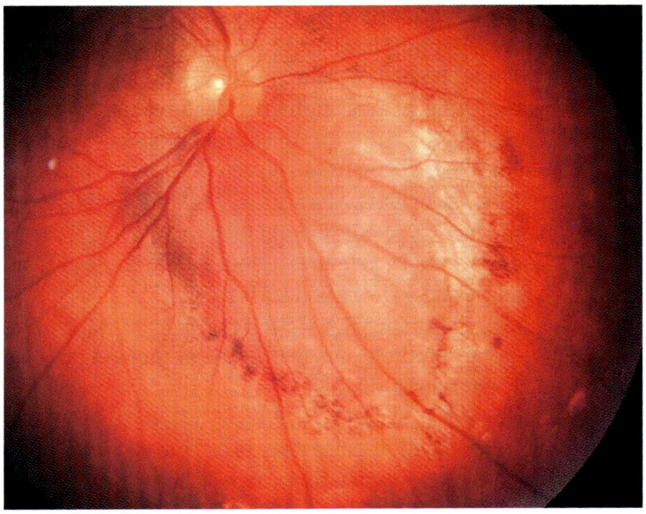

Figure 8–85. Successfully treated choroidal hemangioma.

fluid, overlying photoreceptor degeneration, or cystoid retinal change.[315]

In many centers, including our own, we have altered therapy to use radiation as the first-line approach. The rationale for this is threefold: (1) it appears to flatten the tumor, which, in some cases, will result in better vision; (2) it does not have as high a recurrence rate as with laser, and (3) we believe that the visual results are better, especially if it is a macular tumor.

In patients with a diffuse hemangioma that involves the fovea and produces subretinal fluid (most frequently in Sturge-Weber syndrome), we have successfully dissipated the subretinal fluid with return of vision, using 10 fractions of 200 cGy of photon irradiation.

We have also treated isolated hemangiomas, especially those that have failed with laser, with radiation. The choice of a radiation delivery system and the dose in the latter setting is uncertain. We have preferred to give 20 Gy to the tumor apex, using either protons or brachytherapy, in the belief that we might obtain more vascular closure with this rapid radiation dose delivery. Other workers have used plaques, particles, or photons at doses between 12.5 and 60 Gy.[306–309,316–318]

In some hemangiomas, the fluid dissipates, but vision does not return. In one study, thicker larger tumors had a worse visual outcome.[319] In a study using photon radiation, Schilling noted a lower incidence of fluid resorption than we and others have observed with plaques or protons.[315, 319–322] Zografos and colleagues similarly have evaluated both protons and brachytherapy.[317,323]

In the experience from the group in Switzerland, they have been able to decrease doses to near what we have used; in addition, they have observed that treatment with protons at over 30 Gy may produce visual loss.[317]

A few authors have used TTT. This appears to be a possible option for tumors that are away from the vital visual structures, although the question of local recurrence still remains unanswered.[324] One patient treated with hyperthermia had macular edema 2 years after treatment.[309]

Figure 8–86 shows an additional isolated hemangioma that responded well to low-dose proton radiation.

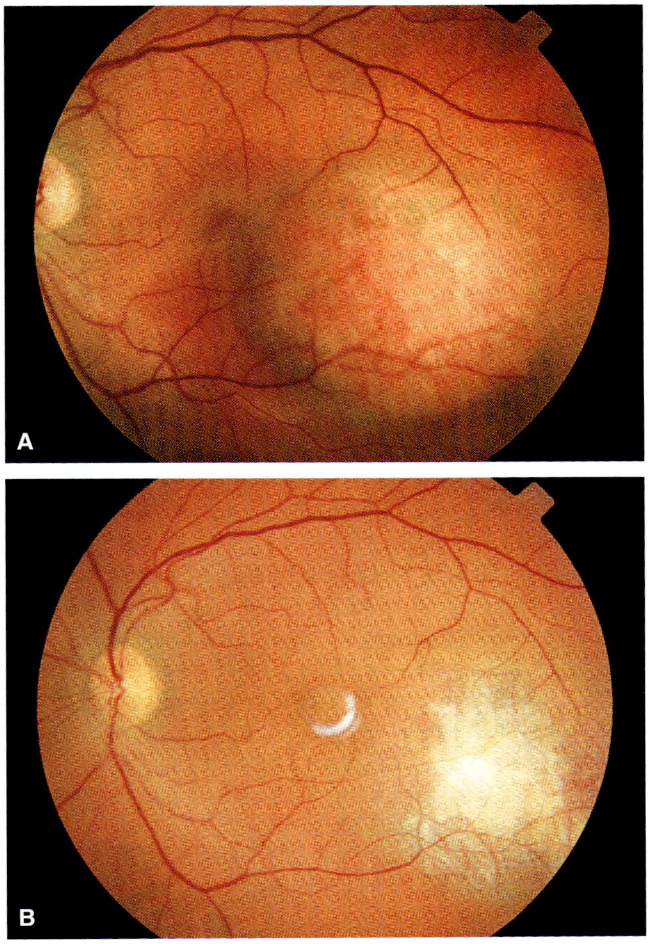

Figure 8–86. Isolated choroidal hemangioma prior to and after low-dose (20-Gy) proton radiation.

THERAPY OF INTRAOCULAR LYMPHOID PROCESSES

Isolated intraocular lymphoid tumors (see Chapter 10) or posterior scleritis can usually be managed with a short-term course of high-dose oral steroids (10 days of 80 mg of daily oral prednisone). Although, rarely, such lesions may not respond to this form of treatment, 20 Gy of photon irradiation can be used to destroy them.

REFERENCES

1. Char DH. Therapeutic options in uveal melanoma. Am J Ophthalmol 1984;98:796–9.
2. Fine SL. Do I take the eye out or leave it in? [editorial]. Arch Ophthalmol 1996;104:653–4.
3. Char DH. Current treatments and trials in uveal melanoma. Oncology 1989;3:113–28.
4. Seddon JM, Albert DM, Lavin PT, Robinson N. A prognostic factor study of disease-free interval and survival following enucleation for uveal melanoma. Arch Ophthalmol 1983;101:1894–9.
5. Leys AM, Dierick HG, Sciot RM. Early lesions of bilateral diffuse melanocytic proliferation. Arch Ophthalmol 1991;109:1590–4.
6. Egan KM, Quinn JL, Gragoudas ES. Childbearing history associated with improved survival in choroidal melanoma. Arch Ophthalmol 1999;117:939–42.
7. Grin CM, Driscoll MS, Grant-Kels JM. Pregnancy and the prognosis of malignant melanoma. Semin Oncol 1996;23:734–6.
8. Gamel JW, McCurdy JB, McLean IW. Ciliochoroidal melanoma: a comparison of prognostic covariates for uveal melanoma. Invest Ophthalmol Vis Sci 1992;33:1919–22.
9. Meecham WJ, Char DH. DNA content abnormalities and prognosis in uveal melanoma. Arch Ophthalmol 1986;104:1626–9.
10. Rennie I. Uveal melanoma: cell cycle and survival. Br J Ophthalmol 1995;79:513–4.
11. Folberg R, Rummelt V, Parys-van Ginderdeuren R, et al. The prognostic value of tumor blood vessel morphology in primary uveal melanoma. Ophthalmology 1993;100:1389–98.
12. De la Cruz PO Jr, Specht CS, McLean IW. Lymphocytic infiltration in uveal malignant melanoma. Cancer 1990;65:112–5.
13. Lattman J, Kroll S, Char DH, et al. Cell cycling and prognosis in uveal melanoma. Clin Cancer Res 1995;1:41–7.
14. Toti P, Greco G, Mangiavacchi P, et al. DNA ploidy pattern in choroidal melanoma: correlation with survival. A flow cytometry study on archival material. Br J Ophthalmol 1998;82:1433–4.
15. Coleman K, Baak JPA, van Diest PJ, Mullaney J. Prognostic value of morphometric features and the Callender classification in uveal melanomas. Ophthalmology 1996;103:1634–41.
16. Ahmad N, Feyes DK, Agarwal R, Mukhtar H. Photodynamic therapy results in induction of WAF1/CIP1/P21 leading to cell cycle arrest and apoptosis. Proc Natl Acad Sci USA 1998;95:6977–82.
17. Foss AJE, Alexander RA, Jefferies LW, et al. Microvessel count predicts survival in uveal melanoma. Can Res 1996;56:2900–3.
18. Mehaffey MG, Folbert R, Meyer M, et al. Relative importance of quantifying area and vascular patterns in uveal melanomas. Am J Ophthalmol 1997;123:798–809.
19. McLean IW. The biology of haematogenous metastasis in human uveal malignant melanoma. Virchows Archiv Pathol Anat 1993;422:433–7.
20. McLean IW, Keefe KS, Burnier MN. Uveal melanoma. Comparison of prognostic value of fibrovascular loops, mean of the 10 largest nucleotide, cell type and tumor size. Ophthalmology 1997;104:777–80.
21. Foss AJE, Alexander RA, Hungerford JL, et al. Reassessment of the PAS patterns in uveal melanoma. Br J Ophthlamol 1997;81:240–6.
22. Alberti W, Pothmann B, Tabor P, et al. Dosimetry and physical treatment planning for iodine eye plaque therapy. Int J Radiat Oncol Biol Phys 1991;20:1087–92.
23. Char DH, Kroll SM, Stoloff A, et al. Cytomorphometry of uveal melanomas: fine needle aspiration biopsy versus standard histology [thesis]. Am Ophthalmol Soc 1989;LXXXVII:197–212.
24. Haynie GD, Shen TT, Gragoudas ES, Young LHY. Flow cytometry analysis of peripheral blood lymphocytes in patients with choroidal melanoma. Am J Ophthalmol 1997;124:357–67.
25. Lawry J, Currie Z, Smith MO, Rennie IG. The correlation between cell surface markers and clinical features in choroidal malignant melanomas. Eye 1999;13:301–8.
26. McCurdy J, Gamel J, McLean I. A simple, efficient, and reproducible method for estimating the malignant potential of uveal melanoma from routine H & E slides. Pathol Res Prac 1991;187:1025–7.
27. Pe'er J, Rummelt V, Mawnlhwang T, et al. Mean often largest nucleoli, microcirculation architecture, and prognosis of ciliary choroidal melanomas. Ophthalmology 1994;101:1227–35.
28. Char DH, Kroll S, Crawford JB, et al. Vascular networks and cell cycling in uveal melanoma. Curr Eye Res 2000 [In press].
29. Keefe KS, McLean IW, George DP, et al. Prognostic

value of closed vascular loops in uveal melanoma. Invest Ophthalmol Vis Sci 1993;34:966.
30. Whelchel JC, Farah SE, McLean IW, Burnier MN. Immunohistochemistry of infiltrating lymphocytes in uveal malignant melanoma. Invest Ophthalmol Vis Sci 1993;34:2603–6.
31. Meecham WJ, Char DH, Kaleta-Michaels S. Infiltrating lymphocytes and antigen expression in uveal melanoma. Ophthal Res 1992;24:20–6.
32. Rennie I. Melanomas, metastases, and survival. Br J Ophthalmol 1993;77:685–6.
33. McLean IW. The biology of haematogenous metastasis in human uveal malignant melanoma. Virchows Arch Pathol Anat Histopathol 1993;422:433–7.
34. Kroll SM, Char DH, Quivey J, Castro J. A comparison of cause-specific melanoma mortality and all-cause mortality in survival analyes after radiation treatment for uveal melanomas. Ophthalmology 1998; 105:2035–45.
35. Foulds WS. Management of intraocular melanoma. Br J Ophthalmol 1990;74:559–60.
36. The Collaborative Ocular Melanoma Study (COMS). Randomized trial of pre-enucleation radiation of large choroidal melanoma III: local complications and observations following enucleation COMS report no. 11. Am J Ophthalmol 1998;126:362–72.
37. Meyer-Schwickerath G, Vogel MH. Malignant melanoma of the choroid treated with photocoagulation. A 10-year follow-up. Mod Probl Ophthalmol 1974;12:544–9.
38. Vogel MH. Treatment of malignant choroidal melanomas with photocoagulation. Evaluation of 10-year follow-up data. Am J Ophthalmol 1972;74: 1–11.
39. Shields JA, Glazer LC, Mieler WF, et al. Comparison of xenon arc and argon laser photocoagulation in the treatment of choroidal melanomas. Am J Ophthalmol 1990;109:647–55.
40. L'Esperance FA Jr. Clinical photocoagulation with the organic dye laser. A preliminary communication. Arch Ophthalmol 1985;103:1312–6.
41. Meyer-Schwickerath G, Vogel M. Treatment of malignant melanomas of the choroid by photocoagulation. Trans Ophthalmol Soc UK 1977;97:416–20.
42. Francois J. Disappearance of pigment after light coagulation of malignant melanoma of the choroid. Am J Ophthalmol 1968;66:443–7.
43. Francois J, Hanssens M, DeLaey JJ. Recurrence of malignant melanoma of the choroid seven and eight years after light coagulation. Ophthalmologica 1971;162:188–92.
44. Barr CC, Norton EW. Recurrence of choroidal melanoma after photocoagulation therapy. Arch Ophthalmol 1983;101:1737–40.
45. Duvall J, Lucas DR. Argon laser and xenon arc coagulation of malignant choroidal melanomata: histological findings in 6 cases. Br J Ophthlamol 1981;65: 464–8.
46. Folk JC, Weingeist TA, Coonan P, et al. The treatment of serous macular detachment secondary to choroidal melanomas and nevi. Ophthalmology 1989;96:547–51.
47. Journee-de Korver JG. Transpupilary thermal therapy: a new laser treatment of choroidal melanoma. The Hague: Kugler; 1998.
48. Oosterhuis JA, Journee-de Korver HG, Keunen JEE. Transpupillary thermotherapy: results in 50 patients with choroidal melanoma. Arch Ophthalmol 1998; 116:157–61.
49. Journee-de Korver JG, Oosterhuis JA, De Wolff-Rouendaal D, Keeme J. Histopathological findings in human choroidal melanomas after transpupillary thermotherapy. Br J Ophthalmol 1997;81:234–9.
50. Oosterhuis JA, Journee-de Korver HG, Kakebeeke-Kemme HM, Bleeker JC. Transpupillary thermotherapy in choroidal melanomas. Arch Ophthalmol 1995;113:315–21.
51. Keunen JEE, Journee-de Korver JG, Oosterhuis JA. Transpupillary thermotherapy of choroidal melanoma with or without brachytherapy: A dillema. Br J Ophthalmol 1999;83:987–8.
52. Shields CL, Shields JA, Cater J, et al. Transpupillary thermotherapy for choroidal melanoma: tumor control and visual results in 100 consecutive cases. Ophthalmology 1998;105:581–90.
53. Robertson DM, Buettner H, Bennett SR. Transpupillary thermotherapy as primary treatment for small choroidal melanomas. Trans Am Ophthalmol Soc 1999;97:407–27.
54. Kim RY, Hu L-K, Foster BS, et al. Photodynamic therapy of pigmented choroidal melanomas of ≥ 3 mm thickness. Invest Ophthalmol Vis Sci 2000 [Submitted]
55. Godfrey DG, Waldro RG, Capone A Jr. Transpupilary thermotherapy for small choroidal melanomas. Am J Ophthalmol 1999;128:88–93.
56. Gerke E, Mackensen D, Bornfeld N. Neovaskularisationen als Komplikationen der Achtkoagulation maligner Aderhautmelanome. Ber Dtsch Ophthal Ges 1981;78:525–7.
57. Shields JA. The expanding role of laser photocoagulation for intraocular tumors. The 1993 H. Christian Zweng Memorial Lecture. Retina 1994;14:310–22.
58. Gomer CJ, Doiron DR, Jester JV, et al. Hematoporphyrin derivative photoradiation therapy for the treatment of intraocular tumors: examination of acute normal ocular tissue toxicity. Cancer Res 1983;43:721–7.
59. Lewis RA, Tse DT, Phelps CD, Weingeist TA. Neovascular glaucoma after photoradiation therapy for uveal melanoma. Arch Ophthalmol 1984;102:839–42.

60. Tse DT, Dutton JJ, Weingeist TA, et al. Hematoporphyrin photoradiation therapy for intraocular and orbital malignant melanoma. Arch Ophthalmol 1984;102:833–8.
61. Panagopoulos JA, Svitra PP, Puliafito CA, Gragoudas ES. Photodynamic therapy for experimental intraocular melanoma using chloroaluminum sulfonated phthalocyanine. Arch Ophthalmol 1989;107:886–90.
62. Winward KE, Dabbs CK, Olsen K, et al. Encircling photothrombotic therapy for choroidal Greene melanoma using rose bengal. Arch Ophthalmol 1990;108:588–94.
63. Ohnishi Y, Murakami M, Wakeyama H. Effects of hematoporphyrin derivative and light on Y79 retinoblastoma cells in vitro. Invest Ophthalmol Vis Sci 1990;31:792–7.
64. Schmidt-Erfurth U, Bauman W, Gragoudas E, et al. Photodynamic therapy of experimental choroidal melanoma using lipoprotein-delivered benzoporphyrin. Ophthalmology 1994;101:89–99.
65. Glatstein E, Rosenthal DJ. Photodynamic therapy: shining light where it is needed. J Clin Oncol 1993; 11:1844–5.
66. McMahon KS, Wieman TJ, Moore PH, Fingar VH. Effects of photodynamic therapy using mono-L-aspartyl chlorin e6 on vessel constriction, vessel leakage, and tumor response. Cancer Res 1994;54: 5374–9.
67. Favilla I, Barry WR, Gosbell A, et al. Phototherapy of posterior uveal melanomas. Br J Ophthalmol 1991;75:718–21.
68. Fingar VH, Wieman TJ, McMahon KS, et al. Photodynamic therapy using a protoporphyrinogen oxidase inhibitor. Cancer Res 1997;57:4551–6.
69. Damato B, Foulds WS. Indications for trans-scleral local resection of uveal melanoma. Br J Ophthalmol 1996;80:1029–30.
70. Shields JA. Local resection of posterior uveal melanoma. Br J Ophthalmol 1996;80:97–8.
71. Damato BE, Foulds WS. Risk factors for metastatic uveal melanoma after trans-scleral local resection. Br J Ophthalmol 1996;80:109–16.
72. Damato BE, Foulds PJ. Risk factors for residual and recurrent uveal melanoma after trans-scleral local resection. Br J Ophthlamol 1996;80:102–8.
73. Char DH, Crawford JB, Miller T. Eyeball resection of uveal tumors. Trans Am Opthalmol Soc 2000 [in press].
74. Peyman GA, Nelson NC Jr, Paris CL, et al. Internal choroidectomy of posterior uveal melanomas under a retinal flap. Int Ophthalmol 1992;16:439–44.
75. Kertes PJ, Johnson JC, Peyman GA. Internal resection of posterior uveal melanomas. Br J Ophthalmol 1998;82:1147–53.
76. Moore RF. Choroidal sarcoma treated by intra-ocular insertion of radon seeds. Br J Ophthalmol 1930; 14:145–52.
77. Gragoudas ES, Seddon J, Goitein M, et al. Current results of proton beam irradiation of uveal melanomas. Ophthalmology 1985;92:284–91.
78. Char DH, Saunders W, Castro JR, et al. Helium ion therapy for choroidal melanoma. Ophthalmology 1983;90:1219–25.
79. Stallard HB. Malignant melanoblastoma of the choroid. Bibl Ophthalmol 1968;75:16–38.
80. Ellsworth RM. Cobalt plaques for melanoma of the choroid. In: Jakobiec FA, editor. Ocular and adnexal tumors, Birmingham, AL: Aesculapius; 1978. p. 76–9.
81. MacFaul PA. Local radiotherapy in the treatment of malignant melanoma of the choroid. Trans Ophthalmol Soc UK 1977;97:421–7.
82. Long RS, Galin MA, Rotman M. Conservative treatment of intraocular melanomas. Trans Am Acad Ophthalmol Otolaryngol 1971;75:84–93.
83. Foerster MH, Fried M, Wessing A, Meyer-Schwickerath G. Tumor regression and functional results in sequential ruthenium therapy and photocoagulation for choroidal melanoma. In: Lommatzsch PK, Blodi FC, editors. Intraocular tumors. Berlin, Germany: Akademie-Verlag; 1983. p. 316–41.
84. Davidorf FH, Makley TA, Lang JR. Radiotherapy of malignant melanoma of the choroid. Trans Am Acad Ophthalmol Otolaryngol 1976;81:849–61.
85. Packer S, Rotman M. Radiotherapy of choroidal melanoma with Iodine-125. Ophthalmology 1980; 87:582–90.
86. Lommatzsch P. Treatment of choroidal melanomas with 106Ru/106Rh beta-ray applicators. Surv Ophthalmol 1974;19:85–100.
87. Kellner U, Foerster MH, Bornfeld N. Calcification-like echographic patterns in uveal melanomas treated with brachytherapy. Br J Ophthalmol 1993;77:827.
88. Shields CL, Shields JA, Karlsson U, et al. Reasons for enucleation after plaque radiotherapy for posterior uveal melanoma. Clinical findings. Ophthalmology 1989;96:919–24.
89. Suit H. Proton beams in clinical radiation therapy. J Jpn Soc Ther Radiol Oncol 1991;3:191–8.
90. Egan KM, Gragoudas ES, Seddon JM, et al. The risk of enucleation after proton beam irradiation of uveal melanoma. Ophthalmology 1989;96:1377–83.
91. Zografos L, Bercher L, Egger E, et al. Treatment of eye tumors by accelerated proton beams. 7 years experience. Klinische Monatsblatter fur Augenheilkunde 1992;200:431–5.
92. Hempel M, Hinkelbein W. Eye sequelae following external irradiation. Cancer Res 1993;130:231–6.
93. Meyer-Schwickerath R, Pfeiffer A, Blum WF, et al. Vitreous levels of the insulin-like growth factors I

and II, and the insulin-like growth factor binding proteins 2 and 3, increase in neovascular eye disease. Studies in nondiabetic and diabetic subjects. J Clin Invest 1993;92:2625–65.

94. Aiello LP. Vascular endothelial growth factor. Invest Ophthalmol Vis Sci 1997;38:1647–52.
95. Char DH, Castro JR, Kroll SM, et al. Five-year follow-up of helium-ion therapy for uveal melanoma. Arch Ophthalmol 1990;108:209–14.
96. Neely KA, Gardner TW. Ocular neovascularization: clarifying complex interactions. Am J Pathol 1998; 153:665–9.
97. Finger PT. Radiation therapy for choroidal melanoma. Surv Ophthalmol 1997;42:215–32.
98. Robertson DM, Earle J, Anderson JA. Preliminary observations regarding the use of iodine-125 in the management of choroidal melanoma. Trans Ophthalmol Soc UK 1983;103:155–60.
99. Sealy R, Buret E, Cleminshaw H, et al. Progress in the use of iodine therapy for tumors of the eye. Br J Radiol 1980;53:1052–60.
100. Finger PT, Buffa A, Mishra S, et al. Palladium 103 plaque radiotherapy for uveal melanoma. Clinical experience. Ophthalmology 1994;101:256–63.
101. Summanen P, Immonen I , Kivela T, et al. Radiation related complications after ruthenium plaque radiotherapy of uveal melanoma. Br J Ophthalmol 1996; 80:732–9.
102. Andreo P. Montecarlo techniques in medical radiation physics. Phys Med Biol 1991;36:861–920.
103. Harnett AN, Thomson ES. An iodine-125 plaque for radiotherapy of the eye: manufacture and dosimetric considerations. Br J Radiol 1988;61:835–8.
104. Karolis C, Frost RB, Billson FA. A thin I-125 seed eye plaque to treat intraocular tumors using an acrylic insert to precisely position the sources. Int J Radiat Oncol Biol Phys 1990;18:1209–13.
105. Poier E, Langmann G, Leitner H, Vidic B. Optimierung der Zielvolumserfassung bei der Bestrahlung intraokylarer melanome mittels Rutheniumapplikatoren. Fortschr der Ophthalmol 1991;88:158–60.
106. Seregard S, Trampe E, Lax I, et al. Results following episcleral ruthenium plaque radiotherapy for posterior uveal melanoma: the Swedish experience. Acta Ophthalmol Scand 1997;75:11–6.
107. Luxton G, Astrahan MA, Liggett PE, et al. Dosimetric calculations and measurements of gold plaque ophthalmic irradiators using iridium-192 and iodine 125 seeds. Int J Radiat Oncol Biol Phys 1988;15: 167–76.
108. Watters D. Molecular mechanism of ionizing radiation-induced apoptosis. Immunol Cell Biol 1999; 77:263–71.
109. Coleman DJ, Silverman RH, Rondeau MJ, et al. Ultrasonic tissue characterization of uveal melanoma and prediction of patient survival after enucleation and brachytherapy. Am J Ophthalmol 1991;112:682–8.
110. Diener-West M, Hawkins BS, Markowitz JA, Schachat AP. A review of mortality from choroidal melanoma. II. A meta-analysis of 5-year mortality rates following enucleation. Arch Ophthalmol 1992;110:245–50.
111. Augsburger JJ, Gamel JW, Sardi VF, et al. Enucleation vs cobalt plaque radiotherapy for malignant melanomas of the choroid and ciliary body. Arch Ophthalmol 1986;104:655–61.
112. Niederkorn JY. Enucleation in consort with immunologic impairment promotes metastasis of intraocular melanomas in mice. Invest Ophthalmol Vis Sci 1984;25:1080–6.
113. Augsburger JJ, Gamel JW, Lauritzen K, Brady LW. Cobalt-60 plaque radiotherapy versus enucleation for posterior uveal melanoma. Am J Ophthalmol 1990;109:585–92.
114. Augsburger JJ, Correa ZM, Freire J, Brady LW. Long-term survival of choroidal and ciliary body melanoma after enucleation versus plaque radiation therapy. Ophthalmology 1998;105:1607–8.
115. Potter R, Janssen K, Prott FJ, et al. Ruthenium-106 eye plaque brachytherapy in the conservative treatment of uveal melanoma: evaluation of 175 patients treated with 150 Gy from 1981-1989. Front Radiat Ther Oncol 1997;30:143–9.
116. Seddon JM, Gragoudas ES, Egan KM, et al. Relative survival rates after alternative therapies for uveal melanoma. Ophthalmology 1990;97:769–77.
117. Summanen P, Immonen I, Heikkonen J, et al. Survival of patients and metastatic and local recurrent tumor growth in malignant melanoma of the uvea after ruthenium plaque radiotherapy. Ophthalmic Surg 1993;24:82–90.
118. Summanen P, Immonen I, Kivela T, et al. Radiation related complications after ruthenium plaque radiotherapy of uveal melanoma. Br J Ophthalmol 1996; 80:732–9.
119. Weenink AC, Van Best JA, Oosterhuis JA, Keunen JEE. Lens transmission by a fluorophotometry after brachytherapy and thermotherapy of choroidal melanoma. Ophthal Res 1998;30:402–6.
120. Seregard S. Long-term survival after ruthenium plaque radiotherapy for uveal melanoma. A meta-analysis of studies including 1,066 patients. Acta Ophthalmol Scand 1999;77:414–7.
121. LeLorier J, Gregoire G, Benhaddad A, et al. Discrepancies between meta-analysis and subsequent large randomized, controlled trials. N Engl J Med 1997;337:536–42.
122. Tjho-Heslinga RE, Kakebeeke-Kemme HM, Davelaar J, et al. Results of ruthenium irradiation of uveal melanoma. Radiother Oncol 1993;29:33–8.
123. Kellner U, Bornfeld N, Foerster MH. Radiation-

induced optic neuropathy following brachytherapy of uveal melanomas. Graefes Arch Clin Exp Ophthalmol 1993;231:267–70.
124. Guthoff R, Haase J, von Domarus D, et al. Das Regressionsveralten des Aderhautmelanoms nach Strahlentherapie - ein neuer prognostischer parameter? Klin Mbl Augenheilk 1990;196:6–10.
125. Karlsson UL, Augsburger JJ, Shields JA, et al. Recurrence of posterior uveal melanoma after 60Co episcleral plaque therapy. Ophthalmology 1989;96:382–8.
126. Brady LW, Markoe AM, Amendola BE, et al. The treatment of primary intraocular malignancy. Int J Radiat Oncol Biol Phys 1988;15:1355–61.
127. Beitler JJ, McCormick B, Ellsworth RM, et al. Ocular melanoma: total dose and dose rate effects with Co-60 plaque therapy. Radiology 1990;176:275–8.
128. Vrabec TR, Augsburger JJ, Gamel JW, et al. Impact of local tumor relapse on patient survival after cobalt 60 plaque radiotherapy. Ophthalmology 1991;98: 984–8.
129. Duker JS, Augsburger JJ, Shields JA. Noncontiguous local recurrence of posterior uveal melanoma after cobalt 60 episcleral plaque therapy. Arch Ophthalmol 1989;107:1019–22.
130. Harbour JW, Char DH, Kroll S, et al. Metastatic risk for distinct patterns of postirradiation local recurrence of posterior uveal melanoma. Ophthalmology 1997;104:1785–93.
131. Abramson DH, Servodidio CA, McCormick B, et al. Changes in height of choroidal melanomas after plaque therapy. Br J Ophthalmol 1990;74:359–62.
132. Lashkari K, Lee KY, Cheng HM, et al. Gadolinium-enhanced magnetic resonance imaging of melanomas treated with iodine plaque and laser coagulation. Ophthalmology 2000 [In press]
133. Ling CC, Li WX, Anderson LL. The relative biological effectiveness of I-125 and Pd-103. Int J Radiat Oncol Biol Phys 1995;32:373–8.
134. Thuomas K-A, Landau I, Kock E, Naeser P. Recurrence of malignant melanoma after irradiation diagnosed by glucose-fructose enhanced by magnetic resonance imaging. Acta Ophthalmol Scand 1996; 74:330–3.
135. Kleineidam M, Augsburger JJ, Hernandez C, et al. Cataractogenesis after Cobalt-60 eye plaque radiotherapy. Int J Radiat Oncol Biol Phys 1993;26: 625–30.
136. Gass JD. Comparison of prognosis after enucleation versus cobalt 60 irradiation of melanomas. Arch Ophthalmol 1985;103:916–23.
137. Ling CC, Chen GT, Boothby JW, et al. Computer assisted treatment planning for 125I ophthalmic plaque radiotherapy. Int J Radiat Oncol Biol Phys 1989;17:405–10.
138. Wu A, Krasin F. Film dosimetry analyses on the effect of gold shielding for iodine-125 eye plaque therapy for choroidal melanoma. Med Phys 1990;17:843–6.
139. Char DH, Quivey JM, Castro J, et al. Helium ions versus iodine 125 brachytherapy in the management of uveal melanoma: a prospective randomized dynamically balanced trial. Ophthalmology 1993;100:1547–54.
140. Quivey JM, Char DH, Phillips TL, et al. High intensity 125-iodine (125I) plaque treatment of uveal melanoma. Int J Radiat Oncol Biol Phys 1993;26: 613–8.
141. Bosworth JL, Packer S, Rotman M, et al. Choroidal melanoma: I-125 plaque therapy. Radiology 1988;169:249–51.
142. Abramson DH, Servodidio CA, McCormick B, et al. Changes in height of choroidal melanomas after plaque therapy. Br J Ophthalmol 1990;74:359–62.
143. Garretson BR, Robertson DM, Earle JD. Choroidal melanoma treatment with iodine 125 brachytherapy. Arch Ophthalmol 1987;105:1394–7.
144. Hill JC, Sealy R, Shackleton D, et al. Improved iodine-125 plaque design in the treatment of choroidal malignant melanoma. Br J Ophthalmol 1992;76: 91–4.
145. Lean EK, Cohen DM, Liggett PE, et al. Episcleral radioactive plaque therapy: initial clinical experience with 56 patients. Am J Clin Oncol 1990;13: 185–90.
146. Char DH, Castro JR, Quivey JM, et al. Uveal melanoma radiation 125I brachytherapy versus helium ion irradiation. Ophthalmology 1989;96:1708–15.
147. Wilson MW, Hungerford JL. Comparison of episcleral plaque and proton beam radiation therapy for the treatment of choroidal melanoma. Ophthalmology 1999;106:1579–87.
148. Nag S, Owen JB, Farnan N, et al. Survey of brachytherapy practice in the United States: a report of the Clinical Research Committee of the American Endocuriethereapy Society. Int J Radiat Oncol Biol Phys 1995;31:103–7.
149. Char DH, Kroll S, Quivey JM, Castro J. Long term visual outcome in eyes eligible for randomization to enucleation versus brachytherapy. Br J Ophthalmol 2000 [In press]
150. Abdel-Dayem HK, Trese MT. A technique for suturing peripapillary radioactive plaques. Am J Ophthalmol 1999;127:224–6.
151. Smiddy WE, Loupe DN, Michels RG, et al. Extraocular muscle imbalance after scleral buckling surgery. Ophthalmology 1989;96:1485–90.
152. Radtke ND, Augsburger JJ, Schmitt T. Management of exudative retinal detachment after plaque therapy for intraocular melanoma. Am J Ophthalmol 1991;112:92–4.
153. Alberti W, Pothmann B, Tabor P, et al. Dosimetry and physical treatment planning for iodine eye plaque

therapy. Int J Radiat Oncol Biol Phys 1991; 20:1087–92.
154. Finger PT, Lu D, Buffa A, et al. Palladium-103 versus Iodine-125 for ophthalmic plaque radiotherapy. Int J Radiat Oncol Biol Phys 1993;27:849–54.
155. Finger PT, Bernson A, Szechter A. Palladium-103 plaque radiotherapy for choroidal melanoma. Ophthalmology 1999;106:606–13.
156. Ling CC, Li WX, Anderson LL. The relative biological effectiveness of I-125 and Pd-103. Int J Radiat Oncol Biol Phys 1995;32:373–8.
157. Weissgold DJ, Gragoudas ES, Green JP, et al. Eye-sparing treatment of massive extrascleral extension of choroidal melanoma. Arch Ophthalmol 1998; 116:531–3.
158. Crawford JB, Char DH. Histopathology of uveal melanomas treated with charged particle radiation. Ophthalmology 1987;94:639–43.
159. Quivey JM, Augsburger J, Snelling L, Brady LW. 125I plaque therapy for uveal melanoma. Anaylsis of the impact of time and dose factors on local control. Cancer 1996;77:2356–62.
160. Boniuk M, Choen JS. Combined use of radiation plaques and photocoagulation in the treatment of choroidal melanomas. In: Jakobiec FA, editor. Ocular and adnexal tumors. Birmingham, AL: Aesculapius; 1978. p. 80.
161. Augsberger JJ, Mullen D, Kleinedidam M. Indirect ophthalmolscope laser treatment as supplement to 125-I plaque therapy for choroidal melanoma. Trans Am Ophthalmol Soc 1992;90:303–16.
162. Lommatzsch PK, Werschnik C, Schuster E. Long-term follow-up of Ru-106/ Rh-106 brachytherapy for posterior uveal melanoma. Graefes Arch Clin Exp Ophthalmol 2000;238:129–37.
163. DePotter P, Shields CL, Shields JA, et al. Plaque radiotherapy for juxtapapillary choroidal melanoma. Arch Ophthalmol 1996;114:1357–65.
164. Missotten L, Dirven W, Van der Schueren A, et al. Results of treatment of choroidal malignant melanoma with high-dose-rate strontium-90 brachytherapy. A retrospective study of 46 patients treated between 1983 and 1995. Graefes Arch Clin Exp Ophthalmol 1998;236:164–73.
165. Brovkina AF, Zarubei GD. Ciliochoroidal melanomas treated with a narrow medical proton beam. Arch Ophthalmol 1986;104:402–4.
166. Egan KM, Ryan LM, Gragoudas ES. Survival implications of enucleation after definitive radiotherapy for choroidal melanoma. Arch Ophthalmol 1998; 116:366–70.
167. Raju MR. Proton radiobiology, radiosurgery and radiotherapy. Int J Radiat Biol 1995;67:237–59.
168. Daftari IK, Char DH, Verhey LJ, et al. Anterior segment sparing to reduce charged particle radiotherapy complications in uveal melanoma. Int J Radiat Oncol Biol Phys 1997;39:997–1010.
169. Lovato AA, Char DH, Castro JR, Kroll SM. The effect of silicone nasolacrimal intubation on epiphora after helium ion irradiation of uveal melanomas. Am J Ophthalmol 1989;108:431–4.
170. Egger E, Zografos L, Munkel G, et al. Results of proton radiotherapy for uveal melanomas. Front Radiat Ther Oncol 1997;30:111–22.
171. Gragoudas ES, Egan KM, Seddon JM, et al. Intraocular recurrence of uveal melanoma after proton beam irradiation. Ophthalmology 1992;99:760–6.
172. Goitein M, Miller T. Planning proton therapy of the eye. Med Phys 1983;10:275–83.
173. Schneider U, Pedroni E. Proton radiography as a tool for quality control in proton therapy. Med Phys 1994;22:353–63.
174. Kindy-Degnan NA, Char DH, Castro JR, et al. Effect of various doses of radiation for uveal melanoma on regression, visual acuity, complications, and survival. Am J Ophthalmol 1989;107:114–20.
175. Gragoudas ES. A randomized control trial of varying radiation doses in the treatment of choroidal melanoma. Trans Am Ophth Soc 1998;96:691–7.
176. Meecham WJ, Char DH, Kroll SM, et al. Anterior segment complications after helium ion radiation therapy for uveal melanoma: radiation cataract. Arch Ophthalmol 1994;112:197–203.
177. Ross RD. Is perception of light useful to the blind patient? Arch Ophthalmol 1998;116:236–7.
178. Gragoudas ES, Egan KM, Seddon JM, et al. Intraocular recurrence of uveal melanoma after proton beam irradiation. Ophthalmology 1992;99:760–6.
179. Glynn RJ, Seddon JM, Gragoudas ES, et al. Evaluation of tumor regression and other prognostic factors for early and late metastases after proton irradiation of uveal melanoma. Ophthalmology 1989;96:1566–73.
180. Guyer DR, Mukai S, Egan KM, et al. Radiation maculopathy after proton beam irradiation for choroidal melanoma. Ophthalmology 1992;99:1278–85.
181. Munzenrider JE, Verhey LJ, Gragoudas ES, et al. Conservative treatment of uveal melanoma: local recurrence after proton beam therapy. Int J Radiat Oncol Biol Phys 1989;17:493–8.
182. Gragoudas ES, Egan KM, Arrigg PG, et al. Cataract extraction after proton beam irradiation for malignant melanoma of the eye. Arch Ophthalmol 1992; 110:475–9.
183. Chinela AB, Zambrano A, Bunge HJ, et al. Gamma knife radiosurgery in uveal melanomas. In: Steiner et al, editors. Radiosurgery: baseline and trends. New York, NY: Raven Press; 1992. p. 161–9.
184. Zehetmayer M, Menapace R, Kitz K, Ertl A. Suction attachment for stereotactic radiosurgery of intraocular malignancies. Ophthalmologica 1994;208:119–21.

185. Logani S, Helenowski TK, Thakrar H, Pothiawala B. Gamma knife radiosurgery in the treatment of ocular melanoma. Stereotactic Funct Neurosurg 1993; 61(Suppl 1):38–44.
186. Mullner K, Langmann G, Pendl G, Faulborn J. Echographic findings in uveal melanomas treated with Leksell gamma knife. Br J Ophthalmol 1998;82: 154–8.
187. Girkin CA, Comey CH, Lunsford LB, et al. Radiation ophthalmolopathy after stereotactic radiosurgery. Ophthalmology 1997;104:1634–43.
188. Zehetmayer M, Menapace R, Kitz K, et al. Stereotactic irradiation of uveal melanoma with the Leksell gamma unit. Front Radiat Ther Oncol 1997;30:47–55.
189. Char DH, Irvine AI, Posner MD, et al. Randomized trial of radiation for age-related macular degeneration. Am J Ophthalmol 1999;127:574–8.
190. Zehetmayer M, Dieckmann K, Kren G, et al. Fractionated stereotactic radiotherapy with linear accelerator for uveal melanoma—preliminary Vienna results. Strahlenther Onkol 1999;175:74–5.
191. Tamat SR, Moore DE, Allen BJ. Determination of the concentration of complex boronated compounds in biological tissues by inductively coupled plasma atomic emission spectrometry. Pigment Cell Res 1989;2:281–5.
192. Larsson BS, Larsson B, Roberto A. Boron neutron capture therapy for malignant melanoma: an experimental approach. Pigment Cell Res 1989;2:356–60.
193. Kroll S, Char DH, Kaleta-Michaels S. A stochastic model for dual label experiments: an analysis of the heterogeneity of S-phase duration. Cell Proliferation 1995;28:545–67.
194. Robertson DM. Choroidal melanomas with a collar-button configuration. Arch Ophthalmol 1999;117: 771–5.
195. Crawford JB, Char DH. Histopathology of uveal melanomas treated with charge particle radiation. Ophthalmology 1987;94:639–43.
196. Goodman DF, Char DH, Crawford JB, et al. Uveal melanoma necrosis following helium ion therapy. Am J Ophthalmol 1986;101:643–5.
197. Coleman DJ, Lizzi FL, Silverman RH, et al. Regression of uveal malignant melanomas following cobalt-60 plaque. Correlates between acoustic spectrum analysis and tumor regression. Retina 1985; 5:73–8.
198. Grizzard WS, Torczynski E, Char DH. Helium ion charged- particle therapy for choroidal melanoma. Histopathologic findings in a successfully treated case. Arch Ophthalmol 1984;102:576–8.
199. Char DH, Lonn LI, Margolis LW. Complications of cobalt plaque therapy of choroidal melanomas. Am J Ophthalmol 1977;84:536–41.
200. Meecham WJ, Char DH, Chen GT, et al. Correlation of visual field, treatment fields, and dose in helium ion irradiation of uveal melanoma. Am J Ophthalmol 1985;100:658–65.
201. Gragoudas ES, Li W, lan AM, et al. Risk factors for radiation maculopathy and papillopathy after intraocular irradiation. Ophthalmology 1999;106:1571–8.
202. Gunduz K, Shields CL, Shields JA, et al. Radiation complications and tumor control after plaque radiotherapy of choroidal melanoma with macular involvement. Am J Ophthalmol 1999;127:579–89.
203. Cappin JM. Malignant melanoma and rubeosis iridis. Histopathological and statistical study. Br J Ophthalmol 1973;57:815–24.
204. Kim MK, Char DH, Castro JL, et al. Neovascular glaucoma after helium ion irradiation for uveal melanoma. Ophthalmology 1986;93:189–93.
205. Gragoudas ES, Egan KM, Walsh SM, et al. Lens changes after proton beam irradiation for uveal melanoma. Am J Ophthalmol 1995;119:157–64.
206. Bacin F, Kwaitkowski F, Dalens H, et al. Long-term results of cobalt 60 curietherapy for uveal melanoma. J Fr Ophthalmol 1998;21:333–44.
207. Decker M, Castro JR, Linstadt DE, et al. Ciliary body melanoma treated with helium particle irradiation. Int J Radiat Oncol Biol Phys 1990;19:243–7.
208. Urano M, Kuroda M, Reynolds R, et al. Expression of manganese superoxide dismutase reduces tumor control radiation dose: gene radiotherapy. Cancer Res 1995;55:2490–3.
209. Weichselbaum RR, Hallahan DE, Beckett MA, et al. Gene therapy targeted by radiation preferentially radiosensitizes tumor cells. Cancer Res 1994;54: 4266–9.
210. Bresnick GH. Excitotoxins: a possible new mechanism for the pathogenesis of ischemic retinal damage. Arch Ophthalmol 1989;107:339–41.
211. Reinhold HS, Fajardo LF, Hopewell JW. The vascular system. Adv Radiat Biol 1990;14:177–223.
212. Casey R, Li WW. Perspective: factors controlling ocular angiogenesis. Am J Ophthalmol 1997;124:521–9.
213. Sinz EH, Kochanek PM, Dixon CE, et al. Inducible nitric oxide synthase is an endogenous neuroprotectant after traumatic brain injury in rats and mice. J Clin Invest 1999;104:647–56.
214. Stieg PE, Sathi S, Warach S, et al. Neuroprotection by the NMDA receptor-associated open-channel blocker memantine in a photothrombotic model of cerebral focal ischemia in neonatal rat. Eur J Pharmacol 1999;375:115–20.
215. Coleman DJ, Lizzi FL, Burgess SE, et al. Ultrasonic hyperthermia and radiation in the management of intraocular malignant melanoma. Am J Ophthalmol 1986;101:635–42.
216. Engin K, Leeper DB, Tupchong L, Waterman FM. Thermoradiotherapy in the management of superfi-

cial malignant tumors. Clin Cancer Res 1995;1: 139–45.
217. Hornback NB. Historical aspects of hyperthermia in cancer therapy. Radio Clin North Am 1989;27:481–8.
218. Blom DJ, De Waard-Sieginga I, Apte RS, et al. Effect of hyperthermia on expression of histocompatibility antigens and heat-shock protein molecules on three human ocular melanoma cell lines. Melanoma Res 1997;7:103–9.
219. Finger PT. Microwave thermoradiotherapy for uveal melanoma. Results of a 10-year study. Ophthalmology 1997;104:1794–803.
220. Overgaard J, Gonzalez D, Hulshof MC, et al. Randomized trial of hyperthermia as adjuvant to radiotherapy for recurrent or metastatic malignant melanoma. European Society for Hyperthermic Oncology. Lancet 1995;345(8949):540–3.
221. Kurhanewicz J, Char DH, Stauffer P, et al. 31P magnetic resonance spectroscopy after combined hyperthermia and radiation. Curr Eye Res 1993;13:151–6.
222. Bollemiher JG, Lagendijk JJ, van Best JA, et al. Effects of microwave-induced hyperthermia on the anterior segment of healthy rabbit eyes. Graefes Arch Ophthalmol 1989;227:271–6.
223. Fuchs E. Das Sarcom des Uvealtractus. Wien: Braumuller; 1882.
224. Sattler H. Die bosartigen Geschwulste des Auges. Leipzig: S. Hirzel; 1926.
225. Jaensch PA. Die Prognose der Enukleation beim Melanosarkom der Uvea. Klin Monatsbl Augenheilk 1930;84:649–62.
226. von Popolzy F. Zur Prognose des Uveasarkoms. Klin Mbl Augenheilk 1937;99:512–27.
227. Zimmerman LE, McLean IW, Foster WD. Does enucleation of the eye containing a malignant melanoma prevent or accelerate the dissemination of tumour cells? Br J Ophthalmol 1978;62:420–5.
228. McLean IW, Foster WD, Zimmerman LE, Martin DG. Inferred natural history of uveal melanoma. Invest Ophthalmol Vis Sci 1980;19:760–70.
229. Seigel D, Myers M, Ferris F III, Steinhorn SC. Survival rates after enucleation of eyes with malignant melanoma. Am J Ophthalmol 1979;87:761–5.
230. Davidorf FH. Treatment of malignant melanoma [letter]. Arch Ophthalmol 1979;97:975–6.
231. Niederkorn JY. Enucleation in consort with immunologic impairment promotes metastasis of intraocular melanomas in mice. Invest Ophthalmol Vis Sci 1984;25:1080–6.
232. Fraunfelder FT, Boozman FW, Wilson RS, Thomas AH. No-touch technique for intraocular malignant melanomas. Arch Ophthalmol 1977;95:1616–20.
233. Blair CJ, Guerry RK, Stratford TP. Normal intraocular pressure during enucleation for choroidal melanoma. Arch Ophthalmol 1983;101:1900–2.
234. Wolter JR. Tenonectomy. Treatment of epibulbar extension of choroidal melanomas. Arch Ophthalmol 1971;86:529–33.
235. Tso MO, Albert DM. Pathological conditions of the retinal pigment epithelium. Neoplasms and nodular non-neoplastic lesions. Arch Ophthalmol 1972;88: 27–38.
236. Smith B, Bosniak SL, Lisman RD. An autogenous kinetic dermis-fat orbital implant: an updated technique. Ophthalmology 1982;89:1067–71.
237. Nunery WR, Hetzler KJ. Dermal-fat graft as a primary enucleation technique. Ophthalmology 1985;92: 1256–61.
238. Hornblass A, Biesman BS, Eviatar JA. Current techniques of enucleation: a survey of 5439 intraorbital implants and a review of the literature. Ophthal Plast Reconstr Surg 1995;11:777–88.
239. Dutton JJ. Coralline hydroxyapatite as an ocular implant. Ophthalmology 1991;98:370–7.
240. Nunery WR, Heinz GW, Bonnin JM, et al. Exposure rate of hydroxyapatite spheres in the anophthalmic socket: histopathologic correlation and comparison with silicone sphere implants. Ophthal Plast Reconstr Surg 1993;9:96–104.
241. Beard C. Remarks on historical and newer approaches to orbital implants. Ophthal Plast Reconstr Surg 1995;11:89–90.
242. Jordan DR, Munro SM, Brownstein S, et al. A synthetic hydroxyapatite implant: the so-called counterfeit implant. Ophthalmol Plast Reconstr Surg 1998;14:244–9.
243. Karcioglu ZA, Al-Mesfer SA, Mullaney PB. Porous polyethylene orbital implant in patients with retinoblastoma. Ophthalmology 1998;105:1311–6.
244. Cartwright MJ. Sculpting of hydroxyapatite orbital implants. Am J Ophthalmol 1992;113:453–4.
245. Char DH, Phillips TL. The potential for adjuvant radiotherapy in choroidal melanoma. Arch Ophthalmol 1982;100:247–8.
246. Char DH, Phillips TL. Pre-enucleation irradiation of uveal melanoma. Br J Ophthalmol 1985;69:177–9.
247. Char DH, Phillips TL, Andejeski Y, et al. Failure of preenucleation radiation to decrease uveal melanoma mortality. Am J Ophthalmol 1988;106: 21–6.
248. Luyten GP, Mooy CM, Eijkenboom WM, et al. No demonstrated effect of pre-enucleation irradiation on survival of patients with uveal melanoma. Am J Ophthalmol 1995;119:786–91.
249. Augsburger JJ, Lauritzen K, Gamel JK, et al. Matched group study of preenucleation radiotherapy versus enucleation alone for primary malignant melanoma of the choroid and cilary body. Am J Clin Oncol 1990;13:382–7.
250. Jordan DR, Brownstein S, Jolly SS. Abscessed hydrox-

yapatite orbital implants. Ophthalmology 1996; 103:1784–7.
251. Edelstein C, Shields CL, de Potter T, Shields JA. Complications of motility peg placement of the hydroxyapatite orbital implant. Ophthalmology 1997; 104:1616–21.
252. Sopakar CNS, Patrinely JP. Abscessed hydroxyapatite orbital implants. Ophthalmology 1997;104:1059.
253. Sloan GH, McNab AA. Complications of hydroxyapatite implants. Ophthalmology 1997;104:1982.
254. Fezza JP, Klippenstein KA, Wessley RE. Use of an orbital epidural catheter to control pain after orbital implant surgery. Arch Ophthalmol 1999;117:784–8.
255. Kreissig I, Rohrbach M, Lincoff H. Irradiation of choroidal melanomas before enucleation? Retina 1989;9:101–4.
256. Bornfeld N, Huser U, Sauerwein W, et al. Preoperative Bestrahlung vor Enukleation bei malignen Melanonom der Uvea: Literaturubersight und erste eigene Erfahrungen. Klin Monatsbl Augenheilkd 1989;194:252–60.
257. Gunlap I, Batioglu F. Effect of pre-enucleation irradiation on the survival of patients with uveal melanoma. Ophthalmologica 1998;212:231–5.
258. The Collaborative Ocular Melanoma Study (COMS). Randomized trial of pre-enucleation radiation of large choroidal melanoma III: local complications and observations following enucleation COMS report no. 11. Am J Ophthalmol 1998;126:362–72.
259. Kersten RC, Tse DT, Anderson RL, Blodi FC. The role of orbital exenteration in choroidal melanoma with extrascleral extension. Ophthalmology 1985;92: 436–43.
260. Eskelin S, Pyrhonen S, Summanen P, et al. Screening for metastatic malignant melanoma of the uvea revisited. Cancer 1999;85:1151–9.
261. Curry BJ, Myers K, Hersey P. Polymerase chain reaction detection of melanoma cells in the circulation: relation to clinical stage, surgical treatment, and recurrence from melanoma. J Clin Oncol 1998; 16:1760–9.
262. Glaser R, Rass K, Seiter S, et al. Detection of circulating melanoma cells by specific amplication of tyrosinase complementary DNA is not a reliable tumor marker in melanoma patients: a clinical two-center study. J Clin Oncol 1995;15:2818–25.
263. Char DH. Metastatic choroidal melanoma. Am J Ophthalmol 1978;86:76–80.
264. Gragoudas ES, Egan KM, Seddon JM, et al. Survival of patients with metastases from uveal melanoma. Ophthalmology 1991;98:383–9.
265. Kath R, Hayungs J, Bornfeld N, et al. Prognosis and treatment of disseminated uveal melanoma. Cancer 1993;72:2219–23.
266. Hall WEB. Malignant melanoma of the uveal tract. Report of a case with death 30 years after enucleation. Arch Ophthalmol 1950;44:381–94.
267. Kirk HQ. Delayed metastasis from choroidal melanoma. Surv Ophthalmol 1966;11:651–6.
268. Coupland SE, Sidiki S, Blark BJ, et al. Metastatic choroidal melanoma in the contralateral orbit 40 years after enucleation. Arch Ophthalmol 1996;114: 751–6.
269. Crowley NJ, Seigler HF. Late recurrence of malignant melanoma. Analysis of 168 patients. Ann Surg 1990;212:173–7.
270. Kath R, Hayungs J, Bornfeld N, et al. Prognosis and treatment of disseminated uveal melanoma. Cancer 1993;72:2219–23.
271. Lorigan JG, Wallace SS, Mavligit GM. Prevalence and location of metastases from ocular melanoma. Imaging studies in 110 patients. AJR Am J Roentgenol 1991;157:1279–81.
272. Young DW, Lever RS, English JS, MacKie RM. The use of BELD combination chemotherapy (bleomycin, vindesine, CCNU, and DTIC) in advanced malignant melanoma. Cancer 1985;55:1879–81.
273. Carrasco CH, Wallace S, Charnsangavej C, et al. Treatment of hepatic metastases in ocular melanoma. Embolization of the hepatic artery with polyvinyl sponge and cisplatin. JAMA 1986;255:3152–4.
274. Glover DJ. New approaches to the chemotherapy of melanoma. Oncology 1991;5:95–104.
275. Bleehen NM, Newland ES, Lee SM, et al. Cancer research campaign phase II trial of temozolomide in metastatic melanoma. J Clin Oncol 1995;13:910–3.
276. Cocconi G, Bella M, Calabresi F, et al. Treatment of metastatic malignant melanoma with dacarbazine plus tamoxifen. N Engl J Med 1992;327:516–23.
277. McClay EF, McClay ME. Systemic chemotherapy for the treatment of metastatic melanoma. Semin Oncol 1996;123:744–53.
278. Houghton AN, Meyers ML, Chapman PB. Medical treatment of metastatic melanoma. Surg Clin North Am 1996;76:1543–54.
279. Creagan ET, Suman VJ, Dalton RJ, et al. Phase III clinical trial of the combination of cisplatin, dacarbazine, and carmustine with or without tamoxifen in patients with advanced malignant melanoma. J Clin Oncol 1999;17:1884–90.
280. Margolin KA, Liu PY, Flaherty LE, et al. Phase II study of carmustine, dacarbazine, cisplatin, and tamoxifen in advanced melanoma: a Southwest Oncology Group study. J Clin Oncol 1998;16:664–9.
281. Bedikian AY, Lagha SS, Mavligit G, et al. Treatment of uveal melanoma metastatic to the liver. Cancer 1995;76:1665–70.
282. Leyvraz S, Spataro V, Bauer J, et al. Treatment of ocular melanoma metastatic to the liver by hepatic arterial chemotherapy. J Clin Oncol 1997;15:2589–95.

283. Rosenberg SA, Lotze MT, Muul LM, et al. A progress report on the treatment of 157 patients with advanced cancer using lymphokine-activated killer cells and interleukin-2 or high-dose interleukin-2 alone. N Engl J Med 1987;316:889–97.
284. Spitler LE, del Rio M, Khentigan A, et al. Therapy of patients with malignant melanoma using a monoclonal antimelanoma antibody-ricin A chain immunotoxin. Cancer Res 1987;47:1717–23.
285. Pyrhonen S, Kouri M, Holsti LR, Cantell K. Disease stabilization by leukocyte alpha interferon and survival of patients with metastatic melanoma. Oncology 1992;49:22–6.
286. Mavligit GM, Charnsangavej C, Carrasco H, et al. Regression of ocular melanoma metastatic to the liver after hepatic arterial chemoembolization with cisplatin and polyvinyl sponge. JAMA 1988;260:974–6.
287. Sznol M, Clark JW, Smith JW II, et al. Pilot study of interleukin-2 and lymphokine-activated killer cells combined with immunomodulatory doses of chemotherapy and sequenced with interferon alfa-2a in patients with metastatic melanoma and renal cell carcinoma. J Natl Cancer Inst 1992;84:929–37.
288. Ma D, Niederkorn JY. Efficacy of tumor-infiltrating lymphocytes in the treatment of hepatic metastases arising from transgenic intraocular tumors in mice. Invest Ophthalmol Vis Sci 1995;36:1067–75.
289. Gunduz K, Shields JA, Shields CL, et al. Surgical removal of solitary hepatic metastasis from choroidal melanoma. Am J Ophthalmol 1998;125:407–9.
290. Keilholz U, Goey SH, Punt CJA, et al. Interferon Alfa-2a and interleukin-2 with or without cisplatin in metastatic melanoma: a randomized trial of the European Organization for Research and Treatment of Cancer Melanoma Cooperative Group. J Clin Oncol 1997;15:2579–88.
291. Eggermont AM. The current EORTC Melanoma Cooperative Group adjuvant trial program on malignant melanoma: prognosis versus efficacy, toxicity and costs. Melanoma Res 1997;2:127–31.
292. Falkson CI, Ibrahim J, Kirkwood JM, et al. Phase III trial of dacarbazine versus dacarbazine with interferon alpha-2b versus dacarbazine with tamoxifen versus dacarbazine with interferon alpha-2b and tamoxifen in patients with metastatic malignant melanoma: an Eastern Cooperative Oncology Group study. J Clin Oncol 1998;16:1743–51.
293. Neale MH, Myatt N, Cree IA, et al. Combination chemotherapy for choroidal melanoma: ex vivo sensitivity to treosulfan with gemcitabine or cytosine arabinoside. Br J Cancer 1999;79:1487–93.
294. Hoon DS, Okamoto T, Wang HJ, et al. Is the survival of melanoma patients receiving polyvalent melanoma cell vaccine linked to the human leukocyte antigen phenotype of patients? J Clin Oncol 1998;16:1430–7.
295. De Vries TJ, Tancikova D, Ruiter DJ, van Muihen GNP. High expression of immunotherapy candidate proteins gp100 MART-1, tyrosinase and TRP-1 in uveal melanoma. Br J Cancer 1998;78:1156–61.
296. Uno T, Chen PW, Murray TG, et al. Gene transfer of the CD80 costimulatory molecule into ocular melanoma cells using a novel episomal vector. Invest Ophthalmol Vis Sci 1997;38:2531–9.
297. Durie FH, George WD, Campbell AM, Damato BE. Analysis of clonality of tumour infiltrating lymphocytes in breast cancer and uveal melanoma. Immunol Lett 1992;33:263–70.
298. Nitta T, Oksenberg JR, Rao NA, Steinman L. Predominant expression of T cell receptor V alpha 7 in tumor-infiltrating lymphocytes of uveal melanoma. Science 1990;249:672–4.
299. Miki S, Kasander B, Streilein JW. Complete elimination ('cure') of progressively growing intraocular tumors by local injection of tumor-specific CD8+ T lymphocytes. Invest Ophthalmol Vis Sci 1993;34:3622–34.
300. Mitchell MS, Liggett PE, Green RL, et al. Sustained regression of a primary choroidal melanoma under the influence of a therapeutic melanoma vaccine. J Clin Oncol 1994;12:396–401.
301. McLean IW, Berd D, Mastrangelo MJ, et al. A randomized study of methanol-extraction residue of bacille Calmette-Guerin as postsurgical adjuvant therapy of uveal melanoma. Am J Ophthalmol 1990;110:522–6.
302. Stephens RF, Shields JA. Diagnosis and management of cancer metastatic to the uvea: a study of 70 cases. Ophthalmology 1979;86:1336–49.
303. Ratanatharathorn V, Powers WE, Grimm J, et al. Eye metastasis from carcinoma of the breast: diagnosis, radiation treatment and results. Cancer Treat Rev 1991;18:261–76.
304. Maor M, Chan RC, Young SE. Radiotherapy of choroidal metastases: breast cancer as primary site. Cancer 1977;40:2081–6.
305. Reddy S, Saxena VS, Hendrickson F, Deutsch W. Malignant metastatic disease of the eye: management of an uncommon complication. Cancer 1981;47:810–2.
306. Zografos L, Gailloud C, Bercher L. Le traitment des hemangiomas de la choroide per radiotherapie. J Fu Ophthalmol 1989;12:797–807.
307. Letson AD, Davidorf FH, Bruce RA Jr. Chemotherapy for treatment of choroidal metastases from breast carcinoma. Am J Ophthalmol 1982;93:102–6.
308. Scott TA, Augsburger JJ, Brady LW, et al. Low dose ocular irradiation for diffuse choroidal hemangiomas associated with bullous nonrhegmatogenous retina detachment. Retina 1991;11:389–93.
309. Chu FC, Huh SH, Nisce LZ, Simpson LD. Radiation

therapy of choroid metastasis from breast cancer. Int J Radiat Oncol Biol Phys 1977;2:273–9.
310. Brinkley JR Jr. Response of a choroidal metastasis to multiple-drug chemotherapy. Cancer 1980;45: 1538–9.
311. Burmeister BH, Benjamin CS, Childs WJ. The management of metastases to eye and orbit from carcinoma of the breast. Austr NZ J Ophthalmol 1990;18:187–90.
312. Minatel E, Trovol MG, Forner L, et al. The efficacy of radiotherapy and the treatment of intraocular metastases. Br J Radiol 1993;66:699–702.
313. Gorin MB, Day R, Constantino JP, et al. Long-term tamoxifen citrate use and potential ocular toxicity. Am J Ophthalmol 1998;125:493–501.
314. Nylen U, Kock E, Lax I, et al. Standardized precision radiotherapy in choroidal metastases. Acta Oncologica 1994;33:65–8.
315. Schilling H, Sauerwein W, Lommatzsch A, et al. Long term results after low dose ocular irradiation for choroidal hemangiomas. Br J Ophthalmol 1997; 81:267–73.
316. Anand R, Augsburger JJ, Shields JA. Circumscribed choroidal hemangiomas. Arch Ophthalmol 1989; 107:1338–42.
317. Zografos L, Egger E, Bercher L, et al. Proton beam irradiation of choroidal hemangiomas. Am J Ophthalmol 1998;126:261–8.
318. Lee V, Hungerford JL. Proton beam therapy for posterior pole circumscribed choroidal haemangioma. Eye 1998;12:925–8.
319. Madreperla SA, Hungerford JL, Plowman PN, et al. Choroidal hemangiomas: Visual and anatomic results of treatment by photocoagulation or radiation therapy. Ophthalmology 1997;104:1773–9.
320. Hannouche D, Frau E, Desjardins L, et al. Efficacy of proton therapy in circumscribed choroidal hemangiomas associated with serous retinal detachment. Ophthalmology 1997;104:1780–4.
321. Gottlieb JL, Murray TG, Gass JDM. Low-dose external beam irradiation for bilateral diffuse choroidal hemangioma. Arch Ophthalmol 1998;166:815–7.
322. Plowman PN, Hungerford JL. Radiotherapy for ocular angiomas. Br J Ophthalmol 1997;81:254–9.
323. Zografos L, Bercher L, Chamot L, et al. Cobalt-60 treatment of choroidal hemangiomas. Am J Ophthalmol 1996;121:190–9.
324. Othmane IS, Shields C, Shields JA, et al. Circumscribed choroidal hemangioma managed by transpupilary thermal therapy. Arch Ophthalmol 1999;117:136–7.

9

Anterior Uveal Tumors

DIAGNOSIS OF IRIS MASS LESIONS

The most common adult iris lesions are nevi, melanomas, and cysts. Other lesions that simulate melanoma include the Cogan-Reese or essential iris atrophy variants of the iridocorneal endothelial (ICE) syndrome, epithelial downgrowth, medulloepithelioma, nodular adenomatosis, leiomyoma, metastasis, iris foreign body, lymphoid tumors, neurofibromatosis, hemangioma, inflammatory lesions, neurofibroma, aberrant lacrimal tissue, peripheral anterior synechiae, and inflammatory iris atrophies.[1–9] In children, and rarely in adults, juvenile xanthogranuloma (JXG) can involve either the iris or the ciliary body.[10–14]

Iris Cysts

The diagnosis of iris cysts is usually straightforward.[15] Patients are often young and have either had trauma or prolonged treatment with topical miotic agents.[16] Nontraumatic lesions, usually within the pigment epithelium, remain stationary, while those associated with trauma often grow; occasionally, after surgery, a free-floating iris cyst can develop. The overlying anterior iris surface is not disrupted in the pigment epithelial cysts (Figure 9–1); in contrast, this is quite common with stromal cysts (Figure 9–2). Iris melanomas alter the anterior iris surface; however, isolated ciliary body melanomas do not.

Iris pigment cysts can occur in any position on the posterior surface of the iris (Figure 9–3). Retroillumination at the slit-lamp or scleral transillumination demonstrates the cystic nature of these lesions and allows differentiation from iris-ciliary body melanomas. Cysts transilluminate easily while melanomas block light. Ultrasonography can demonstrate the cystic nature of both iris and ciliary body cysts; however, we and others have observed histologically confirmed ciliary body melanomas that appeared cystic on ultrasound examination. The newer high-frequency ultrasonography demonstrates these benign posterior pigment cysts very easily (Figure 9–4). What is unclear is how specific the finding of a cystic lesion is, using high-frequency ultrasonography. Certainly, a solid tumor that has a cystic component should still be viewed with suspicion and a biopsy performed.

Recently, a case has been reported of an iris cyst after the use of latanoprost (Xalatan).[17] Rarely, argon or Nd:YAG laser is used to demonstrate the cystic nature of a lesion, which will collapse after a laser burst, versus a solid melanoma which will not.[15–18]

Congenital iris stromal cysts are difficult to manage, since enlargment has occurred in 21 of

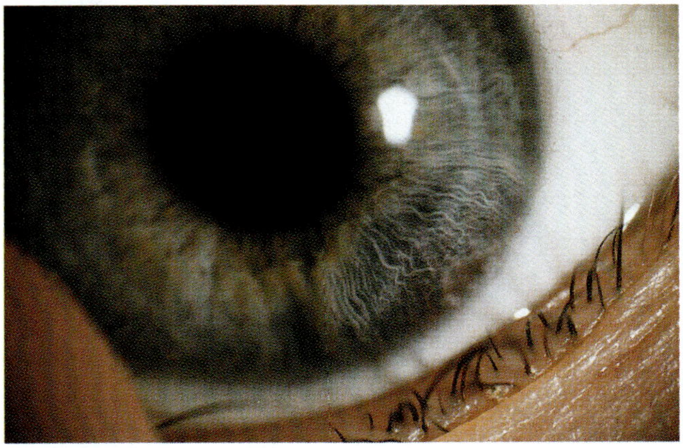

Figure 9–1. Posterior pigmented iris cyst with normal anterior iris surface.

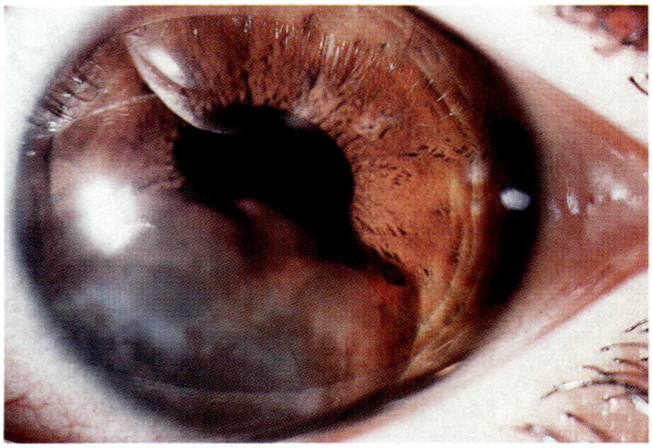

Figure 9–2. Anterior iris stromal cysts with destruction of the iris surface.

25 reported cases.[19] In one report, 8 of 9 children had obstruction of the visual axis, and 7 required multiple treatments.[20] Overall, that group noted that only 3 percent of primary cysts of the iris epithelium were in a central location.[21] While some clinicians have tried trichloroacetic acid, complete surgical removal is the treatment of choice.[17,19,22,23] Rarely, there can be spontaneous collapse of a primary stromal cyst.[24]

Iris Nevi

Typical iris nevi are flat lesions that usually do not involve either the pupil or trabecular meshwork; these tumors are < 4 mm in diameter and generally do not produce glaucoma (Figure 9–5). Occasionally, a large, flat nevoid proliferation can involve substantially greater iris area, and some of these require biopsy. Among dark-skinned patients, a presumably autosomal-dominant pattern of bilateral diffuse nodular nevi has been described in 30 patients.[25] A benign, histologically confirmed,

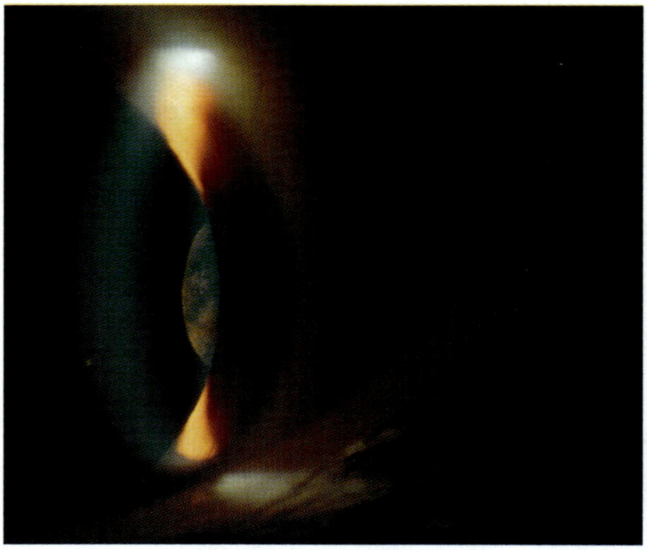

Figure 9–3. Posterior iris pigmentary cyst involving the pupil.

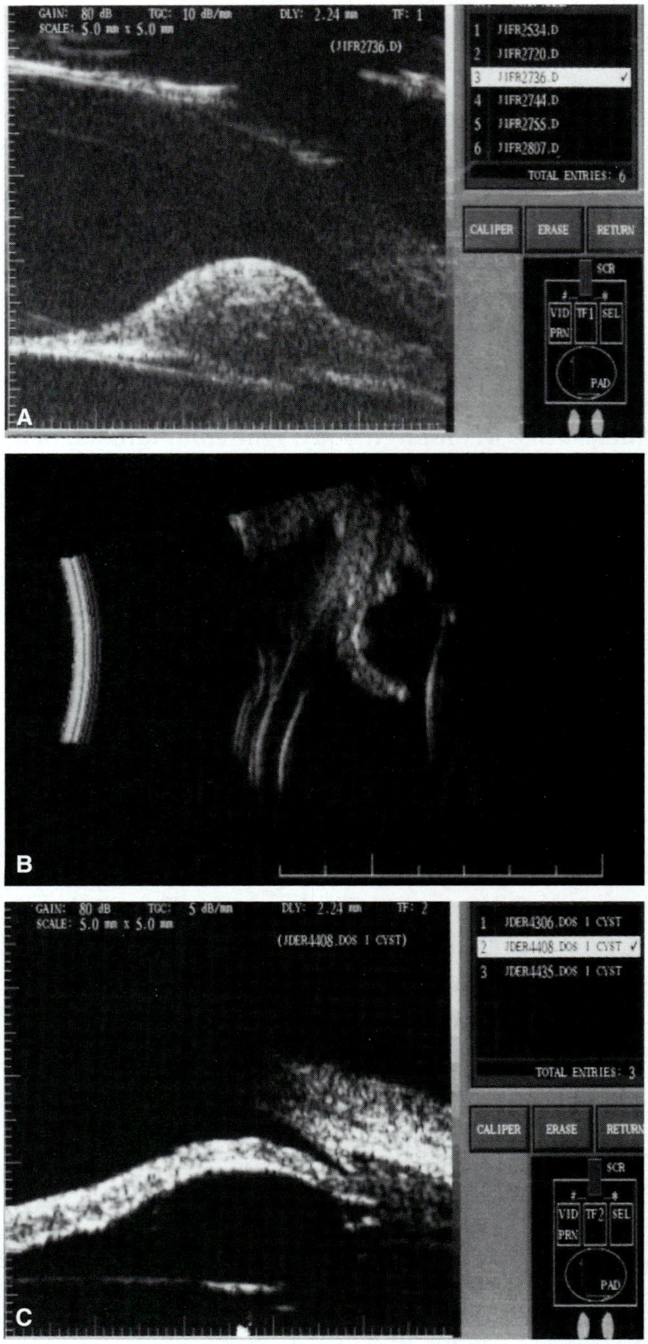

Figures 9–4. *A* to *C*, Three cases of posterior pigment iris cysts shown on high-frequency ultrasonography.

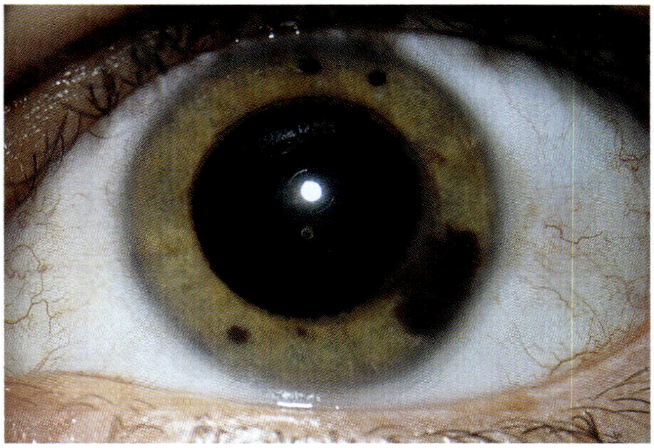

Figure 9–5. Typical iris freckle or nevus. Usually, these do not invade the trabecular network, produce ectropion uveae, or grow.

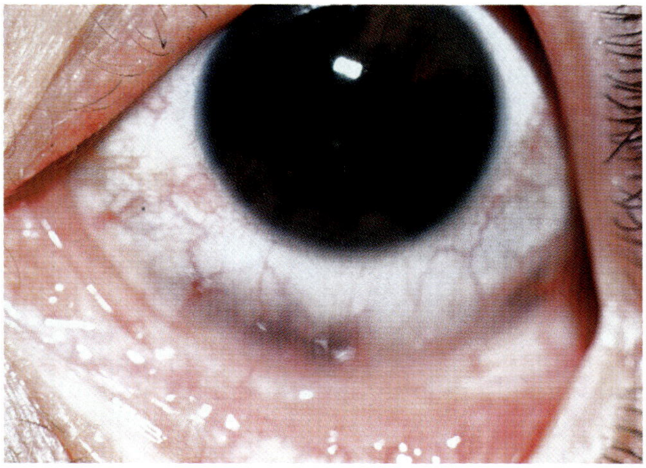

Figure 9–7. Sector melanosis of the iris in a child.

growing iris lesion is shown in Figure 9–6. Unfortunately, 5 years later, the tumor grew further and subsequent sections revealed an area of malignant transformation. In children, a nevoid process, sector melanosis of the iris (Figure 9–7), can occur. We have never observed malignant degeneration in that group of patients. There have been 16 reported cases of familial intraocular melanoma.[26] In one pedigree, two generations of patients with aggressive iris nevi (with apparent extention onto the limbus in one case) were reported.[26] Similarly, melanocytoma, a magnocellular nevus, can also involve the iris or ciliary body. Usually, they are darkly pigmented, but often, they can present an identical clinical and imaging pattern of a melanoma (Figure 9–8 and 9–9).[27–32] Rarely, these can undergo malignant degeneration. Much less often, a leiomyoepithelioma or adenoma of the iris pigmented epithelium can present as a jet black mass.[23] Unfortunately, our experience has shown that we are unable, even with high-frequency ultrasonography, to differentiate a very small histologically documented iris melanoma from an atypical iris nevus (unpublished observations).

Anterior Uveal Melanoma (Ciliary Body and Iris)

Iris and ciliary body melanomas together account for approximately 20 percent of uveal melanomas. Iris color is a risk factor for the development of iris melanocytic lesions. Two studies have demonstrated a statistically significant association between light-

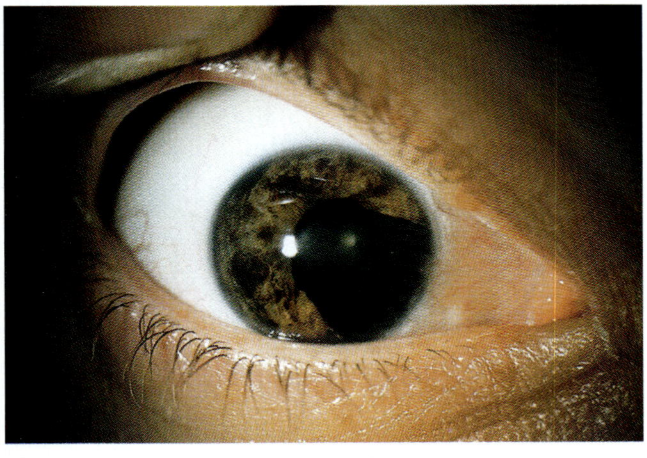

Figure 9–6. Large histologically documented iris nevoid lesion; 5 years later, the pressure became medically uncontrolled and the enucleated specimen showed an iris- ciliary melanoma.

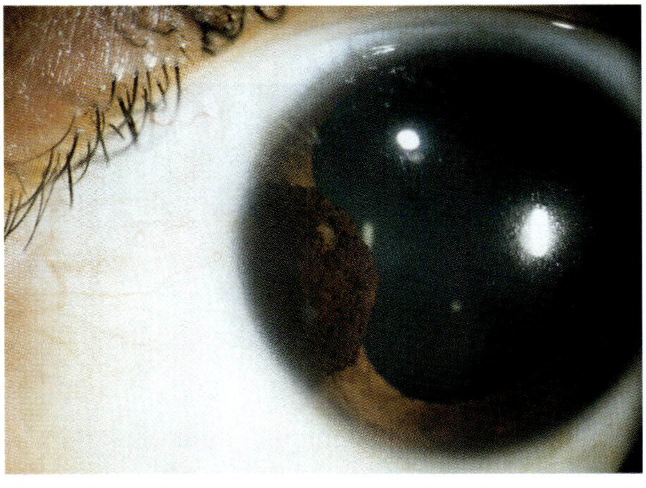

Figure 9–8. Histologically documented iris melanocytoma with growth.

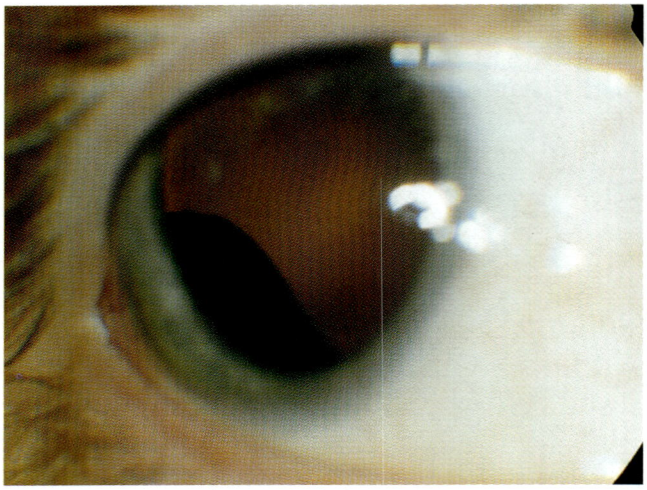

Figure 9–9. Ciliary body melanocytoma that grew and was excised.

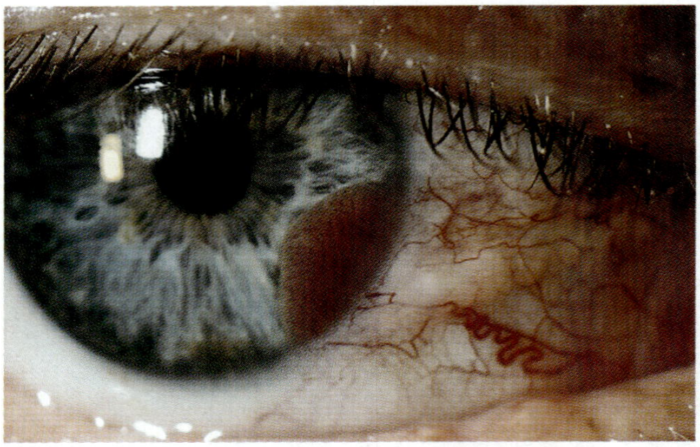

Figure 9–11. Prominent intrinsic vessels in an iris melanoma.

colored irides and the development of both melanomas and nevi of the iris.[33] The ratio of iris to ciliary body and choroidal melanomas is estimated to be between 1:6 and 1:20.[34] There have been approximately 10 cases of uveal melanoma in association with neurofibramatosis type-1 (NF1). In one recent report, the patient had involvement of the iris and cornea by a melanoma.[35] The peak incidence of iris melanomas occurs in patients 10 to 20 years younger than patients with choroidal melanomas. Iris tumors are often detected either as an incidental finding or because of cosmetic change. Patients may have decreased vision due to a sector lens opacity (Figure 9–10) or as a result of astigmatism induced by an iris-ciliary body melanoma pressing against the lens.[36]

Iris melanomas often have prominent intrinsic vessels (Figure 9–11), ectropion iridis (Figure 9–12), secondary cataract, variable pigmentation, and, occasionally, increased intraocular pressure. Sentinel vessels can occur with both iris and ciliary body melanomas (Figure 9–13). Most commonly, melanomas involve the inferior iris.

A diffuse or ring melanoma is a variant of iris melanoma that is extremely difficult to diagnose and manage; it can present as a subtle 360° ring of tumor or can have a focal lesion with a subclinical tumor involving the rest of the angle circumference (Figure 9–14).[37] Usually, the first type of ring melanoma is initially misdiagnosed as a glaucoma of uncertain etiology. Rarely, other tumors, such as lymphomas, can simulate this problem.[38]

Tapioca melanoma is another variant of iris melanoma (Figure 9–15).[39] This tumor is usually a large, irregular, multinodular, lightly pigmented lesion.

The histologic classification of iris melanoma is in flux. Jakobiec reviewed 189 "iris melanoma"

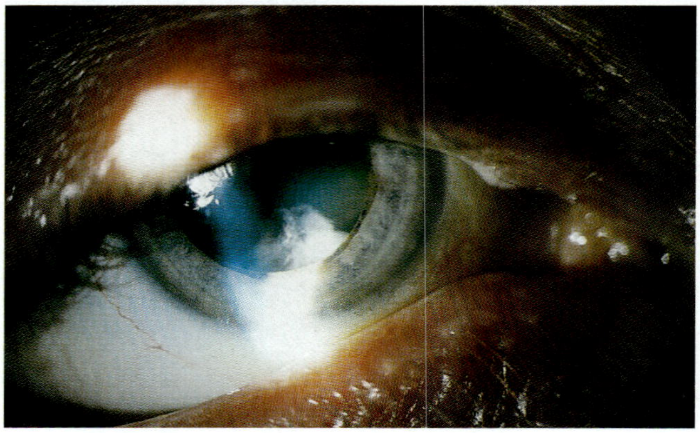

Figure 9–10. Sector lens opacity in association with a peripheral iris-ciliary body tumor.

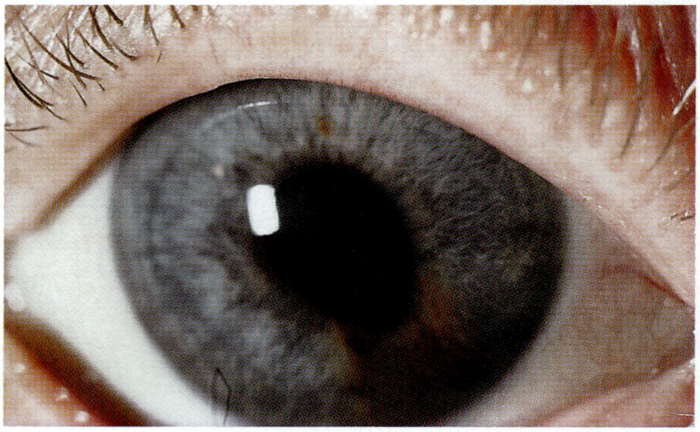

Figure 9–12. Iris melanoma producing pupillary distortion and ectropion iridies.

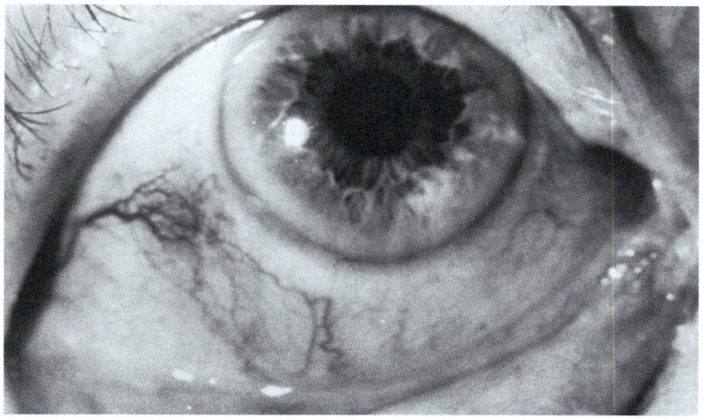

Figure 9–13. Sentinel vessels in association with an anterior uveal melanoma.

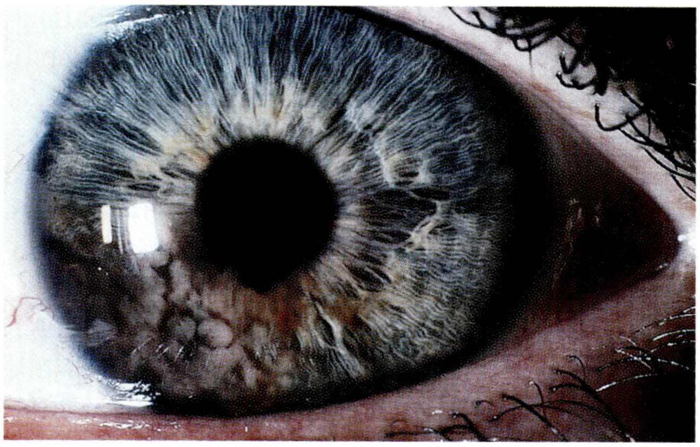

Figure 9–15. Tapioca iris melanoma.

diagnoses and reclassified 87 percent as nevi.[40] Histologically confirmed iris nevi can grow, involve the angle, and produce ectropion iridis. The clinical overlap between benign and malignant iris tumors makes diagnosis sometimes difficult.

All patients with pigmented iris lesions are examined with slit-lamp biomicroscopy and bilateral evaluation with a three-mirror contact lens; fundus examination with 360° scleral depression is also used to ascertain whether the ciliary body or anterior choroid is involved. The presence or absence and the degree of angle-ciliary body involvement (optimally assessed with high-frequency ultrasonography) are noted; it is important to determine angle pigmentation contiguous to and away from the tumor in the involved eye and whether it is or is not present in the contralateral eye. Neither radioactive phosphorus tests nor standard ultrasonography is useful in the evaluation of iris tumors that do not involve the ciliary body. In the past immersion B-scans of iris-ciliary body melanomas did not accurately delineate the ciliary body involvement by the tumor. Fortunately, the development of high frequency ultrasonography has allowed us to demonstrate iris tumors with involvement of the ciliary body quite well (Figure 9–16). These ultrasound probes with 20 to 100 MHz transducers have approximately 10-fold better resolution in the anterior segment than standard echography; however, the diagnostic accuracy of this newer technique and its utility in the management of iris tumors is still uncertain.[41]

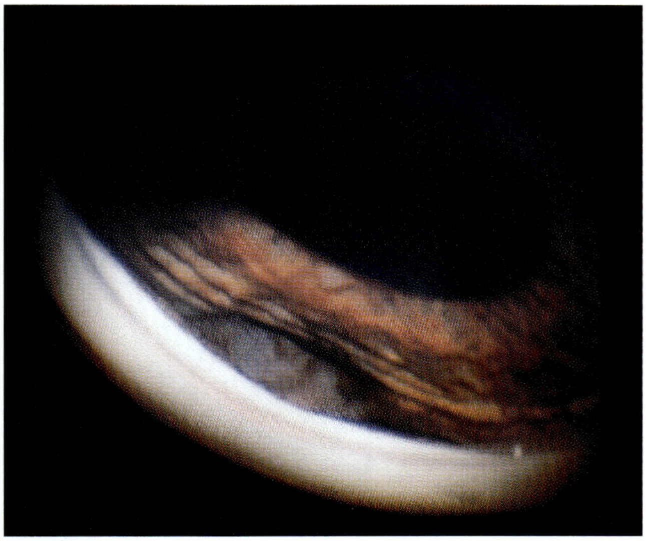

Figure 9–14. Presumed focal melanoma that histologically had 360° angle involvement (ring melanoma).

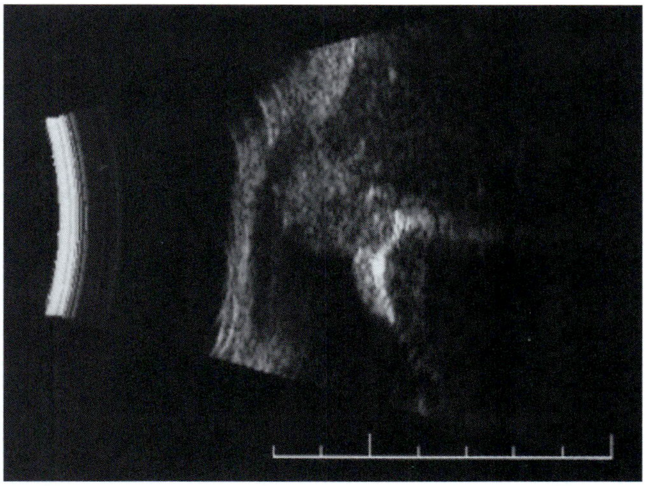

Figure 9–16. High-frequency ultrasonography of an iris-ciliary body melanoma with mass against the posterior cornea. This type of ultrasonography does not demonstrate posterior involvement as well as the standard scan can.

The two signs that are most reliable in the diagnosis of iris melanoma are demonstrable tumor growth, and the presence of an intensely vascular tumor (see Figure 9–11). Figure 9–17 demonstrates a very small melanoma that had documented growth; histologically, it was the mixed-cell type. Ring melanomas are the most difficult to diagnose, if no focal tumor is present.

Anterior segment fluorescein angiography has been advocated by some investigators.[42–45] While obvious iris melanomas often have diffuse confluent fluorescence from ill-defined vascular foci, in indeterminate lesions, angiography has not been helpful. Figure 9–18 shows a fluorescein angiogram of a histologically confirmed iris melanoma with typical leakage. In a series of 26 iris-ciliary body melanomas that underwent iridocyclectomy, we could not differentiate the two benign melanocytic proliferations from the malignant melanomas on the basis of fluorescein angiographic criteria.[45] We were also unable to distinguish spindle cell from either mixed cell or epithelioid melanomas on fluorescein angiographic criteria.[45]

As discussed under management, fine-needle aspiration biopsy (FNAB) can be quite useful in two settings. We have most often used this technique on patients with an apparently focal pigmented tumor and increased intraocular pressure. An FNAB positive for melanoma that is performed 180° away from the main mass is diagnostic for ring melanoma. Rarely, in cases that are suspected of being nonmelanoma malignancies of the iris, this diagnostic assay is also useful.[46]

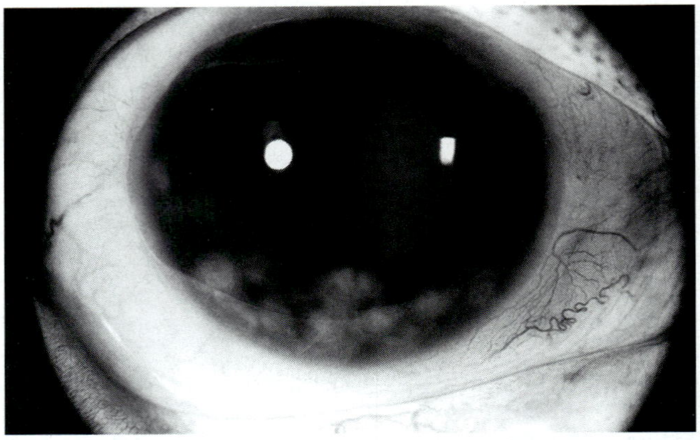

Figure 9–18. Diffuse leakage on fluorescein angiogram of a histologically confirmed iris melanoma.

Other Iris Lesions

Patients with either Cogan-Reese syndrome or the essential iris atrophy spectrum of iridocorneal endothelial syndrome are often referred for evaluation of a suspected iris melanoma.[5] Almost all these patients have peripheral anterior synechiae and corneal endothelial changes, and some have glaucoma; the first two features are not common in melanoma. Patients with essential iris atrophy have a distorted pupil and enlarging areas of iris atrophy; a typical example of this entity is shown in Figure 9–19. The syndrome is more common in females. Probably, there is a viral etiology for these diseases.[47] Cogan-Reese syndrome often has some associated iris atrophy and areas of iris nodules; usually, these nodules are multiple, as shown in Figure 9–20.

Tumors metastatic to the iris, unlike those which involve the choroid, often are detected after the pri-

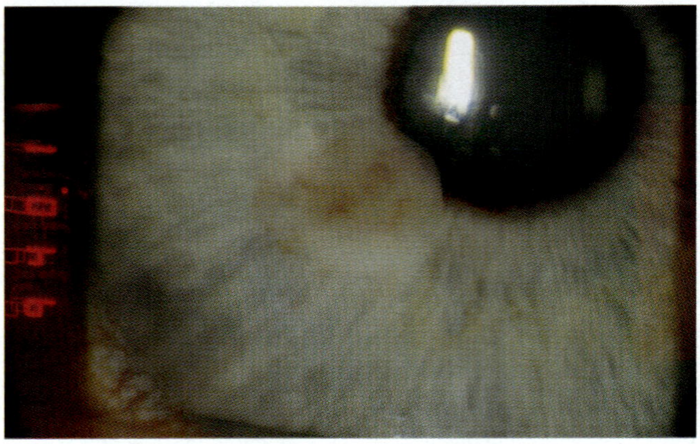

Figure 9–17. Growth in a very small iris tumor that demonstrated mixed cell melanoma in the excised specimen.

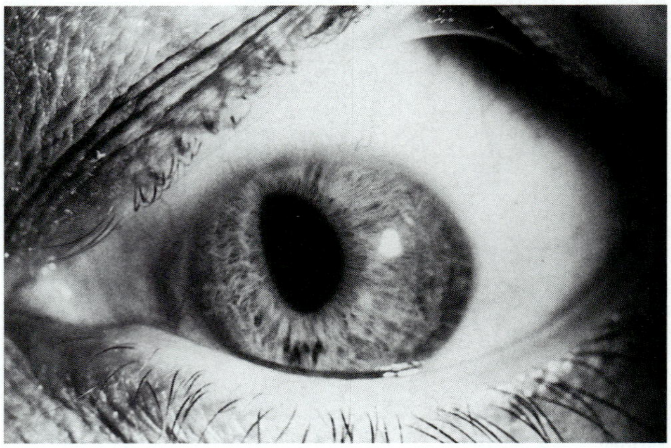

Figure 9–19. Essential iris atrophy with distortion of the pupil.

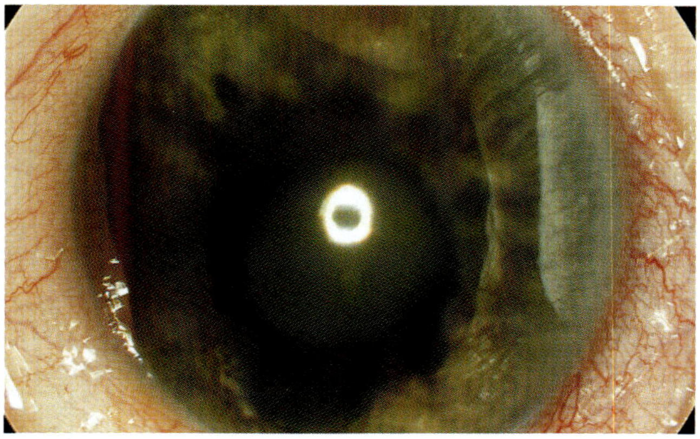

Figure 9–20. Cogan-Reese syndrome with iris nodules, iris atrophy and peripheral anterior synechiae.

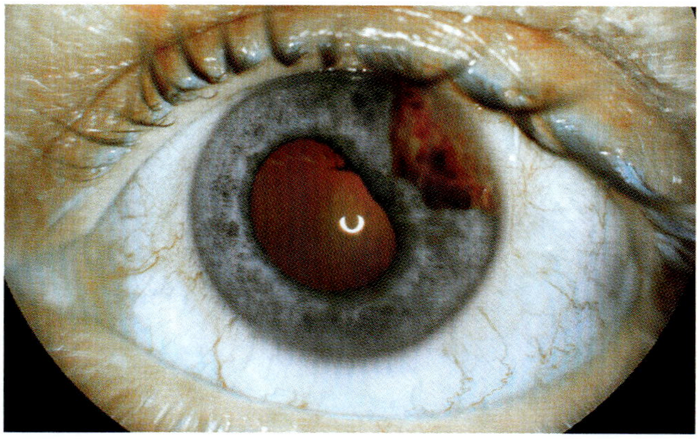

Figure 9–22. A solitary iris metastatic bronchogenic carcinoma.

mary tumor has been discovered. Almost all are amelanotic, and many diffusely involve the iris (Figure 9–21). They are much less frequent than posterior uveal metastases; approximately 10 percent of ocular metastases involve the iris.[48] The most common sites of primary carcinomas are the breast, lung, kidney, and gastrointestinal tract.[49] Less commonly, cutaneous melanoma, thyroid carcinoma, and lymphomas can present in this part of the eye as the initial manifestation of the neoplasm.[38,50–53] Neonatal hepatoblastoma, endometrial carcinoma, Ewing's sarcoma, and renal cell carcinoma have also been described.[36,54–56] As discussed in Chapter 5, many patients with endodermally derived malignancies will have elevated levels (> 10 ng/mL) of plasma carcinoembryonic antigen (CEA); patients with uveal melanomas consistently have lower values.[57] Some of these metastases are solitary as shown in Figures 9–22, 9–23, and 9–24.

Lymphomas or leukemias may produce iris infiltration; this may be the first sign of disease reactivation although it almost never is the first presentation of the malignancy.[2,38,58] In anterior segment lymphoma, a malignant hypopyon is usually present (Figure 9–25). Rarely, other malignancies can produce a pseudohypyon (see Chapter 10).[59] A metastatic cutaneous melanoma may present as a black hypopyon without an obvious mass (Figure 9–26).[53] A presumed breast metastasis presented with bilateral pseudohypopyons (Figure 9–27).

Iris nodules can also occur either with neurofibromatosis or sarcoidosis (Figure 9–28); neither is likely to be confused with a melanoma.[59] Rarely, other diseases, including Cushing's disease, can have Lisch nodules.[60] Other clinical systemic and ocular findings associated with both these conditions allow easy differentiation from a malignant melanoma.

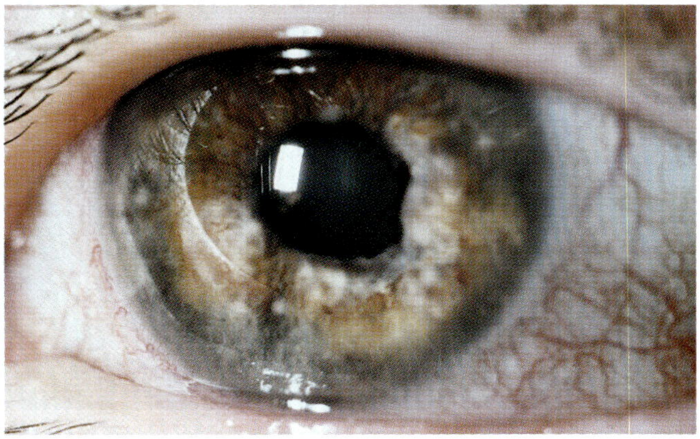

Figure 9–21. Metastatic carcinoma to the iris. These are often diffuse melanocytic lesions.

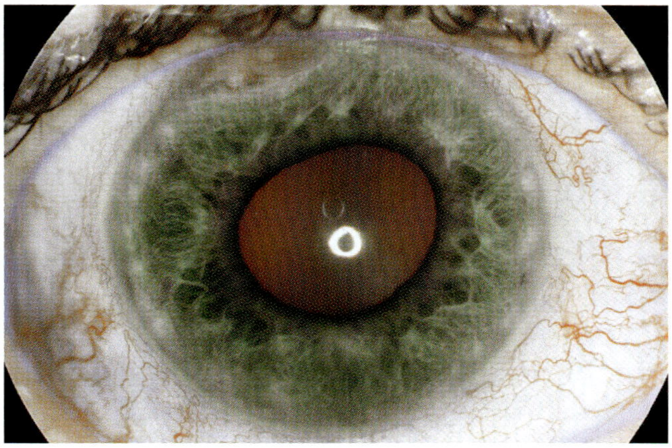

Figure 9–23. A solitary metastatic adenocarcinoma.

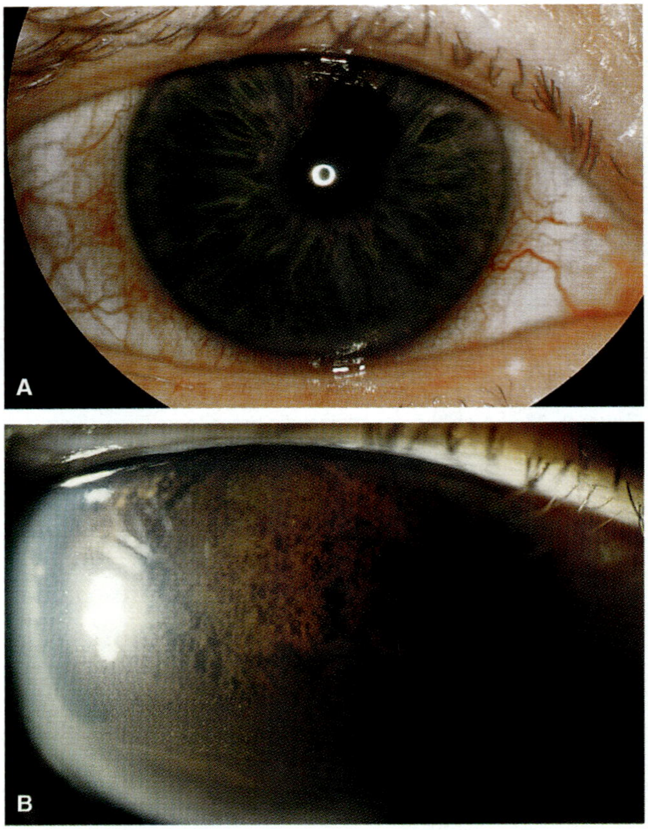

Figures 9–24. *A,* Solitary metastatic cutaneous melanoma in a patient with widespread metastases. *B,* Progression of the iris lesion (that mirrored systemic tumor growth.)

Juvenile xanthogranuloma (JXG) is usually a childhood tumor, occurring rarely in adults.[10–12,61] The lesions are most commonly gray or yellow and have associated heterochromia, hyphema, and glaucoma. While typical skin changes are helpful to establish this diagnosis, they are found in only about one-third of patients with eye lesions.[14,62] Intraocular tumor growth is usually quite rapid. These tumors respond rapidly to either corticosteroids or to as little as 2 Gray (Gy) of photon radiation, although most clinicians have used a slightly higher dose.

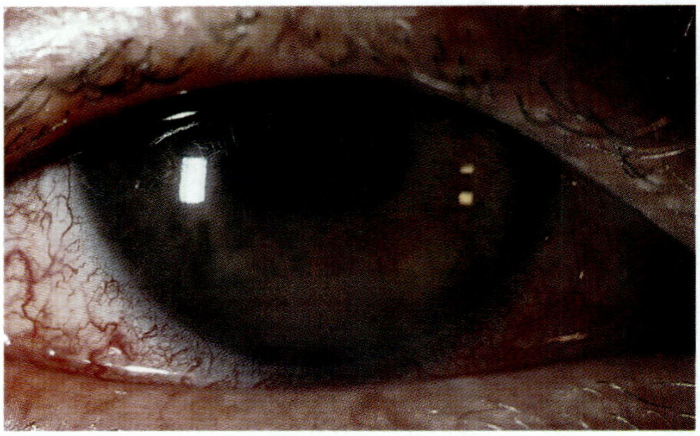

Figure 9–25. Anterior segment lymphoma presented with a malignant hypopyon.

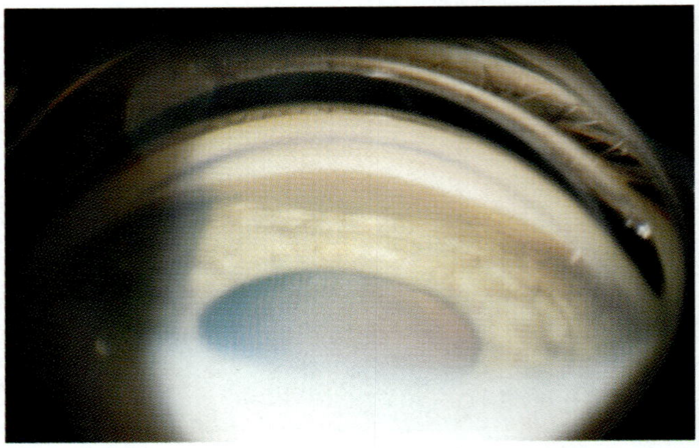

Figure 9–26. Cutaneous melanoma metastatic to the anterior segment, presenting as a black hypopyon.

A number of less common primary iris tumors have been reported. Often, establishing the correct diagnosis, even with conventional light microscopy, has been difficult. Two recent reports emphasize this problem. Kluppel and colleagues reported a 2-month-old girl with a highly vascular 2-clock-hour tumor which was a lacrimal gland choristoma.[63] At the other end of the age spectrum, Spraul reported an 81-year-old with an adeno-carcinoma of the iris epithelium.[64] An especially perplexing group of

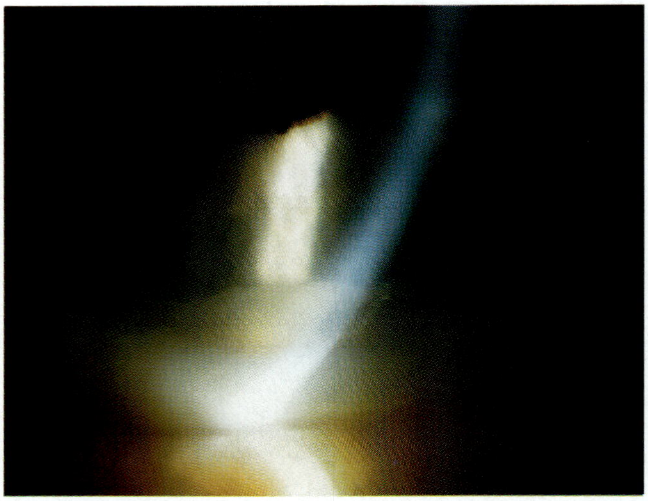

Figure 9–27. Breast carcinoma metastatic to the iris as the initial manifestation of widespread disease with simultaneous bilateral pseudohypopyons.

reported lesions have been iris leiomyomas and leiomyosarcomas. Foss and co-workers showed that 24 cases that had been classified as iris tumors of muscle origin were all melanocytic neoplasms, when studied with appropriate stains and antibodies.[65] Other rare tumors that have been reported to involve the iris include lacrimal choristomas and primary rhabdomyosarcoma.[66,67]

We have very rarely observed some pigmented tumors that enlarged on serial examinations and were shown to be benign when examined after iridocyclectomy. These tumefactions include atypical melanocytic proliferations, adenomas of the ciliary epithelium, and melanocytoma. In an enlarging iris-ciliary body pigment adenoma, we suspected the correct diagnosis on FNAB (Figure 9–29) but performed an iridocyclectomy to be certain. The cytopathology demonstrated benign pigmented cells and large pigment granules. We have also seen a case (see Figure 9–6) in which a substantial iridectomy (approximately 25% of the total iris) showed only benign cells, yet 5 years later, when the eye was blind and painful from medically intractable glaucoma, the enucleated specimen demonstrated melanoma.

MANAGEMENT OF IRIS LESIONS

Iris Melanoma

Iris melanoma management options include observation, iridectomy, iridocyclectomy, and enucleation. The tumor-related mortality associated with iris melanomas has been reported to be extremely small.[6,68] Metastases occur predominantly in three clinical situations: (1) when a partial resection was inadvertently performed, usually during a glaucoma-filtering procedure because the cause of glaucoma was not recognized; (2) when the iris is involved as part of a diffuse uveal melanoma (Figure 9–30) (see Chapter 5); and (3) in tumors with a significant ciliary body component and some iris invasion (Figure 9–31). Less commonly, some investigators have reported a few iris melanomas which have metastasized but do not fit into the above groups. A review of the world's literature found that only 31 of 1,043 (3%) reported iris melanomas developed metastases.[6]

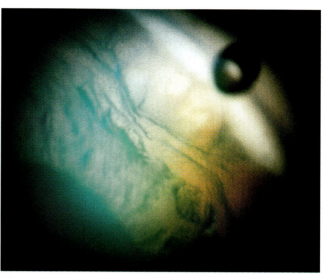

Figure 9–28. Sarcoid granuloma in the angle. The patient had other stigmata of sarcoid, including uveitis, and both a positive gallium scan and an elevated serum ACE.

Shields and colleagues have pointed out that the low death rate which has been reported in retrospective analyses of histologic studies of iris melanomas could be an artifact. Many of the cases that Geisse and Robertson, as well as others, have included in their reports probably would have been reclassified as benign pigmented tumors.[6,40] It is therefore likely that there is a higher metastatic rate with larger tumors, especially those with more malignant cell types or those that recur. In one series, Sunba had noted approximately a 10 percent incidence of metastatic disease associated with iris melanomas.[69]

All elevated iris pigmented tumors are sequentially observed, unless the lesion is highly vascular or glaucoma is present. Figure 9–32 shows an indeterminate pigmented iris tumor followed up for over 10 years, without change. Most possible iris melanomas with normal intraocular pressure are followed up until growth is documented. Figure 9–33 shows a very large iris melanoma in a one-eyed patient who retained 20/30 vision in the affected eye; there had been no growth over a 10-year interval.

In patients with highly vascular lesions that are most consistent with iris melanoma, intervention is indicated. The clinical patterns of iris tumors shown in Figure 9–11 have almost always been associated with melanoma on histologic evaluation, and it has been our clinical impression that the tumor type is

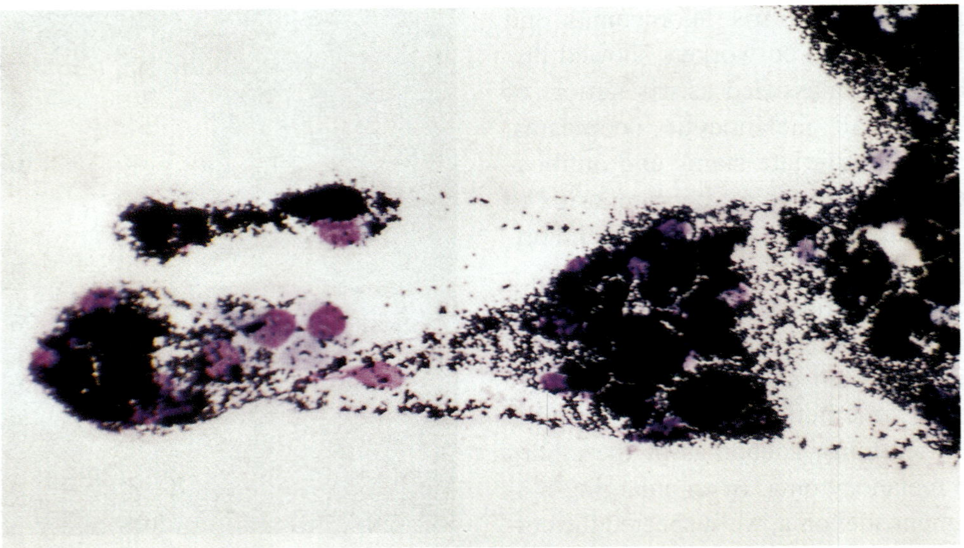

Figure 9–29. Fine-needle biopsy of growing pigmented ciliary epithelial adenoma. Note benign cells, bland nuclei, and pigment granules that are much larger than seen with melanomas. (Original magnification × 190)

more likely to have a more malignant (mixed or epithelioid) cytologic pattern. If the lesion can be adequately excised, a conventional iridectomy is performed. If the angle is involved, an iridocyclectomy is done (see "management of ciliary body melanoma"). Iridectomy is performed through a limbus-based incision. The pupil may be spared if it is not involved. It is crucial to lay the tumor specimen on a piece of sterile filter paper and orient it properly. If the material is just haphazardly placed into a specimen jar, it is virtually impossible to retrospectively ascertain either the margins or the orientation of the specimen.

If glaucoma is present, it is important to determine the cause of the increased intraocular pressure. It may be due to coincident primary glaucoma, malignant cells invading the filtration angle, an iris melanoma with neovascular glaucoma, or tumor pigment (alone or in macrophages) clogging the trabecular meshwork.[70–72] Often, it is impossible to precisely determine the etiology of increased intraocular pressure in a given patient. Clinically undetectable tumor can invade the trabecular meshwork. An FNAB may be useful in such situations (see "invasive diagnostic modalities" in Chapters 8 and 15). The eye in Figure 9–34 had a pressure of 50 mm Hg on maximum

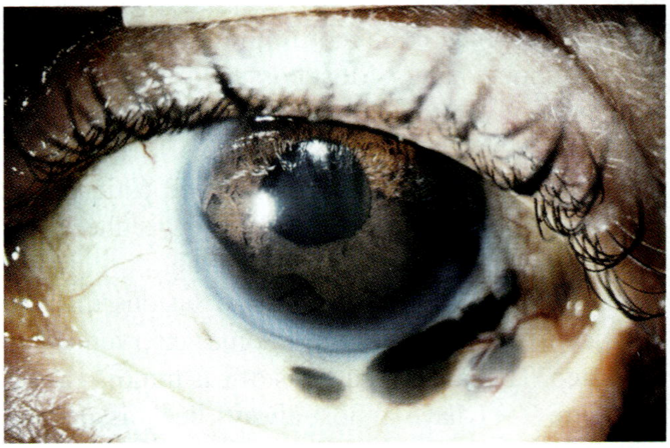

Figure 9–30. Iris melanoma as a component of a diffuse uveal melanoma with extraocular extension.

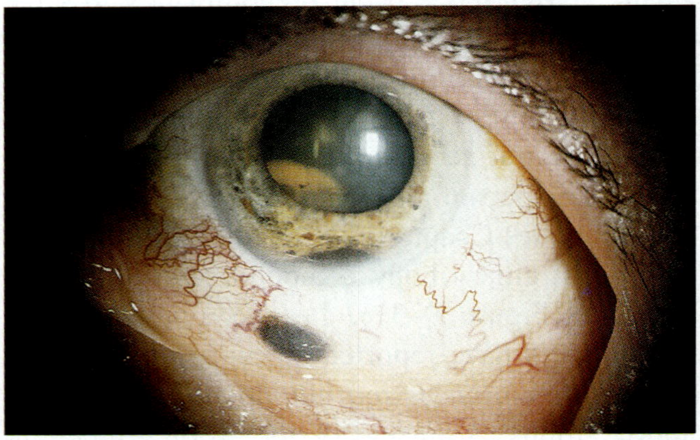

Figure 9–31. Higher mortality is noted in iris-ciliary body melanomas than with pure iris lesions. Tumor-related mortality is further increased with localized extrascleral extension.

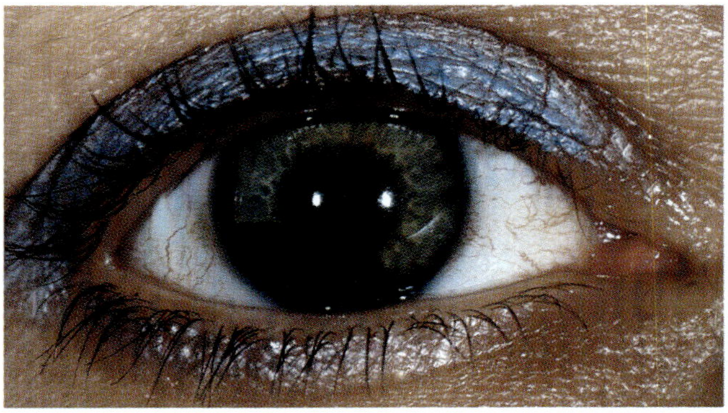

Figure 9–32. Presumed iris melanoma monitored photographically, without change from 1965 to 1986.

medical therapy. There was a focal iris tumor and 360° of angle pigmentation. An FNAB of the angle 180° away from the tumor was used to determine whether pigment-bearing macrophages or tumor cells were present. Only pigmented macrophages were present, and the tumor was removed with an iridocyclectomy. If tumor cells had been noted in the angle 180° from the main mass, enucleation would have been indicated, since a ring melanoma cannot be surgically removed with retention of the eye.[73] A second indication for FNAB in iris tumors is to evaluate a large, growing atypical lesion. In some of these lesions, biopsy has demonstrated malignant cells and thus mandated therapy. Figure 9–35A illustrates an unusual ring iris-ciliary body melanoma; a transcorneal 25-gauge FNAB documented the melanoma (Figure 9–35B). A similar finding was noted in this young woman who had a filtering operation, with no mass noted by the referring doctor

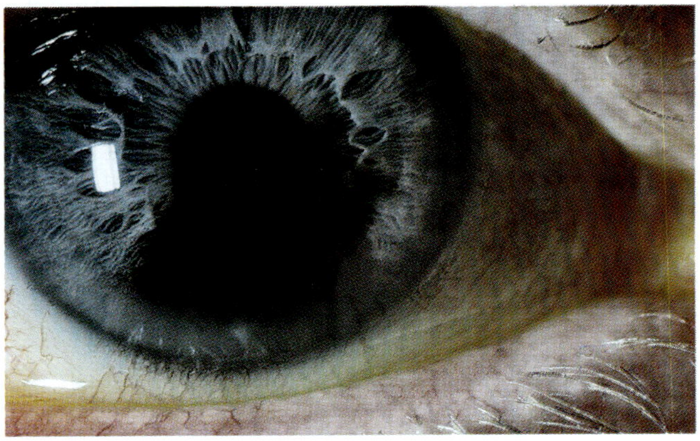

Figure 9–33. Large iris melanoma with corneal touch in a one-eyed patient showing no growth over a 10-year interval, with visual acuity remaining 20/25.

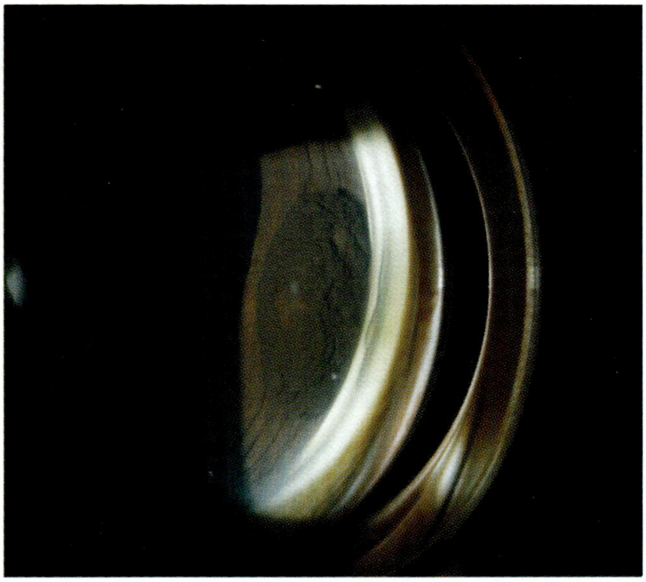

Figure 9–34. Pigmented iris lesion with 4+ anterior segment cells and an intraocular pressure of 50 mm Hg on maximum medical therapy.

and continued increased intraocular pressure (Figure 9–36). FNAB demonstrated the ring melanoma.

Glaucoma management in eyes with possible iris melanomas or atypical iris nevi is difficult. Since tumor-related deaths with iris melanoma can occur after filtering operations inadvertently transect the lesion, we are unwilling to filter these patients. We have only treated the glaucoma medically. If maximum medical therapy does not control the pressure, we allow the glaucoma to progress.[74]

We have not used radiation to treat isolated iris melanomas. Irradiation of the entire anterior segment with either conventional photons or charged particles in sufficient dosage to control the melanoma often destroys the eye. In 14 patients, with very short follow-up, Shields and colleagues have used brachytherapy in tumors that involved < 7 clock hours. Longer follow-up is necessary to determine the efficacy and complications with this approach.[75]

Lesions < 5 clock hours (150° of angle) can be surgically excised. Figure 9–37 shows a patient 5 years after resection of a growing iris melanoma with a large iridectomy; the patient has retained 20/20 vision. There are now five different contact lens companies that make cosmetic lenses to camouflage a sector defect. The role of Lasik or other procedures to correct astigmia as a result of an iridectomy or more commonly after an iridocyclectomy is unclear.

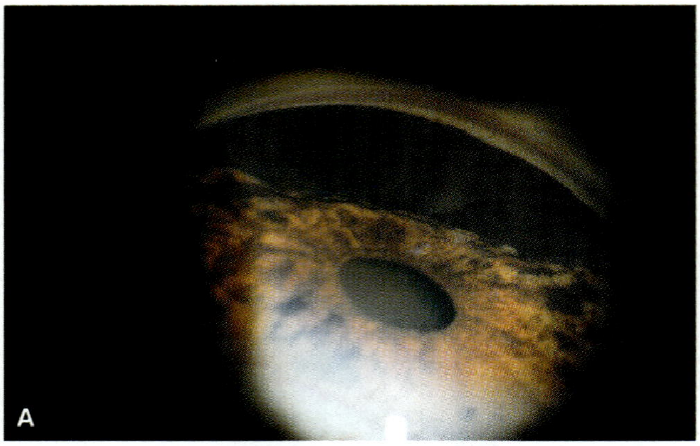

Figure 9–35. *A,* Unusual ring iris-ciliary body ring melanoma. Clinically, this tumor involved approximately 100° of the angle. *B,* Fine-needle biopsy demonstrates melanoma cells 180° from the pigmented lesion shown in Figure 9–35A.

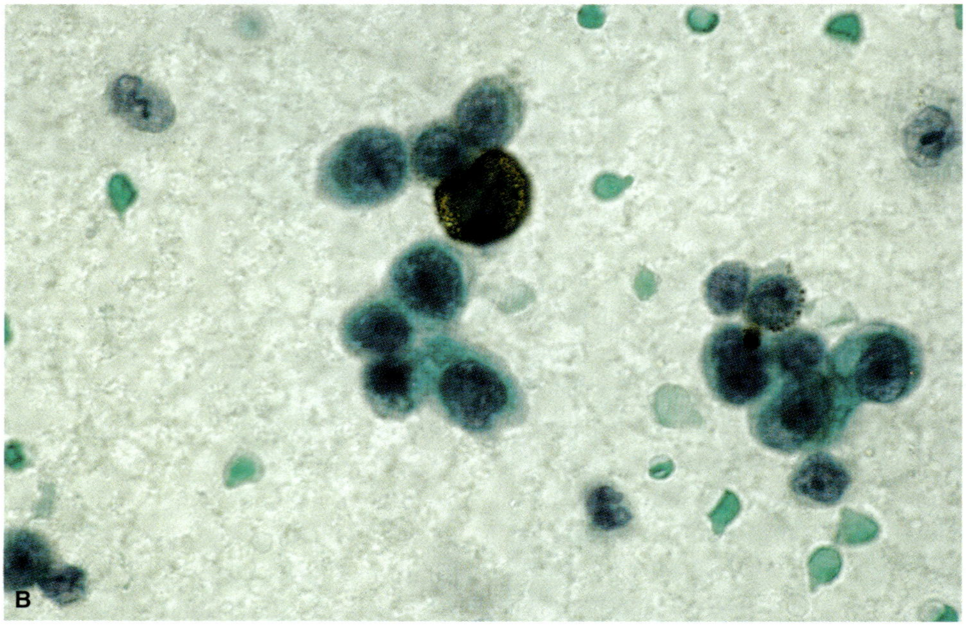

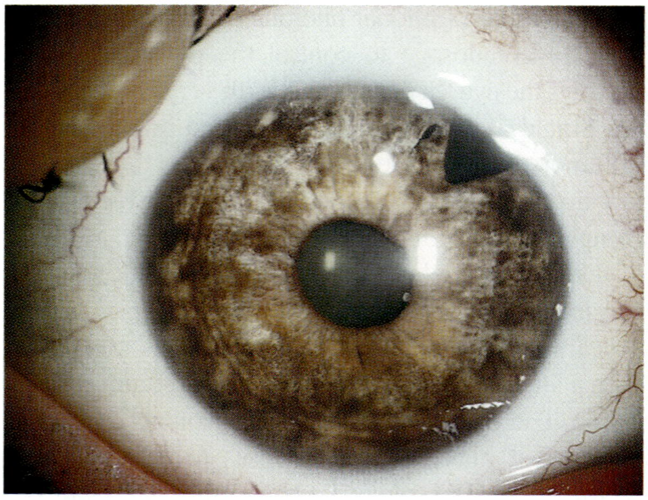

Figure 9–36. Increased pigmentation and pressure without a mass. Trabeculectomy did not control intraocular pressure. On referral, the FNAB was positive for melanoma.

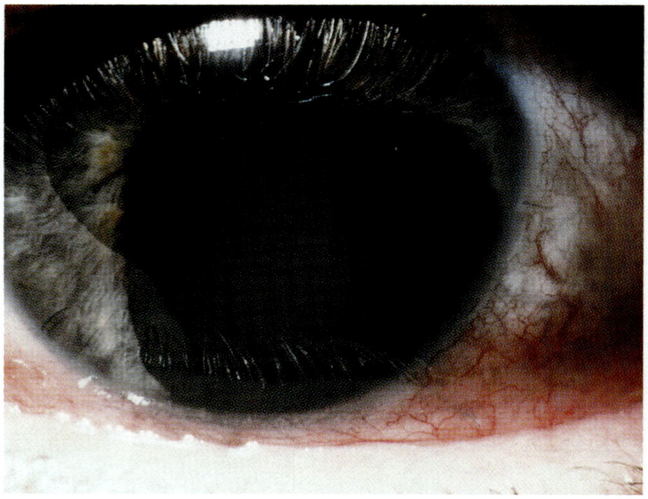

Figure 9–37. Large iridectomy for iris melanoma; the patient remains 20/20 5 years after surgery. Some of these patients prefer a cosmetic contact lens to create an artificial pupil.

Larger lesions (> 5 clock-hours) are usually not amenable to surgical resection; if glaucoma becomes intractable to medical therapy and the eye is painful, enucleation is performed.

Laser therapy has been used to treat local recurrences but has not been used in enough patients to evaluate its efficacy for iris melanoma.[76] In a few patients we treated many years ago, unacceptable complications were noted. There is also a paucity of data regarding photochemotherapy of anterior segment melanomas, using hematoporphyrin-derivative dyes; a number of failures have been reported.[77] A few relatively small iris tumors have been treated with photodynamic therapy.[78] In one report, it appeared that those cases could have been treated surgically with probably no greater complications.

Enucleation is usually recommended for iris ring melanomas with increased pressure and for growing iris melanomas that involve over 60 percent of the circumference of the globe. We have reluctantly followed up a few patients who refused treatment with growing iris melanomas that have eventually spread to involve the entire angle circumference. In one case, after 40 years of follow-up, the lesion grew from 1 to 12 clock-hours with retention of good vision (Figure 9–38). Others have reported similar results.[79] Initially, this patient refused all therapy; eventually the eye was removed because of uncontrolled glaucoma. The patient lived another 5 years and later died of unrelated causes.

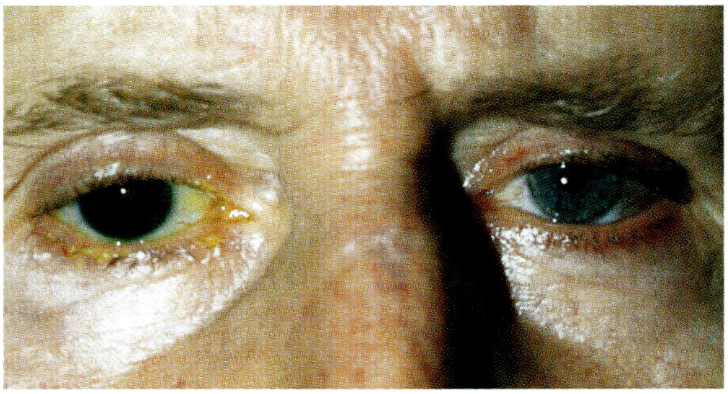

Figure 9–38. Forty years previously this was a 1-clock-hour lesion. It grew in time to involve the entire iris but pressured vision remained good for many years. Melanoma was confirmed histologically 5 years later when the eye became painful and was removed.

Anterior Segment Metastatic Tumor Therapy

The treatment of anterior uveal metastatic tumors is similar to the management of posterior uveal metastatic tumors. If chemotherapy is indicated for management of systemic metastases, an excellent effect often will be observed on the intraocular tumor.[80] Radiation as described for posterior uveal tumors is often effective. At < 30 Gy of photon irradiation, we have usually not seen major posterior segment complications.[53,81]

Juvenile Xanthogranuloma

Many JXG lesions of either the iris or, less commonly, the ciliary body, will spontaneously regress, often after one or two episodes of bleeding. When lesions are large or have produced either serial bleeds or glaucoma, intervention is necessary. Often JXG can be managed with a short course of high-dose systemic steroids.[11] Alternatively, treatment with 2 to 6 Gy of relatively low-dose photon radiation will control these tumors.[14] On those patients whose lesions fail to respond to either steroids or radiation, iridectomy or iridocyclectomy can be performed.

DIAGNOSIS OF CILIARY BODY MELANOMA

Choroidal or choroidal-ciliary body melanomas that involve ocular structures anterior to the equator of the globe carry a worse prognosis than those that do not. The prognosis for patients with an isolated ciliary body melanoma is uncertain.[82] In recent studies, conflicting reports on the effect of ciliary body involvement in melanoma-related prognosis were presented.[83] As discussed in Chapter 5, studies have shown that there are more consistent genomic changes (monosomy of chromosome 3) in ciliochoroidal, compared with posterior, uveal melanomas; however, the etiology and the importance of those genetic alterations remain to be defined.

The differential diagnosis of ciliary body tumors is more concise than that for choroidal tumefactions; however, there is probably a higher incidence of inaccurate diagnoses in tumors in this intraocular location.[84] Peripheral melanocytomas (which are most commonly jet-black), lymphoid tumors, leiomyoma (Figure 9–39) epithelial downgrowth with a cystic configuration, neurilemmoma, rarely

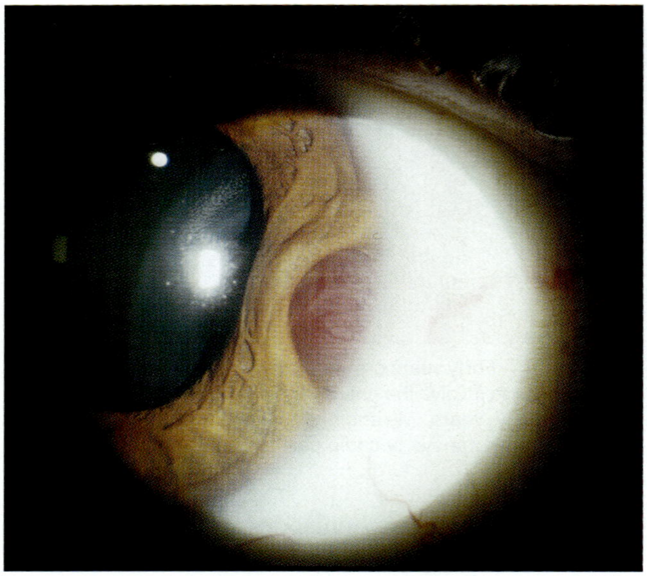

Figure 9–39. A growing benign iris-ciliary body leiomyoma that simulated a melanoma.

metastatic tumors, leiomyoma, xanthogranuloma, tumors of the ciliary epithelium, hemangiopericytoma, lacrimal gland choristoma, and scleral ectasia with uveal staphyloma (Figure 9–40) can simulate ciliary body melanomas.[13,85–100]

Mesectodermal leiomyomas can also simulate a ciliary melanoma.[101] In Figure 9–41, this tumor just appeared to produce forward bowing of the iris. On undilated examination, it perfectly mimicked an iris pigment cyst. There was tumor growth so that despite the benign appearance of the FNAB, we resected it, with a good result.

Ultrasonography is useful in the diagnosis of ciliary body or iris-ciliary body melanomas. The diag-

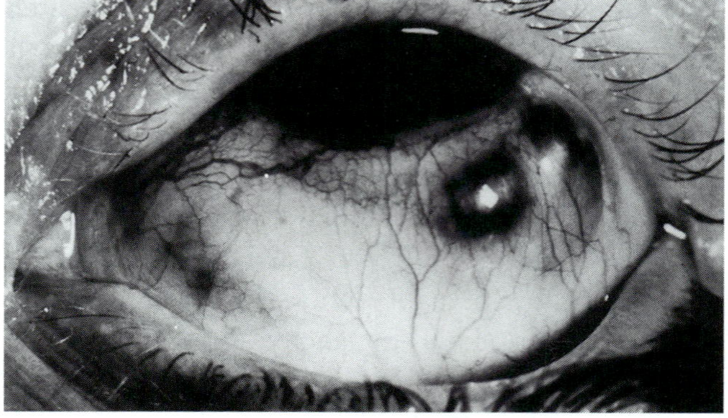

Figure 9–40. Ciliary body staphyloma simulates a melanoma with extraocular extension.

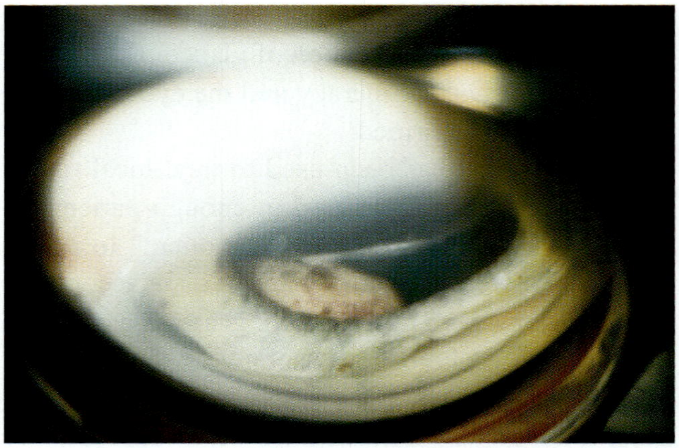

Figure 9–41. Benign, resected ciliary body mesectodermal leiomyoma.

nostic criteria are similar to those used for choroidal melanomas; however, we have observed some lesions that appeared cystic on ultrasonography (Figure 9–42) that histologically were not cysts.[86] Cavitary or cystic melanomas of the ciliary body do occur and can produce large cysts probably due to necrosis or exudation.[102,103] If high-frequency ultrasonography is used, up to 54 percent of normal adults may have small cysts, more commonly in the inferior temporal sector.[20] In difficult diagnostic cases, FNAB can be used. This procedure is described in Chapters 8 and 15. In some reports, however, all tests can be inaccurate, and benign conditions including neurilemmomas, melanocytomas, and adenomas have been mistakenly treated with enucleation.[95,97,101,104] We have not had a false-positive FNAB; although, as previously mentioned, in an almost totally necrotic choroidal melanoma, we recently had one false-negative result.

Tumors of the ciliary epithelium include the following: congenital medulloepithelioma and teratocarcinomas that usually occur in children and adenomas and adenocarcinomas that usually occur in adults.

The majority of medulloepitheliomas arise in childhood, with a median age of 5 years; the oldest reported case is 79-years-old.[90] These tumors can present with glaucoma, cataract, pain, a visible mass, leukocoria, or decreased vision.[61,91] Often, they are white, gray, or yellow; occasionally, a hemorrhage blackens the tumor. There are no established criteria to separate benign from malignant medulloepitheliomas; in one series, 4 of 37 patients died, all with orbital recurrence.[4] An atypical presentation of a

3-year-old with a malignant medulloepithelioma is shown in Figure 9–43. The child had whitish flocculent material in the anterior chamber. Figure 9–44 demonstrates another atypical case. This ciliary body medulloepithelioma was not treated, and the patient presented with a large orbital tumor. We have enucleated all such cases, since they were not focal when we first examined them. The Philadelphia group tried to resect a few, but 5 of 6 had to be enucleated.[105]

Adenomas of the ciliary epithelium can also simulate a ciliary body melanoma, producing cataracts and having associated pigmentation and episcleral sentinel vessels. Radioactive phosphorus uptake tests have been positive with some of these lesions.[92]

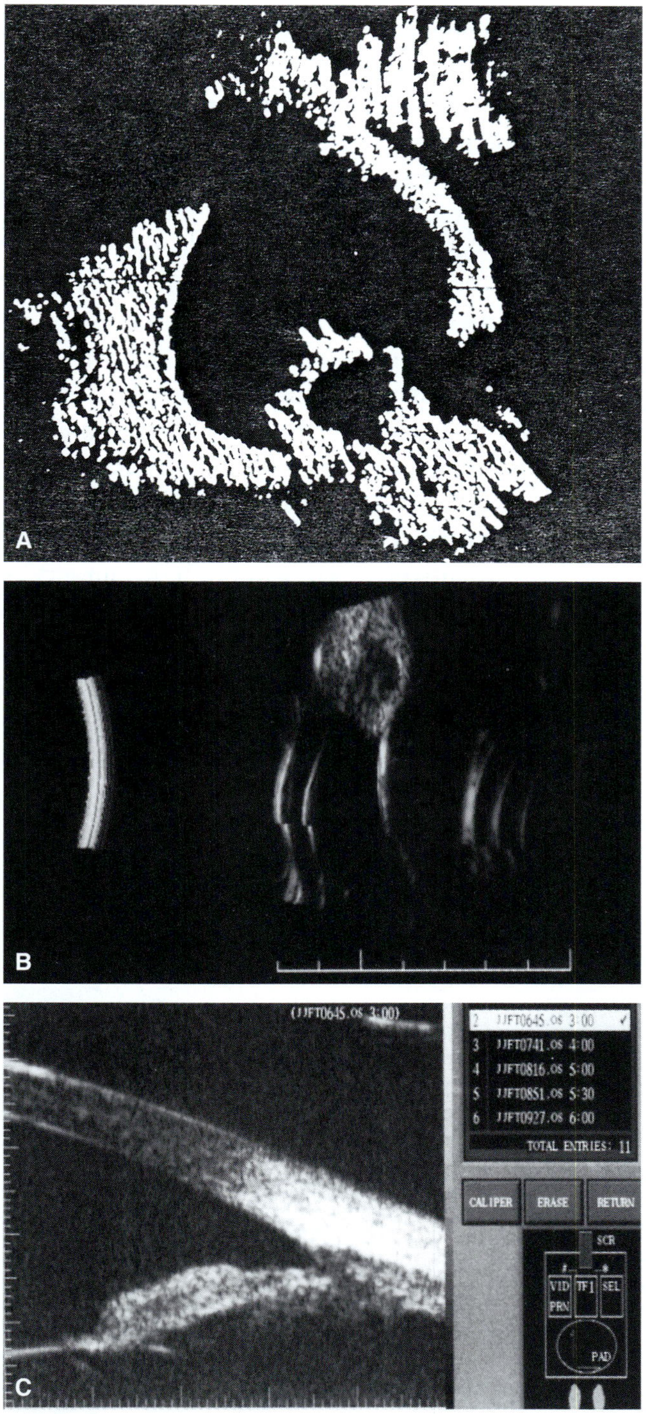

Figure 9–42. *A,* Ciliary body melanoma with ultrasonographically apparent cyst. On histologic examination, no cystic lesions were noted. *B,* Similarly, with high-frequency ultrasonography, there is an apparent cystic component of this iris-ciliary body melanoma. *C,* In contrast, this shows a solid iris melanoma which had documented growth.

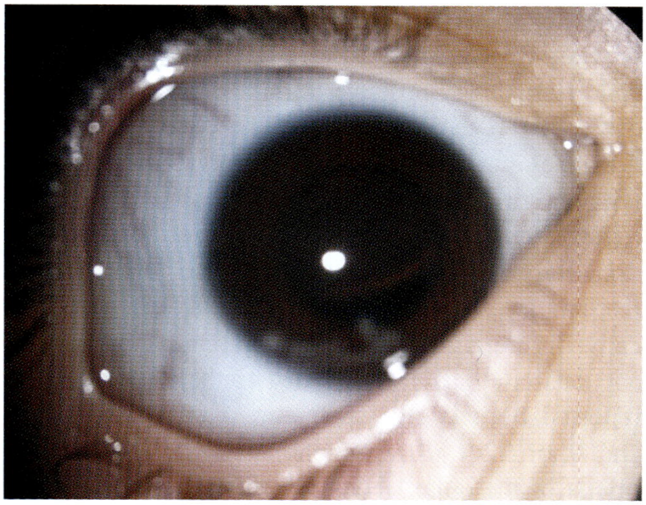

Figure 9–43. Malignant medulloepithlioma presenting 3 years prior to diagnosis with no mass and only flocculent white material in the anterior chamber.

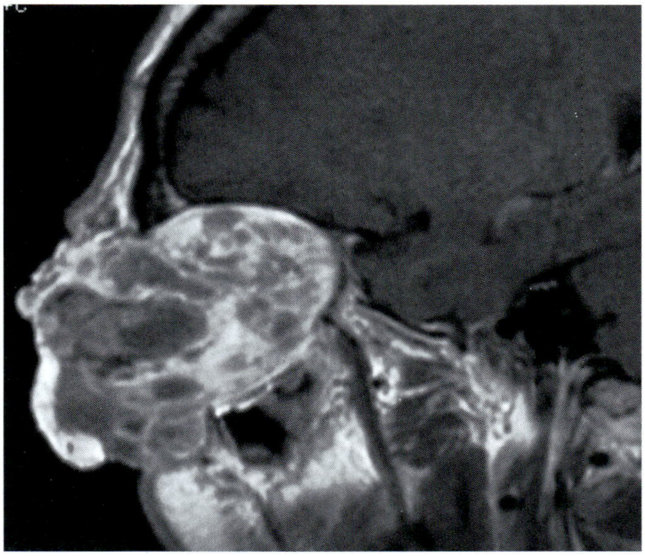

Figure 9–44. Neglected ciliary body medulloepithelioma that presented as an extensive mass and partially necrotic orbital mass.

As Shields has pointed out, usually, these are dark brown or black. Mostly, they are in the periphery and characteristically produce thinning, but not invasion, of the iris. If they are more in the ciliary body location, they have a regular surface, transmit light, and are highly reflective on ultrasonography.[106–108] In one report, a false-positive FNAB was described. As mentioned above, we have resected one of these lesions that had rapid, documented growth and was not clinically differentiated from a melanoma. Pleomorphic adenocarcinomas of the ciliary epithelium have been reported, but they had opaque media with blind eyes, and 9 of 12 eyes were phthisical.[109,110] Neurilemmoma of the ciliary body can simulate a melanoma with increased pigmentation, episcleral vessels, and a homogeneous appearance on ultrasonography.[13]

Shields and colleagues have pointed out that leiomyomas of the cilary body and peripheral choroid have a very typical clinical appearance. They transmit light, unlike melanomas, which block it. These tumors have been reported only in women. On fluorescein angiography, there is a normal uveal vasculature overlying them.[111] On FNAB, we have managed some patients with benign ciliary body lesions that have not grown on serial follow-up, but in whom we have not made a definitive diagnosis even with FNAB (Figure 9–45).

MANAGEMENT OF CILIARY BODY AND IRIS-CILIARY BODY MELANOMAS

General Considerations

There are a number of therapeutic options in the management of ciliary body or iris-ciliary body melanomas. Serial observation, charged particle or radioactive plaque radiation, local resection, and enucleation are indicated in different cases.[82,112–114] Small ciliary body or iris-ciliary body melanomas can be safely monitored, if they are < 10 mm in diameter and < 3 mm in thickness. Growing, small anterior uveal melanomas, those that have eroded through the iris root (Figure 9–46), vascular tumors, and lesions > 10 mm in diameter or > 3 mm in thickness should be treated at the time of diagnosis.

The relative efficacy of surgical removal versus irradiation of these tumors is unclear.[82,115–117] Iridocyclectomy, cyclectomy, cyclochoroidectomy, or iridocyclochoroidectomy has much higher complication rates when melanomas involve > 4 clock-hours of ocular circumference.[114–120] As discussed below, this type of surgery is technically challenging, and results vary widely.

There are no prospective, randomized data on resection versus radiation. Given the variability of surgical techniques, it is doubtful that meaningful data could be generated with that approach.

Our impression has been that two groups of patients are better managed with local resection, compared with radiation. In some focal ciliary body tumors that are 2 to 3 clock-hours in circumference, an experienced surgeon can usually remove them with good margins and preserve excellent vision. Unfortunately, most patients do not have small or small growing tumors isolated to the ciliary body that involve < 3 clock-hours of its circumference. In very thick tumors (generally > 7 mm), especially those with a relatively narrow tumor base, surgery is probably a better option than radiation. The rationale for that last statement is that in irradiated patients, independent of tumor location, tumor thickness (especially > 7 mm) is associated with a poorer ocular outcome. As tumors progressively thicken, there is a more than exponential increase in radiation-associated complications. Similarly, our experience with both brachytherapy and charged particles has shown that eyes with very thick ciliochoroidal

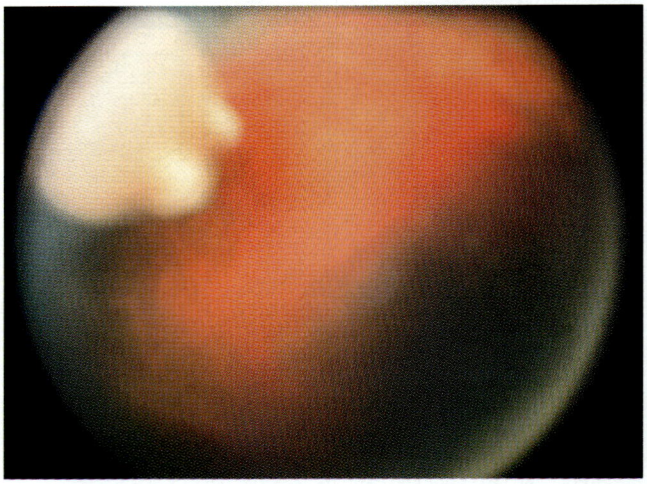

Figure 9–45. The FNAB shows a benign ciliary body spindle cell tumor; 5 years later, the mass is unchanged, and vision remains 20/20.

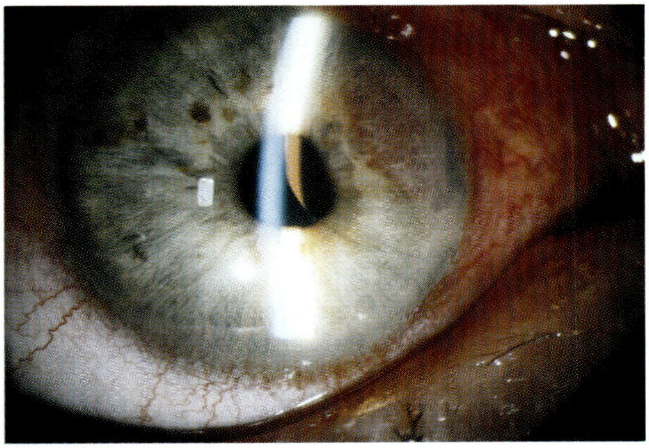

Figure 9–46. Anterior ciliary body melanoma with erosion through the iris root.

melanomas have over a 35 percent incidence of late enucleations from post-treatment complications, mainly neovascular glaucoma, and that < 20 percent retain good vision.[121,122] What has become apparent, however, is that iridocyolochoroidectomies alone are not sufficient, and even with clear surgical margins, patients do better if they have adjunctive radiation, either with particles or a beta-emitting plaque.[123]

The author has done over 150 choroidectomies, iridocyclectomies, and cyclochoroidectomies. What is uncertain is where the equation shifts toward favoring radiation over surgery or vice versa. Certainly a tumor > 15 mm in largest diameter or one that is relatively thin (< 5 mm height) will do better with radiation. It is technically difficult to resect tumors that involve that much of the ocular area, although we have successfully removed some lesions up to 18 mm in diameter. Similarly, eyes with tumors < 5 mm thick will usually have a lower incidence of complications with radiation, compared with surgical resection. As a general rule, while retinal detachment or increased tumor thickness does not pose added technical problems for the surgeon, tumor diameter > 15 mm, a tumor with retinal invasion and collar-button configuration with invasion through the retina, individual variations of orbital anatomy (ocular proptosis, the shape of the nose), and the posterior tumor edge contiguous with the optic nerve are major factors in complications that have been observed. If a ciliochoroidal tumor has broken through Bruch's membrane and has invaded the retina, it is often impossible to peel the inner part of the melanoma off the retina, and part of the tumor unfortunately may be left behind.

Cataract can occur with radiation as well as surgery. An advantage of surgery is that if it is successful, the tumor is removed and there is a lesser incidence of late complications. As discussed later, late recurrences can occur with either type of treatment. Most complications following surgery occur within the first 3 months, while radiation complications continue to develop for years after therapy.

Surgical Resection

Surgical Procedure

The two prevalent techniques for surgical resection of uveal tumors can be divided into (1) those utilizing a full-thickness, en bloc, sclera combined with melanoma resection with placement of an allogeneic corneal or scleral graft, and (2) those in which a 90 percent thickness scleral flap is created, and the tumor and overlying inner sclera are resected.[113–125] We prefer the latter approach and think it is technically easier and as effective as the former. Historically, some surgeons treated the peripheral retina (if the tumor did not involve the choroid) with a row of contiguous cryotherapy 6 weeks prior to resection to decrease the likelihood of retinal detachment. While we initially used this approach, in recent years we have stopped it without observing an increased incidence of retinal detachment. The majority of retinal detachments we have had have occurred either from traction away from the area of tumor resection or from a retinal hole created during surgery and would not have been prevented with this approach. Surgery is performed using hypotensive anesthesia if the patient's cardiovascular status allows it. The use of hypotensive anesthesia decreases bleeding during surgery and simplifies the operation. Unfortunately, the strong technical advantage of hypotensive anesthesia somewhat limits the patients who can be operated on. While one can do an anterior uveal resection without hypotension, we think it is very difficult to get good results for a posterior tumor, and we therefore do not use this treatment in patients who are very old and hypertensive, or have had recent myocardial infarctions or significant cardiovascular disease.

Historically, a modified Flieringa ring or eyewall basket was sutured to the area of resection. We stopped using those when we started to operate on larger tumors. At present, we only use this type of device when we are forced to operate on a young child with a very small tumor; that is quite rare.

Tumor localization techniques are discussed in Chapter 8. We use a corneal diffuse transilluminator as well as indirect ophthalmoscopy with point-source transillumination to localize the tumor. In addition, we use another type of transilluminator that we can hold against the sclera 180° away from the tumor mass. Using these three techniques we take a surgical marker and outline the tumor diameter on the sclera. As mentioned previously, corneal transillumination alone can produce a falsely increased posterior dimension to the tumor, as a result of a shadowing effect of the mass.

The use of an infusion cannula and vitrectomy equipment is optional. Some surgeons perform a vitrectomy in all cases, and often use silicone oil. We have tended not to do this but have instead only used vitrectomy when we felt it was indicated. If vitrectomy is going to be done, an infusion cannula should be sutured approximately 3.5 mm posterior to the limbus in an area 180° degrees away from the tumor. At that point, we also place diathermy marks at other sites 3.5 mm from the limbus that are away from the tumor for possible placement of a light pipe and vitrectomy instrumentation.

In the surgical resection of uveal melanomas, we create a 90 percent thickness scleral flap. If it is an iris-ciliary body tumor, the incision is started at the limbus and carried posteriorly as shown in Figures 9–47A and B. If the tumor is localized just to the choroid or choroid and posterior ciliary body the incision is started approximately 3 mm anterior to and away from the scleral margins of the neoplasm (see Figure 9–48).

A No. 59 Beaver blade is used to create the scleral flap. The edges of the flap should be at least 2 to 3 mm from the transilluminated edges of the tumor. If the sclera remaining over the tumor is too thin (1 to 5 percent thickness), uveal prolapse occurs and makes the dissection more difficult. If this is a problem over a small area, the site may be glued to provide temporary stability. If the scleral flap is too thin, poor closure and/or post surgical hypotony may develop.

A triple row of penetrating diathermy is placed in the resected scleral bed, around the circumference of the tumor as shown in Figure 9–47B. The purpose of the diathermy is threefold: (1) it may prevent a retinal detachment after resection of the tumor; (2) diathermy tends to diminish intraocular bleeding from the cut margins of the uvea at the time of resection. This bleeding is also decreased as a result of hypotensive anesthesia; and (3) if the resection is not complete and there is microscopic extension, it is conceivable that the contiguous rows of diathermy will have destroyed remaining tumor cells. It is likely that diathermy, used by many surgeons, has been partially responsible for the low rate of recurrence noted even when there is a microscopic tumor at the edge of resection following an iridocyclectomy.

As discussed below, the author strongly believes that there is marked difference in the shrinkage of the very thin normal surrounding uveal tissue, compared with the markedly thicker tumor when fixed for histologic sections. As a result, it can often be difficult to be certain if there is sufficient margin between the tumor and the edge of resection even when there is, in fact, a reasonable distance.

After diathermy, but before the tumor is resected, a vitrectomy instrument is placed in the eye, distant from the tumor, and approximately 1 to 1.5 mL of vitreous removed. A diamond knife is used to incise the remaining scleral fibers surrounding the tumor, starting posteriorly and going forward. If the iris is involved, corneal-scleral scissors are used at the limbus to open the wound. Using angled Vannas scissors, the iris portion of the tumor is excised. Using forceps to grasp scleral tissue overlying the tumor, corneal-scleral scissors are used (see Figure 9–47B) to remove the tumor and overlying sclera. If point-source bleeding is noted, a unipolar wet-field cautery is used for hemostasis. Usually, the tumor may be removed en bloc without loss of vitreous. In very thick tumors, often the apex of the lesion must be gently teased and slowly elevated from the retina and vitreous. We have experimented using a laser-scalpel or a CO_2 laser mounted on the microscope for this portion of the resection, but the author remains unconvinced that these techniques are an

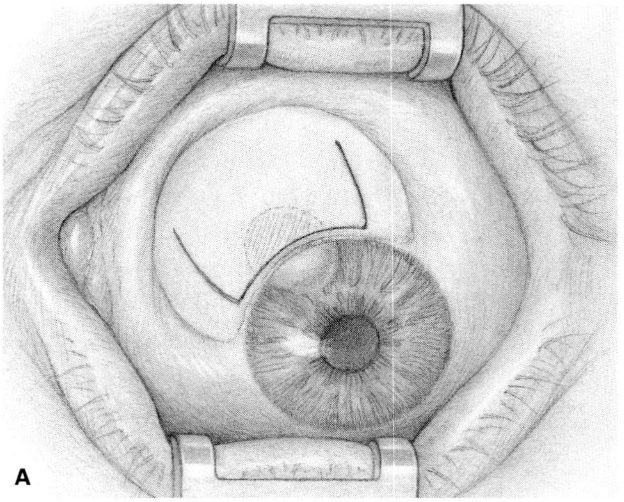

A

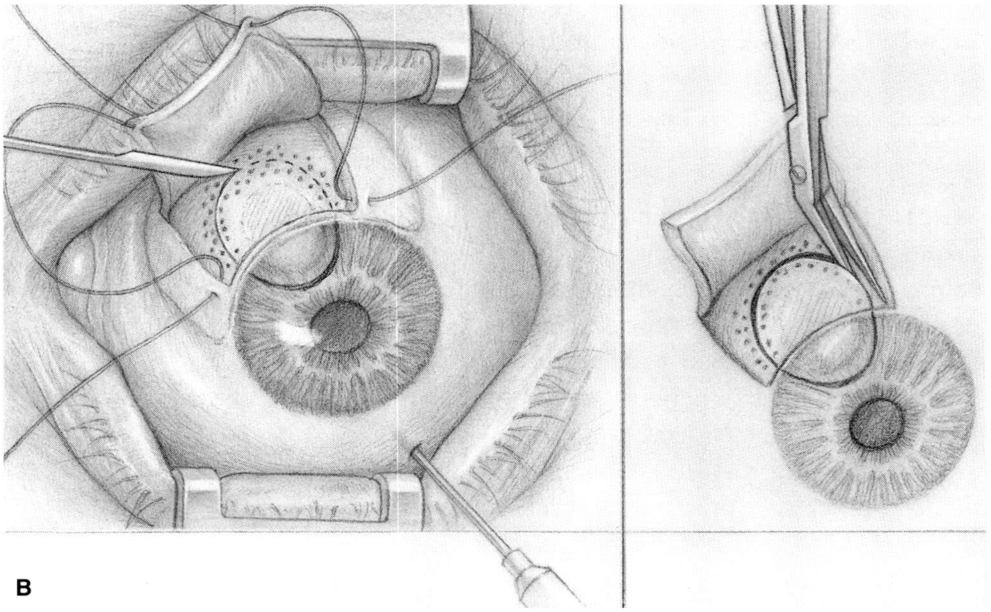

B

Figure 9–47. *A,* A 90 percent thickness scleral flap is created with a "posterior hinge." A few strands of sclera on the uveal surface remain overlying the tumor. *B,* A triple row penetrating diathermy is placed in the scleral bed around the circumference of the tumor. The tumor is resected with a scissors, and it is teased away from the vitreous base.

improvement. Preplaced 8-0 vicryl sutures at the corners of the incision (see Figure 9–47B) are tied. The scleral portion of the incision is closed with interrupted 8-0 vicryl sutures, while the corneal portion is closed with interrupted 10-0 nylon. Either the infusion port is used to refill the vitreous cavity for more posterior resections or for an iridocyclectomy, fluid balanced salt solution (BSS) is introduced through the limbal corneal incision. The suture lines are tested for a tight closure.

Postresection vitrectomy is usually not indicated, unless there is vitreous loss, a retinal detachment, or extensive hemorrhage. There is moderate bleeding at the time of resection in most cases, but usually this does not require intervention. If there is significant vitreous loss at surgery, a modified open-sky vitrectomy through the iridocyclectomy wound is performed to remove vitreous that is adherent to the wound edges. The eye is closed, and a standard, three-port vitrectomy is performed; if the lens is clear, it is not removed.

Results and Complications of Resection

The incidence of ocular complications is highest when larger-diameter (> 15 mm) ciliary body tumors and very large posterior choroidal tumors are resected. Immediate complications of surgery

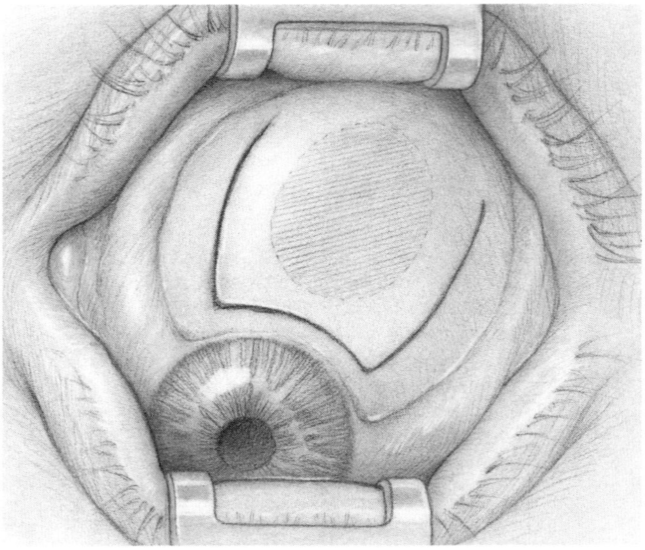

Figure 9–48. Schematic scleral incision for posterior tumors distal to the iris and anterior ciliary body. Scleral incisions are made approximately 3 mm from the tumor margin that was outlined by transillumination and marking pen, on the scleral surface.

include vitreous loss, vitreous hemorrhage, expulsive choroidal hemorrhage, retinal detachment, and intraocular infection. We have had 4 expulsive hemorrhages in over 150 cyclectomies or choriocyclectomies. Almost uniformly, especially if a choroidectomy is performed, an area of peripheral diffuse or focal, hemorrhagic choroidal detachment develops; this slowly resorbs over the first postoperative month. Sometimes, intraocular pressure is transiently elevated and requires a few days antiglaucoma treatment with timolol maleate (Timoptic), carbonic anhydrase inhibitors, or xalatan drops. Hypotony in the immediate postoperative period is associated with a poorer prognosis for retention of the eye. A topical steroid is used for the first 2 weeks to minimize inflammation; this drug may also increase intraocular presssure. Figure 9–49A and B shows an eye with large iris-ciliary body melanoma 2 years after successful resection, but with recurrent tumor (despite negative margins) 5 years later.

Figures 9–50 to 9–52A to C show several cases of large tumors that were resected with reasonable long-term outcome. All these lesions are large and would probably have had significant morbidity had radiation been used. On large tumors that involved the choroid, we routinely reinforced the vitreous base with a relatively high 42 band. The case shown in Figures 9–52A and B initially did well and then had a small recurrence (Figure 9–52C) 4 years later. This tumor was then treated with proton radiation.

The most common late complications after surgical resection include tumor recurrence, retinal detachment, and cystoid macular edema. Cystoid macular edema most commonly occurs following resection of a large tumor with vitreous loss, or persistent intraocular inflammation. This complication is quite difficult to manage, and most patients do not regain better than 20/200 vision.

In the author's experience, late tumor recurrence has been less common, if the surgical margins are clear, if penetrating diathermy was used around the circumference of the tumor, and if postoperative irradiation is given.[123] In one series, almost 40 percent of iridocyclectomy specimens had tumor at the surgical margins, and the majority did not recur.[126] In another series, incomplete resections, as evidenced by posi-

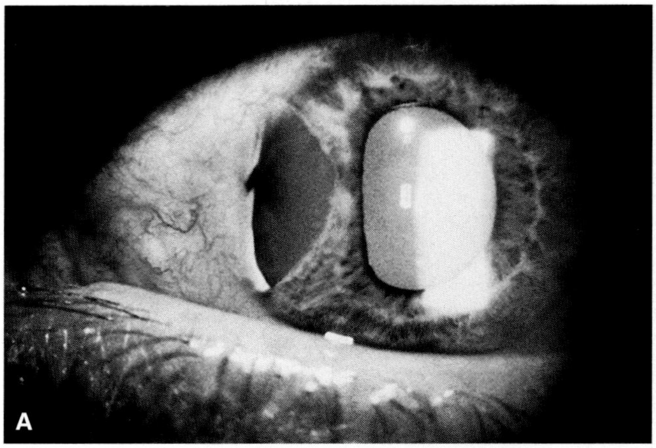

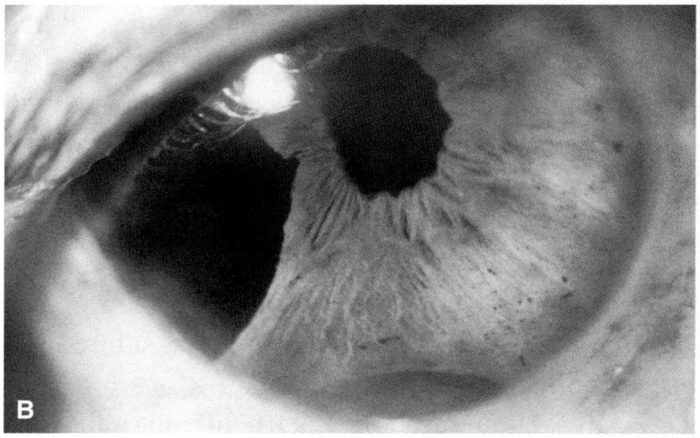

Figure 9–49. *A,* Postoperative appearance of the eye 2 years after resection of a large iris-ciliary body melanoma with good vision. *B,* Patient from Figure 9–49A, 5 years later with recurrent tumor despite clear histologic margins.

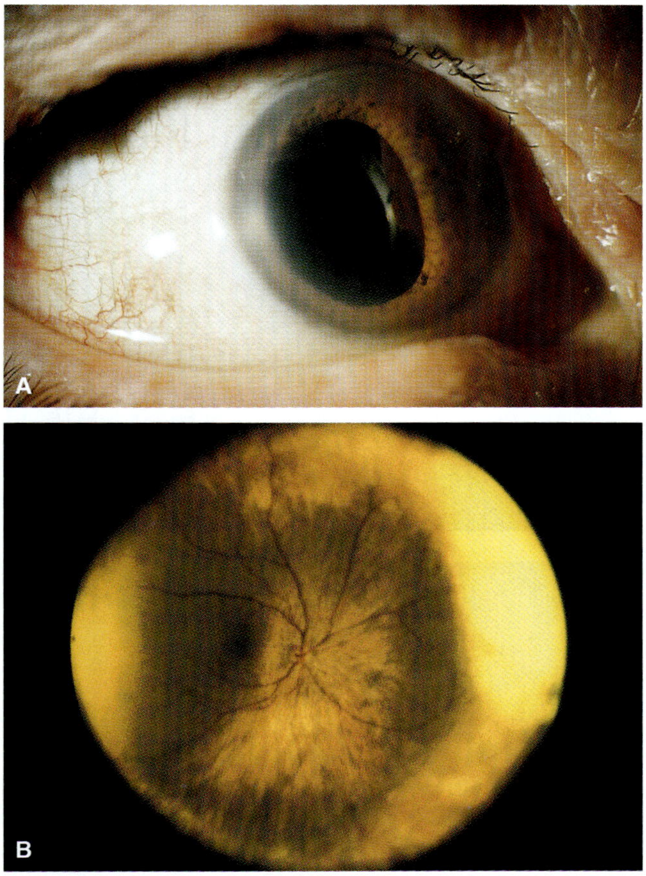

Figure 9–50. *A,* Large ciliochoroidal melanoma (9.5 mm thick) noted after cataract extraction. *B,* Resection of tumor resulted in 20/40 vision. Patient is alive and well 9 years later.

tive margins, was not a major prognostic factor.[119] Given the small specimen size, frozen sections have not been reliable to ascertain the adequacy of tumor margins. If only microscopic extension is noted on permanent histologic sections and there is no clinical evidence of tumor, these eyes irradiated postoperatively are monitored without further intervention. As discussed earlier, we hypothesize that many such cases have been cured by the surrounding diathermy. If there is gross tumor noted on both histologic and clinical examinations after surgery, the eye should be removed or treated with curative radiation with a radioactive plaque or charged particle beam, depending on the amount of residual or recurrent tumor.[119] Data presented by Damato and colleagues is intriguing regarding the beneficial effects of adjuvant radioactive plaques. In their experience, there was significantly less late recurrence when patients received adjuvant plaques; however, it is impossible from that retrospective data analysis to determine if other factors were important in the selection of patients who received radiation therapy.[119]

After surgical resection, all patients require continuing serial observations for possible tumor recurrence. Late retinal detachment usually occurs as a result of vitreous traction, following vitreous loss at surgery. Posterior surgical resections occasionally produce an iatrogenic retinal tear and a late rhegmatogenous retinal detachment.

Radiation Therapy

In eyes with larger-diameter (> 16 mm) ciliochoroidal melanomas, those that involve > 4 clock-hours (120°), or peripheral tumors > 10 mm in diameter and < 5 mm, radiation with either charged in thickness particles or brachytherapy seems to be more effective and has less complications than sur-

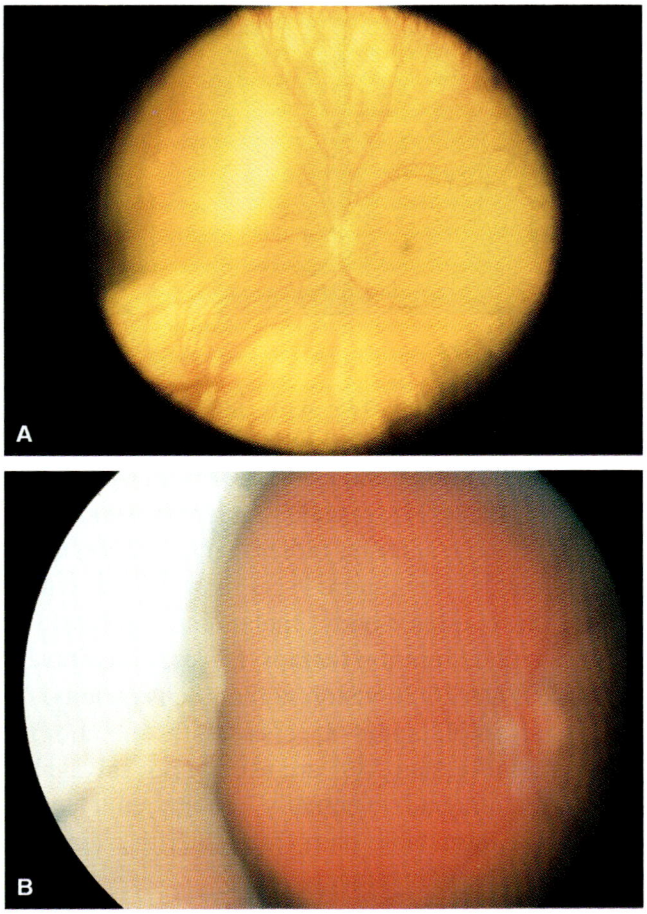

Figure 9–51. *A* and *B,* Large ciliochoroidal melanoma prior to and after resection with 20/25 vision.

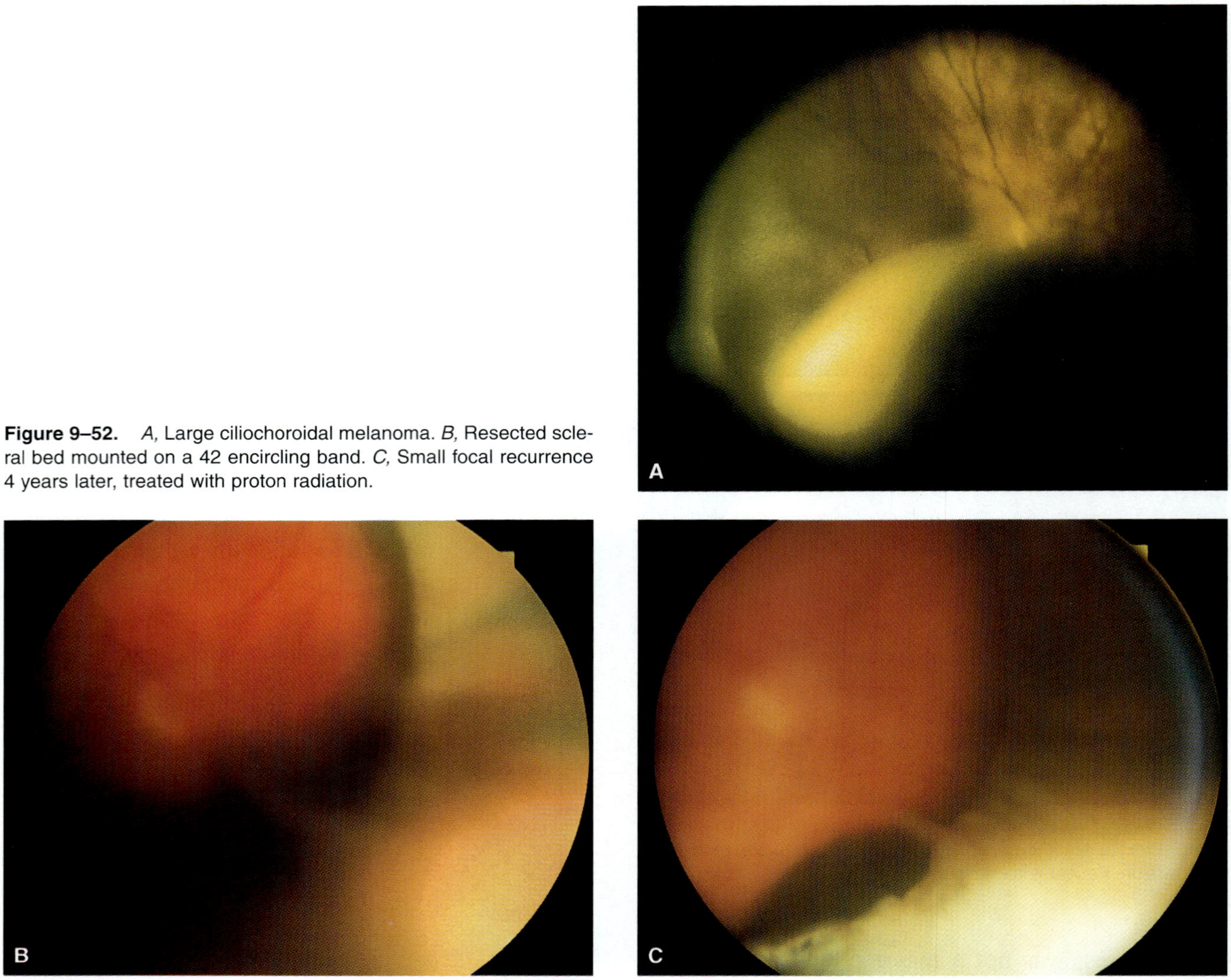

Figure 9–52. *A,* Large ciliochoroidal melanoma. *B,* Resected scleral bed mounted on a 42 encircling band. *C,* Small focal recurrence 4 years later, treated with proton radiation.

gical resection. Patients with larger-area anterior uveal melanomas have a higher incidence of significant complications and of loss of both vision and eye after therapy. Neovascular glaucoma is more frequent with large anterior, rather than posterior, uveal melanomas.[82,119,121] Figure 9–53 shows an eye with a 5-mm thick ciliary-body melanoma successfully treated with helium ion therapy 13 years previously; the patient has 20/20 vision without lens opacity. As discussed in Chapter 8, eyes with melanomas involving more than 180° are usually not salvagable with radiation and eventually require enucleation because of intractable pain from scleritis, keratitis, or neovascular glaucoma.

Anterior uveal melanomas that involve more than 180° of the angle are usually treated with enucleation.

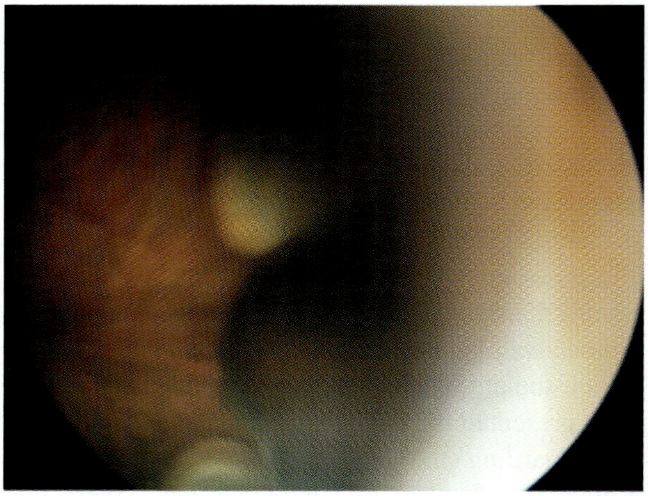

Figure 9–53. Five-millimeter thick ciliary body melanoma 8 years after successful treatment with helium ion irradiation. The lens remains clear and the vision is 20/20.

REFERENCES

1. Ferry AP. Lesion mistaken for malignant melanoma of the iris. Arch Ophthalmol 1965;74:9–18.
2. Gruenewald RL, Perry MC, Henry PH. Leukemic iritis with hypopyon. Cancer 1979;44:1511–3.
3. Bowns GT, Walls RP, Murphree AL, Ortega J. Neonatal neuroblastoma metastatic to the iris. Cancer 1983;52:929–31.
4. Broughton WL, Zimmerman LE. A clinicopathologic study of 56 cases of intraocular medulloepitheliomas. Am J Ophthalmol 1978;85:407–18.
5. Shields MB, Campbell DG, Simmons RJ. The essential iris atrophies. Am J Ophthalmol 1978;85:749–59.
6. Geisse LJ, Robertson DM. Iris melanomas. Am J Ophthalmol 1985;99:638–48.
7. Shields JA, Augsburger JJ, Sanborn GE, Klein RM. Adenoma of the iris-pigment epithelium. Ophthalmology 1983;90:735–9.
8. Ashton N. Primary tumours of the iris. Br J Ophthalmol 1964;48:650–68.
9. Shields JA, Sanborn GE, Augsburger JJ. The differential diagnosis of malignant melanoma of the iris. Ophthalmology 1983;90:716–20.
10. Brenkman RF, Oosterhuis JA, Manschot WA. Recurrent hemorrhage in the anterior chamber caused by a (juvenile) xanthogranuloma of the iris in an adult. Doc Ophthalmol 1977;42:329–33.
11. Bruner WE, Stark WJ, Green WR. Presumed juvenile xanthogranuloma of the iris and ciliary body in an adult. Arch Ophthalmol 1982;100:457–9.
12. Wertz FD, Zimmerman LE, McKeown CA, et al. Juvenile xanthogranuloma of the optic nerve, disc, retina and choroid. Ophthalmology 1982;89:1331–5.
13. Rosso R, Colombo R, Ricevuti G. Neurilemmoma of the ciliary body: report of a case. Br J Ophthalmol 1983;67:585–7.
14. Treacy KW, Letson RD, Summers CG. Subconjunctival steroid in the management of uveal juvenile xanthogranuloma: a case report. Pediatr Ophthalmol Stabisismus 1990;27:126–8.
15. Shields JA, Kline MW, Augsburger JJ. Primary iris cysts: a review of the literature and report of 62 cases. Br J Ophthalmol 1984;68:152–66.
16. Waeltermann JM, Hettinger ME, Cibis GW. Congential cysts of the iris stroma. Am J Ophthalmol 1985; 100:549–54.
17. Krohn J, Hove VK. Iris cyst associated with topical administration of latanorprost. Am J Ophthalmol 1999;127:91–3.
18. Scholz RT, Kelley JS. Argon laser photocoagulation treatment of iris cysts following penetrating keratoplasty. Arch Ophthlmol 1982;100:926–7.
19. Capo H, Palmer E, Nicholson DH. Congenital cysts of the iris stroma. Am J Ophthalmol 1993;116:228–32.
20. Lois N, Shields CL, Shields JA, et al. Primary iris stromal cysts: a report of 17 cases. Ophthalmol 1998; 105:1317–22.
21. Lois N, Shields CL, Shields JA, Mercado G. Primary cysts of the iris pigment epithelium. Ophthalmol 1998;105:1879–85.
22. Albert DL, Brownstein S, Kattleman BS. Mucogenic glaucoma caused by an epithelial cyst of the iris stroma. Am J Ophthalmol 1992;114:222–4.
23. Marigo FA, Finger PT, McCormic SA, et al. Anterior segment implantation cysts. Ultrasound biomicroscopy with histopathologic correlation. Arch Ophthalmol 1998;116:1569–75.
24. Brent DJ, Misler DM, Krishna R, Vaerveld TG. Spontaneous collapse of primary iris stromal cysts. Am J Ophthalmol 1996;122:86–7.
25. Ticho BH, Rosner M, Mets MB, Tso MOM. Bilateral diffuse iris nodular nevi. Ophthalmology 1995;102: 419–25.
26. Paridaen SD, Lyons CJ, McCartney A, Hungerford JL. Familial aggressive nevi of the iris in childhood. Arch Ophthalmol 1991;109:1552–4.
27. Shields JA, Annesley WH, Spaeth GL. Necrotic melanocytoma of iris with secondary glaucoma. Am J Ophthalmol 1977;84:826–9.
28. Thomas CI, Purnell EW. Ocular melanocytoma. Am J Ophthalmol 1969;67:79–86.
29. Howard GM, Forrest AW. Incidence and location of melanocytomas. Arch Ophthalmol 1967;77:61–6.
30. Raichand M, Peyman G, Juarez C, et al. Resection melanocytoma: clinicopathological correlation. Br J Ophthalmol 1983;67:236–47.
31. Shammas HJ, Minckler DS, Hulquist CR, Sherins RS. Melanocytoma of the ciliary body. Ann Ophthalmol 1981;13:1381–3.
32. Shields JA, Augsberger JJ, Bernardino V Jr, et al. Melanocytoma of the ciliary body and iris. Am J Ophthalmol 1980;89:632–5.
33. Rootman J, Gallagher RP. Colors a risk factor in iris melanoma. Am J Ophthalmol 1984;98:558–61.
34. Spencer WH. Ophthalmic pathology. An atlas and textbook, Vol. 3. Philadelphia, PA: WB Saunders Co; 1986.
35. Rahany U, Rumelt S. Iridocorneal melanoma associated with type 1 neurofibromatosis. Ophthalmol 1999;106:614–8.
36. Endo EG, Walton DS, Albert DM. Neonatal hepatoblastoma metastatic to the choroid and iris. Arch Ophthalmol 1996;114:757–61.
37. Litricin O. Diffuse malignant ring melanoma of the iris and ciliary body. Ophthalmologica 1979;178:235–8.
38. Jensen OA, Johansen S, Kiss K. Intraocular T-cell lymphoma mimicking a ring melanoma: first manifestation of systemic disease. Graefe's Arch Clin Exp Ophthalmol 1994;232:148–52.

39. Reese AB, Mund ML, Iwamoto T. Tapioca melanoma of the iris: Part I. Clinical and light microscopy studies. Am J Ophthalmol 1972;74:840–50.
40. Jakobiec FA, Silbert G. Are most iris "melanomas" really nevi? A clinicopathological study of 189 lesions. Arch Ophthalmol 1981;99:2117–32.
41. Pavlin CJ, McWhae JA, McGowan HD, Foster FS. Ultrasound biomicroscopy of anterior segment tumors. Ophthalmology 1992;99:1220–8.
42. Brovkina AF, Chichua AG. Value of fluorescein iridography in diagnosis of tumours of the iridociliary zone. Br J Ophthalmol 1979;63:157–60.
43. Demeler U. Fluorescence angiographical studies in the diagnosis and follow-up of tumors of the iris and ciliary body. Adv Ophthalmol 1981;42:1–17.
44. Jakobiec FA, Depot MJ, Henkind P, Spencer WH. Fluorescein angiographic patterns of iris melanocytic tumors. Arch Ophthalmol 1982;100:1288–99.
45. Fries PD, Char DH. Fluorescein angiography of ciliary body melanomas. Ophthalmologica 1990;201:57–65.
46. Grossniklaus HG. Fine-needle aspiration biopsy of the iris. Arch Ophthalmol 1992;110:969–76.
47. Alvarado JA, Underwood JL, Green WR, et al. Detection of herpes simplex viral DNA in the iridocorneal endothelial syndrome. Arch Ophthalmol 1994;112:1601–9.
48. Wyzinski P, Rootman J, Wood W. Simultaneous bilateral iris metastases from renal cell carcinoma. Am J Ophthalmol 1981;92:206–9.
49. De Rivas P, Marti T, Andreu D, et al. Metastatic bronchogenic carcinoma of the iris and ciliary body. Arch Ophthalmol 1991;109:470.
50. Bowman CB, Guber D, Brown CH, Curtin VT. Cutaneous malignant melanoma with diffuse intraocular metastases. Arch Ophthalmol 1994;112:1213–6.
51. Ainsworth JR, Damato BE, Lee WR, Alexander WD. Follicular thyroid carcinoma metastatic to the iris: a solitary lesion treated with iridocyclectomy. Arch Ophthalmol 1992;110:19–20.
52. Weisenthal R, Brucker A, Lanciano R. Follicular thyroid cancer metastatic to the iris. Arch Ophthalmol 1989;107:494–5.
53. Char DH, Schwartz A, Miller TR, Abele JF. Ocular metastases from systemic melanoma. Am J Ophthalmol 1980;90:702–7.
54. Capeans C, Santos L, Sanchez-Salorio M, Forteza J. Iris metastasis from endometrial carcinoma. Am J Ophthalmol 1998;125:729–30.
55. Gunduz K, Shields JA, Shields CL, et al. Ewing sarcoma metastatic to the iris. Am J Opthalmol 1997;124:550–2.
56. Ware GT, Haik BG, Morris WR. Renal cell carcinoma with involvement of iris and conjunctiva. Am J Ophthalmol 1999;127:460–1.
57. Denslow GT, Kielar RA. Metastatic adenocarcinoma to the anterior uvea and increased carcinoembryonic antigen levels. Am J Ophthalmol 1978;85:363–7.
58. Ninane J, Taylor D, Day S. The eye as a sanctuary in acute lymphoblastic leukaemia. Lancet 1980;I:452–3.
59. Lewis RA, Riccardi VM. Von Recklinghausen neurofibromatosis. Incidence of iris hamartomata. Ophthalmology 1981;88:348–54.
60. Bouzas EA, Mastorakos G, Chrousos GP, Kaiser MI. Lisch nodules in Cushing disease. Arch Ophthalmol 1993;111:439–40.
61. Parmley VC, George DP, Fannin LA. Juvenile xanthogranuloma of the iris in an adult. Arch Ophthalmol 1998;116:377–9.
62. Chang MW, Frieden IJ, Good W. The risk of intraocular juvenile xanthogranuloma: survey of current practices and assessment of risk. J Am Acad Dermatol 1996;34:445–9.
63. Kluppel M, Muler W, Sundmacher R. Lacrimal gland choristoma of the iris. Arch Ophthalmol 1999;117:110–1.
64. Spraul CW, d'Heurle D, Grossniklaus HE. Adenocarcinoma of the iris pigment epithelium. Arch Ophthalmol 1996;114:1512–7.
65. Foss AJE, Pecorella I, Alexander RA, et al. Are most intraocular "leiomyomas" really melanocytic lesions? Ophthalmology 1994;101:919–24.
66. Shields JA, Eagle RC Jr, Shields CL, et al. Natural course and histopathologic findings of lacrimal gland choristoma of the iris and ciliary body. Am J Ophthalmol 1995;119:219–24.
67. Elsas FJ, Mroczek EC, Kelly DR, Specht CS. Primary rhabdomyosarcoma of the iris. Arch Ophthalmol 1991;109:982–4.
68. Arentsen JJ, Green WR. Melanoma of the iris: report of 72 cases treated surgically. Ophthal Surg 1975;6:23–37.
69. Noor Sunba MS, Rahi AHS, Morgan G. Tumors of the anterior uvea: I. Metastasizing malignant melanoma of the iris. Arch Ophthalmol 1990;108:1287–90.
70. Yanoff M. Glaucoma mechanisms in ocular malignant melanomas. Am J Ophthalmol 1970;70:898–904.
71. Shields MB, Klintworth GK. Anterior uveal melanomas and intraocular pressure. Ophthalmology 1980;87:503–17.
72. Shields MB, Proia AD. Neovascular glaucoma associated with an iris melanoma. Arch Ophthalmol 1987;105:672–4.
73. Char DH, Kroll SM, Stoloff A, et al. Cytomorphometry of uveal melanomas: comparison of fine-needle aspiration biopsy samples with histologic sections. Anal Quant Cytol Histol Aug 1991;13:293–9.
74. Char DH, Crawford JB, Kroll S, O'Brien JM. Iris melanoma: diagnostic problems. Ophthalmology 1996;103:251–5.

75. Shields CL, Shields JA, De Potter P, et al. Treatment of non-resectable malignant iris tumors with custom design plaque radiotherapy. Br J Ophthalmol 1995; 79:306–12.
76. Wilson RS, Fraunfelder FT, Hanna C. Recurrent tapioca melanoma of the iris and ciliary body treated with Argon laser. Am J Ophthalmol 1976;82:213–7.
77. Lewis RA, Tse DT, Phelps DC, Weingeist TA. Neovascular glaucoma after photo-irradiation therapy for uveal melanoma. Arch Ophthalmol 1984;102: 839–42.
78. Davidorf J, Davidorf F. Treatment of iris melanoma with photodynamic therapy. Ophthal Surg 1992;23: 522–7.
79. Charteris DG. Progression of an iris melanoma over 41 years. Br J Ophthalmol 1990;74:566–7.
80. Sierocki JS, Charles NC, Schafrank M, Wittes RE. Carcinoma metastatic to the anterior ocular segment: response to chemotherapy. Cancer 1980;45:2521–3.
81. Char DH. Radiation therapy in the management of ocular and adnexal tumors. International Seminar in the Pharmacology of Ocular Surgery. Porvoo, Finland. In: Sears ML, Tarkkanen A, editors. Surgical pharmacology of the eye. New York, NY: Raven Press; 1985. p. 523–36.
82. Char DH. Radiation therapy for uveal melanomas involving the ciliary body. Trans Ophthalmol Soc UK 1986;105:252–6.
83. Ainbinder DJ, Gamel JW, McLean IW, McCurdy JB. Multivariate survival analysis with ciliary body melanoma. Invest Ophthalmol Vis Sci 1994;35:1927.
84. Char DH, Miller T. Accuracy of presumed melanoma diagnosis prior to alternative therapy. Br J Ophthalmol 1995;79:692–6.
85. Karcioglu ZA, Hemphill GL, Wool BM, et al. Granular cell tumor of the orbit: case report and review of the literature. Ophthal Surg 1983;14:125–9.
86. Zakka KA, Foos RY, Spencer WH, et al. Cavitation in intraocular malignant melanoma. Arch Ophthalmol 1982;100:112–4.
87. Croxatto JO, Malbran ES. Unusual ciliary body tumor. Ophthalmology 1982;89:1208–12.
88. Pe'er J, Hidayat AA. Malignant teratoid medulloepithelioma manifesting as a black epibulbar mass with expulsive hemorrhage. Arch Ophthalmol 1984; 102:1523–7.
89. Ryan SJ Jr, Frank RN, Green WR. Bilateral inflammatory pseudotumors of the ciliary body. Am J Ophthalmol 1971;72:586–91.
90. Floyd BB, Minckler DS, Valentin L. Intraocular medulloepithelioma in a 79 year old man. Ophthalmology 1982;89:1088–94.
91. Brownstein S, Barsoum-Homsy M, Conway VH, et al. Nonteratoid medulloepithelioma of the ciliary body. Ophthalmology 1984;91:1118–22.
92. Chang M, Shields JA, Wachtel DL. Adenoma of the pigment epithelium of the ciliary body simulating a malignant melanoma. Am J Ophthalmol 1979;88: 40–4.
93. Smith PA, Damato BE, Ko M-K, Lyness RW. Anterior uveal neurilemmoma: a rare neoplasm simulating malignant melanoma. Br J Ophthalmol 1987;71: 34–40.
94. Brown HH, Brodsky MC, Hembree K, Mrak RE. Supraciliary hemangiopericytoma. Ophthalmology 1991;98:378–82.
95. Campochiaro PA, Gonzalez-Ferandez F, Newman SA, et al. Ciliary body adenoma in a 10-year-old girl who had a rhabdomyosarcoma. Arch Ophthalmol 1992;110:681–3.
96. Kuchle M, Holbach L, Schlotzer-Schrehardt U, Naumann GOH. Schwannoma of the ciliary body treated by block excision. Br J Ophthalmol 1994; 78:397–400.
97. Rummelt V, Naumann GOH, Folberg R, Weingeist TA. Surgical management of melanocytoma of the ciliary body with extraocular extension. Am J Ophthalmol 1994;117:169–76.
98. Dutton JJ, Barbour HL. Hürthle cell carcinoma metastatic to the ciliary body. Cancer 1997;73:163–7.
99. Schalenbourg A, Uffer S, Chamot L, et al. Adenocarcinoma of the nonpigmented ciliary body epithelium: report of a rare case. Bull Soc Belg Ophthalmol 1999;271:29–35.
100. Rowley SA, Karwatowski WSS. Lacrimal gland choristoma of the ciliary body. Arch Ophthalmol 1997;115:1482–3.
101. Yu D-Y, Cohen SB, Peyman G, Tso MOM. Mesectodermal leiomyoma of the ciliary body: New evidence for neural crest origin. J Pediatr Ophthalmol Strabismus 1990;27:317–21.
102. Scott CT, Holland GN, Glasgow AJ. Cavitation in a ciliary body melanoma. Am J Ophthalmol 1997;123: 269–71.
103. Lois N, Shields CL, Shields JA, et al. Cavitary melanomas of the ciliary body: a study of 8 cases. Ophthalmology 1998;105:1091–8.
104. Smith PA, Damato BE, Ko M-K. Bilateral inflammatory pseudotumors of the ciliary body. Am J Ophthalmol 1987;72:586–91.
105. Shields JA, Eagle RC Jr, Shields CL, De Potter P. Congenital neoplasms of the nonpigmented ciliary epithelium (medulloepithelioma). Ophthalmology 1996;103:1998–2006.
106. Shields JA, Shields CL, Mercado G, et al. Adenoma of the iris pigment epithelium: a report of 20 cases. Arch Ophthalmol 117:736–41.
107. Cursiefen C, Schalotzer-Schrehardt U, Holback LM. Adenoma of the non-pigmented ciliary epithelium mimicking a malignant melanoma of the iris. Arch Ophthalmol 1999;117:113–6.

108. Husain SE, Husain N, Boniuk M, Font RL. Malignant nonteratoid medulloepthelioma of the ciliary body in an adult. Ophthalmology 1998;105:596–9.
109. Laver NM, Hidayat AA, Croxatto JO. Pleomorphic adenocarcinomas of the ciliary epithelium. Ophthalmology 1999;106:103–10.
110. Mkunimatsu S, Kraie N, Oharakhamada C. Ultrasound of ciliary body cysts. Am J Ophthalmol 1999;127: 48–55.
111. Shields JA, Shields CL, Eagle RC, De Potter P. Observations on seven cases of intraocular leiomyoma. Arch Ophthalmol 1994;112:521–8.
112. Makley TA Jr. Management of melanomas of the anterior segment. Surv Ophthalmol 1974;19:135–53.
113. Kara GB. Excision of uveal melanomas: a 15-year experience. Ophthalmology 1979;86:997.
114. Naumann GOH, Volcker HE, Gackle D. The blockexcision of malignant melanomas of the ciliary body and peripheral choroid. Doc Ophthalmol 1980;50:43.
115. Robertson DM, Campbell RJ, Weaver DT. Residual intrascleral melanoma. A concern with lamellar sclerouvectomy for uveal melanoma. Am J Ophthalmol 1992;113:467–8.
116. Shields JA, Shields CL, De Potter P: Residual intrascleral and intraretinal melanoma. A concern with lamellar sclerouvectomy for uveal melanoma. Am J Ophthalmol 1992;113:464–7.
117. Peyman GA. Residual intrascleral melanoma. A concern with lamellar sclerouvectomy for uveal melanoma. Am J Ophthalmol 1992;113:467–8.
118. Peyman GA, Apple DJ. Local excision of a choroidal malignant melanoma: full thickness eye wall resection. Arch Ophthalmol 1976;92:216.
119. Damato BE, Paul J, Foulds WS. Risk factors for residual and recurrent uveal melanoma after trans-scleral local resection. Br J Ophthalmol 1996;80:102–8.
120. Shields JA, Shields CL, Shah P, Sivalingam V. Partial lamellar sclerouvectomy for ciliary body and choroidal tumors. Ophthalmology 1991;98:971–83.
121. Decker M, Castro JR, Linstadt DE, et al. Ciliary body melanoma treated with helium particle irradiation. Int J Radiat Oncol Biol Phys 1990;19:243–7.
122. Reese A, Jones I, Cooper W. Surgery for tumors of the iris and ciliary body. Am J Ophthalmol 1968;66: 173–83.
123. Damato BE, Paul J, Foulds WS. Risk factors for metastatic uveal melanoma after trans-scleral local resection. Br J Ophthalmol 1996;80:109–16.
124. Linnic LF. Surgery of tumors of the ciliary body and base of the iris. Br J Ophthalmol 1968;52:289–96.
125. Stallard HB. Partial choroidectomy. Br J Ophthalmol 1966;50:660–2.
126. Forrest AW, Keyser RB, Spencer WH. Iridocyclectomy for melanomas of the ciliary body: a follow-up study of pathology and surgical morbidity. Ophthalmology 1978;85:1237–49.

10

Intraocular Lymphoid and Myeloid Lesions

Lymphoid and myeloid lesions can involve all layers of the eye. While these lesions are rare, leukemias, "ocular reticulum cell sarcoma" (intraocular lymphoma), systemic lymphoma with secondary intraocular deposits, and benign lymphoid proliferations can all simulate either solid intraocular tumors or inflammations of the uvea, vitreous, or optic nerve. Differential diagnosis is discussed in Chapter 6.

LEUKEMIA

The clinical entity of leukemic ophthalmopathy was first described in 1861, and historically, eye findings were an initial diagnostic sign in this malignancy.[1] Most of the retinal findings in leukemia are not due to neoplastic cells but associated hematologic abnormalities, including severe anemia, hypoxia, hyperviscosity, ischemia, and vascular stasis.[2,3] Other retinal findings are hard exudates, cottonwool spots, tortuous veins, and intraretinal hemorrhages.[4] Less commonly, retinal changes from infective processes or peripheral retinal neovascularization can occur in chronic leukemias.[2,5–9] Vascular sheathing is probably due to perivascular infiltrates. Rarely, this simulates a branch angiitis.[10] A number of studies have shown no correlation between retinal involvement, prognosis, and red cell, white cell, or platelet counts.[11–13]

In a postmortem review by Allen and Straatsma, approximately 80 percent of leukemic patients had ocular involvement.[14] Analogous findings were reported by Kincaid and Green; 80 percent of all leukemic cases had some ocular involvement, and in acute leukemia, this incidence did not change from 1920 to 1970.[15] Choroidal involvement is found in over 85 percent of the eyes of leukemia patients, but it is usually not clinically apparent; Kincaid and Green noted this finding in 232 of 257 eyes.[15] Rarely, an exudative retinal detachment in association with choroidal infiltration is the first sign of leukemia. Choroidal detachments due to diffuse leukemic infiltration can occur in adults, and occasionally, a mass can be present.[16–19] In a prospective study, Karesh and colleagues noted intraocular abnormalities in 30 of 53 patients prior to the initiation of systemic therapy.[20] Others have noted a slightly lower incidence of these findings, and this probably reflects a difference in referral patterns.[21] In a study from Malaysia, the authors did not find an association in retinal findings in leukemia with either the hemoglobin or the platelet levels.[22] In adult acute leukemia, there was a correlation between the presence of intraretinal hemorrhages, older age at diagnosis, higher white cell count, and a shorter survival.[23]

When the anterior uvea, especially the iris, is involved with leukemia, there is often a pseudohypopyon (Figure 10–1A and B). Usually, anterior segment involvement is noted either with a systemic leukemic relapse or with central nervous system (CNS) leukemia; it is extremely uncommon for it to be the first sign of the disease.[6,23–28] Rarely, a patient with leukemia can develop malignant transformation and develop lymphoma in one or both eyes.[26] The diagnosis in all these cases can be established with aspiration cytology.[6,24–26,29–31] Iris involvement can also be manifested by color change, mass, or hemorrhage. Often, this is the first sign of leukemic relapse. Rarely, an iris relapse is misdiagnosed as an anterior uveitis and treated with topical steroids; usually, this

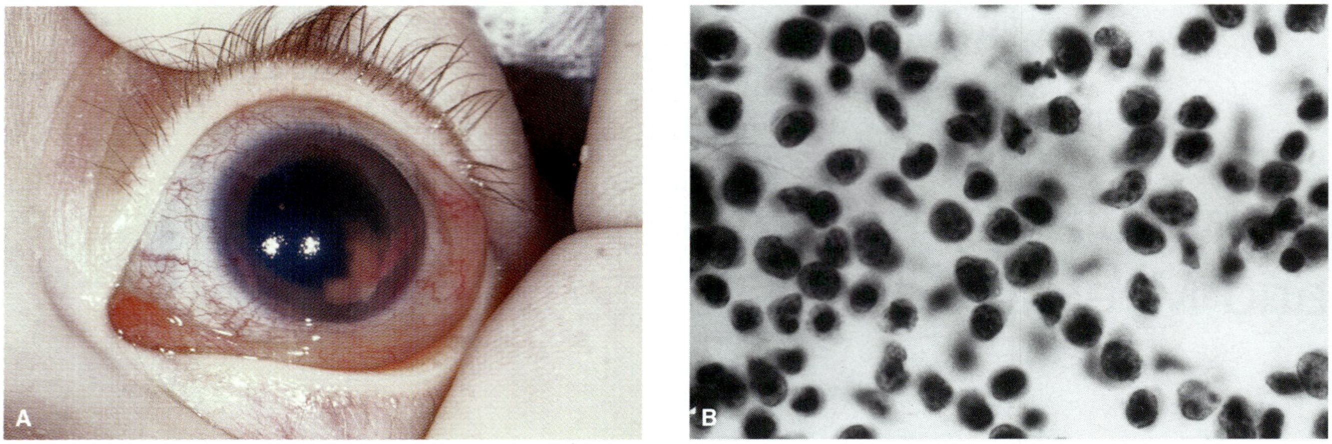

Figure 10–1. Acute lymphocytic leukemia with iris involvement and malignant hypopyon.

occurs if a thorough history was not obtained. The patient shown in Figure 10–2A presented to me with a ciliary body mass and a history of "iridocyclitis" treated with topical prednisolone. Figure 10–2B demonstrates enhancement of the area with gadolinium on T_1-weighted axial magnetic resonance imaging (MRI). This lesion was correctly diagnosed with fine-needle aspiration biopsy (FNAB).

The optic nerve involvement in leukemia can be due to direct extension from the central nervous system, passive swelling by a retrobulbar leukemic infiltration, or increased intracranial pressure. Most patients we have seen with an optic nerve infiltrate (Figure 10–3) have had acute leukemia, but in a large series reported from the Wilmer Institute, the incidence of optic nerve involvement was approximately 18 percent and was similar in both acute and chronic leukemias.[15] Similarly, in another series, optic nerve involvement was noted in 9 of 29 children with leukemia.[29] It most frequently occurs either in a CNS relapse or in a patient with acute lymphocytic leukemia who did not receive prophylactic CNS treatment.[4,32,33] Rarely, it can occur as an isolated sign of relapse, but in one series, most were associated with bone marrow (9 of 11), compared with CNS (3 of 9), relapse.[34] Rarely, optic disc neo-

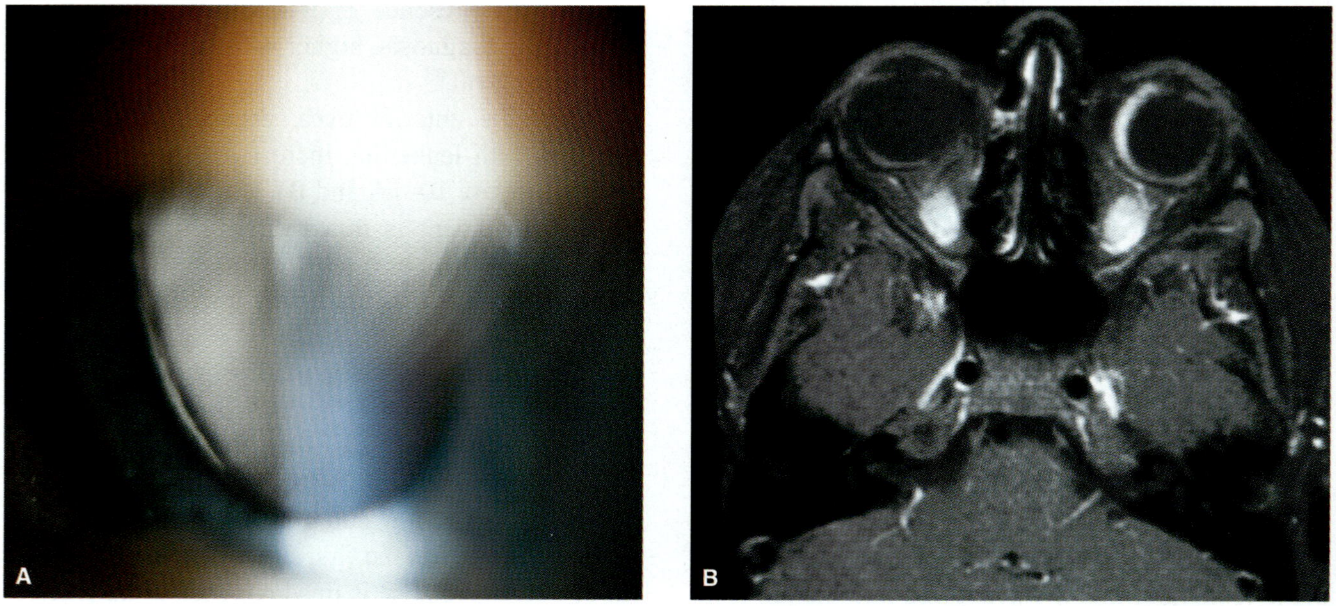

Figure 10–2. *A,* Ciliary body mass and a history of iridocyclitis treated with topical prednisolone; this was undiagnosed recurrent ALL. *B,* Enhancement of the area shown in Figure 10–2A with gadolinium in a T_1-weighted axial MRI.

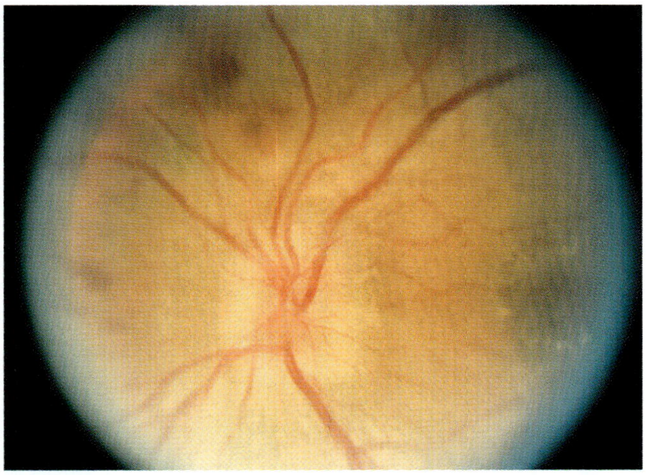

Figure 10–3. Optic nerve infiltration from acute lymphocytic leukemia in a child with CNS relapse.

vascularization develops with leukemia.[35] Usually, intrathecal chemotherapy is not effective for acute optic nerve leukemia.[33] Local radiation with as little as 8 gray (Gy) or 800 rads produces local control in over 90 percent of cases.[8,29]

Hypopyon and iris infiltration are treated with both systemic chemotherapy and irradiation, with good results.[24,26,30,31,36] Generally, 5 to 10 Gy over a 6-day period is sufficient radiation for anterior segment resolution. However, some authors have used lower or higher doses.[6,24,25,32,37] Steroids can also be effective.[38]

There are long-term ophthalmic effects of treatment in children with acute lymphoblastic leukemia (ALL).[39] In 34 patients, 2 developed cataracts, and ocular abnormalities were noted in 4 of the 16 irradiated eyes; however, all had normal vision, and no radiation retinopathy was noted.[31] In 82 survivors with ALL, posterior subcapsular cataracts, probably as a result of steroids, were noted in 52 percent, although most of these patients had good vision at the time of that report.[40] If patients are treated with whole-body irradiation and bone marrow transplantation, depending on the dose and fractionation schedule, ocular radiation complications can vary from 15 to almost 100 percent.[41–44] Ohkoshi and Tsiaras noted that patients who had ocular manifestations with their leukemia had a significantly shorter life span. Among these patients, 27 of 28 died within 21 months.[45] Several series have reported the ocular findings after allogeneic stem or bone marrow transplantation, in patients with leukemia. A Sjögren-like syndrome is observed in approximately 40 percent of cases. Other complications that have been noted include uveitis, retinal hemorrhages, bilateral optic disc edema, and pseudomembranous conjunctivitis.[46–48]

As discussed in Chapter 16, leukemia accounts for 2 to 11 percent of orbital tumors in childhood.[37,49,50] Children with acute myelomonocytic leukemia (AMML), commonly from the Mediterranean basin, often have both eye and orbital leukemia discovered prior to the diagnosis of systemic disease.[4] Figure 16–6 demonstrates such a presentation with diffuse orbital and intraocular involvement.

LYMPHOMA

While the classification of lymphomas continues to evolve, it has not effected the evaluation and management of intraocular lymphoid lesions.[51,52] Intraocular lymphomas can be divided into three broad categories: (1) a group of patients previously described as having ocular reticulum cell sarcoma; usually, these are older patients misdiagnosed as having chronic diffuse uveitis, who have intraocular and CNS lymphoma; (2) a group of patients who present with choroidal-retinal lymphoma and often have systemic involvement; and (3) patients who have systemic lymphoma who mainly develop anterior segment involvement late in their disease course.

Ocular Reticulum Cell Sarcoma

Ocular reticulum cell sarcoma (intraocular lymphoma) is an uncommon intraocular neoplasm usually misdiagnosed as diffuse chronic uveitis.[51] The definition of this condition has not been standardized, and the term is a misnomer. While this tumor was initially thought to be of reticulum cell origin, this idea has been shown to be erroneous. The tumor is composed of malignant lymphocytes (usually of B-cell lineage) or precursors in various stages of differentiation.[51–58]

We have only included patients with primary ocular or ocular and CNS lymphoma under this rubric and have differentiated this disease process from cases of systemic lymphoma with secondary eye involvement. Usually, this neoplastic process develops in older patients, although we have managed patients in their 20s with this malignancy.

Patients are usually referred with diffuse uveitis, for which they have been treated with steroids, with either no response or an exacerbation of their ocular signs and symptoms.[53,59] In one-third of cases, CNS involvement becomes manifest prior to the findings of eye disease.[60]

Approximately 170 cases have been reported.[53–78] As a general rule, any patient over age 50 years with a new onset of bilateral diffuse uveitis should be suspected of having an intraocular lymphoma, although the disease is most frequent in even older patients. Intraocular lymphomas are, however, a rare cause of pseudouveitis in the elderly. In a study from Boston of 138 patients who developed uveitis at age > 60 years, only 2 had the diagnosis of lymphoma.[79] Approximately 85 percent of patients eventually develop CNS lymphoma involvement; however, CNS disease can occur prior to, simultaneous with, or after the development of eye disease.[80] Bilateral ocular involvement is present in over 85 percent of cases, although initially about one-third of patients may present with only one eye involved.[77]

Figures 10–4 and 10–5 show a typical fundus presentation of intraocular lymphoma in a 75-year-old male. Usually, there are diffuse vitreous cells with relatively mild or minimal anterior chamber reaction. The anterior chamber reaction can be either granulomatous or nongranulomatous. The pathognomonic clinical pattern is yellowish white chorioretinal infiltrates with vitritis as shown in Figures 10–5 and 10–6. Rarely, a hemorrhagic retinitis can simulate a cytomegalovirus (CMV) retinitis (Figure 10–7); however, lymphoma deposits are not usually perivascular, and the hemorrhage is isolated. Rarely, this condition can simulate a branch retinal vein occlusion, vasculitis, or acute retinal necrosis.[76,81] Retinal pigment detachments with secondary atrophy and disciform scars can also develop.[82] Exudative detachment is present in 5 percent of cases. Patients with mainly vitreous involvement as opposed to those who have predominantly choroidal lymphoma are more likely to develop central nervous system lymphoma; patients with nonvitreous lesions are more likely to develop systemic lymphoma.[59]

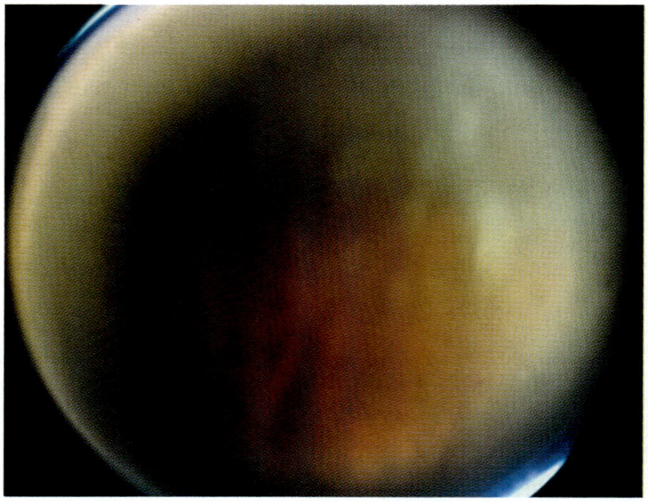

Figure 10–4. Primary intraocular lymphoma (ocular reticulum cell sarcoma) with malignant lymphocytic cellular infiltration of the vitreous presenting as a cellular infiltration of the vitreous cells as part of an intractable chronic diffuse uveitis.

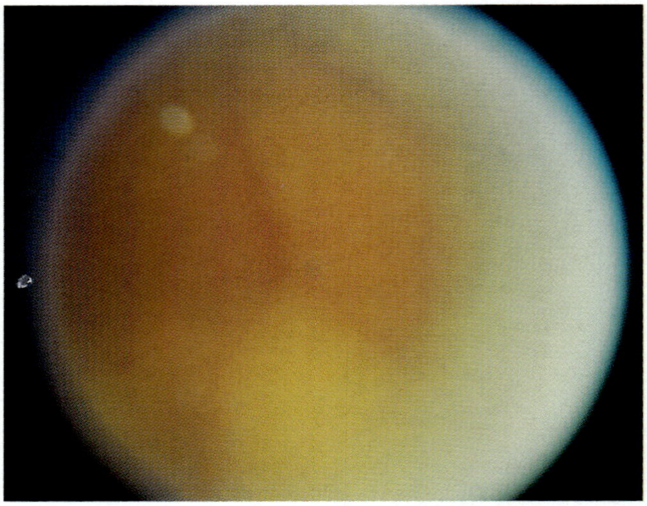

Figure 10–5. Pathognomonic yellowish white chorioretinal infiltrate in "ocular reticulum cell sarcoma."

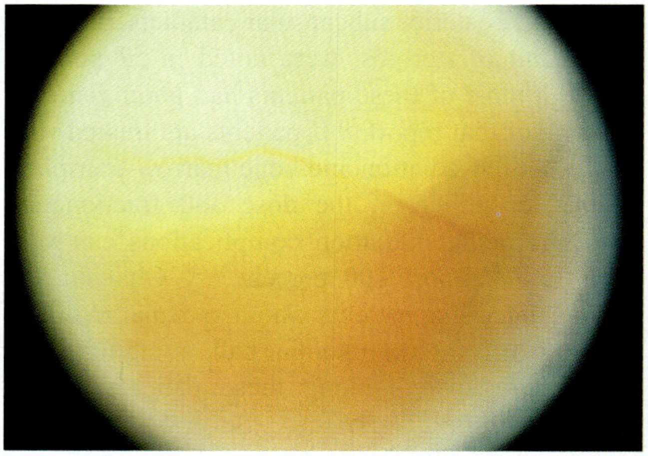

Figure 10–6. Yellowish white infiltrate in "ocular reticulum cell sarcoma."

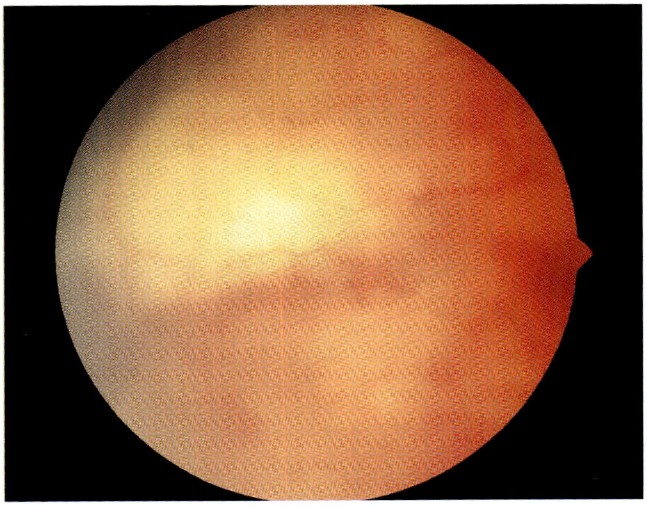

Figure 10–7. Atypical presentation lymphoma with area of hemorrhagic retinitis.

Approximately 10 percent of these intraocular lymphoma patients have a history of a subtle neurologic deficit, usually memory loss or a recent minor cerebral vascular accident. Thirty percent of patients have no neurologic history, physical findings, or laboratory results suggestive of an underlying CNS or systemic lymphoma (see below). In 60 percent of cases, simultaneous eye and CNS lymphomas are documented at the time of presentation. In this latter group of patients, often there are no obvious neurologic findings, and the diagnosis is only established with cerebrospinal fluid cytology or CNS imaging studies.[53,80] As with CNS lymphoma which has increased in the acquired immunodeficiency syndrome (AIDS) population, a few cases of primary ocular lymphoma have been reported in this cohort.[81–89]

Diagnosis

The diagnosis of intraocular lymphoma is usually established on the basis of FNAB of vitreous; rarely a subretinal chorioretinal biopsy is required.[90] There are three important caveats regarding cytopathologic diagnosis for intraocular lymphoma: (1) we have seen three cases in which, despite adequate cytologic material, the diagnosis could not be established on the basis of a single vitreous biopsy.[53] Nussenblatt and co-workers noted similar problems with a negative initial vitreous biopsy in 3 of 10 cases.[57] If clinical suspicion is high, multiple or bilateral vitreous biopsies may be required; (2) the cytopathologic diagnosis is highly dependent on the quality of cytopathologic preparation. Figure 15–5 shows vitreous biopsies from the same patient prepared in different laboratories. In one, it was almost impossible to establish the diagnosis, while the other showed a clear-cut lymphoma; and (3) while some investigators have demonstrated that intraocular lymphomas can be monoclonal, in a small study we have performed, cytomorphology was more sensitive than immunologic techniques to establish a diagnosis.[53] Cytologic features of intraocular lymphoma include cells with irregular nuclear contours and chromatin, lobation of nuclei (Figures 10–8 and 10–9), coarse irregular chromatin, and the presence of nucleoli. Usually, benign inflammatory cells are sparse.

Newer techniques may obviate the above statement. In one study, Davis and colleagues found that flow cytometry was more sensitive than cytology to establish a diagnosis of this disease. In their series, 7 of 10 could be diagnosed on flow cytometry, versus 3 of 10 on histology.[91] We suspect the latter series represents suboptimal cytology rather than the advantage of cytometry. There are two reasons to make that statement: (1) it has not been the experience of major centers that only 30 percent can be diagnosed cytologically; and (2) in a number of cases we have noted with standard flow cytometry a mixed population of lymphoid cells. However, multiparameter flow cytometry, with simultaneous analysis of several cell surface markers can help identify small clonal neoplastic populations among a much larger reactive population. Newer approaches

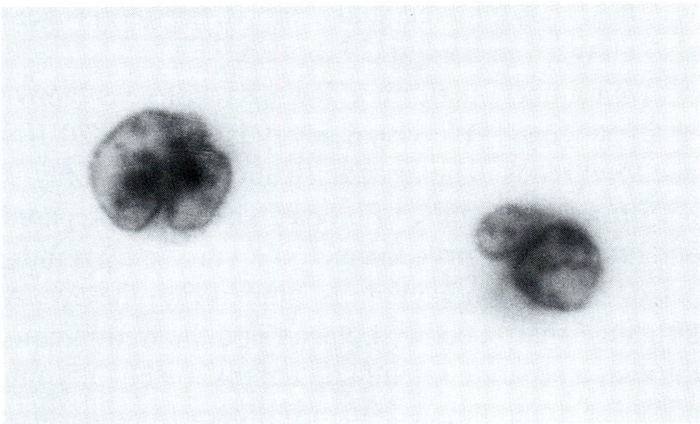

Figure 10–8. Cytopathologic changes in intraocular lymphoma include coarse nuclear chromatin and alterations in nuclear position and shape. Typical "nose"- shaped nuclei are almost pathognomonic for this tumor.

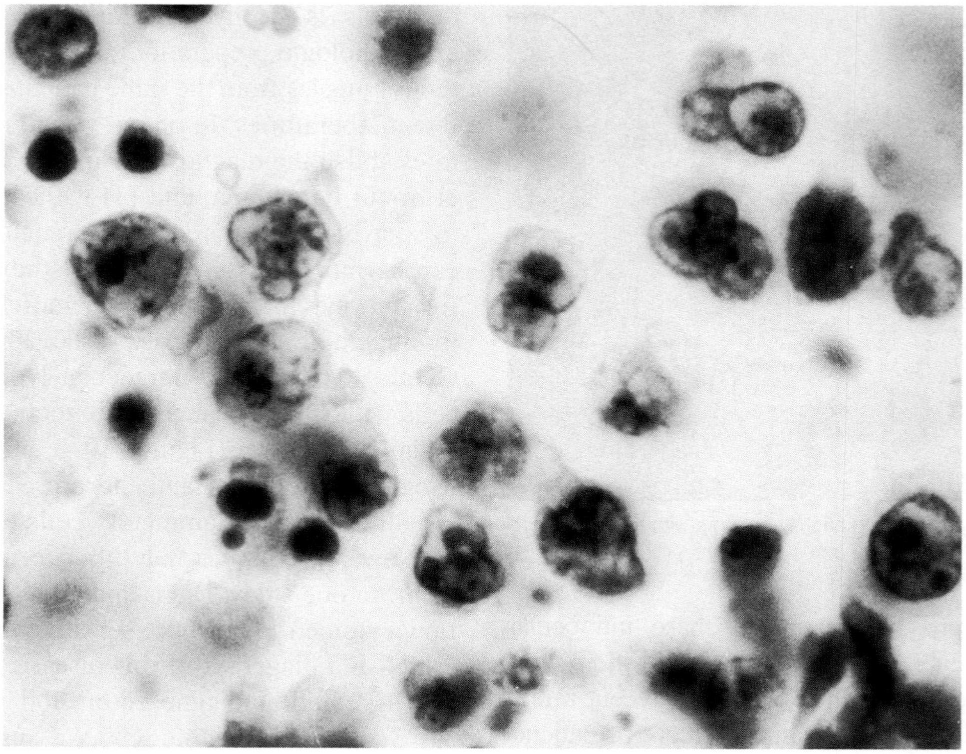

Figure 10–9. Coarse chromatin, nucleoli, and mitoses are often seen in FNAB of intraocular lymphoma.

using polymerase chain reaction (PCR) to detect B- and T-cell gene re-arrangements have shown promise, although as high as 30 percent false-negative rate has been reported.[92–94] While human herpes virus 8 (HHV-8) and Epstein-Barr virus (EBV) have been found in intraocular lymphoma associated with Kaposi's sarcoma (KS), it probably is not very important in the pathophysiology of this disease.[95] Similarly, while some authors have found that interleukin-10 (IL-10) levels tend to be elevated in the vitreous,[96] in another study, the IL-10 levels were also elevated in benign conditions.[97]

We routinely perform a diagnostic vitreous biopsy in all patients. If the visual acuity is less than 20/100 due to vitreous cellular opacification, a vitrectomy is performed at the time of biopsy. The eye is prepared and draped in a sterile manner. If a vitrectomy is indicated, an infusion cannula is sutured into the eye. A 20-gauge sharp needle is placed into the midvitreous through a separate scleral site approximately 3.5 mm posterior to the limbus. One milliliter of liquid vitreous is withdrawn for analysis. The quality of cytologic preparation is superior when vitreous is obtained through a standard needle and syringe, compared with samples of vitreous cells obtained through the vitrectomy instrument and harvested from the balanced salt solution (BSS)-plus reservoir. In the same patient, we have observed significant cytologic deterioration when the latter method is used. We now also save 0.1 mL undiluted vitreous as well as the vitrectomy specimen for molecular biologic studies.

In all cases, at the time of surgery, bilateral bone marrow biopsies are performed along with a lumbar puncture for cerebrospinal fluid cytology. As previously mentioned, approximately 80 percent of patients eventually develop CNS disease, and historically that has led to their death.

All patients in whom the diagnosis of intraocular lymphoma is suspected, we also have complete CNS imaging studies.[98] A T_1-weighted MRI, using thin sections and gadolinium, is more sensitive than brain computed tomography (CT) with contrast. A typical CNS lesion associated with intraocular lymphoma is shown on an MRI scan (Figure 10–10). If CT is used, intravenous contrast is mandatory to optimally visualize the lesion.

The treatment of primary intraocular lymphoma is controversial. In 1980, we reported 9 patients with

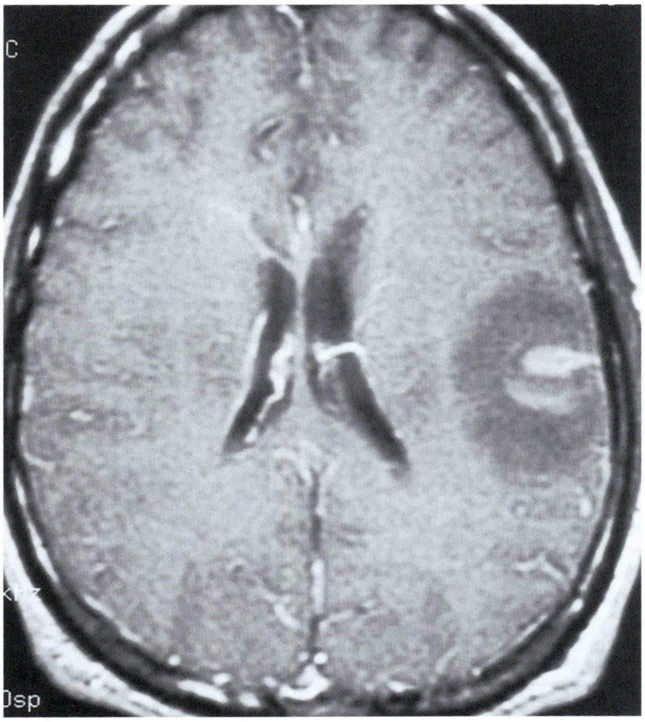

Figure 10–10. MRI with contrast demonstrating a CNS lymphoma in a patient with primary intraocular and CNS lymphoma.

intraocular lymphomas who had been treated with 35 to 45 Gy of ocular and CNS photon irradiation.[71] In 10 of 13 eyes of 8 patients, visual acuity improved. Generally, patients who have initially better vision are more likely to show significant postradiation improvement. Figures 10–11A and B show an intraocular lymphoma before and after radiation treatment. Little ocular morbidity occurred with this dose and fractionation schedule. Unfortunately, most patients treated with just radiation to the eye and CNS had a good initial response but later died of recurrent CNS disease. This led us to treat a series of patients with both eye and CNS disease with a combination of radiation and intrathecal chemotherapy.[80]

Several chemotherapeutic protocols have been used in only a few patients in different centers.[78,99–101] No data have demonstrated the superiority of a given approach. In patients with intraocular and CNS lymphoma, 40 Gy of whole-brain and eye irradiation, with a 5- to 10-Gy boost to the spinal cord, is given along with intrathecal methotrexate. A number of other approaches have been used. Fishburne and colleagues and others have used 400µg intravitreal methotrexate twice weekly to treat intraocular disease, with promising local results.[97,102] Aggressive systemic chemotherapy, with autologous bone marrow transplantation, has also been used with good local control.[96,103] The major problem with the latter approach has been morbidity, where over 80 percent of 1-year survivors > 60 years old developed progressive leukoencephalopathy. A recent report using only chemotherapy showed a lower incidence of progressive leukoencephalopathy.[104]

We have treated a number of patients with long-term (> 10-year) survival. Our best results have been in patients who have minimal CNS disease; vision is restored and life preserved.[53] Patients who are initially referred with gross neurologic disease, often succumb to the CNS lymphoma despite radiation and chemotherapy; some have died during initial evaluation or early treatment.[77] Rarely, we have seen patients treated elsewhere with this regimen develop radiation retinopathy (Figure 10–12), but that has

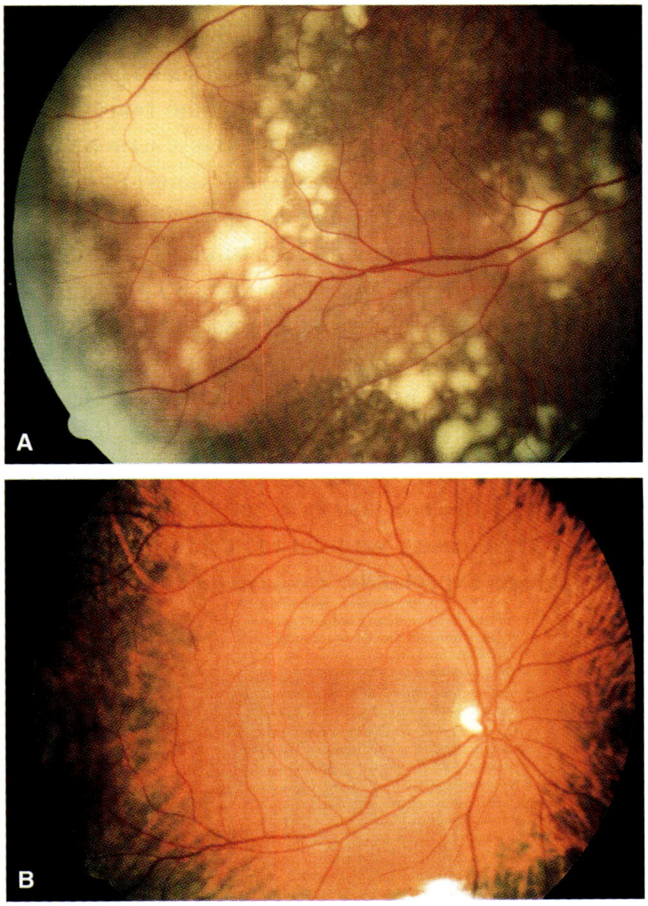

Figure 10–11. *A,* Pretreatment view of a patient with primary intraocular lymphoma. *B,* Postradiation response in the same patient.

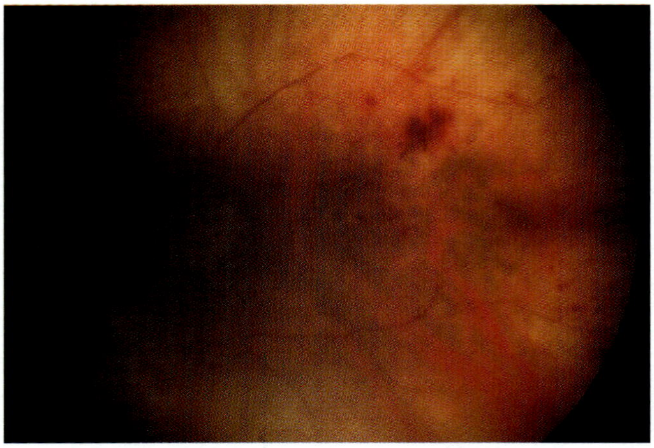

Figure 10–12. Radiation retinopathy without recurrence of intraocular lymphoma in a patient treated elsewhere with eye and brain radiation plus chemotherapy.

not occurred in the approximately 40 patients we have treated at UCSF and Stanford.

A more difficult group of patients to establish treatment guidelines for are those with only intraocular lymphoma.[53] In lymphoma localized to the eye, the two options are to radiate only the eye and serially monitor the CNS with brain MRI scans and cerebrospinal fluid cytologies, or to radiate both the eye and brain with or without adjunctive chemotherapy. Significant morbidity, including deterioration of intellectual function, occurs in up to 30 percent of elderly patients treated with both brain irradiation and intrathecal chemotherapy and in up to 80 percent with aggressive systemic chemotherapy.[80,103–106] As mentioned above, if radiation and systemic chemotherapy are used in older patients, over 80 percent develop significant intellectual deterioration.[97] We, therefore, have been less inclined to aggressively treat very old patients with disease just localized to the eye, and in most of these cases, we treat the eye(s) and monitor such patients expectantly. We have had long-term follow-up of 2 patients treated with only ocular irradiation who are disease-free 7 and 13 years after treatment, respectively.[53] In general, most of these patients do eventually develop CNS disease, and at that point, more treatment is undertaken. We believe that the quality of life is better with that approach, and that a number of those patients can be salvaged when they develop CNS disease (unpublished observations).

In 25 percent of ocular lymphoma patients—predominantly those with choroidal infiltrates, as opposed to vitreous disease—systemic non-CNS lymphoma develops. These patients are treated with ocular radiation and systemic chemotherapy.[59,99–101]

After treatment with radiation, chemotherapy, or both, there is uniform breakdown of the blood-aqueous barrier; all these patients have persistent anterior chamber cell and flare. Similarly, if a central vitrectomy has been performed, the peripheral vitreous opacification remains stationary, despite effective treatment.

All patients are followed up by a medical oncologist. A general physical examination is performed every 3 months, as well as both scans and cerebrospinal fluid cytologic studies on a 6-month basis for the first 5 years after treatment. If relapse or tumor spread occurs, it almost always becomes manifest within 3 years of diagnosis. In our experience, recurrences usually occur within the first year in < 10 percent of treated patients.

Systemic Lymphoma with Secondary Ocular Involvement

We have seen a number of cases in which patients have presented to the ophthalmologist with anterior segment findings as the initial sign of systemic relapse. Figure 10–13 shows a patient previously

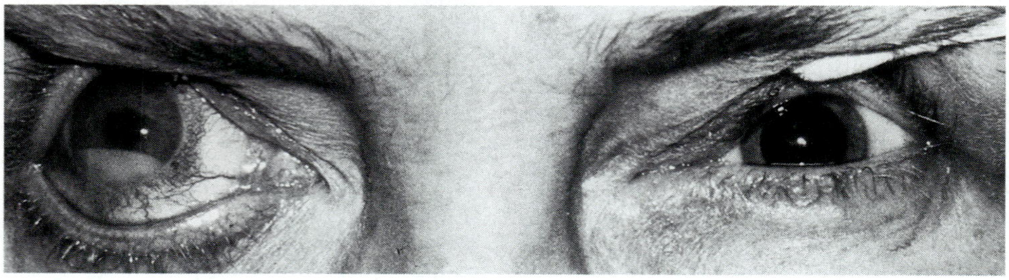

Figure 10–13. Anterior segment relapse as first sign of a systemic lymphoma recurrence.

treated with a combination of chemotherapy and radiation for systemic lymphoma. Approximately 3 years after the initial diagnosis of the disease, she presented with persistent, progressive iridocyclitis and was eventually referred for evaluation of a hypopyon. Fine-needle aspiration of the anterior chamber demonstrated lymphoma that responded rapidly to low-dose (10 Gy) irradiation. In our experience, less commonly, systemic lymphoma symptomatically involves the posterior choroid. Figure 10–14 shows a patient who was initially referred for a uveal melanoma. An FNAB demonstrated that this was a lymphoma.[107] Figure 10–15 shows a patient who presented with ocular findings from a T-cell lymphoma. Others have noted atypical malignant lymphoma presentations in the eye, including a pattern that simulated a ring melanoma.[108,109] A number of rarer lymphomas have been reported, including choroidal infiltrates as an initial manifestation of lymphoma after treatment of arthritis, a primary B-cell lymphoma in a 3-year-old boy, widespread lymphoma in an 11-year-old boy, and T-cell lymphoma involving the anterior chamber.[110–113] Similarly, one case report documented choroidal infiltrates as the initial manifestation of lymphoma in a patient with rheumatoid arthritis on methotrexate.[110]

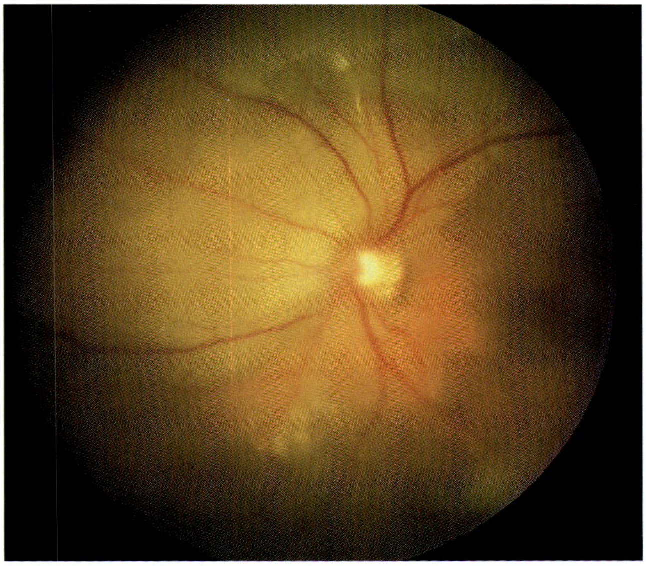

Figure 10–14. Patient presented with a uveal parapapillary tumor that simulated a choroidal melanoma. FNAB was positive for lymphoma.

OTHER INTRAOCULAR LYMPHOID TUMORS

Benign and malignant lymphoid tumors involving the uveal tract have been reported since 1920.[114–116] There have been approximately 50 cases of benign intraocular lymphoid tumors reported.[114] These tumors can be localized choroidal lymphomas, consist of a benign uveal infiltrate, or involve the uveal tract, sclera, optic nerve, and orbit.[116–118] Crookes and Mullaney first reported a case of lymphoid hyperplasia of the uveal tract in 1967.[118] Ryan and co-workers retrospectively analyzed histologic data on 19 cases that exhibited massive lymphoid uveal involvement without inflammation of the sclera.[119] Seventeen of the 19 patients had unilateral disease, and this process simulated a melanoma. The mean age at onset was 55 years, the range being 30 to 94 years. Most patients presented because of decreased vision; however, retinal detachment with glaucoma and/or iridocyclitis occurred, and some patients initially sought care because of inflammation or pain. Histologically, mature lymphocytes were observed in the uveal tract of all cases, and most also had plasma cells. Only one patient had an abnormality on serum protein electrophoresis.[119] A recent Armed Forces Institute of Pathology (AFIP) report reviewed 10 of these cases and, using molecular techniques, noted that 8 of the 10 were well-differentiated small cell lymphomas.[120] None of these patients died from systemic lymphoma; as others have noted, lymphoma was more common in the posterior segment, and the extrascleral component appeared to have a more benign cytology.[120] Rarely, there are intraocular benign EBV driven lymphoproliferative disorder in post-transplant patients.[121] Very few clinical reports of this entity have been published. Usually, there is associated localized extraocular lymphocytic infiltration.[121,122] A case of benign lymphoid hyperplasia of the uveal tract, confirmed with FNAB, is shown in Figure 10–16.

Many patients with benign uveal lymphoid lesions will respond to steroids.[121,123] In a single case report, radiation also appeared effective, and we have had good results in 3 patients treated with 20 Gy of photons.

The benign uveal lymphoid lesions may also occur as part of the spectrum of conditions associated with idiopathic posterior scleritis. Most patients

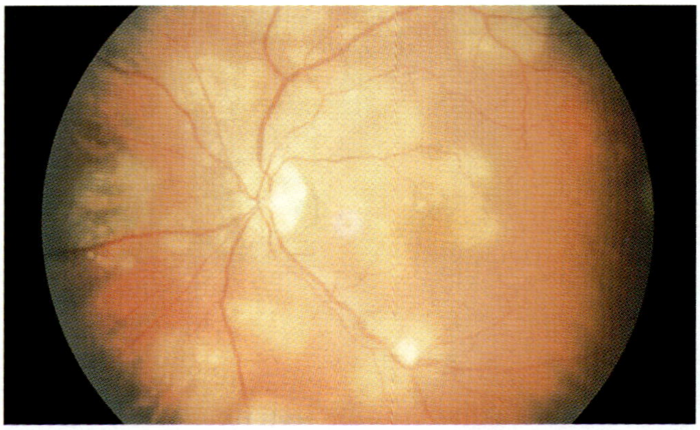

Figure 10–15. Patient with a T-cell lymphoma and diffuse choroidal lesions.

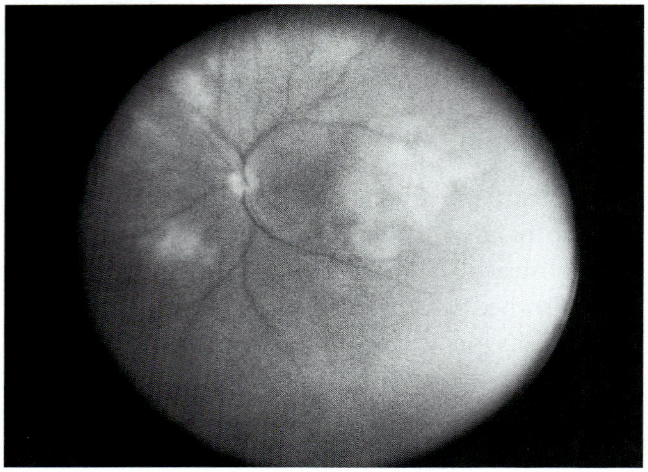

Figure 10–16. Benign lymphoid hyperplasia of the uveal tract confirmed with FNAB.

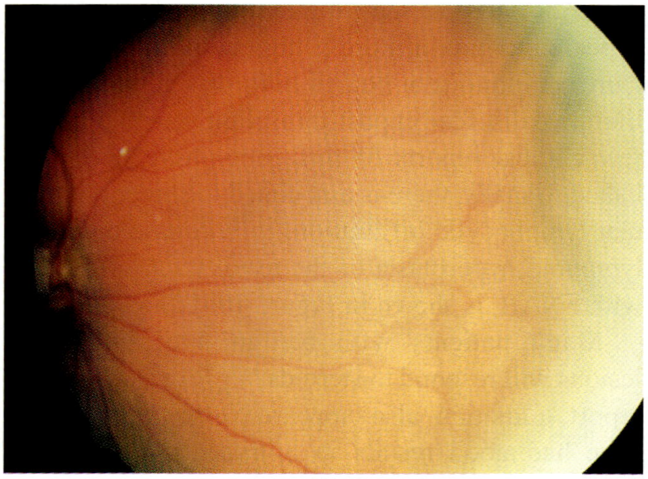

Figure 10–17. Choroidal detachment and transient uveal mass in which the patient had a history of pain without a red eye. Clinical and ultrasound findings simulated a ciliary body melanoma. The presence of a ring of choroidal detachment and pain prompted oral steroid therapy. The eye became completely normal 1 week after treatment.

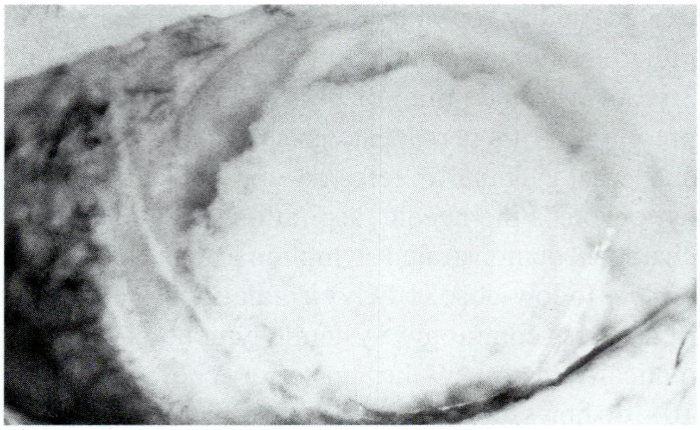

Figure 10–18. Necrotic uveal melanoma with a nondiagnostic ultrasonographic appearance.

have an exudative detachment without an obvious mass. The patient shown in Figure 10–17 was referred with the diagnosis of a ciliary body melanoma. This exudative retinal detachment disappeared during a 2-week course of oral steroids (see Figure 10–17).[124] Many posterior scleritis patients have little anterior segment inflammation; a number have been reported with false-positive radioactive phosphorus uptake tests.[110–129]

The management of either posterior scleritis or benign lymphoid uveal lesions is unclear. Some patients respond to oral steroids.[130] Others have a varied course.[116,123–131]

Finally, it is important to stress that intraocular inflammation does not exclude the diagnosis of a uveal melanoma. A small percentage of patients, generally with large, necrotic uveal melanomas, can have intraocular inflammation as their presenting sign.[132] Figure 10–18 shows a patient who had a negative ultrasound for tumor but had a blind, painful eye that, on histologic examination, had a necrotic melanoma with substantial inflammation.

REFERENCES

1. Libreich R. Uber Retinitis Leucaemica und uber Embolie der Arteria Centralis Retinae. Dtsch Klinik 1861;13:495–7.
2. Frank RN, Ryan SJ Jr. Peripheral retinal neovascularization with chronic myelogenous leukemia. Arch Ophthalmol 1972;87:585–9.
3. Holt JM, Gordon-Smith EC. Retinal abnormalities in diseases of the blood. Br J Ophthalmol 1969;53: 145–60.

4. Rosenthal AR. Ocular manifestations of leukemia. A review. Ophthalmology 1983;90:899–905.
5. Duke JR, Wilkinson CP, Sigelman S. Retinal microaneurysms in leukemia. Br J Ophthlamol 1968;52: 368–74.
6. Masera G, Carnelli V, Uderzo C, et al. Leukaemic hypopyon in acute lymphoblastic leukemia after interruption of treatment. Arch Dis Child 1979;54: 73–4.
7. Jampol LM, Goldberg MF, Busse B. Peripheral retinal microaneurysms in chronic leukemia. Am J Ophthalmol 1975;80:242–8.
8. Newman NM, Smith ME, Gay AJ. An unusual case of leukemia involving the eye: A clinico-pathological study. Surv Ophthalmol 1972;16:316–21.
9. Morse PH, McCready JL. Peripheral retinal neovascularization in chronic myelocytic leukemia. Am J Ophthalmol 1971;72:975–8.
10. Kim TS, Duker JS, Hedges TR III. Retinal angiopathy resembling unilateral frosted branch angiitis in a patient with a relapsing acute lymphoblastic leukemia. Am J Ophthalmol 1994;117:806–8.
11. Culler AM. Fundus changes in leukemia. Trans Am Ophthalmol Soc 1951;49:445–73.
12. Mahneke A, Videboek A. On changes in the optic fundus in leukemia. Acta Ophthalmol 1964;42:201–10.
13. Robb RM, Ervin LD, Sallan SE. A pathological study of eye involvement in acute leukemia of childhood. Trans Am Ophthalmol Soc 1978;76:90–101.
14. Allen RA, Straatsma BR. Ocular involvement in leukemia and allied disorders. Arch Ophthalmol 1961;66:490–508.
15. Kincaid MC, Green WR. Ocular and orbital involvement in leukemia. Surv Ophthalmol 1983;27:211–32.
16. Clayman HM, Flynn JT, Koch K, Israel C. Retinal pigment epithelial abnormalities in leukemic disease. Am J Ophthalmol 1972;74:416–9.
17. Kincaid MC, Green WR, Kelly JS. Acute ocular leukemia. Am J Ophthalmol 1979;87:698–702.
18. Gass JD. Differential diagnosis of intraocular tumors: a stereoscopic presentation. St Louis, MO: CV Mosby; 1974. P. 160–76.
19. Mark LE, Rouhani J, Sawitsky A. Leukemic iris infiltration in a case of meningeal leukemia. Ophthalmology 1974;6:669–74.
20. Karesh JW, Goldman EJ, Kelman SE, et al. A prospective ophthalmic evaluation of patients with acute myeloid leukemia: correlation of ocular and hematologic findings. J Clin Oncol 1989;7:1528–32.
21. Schachat AP, Markowitz JA, Guyer DR, et al. Ophthalmic manifestations of leukemia. Arch Ophthalmol 1989;107:697–700.
22. Jackson N, Reddy SC, Hishamuddin M, Low HC. Retinal findings in adult leukaemia: correlation with leukocytosis. Clin Lab Hematol 1996;18:105–9.
23. Reddy SC, Quah SH, Low HC, Jackson N. Prognostic significance of retinopathy at presentation in adult acute leukemia. Ann Hematol 1998;76:15–8.
24. Ninane J, Taylor D, Day S. The eye as a sanctuary in acute lymphoblastic leukaemia. Lancet 1980;1: 452–3.
25. Tabbara KF, Beckstead JH. Acute promonocytic leukemia with ocular involvement. Arch Ophthalmol 1980;98:1055–8.
26. Zakka KA, Yee RD, Shoor N, et al. Leukemic iris infiltration. Am J Ophthalmol 1980;89:204–9.
27. Abramson DH, Wachtel A, Watson CW, et al. Leukemic hypopyon. J Pediatr Ophthalmol Strabismus 1981;18:42–4.
28. Gruenewald RL, Perry MC, Henry PH. Leukemic iritis with hypopyon. Cancer 1979;44:1511–3.
29. Ridgway EW, Jaffe N, Walton DS. Leukemic ophthalmopathy in children. Cancer 1976;38:1744–9.
30. Engel HM, Green WR, Michels RG, et al. Diagnostic vitrectomy. Retina 1981;1:121–49.
31. Martin B. Infiltration of the iris in chronic lymphatic leukemia. Br J Ophthalmol 1968;52:781–5.
32. Murray KH, Paolino F, Goldman JM, et al. Ocular involvement in leukaemia: report of 3 cases. Lancet 1977;1:829–31.
33. Ellis W, Little HL. Leukemic infiltration of the optic nerve head. Am J Ophthalmol 1973;75:867–71.
34. Schwartz CL, Miller NR, Wharam MD, Leventhal BG. The optic nerve as the site of initial relapse in childhood acute lymphoblastic leukemia. Cancer 1989; 63:1616–20.
35. De Juan E, Green WR, Rice TA, Erozan YS. Optic disc neovascularization associated with ocular involvement in acute lymphocytic leukemia. Retina 1982;2:61–4.
36. Fonken HA, Ellis PP. Leukemic infiltrates in the iris. Successful treatment of secondary glaucoma with x-irradiation. Arch Ophthalmol 1966;76:32–6.
37. Nicholson DH, Green WR. Tumors of the eye, lids and orbit in children. In: Harley RD, editor. Pediatric ophthalmology. Philadelphia, PA: WB Saunders; 1975. p. 923–1067.
38. Bunin N, Rivera G, Goode F, Hustu HO. Ocular relapse in the anterior chamber in childhood acute lymphoblastic leukemia. J Clin Oncol 1987;5:299–303.
39. Weaver RG Jr, Chauvenet AR, Smith TJ, Schwartz AC. Ophthalmic evaluation of long-term survivors of childhood acute lymphoblastic leukemia. Cancer 1986;58:963–8.
40. Hoover DL, Smith LEH, Turner SJ, et al. Ophthalmic evaluation of survivors of acute lymphoblastic leukemia. Ophthalmology 1988;95:151–5.
41. Preti A, Kantarjian HM. Management of adult acute lymphocytic leukemia: present issues and key challenges. J Clin Oncol 1994;12:1312–22.
42. Ozsahin M, Belkacemi Y, Pene F, et al. Total-body irra-

diation and cataract incidence: a randomized comparison of two instantaneous dose rates. Int J Radiat Oncol Biol Phys 1993;28:343–7.
43. Bray LC, Carey PJ, Proctor SJ, et al. Ocular complications of bone marrow transplantation. Br J Ophthalmol 1991;75:611–4.
44. Calissendorff BM, Bolme P. Cataract development and outcome of surgery in bone marrow transplanted children. Br J Ophthalmol 1993;77:36–8.
45. Ohkoshi K, Tsiaras WG. Prognostic importance of ophthalmic manifestations in childhood leukemia. Br J Ophthalmol 1992;76:651–5.
46. Ng JS, Lam DS, Li CK, et al. Ocular complications of pediatric bone marrow transplantation. Ophthalmology 1999;106:160–4.
47. Kerty E, Vigander K, Flage T, Brinch L. Ocular findings in allogeneic stem cell transplantation without total body irradiation. Ophthalmology 1999;106:1334–8.
48. Mencucci R, Rossi Ferrini C, Bosi A, et al. Ophthalmological aspects in allogenic bone marrow transplantation: Sjogren-like syndrome in graft-versus-host disease. Eur J Ophthalmol 1997;7:13–8.
49. Porterfield JF. Orbital tumors in children. A report of 214 cases. Int Ophthalmol Clin 1962;2:319–35.
50. Oakhill A, Willshaw H, Mann JR. Unilateral proptosis. Arch Dis Child 1981;56:549–51.
51. Harris NL, Jaffe ES, Armitage JO, Shipp M. Lymphoma classification: from R.E.A.L. to W.H.O. and beyond. Principles Prac Oncol 1999;13:1–14.
52. Donner LR. Cytogenesis of lymphomas: a brief review of its theoretical and practical significance. Cancer Genet Cytogenet 1997;94:20–6.
53. Char DH, Ljung B-M, Miller TR, Phillips TL. Primary intraocular lymphoma (ocular reticulum cell sarcoma): diagnosis and management. Ophthalmology 1988;95:625–30.
54. Lopez JS, Chan CC, Burnier M, et al. Immunohistochemistry findings in primary intraocular lymphoma. Am J Ophthalmol 1991;112:472–4.
55. Leong AS-Y. Malignant lymphoma: nomenclature, recently recognized subtypes, and current concepts. J Histotechnol 1992;15:175–84.
56. Davis JL, Solomon D, Nussenblatt RB, et al. Immunocytochemical staining of vitreous cells. Indications, techniques, and results. Ophthalmology 1992;99: 250–6.
57. Whitcup SM, de Smet MD, Rubin BI, et al. Intraocular lymphoma. Clinical and histopathologic diagnosis. Ophthalmology 1993;100:1399–1406.
58. Wilson DJ, Braziel R, Rosenbaum JT. Intraocular lymphoma. Immunopathologic analysis of vitreous biopsy specimens. Arch Ophthalmol 1992;110: 1455–8.
59. Klingele TG, Hogan MJ. Ocular reticulum cell sarcoma. Am J Ophthalmol 1975;79:39–47.
60. Char DH, Ljung BM, Deschenes J, Miller TR. Intraocular lymphoma: immunologic and cytologic analysis. Br J Ophthalmol 1988;72:905–11.
61. Cooper EL, Riker JL. Malignant lymphoma of the uveal tract. Am J Ophthalmol 1951;34:1153–8.
62. Littman P, Wang CC. Reticulum cell sarcoma of the brain. A review of the literature and a study of 19 cases. Cancer 1975;35:1412–20.
63. Harstad MK, Arnesen K. Malignant lymphoma of the eye and brain. Report of a case. Acta Ophthalmol 1973;52:211–9.
64. Michels RG, Knox DL, Erozan YS, Green WR. Intraocular reticulum cell sarcoma. Diagnosis by pars plana vitrectomy. Arch Ophthalmol 1975;93:1331–5.
65. Minckler DS, Font RL, Zimmerman LE. Uveitis and reticulum cell sarcoma of brain with bilateral neoplastic seeding of vitreous without retinal or uveal involvement. Am J Ophthamol 1975;80:433–8.
66. Neault RW, Van Scoy RE, Okazaki H, MacCarty SC. Uveitis associated with isolated reticulum cell sarcoma of the brain. Am J Ophthalmol 1972;73:431–6.
67. Nevins RC Jr, Frey WW, Elliott JH. Primary, solitary, intraocular reticulum cell sarcoma (microgliomatosis) (a clinicopathologic case report). Trans Am Acad Ophthalmol Otol 1968;72:867–76.
68. Rubinstein LJ. Tumors of the central nervous system. In: Atlas of tumor pathology. Washington, D.C.: Armed Forces Institute of Pathology; 1972. p. 215–27.
69. Vogel MH, Font RL, Zimmerman LE, Levine RA. Reticulum cell sarcoma of the retina and uvea (report of six cases and review of the literature). Am J Ophthalmol 1968;66:205–15.
70. Volcker HE, Naumann GOH, Rentsch F, Wollensak J. Primares Retikulumzellsarkom der Retina I. Clinico-pathologic study of 5 patients. Klin Mbl Augenheilk 1977;171:489–99.
71. Margolis L, Fraser R, Lichter A, Char DH. The role of radiation therapy in the management of ocular reticulum cell sarcoma. Cancer 1980;45:688–92.
72. Appen RE. Posterior uveitis and primary cerebral reticulum cell sarcoma. Arch Ophthalmol 1975;93:123.
73. Currey TA, Deutsch AR. Reticulum cell sarcoma of the uvea. South Med J 1965;58:919–22.
74. Kim EQ, Zakov ZN, Albert DM, et al. Intraocular reticulum cell sarcoma: a case report and literature review. Albrecht von Graefes Arch Klin Exp Ophthalmol 1979;209:167–78.
75. Sullivan SF, Dallow RL. Intraocular reticulum cell sarcoma: its dramatic response to systemic chemotherapy and its angiogenic potential. Ann Ophthalmol 1977;9:401–6.
76. Gass JD, Trattler HL. Retinal artery obstruction and atheromas associated with non-Hodgkin's large cell lymphoma (reticulum cell sarcoma). Arch Ophthalmol 1991;109:1134–9.

77. Siegel MJ, Dalton J, Friedman AH, et al. Ten-year experience with primary ocular 'reticulum cell sarcoma' (large cell non-Hodgkin's lymphoma). Br J Ophthalmol 1989;73:342–6.
78. Strauchen JA, Dalton J, Friedman AH. Chemotherapy in the management of intraocular lymphoma. Cancer 1989;63:1918–21.
79. Chatzistefanou K, Markomichelakis NN, Christen W, et al. Characteristics of uveitis presenting for the first time in the elderly. Ophthalmology 1998;105:347–52.
80. Char DH, Margolis L, Newman AB. Ocular reticulum cell sarcoma. Am J Ophthalmol 1981;91:480–3.
81. Ridley ME, McDonald HR, Sternberg P Jr, et al. Retinal manifestations of ocular lymphoma (reticulum cell sarcoma). Ophthalmology 1992;99:1153–61.
82. Dean JM, Novak MA, Chan CC, Green WR. Tumor detachments of the retinal pigment epithelium in ocular/central nervous system lymphoma. Retina 1996;16:47–56.
83. O'Neill BP, Illig JJ. Primary central nervous system lymphoma. Mayo Clin Proc 1989;64:1005–20.
84. Grant JW, Issacson PG. Primary central nervous system lymphoma. Brain Pathol 1992;2:97–109.
85. Schanzer MC, Font RL, O'Malley RE. Primary ocular malignant lymphoma associated with the acquired immune deficiency syndrome. Ophthalmology 1991; 98:88–91.
86. Karp JE, Broder S. Aquired immunodeficiency syndrome and non-Hodgkin's lymphomas. Cancer Res 1991;51:4743–56.
87. Matzkin DC, Slamovits TL, Rosenbaum PS. Simultaneous intraocular and orbital non-Hodgkin's lymphoma in the acquired immune deficiency syndrome. Ophthalmology 1994;101:850–5.
88. Stanton CA, Sloan B III, Slusher MM, Greven CM. Acquired immunodeficiency syndrome-related primary intraocular lymphoma. Arch Ophthalmol 1992;110:1614–7.
89. Johnson BL. Intraocular and central nervous system lymphoma in a cardiac transplant recipient. Ophthalmology 1992;99:987–92.
90. Ciulla TA, Pesavento D, Yoo S. Subretinal aspiration biopsy for ocular lymphoma. Am J Ophthalmol 1997;123:420–2.
91. Davis JL, Vichina AL, Ruiz P. Diagnosis of intraocular lymphoma by flow cytometry. Am J Ophtahlmol 1997;124:362–72.
92. Katai N, Kuroiwa S, Fujimori K, Yoshimura N. Diagnosis of intraocular lymphoma by polymerase chain reaction. Arch Ophthalmol 1997;235:431–6.
93. Shen DF, Zhuang Z, Lehoang P, et al. Utility of microdissection of polymerase chain reaction for the detection of immunoglobulin gene rearrangement and translocation in primary intraocular lymphoma. Ophthalmol 1998;105:1664–9.
94. White VA, Gascoyne RD, Paton KE. Use of the polymerase chain reaction to detect B- and T-cell gene rearrangements in vitreous specimens from patients with intraocular lymphoma. Arch Ophthalmol 1999;117:761–65.
95. Chan CC, Shen DF, Whitcup SM, Nussenblatt RB. Detection of human herpes virus-8 and Epstein-Barr virus DNA in primary intraocular lymphomas. Blood 1999;93:2749–51.
96. Whitcup SM, Stark-Vancs V, Wittes RE, et al. Association of interleukin 10 in the vitreous and cerebrospinal fluid and primary central nervous system lymphoma. Arch Ophthalmol 1997;115:1157–60.
97. Fishburne BC, Wilson DJ, Rosenbaum JY, Neuwelt EA. Intravitreal methotrexate as an adjunctive treatment of intraocular lymphoma. Arch Ophthalmol 1997;115:1152–6.
98. Zimmerman RA. Central nervous system lymphoma. Radiol Clin North Am 1990;28:697–721.
99. DeAngelis LM, Yahalom J, Thaler HT, Kher U. Combined modality therapy for primary CNS lymphoma. J Clin Oncol 1992;10:635–43.
100. Brada M, Dearnaley D, Horwich A, Bloom HJG. Management of primary cerebral lymphoma treated with initial chemotherapy: preliminary results and comparison with patients treated with radiotherapy alone. Int J Rad Oncol Biol Phys 1990;18:787–92.
101. Rouwen AJP, Wijermans PW, Boen-Tan TN, Stilma JS. Intraocular non-Hodgkin's lymphoma treated with systemic and intrathecal chemotherapy and radiotherapy. A case report and review of the literature. Graefe's Arch Clin Exp Ophthalmol 1989;227: 355–9.
102. Sandor V, Stark-Vancs V, Pearson D, et al. Phase II trial of chemotherapy alone for primary CNS and intraocular lymphoma. J Clin Oncol 1998;16:3000–6.
103. Soussain C, Merle-Beral H, Reux I, et al. A single-center study of 11 patients with intraocular lymphoma treated with conventional chemotherapy followed by high-dose chemotherapy and autologous bone marrow transplantation in 5 cases. Leuk Lymph 1996;23:339–45.
104. de Smet MD, Vancs VS, Kohler D, et al. Intravitreal chemotherapy for the treatment of recurrent intraocular lymphoma. Br J Ophthalmol 1999;83:448–51.
105. Sagerman RM, Cassady JR, Chang CH. Radiation therapy for intracranial lymphoma. Radiol 1967; 88:552–4.
106. Rosen ST, Makuch RW, Lichter AS, et al. Role of prophylactic cranial irradiation in prevention of central nervous system metastases in small cell lung cancer. Potential benefit restricted to patients with complete response. Am J Med 1983;74:615–24.
107. Fredrick DR, Char DH, Ljung BM, Brinton DA. Solitary intraocular lymphoma as an initial presentation

of widespread disease. Arch Ophthalmol 1989;107: 395–7.
108. Al-Hazzaa SAF, Green WR, Mann RB. Uveal involvement in systemic angiotropic large cell lymphoma. Microscopic and immunohistochemical studies. Ophthalmology 1993;100:961–5.
109. Jensen OA, Johansen S, Kiss K. Intraocular T-cell lymphoma mimicking a ring melanoma. First manifestation of systemic disease. Report of a case and survey of the literature. Graefe's Arch Clin Exp Ophthalmol 1994;232:148–52.
110. Zimmer-Galler L, Ilie JT. Choroidal infiltrates as the initial manifestation of lymphoma in rheumatoid arthritis after frequent low dose methotrexate. Mayo Clin 1994;69:258–60.
111. Wender A, Adar A, Maor E, Yassur Y. Primary B-cell lymphoma of the eyes and brain in a three-year-old boy. Arch Ophthalmol 1994;112:450–1.
112. Stephenson PDG, Duffey RJ, Ferguson JG Jr. Intraocular histiocytic lymphoma: a pediatric case presentation. J Pediatr Opthalmol Strabismus 1989;26:296–8.
113. Goldey SH, Stern GA, Oblon DJ, et al. Immunophenotypic characterization of an unusual T-cell lymphoma presenting as anterior uveitis. A clinicopathologic case report. Arch Ophthalmol 1989;107: 1349–53.
114. Triebenstein O. Ein Beitrag zur Frage der aleukamischen Augenveranderungen. Klin Monatsbl Augenheilkd 1920;64:825–36.
115. Cook C. Uveal lymphosarcoma. Br J Ophthalmol 1954;38:182–5.
116. Zauberman H, Freund M. Pseudolymphoma of the choroid in a patient with senile disciform macular degeneration. Ophthalmologica 1971;163:650–72.
117. Beasley H. Lymphosarcoma of the choroids. Am J Ophthalmol 1961;51:1294–6.
118. Crookes GP, Mullaney J. Lymphoid hyperplasia of the uveal tract simulating malignant lymphoma. Am J Ophthalmol 1967;63:962–7.
119. Ryan SJ, Zimmerman LE, King FM. Reactive lymphoid hyperplasia. An unusual form of intraocular pseudotumor. Trans Am Ophthalmol Otol Soc 1972; 76:652–71.
120. Cockerham GC, Hidayat AA, Bijwaard KE, Sheng ZM. Re-evaluation of reactive lymphoid hyperplasia of the uvea; an immunohistochemical and molecular analysis of 10 cases. Ophthalmology 2000; 107:151–8.
121. Jakobiec FA, Sacks E, Kronish JW, et al. Multifocal static creamy choroidal infiltrates. An early sign of lymphoid neoplasia. Ophthalmology 1987;94:397–406.
122. Grossniklaus HE, Martin DF, Avery R, Shields JA. Uveal lymphoid infiltration. Report of four cases and clinicopathologic review. Ophthalmology 1998; 105:1265–73.
123. Desroches G, Abrams GW, Gass JD. Reactive lymphoid hyperplasia of the uvea. A case with ultrasonographic computed tomographic studies. Arch Ophthalmol 1983;101:725–8.
124. Kannan KA. Lymphomatous pseudotumour of the choroid with secondary retinal detachment. Ind Ophthalmol 1976;23:28–31.
125. Feldon SE, Sigelman J, Albert DM, Smith TR. Clinical manifestations of brawny scleritis. Am Ophthalmol 1978;85:781–7.
126. Goder G. Scleritis posterior pseudotumorosa. Klin Monat 1969;155:200–14.
127. Singh G, Guthoff R, Foster CS. Observation on long-term follow-up of posterior scleritis. Am J Ophthalmol 1986;101:570–5.
128. McGavic JS. Lymphomatoid diseases involving the eye and its adnexa. Arch Ophthalmol 1943;30:179–93.
129. Schwarze E-W, Radaszkiewicz T, Pulhorn G, et al. Maligne and benigne Lymphome des Auges der Lid und Orbitalregion. Virchows Arch Pathol Anat und Histol 1976;370:85–96.
130. Turner L, Howel D. The ocular lymphomas. South Med 1966;J 59:1036–40.
131. Calle R, Zadjdella A, Hay C, Schlienger P. Tumours lymphoides malignes (chrimatives) de l'orbite, de l'oeil et de ses annexes. Bull Cancer 1970;58: 329–59.
132. Fraser DJ Jr, Font RL. Ocular inflammation and hemorrhage as initial manifestations of the uveal malignant melanoma, incidence and prognosis. Arch Ophthalmol 1979;97:1311–4.

11

Retinal Tumors

There are relatively few retinal neoplasms. Retinoblastoma is the most common retinal malignancy and is discussed in the chapters on retinal tumors and retinoblastoma. Metastatic lesions involving the retina are quite rare and much less frequent than uveal tract metastases. Retinal and retinal pigment epithelial (RPE) hamartomas occur, and both neoplasms and malformations of the retinal vasculature and pigment epithelium have been reported. This chapter discusses retinal tumors and simulating lesions that are important in ocular oncology; discussion of other retinal problems can be found in textbooks on retinal disease.

VON HIPPEL-LINDAU SYNDROME AND ISOLATED RETINAL ANGIOMAS

In retrospect, probably the first clinical description of von Hippel-Lindau syndrome (VHL) was by Treacher Collins in 1894.[1] Von Hippel first described vascular tumors of the retina in 1904; Lindau observed their association with cerebellar tumors in 1926.[2–4] In addition to central nervous system (CNS) findings, both visceral carcinomas and cysts occur as part of this syndrome.[5] Renal cell carcinoma, pancreatic carcinoma, pheochromocytoma, endolymphatic sac tumor, islet cell tumor, and meningiomas have been reported with the syndrome, as have cysts in the pancreas, kidney, epididymis, liver, lung, adrenal glands, bone, omentum, and mesocolon.[6–15] The life-time risk of renal cell carcinoma is approximately 70 percent and is the most common cause of death.[15]

Isolated retinal hemangioblastomas (angiomatosis retinae, capillary hemangiomas, or VHL lesions) or those in association with systemic and CNS findings (VHL) occur either as a sporadic, isolated, nonheritable condition or as an autosomal-dominant disease.[16]

Isolated retinal capillary angiomas can be the presenting sign of VHL disease in as many as 43 percent of cases.[17] In one meta-analysis, the authors found that isolated angiomas occurred in statistically significantly older age groups than the retinal hemangioblastoma in association with VHL syndrome (48 years versus 25 years).[18] In contradiction, in a prospective study from the United Kingdom, of 32 patients referred with solitary angiomas, 17 had no evidence in themselves or family members of VHL, nor were there any germline VHL mutations noted.[19] In that latter analysis, the age of the patients with isolated disease was 27.5 years, and the prevalence was less than that of VHL, approximately 1 in 110,000 patients. In a German study of 20 patients with retinal angiomas, 16 had VHL. Interestingly, on the basis of clinical findings or family history, 15 of the 16 could be documented without molecular studies.[20]

Most patients with VHL syndrome have a positive family history. The most common initial presentation is decreased vision in the second or third decade of life. Less frequently, in the VHL syndrome, either CNS involvement or a systemic carcinoma can be the presenting sign; visceral cysts and angioma are usually asymptomatic. Retinal lesions occur in one-half to two-thirds of patients with VHL disease.[12,21]

In a large cross-sectional clinical and molecular study of 183 patients reported from England, the prevalence of ocular lesions in VHL disease was 68 percent (124 of 183) and the mean number of angiomas was 1.85. Neither the occurrence nor number of angiomas appeared to increase with age. They estimated the cumulative probability of vision loss by age 50 years at 35 percent. As would be expected, angiomas were rare in the posterior retina and more common in the supratemporal retina or on the optic disc.[22]

Our understanding of the molecular genetics of this syndrome continues to evolve. The gene for this disease is on chromosome 3 and seems to function as a tumor suppressor. Using a positional cloning strategy, it was located at 3p25-26.[23–27] As we have noted in uveal melanoma, newer methods have shown several other genomic alterations in this condition.[26,27] A study of 93 families all showed germline mutations.[28] A compilation of the VHL mutations is available on the internet at *www.ncicrf.gov/kidney*. This tumor suppressor gene appears to negatively regulate the transcription of elongin.[29,30] Studies of six intraocular angioma tissues demonstrated loss of heterozygosity of the gene in the vacuolated stromal cells but not the vascular or reactive endothelial cells. In addition, vascular endothelial growth factor was also found in these cells.[31] Southern blot analysis, single stranded conformation and polymorphism (SSCP) analysis, and direct sequencing may be used to detect VHL gene mutations. The molecular genetic testing for VHL continues to evolve.[32] Flourescent in situ hybridization (FISH) seems to be a reliable and relatively simple way of testing for deletion of the gene; however, potential complications with a pseudogene located on chromosome 1 may influence the results.[33] FISH is used to delect deletions but does not detect VHL mutations, which are more common.

While for some other VHL lesions, either missense (pheochromocytoma) or nonsense correlations are correlative with systemic bondings, no specific type of genetic changes have correlated with the occular phenotypic expression or severity of eye findings.[15,17,22] A cursory review of the molecular biology of VHL disease has recently been published.[34]

The clinical appearance of a retinal angioma, especially in endophytic tumors which protrude from the inner retina into the vitreous, is usually diagnostic.[35] As shown in Figure 11–1A, endophytic lesions are usually pinkish, with an obvious arterial feeder vessel. Bilateral involvement is common in both isolated retinal angiomas and VHL syndrome. Usually, there are multiple lesions, often of different sizes. On fluorescein angiography, there is rapid perfusion through the feeder vessels, with rapid filling and staining of the hemangioblastoma (Figure 11–2).[36] Less commonly, an exophytic process presents as a pale gray lesion, without an obvious feeder vessel; the fluorescein angiogram identifies the lesion. Rarely, the VHL lesion can mimic a diabetic microaneurysm. A less common presentation includes an exudative detachment and a large pinkish red hemangioblastoma on the optic disc (Figure 11–3).[37,38]

Juxtapapillary exophytic capillary hemangiomas may be isolated or may be part of the VHL syndrome. As discussed below, results of treatment for peripapillary hemangioblastomas have been poor.[5]

Fluorescein angioscopy or angiography can detect lesions before they become clinically appar-

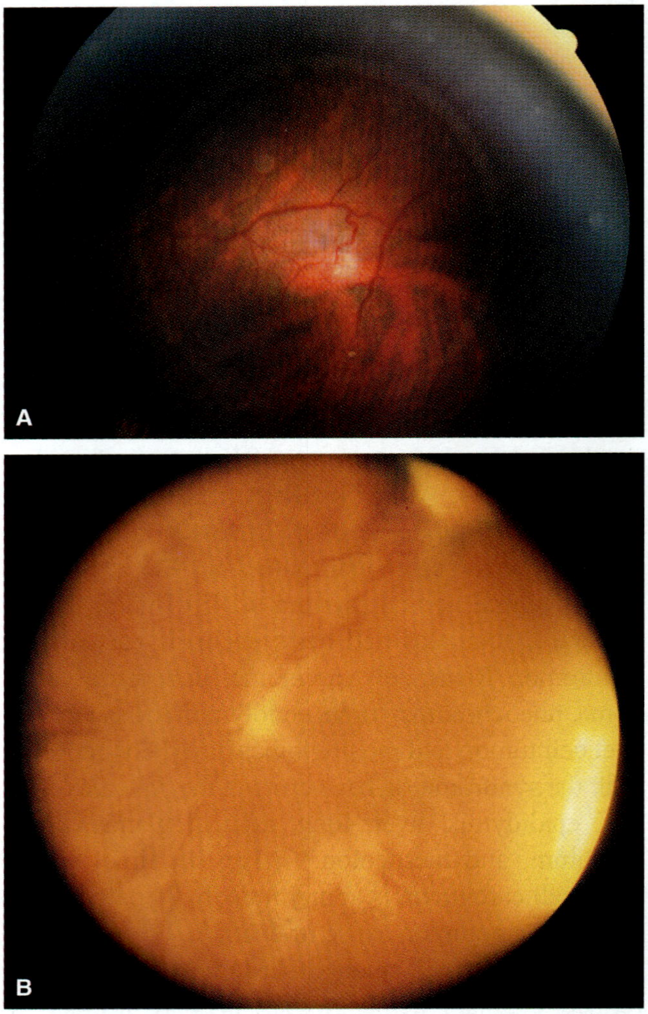

Figure 11–1. *A*, Endophytic von Hippel retinal angioma. *B*, Peripheral angioma with feeder vessels.

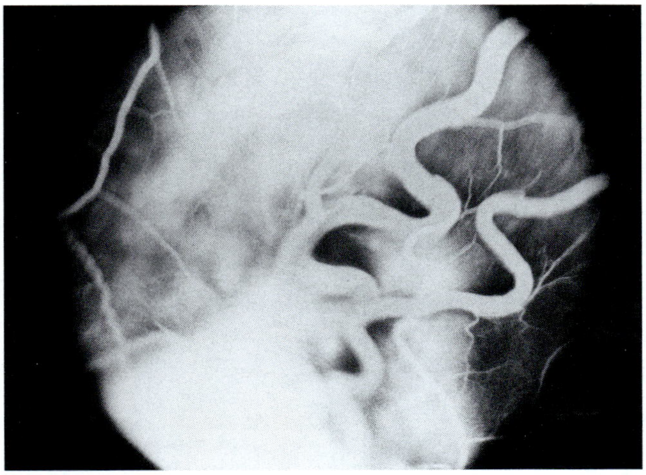

Figure 11–2. Fluorescein angiogram of von Hippel lesion showing rapid perfusion through the feeder vessel and staining in the hemangioblastoma.

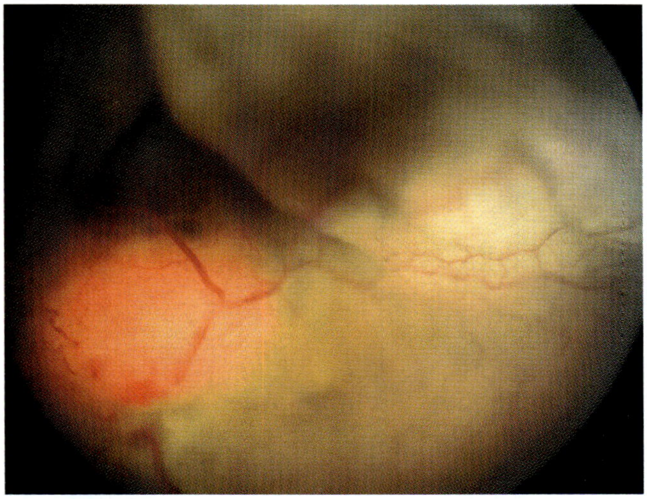

Figure 11–3. Large juxtapapillary hemangioblastoma initially misdiagnosed as a rhegmatogenous retinal detachment.

ent. Other retinal vascular malformations or tumors usually do not have obvious feeder vessels, although they occur occasionally in retinoblastomas and less commonly in melanomas. Figure 11–4 shows an apparent feeder vessel in a child initially misdiagnosed as having a possible retinal angioma that was histologically found to be a retinoblastoma.

Magnetic resonance imaging (MRI) with gadolinium has been shown to be more sensitive than computed tomography (CT) for detecting VHL lesions of the CNS.[39,40] These and body scans should be obtained in any patient with a retinal angioma.[41] MRI of the brain should be performed to establish whether or not there are CNS hemangioblastomas (Figures 11–5A and B); while these tumors are most common in the cerebellum, they can occur in the medulla, other areas of the brainstem, cerebrum, optic chiasm, optic nerve, or spinal cord.[3,4,40,42,43] Abdominal MRI or ultrasonography should be performed to determine if there are angiomas, malignancies, or cysts (Figure 11–6).[41,44,45]

The choice of ocular therapy is dependent on the size and location of the retinal angioma and the presence or absence of overlying fibrosis and hemorrhage. Many small lesions (< 1.5 mm in diameter with minimal elevation) can be monitored and show little growth on serial evaluation.[14,21] Lesions < 4.5 mm in diameter and 1.0 mm in elevation can usually be treated with argon laser or xenon arc photocoagulation; however, especially with thicker lesions, adjunctive cryotherapy, using a double freeze-thaw technique, often is necessary.[16,46–50] Usually, both the tumor and the vessels supplying the mass regress after successful therapy. Figures 11–7A to C show marked regression of the vessel caliber prior to obvious change of the peripheral tumor mass. Treatment complications are most common in lesions with an extensive overlying vitreous and fibrous reaction; the possibility of macular pucker and either exudative or rhegmatogenous detachment in these cases is significant.[51,52] Small

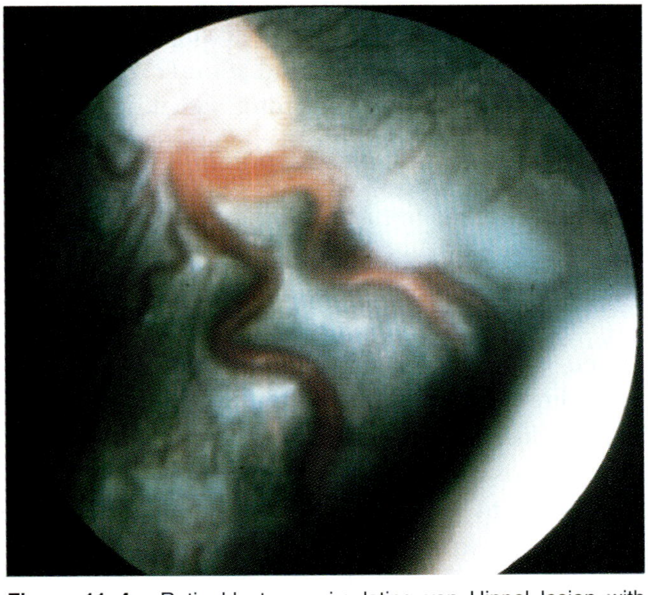

Figure 11–4. Retinoblastoma simulating von Hippel lesion with enlarged "feeder vessels."

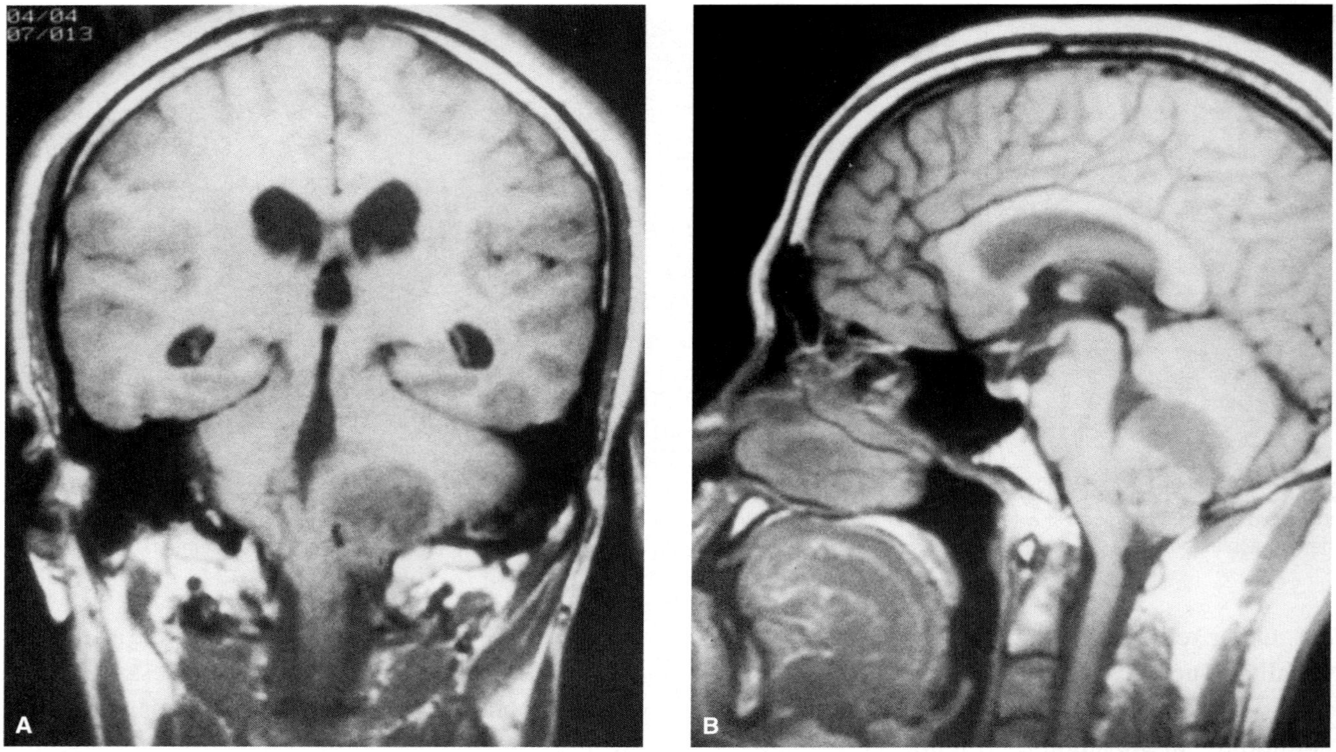

Figure 11–5. *A,* MRI demonstrating CNS cerebellar hemangioblastoma: the coronal view. *B,* MRI demonstrating CNS cerebellar hemangioblastoma: parasagittal view.

lesions without these associated findings generally do well; large lesions, especially on the disc, have a poor visual prognosis. More recently, the use of indirect ophthalmoscopic lasers or dye yellow lasers have been used successfully for lesions < 4 mm in diameter.[53] Vascular tumors on the disc are probably optimally managed with either a single high-dose fraction of Gamma-Knife irradiation (Figure 11–8) or approximately 20 Gy of proton radiation.[54]

Diathermy or eye wall resections have been used to treat very large tumors. In the author's limited experience, it has been found that creating a partial-thickness scleral flap decreases complications when diathermy is used.

New retinal angiomas can occur in the VHL syndrome. Consequently, patients require serial evaluations throughout life. Mortality in this syndrome is usually due to CNS or visceral malignancies. The use of radiosurgery for CNS hemangioblastomas has had excellent results. In one small study, 10 to 15 gray (Gy) resulted in excellent control in most patients without cysts.[55] In another study of 29 tumors in 13 patients, only 3 progressed.[56]

MISCELLANEOUS RETINAL VASCULAR LESIONS

Acquired retinal vascular abnormalities can simulate an isolated VHL lesion; however, they almost

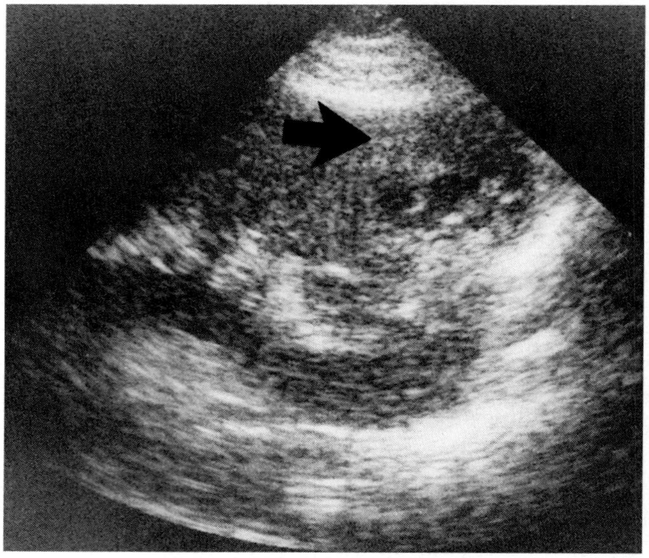

Figure 11–6. Abdominal ultrasound demonstrating renal carcinoma in a patient with von Hippel-Lindau syndrome.

never have feeder vessels. They are yellowish or orange red, and often have exudate and hemorrhage. Figures 11–9A to C show acquired hemangiomas that arose in an area of intermediate uveitis after many years of inflammation. Figure 11–10 shows a spontaneous acquired hemangioma. Most of these tumefactions occur in the inferior temporal periphery. Shields and colleagues described 12 cases; usually, the lesions were peripheral and had an associated exudate and an intraretinal hemorrhage.[57,58] Over 100 such cases have been described, occurring either as primary idiopathic vascular lesions or as complications of intermediate uveitis or retinitis pigmentosa.[59] In a few cases, multiple or bilateral lesions were noted. The etiology remains obscure, although probably angiogenic cytokines are important in their pathophysiology.[60]

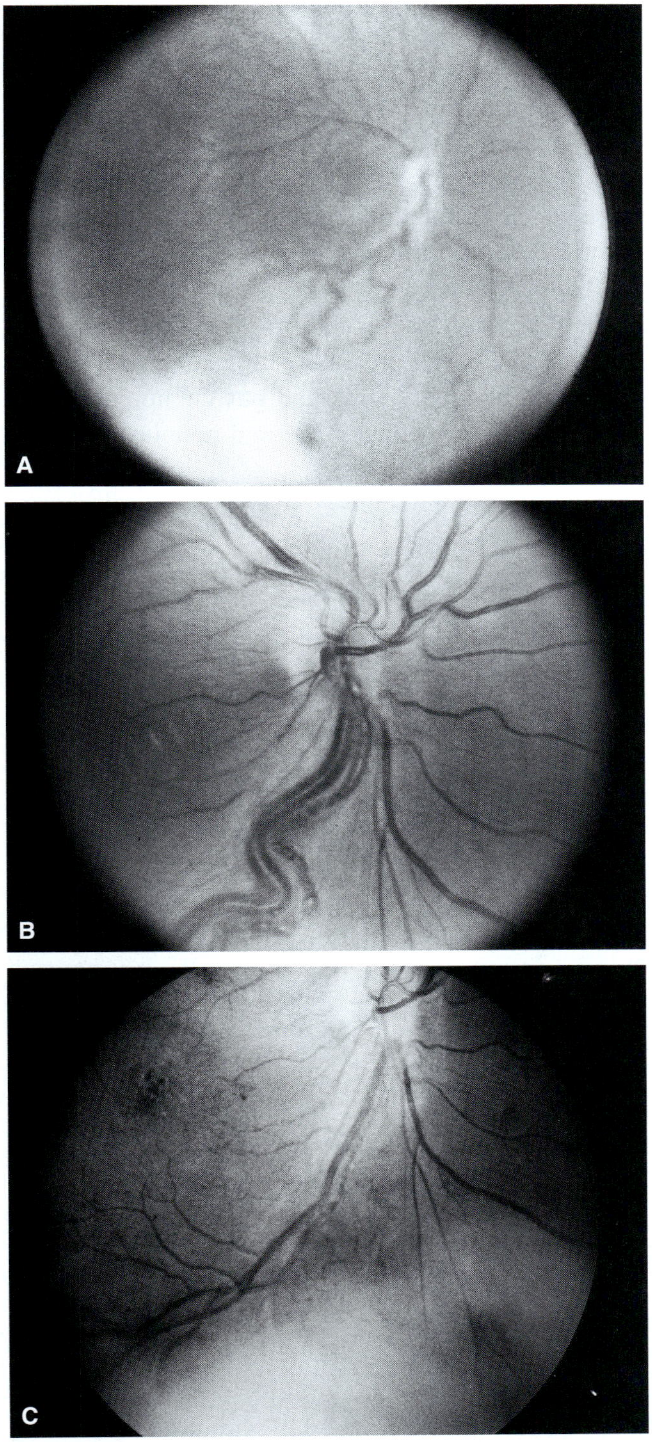

Figure 11–7. *A,* An equator-plus photograph of a large peripheral tumor in a case of von Hippel-Lindau syndrome. *B,* A 30° photograph shows expanded vessels. *C,* Two months after treatment, the tumor remains stationary in size, but vessels are markedly attenuated.

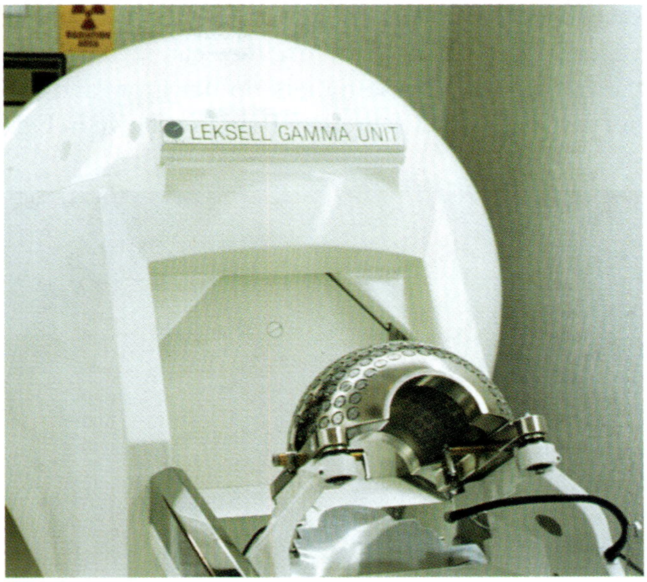

Figure 11–8. Gamma Knife can be used to deliver focused high-dose teletherapy to an angioma on the optic nerve.

If these lesions remain stable, they do not require treatment.[61] If the tumors progress or produce an exudative detachment, cryotherapy, or, if that fails, diathermy through a scleral flap is usually effective. The lesion shown in Figure 11–10A became symptomatic with exudative changes in the fovea, and vision decreased to 20/200. After double freeze-thaw cryotherapy, the lesion slowly regressed, with restoration of vision over a 6-week period to 20/20 (Figure 11–10B).

Retinal cavernous hemangiomas are unusual retinal vascular malformations that occur alone or in association with other CNS and systemic processes.[62–64] Clinically, these lesions usually appear as multiple sacculated aneurysms along the course of a retinal venule (Figure 11–11). Rarely, they can involve only the optic disc.[65] These tumors do not grow and are not associated with subretinal fluid. As shown in Figure 11–11, they occasionally demonstrate fibrotic changes overlying their surface and have been characterized as grape-like clusters with minimal elevation. In Figure 11–12, the angiogram shows the typical pattern with layering out of red cells due to the very slow perfusion through this area.

Most patients with retinal cavernous hemangiomas do not require ocular therapy. Approximately one-third of the patients have evidence of CNS vascular pathology. Approximately 55 cases have been reported, and those which were familial had an autosomal-dominant inheritance, with high penetrance.[64,66]

Racemose hemangioma, a subgroup that is part of the Wyburn-Mason syndrome, has a classic clinical appearance (Figure 11–13); these lesions can be associated with CNS disease but do not clinically simulate the appearance of retinal neoplasms.[67–69]

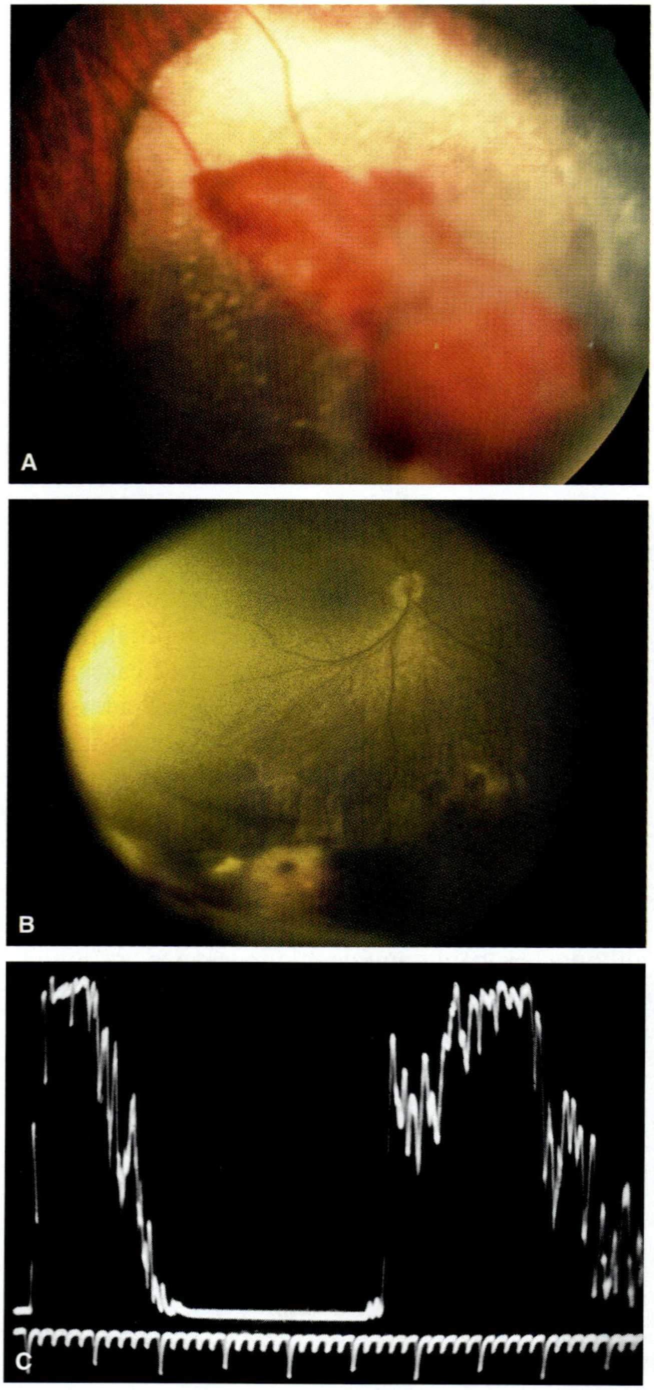

Figure 11–9. *A*, Acquired hemangiomas in patients with long-standing intermediate uveitis. Close up of pinkish lesion in area of scarring. *B*, Equator plus photograph of another small peripheral angioma. *C*, Quantitative echography demonstrated pattern similar to choroidal hemangioma.

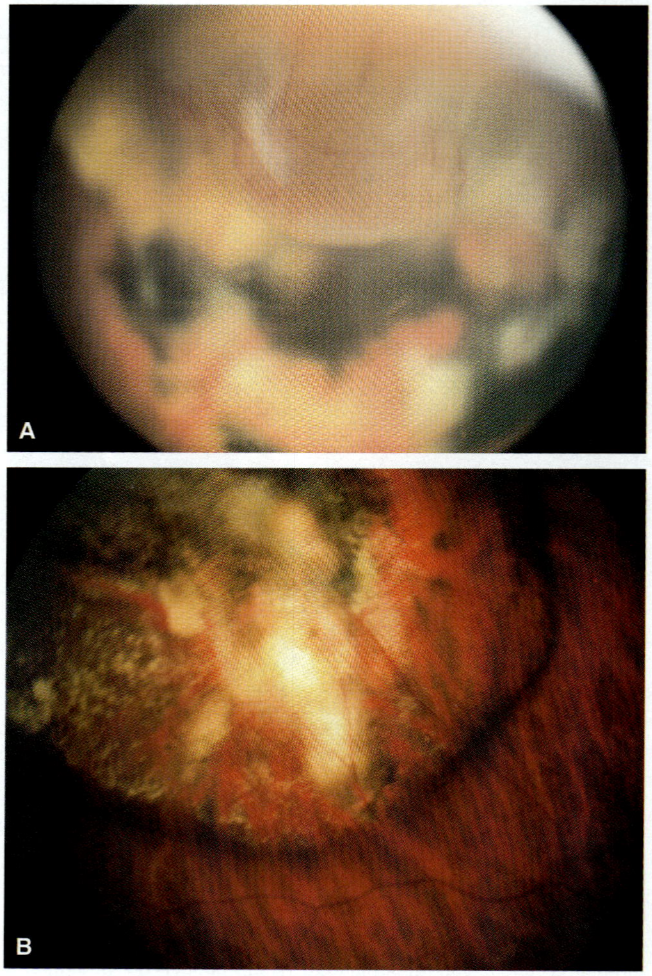

Figure 11–10. *A*, Acquired idiopathic hemangioma. *B*, Lesion shown in Figure 11–10A after cryotherapy.

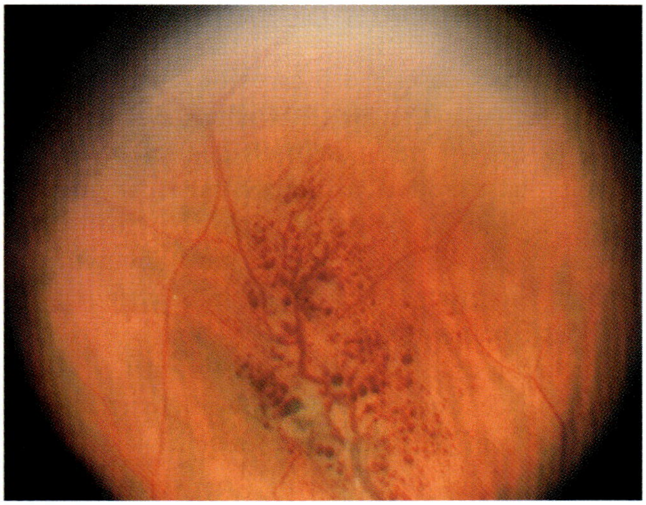

Figure 11–11. Retinal cavernous hemangioma. These tumors have low flow and usually simulate a series of "grape like" microaneurysms along the course of a vein.

MISCELLANEOUS RETINAL LESIONS

Astrocytic hamartoma of the retina can occur as an isolated finding or as a part of tuberous sclerosis or neurofibromatosis.[70-73] These lesions enlarge over time, without evidence of calcification, until late childhood.[74] In one study, with an average follow-up of > 16 years, few of these lesions progressed.[75] Figures 11–14A to C show a 3-month-old patient referred for a retinoblastoma, with several noncalcified astrocytic hamartomas. Fluorescein angiographic findings often demonstrate multiple vessels. The youngest patient diagnosed with a retinal hamartoma in this syndrome was 7 days old.[76] If a child has tuberous sclerosis, other systemic findings may include adenoma sebaceum, shagreen patches most often found in the lumbar area, cutaneous ash-leaf lesions easily visible under Wood's light, subungual fibromas, and cardiac rhabdomyomas.[77] Most patients with tuberous sclerosis are mentally retarded. The retinal mulberry pattern is very uncommon in young patients; calcification is not present until the child is at least 8 years old. Occasionally, a hypopigmented iris spot is also an early sign of tuberous sclerosis.[78] A tuberous sclerosis fundus lesion in an older child is shown in Figures 11–15A and B. As discussed under retinoblastoma in Chapter 12, this calcification does not occur in the age group in which retinoblastoma is most prevalent. Occasionally, these retinal astrocytic hamartomas can be hard to diagnose. There is a case report of a fine-needle aspiration biopsy (FNAB) that showed benign spindle and stellate cells.[79] Rarely, these tumefactions can grow to quite a large size and, less commonly, can appear in an otherwise normal adult.[80,81]

Massive gliosis of the retina is another condition which very rarely can mimic an intraocular neoplasm; in 72 cases reported from the Armed Forces Institute of Pathology, only 4 were thought to have a possible intraocular tumor. While calcification occurs as part of this syndrome, it is a late development.[82]

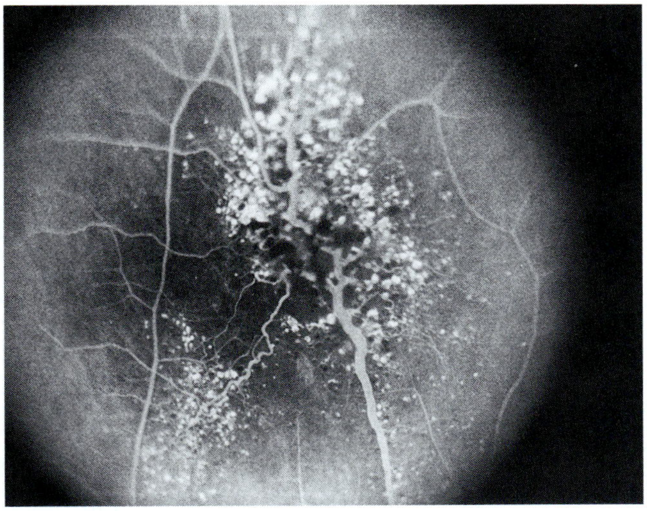

Figure 11–12. Fluorescein angiography showing layering-out of erythrocytes in a retinal cavernous hemangioma.

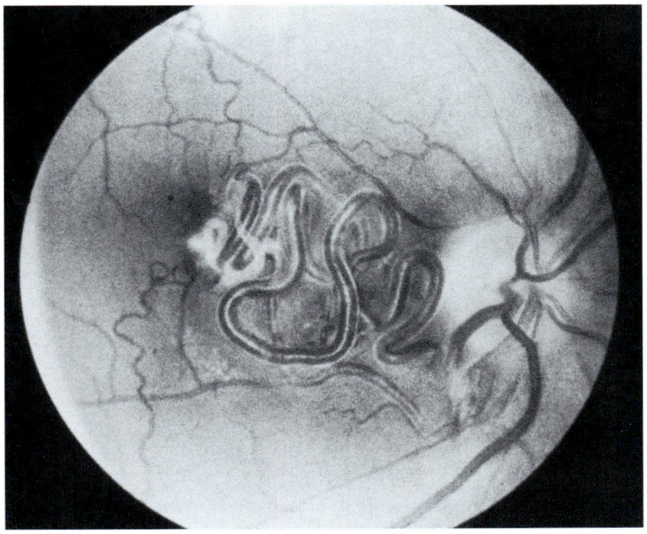

Figure 11–13. Racemose angioma (Wyburn-Mason syndrome).

COATS' DISEASE

George Coats described 6 cases of retinal vascular malformation and reviewed 14 others from the literature in 1908.[83] He initially divided his cases into three groups: group 1 had no vascular hemorrhagic changes, group 2 showed multiple abnormalities of retinal vessels with hemorrhages but without inflammation, and group 3 had both angiomas and arteriovenous communications.

Inclusion criteria for the diagnosis of Coats' disease have been variably defined by different authors.[84] The spectrum of syndromes which Coats initially

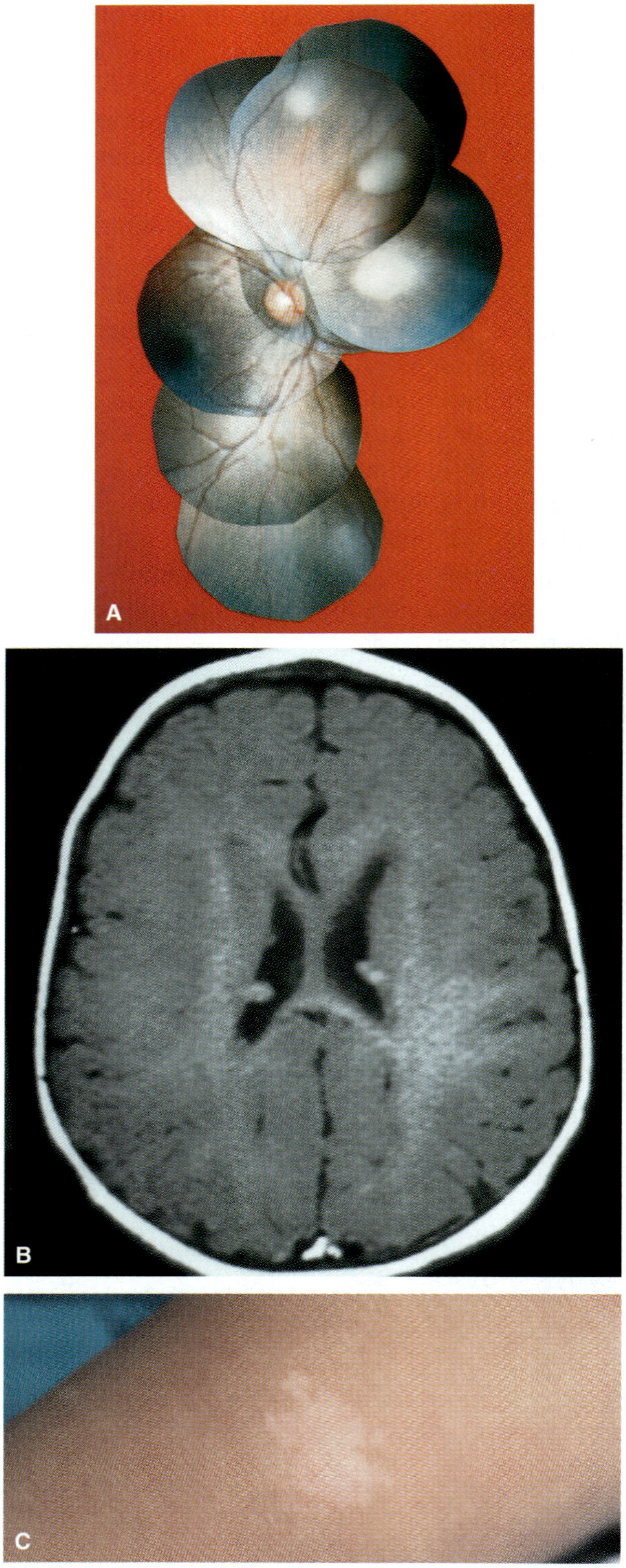

Figure 11–14. *A,* Three-month-old child with nine calcified astrocytic hamartomas. *B,* Tuberous sclerosis evident on axial MRI of brain. *C,* Skin lesion in 3-month-old, consistent with tuberous sclerosis.

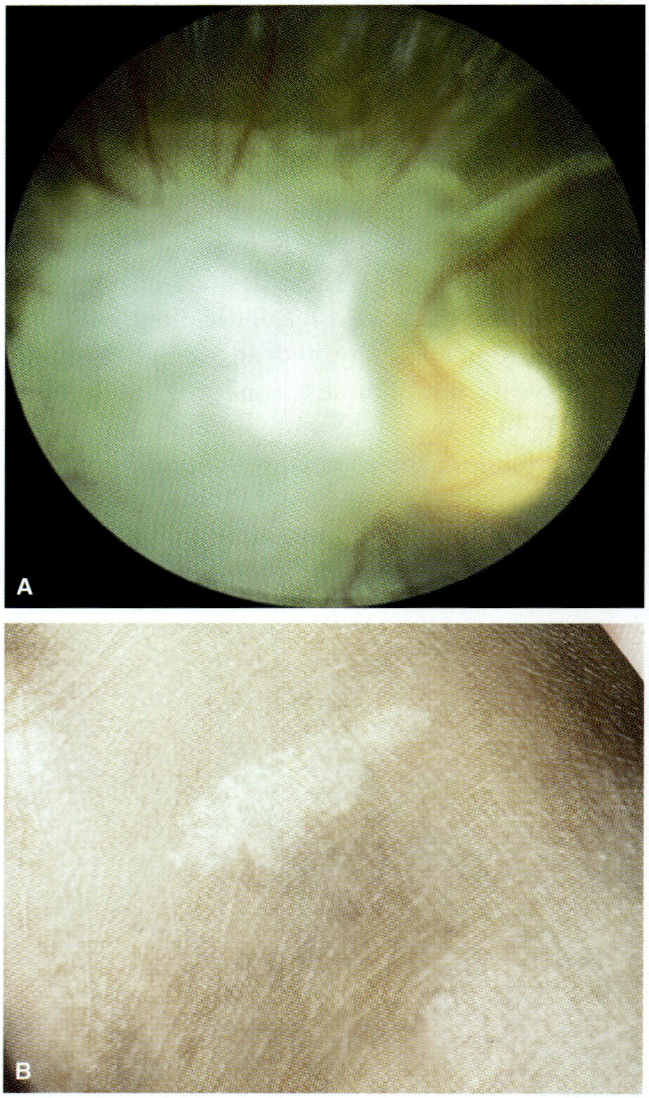

Figure 11–15. *A,* Tuberous sclerosis in an older child. Calcification of these lesions is very unusual < 8 years. *B,* Ash-leaf sign is typical in this disease.

included in his description would encompass Leder's miliary aneurysms, Reese's telangiectasia, VHL disease, racemose aneurysms, and other malformations. Currently, most ophthalmologists restrict the diagnosis of Coats' disease to those entities that have retinal vascular abnormalities with telangiectasia and exudation. Exudation from the vascular abnormalities produces a yellowish tumefaction which can simulate a neoplasm. Over 95 percent of cases are unilateral, and there is a strong male predominance; in one series, 25 of 28 patients were male. Coats' syndrome is not hereditary.[85]

Two variants of Coats' syndrome can simulate a tumor. In children under 3 years old, Coats' syndrome can mimic an exophytic retinoblastoma; in teenage or older patients, the exudation associated with Coats' syndrome can be confused with a metastatic uveal tumor or an amelanotic melanoma.[86]

In very young children, Coats' syndrome usually presents as a total retinal detachment. The subretinal exudate is yellowish in color (Figure 11–16), in contrast to the white or pinkish color observed with retinoblastoma. Examination with scleral depression often reveals telangiectatic changes in the peripheral retina (see Figure 11–16). As discussed in more detail under retinoblastoma, high-resolution thin-section CT evaluation of Coats' syndrome in a child under the age of 4 years never demonstrates intraocular calcification.[87] In contrast, intraocular calcification is almost uniformly present in retinoblastoma > 5 mm thick.[88] Proton magnetic resonance spectroscopy (MRS) can also be used to differentiate Coats' syndrome from retinoblastoma. There is hyperintensity on both T_1- and T_2-weighted images on MRS scans of Coats' disease. In contrast, in retinoblastoma, they are often hyperintense on T_1-weighted scans but hypointense on T_2-weighted scans.[89]

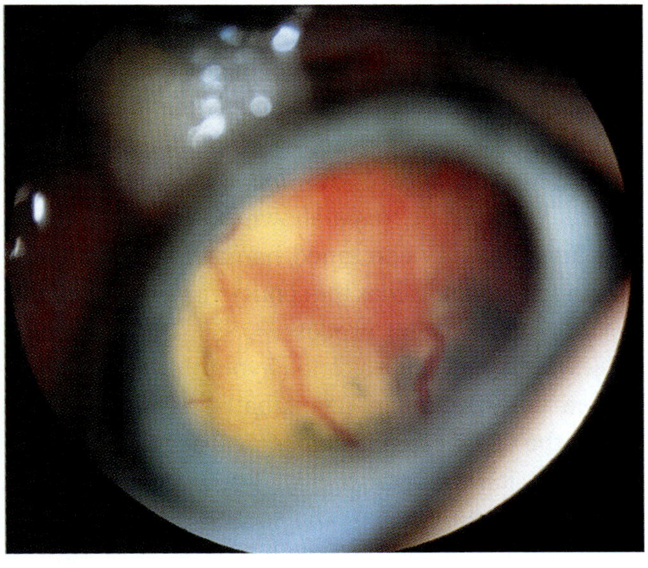

Figure 11–16. Total detachment in Coats' disease. Note the yellowish color of the subretinal exudate and the peripheral retinal telangiectasia.

There is great variation in the presentation patterns and clinical course of Coats' syndrome. The majority of patients at presentation are either < 4 years or > 10 years old.[87] Most untreated young children develop retinal detachment; Morales reported this complication in 17 of 22 cases.[90] In addition, glaucoma occurred in some. Generally, patients < 3 years old had more complications, and the eyes of many of these patients were eventually removed.[85,90,91]

The choice of treatment in Coats' syndrome depends on ocular status and patient age at diagnosis. We and others have used drainage and cryotherapy to treat total detachments, usually in patients < 3 years of age.[91] Microscopic analysis of the subretinal fluid demonstrates lipid-laden macrophages (Figure 11–17). After subretinal fluid drainage, the peripheral retinal telangiectatic areas are treated with double freeze-thaw cryotherapy. Although there is basically no chance of retaining vision in these eyes, the retina remains attached after treatment, and cosmesis is better than if the eye were removed and a prosthesis implanted. In a recent publication, we noted that while we were able to achieve long-term (> 10 years) reattachment in 9 of 10 eyes with Coats' syndrome presenting with possible retinoblastoma, the visual results were dismal.[92]

In older patients, the first symptom in Coats' syndrome is usually decreased vision or visual distortion due to macular exudation with peripheral telangiectasia.[93] These cases are managed with photocoagulation or cryotherapy of the peripheral retinal telangiectasia. In our experience, either ablative modality gives equally good results. The resorption of subretinal exudate is very slow, usually taking between 3 and 12 months following successful treatment. Rarely, after adequate treatment, new retinal telangiectases develop or become apparent in other areas of the peripheral fundus. Despite the rarity of

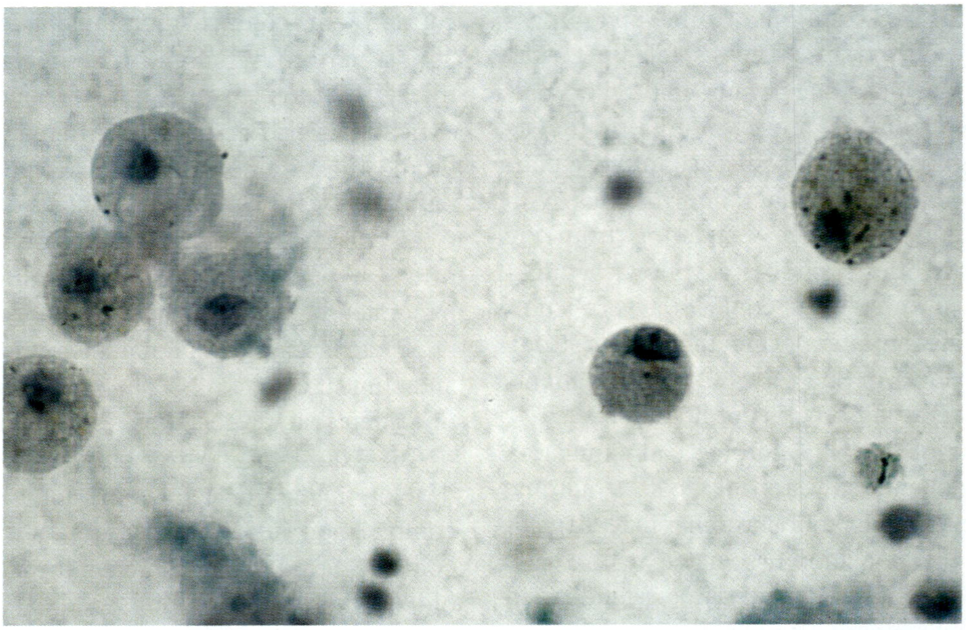

Figure 11–17. Lipid-laden macrophages on fine-needle aspiration biopsy of the subretinal fluid from a patient with Coats' disease.

recurrence, frequent examinations are necessary, and we have observed disease reactivation as late as 5 years after successful treatment. As discussed elsewhere, isolated adult Coats' syndrome in the macular area occurs but usually does not enter into the differential diagnosis of ocular oncologic problems. Occasionally, Coats' syndrome occurs along with other conditions, including retinitis pigmentosa or various systemic syndromes.[93]

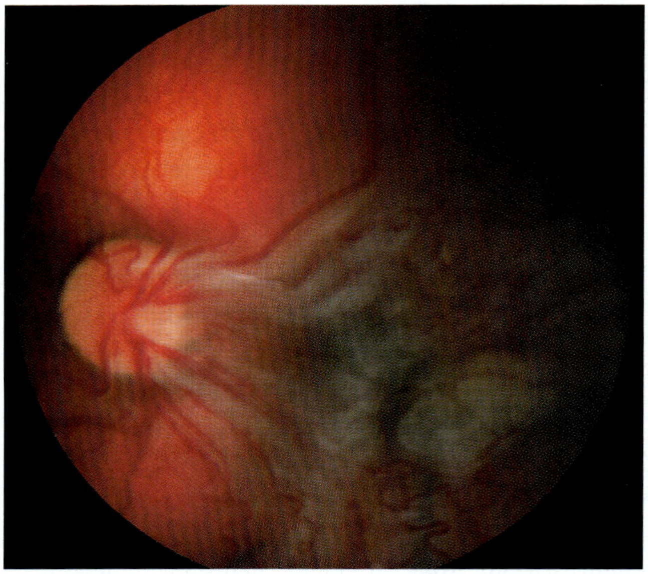

Figure 11–18. Combined retinal-RPE hamartoma in a typical peripapillary location, showing surface contracture and minimum pigmentation.

RETINAL PIGMENTARY LESIONS

Retinal Pigmentary Hamartomas

Combined retinal-RPE hamartomas are quite rare. These lesions have a slight elevation with minimum pigmentation and show contraction of the retinal surface (see Figure 11–18).[94] Their appearance thus produces a pattern consistent with a vascular retinopathy, and they usually do not simulate a neoplasm. Two recent cases of idiopathic reactive hyperplasias of the RPE have shown histologic features that simulate this combined hamartoma, and those authors speculated that this entity may be a reactive not a hamartomatous process.[95]

RPE hypertrophies and hyperplasias are discussed in Chapter 6. They usually are flat and jet-black; the former have rounded or scalloped margins, while the latter have irregular borders. Retinal pigment adenomas are also discussed in Chapter 6. Usually, there is a feeder vessel leading to the lesion as shown in Figures 6–16 and 6–17. Occasionally, RPE adenomas can be mistaken for a uveal melanoma.[96]

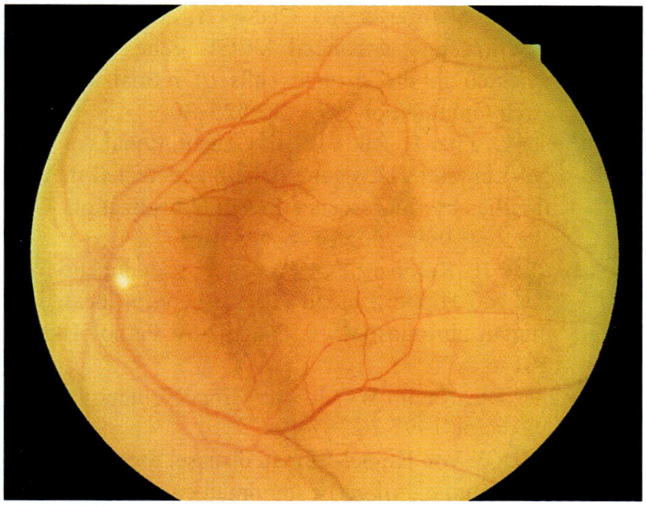

Figure 11–19. Cutaneous melanoma metastatic to the retina.

METASTATIC AND PARANEOPLASTIC SYNDROMES

Approximately 40 cases of metastases to the retina have been reported; about one-half are from cutaneous melanomas and the others from a variety of metastatic carcinomas.[97] The melanomas metastatic to the retina do not simulate a primary uveal melanoma. A case of a cutaneous melanoma metastatic to the retina is shown in Figure 11–19.

Several different carcinomas and melanomas have been shown to produce an autoimmune paraneoplastic syndrome with reactivity toward photoreceptors, other retinal cells, or the optic nerve.[98–101] Usually, these patients have a history of malignancy and present with marked deterioration of their vision. In carcinomas, several antigens and antibodies have been described. The first antigen described in this syndrome was a 23-kDa retinal protein, labeled a cancer-associated retinopathy (CAR) antigen; many of these patients produce antibodies to this protein.[101–103]

Antibodies against recoverin, enolase, and other retinal proteins have also been described.[101–104] The recoverin protein is involved in the activation and regulation of guanylate cyclase that helps to regulate rhodopsin.[105,106] A rare presentation of paraneoplastic syndrome occurs along with retinal vasculitis.[107] The patients with cutaneous melanoma may rarely develop night blindness.[108] Twelve patients with what has been termed melanoma-associated retinopathy have been described with diminished electroretinograms.[109]

REFERENCES

1. Collins ET. Intra-ocular growths (two cases, brother and sister, with peculiar vascular new growth, probably retinal, affecting both eyes). Trans Ophthalmol Soc UK 1894;14:141–9.
2. von Hippel E. Uber eine sehr seltene Erkrankung der Netzhaut: klinisch Beobachtungen. Arch Ophthal 1904;59:83–106.
3. Cushing H, Bailey P. Hemangiomas of the cerebellum and retina (Lindau's disease); with the report of a case. Arch Ophthalmol 1928;57:447–63.
4. Jeffreys R. Clinical and surgical aspects of posterior fossa haemangioblastomata. J Neurol Neurosurg Psychiatry 1975;38:105–11.
5. Hardwig P, Robertson DM. von Hippel-Lindau disease: a familial, often lethal, multi-system phakomatosis. Ophthalmology 1984;91:263–70.
6. Melmon KL, Rosen SW. Lindau's disease: review of the literature and study of a large kindred. Am J Med 1964;36:595–617.
7. Davison C, Brock S, Dyke CG. Retinal and central nervous hemangioblastomatosis and visceral changes (von Hippel-Lindau's disease). Bull Neurol Inst NY 1936;5:72–93.
8. Lee KR, Wilfsberg E, Kepes JJ. Some important radiological aspects of the kidney in Hippel-Lindau syndrome: the value of prospective study in an affected family. Radiology 1977;122:6649–53.
9. Malek RS, Greene LF. Urologic aspects of Hippel-Lindau syndrome. J Urol 1971;106:800–1.
10. Levine E, Lee KR, Weigel FW, Farber B. Computed tomography in the diagnosis of renal carcinoma complicating Hippel-Lindau syndrome. Radiology 1979;130:703–6.
11. Mulholland SG, Atuk NO, Walzak MP. Familial pheochromocytoma associated with cerebellar hemangioblastoma. A case history and review of the literature. JAMA 1969;207:1709–11.
12. Horton WA, Wong V, Eldridge R. von Hippel-Lindau disease: clinical and pathological manifestations in nine families with 50 affected members. Arch Intern Med 1976;136:769–77.
13. Christoferson LA, Gustafson MB, Petersen AG. von Hippel-Lindau's disease. JAMA 1961;178:280–2.
14. Hubschmann OR, Vijayanathan T, Countee RW. Von Hippel-Lindau disease with multiple manifestations: diagnosis and management. Neurosurgery 1981;8: 92–5.
15. Maher ER, Kaelin WG. Von Hippel-Lindau disease. Medicine 1997;76:381–91.

16. Watzke RC, Weingeist TA, Constantine JB. Diagnosis and management of von Hippel-Lindau disease. In: Peyman GA, Apple DJ, Sanders DR, editors. Intraocular tumors. New York, NY: Appleton-Century Crofts; 1977. p. 199–217.
17. Wittebol-Post D, Hes FJ, Lips CJ. The eye in von Hippel-Lindau disease. Long-term follow-up of screening and treatment: recommendations. J Intern Med 1998;243:555–61.
18. Chang JH, Spraul CW, Lynn ML, et al. The two-stage mutation model in retinal hemangioblastoma. Ophthal Genet 1998;19:123–30.
19. Webster AR, Maher ER, Bird AC, et al. A clinical and molecular genetic analysis of solitary ocular angioma. Ophthalmology 1999;106:623–9.
20. Kreusel KM, Bornfeld N, Bender BU, et al. Retinal capillary angioma. Clinical and molecular genetic studies. Ophthalmologe 1999;96:71–6.
21. de Jong PT, Verkaart RJ, van De Vooren MJ, et al. Twin vessels in von Hippel-Lindau disease. Am J Ophthalmol 1988;105:165–9.
22. Webster AR, Maher ER, Moore AT. Clinical characteristics of ocular angiomatosis in von Hippel-Lindau disease and correlation with germline mutation. Arch Ophthalmol 1999;117:371–8.
23. Seizinger BR, Rouleau GA, Ozelius LJ, et al. Von Hippel-Lindau disease maps to the region of chromosome 3 associated with renal cell carcinoma. Nature 1988;332:268–9.
24. Kovacs G, Emanuel A, Neumann HP, Kung HF. Cytogenetics of renal cell carcinomas associated with von Hippel-Lindau disease. Genes Chrom Cancer 1991;3:256–62.
25. Latif F, Tory K, Gnarra J, et al. Identification of the von Hippel-Lindau disease tumor suppressor gene. Science 1993;260:1317–20.
26. Thrash-Bingham CA, Greenberg RE, Howard S, et al. Comparative allelotyping of human renal cell carcinomas using microsatellite DNA probes. Proc Natl Acad Sci USA 1995;92:2854–8.
27. Gordon KB, Thompson CT, Char DH, et al. Comparative genomic hybridization in the detection of DNA copy number abnormalities in uveal melanoma. Cancer Res 1994;54:4764–8.
28. Zbar B, Kaelin W, Maher E, Richard S. Third international meeting on von Hippel-Lindau disease. Cancer Res 1999;59:2251–3.
29. Tsuchiya H, Iseda T, Hino O. Identification of a novel protein (VBP-1) binding to the von Hippel-Lindau (VHL) tumor suppressor gene product. Cancer 1996;56:2881–5.
30. Los M, Aaesman CJM, Terpstra L, et al. Elevated ocular levels of vascular endothelial growth factor in patients with von Hippel-Lindau disease. Ann Oncol 1997;8:1015–22.
31. Chan CC, Vortmeyer AO, Chew EY, et al. VHL gene deletion and enhanced VEGF gene expression detected in the stromal cells of retinal angioma. Arch Ophthalmol 1999;117:625–30.
32. Pack SD, Zbar B, Pak E, et al. Constitutional von Hippel-Lindau (VHL) gene deletions detected in VHL families by fluorescence in situ hybridization. Cancer Res 1999;59:5560–4.
33. Bradley JF, Rothberg PG. Processed pseudogene from the von Hippel-Lindau disease gene is located on human chromosome 1. Diagn Mol Pathol 1999;8:101–6.
34. Maher RE, Kaelin WG Jr. von Hippel-Lindau disease. Medicine 1997;76:381–91.
35. Welch RB. Von Hippel-Lindau disease: the recognition and treatment of early angiomatosis retinae and the use of cryosurgery as an adjunct to therapy. Trans Am Ophthalmol Soc 1970;68:367–424.
36. Goldberg MF, Koenig S. Argon laser treatment of von Hippel-Lindau retinal angiomas. I. Clinical and angiographic findings. Arch Ophthalmol 1974;92:121–5.
37. Jesberg DO, Spencer WH, Hoyt WF. Incipient lesions of von Hippel-Lindau disease. Arch Ophthalmol 1968; 80:632–40.
38. Yimoyines DJ, Topilow HW, Abedin S, McMeel JW. Bilateral peripapillary exophytic retinal hemangioblastomas. Ophthalmology 1982;89:1388–92.
39. Baleriaux-Waha D, Retif J, Noterman J, et al. CT scanning for the diagnosis of the cerebellar and spinal lesions of von Hippel-Lindau's disease. Neuroradiology 1978;14:241–4.
40. Filling-Katz MR, Choyke PL, Patronas NJ, et al. Radiologic screening of von Hippel-Lindau disease: the role of Gd-DTPA enhanced MR imaging of the CNS. J Comput Assist Tomogr 1989;13:743–55.
41. Hes FJ, Feldberg MA. Von Hippel-Lindau disease: strategies in early detection (renal-, adrenal-, pancreatic masses.) Eur Radiol 1999;9:598–610.
42. Otenasek FJ, Silver ML. Spinal hemangioma (hemangioblastoma) in Lindau's disease. J Neurosurg 1961; 18:295–300.
43. Kerr DJ, Scheithauer BW, Miller GM, et al. Hemangioblastoma of the optic nerve: case report. Neurosurgery 1995;36:573–81.
44. Will WL, Lamiell JM, Polk NO. The radiographic manifestations of von Hippel-Lindau disease. Radiology 1979;133:289–95.
45. Wittich G, Czembirek H, Fridrich L, Imhof H. Radiological diagnosis of visceral manifestations in Hippel-Lindau syndrome. Radiologe 1980;20:534–9.
46. Amoils SP, Smith TR. Cryotherapy of angiomatosis retinae. Arch Ophthalmol 1969;81:689–91.
47. Baras I, Harris S, Galin MA. Photocoagulation treat-

ment of angiomatosis retinae. Am J Ophthalmol 1964;58:296–9.
48. Apple DJ, Goldberg MF, Wyhinny GL. Argon laser treatment of von Hippel-Lindau retinal angiomas. II. Histopathology of treated lesions. Arch Ophthalmol 1974;92:126–30.
49. Watzke RC. Cryotherapy for retinal angiomatosis: a clinicopathologic report. Arch Ophthalmol 1974; 92:399–401.
50. Rosa RH Jr, Goldberg MF, Green WR. Clinicopathologic correlation of argon laser photocoagulation of retinal angiomas in a patient with von Hippel-Lindau disease followed for more than 20 years. Retina 1996;16:145–56.
51. Machemer R, Williams JM Sr. Pathogenesis and therapy of traction detachment in various retinal vascular diseases. Am J Ophthalmol 1988;105:170–81.
52. Laatikainen L, Immonen I, Summanen P. Peripheral retinal angiomalike lesion and macular pucker. Am J Ophthalmol 1989;108:563–6.
53. Blodi CF, Russell SR, Pulido JS, Folk JC. Direct and feeder vessel photocoagulation of retinal angiomas with dye yellow laser. Ophthalmology 1990;97:91–7.
54. Patrice JS, Sneed PK, Flickinger JC, et al. Radiosurgery for hemangioblastoma: result of a multiinstitutional experience. Int J Radiat Oncol Biol Phys 1996;35:493–9.
55. Niemela M, Lim YJ, Soderman M, et al. Gamma knife radiosurgery in 11 hemangioblastomas. J Neurosurg 1996;85:591–6.
56. Chang SD, Meisel JA, Hancock SL, et al. Treatment of hemangioblastomas in von Hippel-Lindau disease with linear accelerator-based radiosurgery. Neurosurgery 1998;43:28–35.
57. Shields JA, Decker WL, Sanborn GE, et al. Presumed acquired retinal hemangiomas. Ophthalmology 1983;90:1292–1300.
58. Campochiaro PA, Conway BP. Hemangiomalike masses of the retina. Arch Ophthalmol 1988;106: 1409–13.
59. Shields CL, Shields JA, Barrett J, De Potter P. Vasoproliferative tumors of the ocular fundus. Classification and clinical manifestations in 103 patients. Arch Ophthalmol 1995;113:615–23.
60. Meyer-Schwickerath R, Pfeiffer A, Blum WF, et al. Vitreous levels of the insulin-like growth factors I and II, and the insulin-like growth factor binding proteins 2 and 3, increase in neovascular eye disease. Studies in nondiabetic and diabetic subjects. J Clin Invest 1993;92:2620–5.
61. McCabe CM, Mieler WF. Six-year follow-up of an idiopathic retinal vasoproliferative tumor. Arch Ophthalmol 1996;114:614.
62. Gass JD. Cavernous hemangioma of the retina. A neuro-oculo-cutaneous syndrome. Am J Ophthalmol 1971;71:799–814.
63. Schwartz AC, Weaver RG Jr, Bloomfield R, Tyler ME. Cavernous hemangioma of the retina, cutaneous angiomas, and intracranial vascular lesion by computer tomography and nuclear magnetic resonance imaging. Am J Ophthalmol 1984;98:483–7.
64. Colvard DM, Robertson DM, Trautmann JC. Cavernous hemangioma of the retina. Arch Ophthalmol 1978;96:2042–4.
65. Mansour AM, Jampol LM, Hrisomalos NF, Greenwald M. Case report. Cavernous hemangioma of the optic disc. Arch Ophthalmol 1988;106:22.
66. Bottoni F, Canevini MP, Canger R, Orzalesi N. Twin vessels in familial retinal cavernous hemangioma. Am J Ophthalmol 1990;109:285–9.
67. Archer DB, Deutman A, Ernest JT, Krill AE. Arteriovenous communication of the retina. Am J Ophthalmol 1973;75:224–41.
68. Wyburn-Mason R. Arteriovenous aneurysms of midbrain and retina, facial naevi and mental changes. Brain 1943;66:163–203.
69. Patel U, Gupta SC. Wyburn-Mason syndrome. A case report and review of the literature. Neuroradiology 1990;31:544–6.
70. Reeser FH, Aaberg TM, Van Horn DL. Astrocytic hamartoma of the retina not associated with tuberous sclerosis. Am J Ophthalmol 1978;86:688–98.
71. Landau K, Dossetor FM, Hoyt WF, Muci-Mendoza R. Retinal hamartoma in neurofibromatosis 2. Arch Ophthalmol 1990;108:328–9.
72. Destro M, D'Amico DJ, Gragoudas ES, et al. Retinal manifestations of neurofibromatosis. Diagnosis and management. Arch Ophthalmol 1991;109:662–6.
73. Good WV, Erodsky MC, Edwards MS, Hoyt WF. Bilateral retinal hamartomas in neurofibromatosis type 2. Br J Ophthalmol 1991;75:190.
74. Williams R, Taylor D. Tuberous sclerosis. Surv Ophthalmol 1985;30:143–54.
75. Zimmer-Galler IE, Robertson DM. Long-term observation of retinal lesions in tuberous sclerosis. Am J Ophthalmol 1995;119:318–24.
76. Shami MJ, Benedict WL, Myers M. Early manifestation of retinal hamartomas in tuberous sclerosis. Am J Ophthalmol 1993;115:539–40.
77. Jin F, Wienecke R, Xiao GH, et al. Suppression of tumorigenicity by the wild-type tuberous sclerosis 2 (Tsc2) gene and its C-terminal region. Proc Natl Acad Sci 1996;93:9154–9.
78. Gutman I, Dunn D, Behrens M, et al. Hypopigmented iris spot. An early sign of tuberous sclerosis. Ophthalmology 1982;89:1155–9.
79. Shields JA, Shields CL, Ehya H, et al. Atypical retinal astrocytic hamartoma diagnosed by fine-needle biopsy. Ophthalmology 1996;103:949–52.

80. Gunduz K, Eagle RC, Shields CL, et al. Invasive giant cell astrocytoma of the retina in a patient with tuberous sclerosis. Ophthalmology 1999;106:639–42.
81. Khawly JA, Matthews JD, Machemer R. Appearance and rapid growth of retinal tumor (reactive astrocytic hyperplasia?) Graefes Arch Clin Exp Ophthalmol 1999;237:78–81.
82. Yanoff M, Zimmerman LE, Davis RL. Massive gliosis of the retina. Int Ophthalmol Clin 1971;11:211–29.
83. Coats G. Forms of retinal disease with massive exudation. R London Ophthalmol Hosp Rep 1908;17: 440–525.
84. Campbell FP. Coats' disease and congenital vascular retinopathy. Trans Am Ophthal Soc 1976;74:365–424.
85. Fox KR. Coats' disease. Met Pediatr Ophthalmol 1980;4:121–4.
86. Chang MM, McLean IW, Merritt JC. Coats' disease: a study of 62 histologically confirmed cases. J Pediatr Ophthalmol Strabismus 1984;21:163–8.
87. Sherman JL, McLean IW, Brallier DR. Coats' disease: CT-pathologic correlation in two cases. Radiology 1983;146:77–8.
88. Klintworth GK. Radiographic abnormalities in eyes with retinoblastoma and other disorders. Br J Ophthalmol 1978;62:365-72.
89. Eisenberg L, Castillo M, Kwock L, et al. Proton MR spectroscopy in Coats' Disease. Am J Nucl Radid 1997;18:727–9.
90. Morales AG. Coats' disease. Natural history and results of treatment. Am J Ophthalmol 1965;60:855–65.
91. Ridley ME, Shields JA, Brown GC, Tasman W. Coats' disease: Evaluation and management. Ophthalmology 1982;89:1381–7.
92. Char DH. Coats' disease. Br J Ophthalmol 2000; 84:37–9.
93. Kremer I, Cohen S, Izhak RB, Ben-Sira I. An unusual case of congenital unilateral Coats' disease associated with morning glory optic nerve anomaly. Br J Ophthalmol 1985;69:32–7.
94. Schachat AP, Shields JA, Fine SL, et al. Combined hamartomas of the retina and retinal epithelium. Ophthalmology 1984;91:1609–15.
95. Olsen TW, Frayer WC, Meyer FL, et al. Idiopathic reactive hyperplasia of the retinal pigment epithelium. Arch Ophthalmol 1999;117:50–4.
96. Loose IA, Jampol LM, O'Grady R. Pigmented adenoma mimicking a juxtapapillary melanoma. A 20-year follow-up. Arch Ophthalmol 1999;117:120–2.
97. Leys AM, Van Eyck LM, Nuttin BJ, et al. Metastatic carcinoma to the retina. Clinicopathologic findings in two cases. Arch Ophthalmol 1990;108:1448–52.
98. Weinstein JM, Kelman SE, Bresnick GH, Kornguth SE. Paraneoplastic retinopathy associated with anti-retinal bipolar cell antibodies in cutaneous malignant melanoma. Ophthalmology 1994;101:1236–42.
99. Singh AD, Milam AN, Shields CL, et al. Melanoma-associated retinopathy. Am J Ophthalmol 1995; 119:369–70.
100. Kim RY, Retsas S, Fitzke FW, et al. Cutaneous melanoma—associated retinopathy. Ophthalmology 1994;101:1837–43.
101. Obgruo H, Ogawa KI, Nakagawa T. Recoverin and Hsc-70 are found as autoantigens in patients with cancer associated retinopathy. Invest Ophthal Vis Sci 1999;40:82–99.
102. Thirkill CE, Fitzgerald P, Sergott RC, et al. Cancer-associated retinopathy (CAR syndrome) with antibodies reacting with retinal, optic-nerve, and cancer cells. N Engl J Med 1989;321:1589–94.
103. Guy J, Aptsiauri N. Treatment of paraneoplastic visual loss with intravenous immunoglobulin: report of 3 cases. Arch Ophthalmol 1999;117:471–7.
104. Yamaji Y, Matsubara S, Yamadori I, et al. Characterization of a small-cell-lung-carcinoma cell line from a patient with cancer-associated retinopathy. Int J Cancer 1996;65:671–6.
105. Thirkill CE, Tait RC, Tyler NK, et al. The cancer-associated retinopathy antigen is recoverin-like protein. Invest Ophthalmol Vis Sci 1992;33:2768–72.
106. Adamus G, Guy J, Schmied JL, et al. Role of anti-recoverin autoantibodies in cancer-associated retinopathy. Invest Ophthalmol Vis Sci 1993;34:2626–33.
107. Ohnishi Y, Ohara S, Sakamoto T, et al. Cancer-associated retinopathy with retinal phlebitis. Br J Ophthalmol 1993;77:795–8.
108. Berson EL, Lessell S. Paraneoplastic night blindness with malignant melanoma. Am J Ophthalmol 1988; 106:307–11.
109. Boeck K, Hofmann S, Klopfer M, et al. Melanoma-associated paraneoplastic retinopathy: case report and review of the literature. Br J Derm 1997;137: 457–60.

12

Retinoblastoma: Pathogenesis and Diagnosis

J. WILLIAM HARBOUR, MD

Retinoblastoma is the most common intraocular malignancy in children and is the prototype for inherited cancer predisposition syndromes. Retinoblastoma accounts for about 3 percent of registered cancers in children < 15 years old, and occurs in about 1 in 18,000 live births.[1,2] Some reports have suggested an increase in the incidence of retinoblastoma in the 20th century, but the rate appears to have been stable in recent years.[3] Retinoblastoma has no significant gender or race predilection, and it has not been convincingly linked to any environmental or infectious agents.

Retinoblastoma was first described in 1597, and prognosis was dismal through the nineteenth century, at which time enucleation became more widely accepted.[4] In the 20th century, survival has dramatically increased from around 5 percent to over 95 percent in the developed countries, making retinoblastoma one of the success stories in childhood cancer. Several of the most important challenges that still lie ahead are (1) more sophisticated genetic testing for germline retinoblastoma (*Rb*) gene mutations, (2) new treatments for the intraocular tumors with fewer systemic side effects, and (3) better management of second primary cancers, which are a leading cause of death among survivors of hereditary retinoblastoma.

PATHOLOGY

Retinoblastoma probably arises from primordial retinoblasts, which have the potential to differentiate along the lines of photoreceptors or Mueller cells.[5–7] Histopathologically, retinoblastoma consists of small- to medium-sized round cells with large nuclei and scant cytoplasm.[8] Well-differentiated tumors may have Flexner-Wintersteiner rosettes, Homer-Wright rosettes, and fleurettes, which probably represent photoreceptor differentiation. Tumors may assume an endophytic pattern, in which growth is predominantly into the vitreous cavity, or an exophytic pattern, in which the tumor grows into the subretinal space, often detaching the overlying retina. The growth pattern is not prognostic for survival but can have implications for management (see next chapter). One of the most important histopathologic prognostic features is optic nerve invasion. In one study, 10 percent mortality was observed with superficial invasion of the nerve head, 29 percent with involvement of the lamina cribrosa, 42 percent with extension posterior to the lamina, and 78 percent with tumor cells to the surgical resection line.[9] Other poor prognostic features include extraocular extension and massive choroidal invasion.[10]

PATHOGENESIS

Approximately 35 to 40 percent of patients with retinoblastoma have a germline form of the disease, which can be passed on to offspring by autosomal-dominant transmission (see "genetic forms of retinoblastoma" below). This Mendelian inheritance pattern provided the first clue that retinoblastomas, and indeed many cancers, are caused by mutations in specific genes. Knudsen developed a mathematical model of retinoblastoma inheritance that predicted that a developing retinoblast must acquire mutations in both cellular copies of the *Rb* gene for retinoblastoma to develop. In the hereditary condition, the first mutation is present in the germline, so only one subsequent mutation in a retinal cell is needed. Given the rate of spontaneous mutation during retinal development, the likelihood of a second mutation in the other *Rb* allele in at least one retinoblast is very high, hence the propensity for multiple tumors. In addition, the inherited mutation is present throughout the body, so cancers are more likely to arise in other tissues. In contrast, nonhereditary retinoblastoma occurs only in the unlikely event that both alleles of the *Rb* gene are mutated in the same retinoblast during development. Thus, these patients develop only a single retinal tumor and are not at risk for other systemic cancers. This "two-hit hypothesis" anticipated the existence of the *Rb* gene a decade before its experimental confirmation.[11] This concept also established that "recessive" cancer genes, or the loss of tumor suppressor genes, can predispose to cancer by autosomal-dominant inheritance, although they function in a recessive manner at the cellular level.

Localization of the *Rb* gene was aided by the observation that some patients with retinoblastoma have a visible deletion of chromosome 13 in their constitutional cells.[12] Other studies showed genetic linkage to esterase D, which is located at chromosome 13q14.[13] Taken together, these observations laid the foundation for an intensive search for the *Rb* gene on chromosome 13q14, which culminated in the discovery of a large gene (27 exons spanning 200 kilobases of DNA) which is now known to be mutated in all retinoblastomas, as well as some osteosarcomas and other retinoblastoma-associated cancers.[14–17] Surprisingly, *Rb* gene mutations were also found in some common adult tumors that have no apparent association with retinoblastoma, such as lung cancer.[18]

It is now known that the Rb protein is central to regulating cell division throughout the body and is pathologically inactivated in the vast majority of all cancers.[19] The Rb protein localizes to the nucleus and can exist in both an active hypophosphorylated form and an inactive hyperphosphorylated form.[20] When active, the Rb protein arrests the cell cycle by blocking the expression of genes involved in DNA synthesis and cell division. When the Rb protein is hyperphosphorylated, these cell cycle genes are unopposed in promoting cell division.[21] Cyclin-dependent kinases phosphorylate the Rb protein in a highly regulated manner that normally allows cells to divide only under appropriate physiologic circumstances.[22] In many cancers, however, these kinases are abnormally expressed and inappropriately inactivate the Rb protein. This can happen, for example, when the tumor suppressor $p16^{INK4a}$ is mutated. $p16^{INK4a}$ normally inhibits certain cyclin-dependent kinases; thus, its inactivation allows the Rb protein to become abnormally hyperphosphorylated and inactivated. The proclivity for deregulation of the *Rb* pathway in virtually all cancers has generated intense interest in this pathway for the development of targeted molecular therapies.[23,24]

Since the *Rb* gene is critical for normal cell growth and homeostasis throughout the body, it remains unclear why germline *Rb* gene mutations predispose primarily to the rare eye tumor. In most tissues, loss of *Rb* leads to apoptosis (programmed cell death) by triggering the *p53* pathway, thereby preventing malignant transformation. This explains why both the *Rb* cell cycle pathway and the *p53* apoptosis pathway are disrupted in most cancers.[25,26] Curiously, no consistent mutations in the *p53* pathway or any other genes have been found in retinoblastoma. It is possible that, in developing retinoblasts, there is a unique window of susceptibility in which loss of *Rb* alone can lead to tumor formation without mutations in any other genes. Alternatively, mutations in an apoptosis gene may occur with such high frequency following inactivation of *Rb* that these mutations are not rate limiting for tumorigenesis. In either case, it is likely that the molecular pathophysiology of retinoblastoma will prove to be unique.

GENETIC FORMS OF RETINOBLASTOMA

Somatic/Nonheritable Retinoblastoma

The most common presentation of retinoblastoma is the unilaterally affected child with no family history. These children usually have no germline mutation in the *Rb* gene, they do not develop tumors in the second eye, they are not predisposed to second primary cancers, and they do not transmit the disease to their children. Nonheritable retinoblastoma accounts for about 60 percent of cases and is due to two separate somatic mutations of both cellular copies of the *Rb* gene in the same retinoblast. Since most hereditary retinoblastomas also occur in a "sporadic" fashion (see below), it is best to avoid this term when referring to the nonheritable condition. The mean age at diagnosis of children with this form of retinoblastoma is about 24 months.[27]

Germline/Heritable Retinoblastoma

About 40 percent of all retinoblastoma patients have a germline mutation in the *Rb* gene, although only about 7 percent have a positive family history. Therefore, most patients with heritable retinoblastoma are sporadic cases with a new germline mutation. The heritable form of retinoblastoma is associated with multiple, bilateral eye tumors. In addition, these patients are at risk for second primary cancers throughout the body and transmission of the disease to their offspring in an autosomal-dominant fashion.[28,29] The mean age at diagnosis is about 12 months, significantly younger than of those with nonheritable disease.[27] Importantly, about 15 percent of patients with unilateral disease carry a germline mutation, and they are still at risk for second tumors and hereditary transmission.

CLINICAL PRESENTATION

The two most common presenting signs in patients with retinoblastoma are leukocoria (50 to 60%) and strabismus (20 to 30%) (Figures 12–1 and 12–2), which are most often detected by the family.[30] Less common presentations include an inflamed eye and orbital cellulitis (Figure 12–3). Overall, the mean age at diagnosis is about 18 months, with over 98 percent of cases occurring before age 5 years. However, retinoblastoma can rarely present in adulthood.[31,32]

Obtaining a careful medical history is important for ruling out simulating conditions. For example, a history of prematurity may suggest retinopathy of prematurity; an exposure to puppies, ocular toxocariasis; and neonatal sepsis can produce endogenous endophthalmitis. A family history should be elicited, although this will be negative in the vast majority of retinoblastoma patients. Physical examination is also important in the evaluation of suspected retinoblastoma. Most patients have a normal systemic work-up, but a small minority of patients will have 13q-deletion syndrome, in which retinoblastoma can be associated with moderate growth and mental retardation, broad nasal bridge, short nose, ear abnormalities, muscular hypotonia, microcephaly, and genital abnormalities.[33] Physical signs, such as neurologic deficits or an abdominal mass, may also uncover metastatic disease.

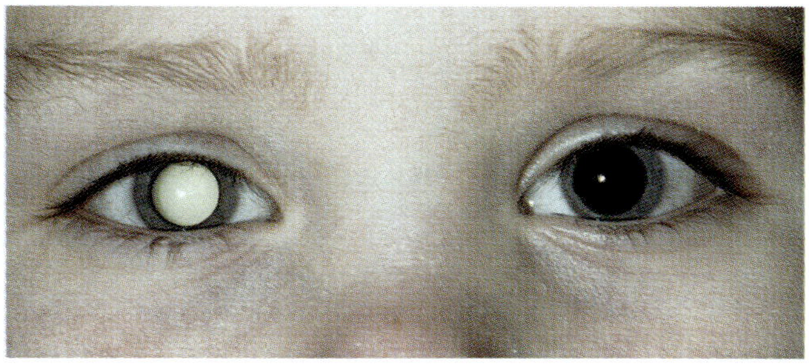

Figure 12–1. Leukocoria is the most common presenting sign of retinoblastoma.

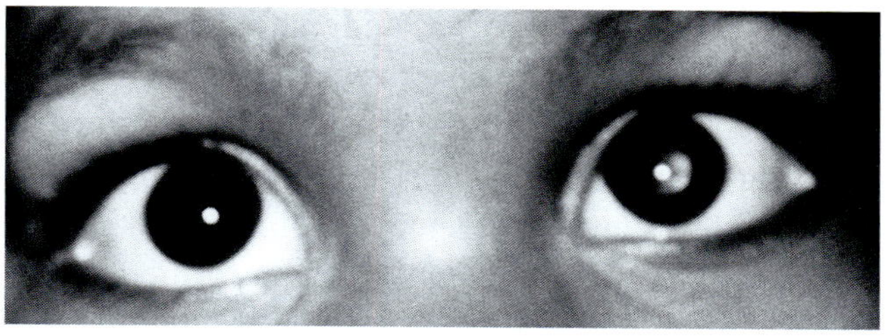

Figure 12–2. Strabismus can be the initial manifestation of retinoblastoma, if central vision is impaired.

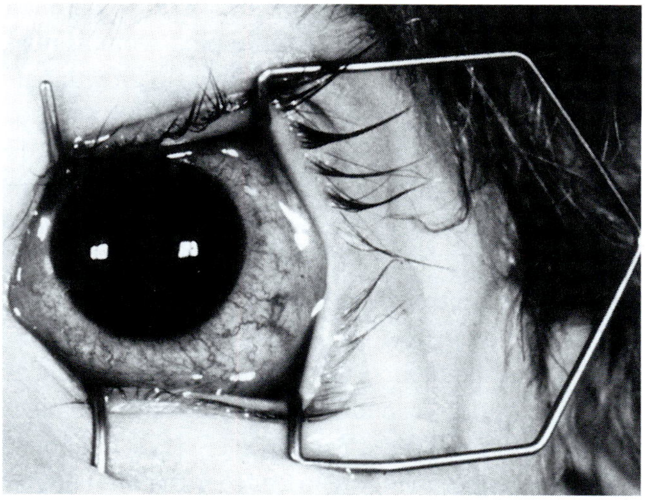

Figure 12–3. Retinoblastoma simulating an intraocular inflammation.

The presentation, type, and natural history of retinoblastoma is highly age dependent. Patients who present with unilateral retinoblastoma before the age of 1 year have a 16 percent risk of developing a new tumor in the same or other eye, compared with a 2 percent risk for older patients.[34] Among patients with bilateral tumors, new tumors develop in a predictable temporal pattern. The earliest tumors tend to develop in the posterior pole, and virtually all macular tumors are present by age 16 months. In contrast, more peripheral tumors develop later.[35] This has important implications for periodic screening examinations. Careful evaluation of the retinal periphery with indirect ophthalmoscopy and scleral depression is needed to rule out new anterior tumors.

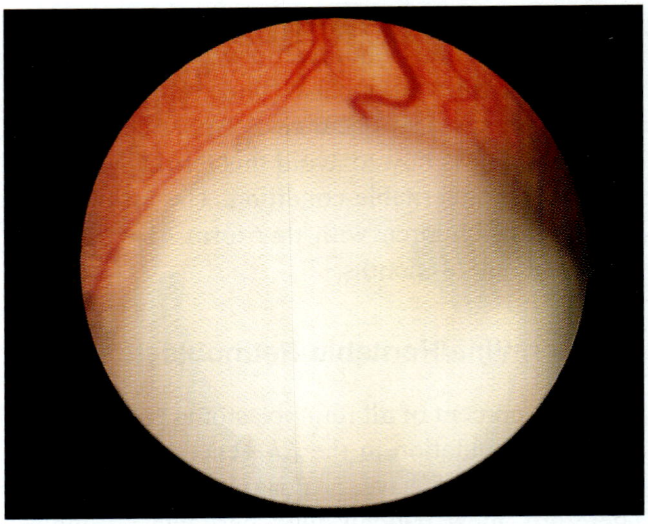

Figure 12–4. Large endophytic retinoblastoma.

CLINICAL FINDINGS

Depending on the age of the patient, an experienced clinician may be able to establish the diagnosis of retinoblastoma with a fair amount of certainty on the basis of an office evaluation. However, a thorough examination under anesthesia is highly recommended to adequately evaluate the child with suspected retinoblastoma. This examination should include inspection of the external eye and adnexa, measurement of intraocular pressure, examination of the anterior segment with the portable slit-lamp examination, and thorough fundus examination with the indirect ophthalmoscope, using scleral depression. Fundus photography and ultrasonography are often needed to document tumor size and appearance.

Clinical examination of an eye with retinoblastoma usually reveals one or more pink/white retinal masses. Tumors may have an endophytic growth pattern (Figure 12–4), often with dispersion of tumor cells into the vitreous (Figure 12–5), or an exophytic growth pattern, in which the tumor grows beneath the retina and causes an overlying retinal detachment (Figure 12–6). Both patterns can be found in the same patient or even the same eye. It is important to look closely for optic nerve involvement, neovascular glaucoma (usually noted as heterochromia) (Figure 12–7), and hyphema, all of which have implications for treatment (see next chapter). Pseudohypopyon (Figure 12–8), vitreous hemorrhage, and total retinal detachment can cause diagnostic difficulties. In tumors with extensive necrosis, preseptal cellulitis may occur, but in most of these cases, there is no extraocular tumor extension into the orbit.

The diffuse infiltrating form of retinoblastoma is an uncommon but important clinical variant. These tumors grow in a relatively flat pattern on the surface of the retina, often with no obvious mass. These tumors are less likely to have calcium and often resemble an inflammatory process due to seeding of tumor cells into the vitreous and anterior chamber.[36,37] These patients are often diagnosed at an older age because of a different pathophysiology or

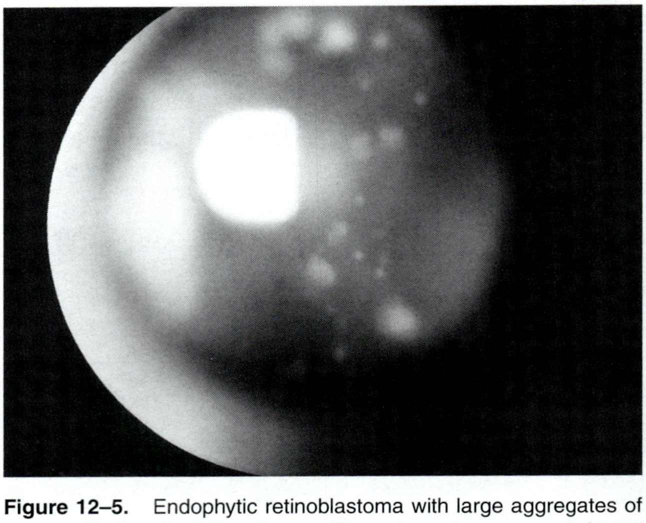

Figure 12–5. Endophytic retinoblastoma with large aggregates of tumor cells "seeding" the vitreous. The aggregates are much larger than the clumps of leukocytes seen in inflammatory processes.

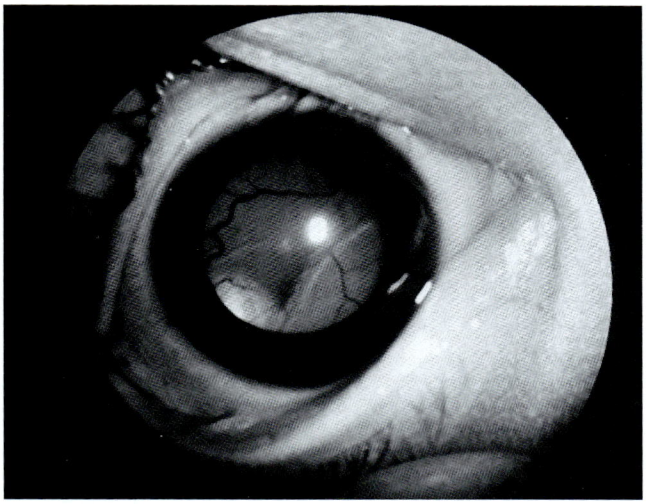

Figure 12–6. Exophytic retinoblastoma associated with overlying retinal detachment. This pattern causes more diagnostic difficulties than endophytic tumors.

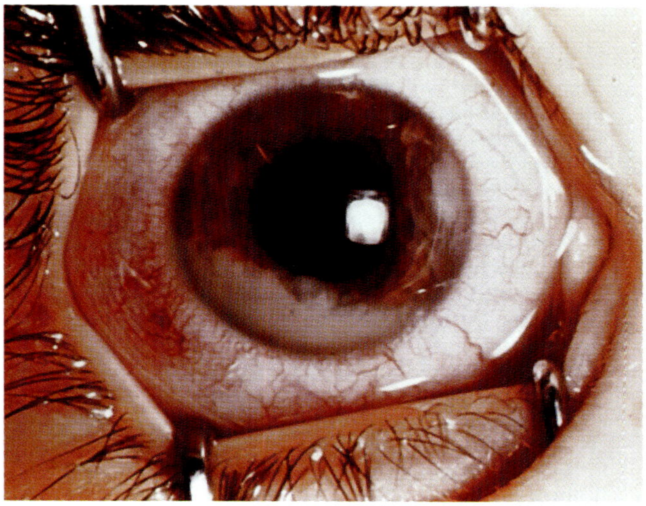

Figure 12–8. Pseudohypopyon due to anterior extension of tumor cells into the anterior chamber.

diagnostic difficulty. Most cases are unilateral, with no family history.

Retinocytoma or "retinoma" is thought to be a benign form of retinoblastoma.[38,39] These tumors are usually small and transluscent with prominent intratumoral calcifications, often with surrounding retinal pigment epithelial (RPE) alterations (Figure 12–9). Histopathologically, these lesions usually have well-differentiated retinoblastoma cells with numerous fleurettes and foci of calcium.[8] They are often found in adults (usually after diagnosing retinoblastoma in an offspring) and usually remain dormant. The etiology of these lesions is unclear, but they may represent either a retinoblastoma that is spontaneously arrested or one in which the second somatic *Rb* gene mutation occurred in a more mature retinoblast. Importantly, the presence of a retinocytoma suggests the presence of a germline *Rb* gene mutation.[38]

DIFFERENTIAL DIAGNOSIS

A large number of childhood ocular conditions can simulate retinoblastoma (Table 12–1). However, the conditions that most commonly present a diagnostic challenge include persistent hyperplastic primary vitreous (PHPV), ocular toxocariasis, and Coats' disease (congenital retinal telangiectasis).

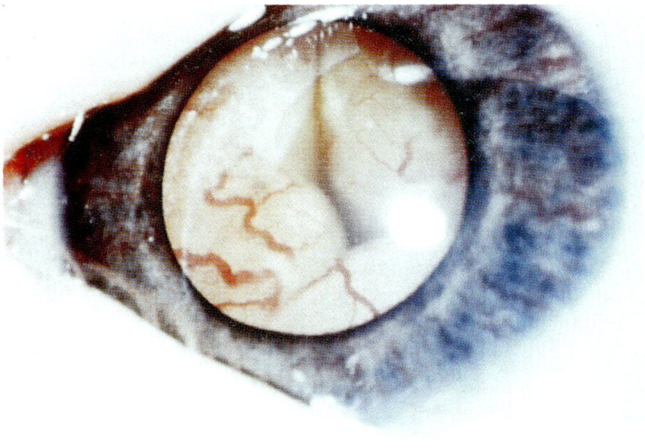

Figure 12–7. Anterior segment neovascularization in association with a large retinoblastoma.

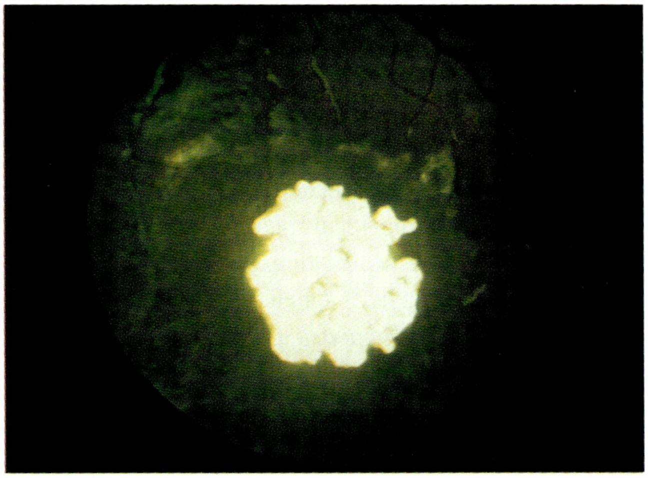

Figure 12–9. Retinocytoma in the parent of a child with bilateral retinoblastoma and no family history of the disease.

Table 12–1. DIFFERENTIAL DIAGNOSIS OF RETINOBLASTOMA

A. Conditions that simulate exophytic retinoblastoma
- Astrocytic hamartoma
- Choroidal hemangioma
- Chorioretinal coloboma
- Coats' disease (congenital retinal telangiectasis)
- Combined hamartoma of the RPE and retina
- Familial exudative vitreoretinopathy
- Incontinentia pigmenti
- Myelinated nerve fibers
- Morning glory disc anomaly
- Norrie's disease
- Retinal capillary hemangioma
- Retinal dysplasia
- Retinopathy of prematurity
- Retinoschisis
- Rhegmatogenous retinal detachment
- PHPV

B. Conditions that simulate endophytic retinoblastoma
- Congenital cytomegalovirus retinitis and other retinitides
- Endophthalmitis
- Juvenile xanthogranuloma
- Leukemia
- Medulloepithelioma
- Pars planitis and other uveitides
- Toxocariasis
- Toxoplasmic retinitis
- Vitreous hemorrhage
- Tuberous sclerosis

C. Other conditions that cause leukocoria
- Congenital cataract
- Congenital corneal opacity
- Persistent hyperplastic primary vitreous

D. Miscellaneous conditions
- Orbital cellulitis
- Traumatic hyphema

RPE = retinal peripheral epithelium; PHPV = persistent hyperplastic primary vitreous.

PHPV is almost always unilateral and is often detected shortly after birth due to leukocoria and microphthalmia. A calcified retinal mass is not found, but rather, the leukocoria is due to an opacified retrolental fibrous plaque and an associated cataract. Ciliary processes are typically elongated. (Figure 12–10) In contrast, retinoblastoma is rarely associated with microphthalmia or cataract. Persistent hyaloid artery, male gender, and anterior tunica vasculosa lentis can also be helpful clues to the diagnosis.

Ocular toxocariasis is caused by a larval form of the canine ascarid *Toxocara canis*. An exposure to puppies can often be elicited. Unlike retinoblastoma, ocular toxocariasis will often cause ocular inflammation, pain, and photophobia. Examination may reveal keratic precipitates, anterior chamber cells, posterior synechia, and other evidence of intraocular

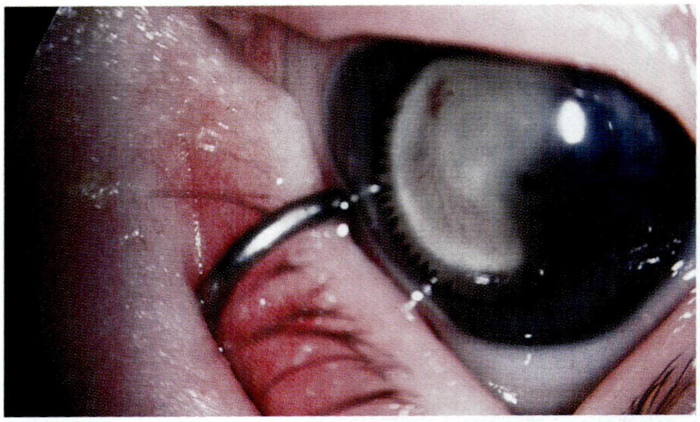

Figure 12–10. Persistent hyperplastic primary vitreous with retrolental fibrous plaque and elongated ciliary processes.

inflammation. The posterior segment manifestations of ocular toxocariasis can take one of several forms. First, an inflammatory retinal mass can produce marked vitreous cells, mimicking endophytic retinoblastoma. Second, a peripheral retinal granuloma may be associated with vitreous bands, traction retinal detachment and a "falciform fold" (Figure 12–11). And third, an isolated macular granuloma may be the only manifestation. The macular lesion will often be found after the inflammatory process has subsided, and these lesions can be distinguished from a small macular retinoblastoma by retinal contraction and dragging of retinal vessels around the lesion, which are usually not seen in retinoblastoma. The most helpful laboratory test is the serum ELISA for *Toxocara canis*, which is positive at 1:8 dilution

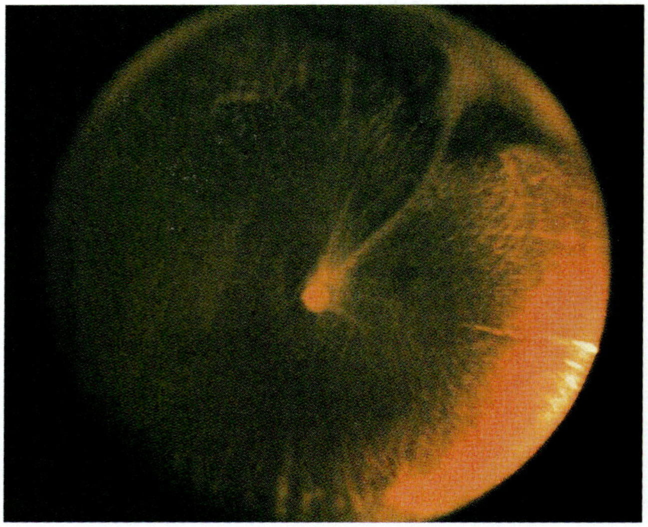

Figure 12–11. Ocular toxocariasis with peripheral inflammatory mass and falciform fold into the posterior pole.

in most patients with ocular toxocariasis but negative in retinoblastoma.[40] Rarely, cytologic evaluation of aqueous or vitreous material is necessary to make the diagnosis, although this is to be strongly discouraged in an eye which may harbor a retinoblastoma. ELISA testing and the presence of eosinophils in the aspirated material can be diagnostic for toxocariasis (Figure 12–12).[41]

Coats' disease is the clinical association of congenital retinal telangiectasis with an exudative retinal detachment (Figure 12–13). It is most frequently diagnosed between ages 4 and 10 years, and the vast majority of patients are males with unilateral tumors. In the retinoblastoma age group, Coats' disease usually presents as a retinal detachment with yellow subretinal exudate, occasionally with glistening cholesterol crystals but no distinct tumor mass. Calcium deposits can rarely be seen, but these are typically in older children who are beyond the retinoblastoma age group. A Coats'-like reaction can sometimes be seen with retinoblastoma, but a yellowish exudate is uncommon, and a tumor can usually be identified. Retinal telangiectatic changes are found most frequently in the temporal periphery and consist of irregular aneurysmal dilatations of retinal vessels, with the intervening regions lacking normal retinal capillaries. These vascular abnormalities are rarely found in retinoblastoma and strongly suggest Coats' disease. Careful clinical examination and the use of appropriate ancillary diagnostic tests can rule out most of the other simulating lesions listed in Table 1.

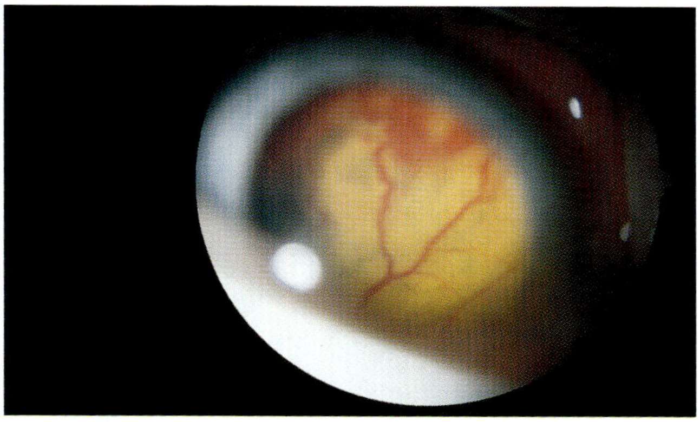

Figure 12–13. Coats' disease presenting as leukocoria in a 2-year-old child. The yellowish exudate along with the peripheral retinal telangiectasis are very characteristic.

ANCILLARY DIAGNOSTIC TESTS

Imaging of the eyes, orbits, and brain with computed tomography (CT) is the most useful noninvasive ancillary diagnostic test in evaluating patients suspected of having retinoblastoma (Figure 12–14).[42] CT demonstrates calcium within the tumor in the vast majority of retinoblastomas, although smaller tumors < 5 mm in thickness may not have detectable calcium. While intralesional calcium can be found in pseudoretinoblastomas in older children, including advanced Coats' disease, chronic ocular toxocariasis, and retinal astrocytoma, it is rare for these conditions to have calcium in the retinoblastoma age group (Figure 12–15).[42] CT is also useful in evaluating optic nerve invasion, orbital tumor extension,

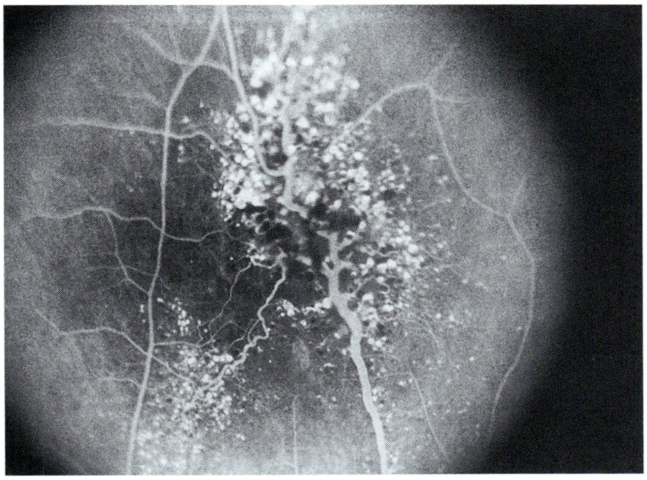

Figure 12–12. Vitreous biopsy in a patient with ocular toxocariasis demonstrating eosinophils.

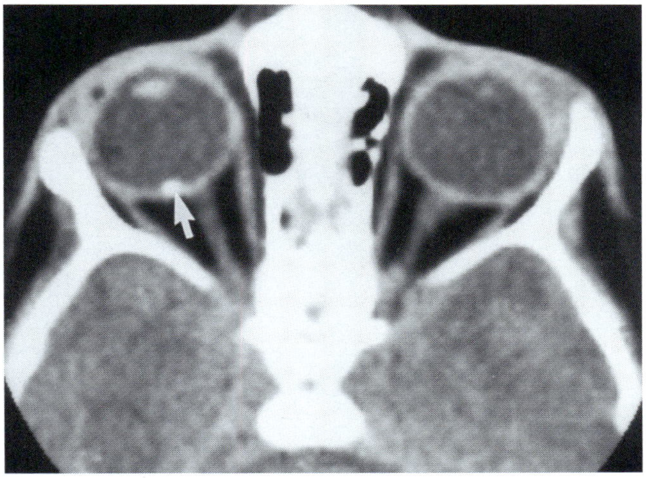

Figure 12–14. Axial computed tomography demonstrating calcification within a small macular retinoblastoma.

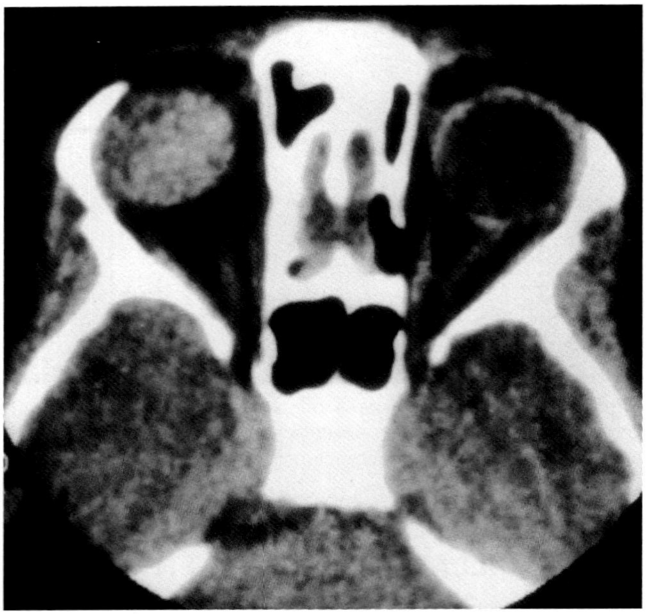

Figure 12–15. Axial computed tomography demonstrating intraocular opacification without calcification in biopsy-proven toxocariasis.

and midline intracranial tumors (Figure 12–16). With modern spiral/helical CT units, most children can be rapidly evaluated without anesthesia.[43]

Ultrasonography is useful as a noninvasive diagnostic test that can be performed in the office. For retinoblastoma, the A-scan mode reveals highly reflective internal echoes and orbital shadowing due to calcium (Figure 12–17). B-scan also shows highly reflective internal signals and orbital shadowing (Figure 12–18). In addition B-scan reveals the topology of the lesion and is helpful in identifying simulating lesions such as PHPV, in which the presence of a retrolental plaque, persistent hyaloidal structures, and absence of a retinal tumor could be diagnostic. Ultrasonography is not as sensitive as CT for detecting calcium or for evaluating the optic nerve, and its utility is highly dependent on the examiner's skill.

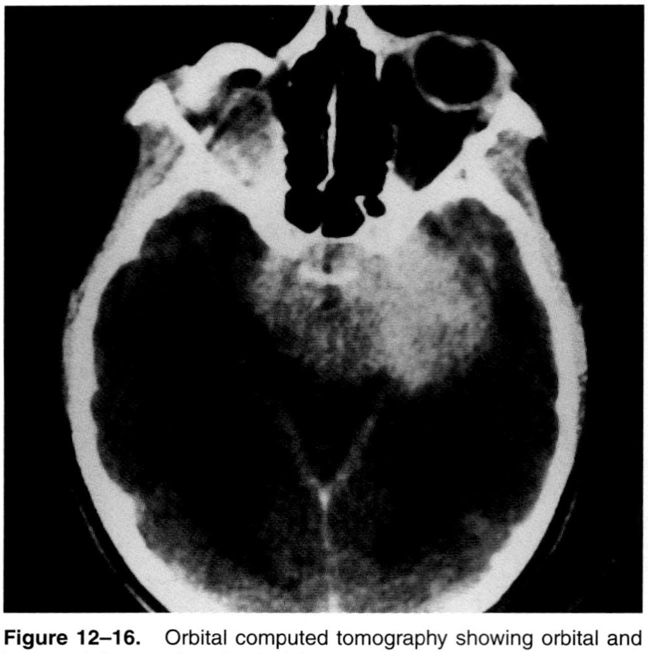

Figure 12–16. Orbital computed tomography showing orbital and intracranial extension of retinoblastoma.

Magnetic resonance imaging (MRI) is not as sensitive as CT for detecting calcium in the initial diagnosis of retinoblastoma. However, MRI is superior for evaluating optic nerve invasion and midline intracranial tumors.

Fluorescein angiography is rarely needed in the evaluation of patients with suspected retinoblastoma. However, this modality may occasionally be useful in ruling out simulating lesions. For example, the characteristic retinal telangiectatic changes of Coats' disease are unambiguously demonstrated with this modality.[44]

Intraocular fine-needle aspiration biopsy (FNAB) for cytologic examination is avoided, whenever possible, in suspected retinoblastomas, due to concern about extraocular tumor spread.[45] However, intraocular FNAB may rarely be necessary in a difficult diagnostic situation in which all noninvasive approaches have failed to achieve the diagnosis (Figure 12–19).[46] To minimize the risk of extraocular spread, such biopsies are usually performed through peripheral clear cornea and should be performed by an experienced ocular oncologist.

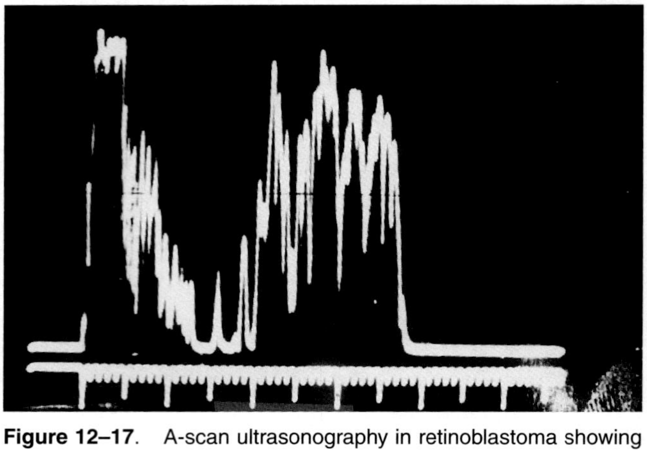

Figure 12–17. A-scan ultrasonography in retinoblastoma showing high internal reflectivity and orbital shadowing.

SYSTEMIC SCREENING

Systemic evaluation for metastatic disease and for second primary cancers is an important component in the overall management of patients with retinoblastoma.

Metastatic Disease

The most common sites of extraocular spread from retinoblastoma include the central nervous system, orbit, bone marrow, and viscera (especially the liver and kidney).[47] Early detection of metastatic spread is critical in order to institute prompt therapy. However, since the incidence of extraocular spread is low in the developed countries (due to early diagnosis and treatment), metastatic testing is not routinely performed in most centers in the United States.[48,49] The presence of clinical or pathologic risk factors for metastasis should prompt an appropriate work-up. If optic nerve invasion is suspected on ophthalmologic examination or imaging studies or if neurologic signs are found on physical examination, lumbar puncture and MRI are indicated.[50] In addition, bone marrow biopsy and bone scan may be indicated when extensive choroidal invasion is present.[51]

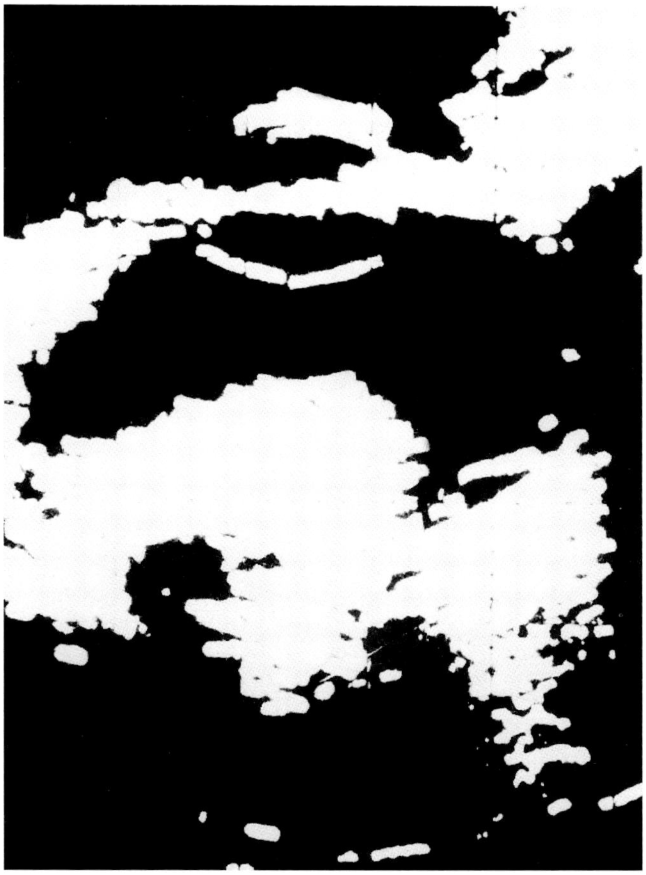

Figure 12–18. B-scan ultrasonography in retinoblastoma showing highly reflective internal signals and marked orbital shadowing.

Second Primary Tumors

With modern diagnostic and therapeutic capabilities, survival for retinoblastoma patients is over 90 percent in the developed countries.[3] Therefore, second primary tumors are now the most common cause of mortality in germline retinoblastoma patients.[52] The germline *Rb* gene mutation in these patients predisposes them to cancers throughout life, including midline intracranial tumors, osteosarcomas, soft tissue sarcomas, melanomas, brain tumors, and other neoplasms.[14,29,53–56] Second tumors can occur even in patients who do not receive radiotherapy, but the risk is much higher within the field of radiation.[57,58] As retinoblastoma survivors live longer, the occurrence of second tumors continues to increase. One study reported a 25 percent rate of second tumors at 40 years after diagnosis.[57] In general, a cancer cell emerges when multiple mutations accumulate in regulatory genes, such as *Rb* and *p53*. The distinctive spectrum of second tumors that occur in retinoblastoma survivors (generally of nonepithelial origin) may reflect a particular susceptibility to loss of *Rb* in these tumors. Since germline retinoblastoma patients already carry one *Rb* mutation in most or all cells of the body, they require fewer additional mutations for cancer to develop. Accumulation of these additional mutations is more likely when the patient has been treated with radiotherapy and some forms of chemotherapy that damage DNA.

The midline intracranial tumors were once called pinealoblastomas due to their proximity to this structure but are now more properly called primitive neuroectodermal tumors (PNETs). Even though they are histopathologically similar to retinoblastoma and are caused by mutations in the *Rb* gene, PNETs are thought to be distinct second neoplasms rather than intracranial spread from the eye tumor.[59] They probably arise from a germinal layer of primitive subependymal neuroblasts and have been observed in transgenic mouse models of hereditary retinoblastoma.[60] PNETs occur in about 6 to 10 percent of germline retinoblastoma patients and are more common in patients with a positive family history.[52,61] The presence of a PNET portends an extremely poor prognosis, and the few patients who have been successfully treated had their PNETs detected before the appearance of clinical symptoms.[62] Therefore, screening for early detection is essential for patients with known or suspected germline disease. CT can detect many of these lesions, since most have calcification.[63] However, MRI has certain advantages in providing higher-resolution images of intracranial structures. Therefore, many centers will initially screen both the eyes and the brain with CT at the initial evaluation, whereas subsequent screenings are performed with MRI every 6 to 12 months, until the child is around 5 years old.

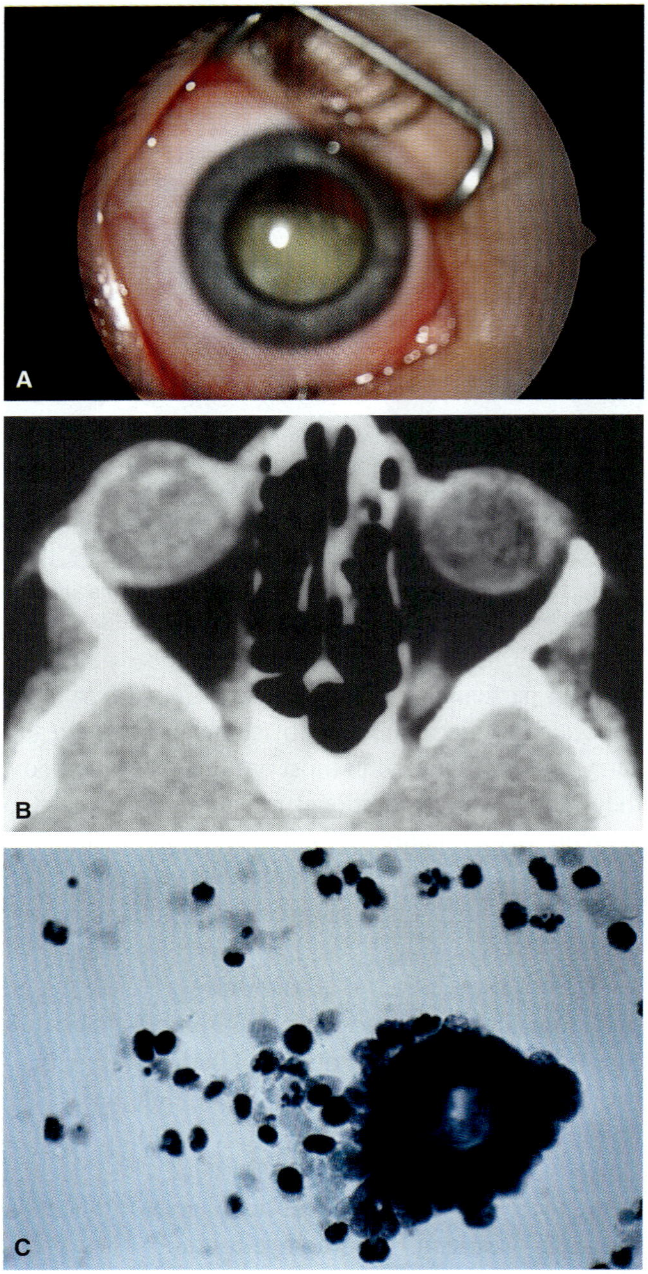

Figure 12–19. *A,* Child with leukocoria in which a solid intraocular tumor was not seen. *B,* Computed tomography failed to demonstrate intraocular calcium. *C,* Cytologic examination of fine-needle aspiration biopsy shows small, round, malignant cells forming rosettes, consistent with retinoblastoma.

Children with germline retinoblastoma continue to be predisposed to second primary cancers throughout life, and the ophthalmologist will to inform the primary-care physician of the spectrum of susceptible cancers.

GENETIC TESTING AND COUNSELING

There are several situations in which genetic testing can be helpful in retinoblastoma. First, in adults with a history of retinoblastoma, it is desirable to determine the genetic status of their children as soon as possible in order to initiate appropriate clinical surveillance and therapy. With chorionic villus sampling, the child's DNA can be analyzed in utero. Second, in children who present with unilateral retinoblastoma and no family history, it is important to determine the germline status. These children have an age-dependent risk that they will develop new tumors in the other eye. In addition, they have a 15 percent chance of carrying a germline mutation despite unilateral involvement.

There are several approaches to genetic testing, depending on the clinical setting. In about 7 percent of retinoblastoma patients, there is a positive family history, which may allow an accurate estimation of risk by performing linkage analysis to study restriction fragment length polymorphisms around the *Rb* locus.[64,65] More commonly, however, direct identification of the causative mutation must be performed. Due to the large size of the *Rb* gene, lack of mutational hot spots and heterogeneity of mutation types, a systematic screening approach is required.[66,67] Cytogenetic analysis is relatively low in resolution and can only detect large chromosomal alterations at chromosome 13q14 in 7 to 8 percent of patients.[68] Southern blot and other techniques for detecting abnormalities in DNA fragment size at the *Rb* locus are relatively rapid and can detect re-arrangements in about 16 percent of hereditary retinoblastoma patients.[69] More sophisticated molecular techniques that can detect smaller mutations have also been employed, including single-strand conformation polymorphism analysis (SSCP), heteroduplex analysis, multiplex fragment length analysis, alteration of restriction fragment length polymorphisms (RFLP), and direct sequencing.[70,71] These techniques can detect small insertions and deletions, or even single base-pair changes, but they are expensive and time consuming, especially if the mutation must be found in peripheral blood leukocytes that also carry a normal *Rb* allele. In most retinoblastomas, the first *Rb* allele is inactivated by mutation, whereas the second allele is lost by mitotic nondysjunction or recombination which results in "loss of heterozygosity."[72] Thus, identifying a mutation is technically easier in tumor tissue, since no normal *Rb* gene is present to interfere with genetic analysis. Therefore, when an eye is enucleated in a patient with unilateral tumor, analysis of tumor tissue may reveal a mutation, and analysis of a blood sample can be performed to determine if this mutation is in the germline. Even with such a multifaceted screening approach, however, current techniques fail to identify the mutation in 17 to 20 percent of patients.[70] Thus, further research is needed to develop more rapid, inexpensive, and clinically useful genetic testing strategies.[66] Several centers offering clinical genetic testing for retinoblastoma can be contacted through the website *www.genetests.com*.

Genetic counseling requires an understanding of the autosomal-dominant inheritance and the implications for the patient, parents, siblings, and offspring.[73] The penetrance (i.e., the percentage of individuals with an inherited mutant *Rb* gene mutation who develop clinical manifestations of the disease) is normally about 85 to 90 percent. Each offspring of a germline retinoblastoma survivor has a 40 to 45 percent chance of developing retinoblastoma. If there is no family history and the germline status is unknown, the parents of a single child with retinoblastoma have a 1 to 6 percent chance that future children will develop the disease. If the parents then have a second affected child, one of the parents must then have a germline mutation, and all future children have a 40 to 45 percent risk. A patient with unilateral retinoblastoma has a 15 percent risk of a germline mutation, so their chance of having an affected child is about 7 percent. When there is a positive family history, normal siblings of an affected patient have a 1 to 6 percent chance of transmitting the disease to their children, since the parent could be a gene carrier.

The genetic counselor must also be familiar with the concept of low penetrance. In retinoblastoma, the penetrance is normally very high, but in a few families, the penetrance may be as low as 30 to 50 percent. Thus, low penetrance should be suspected when more than one individual in a family is affected but there is not a clear autosomal-dominant pattern. The molecular basis for most cases of low penetrance has been elucidated.[74] In some families, there is a mutation in the promoter region of the *Rb* gene which causes a reduced amount of the Rb protein to be produced, whereas in other families a mutation within the coding sequence of the *Rb* gene results in a partial loss of *Rb* function.[75,76] Many of these mutations have been identified and can be detected by genetic testing.

REFERENCES

1. Lennox EL, Draper GJ, Sanders BM. Retinoblastoma: a study of natural history and prognosis of 268 cases. Br Med J 1975;3:731–4.
2. Bishop JO, Madsen EC. Retinoblastoma: review of current status. Surv Ophthalmol 1975;19:342–66.
3. Tamboli A, Podgor MJ, Horm JW. The incidence of retinoblastoma in the United States: 1974 through 1985. Arch Ophthalmol 1990;108:128–32.
4. Albert DM. Historic review of retinoblastoma. Ophthalmology 1987;94:654–62.
5. Bogenmann E, Lochrie MA, Simon MI. Cone cell-specific genes expressed in retinoblastoma. Science 1988;240:76–8.
6. Nork TM, Schwartz TL, Doshi HM, Millecchia LL. Retinoblastoma. Cell of origin. Arch Ophthalmol 1995;113:791–802.
7. Brabec T, Arbizo V, Adamus G, et al. Rod cell-specific antigens in retinoblastoma. Arch Ophthalmol 1989;107:1061–3.
8. McLean IW, Burnier MN, Zimmerman LE, Jakobiec FA. Tumors of the eye and ocular adnexa. In: Rosai J, Sobin LH, editors. Atlas of tumor pathology, 3rd ed. Washington, D.C.: Armed Forces Institute of Pathology; 1994. p. 101–27.
9. Magramm I, Abramson DH, Ellsworth RM. Optic nerve involvement in retinoblastoma. Ophthalmology 1989;96:217–22.

10. Khelfaoui F, Validire P, Auperin A, et al. Histopathologic risk factors in retinoblastoma: a retrospective study of 172 patients treated in a single institution. Cancer 1996;77:1206–13.
11. Knudson AG Jr. Mutation and cancer: statistical study of retinoblastoma. Proc Natl Acad Sci USA 1971; 68:820–3.
12. Turleau C, de Grouchy J, Chavin-colin F, et al. Cytogenic forms of retinoblastoma: their incidence in a survey of 66 patients. Cancer Genet Cytolgenet 1985;16:321–34.
13. Sparkes RS, Murphree AL, Lingua RW, et al. Gene for hereditary retinoblastoma assigned to human chromosome 13 by linkage to esterase D. Science 1983; 219:971–3.
14. Friend SH, Bernards R, Rogelj S, et al. A human DNA segment with properties of the gene that predisposes to retinoblastoma and osteosarcoma. Nature 1986;323:643–6.
15. Fung YK, Murphree AL, T'Ang A, et al. Structural evidence for the authenticity of the human retinoblastoma gene. Science 1987;236:1657–61.
16. Lee WH, Bookstein R, Hong F, et al. Human retinoblastoma susceptibility gene: cloning, identification, and sequence. Science 1987;235:1394–9.
17. Wadayama B, Toguchida J, Shimizu T, et al. Mutation spectrum of the retinoblastoma gene in osteosarcomas. Cancer Res 1994;54:3042–8.
18. Harbour JW, Lai SL, Whang-Peng J, et al. Abnormalities in structure and expression of the human retinoblastoma gene in SCLC. Science 1988;241:353–7.
19. Sherr CJ. Cancer cell cycles. Science 1996;274: 1672–7.
20. Lee WH, Shew JY, Hong FD, et al. The retinoblastoma susceptibility gene encodes a nuclear phosphoprotein associated with DNA binding activity. Nature 1987;329:642–5.
21. Bartek J, Bartkova J, Lukas J. The retinoblastoma protein pathway in cell cycle control and cancer. Exp Cell Res 1997;237:1–6.
22. Harbour JW, Luo RX, Dei Sante A, et al. Cdk phosphorylation triggers sequential intramolecular interactions that progressively block Rb functions as cells move through G1. Cell 1999;98:859–69.
23. Chen YN, Sharma SK, Ramsey TM, et al. Selective killing of transformed cells by cyclin/cyclin-dependent kinase 2 antagonists. Proc Natl Acad Sci USA 1999;96:4325–9.
24. Parr MJ, Manome Y, Tanaka T, et al. Tumor-selective transgene expression in vivo mediated by an E2F-responsive adenviral vector. Nat Med 1997;3: 1145–9.
25. Harbour JW. Tumor suppressor genes in ophthalmology. Surv Ophthalmol 1999;44:235–46.
26. Macleod KF, Hu Y, Jacks T. Loss of Rb activates both p53-dependent and independent cell death pathways in the developing mouse nervous system. EMBO J 1996;15:6178–88.
27. Ellsworth RM. The practical management of retinoblastoma. Trans Am Ophthalmol Soc 1969;67:462–534.
28. Abramson DH, Frank CM, Susman M, et al. Presenting signs of retinoblastoma. J Pediatr 1998;132:505–8.
29. Fontanesi J, Parham DM, Pratt C, Meyer D. Second malignant neoplasms in children with retinoblastoma: the St. Jude Children's Research Hospital experience. Ophthalmic Genet 1995;16:105–8.
30. Moll AC, Imhof SM, Bouter LM, Tan KE. Second primary tumors in patients with retinoblastoma. A review of the literature. Ophthalmic Genet 1994;18: 27–34.
31. Berkeley JS, Kalita BC. Retinoblastoma in an adult. Lancet 1977;2:508–9.
32. Makley TA Jr. Retinoblastoma in a 52-year-old man. Arch Ophthalmol 1963;6:325–6.
33. Allderdice PW, Davis JG, Miller OJ, et al. The 13q-deletion syndrome. Am J Hum Genet 1969;21: 499–512.
34. Abramson DH, Gamell LS, Ellsworth RM, et al. Unilateral retinoblastoma: new intraocular tumours after treatment. Br J Ophthalmol 1994;78:698–701.
35. Abramson DH, Gombos DS. The topography of bilateral retinoblastoma lesions. Retina 1996;16:232–9.
36. Morgan G. Diffuse infiltrating retinoblastoma. Br J Ophthalmol 1997;55:600–6.
37. Nicholson DH, Norton EWD. Diffuse infiltrating retinoblastoma. Trans Am Ophthalmol Soc 1980; 78:265–89.
38. Gallie BL, Ellsworth RM, Abramson DH, Phillips RA. Retinoma: spontaneous regression of retinoblastoma or benign manifestation of the mutation? Br J Cancer 1982;45:513–21.
39. Margo C, Hidayat A, Kopelman J. Retinocytoma: a benign variant of retinoblastoma. Arch Ophthalmol 1983;101:1519–31.
40. Felgberg NT, Shields JA, Federman JL. Antibody to Toxocara canis in the aqueous humor. Arch Ophthalmol 1981;99:1563–4.
41. Shields JA. Ocular toxocariasis: a review. Surv Ophthalmol 1984;28:361–81.
42. Char DH, Hedges TRD, Norman D. Retinoblastoma. CT diagnosis. Ophthalmology 1984;91:1347–50.
43. O'Brien JM, Char DH, Tucker N, et al. Efficacy of unanesthetized spiral computed tomography scanning in initial evaluation of childhood leukocoria. Ophthalmology 1995;102:1345–50.
44. Ohnishi Y, Yamana Y, Minei M. Application of fluorescein angiography in retinoblastoma. Am J Ophthalmol 1982;93:578–88.
45. Karcioglu ZA, Gordon RA, Karcioglu GL. Tumor seeding in ocular fine needle aspiration biopsy. Ophthalmology 1985;92:1763–7.

46. Char DH, Miller TR. Fine needle biopsy in retinoblastoma. Am J Ophthalmol 1984;97:686–90.
47. MacKay CJ, Abramson DH, Ellsworth RM. Metastatic patterns of retinoblastoma. Arch Ophthalmol 1984; 102:391–6.
48. Mohney BG, Robertson DM. Ancillary testing for metastasis in patients with newly diagnosed retinoblastoma. Am J Ophthalmol 1994;118:707–11.
49. Pratt CB, Meyer D, Chenaille P, Crom DB. The use of bone marrow aspirations and lumbar punctures at the time of diagnosis of retinoblastoma. J Clin Oncol 1989;7:140–3.
50. Moscinski LC, Pendergrass TW, Weiss A, et al. Recommendations for the use of routine bone marrow aspiration and lumbar punctures in the follow-up of patients with retinoblastoma. J Pediatr Hematol Oncol 1996;18:130–4.
51. Karcioglu ZA, Al-Mefser SA, Abboud E, et al. Workup for metastatic retinoblastoma. A review of 261 patients. Ophthalmology 1997;104:307–12.
52. Moll AC, Imhof SM, Bouter LM, et al. Second primary tumors in patients with hereditary retinoblastoma: a register-based follow-up study, 1945-1994. Int J Cancer 1996;67:515–9.
53. Albert DM, McGhee CN, Seddon JM, Weichselbaum RR. Development of additional primary tumors after 62 years in the first patient with retinoblastoma cured by radiation therapy. Am J Ophthalmol 1984;97:189–96.
54. Font RL, Jurco SD, Brechner RJ. Postradiation leiomyosarcoma of the orbit complicating bilateral retinoblastoma. Arch Ophthalmol 1983;101:1557–61.
55. Helton KJ, Fletcher BD, Kun LE, et al. Bone tumors other than osteosarcoma after retinoblastoma. Cancer 1993;71:2847–53.
56. Nuutinen J, Karja J, Sainio P. Epithelial second malignant tumours in retinoblastoma survivors. A review and report of a case. Acta Ophthalmol (Copenh) 1982;60:133–40.
57. Eng C, Li FP, Abramson DH, et al. Mortality from second tumors among long-term survivors of retinoblastoma. J Natl Cancer Inst 1993;85:1121–8.
58. Roarty JD, McLean IW, Zimmerman LE. Incidence of second neoplasms in patients with bilateral retinoblastoma. Ophthalmology 1988;95:1583–7.
59. Onadim Z, Woolford AJ, Kingston JE, Hungerford JL. The RB1 gene mutation in a child with ectopic intracranial retinoblastoma. Br J Cancer 1997;76: 1405–9.
60. Marcus DM, Lasudry JG, Carpenter JL, et al. Trilateral tumors in four different lines of transgenic mice expressing SV40 T-antigen. Invest Ophthalmol Vis Sci 1996;37:392–6.
61. Blach LE, McCormick B, Abramson DH, Ellsworth RM. Trilateral retinoblastoma—incidence and outcome: a decade of experience. Int J Radiat Oncol Biol Phys 1994;29:729–33.
62. Paulino AC. Trilateral retinoblastoma: is the location of the intracranial tumor important? Cancer 1999;86: 135–41.
63. Bagley LJ, Hurst RW, Zimmerman RA, et al. Imaging in the trilateral retinoblastoma syndrome. Neuroradiology 1996;38:166–70.
64. Cavenee WK, Murphree AL, Shull MM, et al. Prediction of familial predisposition to retinoblastoma. N Engl J Med 1986;314:1201–7.
65. Wiggs J, Nordenskjold M, Yandell D, et al. Prediction of the risk of hereditary retinoblastoma, using DNA polymorphisms within the retinoblastoma gene. N Engl J Med 1988;318:151–7.
66. Harbour JW. Overview of RB gene mutations in patients with retinoblastoma. Implications for clinical genetic screening. Ophthalmology 1998;105:1442–7.
67. Lohmann DR, Brandt B, Oehlschlager U, et al. Molecular analysis and predictive testing in retinoblastoma. Ophthalmic Genet 1995;16:135–42.
68. Bunin GR, Emanuel BS, Meadows AT. Frequency of 13q abnormalities among 203 patients with retinoblastoma. J Natl Cancer Inst 1989;81:370–4.
69. Kloss K, Wahrisch P, Greger V. Characterization of deletions at the retinoblastoma locus in patients with bilateral retinoblastoma. Am J Med Genet 1991;39:196–200.
70. Lohmann DR, Brandt B, Hopping W, et al. Distinct RB1 gene mutations with low penetrance in hereditary retinoblastoma. Hum Genet 1994;94:349–54.
71. Mastrangelo D, Squitieri N, Bruni S, et al. The polymerase chain reaction (PCR) in the routine genetic characterization of retinoblastoma: a tool for the clinical laboratory. Surv Ophthalmol 1997;41:331–40.
72. Cavenee WK, Dryja TP, Phillips RA, et al. Expression of recessive alleles by chromosomal mechanisms in retinoblastoma. Nature 1983;305:779–84.
73. Carlson EA, Letson RD, Ramsay NK, Desnick RJ. Factors for improved genetic counseling for retinoblastoma based on a survey of 55 families. Am J Ophthalmol 1979;87:449–59.
74. Otterson GA, Chen WD, Coxon AB, et al. Incomplete penetrance of familial retinoblastoma linked to germ-line mutations that result in partial loss of RB function. Proc Natl Acad Sci USA 1997;94: 12036–40.
75. Cowell JK, Bia B, Akoulitchev A. A novel mutation in the promotor region in a family with a mild form of retinoblastoma indicates the location of a new regulatory domain for the RB1 gene. Oncogene 1996; 12:431–6.
76. Lohmann DR, Brandt B, Hopping W, et al. Distinct RB1 gene mutations with low penetrance in hereditary retinoblastoma. Hum Genet 1994;94:349–54.

13

Retinoblastoma: Treatment

J. WILLIAM HARBOUR, MD

Prior to the 20th century, mortality from retinoblastoma approached 100 percent because of delayed diagnosis and ineffective treatments. However, there is now a 95 percent survival rate due to earlier diagnosis and improved treatments. For years, the mainstay of treatment was enucleation. External beam radiotherapy was introduced early in the 20th century. More recently, there has been a resurgent interest in chemotherapy as a means of avoiding some complications of radiation. With a growing number of treatment options, it is increasingly important for the ocular oncologist taking care of retinoblastoma patients to have a thorough knowledge of the risks, benefits, and indications for each modality.

TREATMENT CONSIDERATIONS

The evaluation and treatment of patients with retinoblastoma should be carried out in specialized centers with ophthalmic, pediatric, and radiation oncologists, who have considerable experience with retinoblastoma.

Previously, enucleation was recommended for all unilateral tumors and the worst eye of patients with bilateral tumors. This dictum is no longer appropriate in many settings, since effective alternative therapies are available. However, enucleation is still the best option for many very large tumors. Radiation has been a mainstay of therapy for many years but should be avoided whenever other modalities can yield similar or superior results, since the long-term complications of radiation are becoming increasingly apparent. Systemic chemotherapy, combined with local therapies, has recently re-emerged as a viable treatment option that may replace radiation in many settings. However, the long-term complications of chemotherapy are still undetermined.

Age is a key consideration in treatment of these special patients. Patients with bilateral tumors present earlier than those with unilateral tumors.[1] Children age < 1 year are at considerably higher risk of serious radiation complications than older children.[2] Younger patients are more likely to develop new tumors in the same or other eye.[3] The topographic pattern of tumor development is also age dependent, with macular tumors occurring earlier and peripheral tumors occurring later.[4]

Laterality is another important treatment consideration. Patients with unilateral tumors and no family history usually have at presentation a large tumor that often precludes ocular salvage. In this setting, one must weigh the modest benefit of salvaging an eye with extremely limited vision against the risks of treatment complications and failure. In a minority of cases (20 to 30%), a sporadic unilateral tumor may be amenable to ocular salvage therapy. While the same principles apply to bilateral tumors, one may be more compelled to attempt ocular salvage when vision is threatened in both eyes.

Location, size, and number of tumors are additional treatment considerations. When the fovea or papillomacular bundle are involved, one may wish to avoid locally destructive therapies, whereas these therapies can be highly effective for small equatorial or anterior tumors. When tumors occupy over 50 percent of the retina and intraocular volume, ocular salvage becomes less likely.

TREATMENT MODALITIES

Enucleation

Until recently, the vast majority of unilaterally affected eyes were removed.[5,6] Enucleation is still the treatment of choice in many cases but has become less common with earlier diagnosis and better alternative therapies.[7] In general, enucleation is indicated for large tumors that occupy > 50 percent of the intraocular volume (Figure 13–1). Additional indications include anterior segment tumor extension, neovascular glaucoma, and failure of conservative therapies, usually with extensive, diffuse, vitreous seeding.

The technique for enucleation in children with retinoblastoma is different from that for adults and should be performed by experienced surgeons. Children have smaller orbits than adults do, and standard adult instruments cannot be used. Adult enucleation scissors are often too large to fit in the posterior orbit, so instead, we use the smaller, minimally curved Stevens scissors. We also avoid the use of an optic nerve snare, since this technique creates crush artifact in the optic nerve stump, which is to be avoided, since histopathologic evaluation of the optic nerve is imperative for assessing tumor invasion. It is also imperative to obtain a long segment of the optic nerve, as leaving residual tumor in the optic nerve stump is a poor prognostic indicator.[8,9] Our goal is a 10-mm segment because tumor invasion beyond this point is likely to have seeded the subarachnoid space. If an insufficient stump is obtained, an additional segment can be taken by using Soule retractors to visualize the orbital contents, grasping the nerve stump and cutting an additional segment (Figure 13–2). Use of anterior traction on the globe is critical for obtaining a long nerve segment, but we do not recommend placing traction sutures through the sclera, since this could lead to ocular penetration and extraocular tumor extension. Instead, we cut the horizontal rectus muscles 3 to 4 mm away from the globe to leave long stumps for grasping with hemostats, which can then be used for traction while cutting the optic nerve. Hemostasis is obtained by compression of the orbit with a small test tube. The four rectus muscle stumps are secured to a hydroxyapatite implant wrapped in donor sclera or other materials.

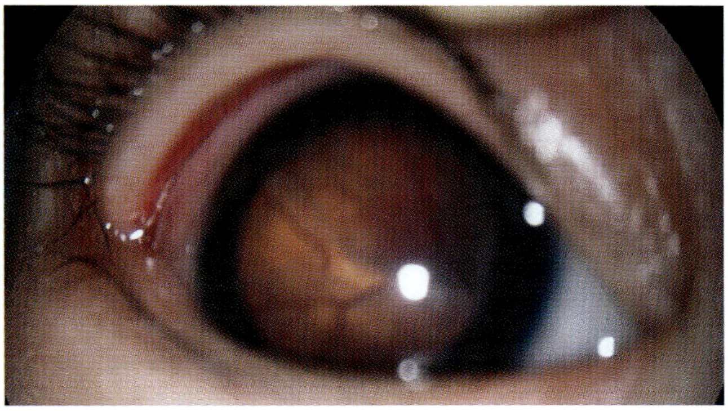

Figure 13–1. Large unilateral exophytic retinoblastoma which is too large for vision-sparing therapy and is best treated by enucleation.

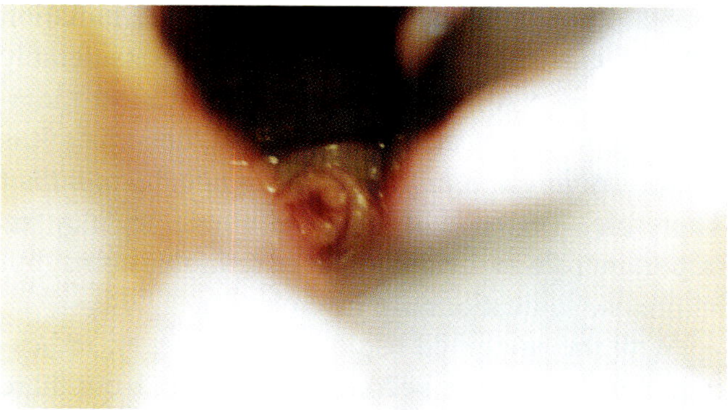

Figure 13–2. Visualization of optic nerve stump after enucleation, using Soule retractors for exposure.

Complications are uncommon but can include conjunctival breakdown and extrusion of the implant. This can be avoided by careful closure of Tenon's layer with two layers of interrupted sutures and closure of the conjunctiva with a separate running suture (see Chapter 8). Orbital cellulitis and hemorrhage can also occur but are rare. The most serious enucleation complication is globe penetration, which could result in extraocular tumor extension.

External Beam Radiotherapy

External beam radiotherapy (EBRT) was first used to treat retinoblastoma in the United States in 1903, but the widespread use of this modality awaited the work of Reese and Martin in the 1930s.[10] EBRT has subsequently become a mainstay of treatment, although the long-term risks of radiation have recently dampened enthusiasm for this modality. Because of these risks, there has been a recent shift to systemic chemotherapy (see below), although the scientific basis for this change is still not firm. It is important to keep in mind that much of the available information on radiation complications is derived from patients treated 30 or more years ago using high-dose orthovoltage therapy, whereas lower doses and megavoltage techniques are now used. Thus, the estimated radiation risks of current techniques have been considerably exaggerated.[11] Also, it is now clear that most radiation complications are age dependent, occurring less frequently in children treated after age 12 months.[2] Therefore, EBRT will likely continue to play an important role in the treatment of retinoblastoma, but its precise indications are in evolution.

With the increased use of chemotherapy, indications for EBRT have become more limited, but there are still situations in which EBRT is superior to chemotherapy, such as when there is substantial vitreous seeding. Other indications vary from center to center but would include large bilateral tumors that have failed chemotherapy. Unilateral tumors will often have a better cosmetic result with enucleation in younger patients. In general, EBRT should be avoided when possible in children age < 12 months, in large tumors that occupy > 50 percent of the intraocular volume, and whenever other modalities are likely to provide similar tumor control.[2]

EBRT can be delivered by several techniques. Most American centers have had better local tumor control with a lateral port, lens-sparing technique, rather than an anterior whole-eye approach (Figure 13–3).[12,13] However, the anterior retina is not adequately treated with lateral ports, so any tumors anterior to the equator need to be treated with local modalities prior to EBRT, and subsequently the anterior retina must be monitored closely with indirect ophthalmoscopy with scleral depression. Radiation is typically delivered using a 4-MeV linear accelerator through lateral fields angled 5° posteriorly to avoid the contralateral lens. If there is a question of optic nerve involvement, the entire orbit is included in the radiation field. Daily fractions of 200 cGy are delivered to a total dose of about 45 Gy. Children are under anesthesia during the treatments.

The complications of EBRT can include lid injury, dry eye, cataract, glaucoma, uveitis, lacrimal gland damage, retinopathy, optic nerve damage, and vitreous hemorrhage, but these are not usually severe at the lower radiation doses used to treat retinoblastoma. The more concerning complications are orbital bone deformities (Figure 13–4) and second primary cancers in the field of radiation (Figure 13–5). The bone orbital deformities are especially disfiguring when treated before age 12 months but are less severe in older children. In germline patients, the risk of second primary cancers increases dramatically within the field of radiation. In one study, patients who did not receive radiation had a 6 percent rate of second tumors, while those receiving radiation had a 35 percent risk.[14] Germline patients are more likely to die of a second cancer than of retinoblastoma itself. It should be re-emphasized, however, that much of our information on orbital bone deformities and second cancers is derived from children treated with older techniques. The risk of these complications is probably lower with modern lower doses, megavoltage equipment, limiting of daily fractionation to < 225 cGy, treatment planning with computed tomography (CT), and other advances.[11,15] In addition, newer intensity-modulated conformal therapies should further decrease local complications.

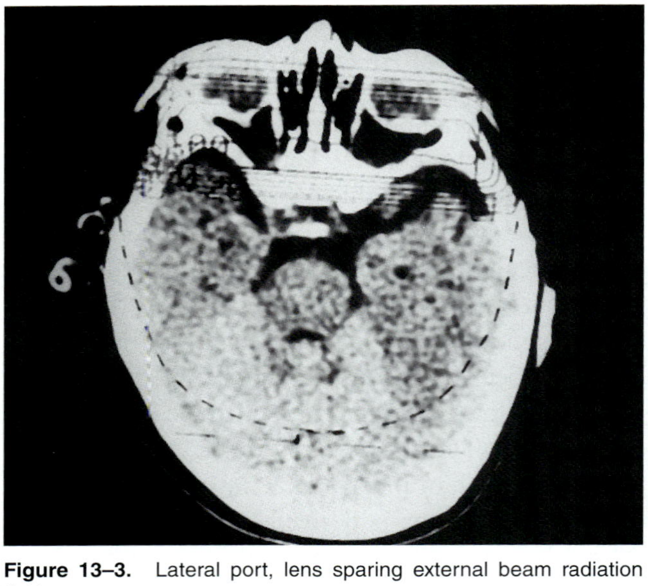

Figure 13–3. Lateral port, lens sparing external beam radiation fields.

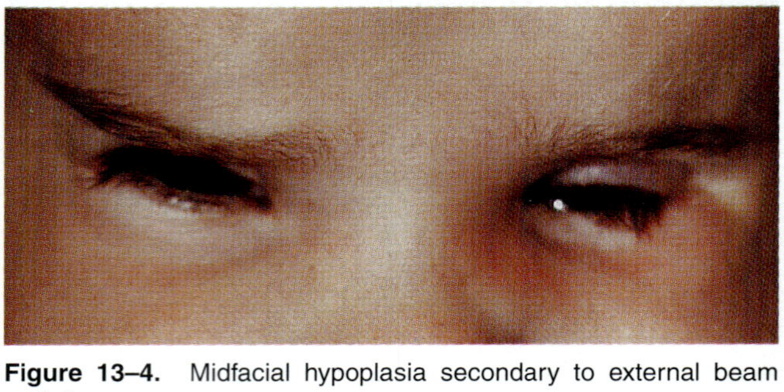

Figure 13–4. Midfacial hypoplasia secondary to external beam radiotherapy.

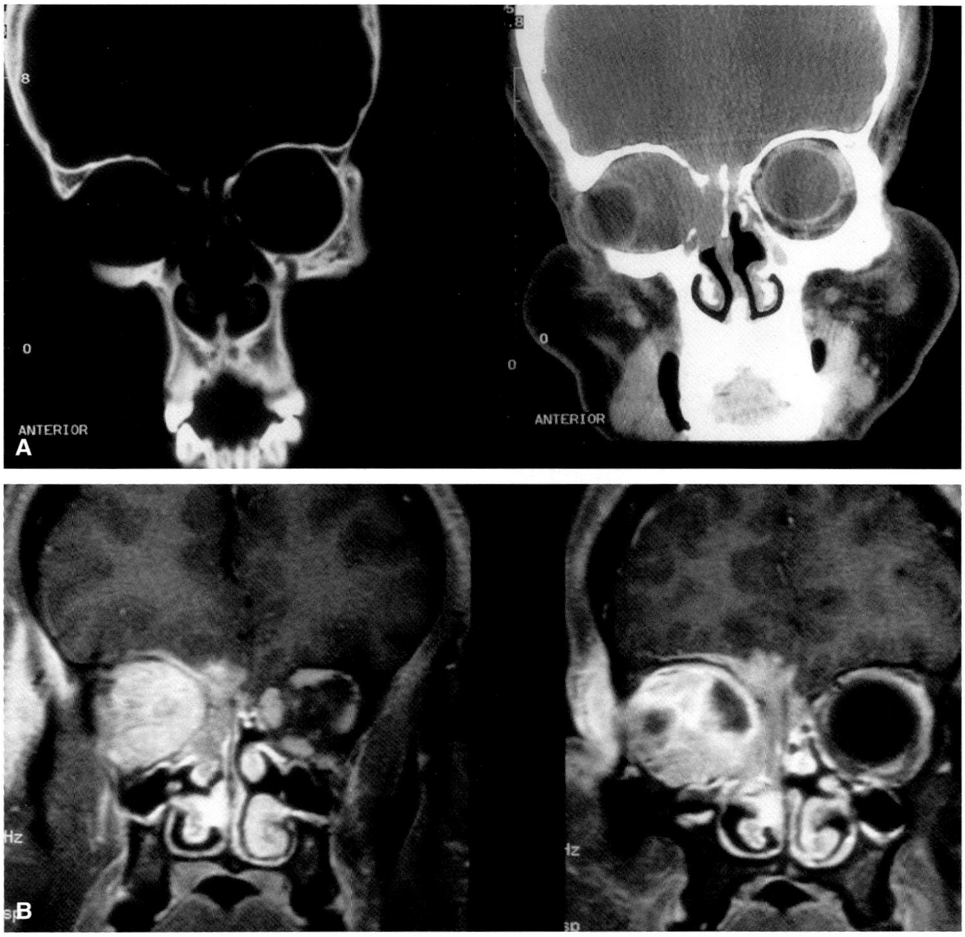

Figure 13–5. Second primary cancer following external beam radiotherapy for bilateral retinoblastoma. Computed tomography (*A*) and magnetic resonance imaging (*B*) of a primitive neuroectodermal tumor in the orbit and sinus 20 years following external beam radiotherapy.

The tumoricidal effect of radiation is largely due to destruction of the reproductive capacity of the neoplasm and subsequent induction of programmed cell death. This often occurs through activation of the *p53* pathway by radiation-induced DNA damage.[16] The visible changes in tumor appearance following EBRT have been well documented and have become the standard for evaluating tumor response following various therapies.[17,18] Five major regression patterns have been described. Type I regression consists of white intratumoral excrescences which resemble cottage cheese (Figure 13–6). Type II is more difficult to distinguish from active tumor. It has been likened to "fish flesh" and looks like active tumor, except that there is a modest shrinkage (25 to 50%) from pretreatment size, and the tumor typically loses its pinkish color due to intratumoral capillaries (Figure 13–7). Type III is a mixture of types I and II (Figure 13–8). Type IV is complete regression with a residual chorioretinal scar. Type 0 is complete disappearance of the tumor. There does not appear to be any correlation between regression pattern and local recurrence.[19]

Exudative retinal detachments usually disappear within 6 months after treatment. Persistent detachment beyond this point suggests either treatment failure or a retinal break. A rhegmatogenous detachment can be repaired once all tumors are well controlled.[20,21] Exudative detachment can also be caused by heavy cryotherapy or laser treatment. A thin serous detachment overlying a regressed tumor does not necessarily indicate tumor activity. Tumor persistence or recurrence will usually be evident within 6 months of initial therapy, and it is rare to have reactivation more than a year after treat-

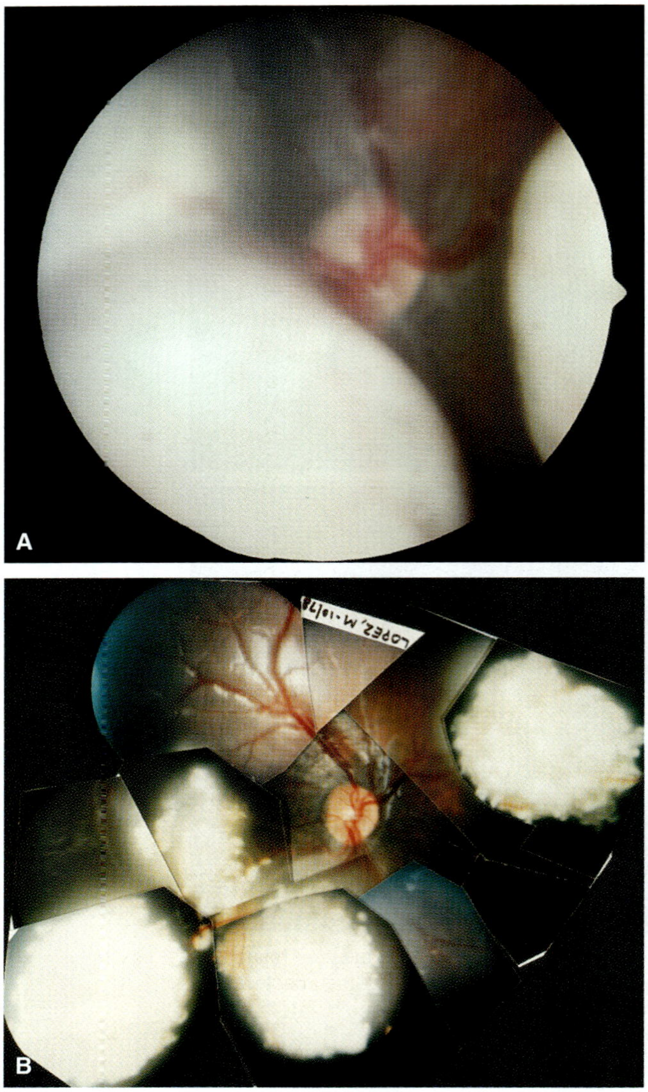

Figure 13–6. *A*, Multiple large tumors in the posterior pole prior to treatment. *B*, Type I "cottage cheese" regression pattern of all tumors following external beam radiotherapy.

ment.[17,19] Larger tumors are more likely to relapse.[19] Reactivation is detected by increased tumor size or new subretinal fluid (Figure 13–9). Vascular changes within the tumor are not a reliable indicator of reactivation, since they may also be due to radiation vasculopathy. Vitreous seeds that are inactive and necrotic usually have a chalky white or gray appearance, but this can be extremely difficult to distinguish from active tumor seeds. Whenever seeds are present, the vitreous base must be monitored indefinitely for activity or tumor implantation.

It is unclear whether the concept that radiation results in "retinal sterilization" is valid. Many patients will acquire new tumors following treatment, although these new tumors may have occurred in anterior areas inadequately treated with radiation. In one study, 16 percent of patients age < 12 months developed new tumors, compared with only 2 percent of older children.[3] When these are detected early, most can be treated with cryotherapy or laser, so it is imperative to continue monitoring the children closely, following treatment, with examination under anesthesia (EUA) using indirect ophthalmoscopy with scleral depression.

Local control rates and visual outcomes vary according to the size and location of tumors, radiation technique, and other factors. With modified lateral ports, the local control rate has been reported to

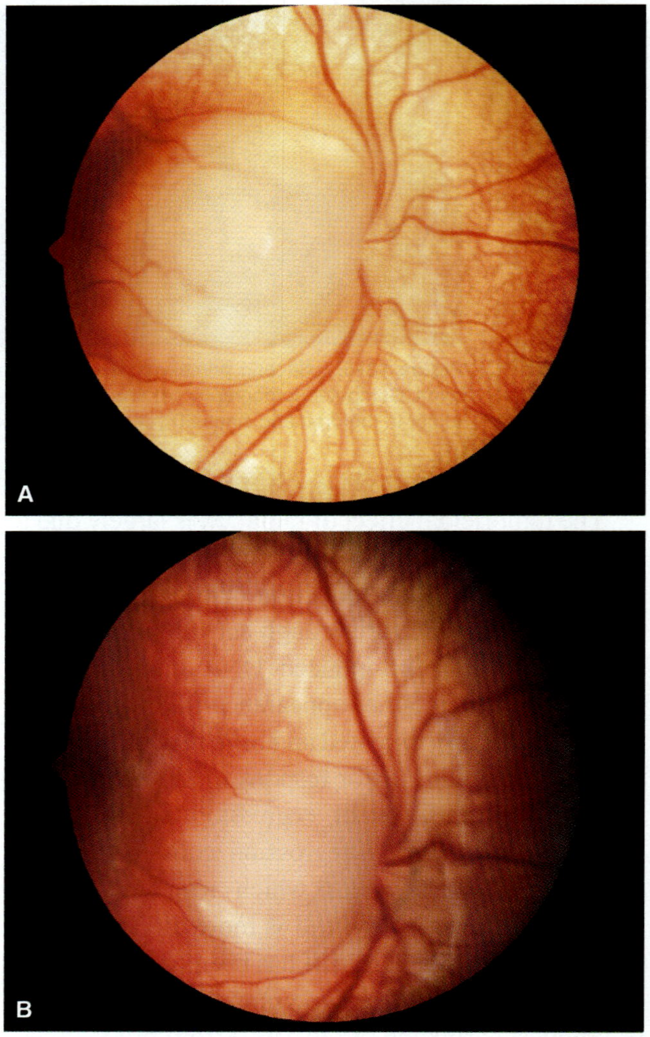

Figure 13–7. *A*, Peripapillary retinoblastoma before treatment. *B*, Type II "fish flesh" differentiated regression pattern following external beam radiotherapy.

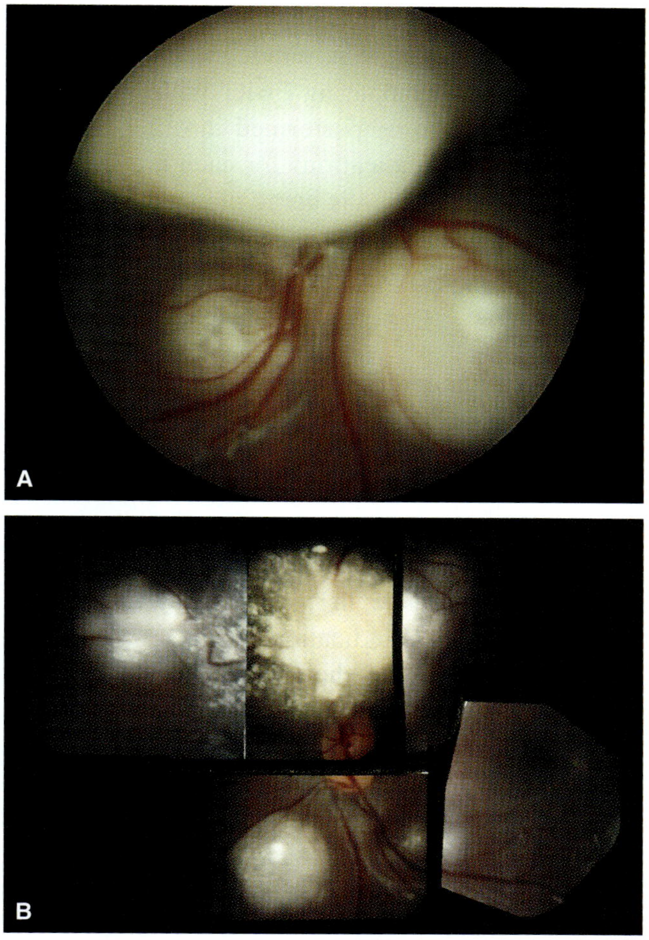

Figure 13–8. *A*, Multiple tumors in the posterior pole prior to therapy. *B*, Type III mixed regression pattern following external beam radiotherapy.

be as high as 84 percent for groups I to III eyes. Around half the patients with bilateral tumors retain at least 20/200 vision in at least one eye, while 20/40 or better is achieved in less than 40 percent.[22,23] Most tumor involving the fovea will result in poor vision.[24] The cure rate is lower for anterior ports and for groups IV to V.[12]

Systemic Chemotherapy

Chemotherapy for retinoblastoma was first attempted in the 1950s using intravenous nitrogen mustard.[25] Although there was often a dramatic initial tumor response, most tumors relapsed and this modality was abandoned. However, the results with chemotherapy have been improved dramatically with the use of adjuvant local therapies, such as cryotherapy and laser photocoagulation.[26] Hence the term chemoreduction, which is chemotherapy used to shrink the tumors to a small enough size to be ablated with other modalities. The interest in chemotherapy has also re-emerged as a result of concern about the long-term complications associated with external beam radiotherapy (see above). While there continues to be controversy regarding the indications for chemotherapy, the agents that should be used, the number of cycles, the long-term risks, and other

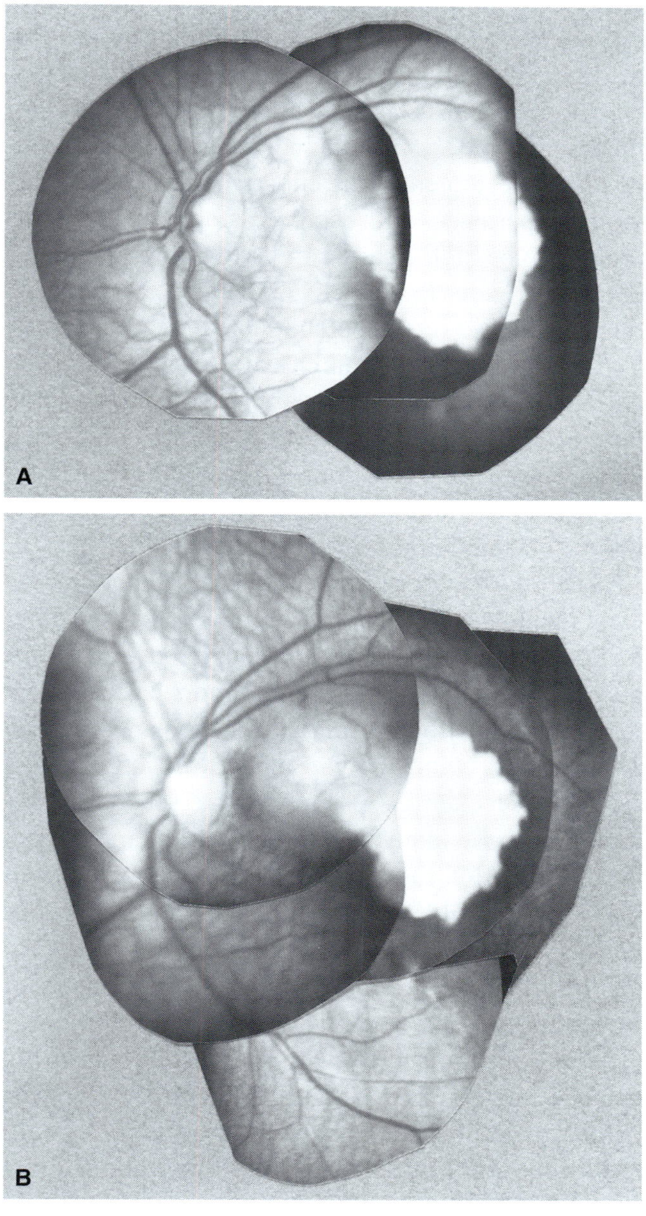

Figure 13–9. *A*, Macular tumor following plaque radiotherapy with type III mixed regression pattern. *B*, Local recurrence of tumor with tumor extension toward the optic nerve 6 months following therapy.

issues, it seems clear that chemotherapy will play an important role in the management of retinoblastoma for the foreseeable future.

For primary therapy of intraocular tumors, the indications for chemotherapy are similar to those described above for external beam radiotherapy. This would include tumors too large to be treated with local therapies. Chemotherapy is also used when there is a risk of metastatic disease, such as when there is pathologic evidence of optic nerve invasion past the lamina cribrosa or massive choroidal invasion. In addition, chemotherapy is used when there is positive cerebrospinal fluid cytology, bone marrow biopsy, or other evidence of frank metastatic disease.[27]

The three most commonly used agents for primary therapy include carboplatin, etoposide, and vincristine. These agents were chosen on the basis of previous experience with neuroblastoma, which was thought to be biologically similar to retinoblastoma.[28] A central venous line for chemotherapy can be placed by the pediatric surgeon at the same time as the EUA. The optimal doses and number of cycles has not been determined, but most centers are using neuroblastoma doses and 5 to 6 cycles. Patients must be examined under anesthesia every 3 to 4 weeks during chemotherapy. Local therapies are used to treat shrunken tumors and any new or recurrent tumors.

The short-term complications of chemotherapy may include bone marrow suppression (especially leukopenia) and line sepsis, although these are infrequent. The incidence of second tumors has been low thus far, but the long-term risk is not clear. Both carboplatin and etoposide can induce second cancers, especially leukemia.[29,30] While the second tumor rate will most likely be lower with chemotherapy than with EBRT, the radiation risk is age related, and many older children may still have a better result with radiotherapy. New techniques for local delivery of chemotherapy are currently being developed to minimize systemic complications.[31,32]

The local control rate with chemotherapy is difficult to compare with that with EBRT because no scientifically valid comparisons have been performed. However, the results with these two modalities appear to be similar for groups I to III.[18,26,33–35] Chemotherapy is not as effective for group V tumors or for vitreous seeding. In these cases, chemotherapy combined with EBRT may allow some patients to avoid enucleation.[28] A multicenter, prospective, randomized trial comparing EBRT with chemotherapy would have to be performed in order to determine the optimal indications for each modality, but at present, no such trial is being planned.

Episcleral Plaque Radiotherapy (Brachytherapy)

For selected tumors, plaque radiotherapy retains the superior tumor response of radiation without the risk of facial bony deformities and second primary cancers (Figure 13–10). Brachytherapy with specially designed eye plaques was introduced by Stallard over 40 years ago.[36] Many improvements have subsequently been made in plaque design, radiation dosage, and clinical indications.

The most common indication for plaque radiotherapy is for solitary tumors < 15 mm in diameter and 3 to 10 mm in thickness.[37] Thinner tumors can often be treated with laser or cryotherapy, while those thicker than 10 mm require higher radiation doses that increase the risk of radiation vasculopathy and damage to orbital structures. Plaque radiotherapy is also effective for localized, overlying vitreous seeding.

The plaque should provide at least a 1-mm margin around the tumor. Currently, most plaques in the United States use gold shielding and Iodine-125 (^{125}I) seeds. This isotope provides acceptable isodose curves while minimizing collateral radiation damage. Plaque insertion is performed in the operating room with the child under general anesthesia. A dummy plaque (same size, identical suture, holes without radiation) may initially be used for localization to reduce radiation exposure to surgical personnel (see Chapter 8). A conjunctival peritomy is performed, and the rectus muscles are looped with silk sutures for control of the globe. The tumor is visualized with the indirect ophthalmoscope, and the tumor margins are marked on the sclera with a marking depressor. The plaque is then sutured to the sclera overlying the tumor, and the plaque edges are checked with indirect ophthalmoscopy to make sure they cover all the tumor margins. A total dose of about 40 Gy is delivered over 3 to 4 days. The plaque is removed in a second procedure.

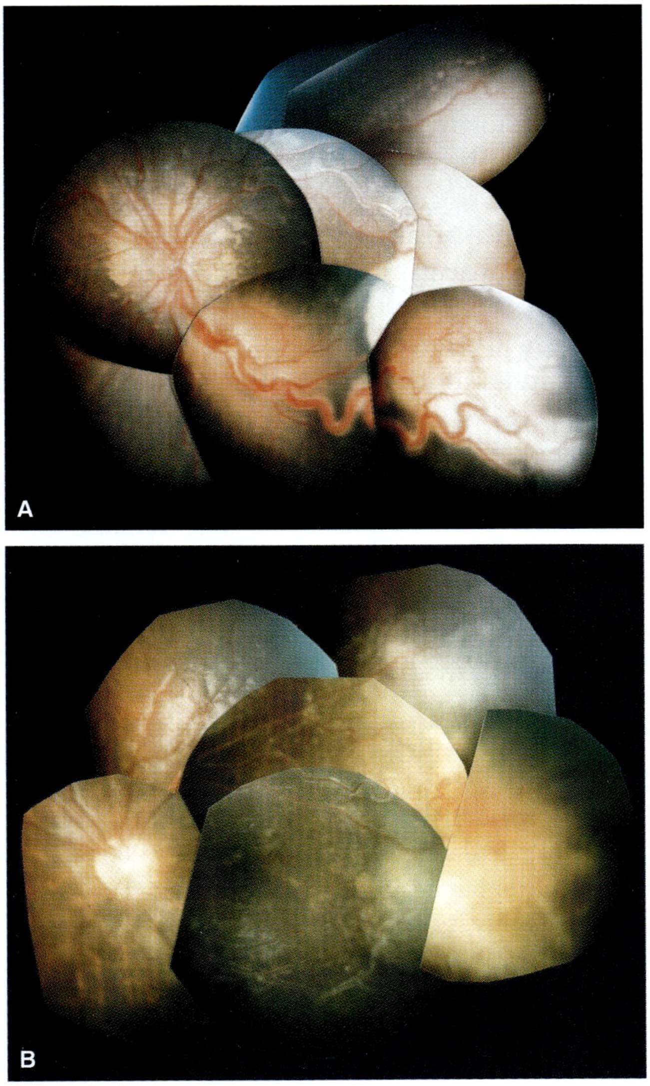

Figure 13–10. *A*, Unilateral, unifocal retinoblastoma in the temporal macula prior to treatment. *B*, Regressed tumor following plaque radiotherapy.

When tumors are properly selected, the success rate can be very high (Figure 13–11). Stallard reported 63 of 69 eyes treated successfully using cobalt plaques.[36] Similar results have been obtained with iodine plaques.[38] In addition, plaque therapy greatly reduces the risk of facial deformity and second primary cancers, compared with EBRT. However, the radiation dose to the retina and optic nerve is much greater with brachytherapy, since there is exponentially more radiation delivered to the tumor base than to the apex. Consequently, the risk of radiation retinopathy and papillopathy is higher and is dependent on both tumor thickness and location. Other unusual complications include scleral necrosis and strabismus.

Laser Therapy

Several forms of laser therapy have been employed for treating retinoblastoma. Xenon arc is highly effective for selected tumors, but it is difficult to use (especially for peripheral tumors) and is no longer available in most centers.[39] Argon laser photocoagulation, usually delivered through an indirect ophthalmoscope, is now the most widely used and convenient laser modality.[40] The mechanism of laser tumor destruction is unclear, although vascular closure probably plays an important role. A technique for delivering heat with the diode laser (810 nm) has enjoyed some popularity, but the advantage of this technique over other laser modalities is unclear.[26]

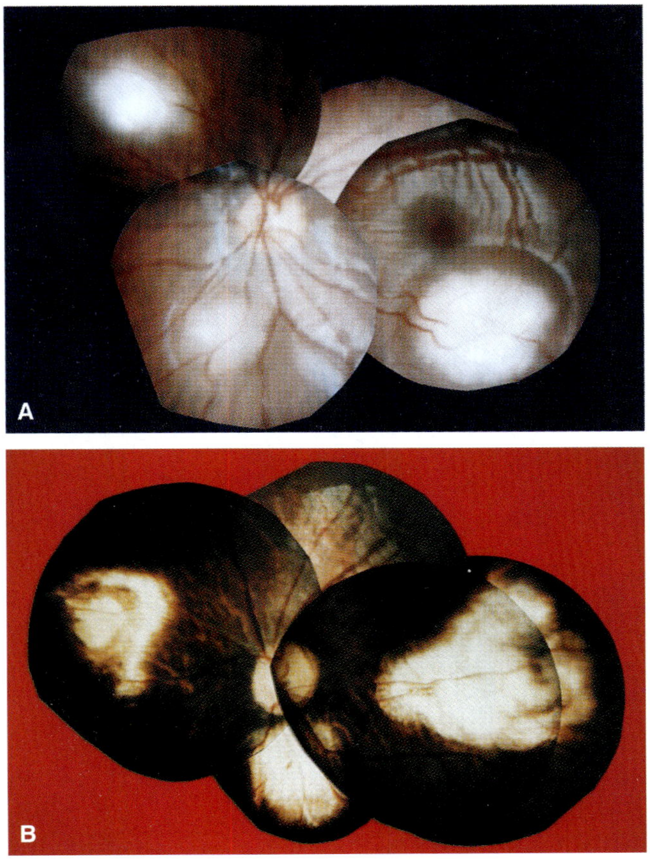

Figure 13–11. Use of plaque brachytherapy after failure of laser therapy. *A*, Unifocal retinoblastoma which has incompletely responded to laser photocoagulation. *B*, Almost complete regression following plaque radiotherapy.

Laser therapy is used mostly for small posterior and equatorial tumors that are < 5 mm in basal dimensions and < 3 mm in thickness (Figure 13–12).[41] More anterior tumors are usually treated with cryotherapy. Overlying vitreous seeds are inadequately treated with laser photocoagulation.

Laser therapy is usually delivered with a portable argon laser mounted on to an indirect ophthalmoscope while the child is under general anesthesia. The tumor surface is treated with multiple overlapping spots until the intratumoral capillaries are observed to blanch. We use a duration of 0.2 seconds and an initial energy of 200 mW. The energy is then increased by 50 to 100 mW intervals until the desired treatment effect is observed. Care should be taken not to use excessively high energies, as this can induce dispersion of the tumor into the vitreous. The energy is then lowered again to treat a 1-mm margin around the tumor. Some clinicians feel that it is also important to treat any feeder vessels, although this increases the risk of hemorrhage. Complications can include retinal breaks, retinal detachment, epiretinal membrane, macular distortion, choroidal neovascularization, subretinal or vitreous hemorrhage, iris damage, and cataract.

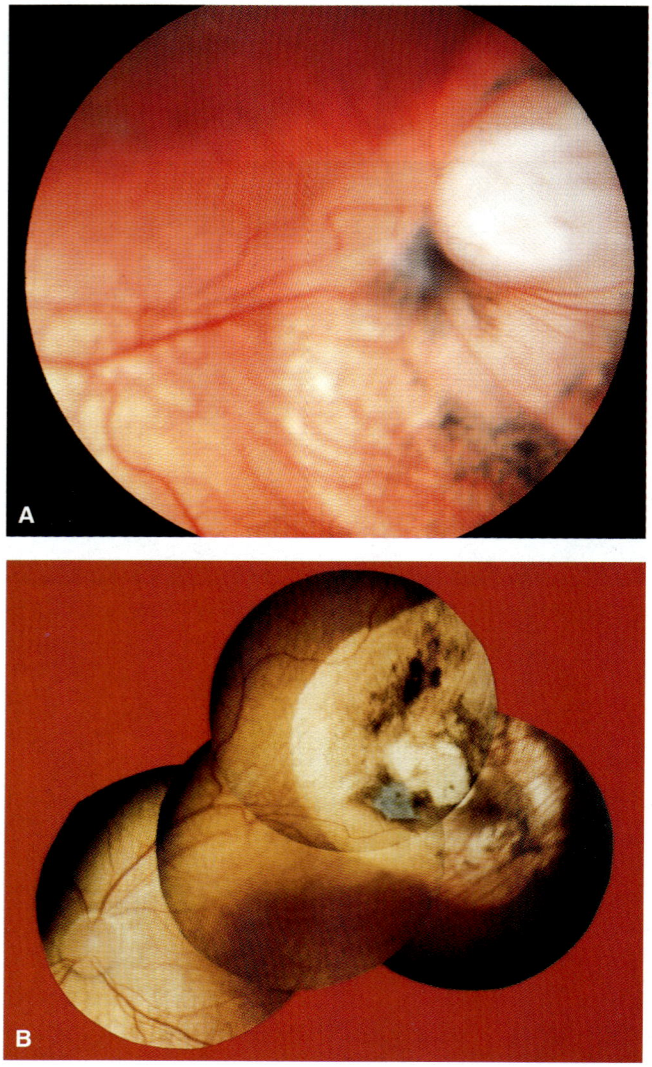

Figure 13–12. *A*, Multiple small retinoblastomas prior to treatment. *B*, Excellent response following laser photocoagulation.

The result of successful treatment is a flat chorioretinal scar. Several laser sessions may be required, but alternative modalities should be considered if the desired treatment goal is not achieved after 2 to 3 sessions. For appropriately selected tumors, laser therapy can be very successful. In one series, there was a 97 percent success rate for tumors < 1.5 mm in thickness, 70 percent for those 1.5 to 3.0 mm, and 29 percent for those > 3 mm.[39]

Cryotherapy

Cryotherapy for the treatment of intraocular tumors was first popularized by Lincoff in the 1960s.[42] The technique and indications have evolved, and cryotherapy is highly effective for appropriately selected tumors. The indications are similar to those for laser therapy (< 5 mm in basal dimensions and < 3 mm in thickness), except that cryotherapy is superior for treating more anterior tumors (Figure 13–13). Like laser therapy, cryotherapy is not effective for vitreous seeds unless they are just above the tumor.

For cryotherapy, the child is under general anesthesia. The retinal cryoprobe is placed on the sclera and visualized with the indirect ophthalmoscope. Various probes are available depending on the size of the eye and the tumor, including pediatric and adult retinal probes (round tip) and a hammerhead probe for larger tumors. For very anterior tumors, the treatment may be delivered with no conjunctival incision, whereas a small peritomy is used to allow the probe to be positioned for more posterior tumors. The whole tumor should be seen to whiten and opacify, with slight freezing of the overlying vitreous. Several treatment applications may be required to cover the entire tumor, and a triple freeze-thaw technique is used. Successfully treated tumors should completely

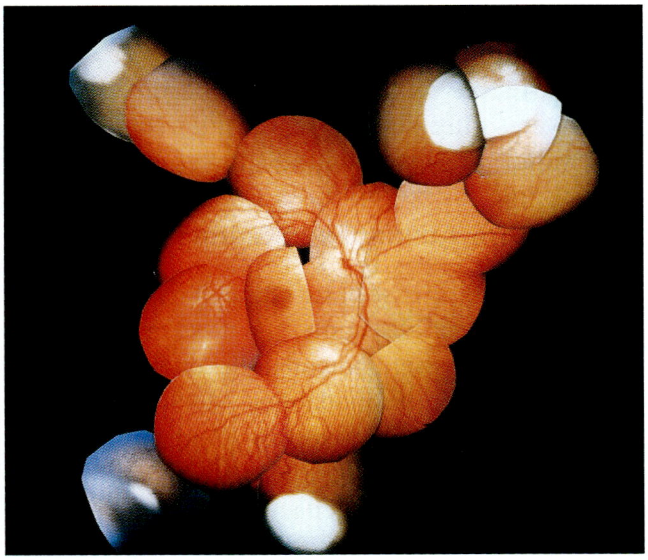

Figure 13–13. Small anterior tumor near the ora serrata with no overlying vitreous seeding. These tumors usually respond well to cryotherapy.

regress to a flat chorioretinal scar within 4 to 6 weeks after treatment (Figure 13–14). If this effect is not achieved, the tumor should be retreated, or a new modality should be chosen.

At least 70 percent of properly selected tumors can be successfully treated with cryotherapy.[43] Our impression is that cryotherapy is somewhat more effective than laser therapy for comparable tumors, but complications are also more common and severe with cryotherapy. These complications can include retinal breaks, rhegmatogenous and exudative retinal detachment, choroidal detachment, uveitis, and theoretic tumor dispersion into the vitreous.

CLASSIFICATION

The most commonly used system for staging retinoblastoma is still the Reese-Ellsworth classification (Table 13–1). This classification scheme is now outmoded since it is based on prognosis for ocular salvage (not patient survival) before the era of modern diagnostic techniques (including indirect ophthalmoscopy) and local therapies. For example, group IVb tumors (a solitary tumor at the ora serrata) previously had a poor prognosis because they were difficult to visualize. Currently, these tumors have a much better prognosis with the availability of indirect ophthalmoscopy and cryotherapy. A new treatment-oriented classification which reflects recent improvements in treatment and local control is currently being developed.

FOLLOW-UP SCHEDULE

The follow-up schedule will vary according to laterality, patient age, treatment, and other factors. In general, younger children require more frequent follow-up, since they are at higher risk for new tumors. This risk starts to decline after 12 months of age. It is also important that children with germline mutations be screened periodically until the age of 5 to 6 years for midline intracranial primitive neuroectodermal tumors (Figure 13–15). In addition, these patients will require systemic monitoring for second primary cancers throughout their life.

Close follow-up is especially important in patients undergoing chemotherapy, since this treatment alone is rarely sufficient to achieve local tumor control. Examination under anesthesia every 3 to 4 weeks is usually required until all tumors have stabilized, with no recurrences or new tumors.

Follow-up can be slightly less frequent with EBRT, although the anterior retina must be watched closely for new tumors, since it is not adequately treated with lateral radiation ports. Initially, examination under anesthesia is recommended every 6 weeks until all tumors are stabilized, then every 2 to 3 months for 1 year, every 4 months for the next year, and slowly extending the follow-up interval thereafter. Recurrences are usually evident within

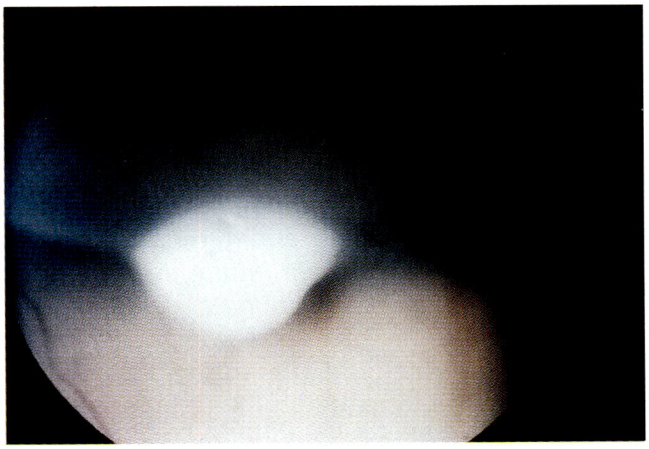

Figure 13–14. Small anterior retinoblastoma before treatment. Two months later there was complete regression

Table 13–1. REESE-ELLSWORTH CLASSIFICATION OF RETINOBLASTOMA

Group	Description	Prognosis for Ocular Salvage
I	a. Solitary tumor, < 6 mm, at or behind equator b. Multiple tumors, none > 6 mm, at or behind equator	Very favorable
II	a. Solitary tumor, 6 to 15 mm, at or behind equator b. Multiple tumors, 6 to 15 mm, behind equator	Favorable
III	a. Any tumor anterior to the equator b. Solitary tumor, > 15 mm, behind equator	Doubtful
IV	a. Multiple tumors, some > 15 mm b. Any tumor extending to ora serrata	Unfavorable
V	a. Massive tumors involving more than half the retina b. Vitreous seeding	Very unfavorable

6 months of treatment, and it is rare to develop a new tumor more than a year after treatment.

PROGNOSIS

With modern diagnostic and therapeutic modalities, the survival rate in the developed countries is around 95 percent. However, a number of risk factors for metastasis and death have been identified, including optic nerve invasion and massive choroidal invasion.[8,9,44–46] Clinically, a suspicion of choroidal or optic nerve invasion (especially when the optic nerve cannot be directly visualized by an overlying tumor) usually necessitates enucleation. Other clinical findings that may portend a poor prognosis include anterior segment rubeosis and tumor extension into the anterior chamber.

Recurrences and death usually occur within the first 2 years after diagnosis.[27,47] Children diagnosed at an older age generally have a better prognosis.[1]

Future Advances in Management

There has been intense basic research on the molecular biology of retinoblastoma, and these investigations are beginning to yield potentially exciting new diagnostic and therapeutic modalities. Much progress has been made in genetic testing for *Rb* gene mutations, and future improvements are likely.[48,49] Better genetic information will allow ocular oncologists to determine whether a patient with unilateral tumor is at risk for new tumors and bilateral involvement, whether a sibling or parent of a patient with bilateral tumor carries the mutation, and whether an offspring of a retinoblastoma survivor carries the mutation. Further, genetic information may allow workers to determine which patients are at higher risk for second cancers and which are likely to be sensitive to chemotherapy or radiotherapy.

Molecular therapy for retinoblastoma and other cancers also appears to be on the horizon. The next generation of antineoplastic agents promises to deliver more potent tumor destruction and better discrimination between tumor and normal cells. Potential approaches include gene replacement therapy, suicide gene therapy, small molecule inhibitors, and other innovative molecular approaches that take advantage of the specific genetic defect in retinoblastoma.[50–53]

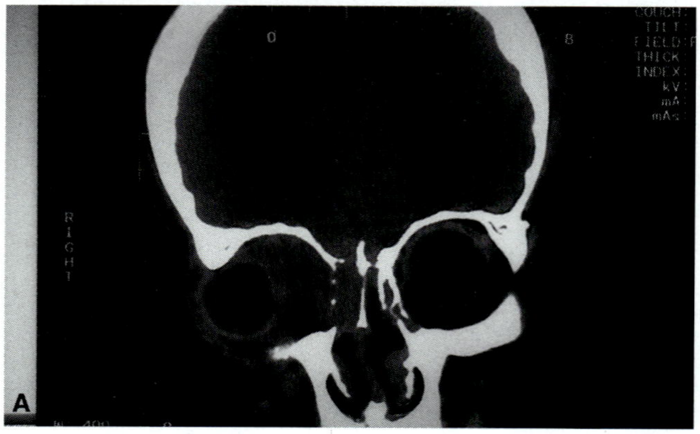

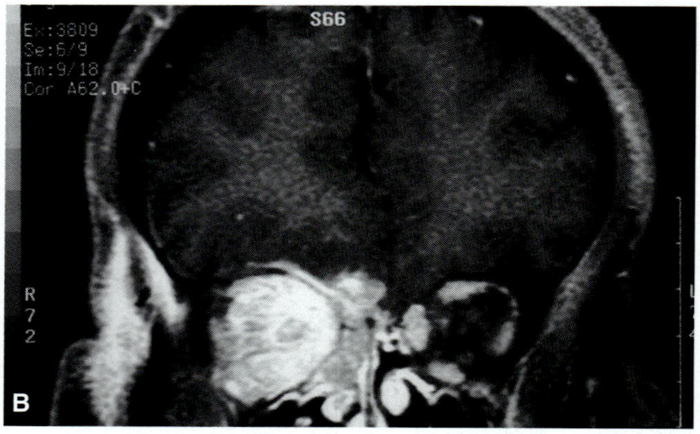

Figure 13–15. Computed tomography (*A*) and magnetic resonance imaging (*B*) of midline intracranial tumor (primitive neuroectodermal tumor) in patient with bilateral germline retinoblastoma.

REFERENCES

1. Rubenfeld M, Abramson DH, Ellsworth RM, Kitchin FD. Unilateral vs. bilateral retinoblastoma. Correlations between age at diagnosis and stage of ocular disease. Ophthalmology 1986;93:1016–9.
2. Abramson DH, Frank CM. Second nonocular tumors in survivors of bilateral retinoblastoma: a possible age effect on radiation-related risk. Ophthalmology 1998;105:573–9.
3. Abramson DH, Gamell LS, Ellsworth RM, et al. Unilateral retinoblastoma: new intraocular tumors after treatment. Br J Ophthalmol 1994;78:698–701.
4. Abramson DH, Gombos DS. The topography of bilateral retinoblastoma lesions. Retina 1996;16:232–9.
5. Hopping W, Schmitt G. The treatment of retinoblastoma. Mod Probl Ophthalmol 1977;18:106–12.
6. Messmer EP, Heinrich T, Hopping W, et al. Risk factors for metastaases in patients with retinoblastoma. Ophthalmology 1991;98:136–41.
7. Shields JA, Shields CL, Sivalingam V. Decreasing frequency of enucleation in patients with retinoblastoma. Am J Ophthalmol 1989;108:185–8.
8. Magramm I, Abramson DH, Ellsworth RM. Optic nerve involvement in retinoblastoma. Ophthalmology 1989;96:217–22.
9. Stannard C, Lipper S, Sealy R, Sevel D. Retinoblastoma: a correlation of invasion of the optic nerve and choroid with prognosis and metastasis. Br J Ophthalmol 1979;63:560–70.
10. Martin HE, Reese AB. Treatment of retinal gliomas by fractionated or divided dose principle of roentgen radiation: preliminary report. Arch Ophthalmol 1936;16:733–61.
11. Wong FL, Boice JJ, Abramson DH, et al. Cancer incidence after retinoblastoma. Radiation dose and sarcoma risk. JAMA 1997;278:1262–7.
12. Blach LE, McCormick B, Abramson DH. External beam radiation therapy and retinoblastoma: long-term results in the comparison of two techniques. Int J Radiat Oncol Biol Phys 1996;35:45–51.
13. Toma NM, Hungerford JL, Plowman PN, et al. External beam radiotherapy for retinoblastoma: II. Lens sparing technique. Br J Ophthalmol 1995;79:112–7.
14. Eng C, Li FP, Abramson DH, et al. Mortality from second tumors among long-term survivors of retinoblastaoma. J Natl Cancer Inst 1993; 85:1121–8.
15. Rosenman J, Chaney EL, Sailer S, et al. Recent advances in radiotherapy treatment planning. Cancer Invest 1991;9:465–81.
16. Nork TM, Poulsen GL, Millecchia LL, et al. P53 regulates apoptosis in human retinoblastoma. Arch Ophthalmol 1997;115:213–9.
17. Abramson DH, Gerardi CM, Ellsworth RM, et al. Radiation regression patterns in treated retinoblastoma: 7 to 21 years later. J Pediatr Ophthalmol Strabismus 1991;28:108–12.
18. Bornfeld N, Schuler A, Bechrakis N, et al. Preliminary results of primary chemotherapy in retinoblastoma. Klin Padiatr 1997;209:216–21.
19. Singh AD, Garway-Heath D, Love S, et al. Relationship of regression pattern to recurrence in retinoblastoma. Br J Ophthalmol 1993;77:12–6.
20. Baumal CR, Shields CL, Shields JA, Tasman WS. Surgical repair of rhegmatogenous retinal detachment after treatment for retinoblastoma. Ophthalmology 1998;105:2134–98.
21. Bovey EH, Fernandez-Ragaz AL, Heon EL, et al. Rhegmatogenous retinal detachment after treatment of retinoblastoma. Ophthalmic Genet 1999;20:141–51.
22. Egbert PR, Donaldson SS, Moazed K, Rosenthal AR. Visual results and ocular complications following radiotherapy for retinoblastoma. Arch Ophthalmol 1978;96:1826–30.
23. Migdal C. Bilateral retinoblastoma: the prognosis for vision. Br J Ophthalmol 1983;67:592–5.
24. Weiss AH, Karr DJ, Kalina RE, et al. Visual outcomes of macular retinoblastoma after external beam radiation therapy. Ophthalmology 1994;101:1244–9.
25. Kupfer C. Retinoblastoma treated with intravenous nitrogen mustard. Am J Ophthalmol 1953;53:505.
26. Murphree AL, Villablanca JG, Deegan WR, et al. Chemotherapy plus local treatment in the management of intraocular retinoblastoma. Arch Ophthalmol 1996;114:1348–56.
27. Pratt CB, Fontanesi J, Chenaille P, et al. Tumor-selective transgene expression in vivo mediated by an E2F- responsive adenoviral vector. Nat Med 1997;3: 1145–9.
28. Kingston JE, Hungerford JL, Madreperla SA, Plowman PN. Results of combined chemotherapy and radiotherapy for advanced intraocular retinoblastoma. Arch Ophthalmol 1996;114:1339–43.
29. Jeha S, Jaffe N, Robertson R. Secondary acute non-lymphoblastic leukemia in two children following treatment with a cis-diamminedichloroplatinum II based regimen for osteosarcoma. Med Pediatr Oncol 1992;20:71–4.
30. Winick NJ, McKenna RW, Shuster JJ, et al. Secondary acute myeloid leukemia in children with acute lymphoblastic leukemia treated with etoposide. J Clin Oncol 1993;11:209–17.
31. Abramson DH, Frank CM, Dunkel IJ. A phase I/II study of subconjunctival carboplatin for intraocular retinoblastoma. Ophthalmology 1999;106:1947–50.
32. Harbour JW, Murray TG, Hamasaki D, et al. Local carboplatin therapy in transgenic murine retinoblastoma. Invest Ophthalmol Vis Sci 1996;37:1892–8.
33. Gallie BL, Budning A, DeBoer G, et al. Chemotherapy with focal therapy can cure intraocular retinoblas-

toma without radiotherapy. Arch Ophthalmol 1996; 114:1321–8.
34. Greenwald MJ, Strauss LC. Treatment of intraocular retinoblastoma with carboplatin and etoposide chemotherapy. Ophthalmology 1996;103:1989–97.
35. Shields CL, Shields JA, Needle M, et al. Combined chemoreduction and adjuvant treatment for intraocular retinoblastoma. Ophthalmology 1997;104: 2101–11.
36. Stallard HB. The treatment of retinoblastoma. Ophthalmologica 1956;Ann:151.
37. Shields CL, Shields JA, De Potter P, et al. Plaque radiotherapy in the management of retinoblastoma. Use as a primary and secondary treatment. Ophthalmology 1993;100:216–24.
38. Hernandez JC, Brady LW, Shields CL, et al. Conservative treatment of retinoblastoma. The use of plaque brachytherapy. Am J Clin Oncol 1993;16:397–401.
39. Abramson DH. The focal treatment of retinoblastoma with emphasis on xenon arc photocoagulation. Acta Ophthalmologica 1989;194:3–63.
40. Shields CL, Shields JA, Kiratli H, De Potter P. Treatment of retinoblastoma with indirect ophthalmoscope laser photocoagulation. J Pediatr Ophthalmol Strabismus 1995;32:317–22.
41. Shields JA, Shields CL, Parsons H, Giblin ME. The role of photocoagulation in the management of retinoblastoma. Arch Ophthalmol 1990;108:205–8.
42. Lincoff H, McLean J, Long R. The cryosurgical treatment of intraocular tumors. Am J Ophthalmol 1967; 63:389–99.
43. Abramson DH, Ellsworth RM, Rozakis GW. Cryotherapy for retinoblastoma. Arch Ophthalmol 1982;100: 1253–6.
44. Khelfaoui F, Validire P, Auperin A, et al. Histopathologic risk factors in retinoblastoma: a retrospective study of 172 patients treated in a single institution. Cancer 1996;77:1206–13.
45. Shields CL, Shields JA, Baez K, et al. Optic nerve invasion of retinoblastoma. Metastatic potential and clinical risk factors. Cancer 1994;73:692–8.
46. Shields CL, Shields JA, Baez KA, et al. Choroidal invasion of retinoblastoma: metastatic potential and clinical risk factors. Br J Ophthalmol 1993;77:544–8.
47. Doz F, Khelfaoui F, Mosseri V, et al. The role of chemotherapy in orbital involvement of retinoblastoma. The experience of a single institution with 33 patients. Cancer 1994;74:722–32.
48. Lohmann DR, Brandt B, Hopping W, et al. The spectrum of RB1 germ-line mutations in hereditary retinoblastoma. Am J Hum Genet 1996;58:940–9.
49. Harbour JW. Overview of RB gene mutations in patients with retinoblastoma. Implications for clinical genetic screening. Ophthalmology 1998;105:1422–47.
50. Huang HJ, Yee JK, Shew JY, et al. Suppression of the neoplastic phenotype by replacement of the RB gene in human cancer cells. Science 1999;242: 1563–6.
51. Hurwitz MY, Marcus KT, Chevez-Barrios P, et al. Suicide gene therapy for treatment of retinoblastoma in a murine model. Human Gene Ther 1998;10:441–8.
52. Chen YN, Sharma SK, Ramsey TM, et al. Selective killing of transformed cells by cyclin/cyclin –dependent kinase 2 antagonists. Proc Natl Acad Sci USA 1999;96:4325–9.
53. Parr MJ, Manome Y, Tanaka T, et al. Tumor-selective transgene expression in vivo mediated by an E2F-responsive adenoviral vector. Nat Med 1997;3: 1145–9.

14

Optic Nervehead Tumors

A number of tumors can involve the optic nerve, including metastases, hemangiomas (Figure 14–1), hamartomas, uveal melanomas, retinoblastomas, melanocytomas (Figure 14–2), hemangioblastomas, medulloepitheliomas, juvenile xanthogranulomas, intraocular extension of either optic nerve sheath meningiomas or optic nerve gliomas, and paraneoplastic neuropathies.[1–7]

MELANOCYTOMA

Melanocytomas of the optic nerve head were probably first visualized shortly after the introduction of the ophthalmoscope in the middle of the 19th century.[8] Many of the early reported cases of optic nerve melanocytomas were erroneously thought to be malignant, although some authors in the late 19th and early 20th centuries believed that these tumors might be benign.[9–13] The definitive articles that established the benign nature of optic nerve melanocytomas were published in 1960 and 1962. Zimmerman and Garron used the term "melanocytoma" to describe these magnocellular nevi of the optic nervehead, and studied 20 enucleated specimens plus 14 clinical cases.[14–15]

Melanocytomas occur most commonly in dark-skinned patients; this tumor has a slight female propensity and is usually detected in middle-aged patients. Melanocytomas are usually unilateral, although bilateral cases have been reported.[16] They are most commonly asymptomatic, although with extensive necrosis decreased vision can occur.[17,18] Retinal vascular alterations have been observed in 30 percent, subretinal fluid in 10 percent, and optic

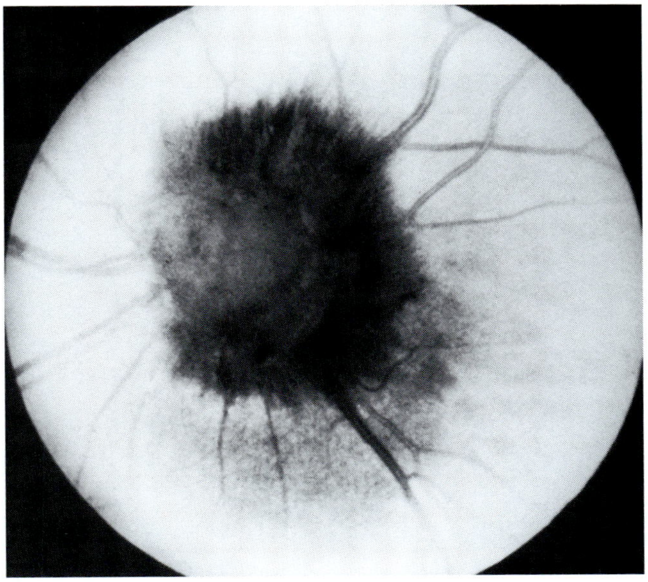

Figure 14–1. Optic disc hemangioma.

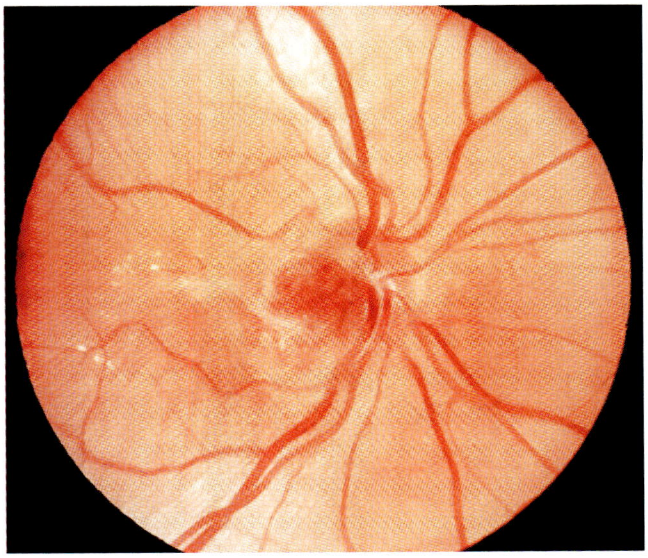

Figure 14–2. An atypical melanocytoma, much larger than is normally seen.

disc edema in 28 percent of cases.[19] On long-term follow-up, approximately 5 percent had some deterioration of vision, 75 percent had an enlarged blind spot, 20 percent had arcuate scotomas, and 30 percent had an afferent pupil defect.[18,19] Clinical examples of optic nerve melanocytomas are shown in Figures 14–2 and 14–3.

Tumor borders may be sharp or, more commonly, fibrillar due to infiltration of the nerve fiber layer. Joffe and colleagues reported on 40 optic disc melanocytomas. The mean age at diagnosis was 50 years. Fifteen of the 40 patients were African American; 29 had a vision of 6/9 or better. In 10 of 40 cases there was overlying orange pigmentation. In 88 percent, the tumor was < 3 mm in diameter. With serial follow-up data, 4 of 27 patients had tumor enlargement.[20] Malignant transformation is extremely rare.[21]

Virtually all optic nerve melanocytomas can be observed without intervention. The author has seen two cases of malignant degeneration. In one case, a mainly amelanotic melanoma arose from a typical melanocytoma and involved a significant area of peripapillary choroid (Figure 14–4). Other authors have reported both melanocytomas with malignant degeneration and primary optic nerve melanomas with posterior extension along the nerve.[22–25] Pigmented adenomas of the optic disc can also sometimes mimic either a melanoma or a melanocytoma.[26,27]

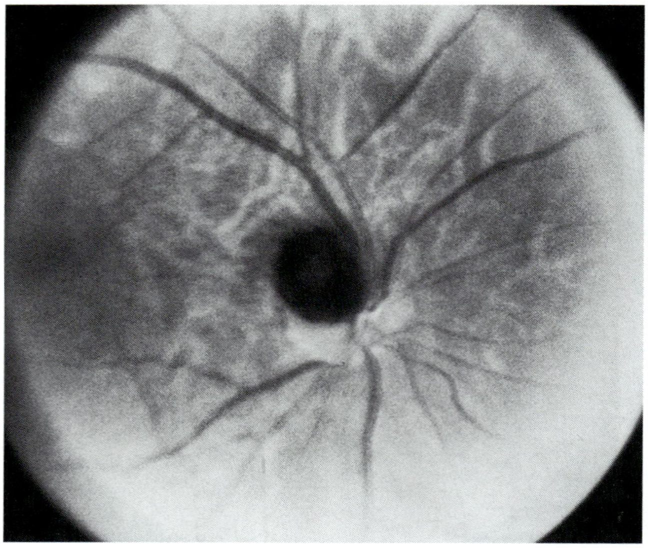

Figure 14–3. Typical optic nervehead melanocytoma in a Japanese female, involving only a portion of the nervehead.

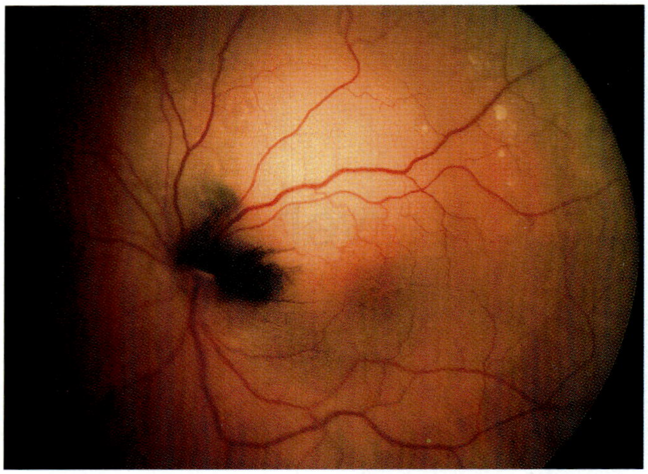

Figure 14–4. Case of malignant degeneration. The amelanotic melanoma appears to have arisen from a typical melanocytoma and there is a significant area of peripapillary choroid involved.

MELANOMA

Juxtapapillary melanomas can simulate an optic nerve inflammation or a primary optic nerve tumor. Figure 14–5 shows a circumferential peripapillary melanoma, initially misdiagnosed as an optic neuritis. While there is a slight statistical increase in tumor-related mortality associated with melanomas around the optic nerve, these tumors are not associated with significantly increased tumor-related mortality, unless the tumor actually compresses the nerve, with marked diminution of vision.[28] The management of these tumors is discussed in Chapter 8 on posterior uveal tumors.[27]

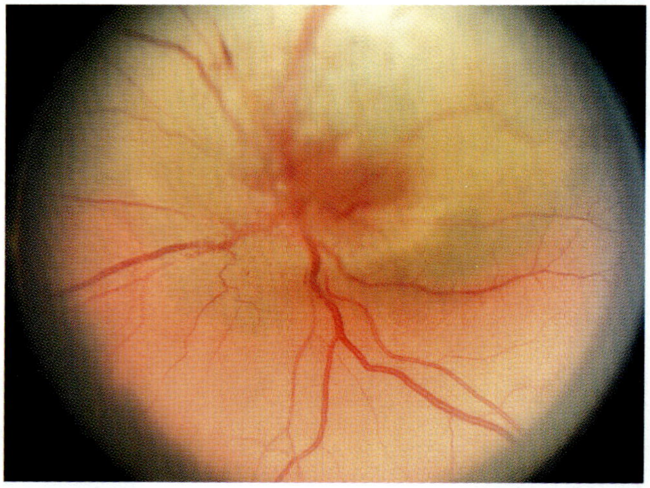

Figure 14–5. Circumferential peripapillar uveal melanoma initially diagnosed as optic neuritis.

METASTASES

Occasionally, metastases will initially involve just the optic nervehead. These are much less common than metastatic deposits in the uveal tract and occur with the same frequency as those involving the vitreous.[29–31] An example of a bronchiogenic carcinoma metastatic to the optic nervehead is shown in Figure 14–6A; the accompanying fluorescein angiogram is shown in Figure 14–6B. Figure 14–7 shows a breast carcinoma metastatic to the optic nerve. As at other sites, optic nerve metastases are often responsive to external beam photon irradiation.

Optic nerve infiltration as a result of acute lymphocytic leukemia is discussed in the chapter on lymphoid lesions.[32,33] Figure 14–8 shows an axial computed tomography (CT) scan of a lymphoma that involved both the optic nerves and clinically simulated the intraocular appearance of leukemic optic nerve infiltrate. As previously discussed, both optic nerve gliomas and optic nerve sheath meningiomas can invade the eye and produce intraocular involvement.[34,35] Juvenile xanthogranuloma and malignant medulloepitheliomas have also rarely involved the optic disc; the latter tumor can produce mortality from contiguous spread to the central nervous system (CNS).[5,36] Figure 14–9 shows a glial proliferation (confirmed on fine-needle aspiration biopsy) in a young boy who had sarcoid involving the eye. Figure 14–10 demonstrates an optic nerve proliferation in a patient with malignant histiocytosis.

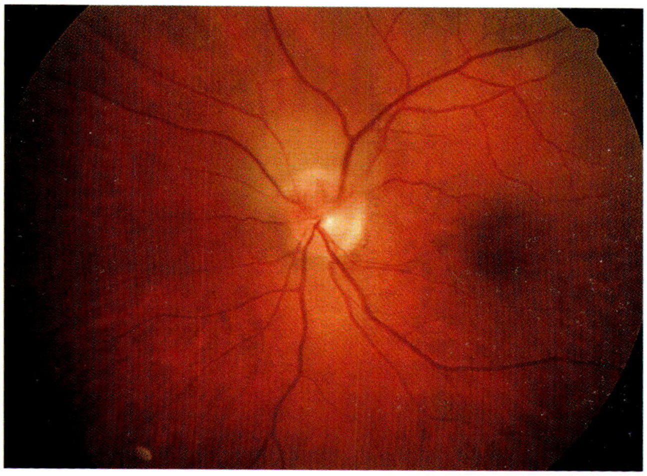

Figure 14–7. Breast carcinoma metastatic to the optic nerve.

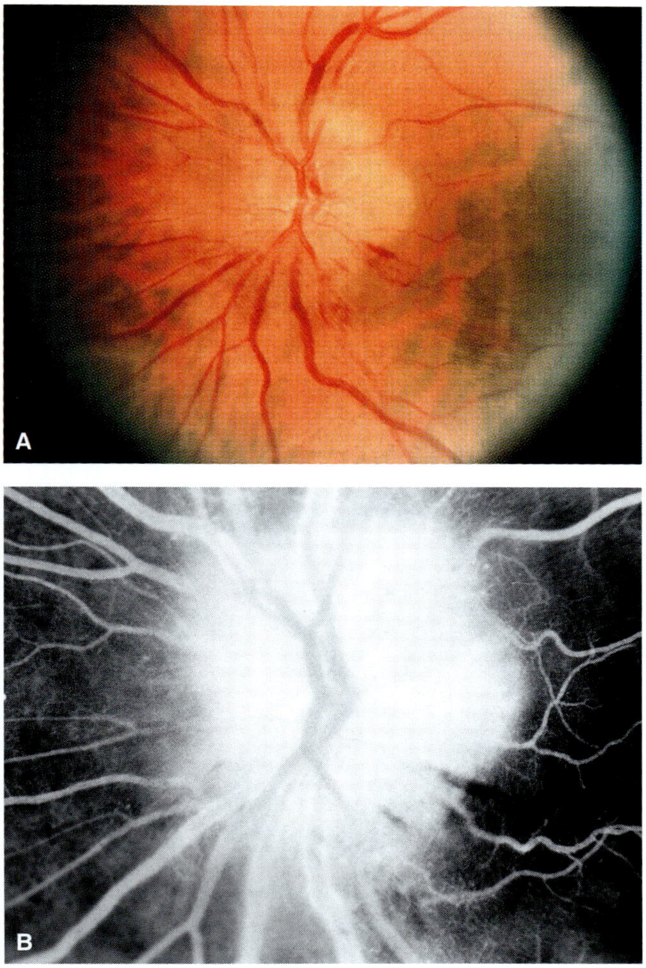

Figure 14–6. *A,* Bronchiogenic carcinoma metastatic to the optic nervehead. *B,* Fluorescein angiogram of the same eye.

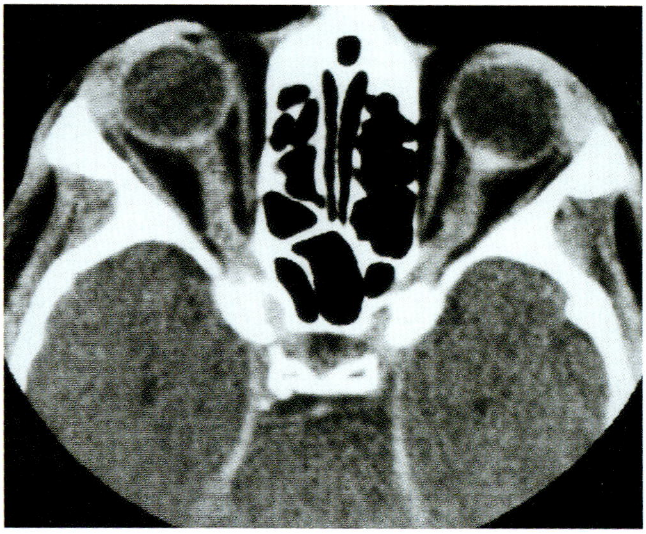

Figure 14–8. Axial CT demonstrates bilateral involvement of the optic nerves. This patient had the fundus pattern that simulated a leukemic optic nerve infiltrate.

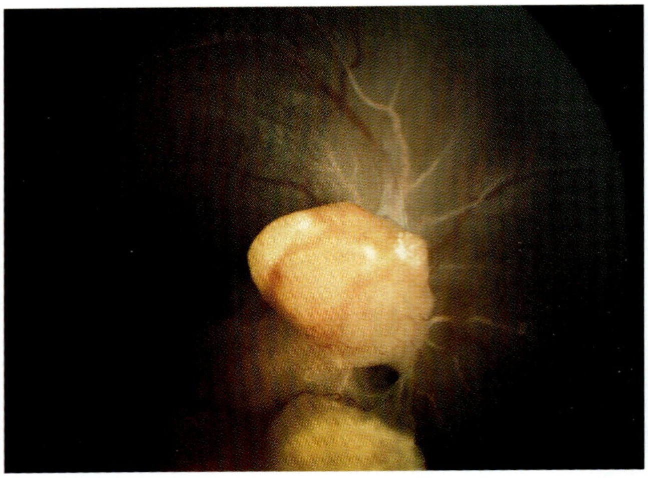

Figure 14–9. Optic nerve glial proliferation in a patient with long-standing sarcoidosis involving the eye.

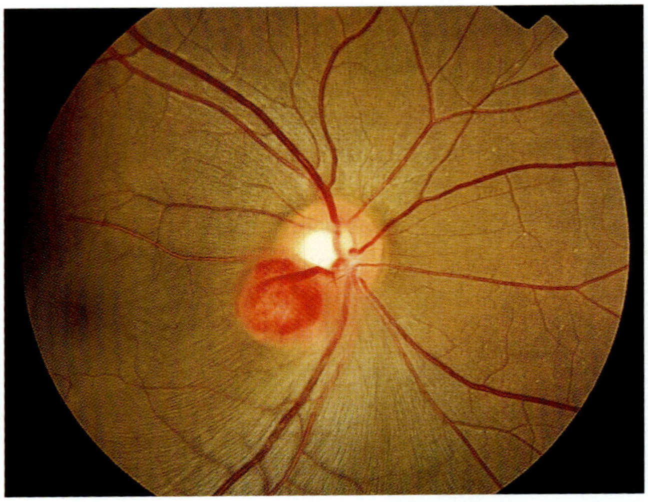

Figure 14–11. Angiogram of disc prior to disc proton irradiation.

ANGIOMAS

Angiomas are discussed in the chapter on retinal tumors. In any patient with either a retinal or optic nerve hemangioma, the diagnosis of von Hippel-Lindau syndrome should be ruled out with CNS magnetic resonance imaging (MRI) scans and either MRI or CT of the abdomen and pelvis. Molecular genetic testing is also helpful, although the optimum strategy of such testing is still uncertain.[37]

Angiomas uncommonly involve the optic disc and in those rare circumstance, most patients have the von Hippel-Lindau syndrome. The diagnosis of an optic disc angioma is straightforward and these lesions have the classic appearance clinically (see Figure 14–1 and Figure 14–11) and have early fluorescence with leakage on angiography. The management of such cases is difficult. Laser has generally not been very effective and is associated with significant morbidity. In patients with CNS hemangioblastomas, various forms of radiation have been effective.[38] We have treated a few optic nerve head angiomas with low-dose, high-fraction radiation either with a Gamma Knife or protons.

A number of other nononcologic processes can produce optic nervehead enlargement, and these are discussed in neuro-ophthalmology textbooks. Other common lesions that could be confused for a neo-

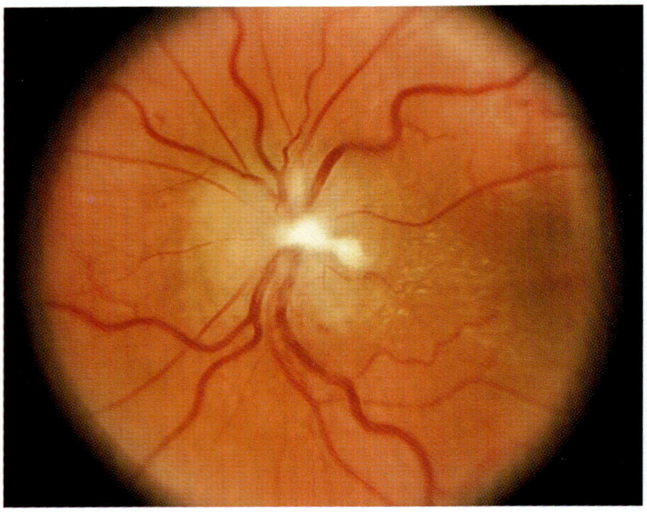

Figure 14–10. Optic nerve abnormality in a young boy with malignant histiocytosis.

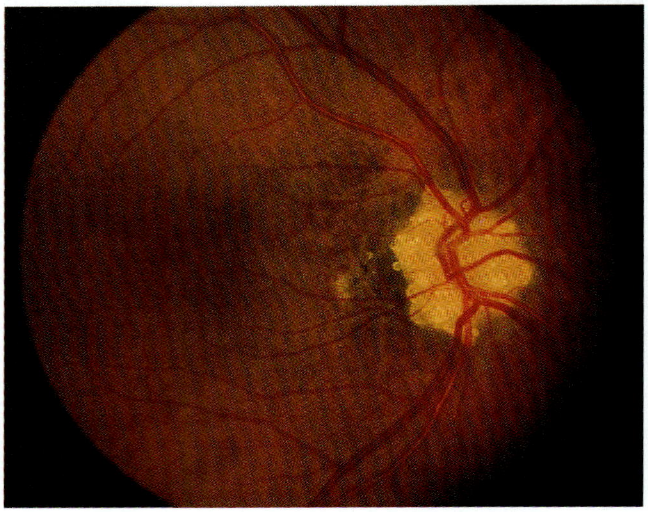

Figure 14–12. Buried optic nerve drusen simulating an optic nerve tumor.

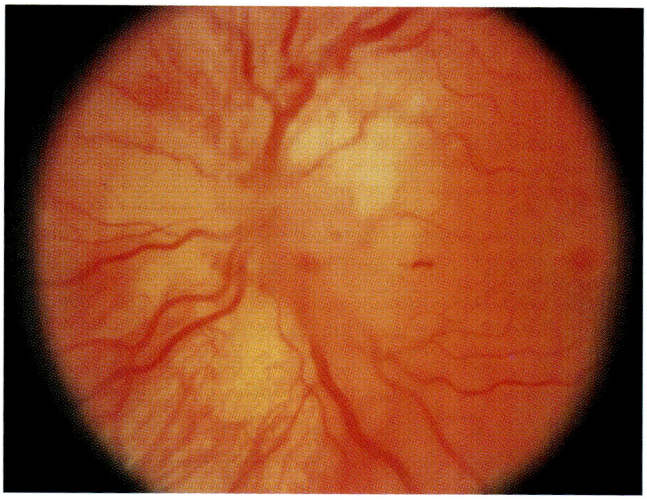

Figure 14–13. Inflammation of the optic disc simulating a neoplasm.

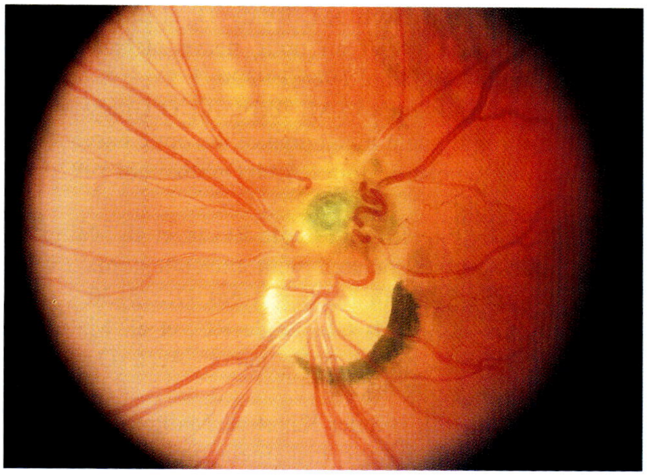

Figure 14–14. Intraocular foreign body simulating an optic nervehead neoplasm.

plastic process include acute anterior optic neuropathy (AION), buried optic nerve drusen (Figure 14–12), and tuberous sclerosis involving the disc. An idiopathic inflammation of the disc is shown in Figure 14–13.[39–41] This lesion spontaneously resolved. Figure 14–14 shows an intraocular foreign body referred to as an optic disc tumor. Rarely, a vascular tumor, such as a cavernous hemangioma, can be localized to the disc.[42]

REFERENCES

1. Wertz FD, Zimmerman LE, McKeown CA, et al. Juvenile xanthogranuloma of the optic nerve, disc, retina, and choroid. Ophthalmology 1982;89:1331–5.
2. Grimson BS, Perry DD. Enlargement of the optic disc in childhood optic nerve tumors. Am J Ophthalmol 1984;97:627–31.
3. Henderson JW, Campbell RJ. Primary intraorbital meningioma with intraocular extension. Mayo Clin Proc 1977;52:504–8.
4. Rosenthal AR. Ocular manifestations of leukemia. A review. Ophthalmology 1983;90:899–905.
5. Reese AB. Medulloepithelioma (of the optic nerve). Am J Ophthalmology 1957;44:4–6.
6. Green WR, Iliff WJ, Trotter RR. Malignant teratoid medulloepithelioma of the optic nerve. Arch Ophthalmol 1974;91:451–4.
7. Luiz, JE, Lee AG, Keltner JL, et al. Paraneoplastic neuropathy and autoantibody production in small-cell carcinoma of the lung. J Neuro-ophthalmol 1998; 18:178–81.
8. Reidy JJ, Apple DJ, Steinmetz RL, et al. Melanocytoma: nomenclature, pathogenesis, natural history and treatment. Surv Ophthalmol 1985;29:319–27.
9. Hirschberg J. Ueber die angeborne Pigmentirung der Sclera und ihre pathogenetische Bedeutung. Albrecht von Graefes Arch Klin Exp Ophthalmol 1883;29:1–12.
10. Coats G. Congenital pigmentation of the papilla. R London Ophthalmol Hosp Rep 1907;17:225–31.
11. Palich-Szanto O. Zwei seltene Befunde am Sehnervenkopfe. Klin Monatsbl Augenheilkd 1915;55: 149–57.
12. Lauber H. Ein Fall von Sarkom der Papille, seit 19 Jahren i Beobachtung. Klin Monatsbl Augenheilkd 1923;71:776.
13. Kreibig W. Das Epipapillaere Melanom. Klin Monatsbl Augenheilkd 1949;115:354–9.
14. Zimmerman LE. Pigmented tumors of the optic nervehead (22nd annual de Schweinitz lecture). Am J Ophthalmol 1960;50:338.
15. Zimmerman LE, Garron LK. Melanocytoma of the optic disc. Int Ophthalmol Clin 1962;2:431–40.
16. Walsh TJ, Packer S. Bilateral melanocytoma of the optic nerve associated with intracranial meningioma. Ann Ophthalmol 1971;3:885–8.
17. Takahashi T. Klinische und histopathologische Beobachtungen beim Melanozytom der Papille. Klin Monatasbl Augenheilkd 1979;175:47–55.
18. Osher RH, Shields JA, Layman PR. Pupillary visual field evaluation in patients with melanocytoma of the optic disc. Arch Ophthalmol 1979;97:1096–9.
19. Brown GC, Shields JA. Tumors of the optic nervehead. Surv Ophthalmol 1985;29:248–64.
20. Joffe L, Shields JA, Osher RH, Gass JD. Clinical and follow-up studies of melanocytomas of the optic disc. Ophthalmology 1979;86:1067–83.

21. Apple DJ, Craythorn JM, Reidy JJ, et al. Malignant transformation of an optic nerve melanocytoma. Can J Ophthalmol 1984;19:320–5.
22. Erzurum SA, Jampol LM, Territo C, O'Grady R. Primary malignant melanoma of the optic nerve simulating a melanocytoma. Arch Ophthalmol 1992;110: 684–6.
23. Shields JA, Shields CL, Eagle RC Jr, et al. Malignant melanoma associated with melanocytoma of the optic disc. Ophthalmology 1990;97:225–30.
24. De Potter P, Shields CL, Eagle RC, et al. Malignant melanoma of the optic nerve. Arch Opthalmol 1996;114:608–12.
25. Meyer D, Ge J, Blinder KJ, et al. Malignant transformation of an optic disk melanomacytoma. Am J Opthalmol 1999;127:710–4.
26. Shields JA, Eagle RC Jr, Shields CL, De Potter P. Pigmented adenoma of the optic nerve head simulating a melanocytoma. Ophthalmology 1992;99:1705–8.
27. Loose IA, Jampol LM, O'Grady R. Pigmented adenoma mimicking a juxtapapillary melanoma. A 20-year follow-up. Arch Ophthalmol 1999;117: 120–2.
28. Weinhaus RS, Seddon JM, Albert DM, et al. Prognostic factor study of survival after enucleation for juxtapapillary melanomas. Arch Ophthalmol 1985; 103:1673–7.
29. Char DH, Schwartz A, Miller TR, Abele JS. Ocular metastases from systemic melanoma. Am J Ophthalmol 1980;90:702–7.
30. Fishman ML, Rosenthal S. Optic nerve metastasis from a mediastinal carcinoid tumor. Br J Ophthalmol 1976;60:583–8.
31. Sung JU, Lam BL, Curtin VT, Tse DT. Metastatic gastric carcinoma to the optic nerve. Arch Ophthalmol 1998;116:692–3.
32. Nikaido H, Mishima H, Ono H, et al. Leukemic involvement of the optic nerve. Am J Ophthalmol 1988;105:294–8.
33. Preti A, Kantarjian HM. Management of adult acute lymphocytic leukemia: present issues and key challenges. J Clin Oncol 1994;12:1312–22.
34. de Keizer RJ, de Wolff-Rouendall D, Bots GT, et al. Optic glioma with intraocular tumor and seeding in a child with neurofibromatosis. Am J Ophthalmol 1989;108:717–25.
35. Miller NR. Primary optic disc tumors. In: Walsh F, Hoyt WF, editors. Clinical Neuro-Ophthalmology. Baltimore, MD: Williams and Wilkins; 1982. p. 265–9.
36. O'Keefe M, Fulcher T, Kelly P, et al. Medulloepithelioma of the optic nerve head. Arch Ophthalmol 1997;115:1325–7.
37. Pack SD, Zbar, B, Pak, E, et al. Consitutional von Hippel-Lindau (VHL) gene deletions detected in VHL families by fluorescence in situ hybridization. Cancer Res 1999;59:5560–4.
38. Patrice SJ, Sneed PK, Flickinger JC, et al. Radiosurgery for hemangioblastoma: results of a multiinstitutional experience. Int J Radiat Oncol Biol Phys 1996;35:493–9.
39. Laties AM, Scheie HD. Sarcoid granuloma of the optic disc: evolution of multiple small tumors. Trans Am Ophthalmol Soc 1970;68:219–33.
40. Beardsley TL, Brown SV, Sydnor CF, et al. Eleven cases of sarcoidosis of the optic nerve. Am J Ophthalmol 1984;97:62–77.
41. Jampol LM, Woodfin W, McLean EB. Optic nerve sarcoidosis. Report of a case. Arch Ophthalmol 1972; 87:355–60.
42. Mansour AM, Jampol LM, Hrisomalos NF, Greenwald M. Case Report. Cavernous hemangioma of the optic disc. Arch Ophthalmol 1988;106:22.

15

Diagnosis and Management of Orbital Tumors

Effective management of orbital neoplasms requires the ophthalmologist to delineate the nature of the lesion, determine whether intervention is necessary, and decide on the optimal therapy. For example, proptosis in children is managed differently from that in adults, since rapid intervention is often necessary in children with exophthalmos. Children are more likely than adults to have either a rapidly growing malignant orbital tumor or contiguous spread of an infectious sinusitis; either can result in blindness or loss of an eye, if the process is not treated rapidly. Conversely, most causes of adult proptosis are relatively chronic and usually do not require rapid intervention.[1,2] The most common orbital tumors are listed in Table 15–1.

In addition to patient age, subjective data (history of present illness, past medical history, and review of systems), physical findings, and tumor location (based on imaging data) are important in establishing a differential diagnosis. Computed tomography (CT) or magnetic resonance imaging (MRI) data can be used to categorize orbital tumefactions into those that involve only a single orbital structure (optic nerve, lacrimal gland, orbital bones, or extraocular muscles) in the intraconal area, the extraconal space, the entire orbit, or both the orbit and contiguous structures. In order to establish an optimal differential diagnosis, extraconal lesions should be divided into those that involve the lacrimal fossa, those that are anterior to the orbital septum, those that involve bone, those that involve multiple orbital compartments and/or adjacent sinuses, globe, and those that involve the central nervous system (CNS). Establishing a differential diagnosis on the basis of the history, clinical findings, and imaging data results in histologic confirmation in over 97 percent of cases.

In children, most orbital lesions occur either prior to age 2 years or after age 6 years and are more likely to have a more fulminant disease course than adult lesions. In the age group < 2 years, capillary hemangiomas, cysts, or malignancies, (orbital metastases, leukemia, or rhabdomyosarcoma) are the most common causes of proptosis. Langerhan's histiocytosis syndromes (uni- or multifocal histiocytosis, including eosinophilic granuloma, Hand-Schuller-Christian, or Letterer-Siwe syndrome), congenital craniofacial abnormalities, and traumatic or developmental cysts occur. Rare tumors, such as contiguous retinoblastoma (rare in the United States), teratomas, orbital cysts or melanocytic proliferations, may also occur. Sinusitis with secondary involvement of the orbit is uncommon in those age < 3 years, since the sinuses are not completely developed or aerated; the author has seen only two children in this younger age group with infective orbital-sinus disease. In the older children, the most common orbital problems are infective sinusitis and rhabdomyosarcoma. Lymphoid lesions, lymphangioma, orbital metastases, and adult tumors can occur in older children.

In adults, the most common cause of unilateral or bilateral proptosis is thyroid eye disease.[2] As discussed elsewhere, many of these patients will have normal serum levels of thyroxine (T_4) and triiodothysonine (T_3) when they present with proptosis.[3] The appropriate first-line tests, if thyroid orbitopathy is suspected, are serum thyroid stimulating hormone (TSH) and thyroid antibodies. Most adult orbital tumors are benign, and orbital pseudotumors, benign cystic lesions (dermoids, mucoceles, inclusion cysts) and cavernous hemangiomas are relatively common.

Table 15–1. COMMON ORBITAL TUMEFACTIONS IN VARIOUS LOCATIONS

- Optic Nerve and Nerve Sheath
  - Optic nerve glioma
  - Optic nerve sheath meningioma
  - Extraocular extension of retinoblastoma
  - Extraocular extension of uveal melanoma
  - Leukemic infiltrate
  - Metastatic carcinoma
  - Inflammatory lesions (pseudotumor)
- Extraocular Muscles
  - Metastatic tumors
  - Rhabdomyoma
  - Rhabdomyosarcoma
  - Lymphoma
  - Alveolar soft part sarcoma
  - Thyroid-related myositis
  - Idiopathic myositis
  - Inflammation as a component of orbital pseudotumor
  - Amyloidosis
  - Carotid artery: cavernous sinus fistula
- Lacrimal Fossa
  - Epithelial tumors
    - Benign mixed tumor ("pleomorphic adenoma")
    - Adenoid cystic carcinoma
    - Mixed carcinoma
    - Adenocarcinoma
  - Lymphoma
  - Metastases
  - Dermoid cysts
  - Infectious inflammation (lues, tuberculosis, mumps, viral)
  - Pseudotumor
- Orbital Bones
  - Developmental bone abnormalities/alterations
    - Axial myopia
    - Fibrous dysplasia
    - Osteopetrosis
    - Craniofacial malformations
    - Neurofibromatosis
  - Mass lesions
    - Epidermoid and dermoid cysts
    - Hematic bone cyst
    - Aneurysmal bone cyst
    - Ossifying fibroma
    - Mucoceles
    - Osteosarcoma
    - Fibrosarcoma
    - Metastases
    - Contiguous sinus malignancies
    - Benign and malignant histiocytosis syndromes
- Intraconal Lesions
  - Benign tumors
    - Cavernous hemangioma
    - Hemangiopericytoma
    - Neurofibroma
  - Neurilemmoma
  - Malignant tumors
  - Malignant hemangiopericytoma
    - Metastases
  - (See optic nerve tumors)
- Extraconal Lesions
  - Lymphoid lesions
    - Lymphoma
    - Pseudotumor
    - Leukemia
  - Metastases
  - Epidermoids
  - Capillary hemangioma
  - Varices
  - Lymphangiomas
  - Inflammation from contiguous sinusitis

The evaluation of any patient suspected of having an orbital neoplasm includes a thorough history of the present illness, past medical history, and a review of systems. Emphasis should be on thyroid disease, systemic malignancies, inflammatory sinus disease, and systemic inflammatory diseases (eg, Sjögren's syndrome, sarcoid, tuberculosis, rheumatoid arthritis, Wegener's granulomatosis). Some nontumefactions, including congenital facial asymmetry, traumatic enophthalmos, unilateral axial myopia, carotid artery-cavernous sinus fistulae, infection, or inflammation, can mimic an orbital tumor and should be ruled out.

In general, I limit my evaluation to a routine ophthalmic examination, unless there are 72 mm of proptosis, significant visual loss, diplopia, conjunctival or lid swelling, or ptosis in conjunction with a lesser degree of exophthalmos.

Most orbital tumefactions with the exception of rhabdomyosarcoma, some metastases, and, rarely, hemorrhagic primary tumefactions have an insidious onset.[4,5] A few physical findings are diagnostically helpful. Bilateral proptosis, in conjunction with scleral show and lid lag, is virtually pathognomonic for thyroid ophthalmopathy. Opticociliary shunt vessels in middle-aged females with minimal proptosis and profound visual loss strongly suggest an optic nerve sheath meningioma. Scleritis, in association with proptosis, is most often observed in orbital pseudotumor, but primary and metastatic malignancies can also produce this finding. Arteriolarization of conjunctival vessels in association with acute unilateral proptosis in an adult is characteristic of a dural or carotid-cavernous sinus fistula.[6,7] Most signs of orbital disease are not diagnostic for a specific type of orbital tumor. The location of a tumor, the presence or absence of exophthalmos or enophthalmos, choroidal folds, anterior chamber angle neovascularization, optic nerve inflammation or atrophy, or most other physical findings do not establish a specific diagnosis.[8,9]

Choroidal folds were first described clinically in 1884, and initially most investigators felt they were a sign of orbital disease (Figure 15–1).[10] Norton differentiated between retinal and choroidal folds; Cangemi and co-workers found that only 10 of 53 patients with choroidal folds had them on the basis of an orbital etiology.[8,11] Other causes of choroidal folds include hypermetropia, macular degeneration, retinal detachment, hypotony, trauma, scleritis, uveitis, and ocular tumors of unknown etiology.[8]

Enophthalmos is associated with < 5 percent of orbital problems.[12] The mechanisms of orbital retraction are fat atrophy, traction or structural abnormalities. Most frequently, enophthalmos is due to trauma followed by scirrhous carcinoma and less commonly microphthalmos, orbital varices, barotrauma, mucoceles, sinusitis, or prior orbital surgery.

Displacement of the globe (straight ahead, inferior-medial, lateral) may help to ascertain the location of an orbital tumor (intraconal, lacrimal fossa, and sinuses, respectively) and hence establish a differential diagnosis on the basis of location; either CT or MRI is much more accurate than physical examination to delineate the tumor's relationship to normal structures. Alterations in proptosis as a function of bending over, vascular pulsations, or a positive Valsalva maneuver may help to ascertain the vascular nature of the lesion. The mass itself may be palpable, depending on its location in the orbit. Generally, palpation of the mass is not too helpful in ascertaining its histologic nature. Pseudotumors, fibrous tumors, and malignancies are generally firm, while vascular or cystic lesions are compressible.

An overview of orbital diagnosis and management is presented here and in detail in the following chapters. This chapter reviews the use of imaging techniques and fine-needle aspiration biopsy (FNAB) in the diagnosis, evaluation, and management of patients with orbital tumefactions. The following chapter discusses the diagnosis and management of the most common pediatric orbital diseases. Chapters after that summarize data available regarding the presentation and management of the most common adult orbital neoplasms. In those chapters, adult orbital tumefactions have been arbitrarily organized into lesions involving the optic nerve alone, intraconal space, and extraconal space. Those in the extraconal space have been divided into lesions which involve predominantly the sinuses, lacrimal fossa, and lacrimal sac. Orbital metastases and orbital lymphoid lesions that most commonly involve the extraconal space but can involve any area of the orbit are discussed separately. Orbital radiation and surgical approaches are covered at the end of the book.

ORBITAL IMAGING

General Principles

There are several areas where orbital imaging techniques have improved the management of orbital diseases. First, CT, MRI, and ultrasonography (US) scans have markedly improved diagnostic accuracy in the evaluation of orbital masses. Second, these cross-sectional imaging techniques (CT and MRI) are useful to determine whether any therapeutic intervention is necessary and, if so, the rapidity of treatment. Third, multiplanar CT or MRI data are helpful in determining the optimal surgical or radiation therapy by delineating the relationship of the lesion to contiguous orbital and adjacent eye, sinus,

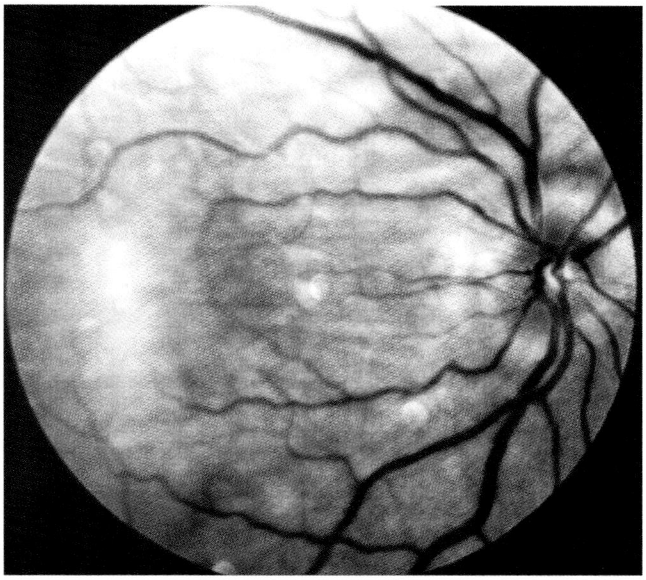

Figure 15–1. Choroidal folds.

or CNS structures. Fourth, these techniques can be amalgamated with FNAB to improve diagnostic accuracy. Finally, noninvasive imaging techniques are invaluable for the serial evaluation of a patient prior to or after treatment.

CT and MRI are cross-section imaging techniques. One-to two-millimeter thick axial and/or coronal CT sections provide superb anatomic detail (spatial resolution). Data from sections obtained in one plane, usually axial, can be reformatted in any other plane through computer manipulation of the data to further increase diagnostic accuracy and more accurately predict the lesion location and histology.[2,4] Prior to the availability of CT, the ability to detect an orbital mass with plain radiography was between 21 and 39 percent.[6,7,13] The accuracy of CT diagnosis has progressively increased with newer equipment and better techniques from 60 to over 95 percent.[2,6,8] The CT image is often sufficiently characteristic to obviate the need for orbital biopsy.

In contrast to projection radiographs (plain films) that image bone, CT can directly image orbital soft tissue abnormalities. On CT, structures of varying tissue density can be distinguished on the basis of differential X-ray absorptions. These densities are imaged relative to the density of water. Retro-orbital fat absorbs X-rays to a lesser degree than water; it is displayed on the CT as a black (low-density) area that contrasts with the whiter (higher-density) extraocular muscles and the optic nerve. The ability of CT to differentiate these tissues is due to their relative contrast differences, which range as high as 14 percent. Modern scanners can distinguish tissues with < 1 percent contrast difference.

The presence of retrobulbar fat allows high spatial and density resolution of orbital structures on CT, often without the need for intravenous contrast material. Orbital fat has required the use of fat saturation techniques combined with contrast (gadolinium) to allow similar enhancement and contrast of orbital tumors with fat in MRI scans. In lesions of the optic nerve, its sheath, or processes that involve the contiguous CNS, MRI, often with fat saturation and gadolinium enhancement, has improved detection rates over CT.

Orbital CT scans are routinely performed using 1- to 1.5-mm thick sections at 1-mm intervals in the axial plane. This provides high spatial detail in the X, Y, and Z axes. The individual picture or volume elements (voxels) in these axial slices can then be reformatted (re-arranged) in any plane to provide coronal, sagittal, and para-axial or parasagittal oblique images. These reformatted images are generated after the patient has left the scanner. They do not require additional patient exposure to ionizing radiation. In most centers, the lens dose from orbital CT is approximately 18.5 mGy.[14] Coronal re-formations decrease the high spatial frequency artifacts (eg, from dental appliances) that are often encountered with direct coronal scans. The use of multiplanar re-formations enables the radiologist and ophthalmologist to view a lesion of interest in an optimal anatomic plane and to assess its location relative to contiguous orbital, bone, sinus, and CNS structures. A basic principle of both geometric and computed tomography is that an object should be imaged perpendicular to the plane in which it lies; this can be readily accomplished with multiplanar re-formation techniques. There are occasions when direct coronal scans are useful, such as orbital blow-out fractures and craniofacial neoplasms. In orbital series, the false-negative and false-positive rates with CT scans were < 3 percent and < 5 percent, respectively.[2,5–9] CT scanning of the orbits is usually performed without the use of intravenous contrast agents. However, contrast enhancement may be useful in delineating intracranial spread of malignancies. As discussed below, this appears to be the optimal accuracy available with this technology.

Figure 15–2 demonstrates, on a modern scanner, the anatomic detail which is obtained routinely with 1-mm thick sections. In this axial scan through the superior portion of the orbit, one can discern the globe, lacrimal gland, superior ophthalmic vein, and supratrochlear vein.

Older equipment yields suboptimal images with inferior spatial and density resolution. A normal CT study performed on inferior equipment provides only a false sense of security. Optimum CT data are also dependent on proper examination technique; the entire orbit, or at least the area of interest, must be scanned using thin sections at the correct angulation to obtain useful data. Neuroradiologists and ophthalmic surgeons can use these scanners to increase diagnostic accuracy.

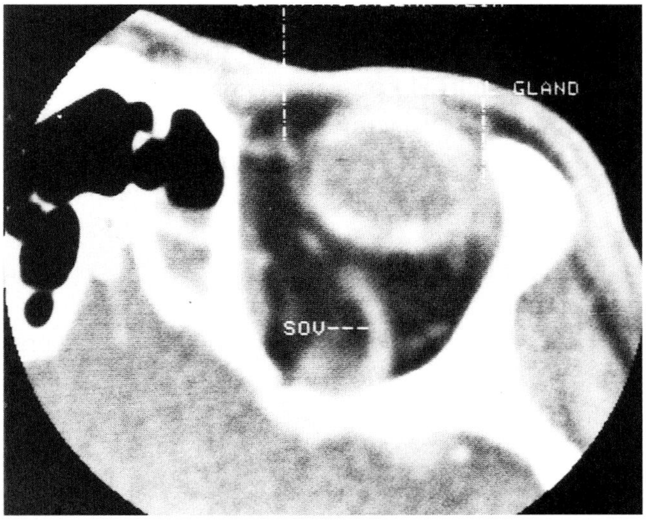

Figure 15–2. Anatomic detail on a 1.5 mm axial section. Superior ophthalmic vein (SOV). (From Char DH, Norman D. The use of computed tomography and ultrasonography in the evaluation of orbital masses. Surv Ophthalmol 1982;2:49–63.)

Improvement in both resolution and the ability to perform multiplanar re-formations has increased the importance of CT and has diminished our use of ultrasonography (US).[3] The addition of MRI has further limited the role of US in these diseases. CT has also had a major impact on treatment planning. As discussed in the final chapter of the book, especially for external beam radiation simulation, CT has probably resulted in as high as a 30 percent improvement in the accuracy of field placement.

The development of spiral (helical) CT techniques have been very helpful, especially in pediatric cases where the rapid data collection results in being able to obtain scans without anesthesia.[15,16] This technique is also quite important in some orbital lesions in which the effect of a Valsalva maneuver is to be assessed or in those patients who are quite ill and require a rapid scan.

Optimal visualization of the relationship of tumor with contiguous normal structures is vital in determining both the surgical approach and the need for ancillary therapy. In orbital lesions that require surgical intervention, CT re-formations or multiplanar MRI sequences permit a more accurate preoperative determination of the extent of tumor involvement. They also facilitate planning for the most appropriate surgical approach as well as the extent of surgery required.

Ultrasonography

We have almost eliminated the use of orbital US due to improvements in CT and MRI. A combination of quantitative echography with a Kretz A-scan and immersion B-scan ultrasound can be used to detect the presence of some orbital lesions and predict their histologic pattern on the basis of US characteristics of a tumor's surface and shape. The characteristics shown could be regular, irregular, with smooth or ragged edges, encapsulated or nonencapsulated, infiltrative, or focal, and the internal tumor pattern could be cystic, vascular, or solid with various patterns of internal reflectivity.

If a superb ultrasonographer is present, then US is a cost-effective screening test for some anterior and midorbit disease.[11] While some authors have felt that US might be as good as or better than CT or MRI in the diagnosis of midorbital changes, a study by Demer and Kerman outlined some of the limitations of US, compared with MRI.[11] In anterior orbital and intraconal lesions, US appears to be as accurate as CT or MRI in detecting and predicting the histology of an orbital mass.[17–22] Unfortunately, in a proptotic patient, a major reason to obtain a scan is to plan therapy, and for that purpose, US is distinctly inferior to both MR and CT.

There are a number of other disadvantages of US, compared with either CT or MRI. The quality of US examination is directly related to the orbital experience of the ultrasonographer. First, most CT and some MRI protocols are now sufficiently automated so that if good equipment is available, an excellent scan will be uniformly produced. Second, we previously obtained both US and CT in all orbital tumor cases, and US was not found to add significant information to high-resolution, thin-section CT. Third, the anatomic detail available with either CT or MRI, especially the graphic demonstration of the relationships between the tumor and adjacent structures is far superior and easier for the clinician to use than US. Fourth, for many orbital lesions, especially those that involve contiguous bone, brain, sinus, or lesions in the orbital apex, US is far less sensitive and accurate than CT or MRI. While the predictive accuracy of tissue characterization with echography has been highly touted, it is not useful as has been suggested.[23,24] As an example, on US the soft tissue mismatch and impedance characteristics of lymphoma, pseudotumor, and metastases are similar; placing a patient correctly in this broad diagnostic category is not specific enough for most management decisions. Similarly, while US would substantiate the CT diagnosis of a cystic lesion, it cannot distinguish between a mucocele and a dermoid; an MRI or CT scan can usually be used to do so.[3,9,22]

Magnetic Resonance Imaging

MRI was derived from nuclear magnetic resonance experiments performed at analytical chemistry laboratories since the late 1940s.[25] It is based on the principle that nuclei with an odd number of nucleons (protons and neutrons) behave as small magnets or dipoles. In the human body, hydrogen nuclei (protons) are ubiquitous, and their resonance is the basis of clinical MRI techniques. When the object under study is placed in a magnetic field, there is a net alignment of protons within the field. When exposed to a radiofrequency (RF) excitation, there is a reversal of polarity of some of these hydrogen nuclei and they are raised to a higher energy level. When the RF is terminated, the proton returns to the original polarity, or is remagnetized, and the emitted energy can be measured. This phenomenon is called T_1 relaxation, vertical relaxation, or spin lattice relaxation. It is an event that is best measured immediately after the RF is terminated. Differences in the rates of repolarization vary with the molecular environment and are partially the basis for tissue contrast in MRI. Exposure to RF excitation also initiates a uniform synchronous precession, or spin, among the protons. When the RF is terminated, this precession diminishes at differing rates for protons in different molecular environments. The energy emission measured from this event is called T_2 relaxation, horizontal relaxation, or spin-spin relaxation time. Since the RF-initiated events are dependent on the frequency and magnetic field strength, the location of these events in three-dimensional space can be determined by imposing a gradient (approximately 1 kilogauss per centimeter) on the magnetic field and varying the RF.

Field strengths used for clinical imaging range from 0.15 to 4.5 tesla.[26–33] Presently, optimal orbital or intraocular anatomic detail is obtained with 1.5T MRI units, usually with surface coils and thin-section scans. Signal-to-noise ratio improves with increasing field strength. The components of the magnetic resonance signal that form an image reflect proton density, T_1 relaxation, T_2 relaxation, and vascular flow, if present.

There are a number of similarities in the generation of a CT and an MR image. The relative intensity of the MRI signal is displayed as a pixel matrix on a gray scale similiar to that of CT. The major differences are the techniques and tissue properties that are imaged. In CT, tissue density is related to the attenuation of X-rays coursing through that area of the body. In MRI, relative rates of remagnetization and loss of precessional frequency and proton density are responsible for signal intensity differences. These are influenced by imaging techniques, field strength and tissue magnetic susceptibility. Because of this host of variables, MRI intensity values are not related to a standard reference but, rather, to other tissues in the volume being imaged with a given set of imaging parameters.

In the generation of a CT image, numbers are produced that are directly related to the X-ray attenuation in a finite volume of tissue; represented by an individual number, termed a "voxel." The numerical representation of the MR image is the same as for CT; however, the physical property that results in the MRI numerical value of a voxel is the intensity of the radiowave signal of the perturbed hydrogen nuclei in a given volume of tissue.

Unlike the photon–tissue interaction, which can be characterized as a single-moment event, an MRI signal has two major temporal factors that influence it: (1) the alignment of protons in tissue varies at the time they are stimulated by both the radiowaves and the magnetic field, and their initial status affects both initial signal intensity and decay; and (2) once the tissue protons are perturbed, they have a characteristic decay envelope.

Retrobulbar fat which has both a short T_1 and medium T_2 relaxation will produce a relatively strong signal. Muscle is intermediate in signal intensity, and cerebrospinal fluid and vitreous have long

T_1 and long T_2 relaxation times. Cortical bone is displayed as black (signal void), as there is no mobile hydrogen, and therefore no MRI signal.

Instrument parameters (repetition time [TR] and echo delay [TE]) can be varied to emphasize T_1 or T_2 relaxation. The TR indicates the time interval between excitations and usually ranges from 50 to 4,000 milliseconds (msecs). TE is the time after excitation at this resonant energy, and can range from 2.5 to 120 msec. Images with relatively short TRs (< 500 msec) and short TEs (< 40 msec) are T_1 weighted. Images obtained with long TRs (approximately 2,000 msec) and long TEs (> 60 msec) are T_2 weighted. T_1 and T_2 can also be measured as an absolute number. It has been hoped that these objective values would be useful in developing a tissue specificity.[34–36] Thus far, it appears that there is substantial overlap, as discussed in the following chapters between benign and malignant orbital processes.

In the years since the first edition of *Clinical Ocular Oncology*, there has been substantial MRI data published on orbital tumors.[26–46] Several modifications and scan techniques have improved the quality and utility of orbital MRI.[43–46] T_1-weighted images (TR < 500 msec) and TE (< 40 msec) optimally display anatomic features. Newer MRI approaches have not yet shown a marked impact on the management of orbital tumors. Some of these include fluid-attenuated inversion recovery and diffusion-weighted imaging.[47] In addition, a number of cases have been reported in which poor quality MRI, especially those due to chemical shift artifacts, has resulted in incorrect diagnosis and uninterpretable scans.[48]

In addition to observing TR values displayed alongside the MR image, orbital fat is bright (white) on T_1, and these images will be best for assessing anatomic relationships of an orbital tumor. T_2 features of a lesion are best displayed on scans with a long TR (> 2,000 msec) and these scans can be identified by the relatively dark orbital fat. Table 15–2 lists T_1 and T_2 patterns of some orbital tumors. Unfortunately, there are limitations with MRI scans. For patients, these scans take longer and are more costly. In young children, sedation or anesthesia is necessary. In some patients, a large amount of dental hardware can also produce an MRI scan with insufficient artifact to obviate its usefulness as shown in Figure 15–3.

Table 15–2. MRI T1 AND T2 CHARACTERISTICS OF ORBITAL TUMORS

Tumor Type	T1	T2
Pseudotumor	ISD—muscle (dark)	ISD—fat (dark)
Lymphoma	ISD—muscle (dark)	Bright or dark
Cavernous hemangioma	ISD—muscle (dark)	HPD—CNS (bright)
Lymphangioma	ISD—fat (bright)*	HPD—CNS (bright)*
Dermiod	ISD—fat (bright)†	ISD—fat (dark)†
Metastases	ISD—muscle	HPD—CNS (bright)
Extraconal meningioma, schwannoma, neurofibroma	ISD—muscle (dark)	HPD—CNS (bright)
Nerve sheath meningioma	ISD—muscle (dark)	ISD—fat (dark)
Optic nerve glioma	ISD—muscle/nerve	ISD—nerve (dark)
Hematic cyst	ISD—fat (bright)	HPD—CNS (bright)
Lacrimal tumors	ISD—muscle (dark)	HPD—CNS (bright)

CNS = central nervous system; ISD = isodense to tissue listed;
HPD = hyperdense to tissue listed.
*Usually a mixed, heterogeneous pattern.
†May have fluid level; if none is present, fat is isodense to muscle.

SUMMARY OF SCAN FINDINGS

As discussed in subsequent chapters, there are a few situations where MRI scans are superior to CT, and a few clinical settings where CT data are more useful. Generally, for intraocular tumors, only in three settings is MRI definitely superior to US: (1) as

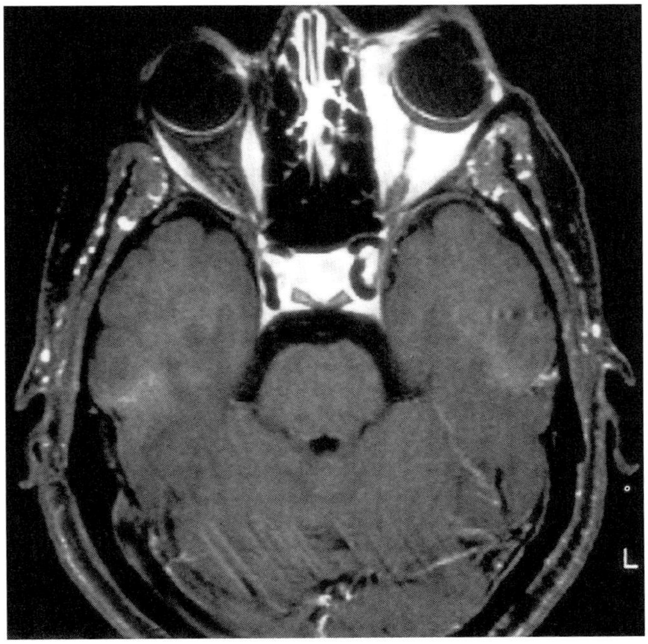

Figure 15–3. Large amount of dental hardware has resulted in a bizarre appearance of this axial MRI scan.

described in the chapter on posterior uveal tumor diagnosis, in some cases of extramacular disciform lesions, bright signal on both T_1-weighted and T_2-weighted images is distinct from the pattern of a uveal melanoma; (2) in patients in whom there is suspected localized extrascleral extension of a melanoma, MRI as, discussed in that chapter, is probably a more accurate technique; and (3) in retinoblastomas with optic nerve extension, MRI may be more sensitive at detecting localized extraocular spread than US or CT.

In orbital tumor diagnosis, MRI with fat saturation and gadolinium contrast should be used in patients with suspected meningiomas of the optic nerve sheath or of the sphenoid wing, or those with possible compressive optic neuropathy due to thyroid orbitopathy. As discussed in the chapter on optic nerve tumors, this technique is much more sensitive than CT for detecting the tumor. MRI also is more sensitive in the detection of soft tissue orbital apical tumors or those that invade the CNS. In some atypical vascular orbital lesions, MRI and the ability to obtain MR angiography have been diagnostically helpful. In other cases, such as an orbital varix (see chapter on intraconal tumors), spiral CT, performed with and without Valsalva maneuver, established the diagnosis when it was not clear on MRI. As is the case with CT, the quality of equipment (field strength, surface coils, ability to perform thin sections) and personnel are integral to the quality of the scan produced.[49]

In a cost-conscious era, as a general rule, a good-quality, thin-section CT is the imaging test of choice in a patient with orbital disease that does not produce decreased vision. While exceptions occur, with the caveats listed above, in most cases MRI has not increased the accuracy of our diagnosis or changed the management of orbital tumors. We have evaluated many orbital tumor patients who were referred with MRI and CT scans; the results have usually been concordant. In patients with benign and malignant lacrimal gland masses of various etiologies, we did not observe any improvement in diagnostic accuracy with MRI, compared with CT.[34] In addition to being less expensive, CT is probably still superior to MRI for orbital diagnosis in two areas: (1) CT is the imaging technique of choice in patients with orbital bone involvement; and (2) in young children, a spiral CT can be obtained without anesthesia, and if the data are adequate, CT presents a safer method of evaluation than MRI on a sleeping child. In cases in which we are going to use an endoscopic approach to an apical tumor through the nasal sinuses, the direct visualization of bone on CT (as contrast with the signal void noted on MRI) allows us to plan surgery more precisely.

MRI does have a potential additional unique quality in that an image may be obtained directly in any plane, simply by altering the orientation of the gradients. This means that images in any plane will have identical spatial and contrast detail. Surface coil techniques have facilitated a significant improvement in the spatial detail that appears to be superior to that of CT.[50]

A number of publications discuss basic principles of CT, MRI, and US.[18,20,22,25,36,43,46] The reader is referred to those reports for more technical information on these imaging techniques. In the chapters on orbital tumors, CT and MR images have been incorporated to show our use of these modalities in the management of orbital lesions.

We prefer, for the most part, multiplanar MRI scans, if they are available from machines utilizing high-magnetic-field, thin-section, and surface coils. Multiplanar scans or CT scans with computer reconstruction are crucial if that modality is used. Figure 15–4 shows the axial MRI scan of a patient referred with bilateral apical tumors; this patient had compressive thyroid neuropathy due to enlarged extraocular muscles, especially the inferior recti. The diagnosis would have been obvious on CT with computer re-formation or on multiplanar MRI scans but was not apparent to the referring ophthalmologist or the radiologist on the basis of only an axial MRI scan.

FINE-NEEDLE BIOPSY

The concept of needle biopsy is not new. This technique was first attempted in the 1880s and had transient use in major American cancer centers in the 1920s and 1930s.[51–53] Early needle aspiration biopsies were performed with large needles, generally between 15- and 18-gauge, and some tumor dissemination did occur.[54]

In the 1950s, a number of European centers adopted the use of a smaller-gauge FNAB technique with excellent results.[55] Using a 22-gauge or smaller needle, there have been very few documented cases of local or distant tumor dissemination.[56–60]

Much data support the concept that FNAB is a safe procedure. Berg and Robbins retrospectively analyzed a matched group of breast carcinoma patients with 15-year actuarial survival, who either had or did not have FNAB. There was no difference in the incidence of local disease, metastases, or tumor-related mortality.[61] Similarly, a number of investigators have used highly malignant animal models to study the effects of FNAB on tumor dissemination. Most investigators have demonstrated a small number of tumor cells in the needle track, but those cells are too small in number to form a viable colony and develop a tumor nodule.[62,63] Eriksson and co-workers used five different types of highly malignant animal tumors and were unable to establish a difference in tumor metastases or tumor-related mortality among those animals that had excisional biopsy, incisional biopsy, or FNAB of a limb tumor.[62]

Lalli and colleagues studied 157 salivary gland pleomorphic adenomas that had received FNAB and found no evidence of tumor dissemination.[58] The safety in over 500,000 nonophthalmic FNABs has been demonstrated. Less than 10 reports of local spread have been published, and almost all were with a 20-gauge or larger needle.[56,59,60] It is highly doubtful that orbital or ocular tumor dissemination would be different from that of systemic tumors.

We recently reported our results with 731 patients with uveal melanoma who did or did not have an FNAB. With Cox multivariate analysis, there is no adverse affect on survival in patients who received FNAB.[64]

The detection of a lesion and the accuracy of diagnosis with FNAB are highly dependent on the correct placement of the needle and, equally importantly, experience in cytopathologic interpretation.[53] Some series have noted improvement in accuracy from 73 to 92 percent with increased experience.[65] In a series from Toronto of 259 nonophthalmic FNABs, detection of malignancy increased from 83 to 93 percent in a 10-year interval.[66] In addition to expertise in correctly placing the needle into a lesion, and cytopathologic interpretation, technical factors in handling the specimen, and slide preparation can have a major impact on the accuracy of diagnosis. In our experience, the quality of cytologic preparation can markedly influence the sensitivity of the technique. Figures 15–5A and B show samples from the same eye prepared in different laboratories. The difference in cytologic detail graphically illustrates this point.

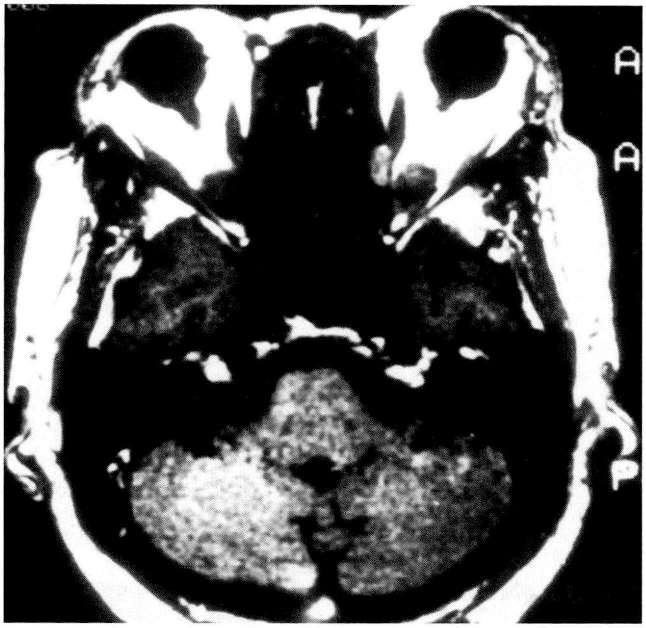

Figure 15–4. Axial MR image in a patient referred with an apical tumor. CT with re-formation would have demonstrated enlarged apical muscles and compressive thyroid optic neuropathy as the correct diagnosis.

Cytologic interpretation is different from analysis of standard histologic materials. We have examined three cases of intraocular lymphoma in which a definitive diagnosis could be made on the cytologic material; all had been misdiagnosed at other institutions because inexperienced people had attempted to render a cytopathologic diagnosis (unpublished data).

The use of FNAB of orbital lesions was pioneered in Europe in the late 1970s.[66,67] In the United States, Kennerdell and associates have been responsible for popularizing this technique.[68–70] In their experience with 156 cases, a correct diagnosis was possible in 80 percent.[70] They have stressed that fibrous tumors, lymphoid lesions, and apical masses are often difficult to diagnose correctly, but especially in the latter group, this technique can be very helpful.[70]

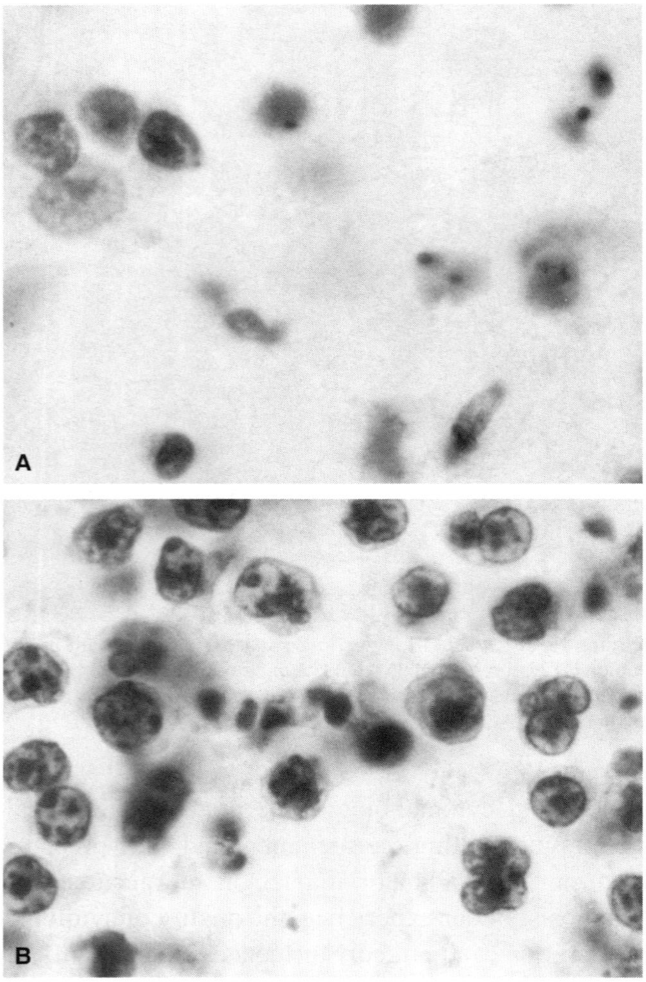

Figure 15–5. *A,* Vitreous biopsy prepared in one laboratory; diagnosis is not clear, and cellular detail is not optimal. *B,* Second vitreous biopsy obtained 72 hours later from the same eye, but prepared in another laboratory. This shows better cellular detail due to superior preparation technique.

We have used orbital FNAB in approximately 300 cases with excellent results. We have had no significant morbidity with this technique in properly selected cases. While an easily palpable lesion does not require CT-directed biopsy, lesions in the intraconal or posterior orbital areas should be biopsied with CT confirmation. As Czerniak and co-workers have demonstrated, marked improvement in diagnostic accuracy was noted when CT was used to confirm needle placement, in contrast to those performed before the amalgamation of these two techniques.[71]

We routinely perform orbital FNAB using a 25-gauge needle. The needle is placed into the orbital lesion and a single CT scan is performed to localize its tip (Figure 15–6). Optimal placement of a needle is in the middle to outer one-third of a tumor. In this area, necrosis should be minimal. It should be noted that if the needle position is not confirmed by CT, it is impossible to determine whether the lesion has been sampled, and a negative biopsy finding will not be meaningful or may be deceptive. Once the needle position is confirmed by CT, a syringe or suction apparatus is attached to the needle. Suction is applied with a slight anteroposterior movement (1 to 2 mm) of the needle. A suction-cutting technique is used because aspiration is sometimes not sufficient to obtain biopsy material from solid tumors. We attempt to cut some tissue with the edge of the needle and aspirate it into the needle, but not the syringe. Greater anteroposterior movement (up to 5 mm) is most effective for obtaining a good sample in large tumors. In small orbital lesions, tumors near the orbital apex, those contiguous with the CNS with orbital roof defects, or intraocular masses, we limit the anteroposterior movement to 1 to 2 mm. Suction is released after three or four gentle movements of the needle, and the needle is withdrawn from the orbit. The needle is disconnected, air is drawn into the syringe and then used to expel the material from

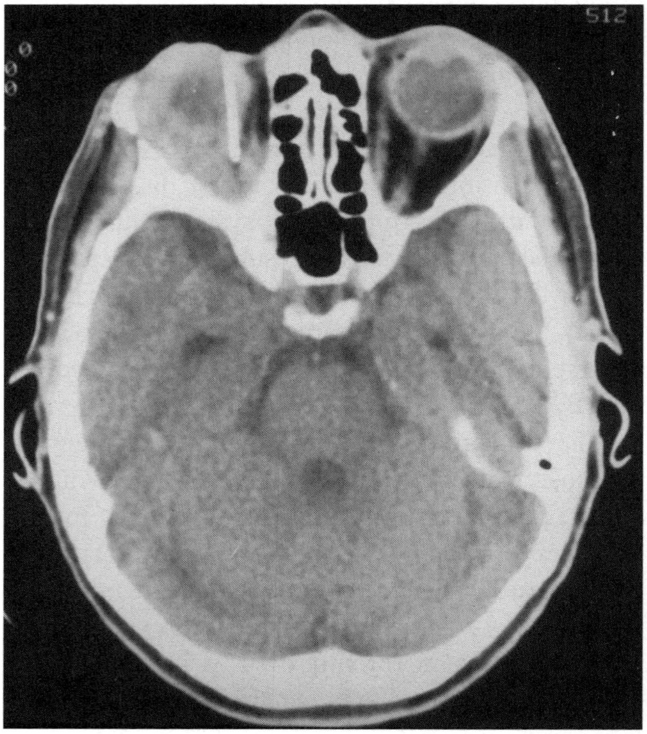

Figure 15–6. CT scan demonstrating needle tip as evidenced by the dark shadow that shows the tip in a posterior orbital tumor.

the tip of the needle onto slides for cytologic evaluation. In a large series of intraocular cases, we have routinely obtained 0.5 to 2.0×10^6 cells from a 25-gauge FNAB (Figure 15–7). In some centers, the use of just a needle with capillary action rather than aspiration has been shown to be adequate to obtain an excellent specimen.[72]

One of the major requirements for CT-guided FNAB is the presence of an expert cytopathologist. We routinely perform all our orbital needle biopsies in the neuroradiology CT scanner with a cytopathologist in attendance. The availability of a cytopathologist in the neuroradiology suite allows us to immediately rebiopsy the lesion if the initial biopsy was negative, without removing the patient from the scanner.

As Kennerdell, Czerniak, and others have noted, the major indication for FNAB is in patients who require cytologic diagnosis of an orbital mass or lesion, but do not require surgical therapy. As an example, Figure 15–8 demonstrates the axial CT pattern in an older patient with a diffuse orbital mass. A metastasis to the orbit was suspected, even though the patient had no history, radiologic evidence, or laboratory findings of a primary malignancy. Aspiration cytology demonstrated an adenocarcinoma, and this patient was treated with irradiation. Figure 15–9 demonstrates the CT scan of a probable sphenoid ridge meningioma; diagnosis was confirmed with FNAB. Other workers have similarly duplicated these results.[73]

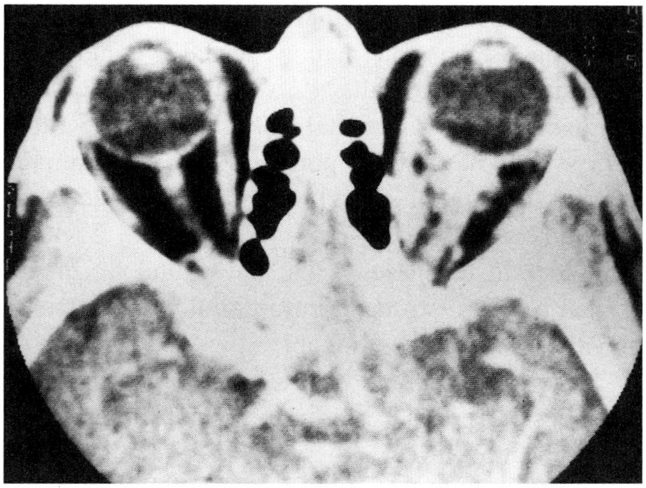

Figure 15–8. Axial orbital CT demonstrating diffuse orbital mass consistent with but not diagnostic of a metastatic tumor.

We do not use FNAB in lesions that are going to be watched regardless of the outcome or in those in which orbitotomy is going to be performed regardless of the aspiration cytology results. In one orbital FNAB series, a very low incidence of correct diagnoses was obtained, probably because in many cases, the indications for FNAB were inappropriate.[74,75] In several series with small numbers of cases, there is approximately an 80 percent diagnostic accuracy.[76,77]

We have not observed significant morbidity due to intraocular or orbital FNAB. Others have noted similar findings.[78–80] However, the possibility of complications, including death from FNAB, has

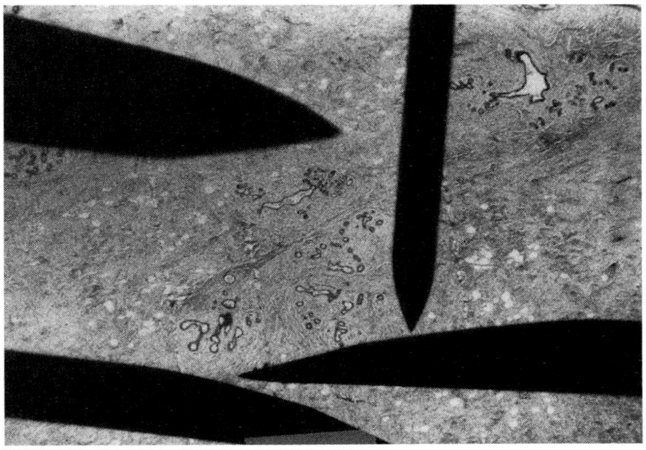

Figure 15–7. Overlay of 22-, 23-, and 25-gauge needles on fine-needle aspirate. An average of 10^6 cells are obtained. (Photo courtesy of T. Miller, MD, San Francisco, CA.)

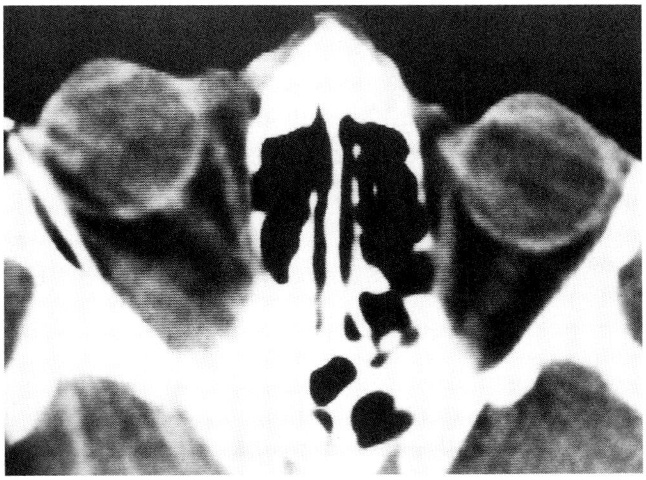

Figure 15–9. Needle positioned just anterior to probable sphenoid ridge meningioma. Biopsy confirming meningioma.

been demonstrated in other sites, and in inexperienced hands, possible damage to the eye and brain or death could result.[75,76] We have particularly avoided the use of orbital endoscopy, since these instruments have more potential to cause damage and possible tumor spread.[81] Using an endoscope in the combined orbital sinus surgery, it is obvious, with current technology, that the orbital fat makes the use of this instrument intraorbitally cumbersome and significantly less valuable.

Over 1,000 orbital FNABs have been reported in meetings or in print.[81–94] We have had two worrisome hemorrhages, but in neither case was vision lost nor was an invasive maneuver required after FNAB. In most cases, needle biopsies have obviated the need for an open surgical procedure. In some cases, FNAB does not adequately sample a tumor due to small size, poor technique, or a fibrous matrix. In some settings, a clear case of false-negative diagnosis occurs. FNAB accuracy is also dependent on the experience in the unit and the type of tumor studied. In one analysis, only 22 of 36 malignancies were diagnosed using this technique.[95] In the chapter on anterior uveal tumors, a patient with orbital and CNS extension from an untreated malignant medulloepithelioma is shown (see Figure 9–44). In that case, it appears clinically that the tumor had destroyed the eye; an orbital FNAB showed a pattern most consistent with a lymphoid lesion. Flow cytometry was not consistent with that diagnosis. Open biopsy of orbital tissue was also nondiagnostic, but when the eye was decalcified, the true nature of the lesion and the secondary nature of the lymphoid component were appreciated. Similarly, in rare cases, we have only obtained lymphoid reactivity surrounding a neoplastic process.

The appropriate use of the above diagnostic modalities, with examples, is discussed in the subsequent chapters on orbital tumors.

Summary

It is difficult to provide a short, lucid overview of the diagnosis and management of adult orbital tumefactions discussed in the following chapters. Adult proptosis usually has an insidious onset, chronic course, and does not require rapid therapeutic intervention. The rapid onset of proptosis is more common with infectious processes or hemorrhage; occasionally, hemorrhage is associated with an orbital neoplasm, most commonly a metastasis.

Thyroid orbitopathy is the most common cause of either unilateral or bilateral proptosis in adults.[3] The extraocular muscles are the major site of orbital involvement in thyroid eye disease.[96]

The discussion of adult orbital tumors has been arbitrarily divided on the basis of the orbital areas they most frequently involve. Usually, an optimal differential diagnosis of an orbital tumor cannot be established from clinical evaluation; it can be proposed on the basis of the orbital area involved, as revealed by either CT or MRI studies. The discussion of adult orbital tumors is divided into lesions in the extraconal area (lacrimal fossa, extraocular muscles, and other extraconal tumors), those lesions involving the contiguous sinuses and orbital walls, and tumefactions of the intraconal space and optic nerve neoplasms.

As in other sections of this book, very rare lesions that can only be diagnosed after complete histologic evaluation have not been discussed. A discussion of most of these entities can be found in other books.[96,97]

Both positron emission tomography (PET) and magnetic resonance spectroscopy (MRS) have been described by us and others in orbital processes, but they are currently research tools.[98–100] We have recently reported a case in which PET data helped us establish the diagnosis of a recurrent fibrous histiocytoma. It is doubtful that this technology will be useful in most orbital conditions. Some patients who are being followed up after nonsurgical treatment may benefit by this PET technology, especially as cameras allow us to accurately image lesions < 7 mm in maximum diameter.[99] Similarly, while color Doppler imaging can demonstrate orbital vessels, it is uncertain whether this will have any application in the diagnosis or management of eye tumors.[101,102] In thyroid orbitopathy, MRS data have the intriguing possibility to more accurately delineate when this orbital process changes from a predominantly inflammatory to a fibrotic one.[103] This type of MRS data might be helpful to monitor chemotherapy or radiation of some orbital processes.[100] While three-dimensional radiologic studies have been used in plastic surgery, their efficacy in tumor diagnosis remains uncertain.[98]

REFERENCES

1. Grove AS Jr. Evaluation of exophthalmos. N Engl J Med 1975; 292:1005–13.
2. Char DH, Norman D. The use of computed tomography and ultrasonography in the evaluation of orbital masses. Surv Ophthalmol 1982;2:49–63.
3. Char DH. Thyroid eye disease, 3rd ed. Boston, MA: Butterworth Heinemann, Inc; 1997.
4. Lederman M, Wybar K. Embryonal sarcoma. Proc R Soc Med 1976;69:895–903.
5. Hilal SK. Computed tomography of the orbit. Ophthalmology 1979;86:864–70.
6. Perlmutter JC, Klingele TG, Hart WM Jr, Burde RM. Disappearing optico-ciliary shunt vessels and pseudotumor cerebri. Am J Ophthalmol 1980;89: 703–7.
7. Dallow RL. Reliability of orbital diagnostic tests: ultrasonography, computerized tomography, and radiography. Ophthalmology 1978;85:1218–28.
8. Cangemi FE, Trempe CL, Walsh JB. Choroidal folds. Am J Ophthalmology 1978;86:380–7.
9. Forbes GS, Sheedy PF, Waller RR. Orbital tumors evaluated by computed tomography. Radiology 1980;136:101–11.
10. Nettleship E. Peculiar lines of the choroid in a case of post-papilliptic atrophy. Trans Ophthalmol Soc UK 1994;4:167–9.
11. Demer JL, Kerman BM. Comparison of standardized echography with magnetic resonance imaging to measure extraocular muscle size. Am J Ophthalmol 1994;118:351–61.
12. Kline RA, Rootman J. Enophthalmos: a clinical review. Ophthalmology 1984;91:229–37.
13. Taveras JL, Haik BG. Radiography of the eye and orbit: a historical review. Surv Ophthalmol 1988; 32:361–8.
14. Maslenan AC, Hadley D. Radiation dose to the lens from computed tomography scanning in a neuroradiology department. Br J Radiol 1995;68:19–22.
15. Maya MM, Heier LA. Orbital CT. Current use in the MR era. Neuroimaging Clin North Am 1998;8: 651–83.
16. Char DH, Miller T, O'Brien JM. Intraocular lymphomas: diagnosis and therapy. Semin Ophthalmol 1993;8:17.
17. Li KC, Poon PY, Hinton P, et al. MR imaging of orbital tumors with CT and ultrasound correlations. J Comput Assist Tomograph 1984;8:1039–47.
18. Byrne SF, Glaser JS. Orbital tissue differentiation with standardized echography. Ophthalmology 1983;90: 1071–90.
19. Hodes BL, Weinberg P. A combined approach for the diagnosis of orbital disease: computed tomography and standardized A-scan echography. Arch Ophthalmol 1977;95:781–8.
20. Ossoinig K. Echography of the eye, orbit, and periorbital region. In: Arger PH, editor. Orbit roentgenology. New York, NY: John Wiley; 1977. p. 223–69.
21. Coleman DJ, Jack RL, Jones IS, Franzen LA. II. Hemangiomas of the orbit. Arch Ophthalmol 1972; 88:368–74.
22. Coleman DJ, Lizzi FL, Jack RL. Ultrasonography of the eye and orbit. Philadelphia, PA: Lea & Febiger; 1977.
23. Balchunas WR, Quencer RM, Byrne SF. Lacrimal gland and fossa masses: evaluation by computed tomography and A-mode echography. Radiology 1983;149:751–8.
24. Bernardino ME, Zimmerman RD, Citrin CM, Davis DO. Scleral thickening: a CT sign of orbital pseudotumor. AJR Am J Roentgenol 1977;129:703–6.
25. Kramer DM. Basic principles of magnetic resonance imaging. Radiol Clin North Am 1984;22:765–78.
26. Sobel DF, Mills C, Char DH, et al. NMR of the normal and pathologic eye and orbit. Am J Nucl Radiol 1984;5:345.
27. Hawkes RC, Holland GN, Moore WS, et al. NMR imaging in the evaluation of orbital tumors. Am J Nucl Radiol 1983;4:254–6.
28. Crooks LE, Hoenninger J, Arakawa M, et al. High-resolution of magnetic resonance imaging. Radiology 1984;150:163–71.
29. Crooks LE, Ortendahl DA, Kaufman L, et al. Clinical efficiency of nuclear magnetic resonance imaging. Radiology 1983;146:123–38.
30. Morrice GD, Smith FW. Early experience with nuclear magnetic resonance (NMR) imaging in the investigation of ocular proptosis. Trans Ophthalmol Soc UK 1983;103:143–54.
31. Moseley I, Brant-Zawdski M, Mills C. Nuclear magnetic resonance imaging of the orbit. Br J Ophthalmol 1983;67:333–42.
32. Smith FW, Cherryman GR, Singh AK, Forrester JV. Nuclear magnetic resonance tomography of the orbit at 3.4 MHz. Br J Radiology 1985;58:947–57.
33. Han JS, Benson JE, Bonstelle CT, et al. Magnetic resonance imaging of the orbit: preliminary experience. Radiology 1984;150:755–9.
34. Char DH, Sobel D, Kelly WM. Nuclear magnetic resonance scanning in orbital and intraocular tumor diagnosis. Ophthalmology 1985;92:1305–10.
35. Sacks E, Worgul BV, Merriam GR Jr, Hilal S. The effects of nuclear magnetic resonance imaging on ocular tissues. Arch Ophthalmol 1986;104:890–3.
36. Paushter DM, Modic MT, Borkowski GP, et al. Magnetic resonance: principles and applications. Med Clin North Am 1984;68:1393–1421.

37. Virapongse C, Mancuso A, Fitzsimmons J. Value of magnetic resonance imaging in assessing bone destruction in head and neck lesions. Laryngoscope 1986;96:284–91.
38. Holman RE, Grimson BS, Drayer PB, et al. Magnetic resonance imaging of optic gliomas. Am J Ophthalmol 1985;100:596–601.
39. Edwards JH, Hyman RA, Vacirca SJ, et al. 0.6 T magnetic resonance imaging of the orbit. AJR Am J Roentgenol 1985;144:1015–20.
40. Schenck JF, Hart HR Jr, Foster TH, et al. Improved MR imaging of the orbit at 1.5T with surface coils. AJR Am J Roentgenol 1985;144:1033–6.
41. Zimmerman RA, Bilaniuk LT, Yanoff M, et al. Orbital magnetic resonance imaging. Am J Ophthalmol 1985;100:312–7.
42. Daniels DL, Herfkins R, Gager WE, et al. Magnetic resonance imaging of the optic nerves and chiasm. Radiology 1984;152:79–83.
43. Jay WH. Advances in magnetic resonance imaging. Am J Ophthalmol 1989;108:592–6.
44. Hendrix LE, Kneeland JB, Haughton BM, et al. MR imaging of optic nerve lesions: value of gadopentetate dimeglumine and fat- suppression technique. Am J Nucl Radiol 1990;11:749–54.
45. Tien RD. Fat-suppression MR imaging and neuroradiology: techniques and clinical application. AJR Am J Roentgenol 1992;158:369–79.
46. Weber AL. Comparative assessment of diseases of the orbit using computed tomography and magnetic resonance imaging. Isr J Med Sci 1992;28:153–60
47. Eastwood JD, Hudgins PA. New techniques in magnetic resonance imaging. Curr Opin Ophthalmol 1998;9:54–60.
48. Herrick RC, Hayman LA, Taber KH, et al. Artifacts and pitfalls in MR imaging of the orbit: a clinical review. Radiographics 1997;17:707–24.
49. Mintz E, Kline LB, Dubal ER. Diagnostic misinterpretation of fat suppression orbital magnetic resonance scanning. Am J Ophthalmol 1993;115:262–4.
50. Sullivan JA, Harms SE. Surface-coil MR imaging of orbital neoplasms. Am J Nucl Radiol 1986;7:29–34.
51. Orell SR. Fine-needle aspiration biopsy and perspective. Pathology 1982;14:113–4.
52. Martin HE, Ellis EB. Biopsy by needle puncture and aspiration. Ann Surg 1930;92:169–81.
53. Martin HE, Stewart FW. The advantages and limitation of aspiration biopsy. AJR Am J Roentgenol 1936; 35:245–7.
54. Moloo Z, Finley RJ, Lefcoe MS, et al. Possible spread of bronchogenic carcinoma to the chest wall after a transthoracic fine-needle aspiration biopsy. Acta Cytol 1985;29:167–9.
55. Tao LC, Pearson FG, Delarue NC, et al. Percutaneous fine-needle aspiration biopsy. Cancer 1980;45: 1480–5.
56. Wehle MJ, Grabstald H. Contraindications to needle aspiration of a solid renal mass: tumor dissemination by renal needle aspiration. J Urol 1986;136: 446–8.
57. Sterrett G, Whitaker D, Glancy J. Fine-needle aspiration of the lung. Pathol Ann 1982;17:197–228.
58. Lalli AF, McCormack LJ, Zelch M, et al. Aspiration biopsies of chest lesions. Radiology 1978;127: 35–40.
59. Sinner WN, Zajicek J. Implantation metastasis after percutaneous transthoracic needle aspiration biopsy. Acta Radiol Diagn 1976;17:473–80.
60. Gibbons RP, Bush WH Jr, Burnett LL. Needle tract seeding following aspiration of renal carcinoma. J Urol 1977;8:865–7.
61. Berg JW, Robbins GF. A later look at the safety of aspiration biopsy. Cancer 1962;15:826–9.
62. Eriksson O, Hagmar B, Ryd W. Effects of fine-needle aspiration and other biopsy procedures on tumor dissemination in mice. Cancer 1984;54:73–8.
63. Engzell U, Espositi PL, Rubio C, et al. Investigation on tumour spread in connection with aspiration biopsy. Acta Radiol 1971;10:385–98.
64. Char DH, Miller T, Kroll SM. Orbital metastases: Diagnosis and course. Br J Ophthalmol 1997;81: 386–90.
65. Tao L-C, Sanders DE, McLoughlin MJ, et al. Current concepts in fine needle aspiration biopsy cytology. Hum Pathol 1980;11:94–6.
66. Westman-Naeser P. Tumours of the orbit diagnosed by fine-needle biopsy. Acta Ophthalmolo 1978;56: 969–76.
67. Schyberg E. Fine-needle biopsy of orbital tumours. Acta Ophthalmol 1975;125:11.
68. Kennerdell JS, Dubois DJ, Dekker A, Johnson BL. CT-guided fine-needle aspiration biopsy of orbital optic nerve tumor. Ophthalmology 1980;87:491–6.
69. Spoor TC, Kennerdell JS, Dekker A, et al. Orbital fine-needle aspiration biopsy with B-scan guidance. Am J Ophthalmol 1980;89:274–7.
70. Kennerdell JS, Slamovits TL, Dekker A, Johnson BL. Orbital fine-needle aspiration biopsy. Am J Ophthalmol 1985;99:547–51.
71. Czerniak D, Woyke S, Daniel B, et al. Diagnosis of orbital tumors by aspiration biopsy guided by computerized tomography. Cancer 1984;54:2385–9.
72. Dey P, Ray R. Comparison of fine-needle sampling by capillary action and fine-needle aspiration. Cytopathology 1993;4:299–303.
73. Mehrotra R, Kumar S, Singh K, et al. Fine-needle aspiration biopsy of orbital meningioma. Diagn Cytopathol 1999;21:402–4.

74. Krohel GB, Tobin DR, Chavis RM. Inaccuracy of fine-needle aspiration biopsy. Ophthalmology 1985;92:666–70.
75. Karcioglu ZA, Gordon RA, Karcioglu GL. Tumor seeding in ocular fine-needle aspiration biopsy. Ophthalmology 1985;92:1763–7.
76. Zeppa P, Tranfa F, Errico ME, et al. Fine-needle aspiration (FNA) biopsy of orbital masses: a critical review of 51 cases. Cytopathology 1997;8:366–72.
77. Gupta S, Sood B, Gulati M, et al. Orbital mass lesions: US-guided fine-needle aspiration biopsy—experience in 37 patients. Radiology 1999;213:568–72.
78. Berquist TH, Bailey PB, Cortese D, Miller WE. Transthoracic needle biopsy: accuracy and complications in relation to location and type of lesion. Mayo Clin Proc 1980;55:475–81.
79. Liu D. Complications of fine-needle aspiration biopsy of the orbit. Ophthalmology 1985;92:1768–70.
80. Arora R, Rewari R, Betharia SM. Fine-needle aspiration cytology of orbital and adnexal masses. Acta Cytol 1992;36:483–91.
81. Norris JL, Stewart WB. Bi-manual endoscopic orbital biopsy. Ophthalmology 1985;92:34–8.
82. Das DK, Das J, Bhatt NC, et al. Orbital lesions: Diagnosis by fine-needle aspiration cytology. Acta Cytol 1994;38:158–64.
83. O'Hara BJ, Ehya H, Shields JA, et al. Fine-needle aspiration biopsy in pediatric ophthalmic tumors and pseudotumors. Acta Cytol 1993;37:125–30.
84. Slamovits TL, Rosen CE, Suhrland MJ. Neuroblastoma presenting as acute lymphoblastic leukemia but correctly diagnosed after orbital fine-needle aspiration biopsy. J Clin Neuro-ophthalmol 1991;11:158–61.
85. Palma D, Canall N, Scaroni P, Torri AM. Fine-needle aspiration biopsy: its use in the management of orbital and intraocular tumors. Tumor 1989;75:593–8.
86. Zeppa P, Tranfa F, Errico MF, et al. Fine needle aspiration (FNA) biopsy of orbital masses: a critical review of cytopathology 1997;8:366–72.
87. Cristallini EG, Bolis GB, Ottaviano P. Fine-needle aspiration biopsy of orbital meningioma. Acta Cytol 1990;34:236–8.
88. Dey P, Radhika S, Rajwanshi A, et al. Fine-needle aspiration biopsy of orbital and eyelid lesions. Acta Cytol 1993;37:903–7.
89. Zajdela A, Vielh P, Schlienger P, Haye C. Fine-needle cytology of 292 palpable orbital and eyelid tumors. Am J Clin Pathol 1990;93:100–4.
90. Geisinger KR, Silverman JF, Cappellari JO, Dabbs DJ. Fine needle aspiration cytology of malignant hemangiopericytomas with ultrastructural and flow cytometric analyses. Arch Pathol Lab Med 1990;114:705–10.
91. Arora R, Betharia SM. Fine-needle aspiration biopsy of pediatric orbital tumors: an immunocytochemical study. Acta Cytol 1994;38:5110–6.
92. Tiji JWM, Koornneef L. Fine-needle aspiration biopsy in orbital tumours. Br J Ophthalmol 1991;75:491–2.
93. Char DH, Miller T. Orbital pseudotumor: fine-needle aspiration biopsy and response to therapy. Ophthalmology 1993;100:1702–10.
94. Teng CS, Yeo PP. Ophthalmic Graves' disease: natural history and detailed thyroid function studies. Br Med J 1977;1:273–5.
95. Zurrida S, Alasio L, Tradati N, et al. Fine-needle aspiration of parotid masses. Cancer 1993;72:2306–11.
96. Jakobiec FA, Font RL. Orbit. In: Spencer WH, editor. 3rd ed. Ophthalmic Pathology. Philadelphia, PA: WB Saunders; 1986.
97. Henderson JW. Metastatic carcinoma. In: Orbital tumors. Philadelphia, PA: Raven Press; 1994. p. 473–83.
98. Hosokawa C, Kawabe J, Okamura T, et al. Usefulness of 99mTc-PMY SPECT and 18F-FDG PET in diagnosing orbital metastasis of hepatocellular carcinoma. Kaku Igaku Jap J Nucl Med 1994;31:1237–42.
99. Char DH, Caputo G, Miller T. Orbital fibrous histiocytomas. Orbit 2000 [in press].
100. Cousins JP. Clinical MR spectroscopy: fundamentals, current applications, and future potential. AJR Am J Roentgenol 1995;164:1337–47.
101. Senn BC, Kaiser HJ, Schotzau A, Flammer J. Reproducibility of color Doppler imaging in orbital vessels. Ger J Ophthalmol 1996;5:386–91.
102. Mendivil A, Cuartero V. Color doppler image of central retinal artery of eyes with an intraconal mass. Curr Eye Res 1999;18:104–9.
103. Fries PD, Char DH, Swift P. Experimental orbital myositis: evaluation of therapeutic modalities. Orbit 1991;10:125–32.

16

Pediatric Orbital Tumors

The presentations and differential diagnoses of orbital tumefactions in children are quite different from those observed in adults. Even among children of different age groups, there is a marked variation in the frequency of different orbital tumors.

Children with orbital lesions should be evaluated in an urgent manner. While a number of series on pediatric orbital tumors have stressed that most lesions are not malignant, treatable primary orbital malignancies are not rare in childhood, and some histologically benign processes can produce profound ocular morbidity with visual loss, if not treated promptly.[1–4]

A list of the most frequent orbital tumors in childhood is shown in Table 16–1. The list is deliberately not all-inclusive; very rare tumors are not listed, and lesions that only involve older teenagers are discussed under adult orbital disease in other chapters.

As has been discussed by others, the frequency of orbital tumors is a function of the geographic location of the survey, the authors' interest, and local referral patterns.[3,5] As Moss pointed out in adult orbital tumefactions, depending on the series, the most frequent tumors had been described as mixed tumors of the lacrimal gland, meningiomas, hemangiomas, or as thyroid eye disease.[5] Similarly, a recent histologic series by Shields and co-workers of 250 pediatric orbital biopsies seemed skewed toward cystic lesions, with 46 percent of biopsies being dermoid cysts, 16 percent inflammatory lesions, 7 percent vascular tumors (hemangioma or lymphangioma), 7 percent mainly adipose tissue (either orbital fat or dermolipomas), 4 percent rhabdomyosarcomas or secondary orbital malignancies, and lymphoid tumors and optic nerve tumors accounted for 2.4 percent of cases.[4] In a Turkish series, the most common pediatric orbital tumor was rhabdomyosarcoma, and dermoid cysts were the most common benign lesions.[6] Kodsi and colleagues reviewed 340 childhood orbital lesions examined over a 60-year period at the Mayo Clinic.[7] They noted the following frequencies of orbital tumefactions: cystic lesions 23 percent, vascular processes (hemangiomas and lymphangiomas) 18 percent, optic nerve and central nervous system (CNS) 16 percent, bone lesions 9 percent, and rhabdomyosarcoma 7 percent.[7] Bullock and colleagues analyzed 141 cases of their own and reviewed 1,370 pediatric orbital tumors already in the literature.[8] Overall, approximately 24 percent of the reported cases of orbital tumors were malignant.[8] In the author's experience in an ophthalmic oncology practice, I have managed a higher percentage of malignant pediatric orbital tumors. The author has arbitrarily divided pediatric orbital tumors into those that occur in infancy and those that occur in childhood. Teenagers are more prone to have the adult pattern of orbital disease, and those lesions are discussed under adult orbital tumors.

In infants, the most common causes of proptosis are hemangioma, metastatic neuroblastoma, superficial dermoids, and leukemia.[9]

NEUROBLASTOMA

Neuroblastoma is the most common tumor in early childhood and has an incidence of approximately 10 per 12 million live births.[10] In a study of 9,308 systemic childhood malignancies, neuroblastoma accounted for approximately 7 percent of cases.[11,12] These tumors are derived from sympathetic ganglion tissue. Approximately 70 percent develop in the upper abdomen; however, they can rarely occur as a result of a cervical sympathetic ganglion chain tumor.[12,13] Approximately 500 new cases of neuroblastoma are diagnosed in the United States each year.[14] At the time of diagnosis, approximately 70 percent of neuroblastoma patients have metastatic disease.[15]

Table 16–1. COMMON PEDIATRIC ORBITAL TUMEFACTIONS

Primary orbital malignancies
Rhabdomyosarcoma
Alveolar soft part sarcoma
Fibrosarcoma
Malignant fibrous histiocytoma
Leiomyosarcoma
Osteosarcoma
Systemic malignancies with orbital involvement
Burkitt's lymphoma
Chloroma (myeloblastoma or myeloid sarcoma)
Neuroblastoma
Ewing's sarcoma
Wilm's tumor
Secondary orbital involvement from contigious malignancies
Retinoblastoma
Esthesioneuroblastoma
Cystic lesions
Dermoid and epidermoid cysts
Hematic cysts
Aneurysmal bone cyst
Choristomatous cyst
Traumatic inclusion cyst
Microphthalmos with orbital cyst
Ecchinococcus cyst
Congenital teratoma
Vascular lesions
Hemangioendothelioma (hemangioma)
Lymphangioma
Orbital varix
Benign fibrous tumors
Fibrous dysplasia
Neurofibroma
Cartilaginous hamartoma
Juvenile ossifying fibroma
Inflammatory lesions
Pseudotumor
Histiocytosis syndromes
Pseudorheumatoid nodule
Thyroid orbital disease
Infectious processes
Contiguous orbital involvement from sinusitis
Orbital tuberculosis
Viral and bacterial lacrimal gland inflammation
Optic nerve tumors
Optic nerve glioma
Leukemic infiltrate
Pseudotumor
Meningioma
Sarcoid
Miscellaneous
Brown tumor
Melanocytic neuroectodermal tumor of infancy (retinal anlage tumor)

Molecular studies in neuroblastoma have demonstrated serial cumulative genomic alterations. Early changes may include loss of chromosome 1p (del-1p); probably, this represents the loss of a tumor suppressor gene at 1p36.[16] Overexpression of the *N-myc* on 2p24 is associated with rapid disease progression, poor prognosis, and/or advanced disease.[16–19] However, the exact prognostic relevance of different genomic changes has been subject to ultimate interpretation.[20] Approximately 85 percent of patients have a deletion or rearrangement of chromosome 1p.[21] *N-myc* has previously been shown to correlate with metastatic disease.[22,23] A number of other genomic changes have also been noted in this tumor.[24]

Approximately 20 percent of children with neuroblastoma have evidence of ophthalmic involvement, either with proptosis, Horner's syndrome, or opsoclonus.[25] In a group of 648 children with metastatic neuroblastoma, 18 percent had either intracranial or orbital metastases.[26] Patients with orbital metastases in this series had a decreased survival. In a retrospective study from St. Jude's Hospital of 450 neuroblastoma patients, 47 had some physical abnormality of the eye.[27] Often, ophthalmic signs are the first manifestation of neuroblastoma, and many of these patients present to the ophthalmologist with orbital metastases prior to the discovery of the primary neoplasm. Characteristic clinical findings of metastatic orbital neuroblastoma are the rapid onset of swelling and proptosis. Often, these signals are misdiagnosed as being of either inflammatory or traumatic origin, especially when children present with ecchymosis of the lower lids.[28] Figure 16–1 demonstrates a child who presented with unilateral orbital proptosis after returning from a camping trip. Two days prior to presentation, he had had subtle ecchymosis of the lower lid.

A number of other presentations of neuroblastoma in the eye include squint, dilated or fixed pupils, edema or atrophy of the optic nerve, retinal edema, exudates and hemorrhages, or Horner's syndrome. The latter presentation is most commonly seen in patients under 2 years old who have mediastinal or cervical primary neuroblastomas.[25] A unilateral Horner's syndrome is often associated with localized cervical disease; it has a relatively favorable outcome. Eight of 11 cases had long-term survival. Similarly, opsoclonus was a feature of only localized disease, and these children also fared better.[29]

Almost all children with metastatic orbital neuroblastoma have bone involvement with diffuse orbital, bone, and brain metastases demonstrable on either computed tomography (CT) or magnetic resonance imaging (MRI). Figure 16–2A shows a plain skull radiograph of a child initially referred for a tripod fracture felt to be due to parental abuse. Figure 16–2B shows the extent of tumor involvement on CT with bony destruction and contiguous CNS disease. On fine-needle aspiration biopsy (FNAB), a small, malignant, round cell, nonlymphocytic tumor was diagnosed (Figure 16–2C). Rarely, as shown in Figure 16–3, the orbital bone changes associated with a metastatic neuroblastoma can be minimal.

We have found FNAB useful in establishing the correct diagnosis in many of these patients with orbital neuroblastoma. Unfortunately, it can sometimes be difficult to differentiate other small round cell neoplasms, such as Wilm's tumor, rhabdomyosarcoma, lymphoma or Ewing's sarcoma on the basis of FNAB.[30,31] As discussed elsewhere in

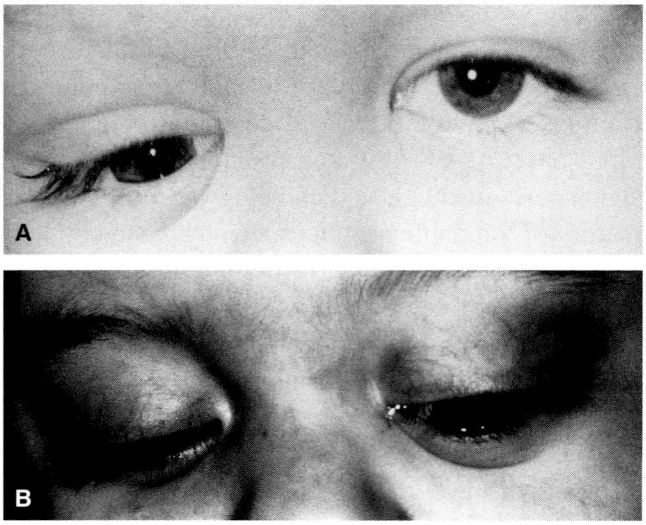

Figure 16–1. *A* and *B*, Clinical photographs of orbital neuroblastoma. Lid ecchymoses are often associated with this tumor and may mimic trauma.

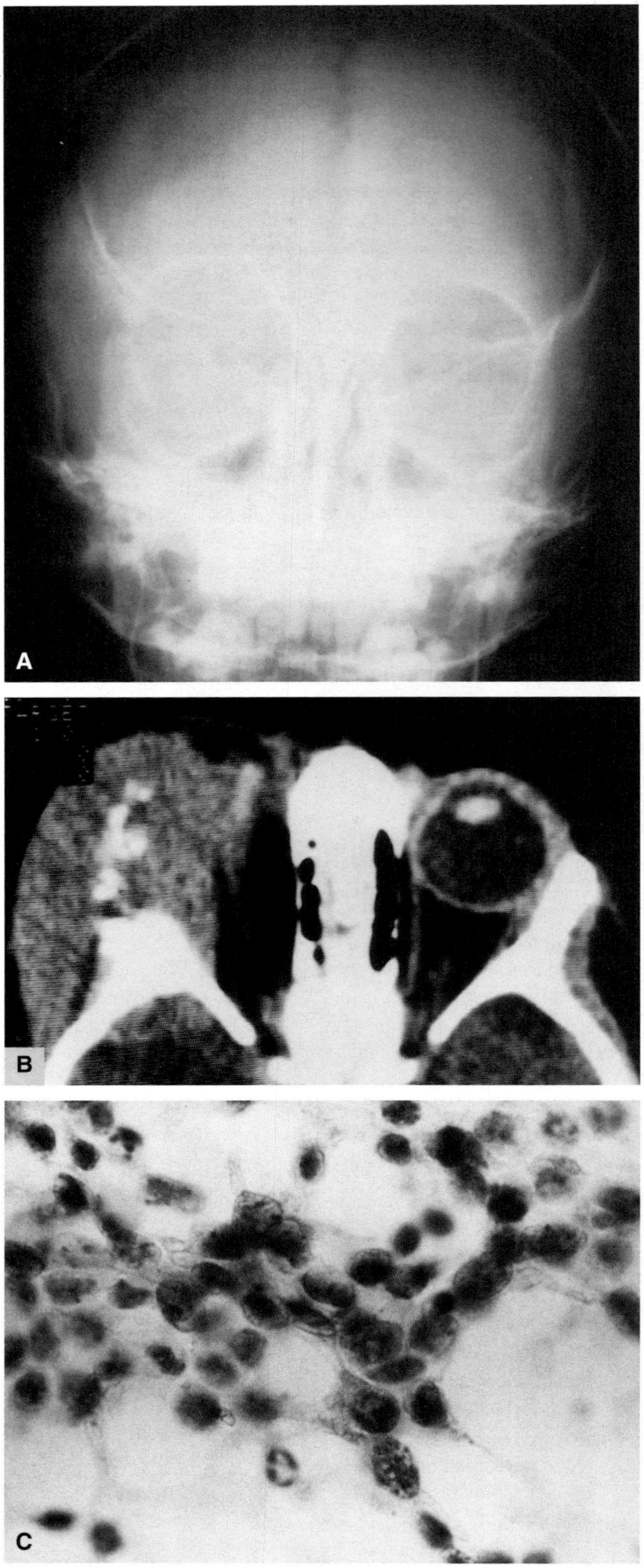

Figure 16–2. *A*, Plain skull radiograph, showing bone involvement from metastatic neuroblastoma that simulates trauma. *B*, Axial CT scan demonstrating neuroblastoma responsible for the bony lesion. *C*, Fine-needle biopsy shows a small round-cell malignant neoplasm consistent with neuroblastoma.

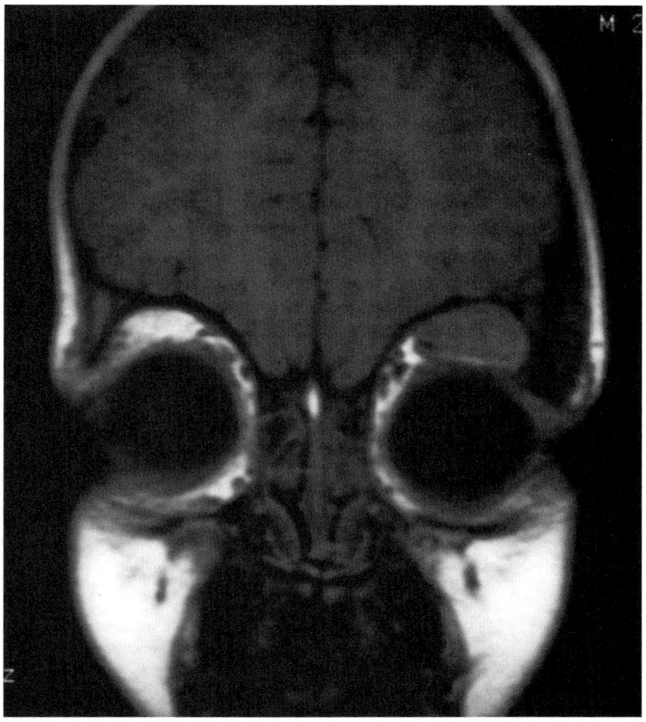

Figure 16–3. Direct coronal MRI of neuroblastoma with minimal bone involvement.

this book, modifications have allowed us to use FNAB samples to perform fluorescent in situ hybridization (FISH) and other molecular biologic techniques.

The evaluation of patients with possible metastatic orbital neuroblastoma involves multimodality examinations with pediatric and ocular oncologists. In patients < 2 years, destructive osseous lesions of the orbit are most likely due to neuroblastoma, although, rarely, one of the Langerhan's histiocytosis syndromes can produce some similar features (see below). Often, on general physical examination, an abdominal mass can be palpated. Patients should have a careful physical and neurologic evaluations. Ancillary studies, in addition to orbital and brain CT or MRI, include bone marrow studies, complete skeletal survey, intravenous pyelogram, and urinary catecholamines. In one study of 145 metastatic neuroblastoma patients, single bone marrow aspirates underestimated the prevalence of marrow involvement by as much as 83 percent.[32] In patients with widespread disease, elevation of the urinary catechol are found in over 80 percent of cases.[33] Bone scan is useful, since approximately 15 percent of patients with negative skeletal surveys will have a positive radionucleide study.[10] The use of metaiodobenzylguanidine is another imaging study which appears to increase prognostic accuracy in metastatic disease.[34]

There is limited evidence to suggest that debulking of an orbital neuroblastoma metastasis improves prognosis.[35–36] Generally, survival is best in children < 11 months of age. In one study, there was 72 percent survival for all stages of neuroblastoma in children < 11 months of age, versus 12 percent in children 2 years and older.[37] Disseminated disease, including involvement of the orbit, has historically been almost uniformly fatal although newer combined multimodality regimens (surgery, chemotherapy, bone marrow transplantation) have increased the length of survival.[35,38] In one series, 4 of 46 patients with metastases (stage IV disease) had survival of over 1 year.[39] In contrast, infants with stage IV disease often do well; in another series, 10 of 11 were disease free between 2.5 and 13 years after diagnosis.[40]

Intensive chemotherapy with autologous bone marrow transplantation has increased the event-free 4-year survival to approximately 40 percent in some series.[41–49] The therapeutic paramenters used in these trials are undergoing evolution.[45,46] There have been some molecular pilot treatment studies, including a new agent reactive with topoisomerase.[47,48]

OTHER PRIMARY ORBITAL MALIGNANCIES

Wilm's tumor rarely metastasizes to the orbit in the same age group. It is much less frequent than orbital neuroblastoma but can be difficult to differentiate, either by clinical presentation or sometimes even on histologic examination.[49]

In a slightly older pediatric or an adult population, esthesioneuroblastoma, a tumor similar to neuroblastoma, occurs. This tumor was first recognized in 1924 and approximately 250 cases have now been reported.[50] The peak incidence appears to be in the second and third decades of life. Often, these lesions can be difficult to diagnose. Most commonly, they involve the sinuses, but in approximately 10 percent of cases, ophthalmic symptoms are the first sign of this tumor. More commonly, nasal blockage or a bloody nasal discharge are the initial presentation. Figure 16–4 demonstrates a CT scan of an esthesioneuroblastoma with secondary orbital involvement in a teenage boy. Often, these patients do quite well with a combination of resection, chemotherapy, and radiation.

Leukemic involvement of the orbit is another common cause of proptosis in infants (Figure 16–5). Most commonly, leukemic orbital involvement is observed in children from the Mediterranean basin or Africa. In the latter group of patients, it is the second most common cause of orbital proptosis after Burkitt's lymphoma.[9,51] Rarely, a neuroblastoma can be confused with a leukemic orbital lesion. In one report, this diagnostic uncertainty was resolved using special stains on a fine-needle aspirate.[52] Occasionally, a combination of chromosomal and immunophenotypical analysis of tumor specimens can be helpful to differentiate these.[53]

ACUTE MYELOMONOCYTIC LEUKEMIA

Acute myelomonocytic leukemia (AMML) often produces a greenish orbital tumor which has been termed, because of the color, a chloroma. Other terms for this tumor are ocular granulocytic sarcoma, myeloblastoma, or myeloid sarcoma. In one Turkish series, 20 of 56 children with AMML had ocular involvement. Seventeen of these children were males, and bilateral involvement occurred in 9 patients.[51,54] A more recent report noted that 33 of 121 such patients had ocular involvement.[55] In that latter publication, the mean survival with ophthalmic manifestations was 8.7 months, compared with 28.6 months when the eye and adnexa were not involved.[55] The hematologic diagnosis was made before the onset of ocular disease in only 1 of the 20 cases, and the orbital manifestations responded earlier to chemotherapy than the hematologic manifestations.[54] A child with orbital and intraocular involvement from AMML is shown in Figure 16–6. Zimmerman and Font collected 33 cases of this tumor at the Armed Forces Institute of Pathology (AFIP), and the median age in that series was 7 years.[56] Pui and colleagues noted that approximately 5 percent of children with AMML developed granulocytic sarcomas. In orbital granulocytic sarcoma, there was homogenous gadolinium uptake MRI scans. In contrast, an intraorbital hemorrhage usually gives heterogeneous results, and an orbital

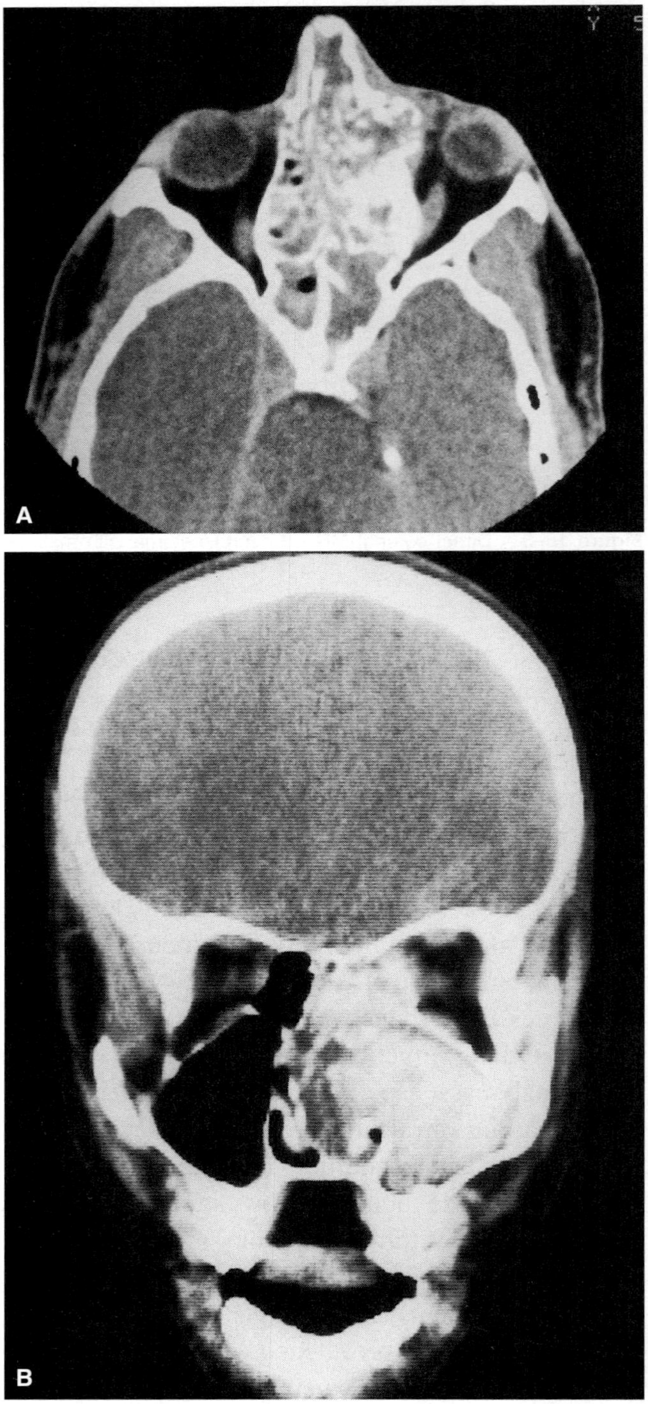

Figure 16–4. *A,* Axial CT scan of an esthesioneuroblastoma with secondary orbital involvement in a teenage boy. Posterior orbital involvement is shown. *B,* The extent of sinus involvement of the lesion shown in Figure 16–4A.

abscess is usually either hypointense or isointense on T_1-weighted images and hyperintense on T_2-weighted scans.[57] Overall, in a pediatric group, leukemias, including the more common acute lymphocyte type, account for 2 to 10 percent of orbital tumors.[58–61] Clinically, we have noted two types of typical presentations with infants having leukemia in the orbit. Sometimes, these children present with only orbital disease, often in a preseptal location. An example of this pattern is shown in Figure 16–5. This child presented with a medial canthal mass. After orbital biopsy, a bone marrow biopsy confirmed systemic leukemia. Rarely, leukemia can present as an acute dacryocystitis.[62] Figure 16–6 shows a child with AMML with panophthalmitis as a result of leukemic involvement. Figure 16–7 shows another acute leukemia patient with orbital involvement by this neoplasm. Some children have developed leukemic relapse in the orbit. As discussed above, the MRI pattern in leukemic children with orbital findings is quite useful, since the differential diagnosis includes neoplasm, infection, or hemorrhage, and often, these can be distinguished on the basis of MRI characteristics.[57]

The management of leukemia is outside the purview of this book. Better results have been obtained with more aggressive treatment, and this is being performed in several centers around the world.[63–67] As discussed above with AMML, and acute leukemia in general, ophthalmic involvement is associated with a poorer prognosis. In one report, 27 of 28 patients with ophthalmic manifestations of acute leukemia died within 28 months.[67] Rarely, in children, a lymphoma can involve the orbit.[68]

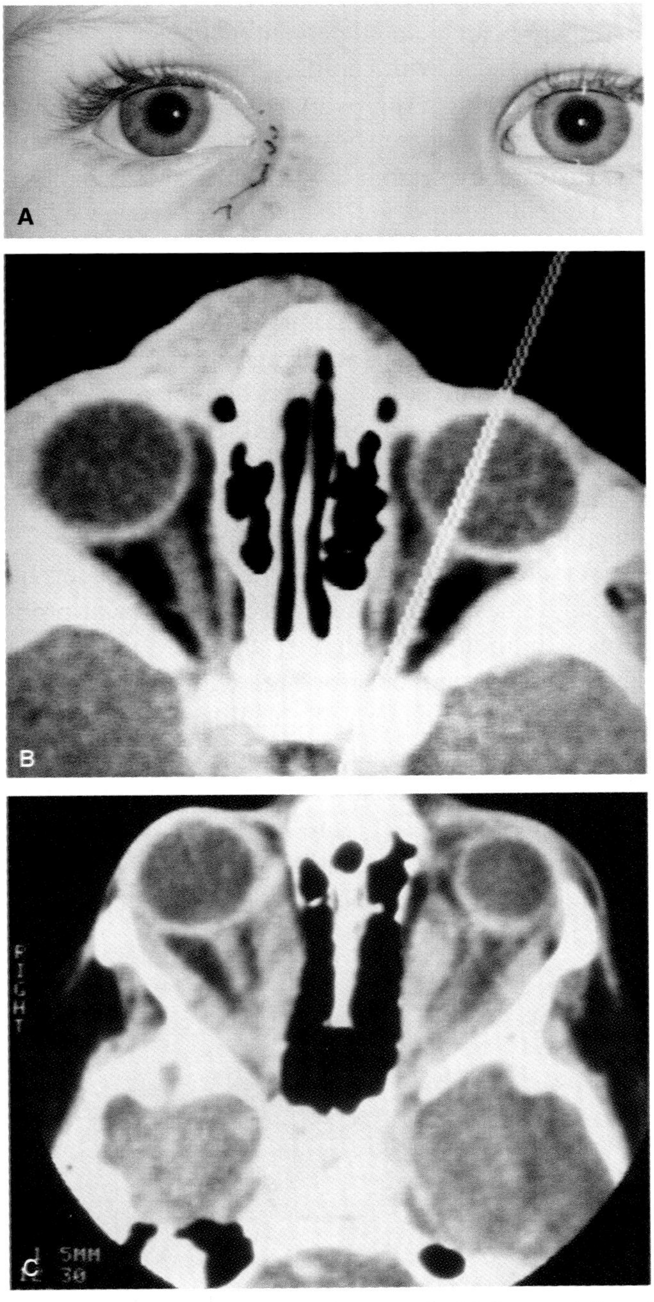

Figure 16–5. *A,* Clinical view of preseptal orbital presentation of acute leukemia. *B,* Axial CT scan of preseptal orbital presentation of acute leukemia. *C,* Relapse of acute leukemia manifested as an orbital myositis.

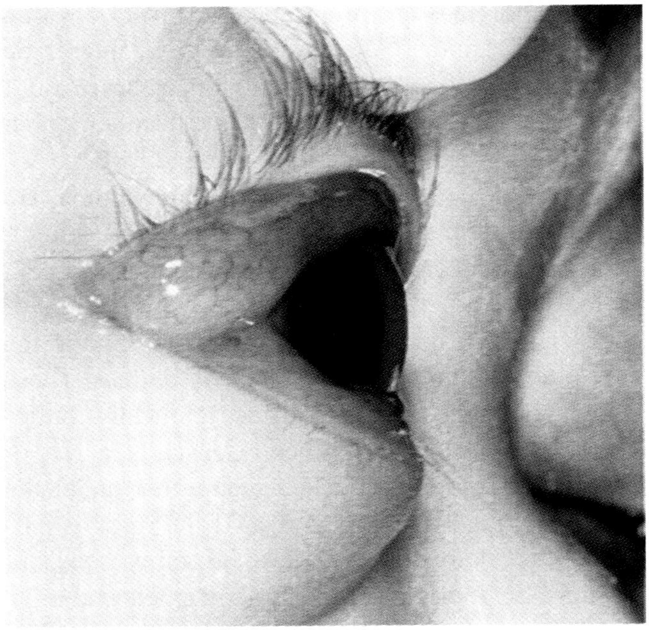

Figure 16–6. Child with panophthalmitis and orbital mass secondary to acute myelomonocytic leukemia (AMML)

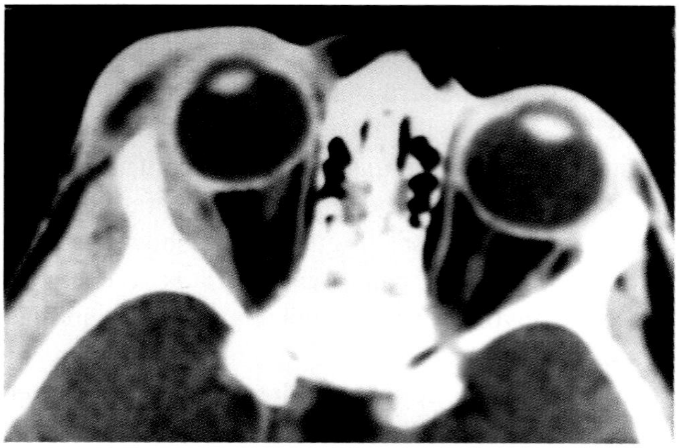

Figure 16–7. Axial CT scan demonstrates orbital involvement in a 1-year-old child with acute leukemia.

Rhabdomyosarcoma can also present in the < 2-year age group, but it is more commonly seen in slightly older children, as discussed later.

BENIGN ORBITAL TUMORS OF INFANCY

Capillary Hemangiomas

The most common benign ocular tumor of infancy is capillary hemangioma; it may involve the lid, conjunctiva, orbit, or simultaneously more than one of these areas. Most commonly, capillary hemangiomas present in the first year of life, and orbital or lid hemangiomas are often noted at birth or within the first 2 months.[69] As discussed in Chapter 1 on eyelid tumor diagnosis, hemangiomas have a 3:1 female-to-male ratio, and there have been a number of interesting animal models developed.[70]

Ninety-five percent of capillary hemangiomas are evident before 6 months of life. Figure 16–8 demonstrates a typical case of a lid-orbital capillary hemangioma, with progression over the first 9 months of life.[70] Usually, these tumors grow rapidly for the first 6 to 12 months and then slowly regress. These lesions are almost always diffuse clinically, radiologically, or at surgery. There is usually a red or bluish hue to the mass, when seen either under the skin or through the conjunctiva. If the mass is palpable, it is relatively soft and can be compressed, but margins are poorly defined. As shown below, the CT or MRI patterns are characteristic, and usually they are in both the intraconal and extraconal areas of the orbit. The orbit may be expanded, but bone invasion is rare; that latter finding mandates a biopsy to rule out a malignancy. As Henderson has pointed out, however, the course of hemangiomas can be unpredictable.[71] Regression usually occurs between the ages of 5 and 7 years but may continue until age 18 years, and sometimes they spontaneously resolve during infancy.[72]

A number of previous series have demonstrated that there is up to an 80 percent incidence of serious ocular sequelae with capillary hemangiomas of the orbit and eyelids. Approximately 60 percent develop amblyopia and a significant number develop asymmetric refractive errors.[73–75] Kushner and others (see pediatric lid tumors in Chapters 1 to 3) reviewed the rationale and results of intralesional steroid injection for infantile adnexal hemangiomas.[76] He reported on 10 patients treated with intralesional steroids and found that reasonable shrinkage of the tumor was noted in 9. Others have noted similar responses.[77] Significant complications have been reported with intralesional steroids.[78] In the author's personal experience, intralesional steroids are used and there has not been a major complication.

We do not intervene in infantile orbital or lid hemangiomas, unless they are causing visual problems. Children are evaluated clinically and, if the lesion is unusual or growing, with MRI (Figure 16–9). The MRI pattern of a capillary hemangioma usually shows an isodense lesion on T_1-weighted images and a tumor that is hyperintense to brain on T_2-weighted images (Figure 16–10).

Infantile capillary hemangiomas should be treated when definite growth has a possible effect on vision.

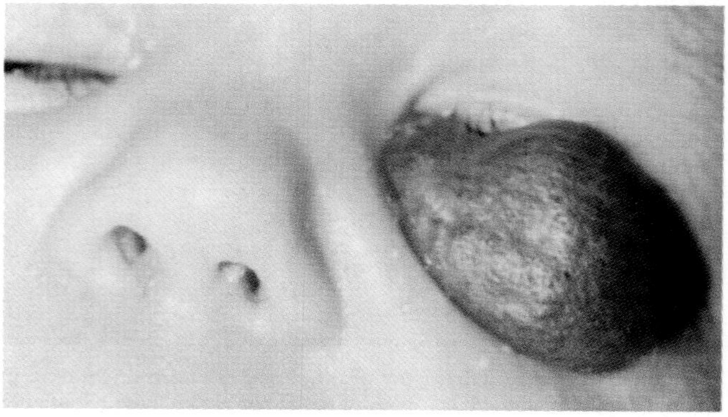

Figure 16–8. Orbital and lid capillary hemangioma. Presenting as a small lesion, this tumor showed growth on serial observation.

Our first mode of therapy is intralesional steroids. We inject 1 mL of methylprednisolone sodium succinate (SoluMedrol) (40 mg/mL) diffusely throughout the lesion with a 25-gauge needle. We do not use general anesthesia and have not seen complications with this approach, although they have been described (see Chapter 2).[78] Usually, tumor regression begins in 2 to 3 days, and maximum effect is seen within 1 week. In the author's experience, if two injections spaced 1 week apart yield no results, surgery is necessary.

Other authors have been more impressed with the use of oral steroids at 3 to 5 mg/kg of prednisone daily. In the author's experience, injectable steroids are preferred, but there is a paucity of data that support one approach versus the other.[79] The "clinical trade-off" is between more likely systemic complications with oral agents, compared with local complications with rejection.

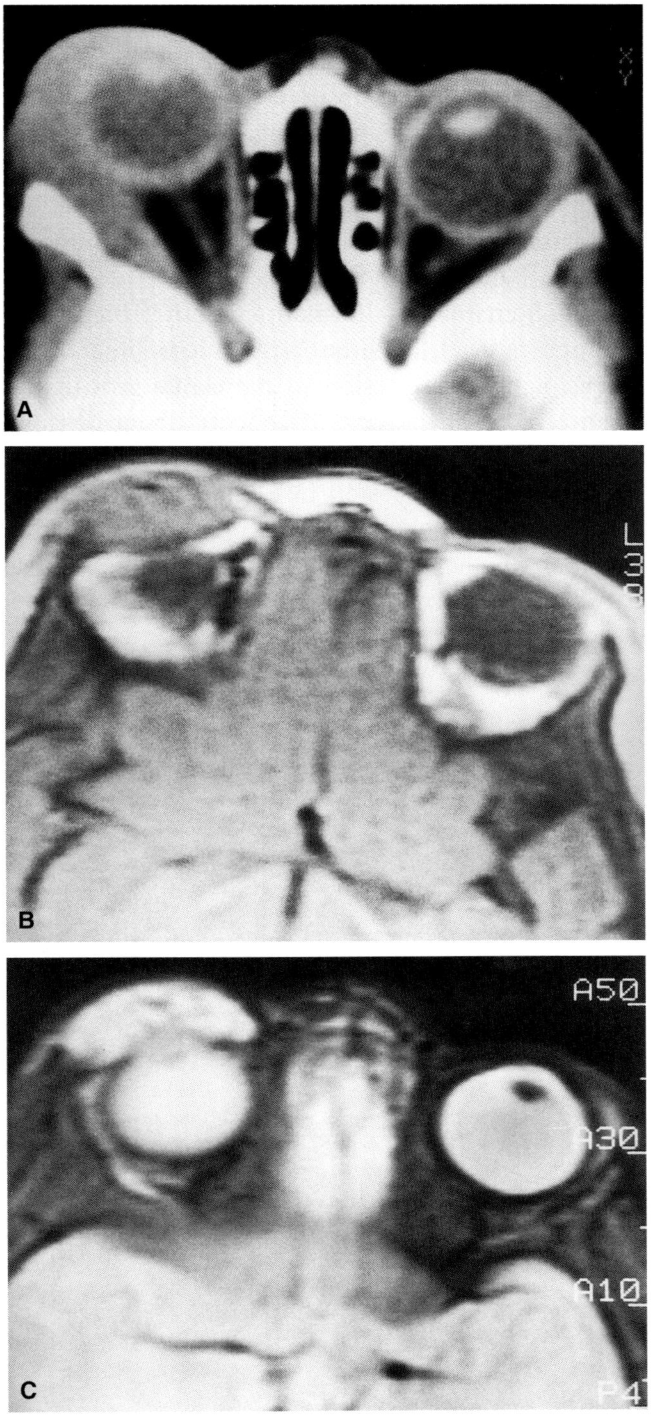

Figure 16–9. *A,* Axial CT scan of biopsy-proven capillary hemangioma. *B,* T_1-weighted axial MRI scan of capillary hemangioma of the lid and anterior orbit. *C,* T_2-weighted axial MRI scan. The T_1 and T_2 MRI patterns demonstrate the vascular nature of the lesion (see Table 15–2)

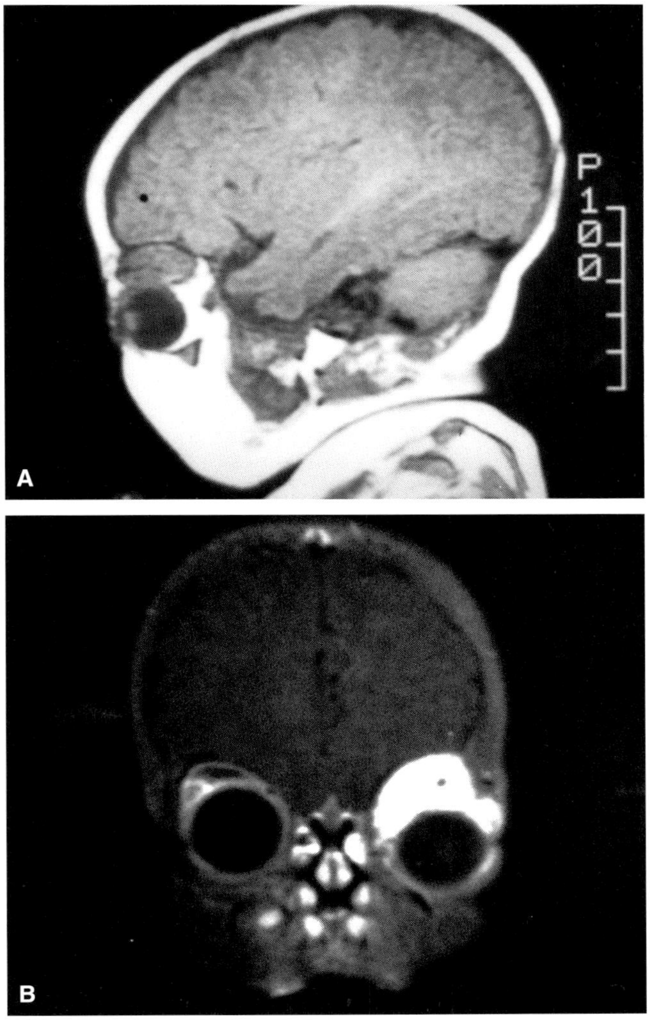

Figure 16–10. *A,* T_1-weighted axial MRI scan shows an isodense tumor. *B,* T_2-weighted direct coronal scan shows that the capillary hemangioma is hyperintense with regard to brain.

Although capillary hemangiomas are usually relatively diffuse, occasionally we and others have been able to remove most of the tumor with excellent cosmetic and visual results.[80] Figures 16–11A and B demonstrate a growing capillary hemangioma producing amblyopia. The tumor was resected (Figure 16–11C); after aggressive patching, the patient had good return of vision (Figure 16–11D). Plager and Sneider reported three patients who had total resections of their hemangiomas with resolution of the astigmia. Others had noted that approximately 16 percent had marked reduction of astigmia after intralesional steroids.[81]

An intriguing report of treatment using interferon alpha-2b in a massive tumor that had not responded to oral steroids was published.[82] This agent has been effective for hemangiomas in the respiratory system, but serious side effects have been reported.[83] We would use it only if the above options were not effective.[82] Very rarely, hemangiomas can involve the orbital bones; but only approximately a dozen cases have been reported.[83]

Cystic Infant Lesions

Cystic lesions of the orbit more commonly occur in slightly older children. We have seen 5 children who presented with neonatal hematic cysts.[84] Figure 16–12 demonstrates such a cyst on a direct parasagittal MRI scan. In all the neonatal deep orbital cysts we have observed, there was a history of either birth trauma, poor Apgar scores, or a hematologic abnormality. In 4 of the 5 cases, simple aspiration with a needle resulted in complete resolution. One case recurred and eventually required removal of the cyst and its lining.

Colobomatous malformations with orbital cysts are not rare in children with microphthalmos.[85] Occasionally, these lesions demonstrate growth and require removal because of concern about possible malignancy. Figure 16–13 shows the MRI and CT patterns of such a lesion in a child with microphthalmos with coloboma. While it is not always discernible whether or not an open connection exists between the microphthalmic eye and the contiguous

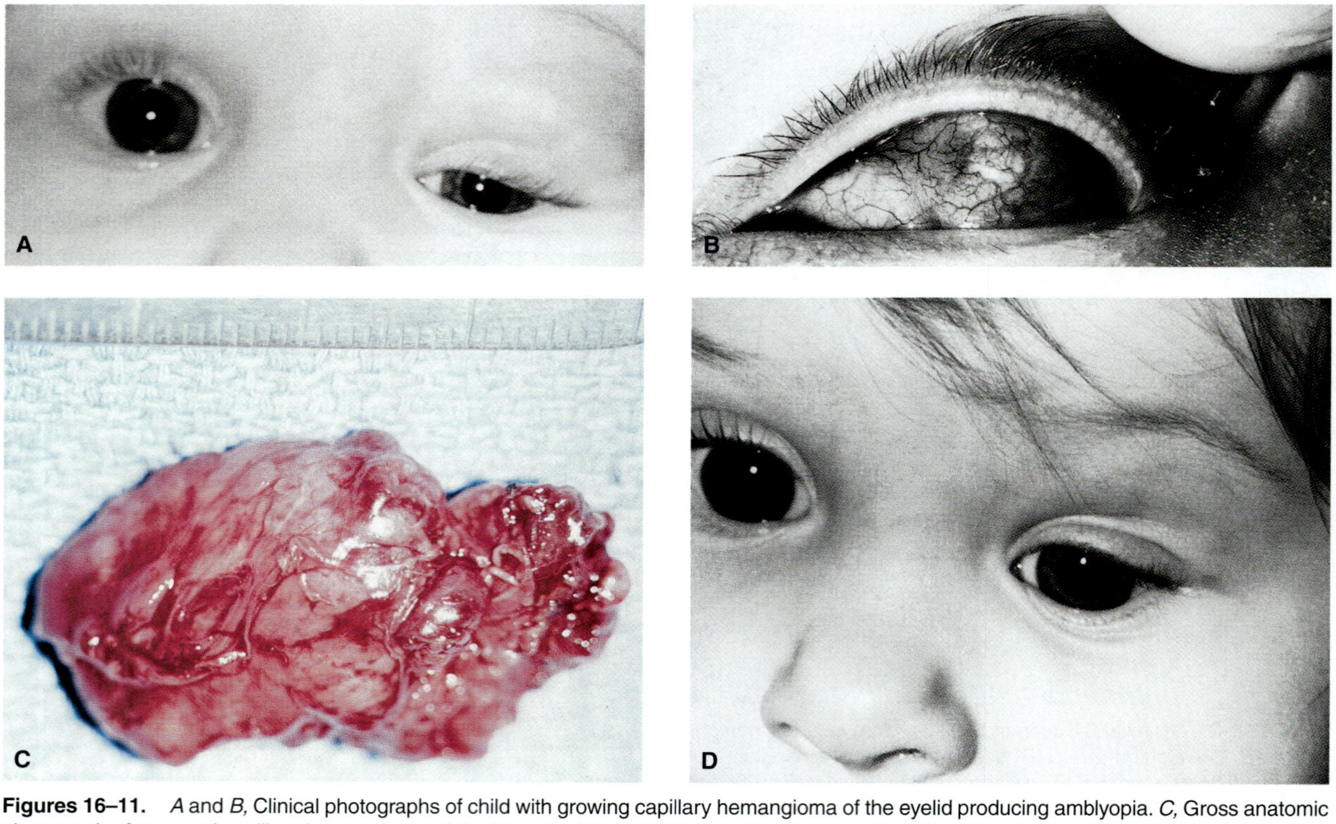

Figures 16–11. *A* and *B*, Clinical photographs of child with growing capillary hemangioma of the eyelid producing amblyopia. *C*, Gross anatomic photograph of removed capillary hemangioma of the lid and orbit. *D*, Child 1 month after resection of capillary hemangioma of the orbit.

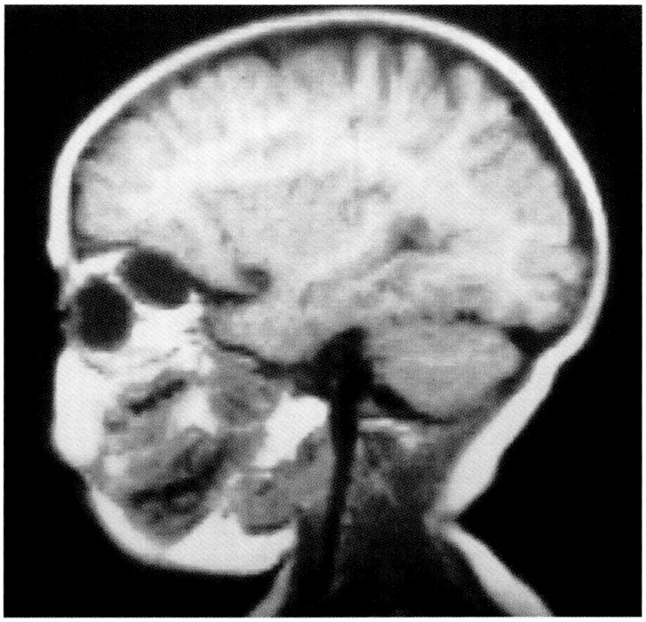

Figure 16–12. Direct sagittal MRI scan of a congenital neonatal orbital cyst.

cyst, we have been able to remove the cyst surgically and leave an intact eye (in terms of retaining space and not developing phthisis). Figure 16–14 shows an optic nerve coloboma, microphthalmos, and orbital cyst. Figure 16–15 shows an axial CT scan of a child thought to have the above clinical findings; however, both CT and histology demonstrated an enlarged cystic eye.

Orbital teratomas are relatively uncommon; only 60 cases have been reported.[86–90] This group of conditions is reviewed well elsewhere.[90,91] These teratomas are congenital tumors that consist of tissue derived from more than one layer. They usually present with sudden onset of proptosis in the neonatal or infant periods (Figure 16–16).[85–89] Teratomas of the orbit are usually benign but should be removed surgically to decrease the likelihood of continued orbital expansion or malignant transformation (a rare occurrence).[92] Even more rarely, ectopic brain tissue can occur in the orbit.

Encephaloceles can also present as orbital proptosis. However, on imaging, the direct connection with the CNS should be obvious.[93] A child with a meningocele and typical downward displacement of the globe is shown in Figure 16–17.

In older children, orbital dermoids most commonly occur in the lacrimal fossa. In young children, more often, there are anterior epidermoid cysts or superficial dermoids. An axial MRI scan shows such a lesion (Figure 16–18). These are almost always relatively hard, not fixed to bone, and not freely mobile (Figure 16–19). Most children with

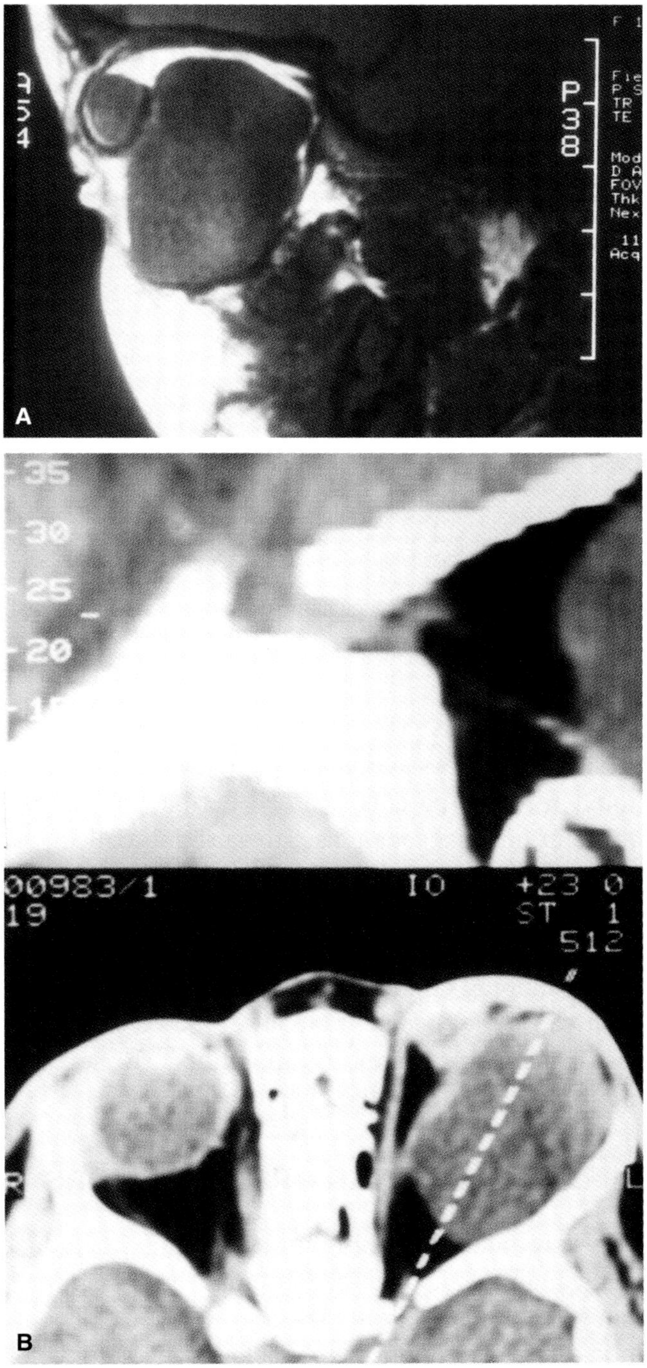

Figure 16–13. *A,* Parasagittal T_1-weighted MRI scan demonstrating large orbital cyst in a microphthalmic eye with coloboma. *B,* Axial CT scan with parasagittal reconstruction demonstrates large colobomatous cyst with microphthalmos.

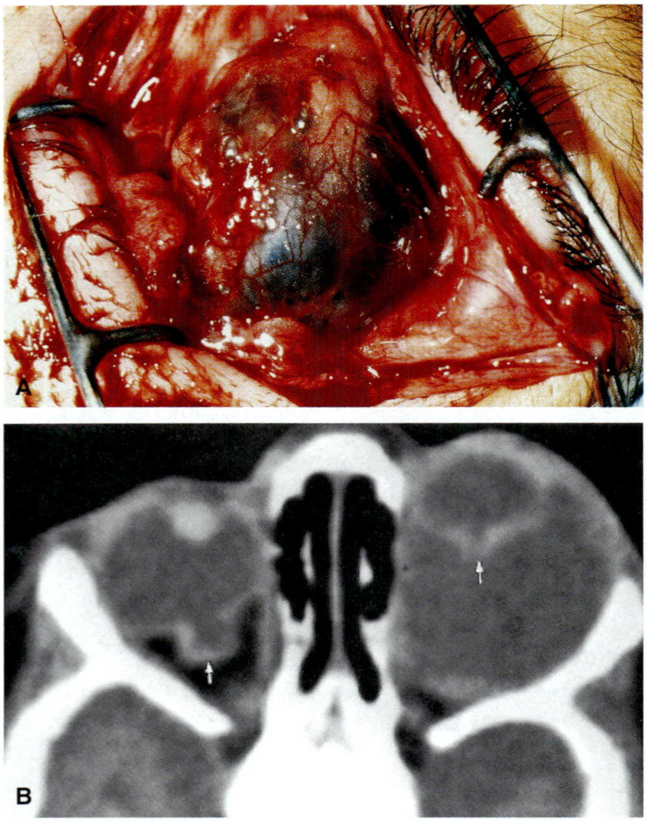

Figure 16–14. Operative photograph (*A*) and axial CT (*B*) showing bilateral ocular colobomas with a left retro-orbital cyst. Both optic nerves have a funnel-shaped abnormality (*arrows*). (From Char et al.,[226] with permission)

these lesions are asymptomatic and the lesions are noted by their parents. Rarely, dermoid cysts can occur in unusual locations; Howard and colleagues reported two cases where the tumor involved the lateral rectus muscle.[94] These can be removed with a simple excision.[95] In older children, especially from the developing countries, *Echinococcus* cysts of the orbit can rarely occur; in about 25 percent of these cases, there is systemic eosinophilia.[96] Bone cysts are discussed later in the chapter.

RARE PIGMENTED ORBITAL TUMORS

Very rare benign infantile orbital tumors, including congenital melanocytic hamartomas, have been previously reported (Figure 16–20).[97] Another uncommon pigmented tumor is the melanocytic neuroectodermal tumor of infancy (retinal anlage tumor).[98,99] These tumors usually arise in the anterior maxilla, and while they can be locally invasive, they do not

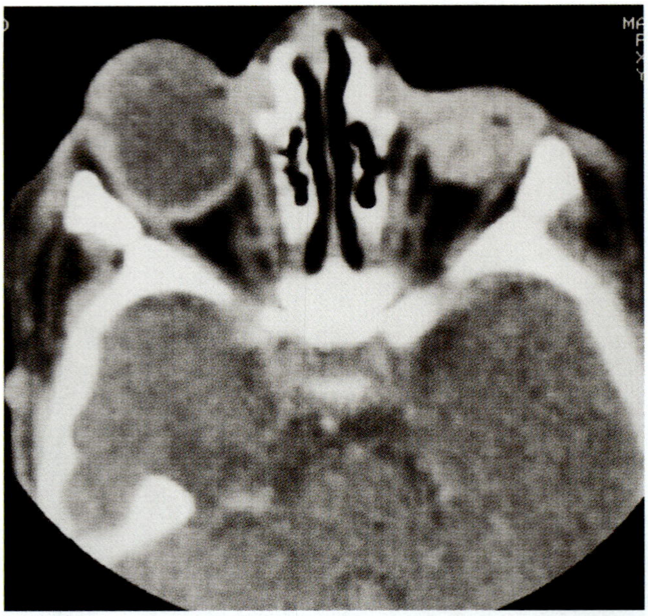

Figure 16–15. Axial CT scan of enlarged cystic eye in a neonate; the opposite eye is microphthalmic.

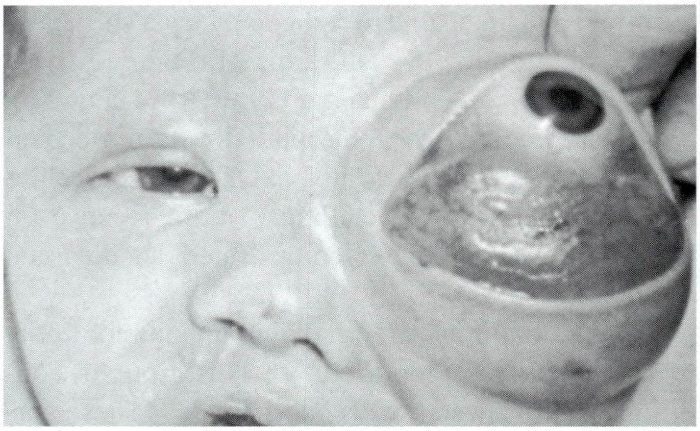

Figure 16–16. Orbital teratoma. (From Walsh FB, Hoyt WF. Clinical neuro-ophthalmology, 3rd ed. Baltimore, MD: Williams and Wilkins; 1969.)

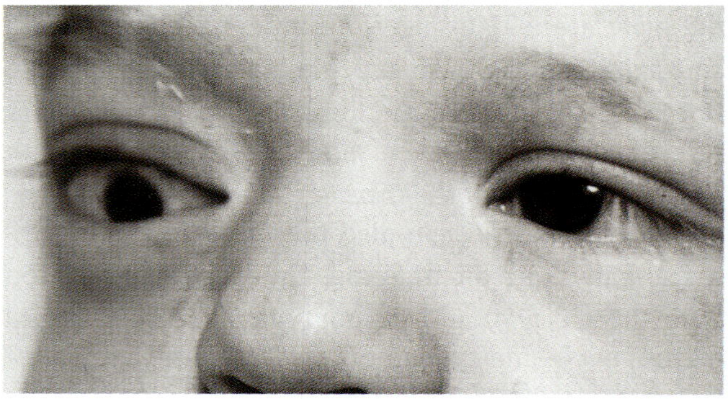

Figure 16–17. Meningoencephalocele produced inferior placement of the right globe. Typically, these lesions involve the superior nasal portion of the orbit.

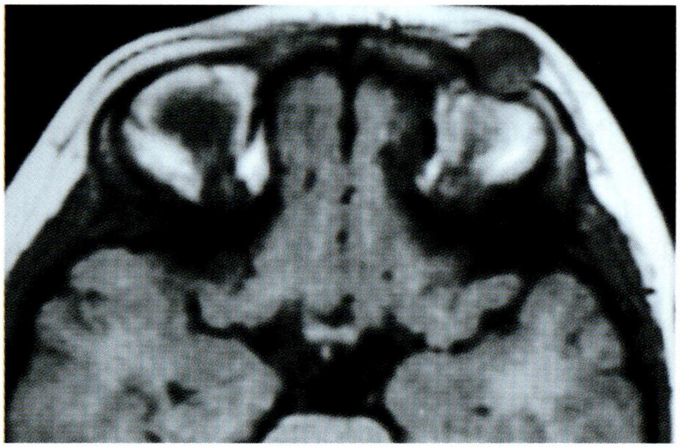

Figure 16–18. Axial MRI scan shows an anteriorly located dermoid cyst.

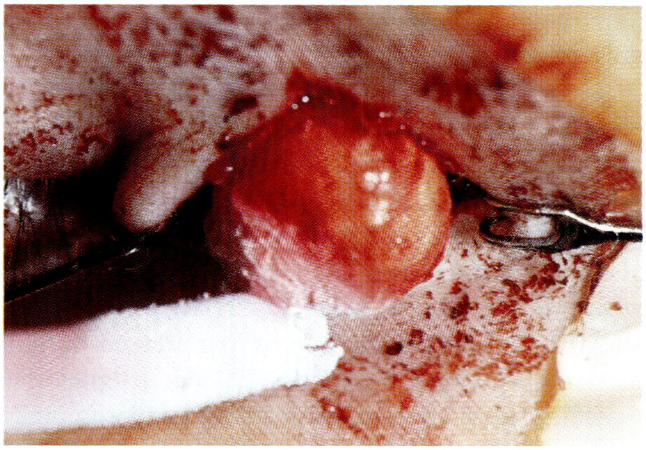

Figure 16–19. Anterior superficial dermoids.

metastasize. They occur almost exclusively in infants and can be cured with total resection. Rarely, congenital malignant melanomas can occur, and there have been 23 such reports at various body sites. A recent report documented a congenital melanoma that involved the orbit with multiple metastases.[100]

A number of other rare orbital tumors occur but are almost always diagnosed only on histologic examination. These include primitive neuroectodermal tumors, lipomas, hamartomas, giant cell tumors, efferent fibroglial choristomas, Zimmerman's tumor, malignant nerve sheath tumors, and primary endodermal sinus tumors.[101–107]

CHILDHOOD ORBITAL MALIGNANCIES

Rhabdomyosarcoma

Rhabdomyosarcoma is the most common primary orbital malignancy, and it accounts for 5 percent of all childhood malignancies.[108] It is the sixth most common cancer of childhood with an incidence of approximately four per million per year.[109] It is more common in Caucasian males. This tumor was first recognized to occur in the orbit in 1882.[110] The incidence of orbital involvement is variable.[111] Approximately 15 to 20 percent of rhabdomyosarcomas develop in the orbit, but some reports shows that as few as 7 percent or as many as 25 percent of primaries occur at this site.

A number of molecular biologic investigations have been performed on rhabdomyosarcoma. Often, there is a gene rearrangement between chromosomes 2 and 13, which involves the *PAX3* gene located on 2q35.[112] Other genomic changes have always been noted on chromosome 11.[113]

The mean age of presentation in orbital rhabdomyosarcoma is approximately 7.5 years, the range being birth to age 78 years.[114] In our experience, orbital rhabdomyosarcoma has a bimodal pattern, it presents at either < 3 years or > 6 years.

The most common presentations of orbital rhabdomyosarcoma are ptosis or lid mass in 48 percent, proptosis in 27 percent, suspected trauma in 13 percent, or conjunctival mass in 5 percent (Figure 16–21).[115,116] Most often, a mass develops in the superior nasal quadrant of the orbit, and the tumor on CT or MRI usually appears to be in or contiguous to an orbital muscle.[117] Palpation of the mass is not revealing; some are fibrous or compressible from

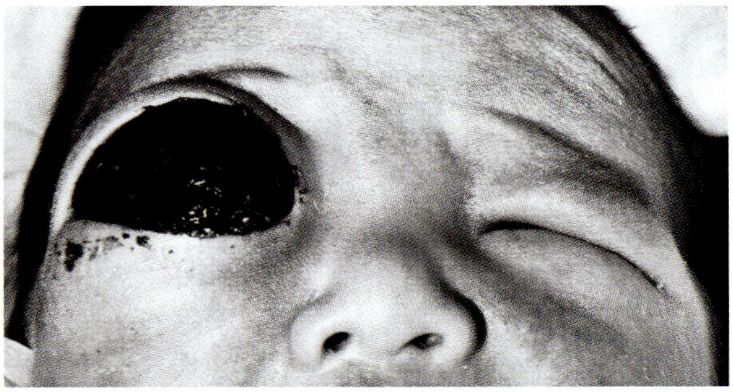

Figure 16–20. Congenital melanocytic hamartoma that enlarged the orbit and destroyed the eye. (With permission from Char DH, Crawford JB, Ablin AR, et al. Orbital melanocytic hamartoma. Am J Ophthalmol 1981;91:357–61).

intratumor hemorrhage. Rarely, these tumors can present with nasolacrimal duct obstructions.[118]

Most rhabdomyosarcomas have both rapid onset and progression of orbital proptosis. Figure 16–22 demonstrates how rapidly these tumors can grow. The CT scans in Figures 16–22A and B, taken when the patient first presented to the local ophthalmologist, demonstrate an orbital mass. Three days later, when we first saw the child (Figure 16–22C and D), an MRI showed the eye almost compressed to half its normal volume. Figure 16–23 demonstrates the typical surgical appearance of a rhabdomyosarcoma. Its texture and color are quite different from those of either lymphangioma (see Figure 16–35) or capillary hemangioma (Figure 16–11C).

The evaluation of patients with suspected orbital rhabdomyosarcoma includes either CT with computer reconstruction or MRI. At present, high-quality MRI or CT scans are appropriate.[117] We still prefer to detect bone invasion with CT. Vascular channels are often present in rhabdomyosarcomas and can result in enhancement on CT.[119] Bone windows on CT are essential because they can demonstrate bony involvement. Figure 16–24 shows a case of rhabdomyosarcoma involving the orbital roof. Most commonly, tumor-related mortality associated with orbital rhabdomyosarcoma occurs as a result of contiguous spread into the CNS.[120] Involvement of the orbital bones is a poor prognostic sign.[116,121] In a historic series of 29 cases reported by Letterman in 1976, 17 died, and the most common cause of death was contiguous spread of tumor into the middle fossa and the cranium.[121] As discussed below, survival has improved even in these patients.[122] Occasionally, the tumor can metastasize to the lung.

Treatment has markedly improved over the last 25 years.[122–125] In 1966, Jones and co-workers reported a 45 percent cure rate of orbital rhabdomyosarcoma with aggressive surgery, usually exenteration.[126] More recently, over 90 percent of tumors can be controlled with a combination of surgical debulking, approximately 50 gray (Gy) of external beam megavoltage photon irradiation and chemotherapy, depending on stage, using vincristine, cyclophosphamide, and Adriamycin.[111,116,127–133] If the patient remains tumor free for over 3 years after diagnosis, recurrence is extremely unlikely.[128] Even with refractory orbital rhabdomyosarcomas, long-term survival can be excellent.[134] The most recent intergroup rhabdomyosarcoma study showed equally good survival without the use of alkalizing agents.[122,133]

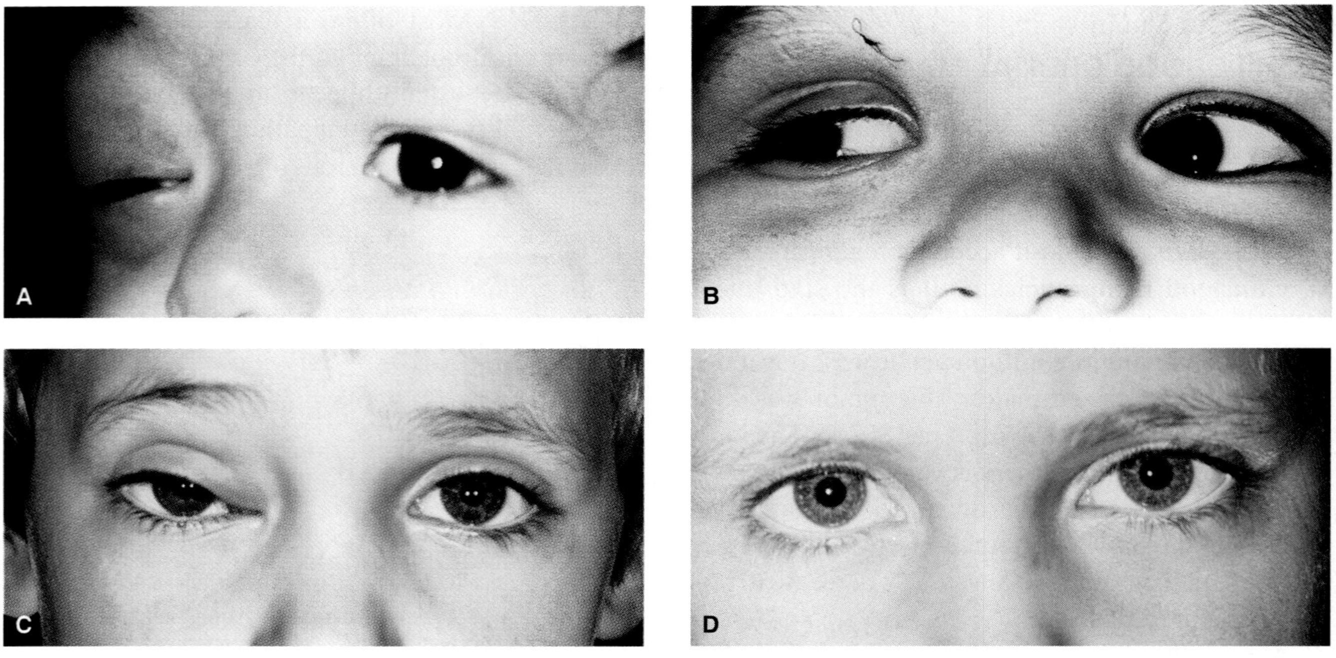

Figure 16–21. *A,* Pretherapy view of proptosis and lid swelling as initial manifestations of orbital rhabdomysarcoma. *B,* View after debulking, irradiation, and chemotherapy. *C,* Pretreatment photograph. *D,* Post-treatment photograph of another case treated in a similar fashion.

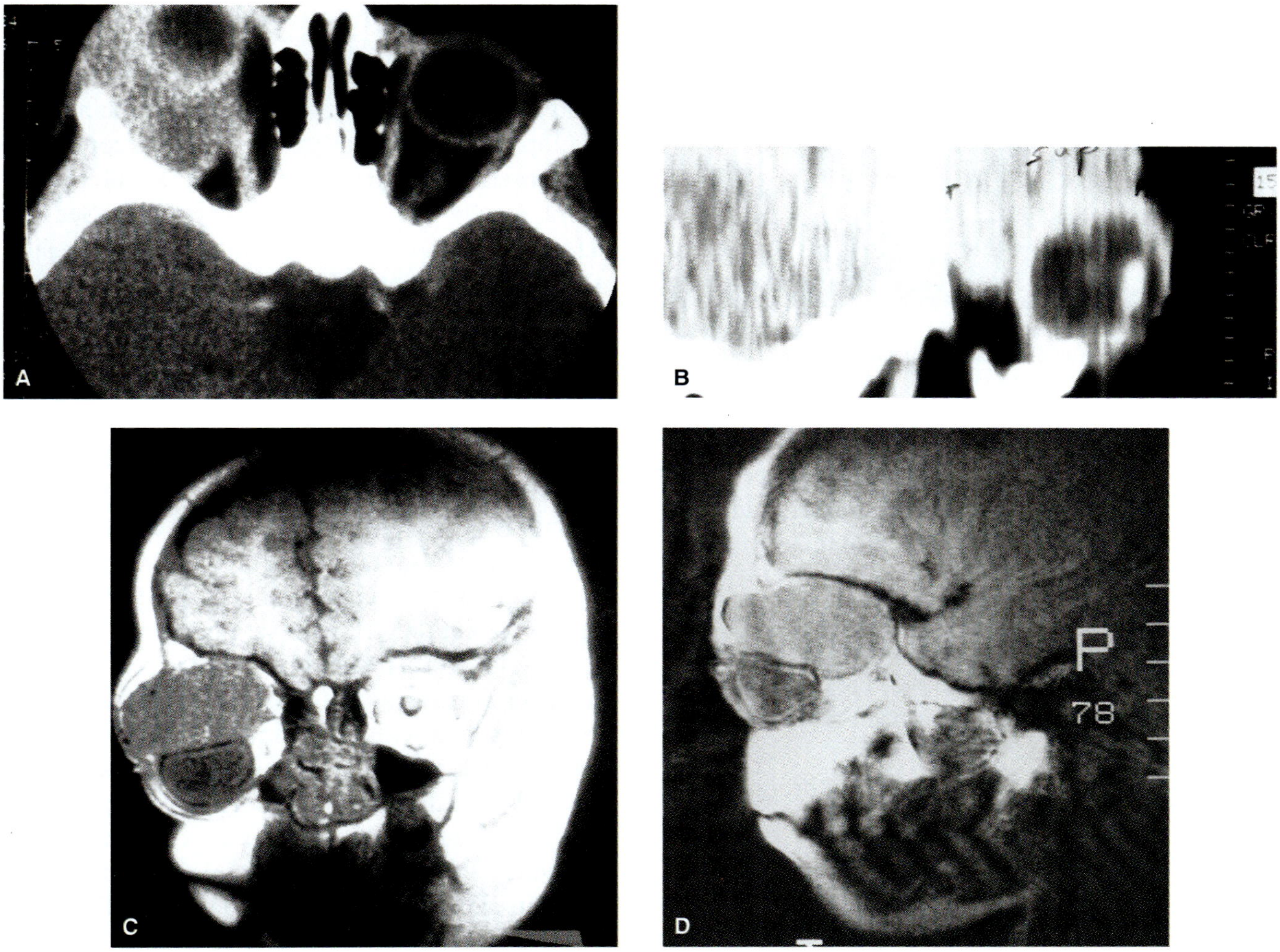

Figure 16–22. *A*, Axial CT scan from referring institution demonstrating rhabdomyosarcoma of the orbit. *B*, Re-formation of the scan demonstrating rhabdomyosarcoma of the orbit. *C*, Direct coronal T_1-weighted MRI scan 3 days later. *D*, Parasagittal MRI scans were obtained 3 days after the CT scan in *A* and *B* demonstrating very rapid development of globe compression by the rhabdomyosarcoma.

Treatment of orbital rhabdomyosarcoma with a combination of surgical debulking, chemotherapy, and radiation, has historically been associated with a significant morbidity.[124,135–139] In one series, 3 of 9 patients developed significant corneal ulcers.[127] Abramson and co-workers reported that approximately 33 percent of eyes eventually were enucleated.[116] In a later report, this group noted that 21 of 32 eyes were functionless (enucleated or blind), and only 2 had 20/50 or better vision.[138] Heyn and colleagues observed 95 percent survival with orbital rhabdomyosarcoma, but cataract and lacrimal duct stenosis were common complications.[135] Ninety percent of patients developed cataracts on long-term follow-up, and 50 percent developed bony orbital

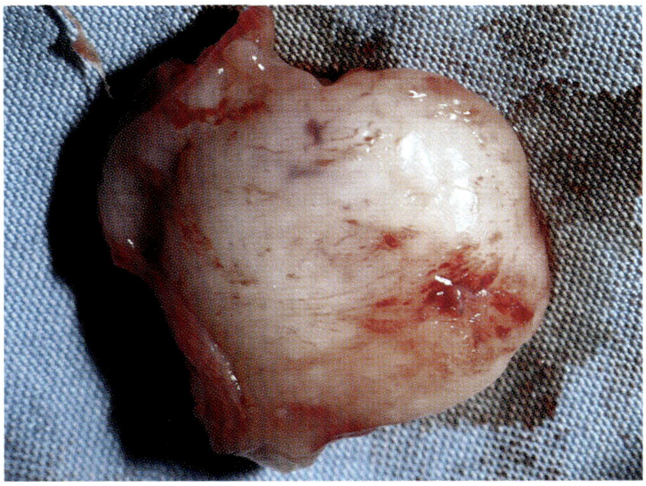

Figure 16–23. View of a resected rhabdomyosarcoma. These tumors are typically whitish fibrous masses.

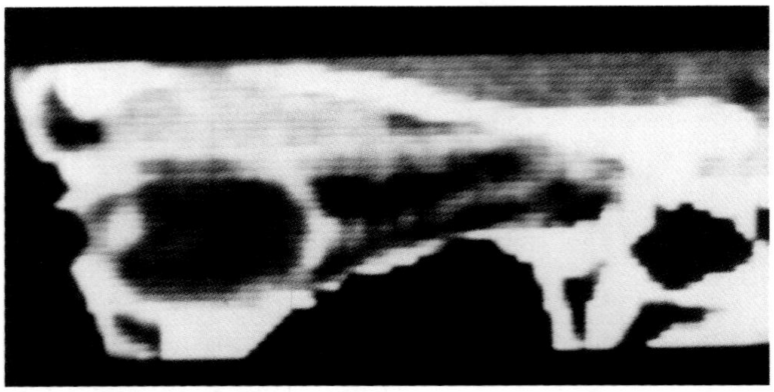

Figure 16–24. Parasagittal re-formation of orbital CT showing rhabdomyosarcoma with erosion through the bony orbital roof.

hypoplasia.[139] Radiation retinopathy can also develop. While cataracts eventually occurred in almost all cases of rhabdomyosarcoma, radiation retinopathy is less common (approximately 33%). Orbital bone hypoplasia is common only in young children (and less so in children > 7 years old at the time of diagnosis). While some favorable prognostic groups, including orbital tumors, have been treated without irradiation, there have been more treatment failures in those cases.[140]

We have not lost any eyes with orbital rhabdomyosarcoma. Additive ocular morbidity associated with the use of both chemotherapy and irradiation must be borne in mind when planning treatment of these patients.[135,138] As discussed in later chapters, the use of newer radiation approaches, including intensity modulated, conformal therapy, should markedly decrease the incidence of complication noted by Heyn and others. In some of these difficult cases, the use of brachytherapy has been advocated, although the author has not had experience with it in this setting and believes that conformal therapy will be much more applicable.[141,142.]

Some young children have undifferentiated sarcomas that may be rhabdomyosarcoma but which cannot be definitely diagnosed on either light or electron microscopy.[143] These neoplasms are treated like rhabdomyosarcoma. Rarely, a rhabdomyosarcoma will metastasize to the orbit or develop in another intraocular site.[144,145,150] A malignant ectomesenchymoma is a variant of this tumor.[146] A few cases of malignant rhabdoid tumors have been described in young children.[147] A few reports of FNAB diagnosis for recurrent sarcomas in the orbit have been published.[148]

Miscellaneous Sarcomas

In the pediatric age group, other sarcomas rarely involve the orbit. Most commonly, children who develop either orbital osteogenic sarcomas or leiomyosarcomas have had bilateral retinoblastoma approximately 10 years previously.[149–151] (See the chapter on retinoblastoma treatment for discussion of osteogenic sarcoma.) Any child with a history of a bilateral retinoblastoma should have yearly bone scans and evaluation by a pediatric oncologist. Any orbital swelling or pain in these children should call for prompt evaluation with either CT or MRI and, if a lesion is noted, a biopsy. Juvenile fibrosarcoma has been reported in the orbit, but it is much less common.[152] The mean age of these patients is approximately 4 years. In contradistinction to the adult fibrosarcoma, in the pediatric age group, most patients fare quite well with surgical resection.

Alveolar soft part sarcoma usually occurs in the second or third decade of life, and we have managed some teenagers with this tumor. A review by Font and co-workers noted that the mean age was 23 years.[153] In that series, 3 of the 17 patients developed metastases, and the preferred treatment for disease confined to the orbit was surgical resection. We have had experience with one such case. Typically, these lesions are firmly attached to a muscle and are yellowish-white in color with overlying engorged vasculature.[154–156] They are managed with a combination of surgical debulking and radiation. On CT, these lesions can simulate cavernous hemangioma, as seen in Figure 16–25.[157]

Malignant fibrous histiocytomas can also occur in the orbit in pediatric patients. These lesions generally are relatively diffuse, and clinically, they are not diagnosed until histologic inspection of the tumor.[158] (See chapter on intraconal tumors for a discussion of histiocytomas.) A benign variant, nodular fasciitis, has been reported in children, although it is more common in adults.[159]

CHILDHOOD SECONDARY ORBITAL MALIGNANCIES

Retinoblastoma can occasionally present either primarily as an orbital cellulitis or as a recurrence in the orbit. Figure 12–25 in the retinoblastoma chap-

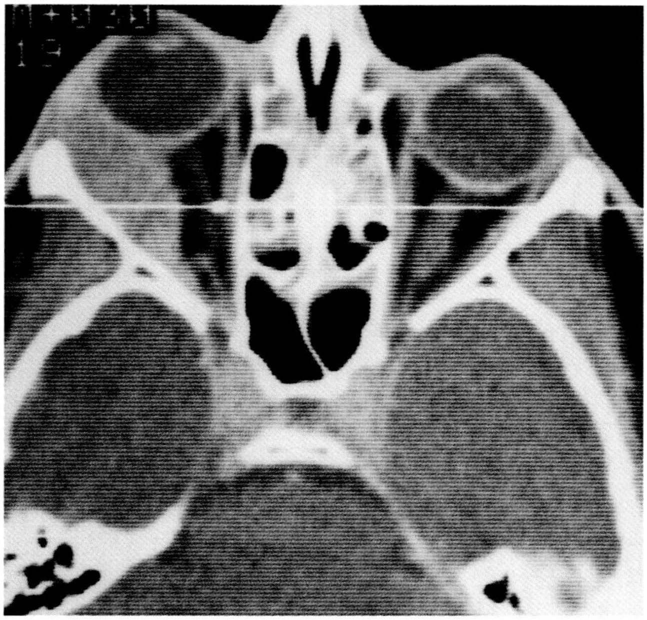

Figure 16–25. Orbital axial CT scan of biopsy-proven alveolar soft part sarcoma.

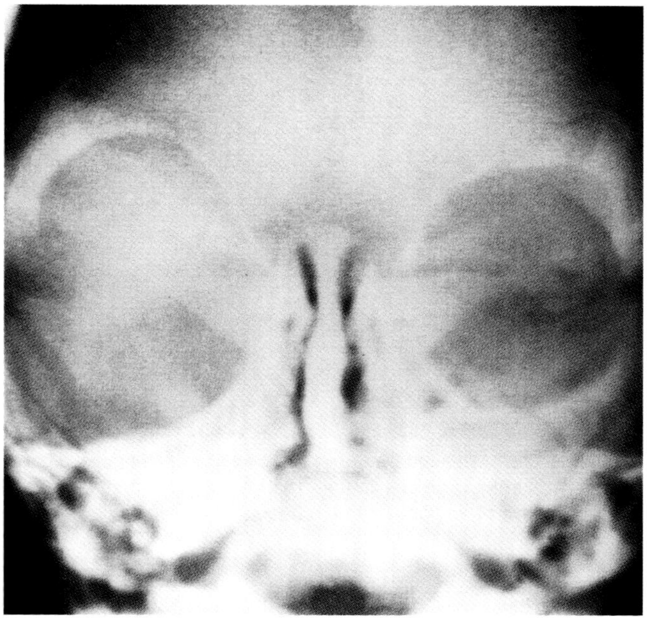

Figure 16–26. Orbital expansion secondary to lymphangioma. Any chronic expansile benign childhood orbital tumor can produce this pattern.

ter shows an orbital recurrence of retinoblastoma. As mentioned previously, esthesioneuroblastoma can secondarily involve the orbit. We have also observed children with systemic lymphomas and leukemias who developed preseptal orbital involvement (see Figure 16–5). As previously discussed, a number of metastases can develop in the orbit.

Benign Vascular Tumors of Childhood

Capillary hemangiomas of the orbit usually present within the first few months of life, although rarely they can become manifest at a slightly older age. In a patient > 2 years old, this diagnosis is extremely unlikely. Cavernous hemangiomas are rarely diagnosed in the first decade of life; this tumor occurs much more often in older patients (see chapter on intraconal tumors). The most frequent orbital vascular tumor presenting in children is lymphangioma. This orbital tumor was first recognized in 1868, and it accounts for 1.5 to 7 percent of orbital lesions.[71,160,161] Often, the orbit is expanded as shown in Figure 16–26; any longstanding benign orbital process in early childhood can produce this picture.

The etiology, pathogenesis, and pathophysiology of orbital lymphangiomas are controversial, and Wright has questioned the terminology used to discuss this entity.[162] What have been called lymphangiomas probably include some of these tumors and also some cases of orbital varices or other venous system malformations.[163–166]

An orbital varix with bleeding after trauma is shown in Figure 16–27. Usually such children present with acute proptosis after sustaining relatively minor facial trauma. Similarly, children with orbital varices often have marked increase in exophthalmos, with a Valsalva maneuver. Figure 16–28 shows a

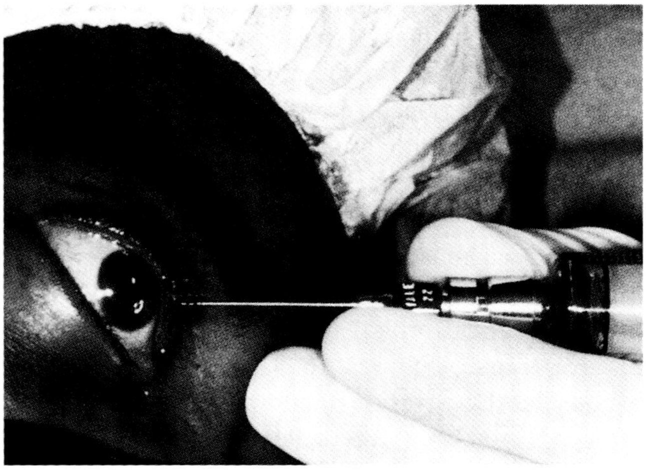

Figure 16–27. Evacuation with a syringe of an orbital varix with bleeding secondary to trauma.

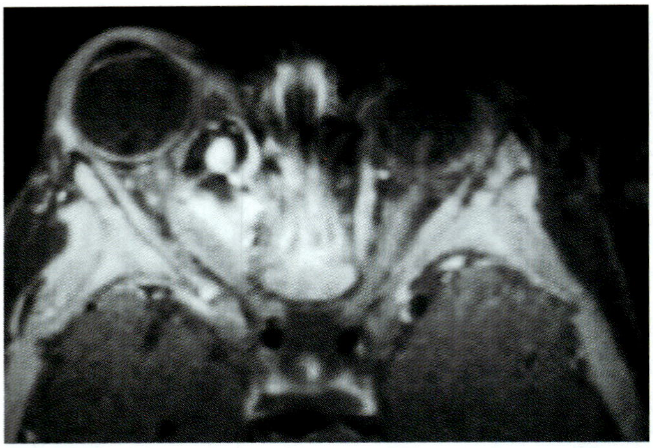

Figure 16–28. This was a large, high flow, arteriovenous malformation. At surgery portions of the orbit had findings that were very typical for a lymphangioma with a "chocolate- like" lobulated cysts.

large arteriovenous malformation that had some orbital features of a lymphangioma noted at surgery. Specifically the "chocolate-filled" cysts can be a secondary effect of massive bleeding or can develop in a lesion that has lymphoid elements.

Prior to 1959, only 34 cases of lymphangiomas were reported; Jones added 62 cases to the literature at that time.[167] He noted that approximately 25 percent of orbital lymphangiomas involved only the orbit, 33 percent only the conjunctiva, and 21 percent more than one adnexal structure.

Lymphangiomas occur three times more frequently in females than in males, and all 19 cases reported by Iliff and Green occurred in the first decade of life.[168] Lymphangiomas are usually diffuse and often start either in the superior nasal or inferior orbit, presenting either as a gradual onset of orbital proptosis or as acute orbital swelling during or after a viral upper respiratory infection.[169]

In our experience, lymphangiomas are usually diffuse lesions with multiloculated orbital chocolate-colored cysts. An example of an axial CT scan of an orbital lymphangioma is shown in Figure 16–29. Occasionally, these lesions are either confined to the conjunctiva (Figure 16–30), or they may produce a focal orbital tumor, if seen early in the disease course (Figures 16–31 and 16–32). These lesions can have various patterns on MRI scans. If there has not been recent hemorrhage, they often enhance with gadolinium and are hyperintense to brain on T_2-weighted images. If there is hemorrhage,

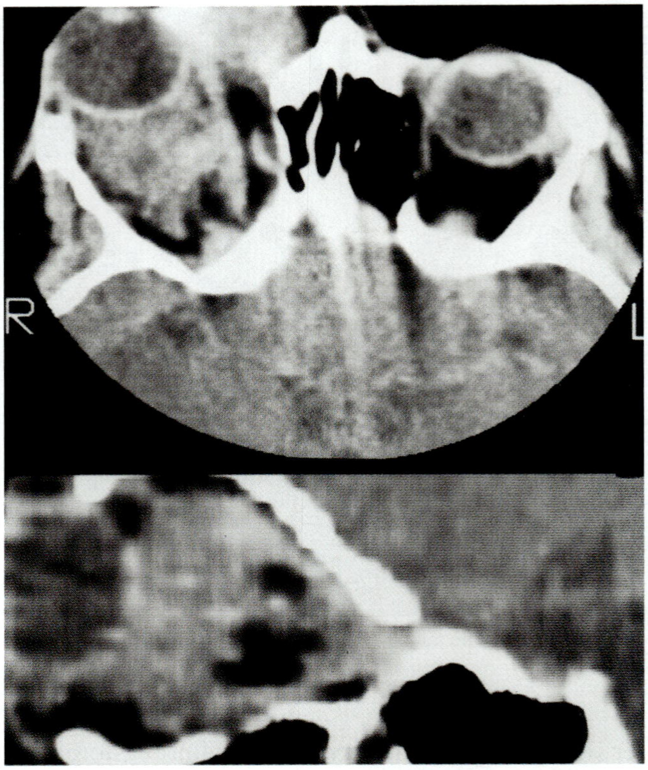

Figure 16–29. Axial CT scan and parasagittal reconstruction showing diffuse orbital lymphangioma with intraconal and extraconal involvement but without invasion of bone.

often there is a variegated color in areas, and the pattern depends on when the bleeding occurred in relationship to the scan. (Figure 16–33). The author has removed three focal orbital lymphangiomas without recurrence. It has been the author's clinical impression that these generally present more often in younger patients than do diffuse lymphangiomas. All three patients presented with proptosis. Rarely, these are first seen in older patients, as in the 60-year-old female shown in Figure 16–34.

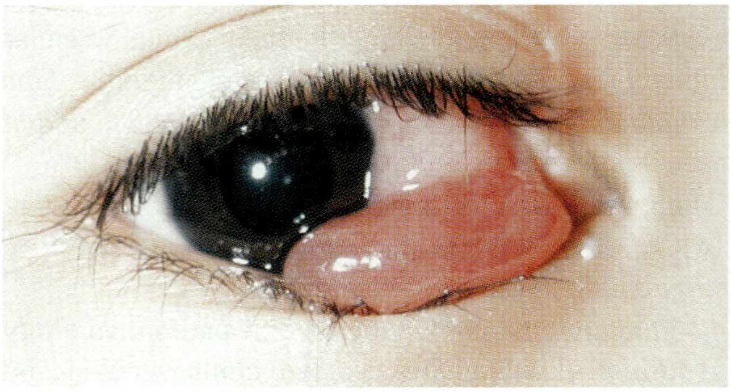

Figure 16–30. Conjunctival lymphangioma.

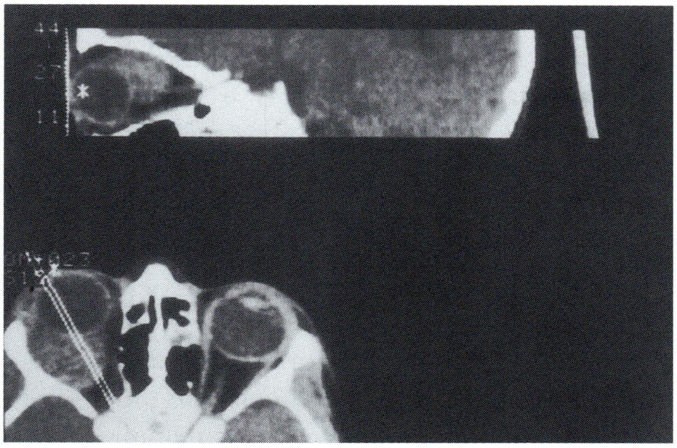

Figure 16–31. Focal biopsy-proven lymphangioma of the orbit on axial CT scan and parasagittal reconstruction.

Rootman and co-workers classified their orbital lymphangiomas into those which are superficial, deep, or diffuse. Most lymphangiomas are diffuse at the time of presentation.[170] Some of these diffuse lesions can be surgically debulked, and in some cases, the carbon dioxide laser has been used to remove portions of the tumor.[171] MRI has been helpful in these cases to determine whether there is an active flow component or varix associated with the lymphangiomas.[172,173] On MRI scans, in a case with hemorrhage, there are areas that are both hyperintense and hypointense to brain on T_1- and T_2-weighted images (Figures 16–35A and B).

Rarely, as discussed above, a lymphangioma-like pattern can also be associated with a large arteriovenous malformation.[174] In the author's experience, the management of children with diffuse orbital lym-

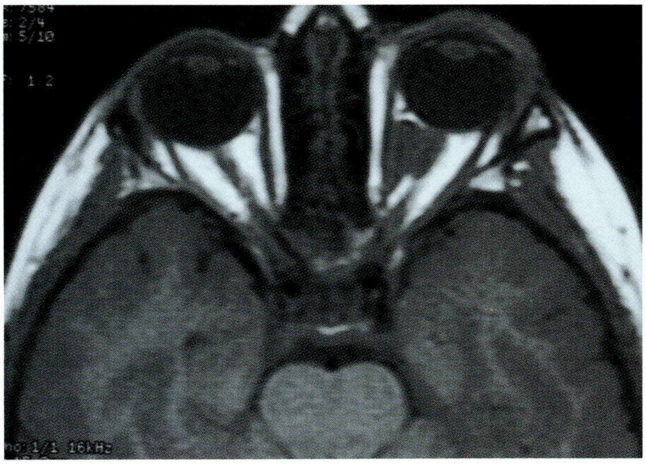

Figure 16–32. Axial MRI scan shows a focal lymphangioma.

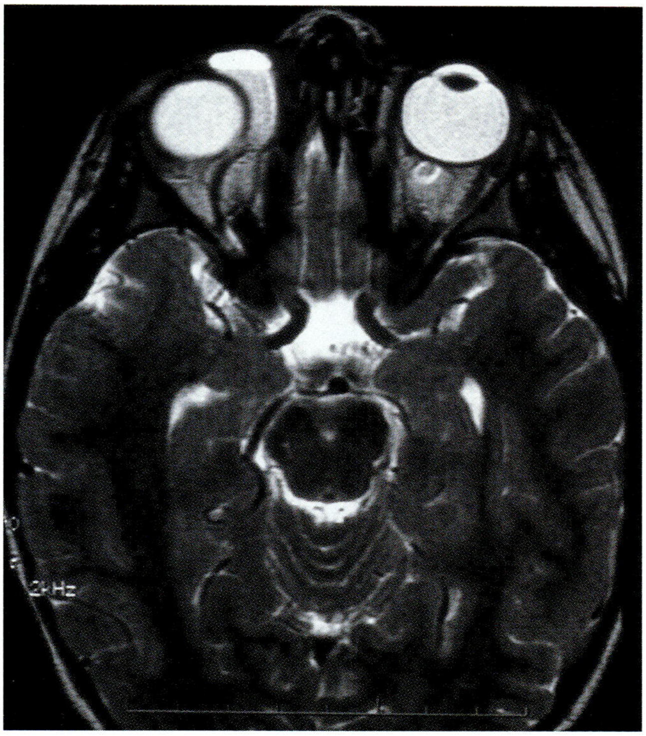

Figure 16–33. Lymphangiomas that have not recently bled often enhance with gadolinium and are hyperintense to brain on T_2-weighted images, as shown here.

phangiomas is often unsatisfactory. The tumor shown in Figure 16–36 was so diffuse and loculated that only portions could be removed. The presence of this lesion almost invariably results in bony enlargement of the orbit and significant cosmetic defect.

We have recently published our results with 26 orbital lymphangioma patients. These cases excluded any patient who had a vascular flow abnormality on imaging.[175] In approximately 75 percent, cosmetically satisfactory results were obtained. Patients who presented with restriction of extraocular movement often had more diffuse lesions and a poorer outcome.

Occasionally, orbital lymphangiomas become so massive that they destroy the eye and produce intractable pain necessitating exenteration. Rose and Wright described 16 benign orbital lesions that required exenteration for either pain or exposure.[176] An example of such a poor prognosis lymphangioma is shown in Figure 16–37. This patient had a 10-year history of a growing lymphangioma. Despite multiple resections, eventually the eye became painful and lost all light perception, and an exenteration was performed. The preoperative CT scan is shown in

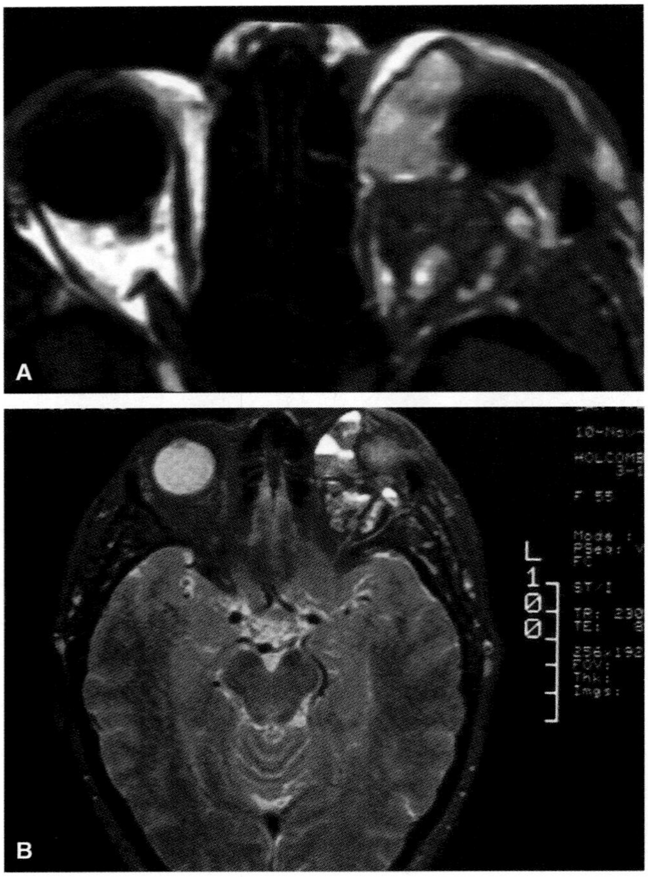

Figure 16–34. Lymphangioma presented at age 60 years. *A,* T_1-weighted axial MRI scan. *B,* T_2-weighted axial MRI scan.

Figure 16–38. After exenteration and closure with a temporalis skin flap, the patient and her family were much relieved and the patient's personality improved markedly. More commonly, orbital lymphangiomas either stabilize or show some regression in the second decade of life.

INFLAMMATORY LESIONS

Orbital pseudotumor is discussed in the chapter on orbital pseudotumors. We have seen children as young as age 6 years present with orbital myositis, a diffuse lymphoid lesion, or a lacrimal mass (Figure 16–39). The evaluation of these children is similar to that of adults. Pseudorheumatoid nodule is another variant of orbital inflammatory disease, which can present in children in the first decade of life. On ultrasonography, these lesions have a pattern consistent with a pseudotumor, and the diagnosis can be confirmed on histologic evaluation. Usually, these involve the lateral aspect of the upper lid.[177] Pediatric pseudotumors diagnosed by FNAB biopsy have been reported.[178] Rarer lesions which have some inflammatory component include nodular fasciitis, periorbital inflammatory myofibromatosis, and a giant cell repair of granuloma.[179–181]

LANGERHANS' CELL HISTIOCYTOSIS

Histiocytic disorders of the orbit involve a spectrum of Langerhans' cell proliferations. The older terminology, including eosinophilic granuloma, Hand-Schuller-Christian disease, and Letterer-Siwe disease, has been replaced by the classification into unifocal or multifocal eosinophilic granuloma of bone, diffuse histiocytosis-X, and malignant histiocytosis.[182,183] More recently the Histiocyte Society has suggested the term Langerhans' cell histiocytosis to encompass all these diseases.[184] The etiology

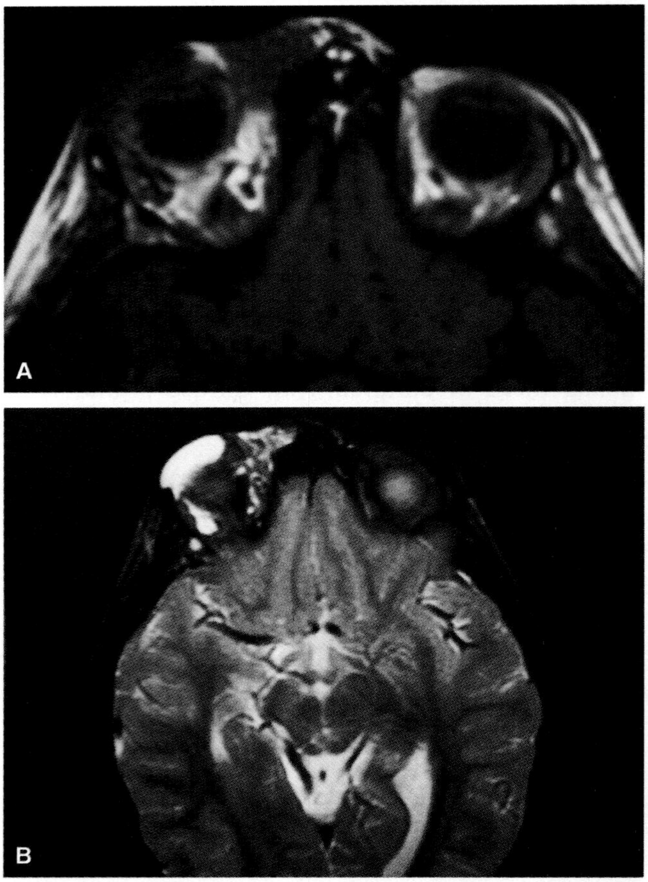

Figure 16–35. *A,* T_1-weighted image of a lymphangioma that had hemorrhage associated with tumor. *B,* T_2-weighted image of the case shown in Figure 16–35A.

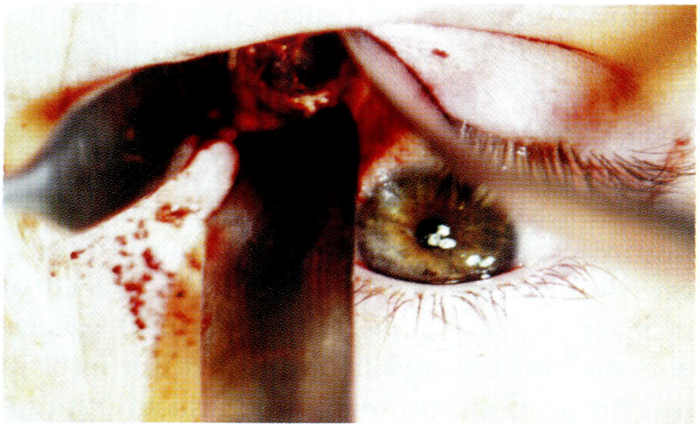

Figure 16–36. Loculated chocolate cysts diffusely involve the orbit in most lymphangiomas.

for these abnormal proliferations of Langerhans' cells is unknown.

The entire group of histiocytic disorders of the orbit account for < 1 percent of orbital tumors.[182,185–189] Unifocal eosinophilic granuloma consists of a single bone lesion. Often, this involves the lacrimal fossa area.[173,182] Clinically, the presentation of an eosinophilic granuloma is relatively typical. Usually, these patients present with an upper outer quadrant orbital swelling with pain (Figure 16–40). The differential diagnosis would include a ruptured dermoid cyst producing inflammation, an orbital pseudotumor, or metastasis; either CT or plain film radiography demonstrates a focal lytic bone lesion. The radiographic pattern is relatively typical and is characterized by smooth, clearly punched-out areas with surrounding sclerosis (Figure 16–41A). These radiographic findings are distinct from osteomas, metastatic tumors, rhabdomyosarcoma, dermoid cysts, or osteomyelitis.[189]

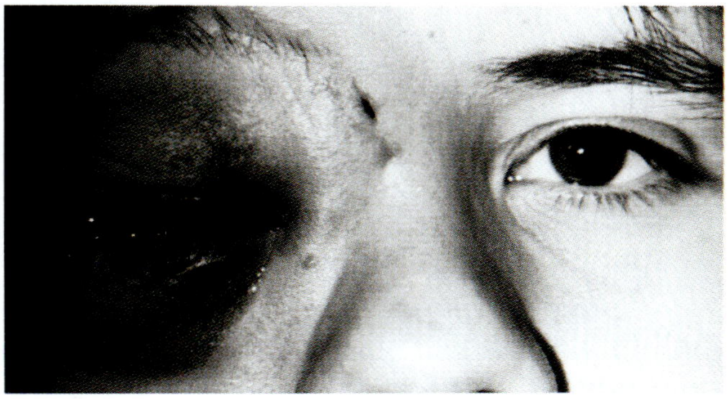

Figure 16–37. A poor-prognosis lymphangioma; this lesion evidently destroyed vision and the eye.

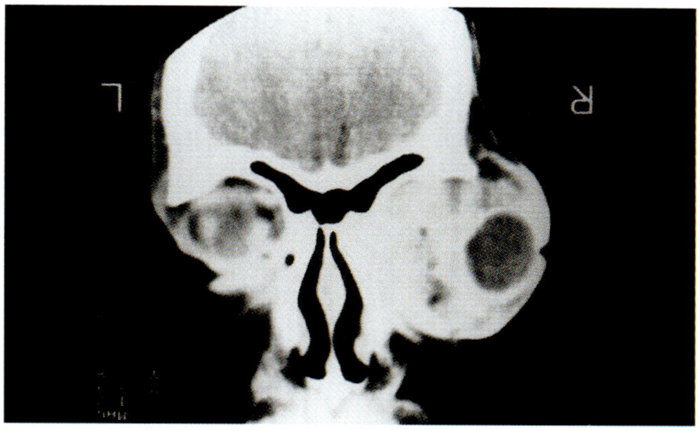

Figure 16–38. CT scan of the case shown in Figure 16–37, demonstrating a very large lymphangioma that destroyed vision and became painful, necessitating exenteration.

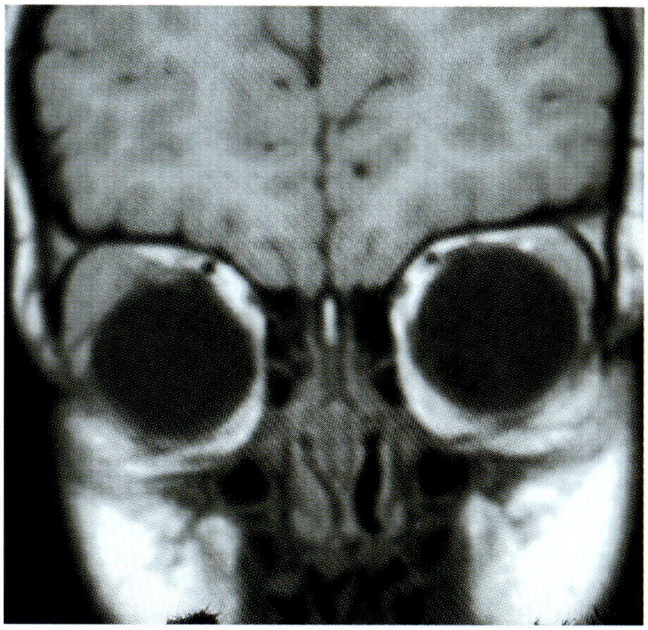

Figure 16–39. Direct coronal MRI scan demonstrating lacrimal gland involvement by a lymphoid process in a 6-year-old child.

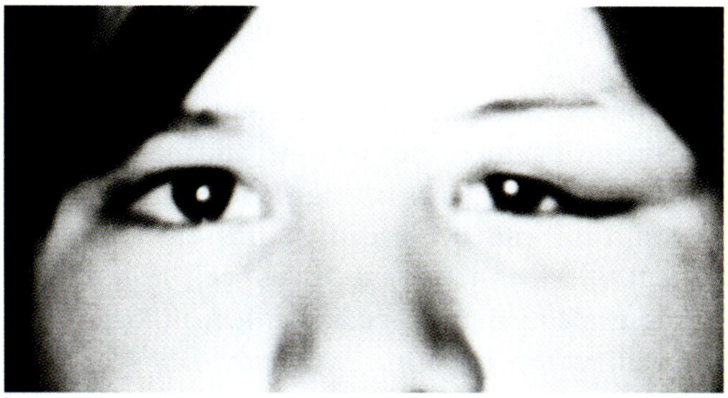

Figure 16–40. Clinical photograph of unifocal eosinophilic granuloma of bone involving the lateral orbital rim.

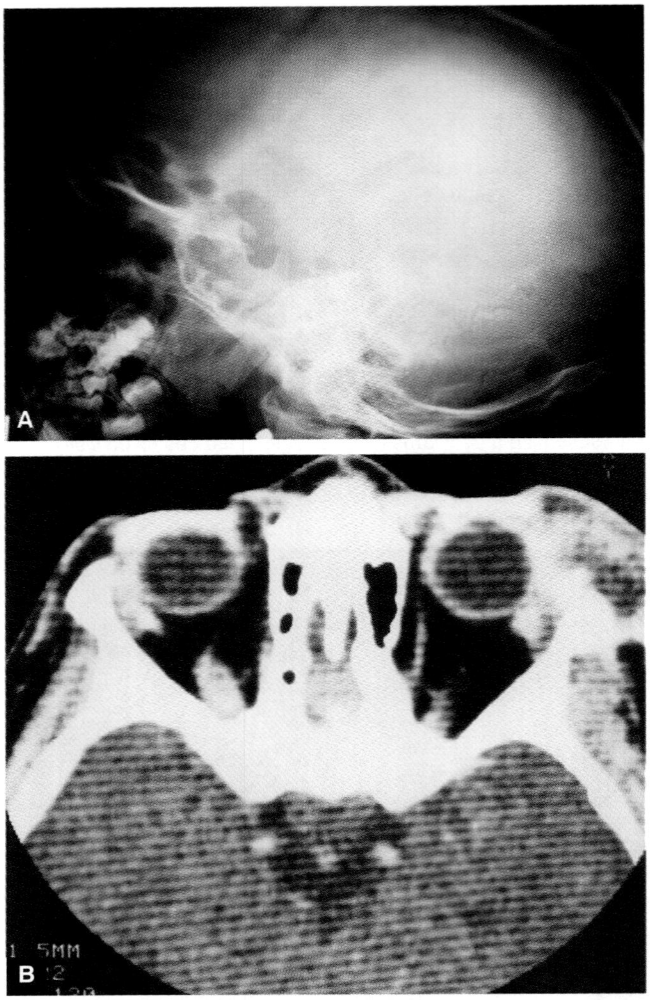

Figure 16–41. *A,* Plain skull film demonstrates smooth punched-out area with surrounding sclerosis, typical of unifocal eosinophilic granuloma. *B,* CT scan demonstrating bone destruction with lateral orbital swelling.

The CT pattern of a unifocal eosinophilic granuloma is shown in Figure 16–41B. Occasionally, the bone destruction is more widespread, as shown in Figure 16–42, in a patient with diffuse or multifocal eosinophilic granuloma. Rarely, these have expanded into the middle cranial fossa.[190]

Multifocal eosinophilic granuloma has bony involvement at more than one site, and many patients previously classified as having Hand-Schuller-Christian disease can be placed in this category. Any patient with possible Langerhans' cell histiocytosis needs evaluation by a pediatric hematologist with skeletal survey, bone marrow, body CT, and blood studies (complete blood count, liver function tests, sedimentation rate). Diffuse histiocytosis, which has previously been termed Letterer-Siwe disease, has multisystem involvement, including skin, middle ear, lungs, or abdominal viscera, and often occurs in younger patients. We have seen orbital involvement in these children, and in patients < 2 years of age with Langerhans' cell histiocytosis syndrome, diffuse systemic involvement is quite common. A typical skin and orbital lesion prior to and after 6 Gy of radiation is shown in Figure 16–43. Unlike patients with unifocal eosinophilic granuloma that involves only the orbit, patients with diffuse histiocytosis usually present because of systemic illness.[184]

A number of therapeutic options can be used to manage Langerhans' cell histiocytosis that involves the orbit.[191] If the child has diffuse systemic disease, these lesions respond to low-dose orbital radiation and chemotherapy.[182,192–194] If only the orbit is involved, curettage, intralesional steroid injection, or low-dose radiation are all effective.[182] Figures 16–44A and B show a 2-year-old child with a unifo-

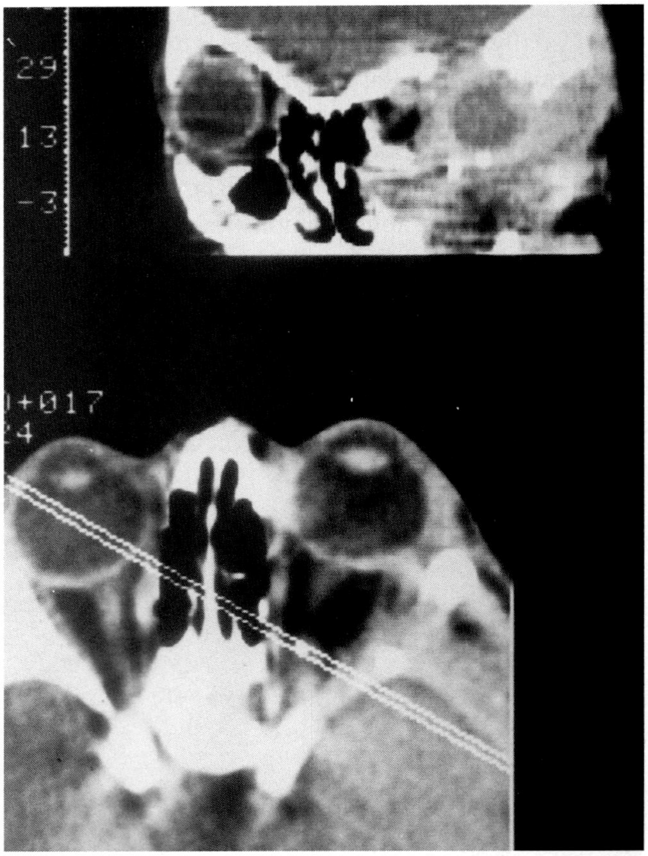

Figure 16–42. Axial CT scan with coronal reconstruction demonstrates diffuse bone destruction in multifocal eosinophilic granuloma with orbital involvement.

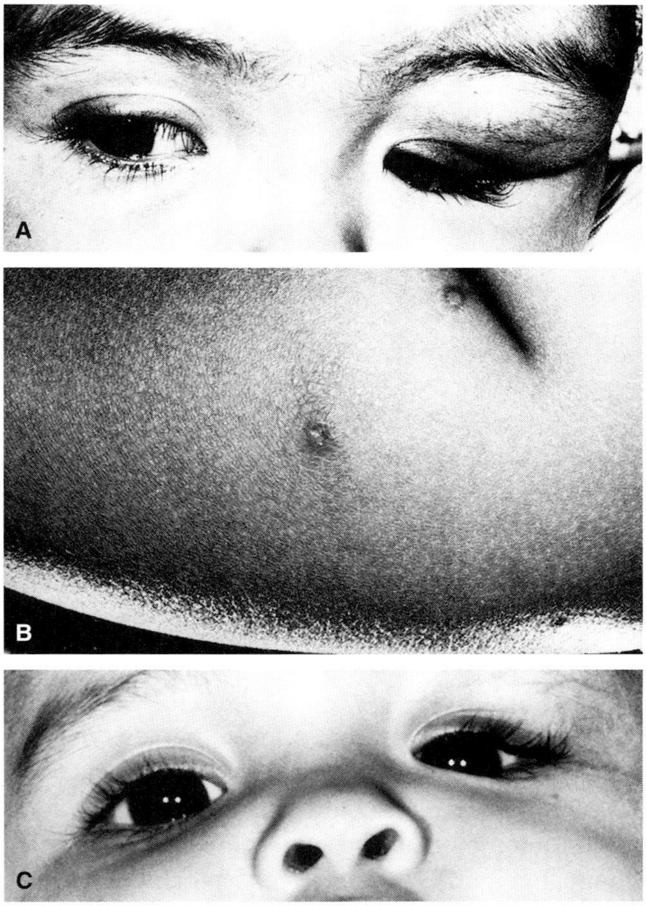

Figure 16–43. *A* and *B,* Cutaneous and orbital involvement in a child with diffuse histiocytosis. *C,* After 6 Gy (600 rads) of photon irradiation.

cal histiocytosis lesion in the lacrimal fossa prior to and after FNAB, which documented diagnosis, and injection of steroid. Usually, there is a 6- to 12-week interval between injection and complete resolution. We and others have made the diagnosis with FNAB and then treated it with local steroid injection.[195] The trend in patients with more advanced disease has been to use less radiation and more etoposide.[194] The long-term sequelae after Langerhans' cell treatment are not innocuous. In a series of 71 patients, some of whom the author managed, 10 died of multisystem disease, and late sequelae were noted in 64 percent.[196]

Orbital involvement in malignant histiocytosis is rare. We have seen 2 patients who developed this picture. As is typical with malignant histiocytosis, our patients first presented in their late teenage years with fever and weight loss.[182,197,198]

Contiguous orbital inflammation or infection from sinusitis is discussed elsewhere. It is a frequent cause of acute proptosis in children, usually between the ages of 5 and 10 years.

OPTIC NERVE TUMORS

Orbital optic nerve tumors in children are most commonly due to glioma (pilocytic astrocytomas). Much less commonly, meningioma, sarcoidosis, metastases, idiopathic inflammation, or leukemia can involve the pediatric optic nerve. Optic nerve glioma was first described in 1816 by Scarpa, and there have been over 2,300 optic nerve gliomas described in the literature.[199–206] Approximately 75 percent of cases have occurred in patients < 10 years of age; most present between the ages of 5 and 8 years. Optic nerve gliomas account for approximately 5 to 10 percent of pediatric orbital tumors.[2] Optic nerve glioma occurs as an isolated finding or as part of neurofibromatosis (NF).

The *NF1* gene spans 350 kb in the region of 17q 11.2.[207,208] It encodes a protein, neurofibromin, which is part of the GTPase activating family, and downregulates *ras* activity. Loss of this tumor suppressor gene is probably important in disease.

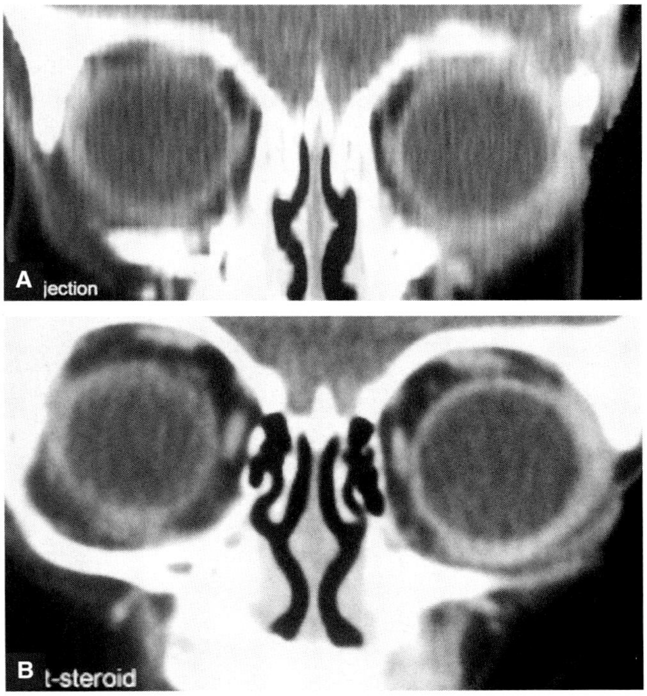

Figure 16–44. *A,* A unifocal histiocytosis of the lacrimal fossa. The diagnosis was made by FNAB. *B,* Approximately 12 weeks after steroid injection, the area appears normal.

In NF, the incidence of optic nerve glioma is between 12 and 38 percent.[209] Conversely, approximately 25 to 50 percent of patients with optic nerve gliomas have NF. In a review by Dutton, 29 percent of optic nerve glioma patients had stigmata of *NF1*.[206]

NF is an autosomal-dominant disease that occurs in approximately 1 of 3,000 people.[209] Lisch nodules, which are iris hamartomas, are noted in 94 percent of patients > 6 years, but only 28 percent of younger patients.[209] Lewis and co-workers studied 217 patients with NF and found that 15 percent had anterior pathway tumors.[210,211] Often, optic gliomas are asymptomatic in neurofibromatosis. Less than one-third of optic nerve tumors were suspected either on clinical or histologic evaluation in these patients, although MRI detects a greater number of cases.[212–215] In one interesting report of 2 cases with asymptomatic chiasmal and hypothalamic lesions, MRI demonstrated spontaneous partial regression.[216] Gadolinium with MRI increases the detection of CNS extension.[214] The MRI signs of optic nerve gliomas in NF type 1 (NF1) have been well described by Imes and Hoyt.[215,217] Optic nerve gliomas that are found in association with NF1 are usually fusiform, with a high signal intensity surrounding a core of lower signal intensity due to the perineural arachnoidal gliomatosis (Figure 16–45). In addition, there is often the double intensity tubular thickening with the downward kinking of the nerve in the NF1 population (Figure 16–46). This is rarely seen in those who have the idiopathic form of optic nerve gliomas.[211–215]

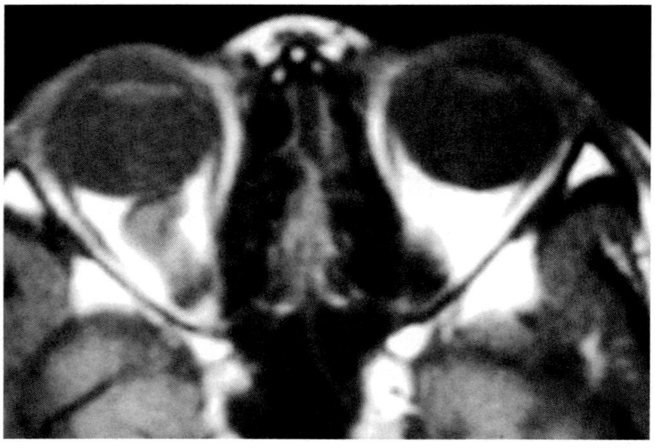

Figure 16–45. Axial T_1-weighted MRI scan shows a fusiform enlargement of an optic nerve glioma.

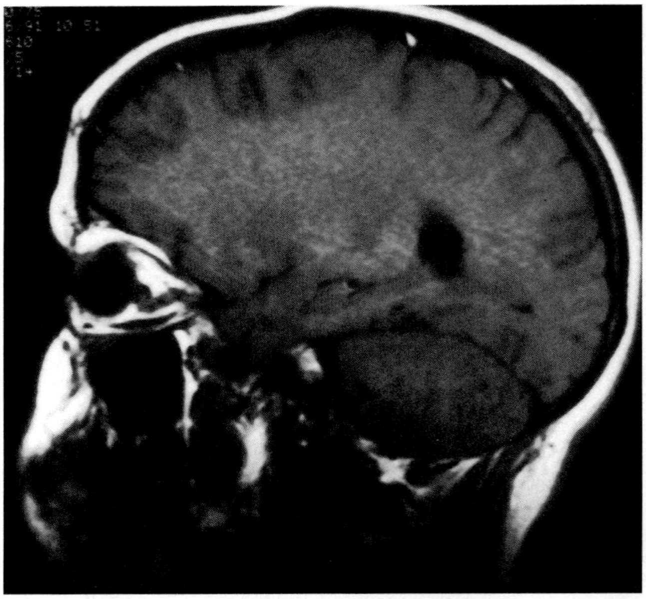

Figure 16–46. A parasagittal T_1-weighted MRI scan shows downward kinking of the optic nerve in NF1.

Most patients with optic nerve gliomas initially present with decreased vision and field loss.[212,213] Proptosis is usually < 3 mm; protrusion of the globe is more common in the optic nerve than chiasmal gliomas (Figure 16–47). Rarely, patients can have other ophthalmic signs or symptoms, including strabismus, nystagmus, optic neuritis, optic atrophy, or hypothalamic syndromes. Rarely, these tumors can calcify and produce acute visual loss.[218] Even more rarely, patients can develop other findings, including venous stasis retinopathy, neovascular glaucoma, intraocular invasion, or enlarged optic disc. Pain is rare.[219–220] Optic nerve gliomas are distinctly uncommon in NF type 2 (NF2).[221]

The location and degree of optic nerve and anterior visual pathway involvement are often difficult to ascertain, on either clinical or imaging examinations. It is estimated that < 15 percent of optic nerve

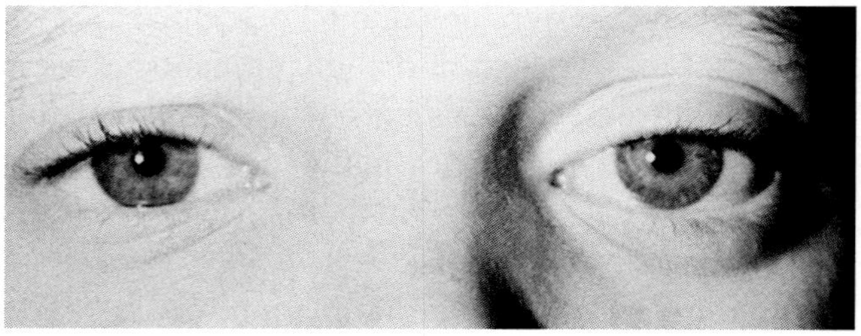

Figure 16–47. Axial proptosis in a young boy with optic nerve glioma.

gliomas involve only the orbital portion of the nerve, 60 percent involve the chiasm, and 25 percent involve the intracranial structures.[206,222,223] Optic nerve gliomas confined to the orbit are more common in NF1 patients versus those who do not have that disease. When patients have involvement in the hypothalamic area, they usually present with a diencephalic syndrome that is manifested as changes in alertness, lethargy, or seizures.[224]

MRI evaluations are the radiologic methods of choice in patients with optic nerve gliomas.[217] It is important to determine the intracanalicular, chiasmal and postchiasmal extension of the lesion.[214,224] There is usually enlargement and asymmetry of the optic foramen, without erosion or hyperostosis. Images of these lesions will be enhanced with contrast. On CT, gliomas will present with uniform thickening of the entire nerve, a solitary fusiform enlargement, or irregular thickening (Figures 16–48 to 16–50).[225,226] Occasionally, the glioma has a kink in its appearance, which is very typical. Some of these tumors will not been seen to grow on long-term follow-up.[227,228] In an atypical case, CT-directed FNAB can be diagnostic.[229] Figure 16–51 shows the axial MRI scan of a 25-year-old male with recently decreased vision and an optic nerve mass. Cytopathology is shown in Figure 16–52, and it was diagnostic for a glioma. The patient's vision improved after radiation.

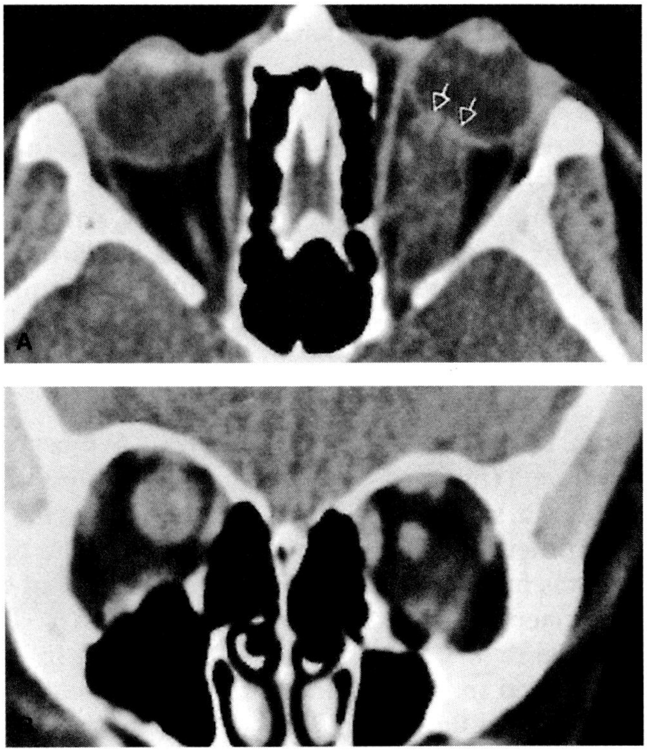

Figure 16–48. *A,* A case of blurred vision caused by left fusiform optic nerve glioma in a 15-year-old girl. On axial CT scan, the posterior of the proptotic left globe is indented (*arrows*). *B,* On coronal CT scan, the nerve is enlarged. (From Char et al.,[226] with permission)

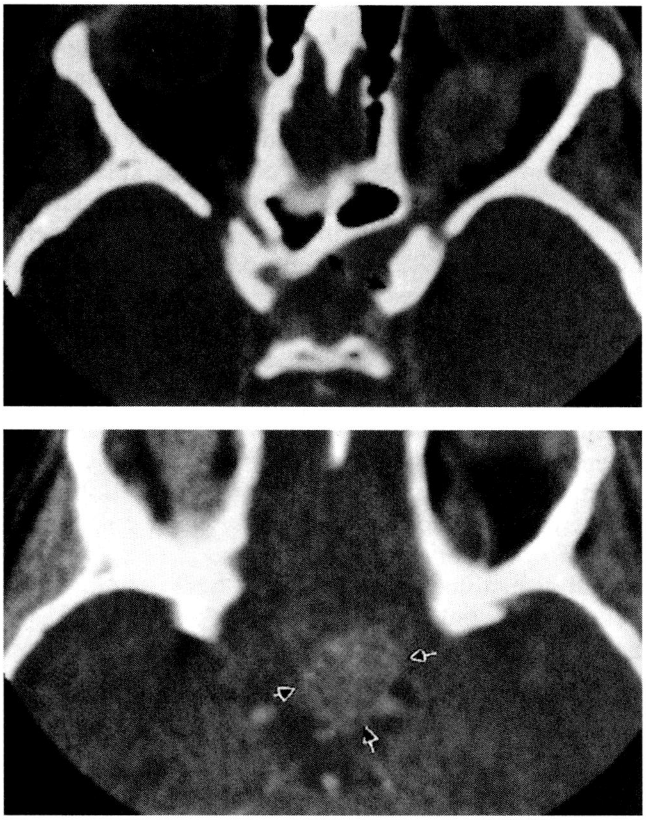

Figure 16–49. *A,* Neurofibroma ptosis and an optic nerve and chiasmal glioma in a 13-year-old girl. Axial CT scan showing a fusiform enlarged optic nerve that extends through the optic canal (*arrows*). *B,* Axial scan at a higher level showing the mass involving the chiasm (*open arrows*). (From Char et al.,[226] with permission).

The management of optic nerve gliomas is controversial. Some authors believe that many of these tumors confined to the optic nerve and chiasm are congenital hamartomas and should be merely watched.[230] Other authors believe all optic nerve gliomas require aggressive intervention with either surgery or radiation.[231–233] In reviewing a number of different series, it is obvious that the disease can run a full spectrum from benign proliferation to extremely aggressive and malignant behavior. Gliomas posterior to the chiasm have greater malignant potential than have anterior lesions, but this is not always the case.[234–236] Increased intracranial pressure is a poor

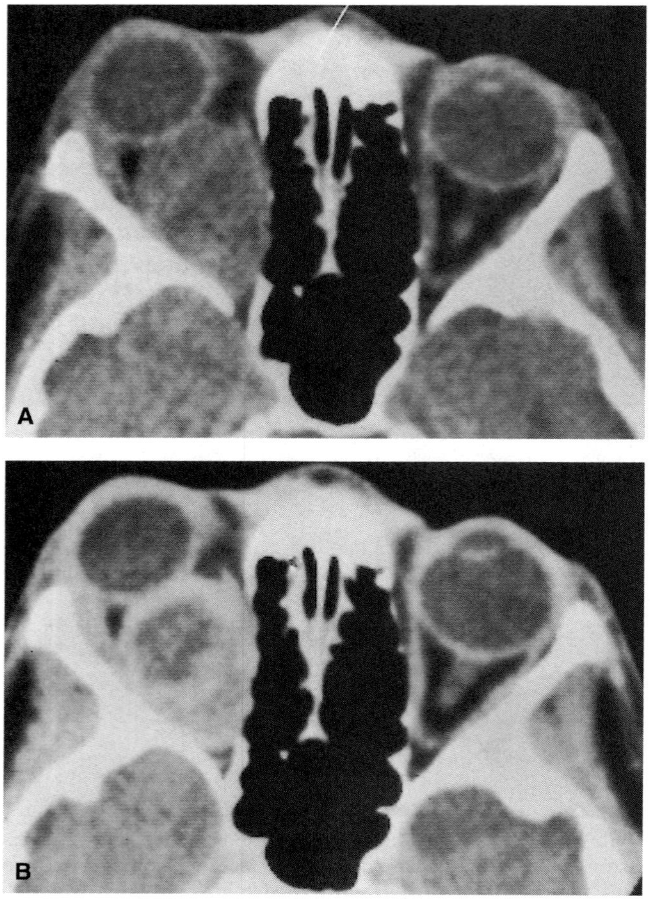

Figure 16–50. *A,* This child had progressive proptosis with loss of vision. The scans were obtained shortly before a debulking procedure was done through a lateral orbitotomy. Axial CT scan demonstrates a fusiform enlargement of the optic nerve. *B,* On postcontrast axial CT scan, the tumor shows peripheral enhancement, and a central radiolucent zone secondary to necrosis. This pattern was histologically confirmed. (From Char et al.,[226] with permission).

prognostic sign.[237] In a small series from London of about 69 patients treated from 1977 to 1994, using multivariate analysis, relapse-free survival was shown to have improved with older age, NF1, and treatment with chemotherapy and radiation.[238]

Review of the natural history of this tumor is confusing. Spontaneous regressions occur, and many papers presenting strong opinions on management probably have an inadvertent referral bias, in that their cases may not represent the usual pattern of disease course for this tumor. In 1969, Hoyt and Baghdassarian reviewed 36 patients with optic glioma.[230] Twenty-nine had chiasmal hypothalamic involvement, and only 6 patients died, 1 as a complication of intervention.[230] In 41 eyes in 23 patients, when no intervention was undertaken, 25 percent progressed, while in the 28 eyes which received radiation, a similar number appeared to progress. This series was updated in 1986.[239] Sixteen of the 28 patients originally reviewed in 1969 are dead, 5 from chiasmal gliomas. The mortality in patients with or without NF were similar. Nine of the 16 deaths occurred in patients with NF; 2 were from chiasmal tumors, 2 died as a result of surgery, and 3 died of other causes. The 12 surviving patients have not had any visual deterioration since 1969. The overall death rate was 57 percent; most deaths occurred within 3 years of diagnosis. Similarly, Listernick and colleagues noted that many of these lesions should be watched, and in a large series only 3 patients developed loss of vision.[240]

The roles of surgery, chemotherapy, and radiation in gliomas of the optic nerve tumors are evolving. In almost all series, survival in all tumors isolated to the orbit is excellent.[206,23,241] In these anterior optic nerve gliomas that do not involve the chiasm, observation is indicated if visual acuity is good and the tumor remains stable. If the neoplasm starts to grow or vision decreases, treatment is advocated. The choice of treatment is uncertain. Historically, irradiation or surgery was used; however, there was significant morbidity, especially in young irradi-

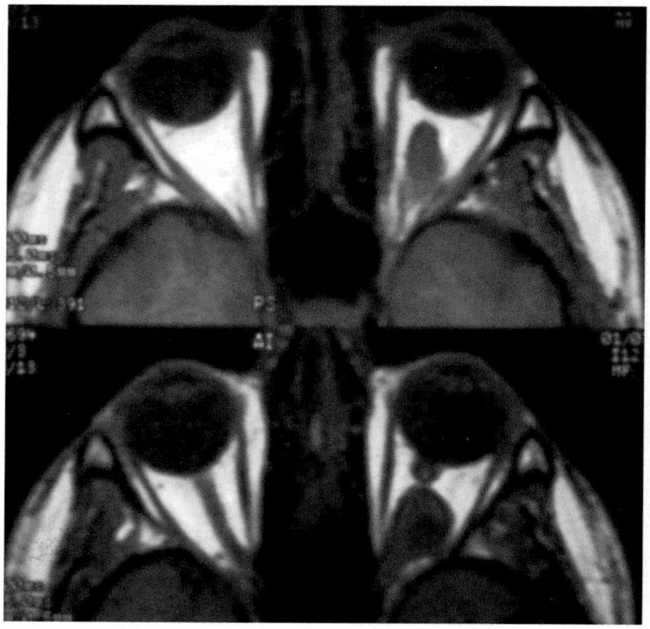

Figure 16–51. Axial MRI scan shows an optic nerve mass in a 25-year-old patient who presented with decreased vision.

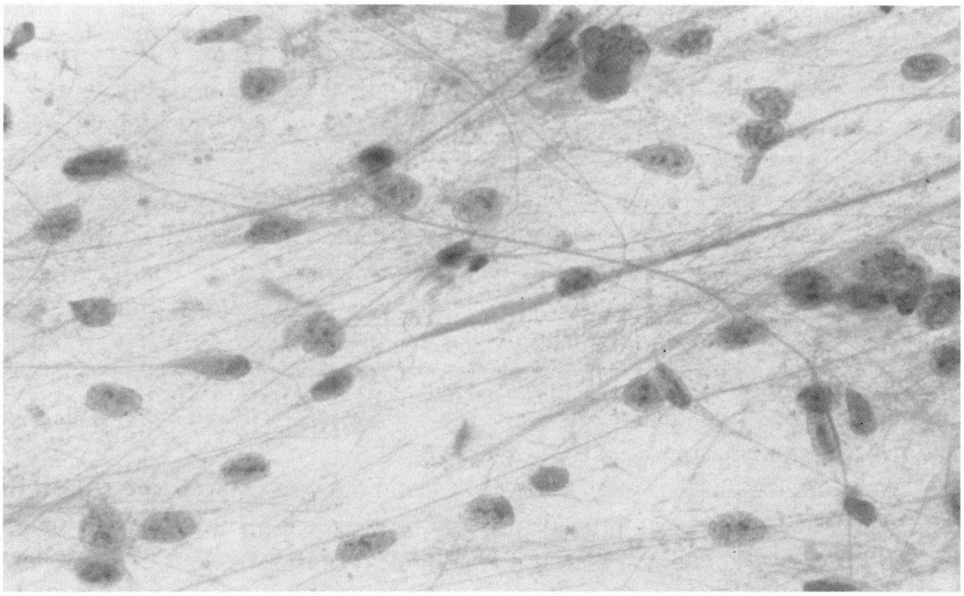

Figure 16–52. Shows the cytopathology of the optic nerve glioma demonstrated in Figure 16–51. Vision, at presentation, was decreased to 20/50. Visual acuity and field remained stationary after biopsy; his visual symptoms improved after radiation.

ated patients.[240,242–244] Several groups have treated these gliomas and more posterior tumors with chemotherapy, with retention of vision.[243–246] While a high percentage of patients who received chemotherapy relapsed and required radiation salvage, several clinicians believe that by delaying radiation, neurotoxicity may be diminished.[243,247] Surgical intervention in orbital cases is usually limited to blind eyes with marked proptosis (Figure 16–53A). In such cases, we have removed the bulk of the tumor through a lateral orbitotomy with retention of the eye (Figure 16–53B).[229] While local recurrences can occur, they are uncommon.[200,248–250]

Lesions isolated to the chiasm or to the chiasm and optic nerve are usually serially observed, unless there is visual loss or growth is documented. Some authors have advocated surgery, radiation, or chemotherapy.[206,232,233,247] We have limited the use of intracranial surgery, chemotherapy, or radiation to enlarging tumors with marked visual and CNS symptoms.[251] Kuenzle studied 21 optic nerve pathway gliomas in association with NF. Ten remained stable. Significantly 11 of the 21 developed other nonpathway CNS tumors within 4 years.[252]

Other clinicians have advocated radiation therapy for all chiasmal gliomas.[253,254] In a report from the

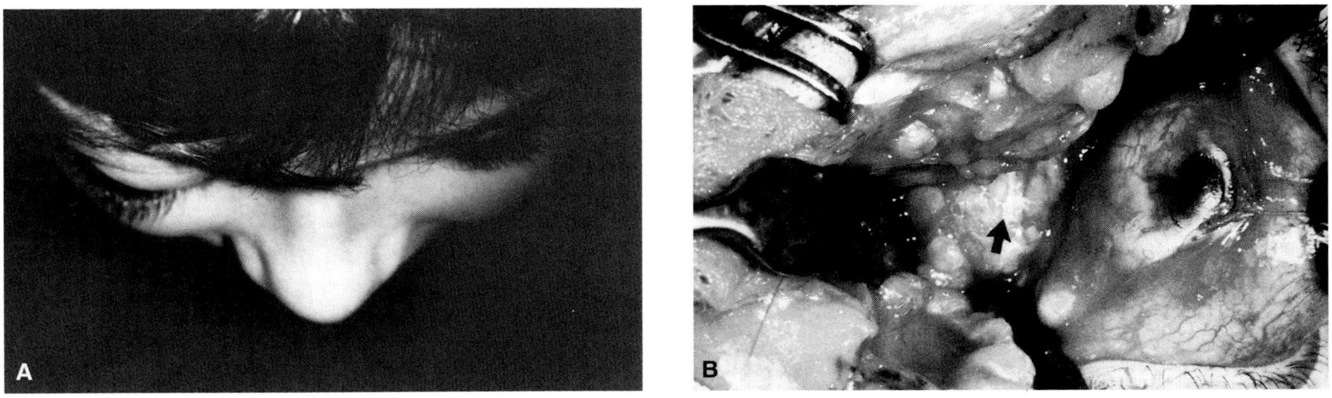

Figure 16–53. *A,* Progressive proptosis secondary to an optic nerve glioma led to surgical removal with retention of the eye. *B,* Intraoperative photograph of case shown in Figure 16–53A demonstrates enlarged optic nerve (*arrow*).

Curie Institute, between 1970 and 1986, 57 patients with chiasmal tumors were irradiated.[255] These were a slightly older population than usual with a mean age of 17 years at presentation. Forty percent of the patients had NF. In those cases where the tumors were confined to the anterior chiasm, the relapse-free survival rate was 100 percent at 5 years and 88 percent at 10 years. When the tumor involved the adjacent structures the 10-year survival rate was 72 percent. Long-term visual results were evaluable in approximately 35 patients, and 21 had improved visual acuity after radiation.[236] Pierce and colleagues irradiated 24 optic nerve gliomas that involved the chiasm.[256] Sixteen of 24 had decreased vision; after radiation, only 3 had tumor progression. Vision stabilized or improved in 21 patients.[256] Jenken and co-workers noted that 5 of 28 irradiated patients died of second tumors versus none of the 49 who did not receive radiation.[242]

In contrast, in another series, 85 patients were treated after histologic confirmation; only 2 had visual acuities of better than 20/50.[257] Six of 33 tumors confined to the optic nerve had recurrences after treatment versus 19 of 52 chiasmal tumors.[257] Five of the 33 patients with optic nerve gliomas died, as did 29 of 52 of those with chiasmal tumors. Some authors believe that patients with NF may have had a better prognosis.[258]

Radiation treatment of optic nerve gliomas generally is most effective, if at least 50 Gy is given, but as discussed above, it is uncertain how many of these lesions would have remained stable without therapy.[259,260] Radiation is probably the treatment of choice for hypothalamic involvement.[261–263] There are, however, no definitive data showing improved survival with radiation.[206,264–266]

The prognosis in patients with optic nerve glioma is a function of the location of the tumor, the presence of hydrocephalus and the histologic tumor grade.[247,267] Lower radiation complications were noted when the fraction size was < 200 cGy, and the total dose was < 54 Gy.[268,269]

Less commonly, other tumors can involve the optic nerve in children. Leukemic infiltrates are discussed in the chapter on intraocular lymphoma. While optic nerve sheath meningiomas are much more frequent in adults, they can occur in children, especially in those with NF.[270] Two cases of non–optic nerve intraorbital meningiomas have been reported in young males at ages 7 and 10 years.[271] Malignant teratomas of the optic nerve have also been reported, as have diffuse hyperplasia of the optic nerve in association with NF.[272, 273] Other rarer optic nerve tumefactions in childhood include ganglionomas, hemangioblastomas, and optic nerve sheath meningoceles.[273–276] Similarly, there can be multiple focal neurofibromas in the orbit in patients with NF.[277] Rarely, acute optic nerve gliomas can occur.[278]

FIBROUS AND BONY LESIONS

Dermoid cysts that involve the orbital bones are more frequent in adults (see chapter on lacrimal gland tumors). A number of uncommon bony lesions can involve the pediatric orbit, including aneurysmal bone cysts, giant cell granulomas, intraosseous hemangioma, and brown tumors.[279–282] Brown tumors occur in hyperparathyroidism and result in lytic destruction of bone with local hemorrhage.[283] Often, the skull has a salt-and-pepper appearance on imaging studies secondary to the hyperparathyroidism.[1,284] Less than 20 of reported cases of aneurysmal bone cysts involved the orbit, and most occurred in the orbital roof.[279,285,286] Occasionally, these lesions can cause optic nerve compression, with loss of central vision.[287] Usually, these lesions are hyperintense on T_2–weighted MRI scans.[286] Differentiation between a giant cell reparative granuloma, brown tumor, and aneurysmal bone cyst is relatively straightforward. Brown tumor is part of the osteitis fibrosis of hyperparathyroidism. Aneurysmal bone cysts versus orbit giant cell granulomas are diagnosed on the basis of histologic examination. The latter lesion is less common.[288]

A number of fibrous processes can involve the orbit, either primarily or secondarily. As discussed in the chapter on orbital pseudotumors, an inflammatory process can eventually become fibrotic. Juvenile ossifying fibroma of the orbit is a misnomer, since it can also occur in the adult.[280,281] This entity, first described in 1949 by Gogl, has had a number of different terms and has occasionally been lumped with fibrous dysplasia.[289] Patients usually present with proptosis and occasional visual complaints in the second decade of life. Most commonly, juvenile ossifying fibromas arise in either the ethmoid or frontal sinuses and produce inferior displacement of the eye.[288]

In contradistinction to fibrous dysplasia, ossifying fibromas usually have well-defined margins and ovoid expansion of overlying bone.[290] Juvenile nasopharyngeal angiofibromas are most commonly found in the second decade of life in young Caucasian males.[291] These can have aggressive local growth, and rarely either develop spontaneous regression or malignant transformation. In approximately 12 percent of cases, orbital extension can occur with decreased vision.[291,292] Sinus tumors secondarily involving the orbit are discussed in the chapter on lacrimal sac tumors.

Figure 16–54 shows a child with congenital orbital fibrosis of undetermined etiology.

Katz and Nerad recently reviewed 20 patients with fibrous dysplasia of the orbit. Eleven were older than 18 years at the time of presentation. Multiple bones of the orbit are involved, and in some cases, multiple transformations have occurred.[293]

LACRIMAL GLAND TUMORS

Lacrimal fossa tumors, with the exception of dermoid cysts or unifocal eosinophilic granulomas, are unusual in children. As discussed in the adult section, we have seen 2 teenagers (and 1 preteenager) with adenoid cystic carcinomas, but these are distinctly uncommon.

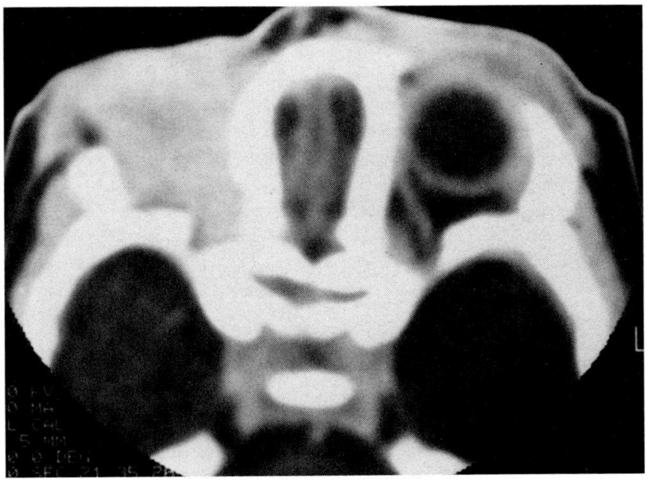

Figure 16–54. Congenital orbital fibrosis of undetermined etiology in a child.

We had one child who presented with an adenoid cystic carcinoma and rapidly developed widespread disease. The group from the AFIP presented 11 such cases under the age of 18 years. They noted that, in general, these younger patients fared better than did older patients with this disease, probably because of histologic variation.[294] While benign epithelial lacrimal gland tumors are much more common in adults, we have managed one 5-year-old who presented with a pleomorphic adenoma of the lacrimal gland.[295] More commonly, children and teenagers with lacrimal gland enlargement have a chronic or acute dacryadenitis secondary to viral infection. Figure 16–55A and B shows a young girl with an acute S-shaped lid swelling typical of lacrimal gland inflammation. The patient had a history of a viral upper respiratory tract infection approximately 1 week prior to the development of the lacrimal gland swelling, and the lesion resolved spontaneously over 2 weeks. Figure 16–55B shows an axial CT demonstrating chronic dacryadenitis, without bone involvement in this patient. Occasionally, a lipoma or lipo-

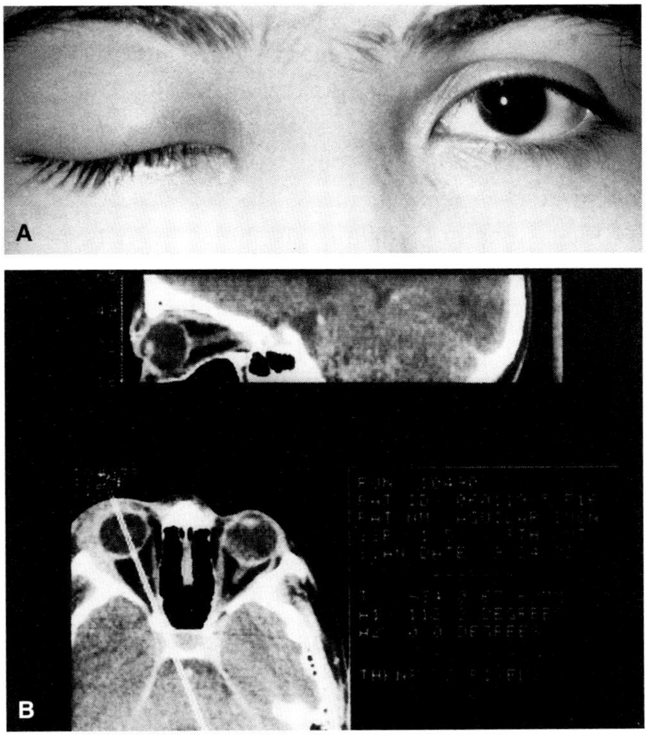

Figure 16–55. *A,* Young girl with chronic dacryoadenitis, presumably of viral etiology. *B,* Axial CT scan with parasagital reconstruction showing inflammation of the lacrimal gland with "spill-over" into contiguous areas.

dermoid can occur in the area of the palpebral portion of the lacrimal gland, as shown in Figure 16–56.

SINUSITIS WITH CONTIGUOUS INVOLVEMENT OF THE ORBIT

A problem that requires rapid surgical intervention in children is the development of bacterial sinusitis with secondary involvement of the orbit. Most of these children are between 6 and 10 years of age. Development of sinusitis at age $>$ 2 years is very uncommon, since the sinuses are not completely aerated. Figure 16–57 shows a case in a 1-year-old child who presented with orbital cellulitis due to contigous ethmoid infection. Figure 16–58A demonstrates an 8-year-old boy with the onset of an upper respiratory tract infection with high fever approximately 2 days prior to the sudden development of proptosis and decreased vision. On axial CT evaluation, opacification of the ethmoid sinus is present with contiguous extension in the orbit (Figure 16–58B). Bacterial sinusitis with secondary orbital involvement will often cause loss of vision; patients with these symptoms should be treated on an urgent basis.[296] In patients with severe orbital proptosis, paresis of extraocular movement, and inflammatory orbital signs that are progressive despite high-dose intravenous antibiotics, surgical drainage of the sinuses and orbital abscess is usually required in addition to medical therapy.

Occasionally, sinusitis associated with contiguous orbital disease can be quite subtle, and the presentation may mimic a primary orbital tumor (Figure 16–59A). The axial CT scan shown in Figure 16–59B was initially thought most likely to represent an orbital rhabdomyosarcoma; the patient was a young afebrile girl, whose only symptoms and signs were related to her orbital problem. At surgery, orbital and sinus abscesses were found, and they responded nicely to drainage and antibiotics.

Other sinus diseases that can involve the orbit are discussed in the section on adult orbital tumors.

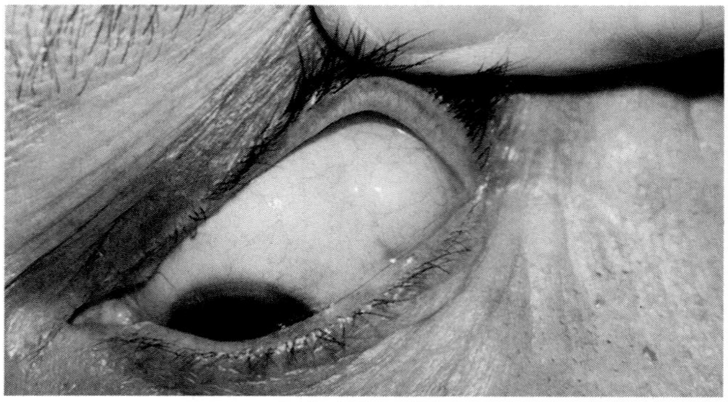

Figure 16–56. Lipoma in the superior-temporal quadrant

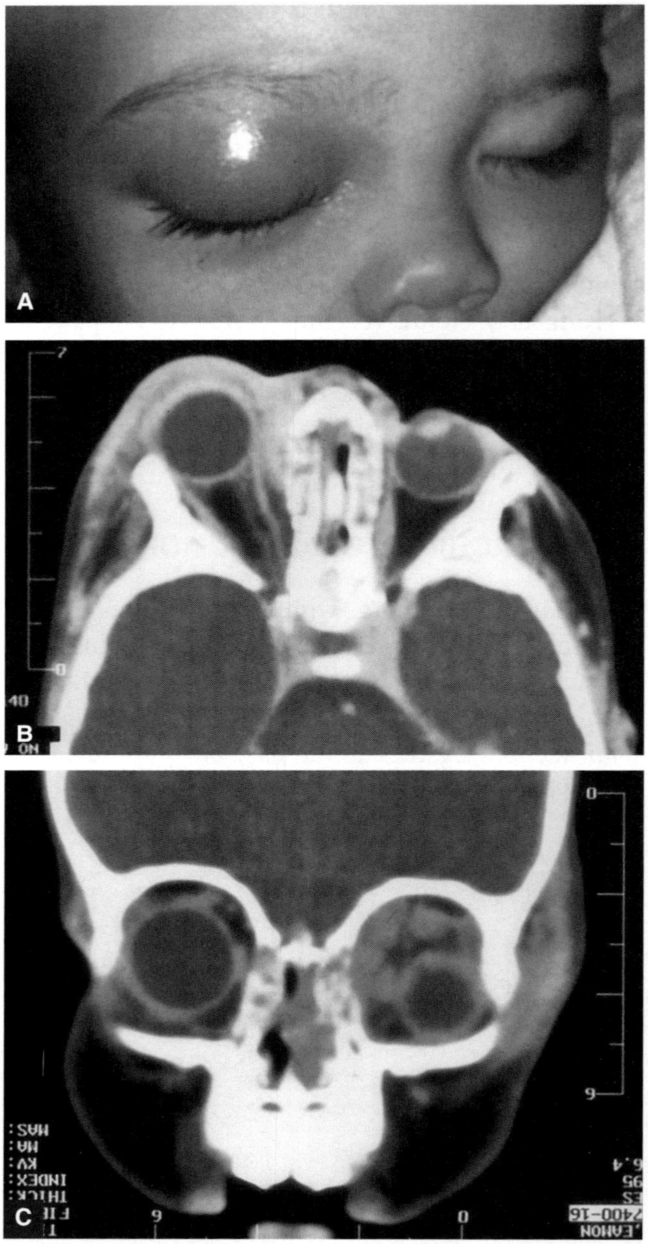

Figure 16–57. *A,* Clinical photograph of a 1-year-old child who presented with an orbital abscess. Usually, orbital abscess from contiguous sinus disease does not occur until after age 3 years, when the sinuses are aerated. *B,* Axial CT scan demonstrates orbital abscess from contiguous ethmoid sinusitis. *C,* Coronal CT scan of the case shown in Figure 16–57A and B.

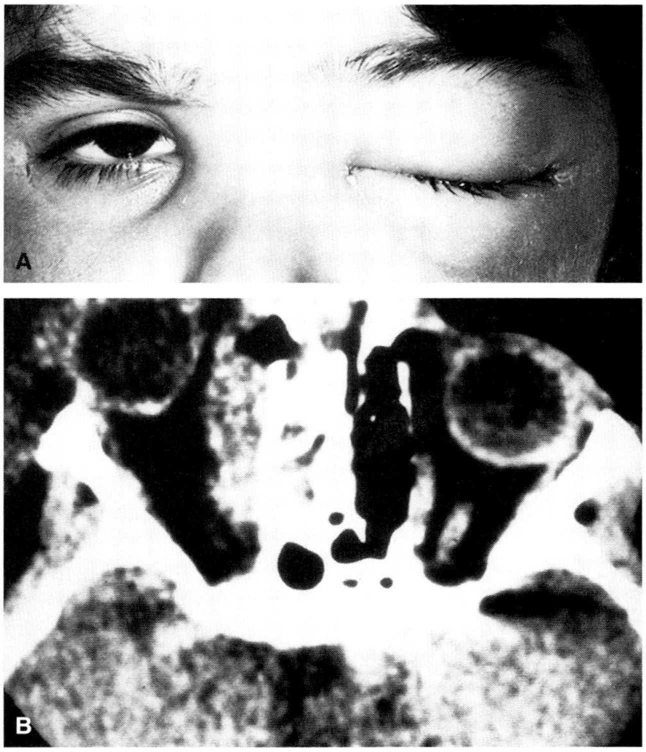

Figure 16–58. *A,* Eight-year-old boy with bacterial sinusitis secondarily involving the orbit. *B,* CT scan demonstrating ethmoid sinusitis with contiguous involvement of the orbit.

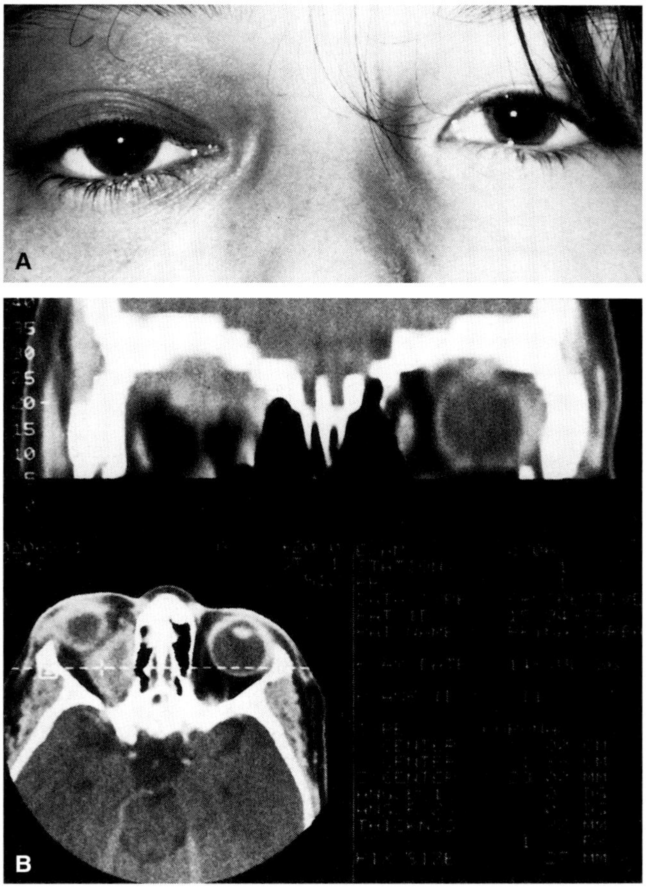

Figure 16–59. *A,* Clinical photograph of a child initially seen with what was thought to be a rhabdomyosarcoma. She was afebrile and had no history of upper respiratory tract infection. *B,* Axial CT scan with coronal reformation of subtle sinusitis with orbital extension simulating an orbital rhabdomyosarcoma.

REFERENCES

1. Eldrup-Jorgensen P, Fledelius H. Orbital tumours in infancy. An analysis of Danish cases from 1943-1962. Acta Ophthalol 1975;53:887–93.
2. Porterfield JF. Orbital tumors in children: a report on 214 cases. Int Ophthalmol Clin 1962;2:319–35.
3. Templeton AC. Orbital tumours in African children. Br J Ophthalmol 1971;55:254–61.
4. Shields JA, Bakewell B, Augsburger JJ, et al. Space-biopsies occupying orbital masses in children. A review of 250 consecutive cases. Ophthalmology 1986;93:379–84.
5. Moss HM. Expanding lesions of the orbit. A clinical study of 230 consecutive cases. Am J Ophthalmol 1962;54:761–70.
6. Gunalp I, Gunduz K. Biopsy-proven orbital lesions in Turkey. Orbit 1994;13:67–79.
7. Kodsi SR, Shetlar DJ, Campbell RJ, et al. A review of 340 orbital tumors in children during a 60-year period. Am J Ophthalmol 1994;117:177–82.
8. Bullock JD, Goldberg HS, Rakes SM. Orbital tumors in children. Ophthal Plast Reconstr Surg 1989;5:13–6.
9. Dock G. Chloroma and its relation to leukemia. Am J Med Sci Philadelphia, 1893;56:152–85.
10. Evans AE. Staging and treatment of neuroblastoma. Cancer 1980;45:1799–802.
11. Miller RW, Young JL, Nobakobic B. Childhood cancer. Cancer 1994;75:395–405.
12. Lopez-Ibor B, Schwartz AD. Neuroblastoma. Pediatr Clin North Am 1985;32:755–78.
13. Apple DJ. Metastatic orbital neuroblastoma originating in the cervical sympathetic ganglionic chain. Am J Ophthalmol 1969;68:1093–5.
14. Ungerleider RS. Working conference on neuroblastoma treatment trials. Cancer Treat Rep 1981;65:719–23.
15. Maurer HM. Current concepts in cancer. Solid tumors in children. N Engl J Med 1978;199:1345–8.
16. Tonini P. Neuroblastoma: a multiple biological disease. Eur J Cancer 1993;29A:802–4.
17. Brodeur GM, Fong CT, Morita M, et al. Molecular analysis and clinical significance of N-myc amplification and chromosome 1 abnormalities in human neuroblastoma. Prog Clin Biol Res 1988;271:3–15.
18. Bourhis J, Dominici C, McDowell H, et al. N-myc

genomic content and DNA ploidy in stage IVS neuroblastoma. J Clin Oncol 1991;9:1371–5.

19. Avet-Loiseau H, Venuat A-M, Benard J, et al. Morphologic and molecular cytogenetics in neuroblastoma. Cancer 1995;75:1694–9.
20. Gershenwald JE, Buzaid AC, Ross MI. Classification and staging of melanoma. Melanoma 1998;12: 737–65.
21. Ramani P, Shipley J. Recent advances in the diagnosis, prognosis and classification of childhood solid tumours. Br Med Bull 1996;52:724–41.
22. Goodman LA, Lui BCS, Thiele CJ, et al. Modulation of N-myc expression alters the invasiveness of neuroblastoma. Clin Exp Metastasis 1997;15:130–9.
23. Hiyama E, Hiyama K, Ohtsu K, et al. Telomerase activity in neuroblastoma: is it a prognostic indicator of clinical behavior. Eur J Cancer 1997;33:1932–6.
24. Takita J, Hayashi Y, Yokota J. Loss of heterozygosity in neuroblastomas—an overview. Eur J Cancer 1997; 33:1971–3.
25. Musarella MA, Chan HSL, DeBoer G, Gallie BL. Ocular involvement in neuroblastoma: prognostic implications. Ophthalmol 1984;91:936–40.
26. DuBois SG, Kalika Y, Lukens JN, et al. Metastatic sites in stage IV and IVS neuroblastoma correlate with age, tumor biology, and survival. J Pediatr Hematol Oncol 1999;21:181–9.
27. Belaumi AF, Kauffman WM, Jenkins JJ, et al. Blindness in children with neuroblastoma. Cancer 1997; 80:1997–2004.
28. Mortada A. Clinical characteristics of early orbital metastatic neuroblastoma. Am J Ophthalmol 1967; 63:1787–93.
29. Alfano JE. Ophthalmological aspects of neuroblastomatosis: a study of 53 verified cases. Trans Am Acad Ophthalmol Otolaryngol 1968;72:830–48.
30. Tiche TJ, Askin FB. Neuroblastoma and differential diagnosis of small-round, blue cell tumors. Human Pathol 1983;14:569–95.
31. Silverman JF, Joshi VV. FNA biopsy of small round cell tumors of childhood: cytomorphologic features and the role of ancillary studies. Diag Cytopathol 1994;10:245–55.
32. Cheung N-KV, Heller G, Kushner BH, et al. Detection of metastatic neuroblastoma in bone marrow: when is routine marrow histology insensitive? J Clin Oncol 1997;15:2807–17.
33. Exelby PR. Retroperitoneal malignant tumors: Wilms' tumor and neuroblastoma. Surg Clin North Am 1981;61:1219–37.
34. Suc A, Lumbroso J, Rubie H, et al. Metastatic neuroblastoma in children older than one year. Cancer 1996;77:805–11.
35. Chamberlain RS, Quinones R, Dinndorf P, et al. Complete surgical resection combined with aggressive adjuvant chemotherapy and bone marrow transplantation prolongs survival in children with advanced neuroblastoma. Ann Surg Oncol 1995;2:93–100.
36. Haase GM. Metastatic neuroblastoma—Does combining several "magic bullets" make a difference? Ann Surg Oncol 1995;21:91–2.
37. Breslow N, McCann B. Statistical estimation of prognosis for children with neuroblastoma. Cancer Res 1971;31:2098–2103.
38. Garaventa A, Ladenstein R, Chauvin F, et al. High-dose chemotherapy with autologous bone marrow rescue in advanced stage IV neuroblastoma. Eur J Cancer 1993;29A:487–91.
39. Simone JV. The treatment of neuroblastoma. J Clin Oncol 1984;2:717–8.
40. Kretschmar CS, Frantz CN, Rosen EM, et al. Improved prognosis for infants with stage IV neuroblastoma. J Clin Oncol 1984;2:799–803.
41. Stram DO, Matthay KK, O'Leary M, et al. Consolidation chemoradiotherapy and autologous bone marrow transplantation versus continued chemotherapy for metastatic neuroblastoma: a report of two concurrent Children's Cancer Group Studies. J Clin Oncol 1996;14:2417–26.
42. Hartmann, O, Valtau-Couanet D, Benhamou E, et al. Stage IV neuroblastoma in patients over 1 year of age at diagnosis: Consolidation of poor responders with combined Busulfan, Cyclophosphamide and Melphalan followed by in vitro Mafosfamide-purged autologous bone marrow transplantation. Eur J Cancer 1997;33:2126–29.
43. Kamani NR. Autotransplants for neuroblastoma. Bone Marrow Transpl 17:301–4, 1996.
44. Sibley GS, Mundt AJ, Goldman S, et al. Patterns of failure following total body irradiation and bone marrow transplantation with or without a radiotherapy boost for advanced neuroblastaom. Int J Radiation Oncology Biol Phys 1995;32:1127–1135.
45. Ladenstein R, Philip T, Gardner H. Autologous stem cell transplantation for solid tumors in children. Curr Opin Ped 1997;9:55–69.
46. Coze C, Hartmann O, Michon J, et al. NB87 induction protocol for stage 4 neuroblastoma in children over 1 year of age: a report for the French Society of Pediatric Oncology. J Clin Oncol 1997;15:3433–40.
47. Vassal G, Pondarre C, Cappelli C, et al. DNA topoisomerase 1, a new target for the treatment of neuroblastoma. Eur J Cancer 1997;33:2011–5.
48. Pardo N, Marti F, Fraga G, et al. High-dose systemic interleukin-2 therapy in stage IV neuroblastoma for one year after autologous bone marrow transplantation: pilot study. Med Pediatr Oncol 1996;27:534–9.
49. Fratkin JD, Purcell JJ, Krachmer JH, Taylor JC. Wilms' tumor metastatic to the orbit. JAMA 1977;238: 1841–2.

50. Rakes SM, Yeatts RP, Campbell RJ. Ophthalmic manifestations of esthesioneuroblastoma. Ophthalmol 1985;92:1749–53.
51. Davies JN, Owor R. Chloromatous tumours in African children in Uganda. Br Med J 1965;2:405–7.
52. Slamovits TL, Rosen CE, Suhrland MJ. Neuroblastoma presenting as acute lymphoblastic leukemia but correctly diagnosed after orbital fine-needle aspiration biopsy. J Clin Neuro-ophthalmol 1991;11:158–61.
53. Tanigawa M, Tsuda Y, Amemiya T, et al. Orbital tumor in acute myeloid leukemia associated with karyotype 46, XX, t(8:21) (q22;q22): a case report. Ophthalmologica 1998;212:202–5.
54. Cavdar AO, Arcasoy A, Babacan E, et al. Ocular granulocytic sarcoma (chloroma) with acute myelomonocytic leukemia in Turkish children. Cancer 1978;41:1606–9.
55. Cavar AO, Babacan E, Gozdasoglu S, et al. High risk subgroup of acute myelomonocytic leukemia (AMML) with orbito-ocular granulocytic sarcoma (OOGS) in Turkish children. Acta Haematol 1989; 81:80–5.
56. Zimmerman LE, Font RL. Ophthalmologic manifestations of granulocytic sarcoma (myeloid sarcoma or chloroma). Am J Ophthalmol 1975;80:975–90.
57. Pui MH, Fletcher BD, Langston JW. Granulocytic sarcoma in childhood leukemia: imaging features. Radiology 1994;190:698–702.
58. Davis JL, Parke DW II, Font RL. Granulocytic sarcoma of the orbit. A clinicopathologic study. Ophthalmology 1985;92:1758–62.
59. Nicholson DH, Green WR. Tumors of the eye, lids and orbit in children. In: Harley RD, editor. Pediatric ophthalmology. Philadelphia, PA: WB Saunders; 1975. p. 923–1067.
60. Abiose A, Adido J, Agarwal SC. Childhood malignancies of the eye and orbit in northern Nigeria. Cancer 1985;55:2889–93.
61. Oakhill A, Willshaw H, Mann JR. Unilateral proptosis. Arch Dis Child 1981;56:549–51.
62. Wirostko WJ, Garcia GH, Cory S, Harris GJ. Acute dacryocystitis as presenting sign of pediatric leukemia. Am J Ophthalmol 1999;127:734–6.
63. Preti A, Kantarjian H. Management of adult acute lymphocytic leukemia: present issues and key challenges. J Clin Oncol 1994;12:1312–22.
64. Ozsahin M, Belkacemi Y, Pene F, et al. Total-body irradiation and cataract incidence: a randomized comparison of two instantaneous dose rates. Int J Radiat Oncol Biol Phys 1993;28:343–7.
65. Nachman J, Sather HN, Cerlow JM, et al. Response of children with high risk acute lymphoblastic leukemia treated with and without cranial irradiation: a report from the children's cancer group. J Clin Oncol 1998;16:920–30.
66. Cunningham ET, Irvine AR, Rugo HS. Bone marrow transplantation retinopathy in the absence of radiation therapy. Am J Ophthalmol 1996;122:268–70.
67. Oshkishi K, Tsiaras WG. Prognostic importance of ophthalmic manifestations in childhood leukaemia. Br J Ophthalmol 1992;76:651–5.
68. Leidenix MJ, Mamalis N, Olson RJ, et al. Primary T-cell immunoblastic lymphoma of the orbit in a pediatric patient. Ophthalmology 1993;100:998–1002.
69. Flanagan JC. Vascular problems of the orbit. Ophthalmology 1979;86:896–913.
70. Smith SW, Carruthers JD. Intractable periocular hemangioma of infancy. Can J Ophthalmol 1985; 20:220–4.
71. Henderson JW. Orbital tumors, 3rd ed. New York, NY: Raven Press; 1994.
72. Basta LL, Anderson LS, Acers TE. Regression of orbital hemangioma detected by echography. Arch Ophthalmol 1977;95:1383–6.
73. Stigmar G, Crawford JS, Ward CM, Thomson HG. Ophthalmic sequelae of infantile hemangiomas of the eyelids and orbit. Am J Ophthalmol 1978;85: 806–13.
74. Haik BG, Jakobiec FA, Ellsworth RM, Jones IS. Capillary hemangioma of the lids and orbit: an analysis of the clinical features and therapeutic results in 101 cases. Ophthalmol 1979;86:760–92.
75. Robb RM. Refractive errors associated with hemangiomas of the eyelids and orbit in infancy. Am J Ophthalmol 1977;83:52–8.
76. Kushner BJ. Intralesional corticosteroid injection for infantile adnexal hemangioma. Am J Ophthalmol 1982;93:496–506.
77. Brown BZ, Huffaker G. Local injection of steroids for juvenile hemangiomas which disturb the visual axis. Ophthal Surg 1982;13:630–3.
78. Egbert JE, Schwartz GS, Walsh AW. Diagnosis and treatment of an ophthalmic artery occlusion during an intralesional injection of corticosteroid into an eyelid capillary hemangioma. Am J Ophthalmol 1996;121:638–42.
79. Achauer BM, Chang CJ, Vanderkamp BM. Management of hemangioma of infancy: review of 245 patients. Plast Reconstr Surg 1997;99:1301–8.
80. Walker RS, Custer PL, Nerad JA. Surgical excision of periorbital capillary hemangiomas. Opthalmology 1994;101:1333–40.
81. Plager DA, Snyder SK. Resolution of astigmatism after surgical resection of capillary hemangiomas in infants. Ophthalmology 1997;104:1102–6.
82. Loughnan MS, Elder J, Kemp A. Treatment with a massive orbital-capillary hemangioma with interferon alpha-2b: short-term results. Arch Ophthalmol 1992;110:1366–7.
83. Friendly DS, Font RL, Milhorat TH. Hemangioen-

dothelioma of the frontal bone. Am J Ophthalmol 1982;93:482–90.
84. Skalka HW, Callahan MA. "Congenital" hematic cyst of the orbit. Ann Ophthalmol 1979;11:1103–7.
85. Ide CH, Davis WE, Black SP. Orbital teratoma. Arch Ophthalmol 1978;96:2093–6.
86. Hoyt WF, Joe S. Congenital teratoid cyst of the orbit. A case report and review of the literature. Arch Ophthalmol 1962;68:196–201.
87. Levin ML, Leone CR Jr, Kincaid MC. Congenital orbital teratomas. Am J Ophthalmol 1986;102:476–81.
88. Barber JC, Barber LF, Guerry D III, et al. Congenital orbital teratoma. Arch Ophthalmol 1974;91:45–8.
89. Kivela T, Merenmies L, Ilveskoski I, Tarkkan N. A congenital intraocular teratoma. Ophthalmology 1993; 100:782–91.
90. Kivela T, Tarkkanen A. Orbital germ cell tumors revisited: a clinicopathological approach to classification. Surv Ophthalmol 1994;38:541–54.
91. Bilgic S, Dayanir V, Kiratli H, Gungen Y. Congenital orbital teratoma: a clinicopathologic case report. Ophthal Plast Reconstr Surg 1997;13:142–6.
92. Garden JW, McManis, JC. Congenital orbital-intracranial teratoma with subsequent malignancy: case report. Br J Ophthalmol 1986;70:111–3.
93. Pollock JA, Newton TH, Hoyt WF. Transsphenoidal and transethmoidal encephaloceles. A review of clinical and roentgen features in 8 cases. Radiol 1968;90:442–53.
94. Howard GR, Nerad JS, Bonavolonta G, Tranfa F. Orbital dermoid cysts located within the lateral rectus muscle. Ophthalmology 1994;101:767–71.
95. Sherman RP, Rootman J, LaPointe JS. Orbital dermoids: clinical presentation and management. Br J Ophthalmol 1984;68:642–52.
96. Mohammad AENA, Ray CJ, Karcioglu ZA. Echinococcus cysts of the orbit and substernum. Am J Ophthalmol 1994;118:676–8.
97. Char DH, Crawford JB, Ablin AR, et al. Orbital melanocytic hamartoma. Am J Ophthalmol 1981; 91:357–61.
98. Hall WC, O'Day DM, Glick AD. Melanotic neuroectodermal tumor of infancy. An ophthalmic appearance. Arch Ophthalmol 1979;97:922–5.
99. Lamping KA, Albert DM, Lack E, et al. Melanotic neuroectodermal tumor of infancy (retinal anlage tumor). Ophthalmology 1985;92:143–9.
100. Broadway D, Lang S, Harper J, et al. General malignant melanoma of the eye. Cancer 1991;67:2642–52.
101. Singh AD, Husson M, Shields CL, et al. Primitive neuroectodermal tumor of the orbit. Arch Ophthalmol 1994;112:217–21.
102. Brown HH, Kersten RC, Kulwin DR. Lipomatous hamartoma of the orbit. Arch Ophthalmol 1991; 109:240–3.
103. Vernet O, Ducrey N, Deruaz J-P, De Tribolet N. Giant cell tumor of the orbit. Neurosurgery 1993;32: 848–51.
104. Grossniklaus HE, Wojno T. Orbital aberrant fibroglial tissue (fibroglial choristoma) associated with microphthalmos. J Pediatr Ophthalmol Strabismus 1994;31:338–40.
105. Ellis J, Eagle RC, Shields JA, et al. Phakaomytosis choristoma (Zimmerman's tumor). Ophthalmology 1993;100:955–60.
106. Eviatar JA, Hornblass A, Herschorn B, Jakobiec FA. Malignant peripheral nerve sheath tumor of the orbit in a 15-month-old child. Ophthalmology 1992; 99:1595–9.
107. Appignani BA, Jones KM, Barnes PD. Primary endodermal sinus tumor of the orbit: MR findings. AJR Am J Roentgenol 1992;159:399–401.
108. Miser JS, Pizzo PA. Soft tissue sarcomas in childhood. Pediatr Clin North Am 1985;32:779–800.
109. Grufferman S, Wang HH, Delong ER, et al. Environmental factors in the etiology of rhabdomyosarcoma in childhood. J Natl Cancer Inst 1982;68:107–13.
110. Bayer S. Rhabdomyoma orbitae. Nord Med Ark 1882; 14:1–7.
111. Kingston JE, McElwain TJ, Malpas JS. Childhood rhabdomyosarcoma: experience of the Children's Solid Tumor Group. Br J Cancer 1983;48:195–207.
112. Pappo AS, Shapiro DN, Crist WM. Rhabdomyosarcoma: biology and treatment. Pediat Clin North Am 1997;44:953–72.
113. Sabbioni S, Barbanti-Brodano G, Croce CM, et al. A gene at 11p15 involved in rhabdomyosarcoma and rhabdoid tumor development. Cancer Res 1997;57: 4493–7.
114. Knowles DM, Jakobiec FA, Potter GD, Jones IS. Ophthalmic striated muscle neoplasms. Surv Ophthalmol 1976;21:219–61.
115. Cameron JD, Wick MR. Embryonal rhabdomyosarcoma of the conjunctiva. A clinicopathologic and immunohistochemical study. Arch Ophthalmol 1986;104:1203–4.
116. Abramson DH, Ellsworth RM, Tretter P, et al. The treatment of orbital rhabdomyosarcoma with irradiation and chemotherapy. Ophthalmology 1979;86: 1330–5.
117. Mafee MF, Pai E, Philip B. Rhabdomyosarcoma of the orbit. Evaluation with MR imaging and CT. Radiol Clin North Am 1998;36:1215–27.
118. Baron EM, Kersten RC, Kulwin DR. Rhabdomyosarcoma manifesting as acquired nasolacrimal duct obstruction. Am J Ophthalmol 1993;115:239–42.
119. Lueder GT, Burrows PE, Hurwitz JJ, et al. Vascular patterns in orbital rhabdomyosarcoma. J Pediatr Ophthalmol Strabismus 1994;31:46–9.
120. Jereb B, Haik BG, Ong R, Ghavimi F. Parameningeal rhabdomyosarcoma (including the orbit): results of

orbital irradiation. Int J Radiat Oncol Biol Phys 1985;11:2057–65.
121. Lederman M, Wybar K. Ocular malignant diseases. Proc Royal Soc Med 1976;69:895–903.
122. Pappo AS, Shapiro DN, Crist WM, Maurer HM. Biology and therapy of pediatric rhabdomyosarcoma. J Clin Oncol 1995;13:2123–39.
123. Flamant F, Hill C. The improvement in survival associated with combined chemotherapy in childhood rhabdomyosarcoma. A historical comparison of 345 patients in the same center. Cancer 1984;53:2417–21.
124. Wharam M, Beltangady M, Hays D, et al. Localized orbital rhabdomyosarcoma. Ophthalmology 1987; 94:251–4.
125. Akyuz C, Sancak R, Buyukpamukcu N, et al. Turkish experience with rhabdomyosarcoma: an analysis of 255 patients for 20 years. Turk J Pediatr 1998;40: 491–501.
126. Jones IS, Reese AB, Kraut J. Orbital rhabdomyosarcoma. An analysis of 62 cases. Am J Ophthalmol 1966;61:721–36.
127. Razek AA, Perez CA, Lee FA, et al. Combined treatment modalities of rhabdomyosarcoma in children. Cancer 1977;39:2415–21.
128. Sutow WW, Lindberg RD, Gehan EA, et al. Three year relapse-free survival rates in childhood rhabdomyosarcoma of the head and neck: report from the Intergroup Rhabdomyosarcoma Study. Cancer 1982; 49:2217–21.
129. Mandell LR. Ongoing progress in the treatment of childhood rhabdomyosarcoma. Oncology 1993;7:71–81.
130. Van Manen SR, De Kraker J, Voute PA. The role of chemotherapy, surgery, and radiotherapy in rhabdomyosarcoma of the orbit. Pediatr Hematol Oncol 1991;8:273–6.
131. Fiorillo A, Migliorati R, Grimaldi M, et al. Multidisciplinary treatment of primary orbital rhabdomyosarcoma. A single-institution experience. Cancer 1991; 67:560–3.
132. Rodary C, Gehan EA, Flamant F, et al. Prognostic factors in 951 nonmetastatic rhabdomyosarcoma in children: a report from the international rhabdomyosarcoma workshop. Med Pediatr Oncol 1991;19:89–95.
133. Crist W, Gehan EA, Ragab AH, et al. The Third Internatur Group Rhabdomyosarcoma. J Clin Oncol 1995;13:610–30.
134. Mannor GE, Rose GE, Plowman PN, et al. Multidisciplinary management of refractory orbital rhabdomyosarcoma. Ophthalmology 1997;104:1198–201.
135. Heyn R, Ragab A, Raney RB Jr, et al. Late effects of therapy in orbital rhabdomyosarcoma in children. A report from the Intergroup Rhabdomyosarcoma Study. Cancer 1986;57:1738–43.
136. Jereb B, Ghavimi F, Exelby P, Zang E. Local control of embryonal rhabdomyosarcoma in children by radiation therapy when combined with chemotherapy. Int J Radiat Oncol Biol Phys 1980;6:827–33.
137. Donaldson SS, Castro JR, Wilbur JR, Jesse RH Jr. Rhabdomyosarcoma of head and neck in children: combination treatment by surgery, irradiation, and chemotherapy. Cancer 1973;31:26–35.
138. Abramson DH, Notis CM. Visual acuity after radiation for orbital rhabdomyosarcoma. Am J Ophthalmol 1994;118:808–9.
139. Sagerman RH. Orbital rhabdomyosarcoma: a paradigm for irradiation. Radiology 1993;187:605–7.
140. Rousseau P, Flamant F, Quintana E, et al. Primary chemotherapy in rhabdomyosarcomas and other malignant mesenchymal tumors of the orbit: results of the International Society of Pediatric Oncology MMT 84 study. J Clin Oncol 1994;12:516–21.
141. Kingston JE, Plowman PN, Wright J. Radiotherapy still has a major role in the management of localized orbital rhabdomyosarcoma. J Clin Oncol 1995;13: 798–9.
142. Nag S, Olson T, Ruymann F, et al. High dose rate brachytherapy in childhood sarcomas: a local control strategy preserving bone growth and function. Med Pediatr Oncol 1995;25:463–9.
143. Elias AD. Advances in the diagnosis and management of sarcomas. Curr Opin Oncol 1992;4:681–8.
144. Fekrat S, Miler NR, Loury MC. Alveolar rhabdomyosarcoma metastasized to the orbit. Arch Ophthalmol 1993;111:1662–4.
145. Elsas FJ, Morczek EC, Kelly DR, Specht CS. Primary Rhabdomyosarcoma of the iris. Arch Ophthalmol 1991;109:982–4.
146. Matsko TH, Schmidt RA, Milam AH, Orcutt JC. Primary malignant ectomesenchymoma of the orbit. Br J Ophthalmol 1992;76:1438–41.
147. Gunduz K, Shields JA, Eagle RC, et al. Malignant rhabdoid tumor of the orbit. Arch Ophthalmol 1998; 116:243–6.
148. Das DK, Das J, Kumar D, et al. Leiomyosarcoma of the orbit. Diagnosis of its recurrence by fine-needle aspiration cytology. Diagn Cytopathol 1992;8:609–13.
149. Font RL, Jurco S III, Brechner RJ. Postradiation leiomyosarcoma of the orbit complicating bilateral retinoblastoma. Arch Ophthalmol 1983;101:1557–61.
150. Wojno T, Tenzel RR, Nadji M. Orbital leiomyosarcoma. Arch Ophthalmol 1983;101:1566–8.
151. Folberg R, Cleasby G, Flanagan JA, et al. Orbital leiomyosarcoma after radiation therapy for bilateral retinoblastoma. Arch Ophthalmol 1983;101:1562–5.
152. Weiner JM, Hidayat AA. Juvenile fibrosarcoma of the orbit and eyelid. A study of five cases. Arch Ophthalmol 1983;101:253–9.
153. Font RL, Jurco S III, Zimmerman LE. Alveolar soft-part sarcoma of the orbit: a clinicopathologic analysis of seventeen cases and a review of the literature. Hum Pathol 1982;13:569–79.

154. Altamirano-Dimas M, Albores-Saavedra J. Alveolar soft part sarcoma of the orbit. Arch Ophthalmol 1966;75:496–9.
155. Moriarty P, Garner A, Wright JE. Case report of granular cell myoblastoma arising within the medial rectus muscle. Br J Ophthalmol 1983;67:17–22.
156. Nirankari MS, Greer CH, Chaddah MR. Malignant non-chromoffin paraganglioma in the orbit. Br J Ophthalmol 1963;47:357–63.
157. Grant GD, Shields JA, Flanagan JC, Horowitz P. The ultrasonographic and radiologic features of a histologically proven case of alveolar soft-part sarcoma of the orbit. Am J Ophthalmol 1979;87:773–7.
158. Caballero LR, Rodriguez AC, Sopelana AB. Angiomatoid malignant fibrous histiocytoma of the orbit. Am J Ophthalmol 1981;92:13–5.
159. Kaw YT, Ruesta RA. Nodular fasciitis of the orbit diagnosed by fine needle aspiration cytology. Acta Cytologica 1993;37:957–60.
160. Wecker L. Die Cavernosem Tumoren der Orbita. Klin Monatsbl Augenheilkd 1868;6:47–9.
161. Reese AB. Expanding lesions of the orbit. Trans Ophthalmol Soc UK 1981;91:85–104.
162. Wright JE. Orbital vascular anomalies. Trans Am Acad Ophthalmol Otolaryngol 1974;78:606–16.
163. Bilaniuk LT. Orbital vascular lesions. Role of imaging. Radiol Clin North Am 1999;37:169–83.
164. Rootman J. Orbital venous abnormalities. Ophthalmology 1998;105:387–8.
165. Harris GJ. Orbital venous anomalies. Ophthalmology 1998;105:388–9.
166. Katz SE, Rootman J, Vangveeravong S, Graeb D. Combined venous lymphatic malformations of the orbit (so-called lymphangiomas): association with noncontiguous intracranial vascular anomalies. Ophthalmology 1998;105:176–84.
167. Jones IS. Lymphangiomas of the ocular adnexa. An analysis of sixty-two cases. Am J Ophthalmol 1961; 51:481–509.
168. Iliff WJ, Green WR. Orbital lymphangiomas. Ophthalmology 1979;86:914–29.
169. Harris GJ, Sakol PJ, Bonavolonta G, De Conciliis C. An analysis of thirty cases of orbital lymphangioma. Ophthalmology 1990;97:1583–92.
170. Rootman J, Hay E, Graeb D, Miller R. Orbital-adnexal lymphangiomas. Ophthalmology 1986;93:1558–70.
171. Kennerdell JS, Maroon JC, Garrity JA, Abla AA. Surgical management of orbital lymphangioma with the carbon dioxide laser. Am J Ophthalmol 1986; 102:308–14.
172. Bond JB, Haik BG, Tavaras JL, et al. Magnetic resonance imaging of orbital lymphangioma with or without gadolinium contrast enhancement. Ophthalmology 1992;99:1318–24.
173. Kazim N, Kennerdell JS, Rothfus W, Marquardt M. Orbital lymphangioma: correlation of magnetic resonance images and intraoperative findings. Ophthalmology 1992;99:1588–94.
174. Coll GE, Goldberg RA, Krauss H, Bateman BJ. Concomitant lymphangioma and arteriovenous malformation of the orbit. Am J Ophthalmol 1991;112: 200–5.
175. Tunc M, Sadri E, Char DH. Orbital lymphangioma: an analysis of 26 patients. Br J Ophthalmol 1999;83: 76–80.
176. Rose GE, Wright JE. Exenteration for benign orbital disease. Br J Ophthalmol 1994;78:14–8.
177. Floyd BB, Brown B, Isaacs H, Minckler DS. Pseudorheumatoid nodule involving the orbit. Arch Ophthalmol 1982;100:1478–80.
178. Arora R, Betharia SM. Fine-needle aspiration biopsy of pediatric orbital tumors. An immunocytochemical study. Acta Cytologica 1994;38:511–6.
179. Kaw YT, Cuesta RA. Nodular fasciitis of the orbit diagnosed by fine-needle aspiration cytology: a case report. Acta Cytologica 1993;37:957–60.
180. Linder JS, Harris GJ, Segura AD. Periorbital infantile myofibromatosis. Arch Ophthalmol 1996;114: 219–22.
181. Hyver SW, Ellis DS, Stewart WB, et al. Sino-orbital giant cell reparative granuloma. Ophthal Plast Reconstr Surg 1998;14:178–81.
182. Char DH, Ablin A, Beckstead J. Histiocytic disorders of the orbit. Ann Ophthalmol 1984;16:867–73.
183. Broadbent V, Gadner H. Current therapy for Langerhans' cell histiocytosis. Hematol Oncol Clin North Am 1998;12:327–38.
184. Writing Group of the Histiocyte Society. Histiocytosis syndromes in children. Lancet 1987;1:208–9.
185. Baghdassarian SA, Shammas HF. Eosinophilic granuloma of the orbit. Ann Ophthalmol 1977;9:1247–51.
186. Heuer HE. Eosinophilic granuloma of the orbit. Acta Ophthalmol 1972;50:160–5.
187. Mittelman D, Apple DJ, Goldberg MF. Ocular involvement in Letterer-Siwe disease. Am J Ophthalmol 1973;75:261–5.
188. Jakobiec FA, Trokel SL, Aron-Rosa D, et al. Localized eosinophilic granuloma (Langerhans'-cell histiocytosis) of the orbital frontal bone. Arch Ophthalmol 1980;98:1814–20.
189. Nesbit ME Jr, Wolfson JJ, Kieffer SA, et al. Orbital sclerosis in histiocytosis X. AJR Am J Roentgen 1970;110:123–8.
190. Furuta S, Sakaki S, Hatakeyama T, et al. Pediatric orbital eosinophilic granuloma with intra- and extracranial extension. Neurol Med Chir 1991;31: 590–2.
191. Arceci RJ, Brenner MK, Pritchard J. Controversies and new approaches to treatment of Langerhans' cell histiocytosis. Hematol Oncol Clin North Am 1998;12:339–57.

192. Greenberger JS, Crocker AC, Vawter G, et al. Results of treatment of 127 patients with systemic histiocytosis (Letterer-Siwe syndrome, Schuller-Christian syndrome and multifocal eosinophilic granuloma). Medicine 1981;60:311–38.
193. Geiser SF. The histiocytosis syndromes. Pediatr Ann Als 1964;8:54.
194. Ladisch S, Gadner H. Treatment of Langerhans' cell histiocytosis—evolution in current approaches. Br J Cancer 1994;78:S241–6.
195. Ghazi I, Phillippe J, Portas M, et al. Granulome eosinophile isole de la paroi externe de l'orbite. J Fr Ophthalmol 1991;14:189–94.
196. Willis B, Ablin A, Weinberg V, et al. Disease course and late sequelae of Langerhans' cell histiocytosis. 25 year experience at the University of California, San Francisco. J Clin Oncol 1996;14:2073–82.
197. Nezelof C, Frileux-Herbert F, Cronier-Sachot J. Disseminated histiocytosis X: analysis of prognostic factors based on a retrospective study of 50 cases. Cancer 1979;44:1824–38.
198. Gonzalez CL, Jaffe ES. The histiocytoses: clinical presentation and differential diagnosis. Oncology 1990;4:47–60.
199. Panizza B. Fungo midollare dell'occhio. Pavia: Pietro Bizzoni s. Bolzani; 1821.
200. Hudson AC. Primary tumours of the optic nerve. Royal London Ophthalmol Hosp Rep 1912;18:317–439.
201. Byers WGM. Primary intradural tumors of the optic nerve (Fibromatosis nervi Optici). Stud Royal Victoria Hosp, Montreal 1901;1:3.
202. Dodge HW Jr, Love JG, Craig WM, et al. Gliomas of the optic nerves. Arch Neurol Psychiatr 1958;79: 607–21.
203. Lloyd L. Gliomas of the optic nerve and chiasm in childhood. Trans Am Ophthalmol Soc 1973;72:488.
204. Liss L, Wolter JR. The histology of the glioma of the optic nerve; a study with silver carbonate. Arch Ophthalmol 1957;58:689–94.
205. Alvord EC Jr, Lofton S. Gliomas of the optic nerve or chiasm. Outcome by patients' age, tumor site, and treatment. J Neurosurg 1988;68:85–98.
206. Dutton JJ. Gliomas of the anterior visual pathway. Surv Ophthalmol 1994;38:427–52.
207. Shen MH, Harper PS, Upadhyaya M. Molecular genetics of neurofibromatosis type 1 (NF1). J Med Genet 1996;33:2–17.
208. Goldgar DE, Green P, Parry DM, Mulvihill JJ. Multipoint linkage analysis in neurofibromatosis type I: an international collaboration. Am J Hum Genet 1989;44:6–12.
209. Listernick R, Charrow J, Greenwald M, Mets M. Natural history of optic pathway tumors in children with neurofibromatosis. J Pediatr 1994;125:63–6.
210. Riccardi VM. Von Recklinghausen neurofibromatosis. N Engl J Med 1981;305:1617–27.
211. Lewis RA, Gerson LP, Axelson KA, et al. von Recklinghausen neurofibromatosis. II. Incidence of optic gliomata. Ophthalmology 1984;91:929–35.
212. Listernick R, Charrow J, Greenwald MJ, Esterly NB. Optic gliomas in children with neurofibromatosis type I. J Pediatr 1989;114:788–92.
213. Curatolo P, Cusmai R. Optic glioma in children with neurofibromatosis. Lancet 1987;1:1140.
214. Zimmerman CF, Schatz NJ, Glaser GS. Magnetic resonance imaging of optic nerve meningiomas. Ophthalmology 1990;97:585–91.
215. Imes RK, Hoyt WF. Magnetic resonance imaging signs of optic nerve gliomas in neurofibromatosis I. Am J Ophthalmol 1991;111:729–34.
216. Gottschalk S, Tavakolian R, Buske A, et al. Spontaneous remission of chiasmatic/hypothalamic masses in neurofibromatosis type 1: report of two cases. Neuroradiology 1999;41:199–201.
217. Hollander MD, FitzPatrick M, O'Conner SG, et al. Optic gliomas. Radiol Clin North Am 1999;37: 59–71.
218. Jordan DR, Anderson RL, White GL Jr, Mamalis N. Acute visual loss due to a calcified optic nerve glioma. Can J Ophthalmol 1989;24:335–9.
219. Buchanan TA, Hoyt WF. Optic nerve glioma and neovascular glaucoma: report of a case. Br J Ophthalmol 1982;66:96–8.
220. Grimson BS, Perry DD. Enlargement of the optic disk in childhood optic nerve tumors. Am J Ophthalmol 1984;97:627–31.
221. Dossetor FM, Landau K, Hoyt WF. Optic disc glioma in neurofibromatosis type II. Am J Ophthalmol 1989;108:602–3.
222. DeSousa AL, Kalsbeck JE, Mealey J Jr, et al. Optic chiasmatic glioma in children. Am J Ophthalmol 1979;87:376–81.
223. Reese AB. Glioma of the optic nerve, retina and orbit. In: Tumors of the eye, 3rd ed. Hagerstown, MD: Harper & Row: 1976. p. 134–45.
224. Haik BG, Saint Louis L, Bierly J, et al. Magnetic resonance imaging in the evaluation of optic nerve gliomas. Ophthalmology 1987;94:709–7.
225. Byrd SE, Harwood-Nash DC, Fitz CR, et al. Computed tomography of intraorbital optic nerve gliomas in children. Radiology 1978;129:73–8.
226. Char DH. Ocular and orbital pathology — clinical aspects. In: Newton TH, Norman D, editors. Modern neuroradiology, Vol 3: Computed tomography of the head and neck. Clavadel Press 1992.
227. Holman RE, Grimson BS, Drayer BP, et al. Magnetic resonance imaging of optic gliomas. Am J Ophthalmol 1985;100:596–601.
228. Glaser JS, Hoyt WF, Corbett J. Visual morbidity with chiasmal glioma. Long-term studies of visual fields in untreated and irradiated cases. Arch Ophthalmol 1971;85:3–12.

229. Pennelli N, Lontaguti A, Carteri A, et al. Juvenile pilocytic astrocytoma of the optic nerve diagnosed by fine needle aspiration biopsy. Acta Cytologica 1988;32:395–8.
230. Hoyt WF, Baghdassarian SA. Optic glioma of childhood. Natural history and rationale for conservative management. Br J Ophthalmol 1969;53:793–8.
231. Housepian EM. Surgical treatment of unilateral optic nerve gliomas. J Neurosurg 1969;31:604–7.
232. MacCarty CS, Boyd AS Jr, Childs DS Jr. Tumors of the optic nerve and optic chiasm. J Neurosurg 1970;33:439–44.
233. Richards RD, Lynn JR. The surgical management of gliomas of the optic nerve. Am J Ophthalmol 1966; 62:60–5.
234. Dosoretz DE, Blitzer PH, Wang CC, Linggood RM. Management of glioma of the optic nerve and/or chiasm and analysis of 20 cases. Cancer 1980;45: 1467–71.
235. Nishio S, Takeshita I, Fujiwara S, Fukui M. Opticohypothalamic glioma: an analysis of 16 cases. Child's Nerv Syst 1993;9:334–8.
236. Bruggers CS, Friedman HS, Phillips PC, et al. Leptomeningeal dissemination of optic pathway gliomas in three children. Am J Ophthalmol 1991; 111:719–23.
237. Chutorian AM, Carter S. Glioma of the optic nerve. Lancet 1970;1:786.
238. Chan MY, Foong AP, Heisey DM, et al. Potential prognostic factors of relapse-free survival in childhood optic pathway glioma: a multivariate analysis. Pediatr Neurosurg 1998;29:23–8.
239. Imes RK, Hoyt WF. Childhood chiasmal gliomas: update on the fate of patients in the 1969 San Francisco study. Br J Ophthalmol 1986;70:179–82.
240. Listernick R, Charrow J, Greenwald M, Mets M. Natural history of optic pathway tumors in children with neurofibromatosis type 1: a longitudinal study. J Pediatr 1994;125:63–6.
241. Kovalic JJ, Grigsby PW, Shepard MJ, et al. Radiation therapy for gliomas of the optic nerve and chiasm. Int J Radiat Oncol Biol Phys 1990;18:927–32.
242. Jenken D, Angyalfi S, Becker L, et al. Optic glioma in children: surveillance, resection, or irradiation? Int J Radiat Oncol Biol Phys 1993;25:215–25.
243. Kretschmar CS, Linggood RM. Chemotherapeutic treatment of extensive optic pathway tumors in infants. J Neuro-oncol 1991;10:263–70.
244. Regueiro CA, Ruiz MV, Millan I, et al. Prognostic factors and results of radiation therapy in optic pathway tumors. Tumors 1996;82:353–9.
245. Janss AJ, Grundy R, Cnaan A, et al. Optic pathway and hypothalamic/chiasmatic gliomas in children younger than age 5 years with a 6-year follow-up. Cancer 1995;75:1051–9.
246. Petronio J, Edwards MS, Prados M, et al. Management of chiasmal and hypothalamic gliomas of infancy and childhood with chemotherapy. J Neurosurg 1991;74:701–8.
247. Capo H, Kupersmith MJ. Efficacy and complications of radiotherapy of anterior visual pathway tumors. Neurol Clin 1991;9:179–201.
248. Chutorian AM, Schwartz JF, Evans RA, Carter S. Optic gliomas in children. Neurology 1964;14:83–95.
249. Posner M, Horrax G. Tumors of the optic nerve; long survival in 3 cases of intracranial tumor. Arch Ophthalmol 1948;40:56–76.
250. Spencer WH. Primary neoplasms of the optic nerve and its sheaths: clinical features and current concepts of pathogenetic mechanisms. Trans Am Ophthalmol Soc 1972;70:490–528.
251. Oxenhandler DC, Sayers MP. The dilemma of childhood optic gliomas. J Neurosurg 1978;48:34–41.
252. Kuenzle C, Weissert M, Roulet E, et al. Follow-up of optic pathway gliomas in children with neurofibromatosis type 1. Neuropediatrics 1994;25:295–300.
253. Horwich A, Bloom HJG. Optic gliomas: radiation therapy and prognosis. Int J Radiat Oncol Biol Phys 1979;11:1067–79.
254. Taveras JM, Mount LA, Wood EH. The value of radiation therapy in the management of glioma of the optic nerves and chiasm. Radiology 1956;66:518–28.
255. Bataini JP, Delanian S, Ponvert D. Chiasmal gliomas: results of irradiation management in 57 patients and review of literature. Int J Radiat Oncol Biol Phys 1991;21:615–23.
256. Pierce SM, Barnes PD, Loeffler JS, et al. Definitive radiotherapy in the management of symptomatic patients with optic glioma. Cancer 1990;65:45–52.
257. Wagener HP. Gliomas of the optic nerve. Am J Med Sci 1959;237:238–61.
258. Rush JA, Younge BR, Campbell RJ, MacCarty CS. Optic glioma. Long-term follow-up of 85 histopathology verified cases. Ophthalmology 1982;89: 1213–9.
259. Montgomery AB, Griffin T, Parker RG, Gerdes AJ. Optic nerve glioma: the role of radiation therapy. Cancer 1977;40:2079–80.
260. Danoff BF, Kramer S, Thompson N. The radiotherapeutic management of optic nerve gliomas in children. Int J Radiat Oncol Biol Phys 1980;6:45–50.
261. Robertson AG, Brewin TB. Optic nerve glioma. Clin Radiol 1980;31:471–4.
262. Harter DJ, Caderao JB, Leavens ME, Young SE. Radiotherapy in the management of primary gliomas involving the intracranial optic nerves and chiasm. Int J Radiat Oncol Biol Phys 1978;4:681–6.
263. Brand WN, Hoover SV. Optic glioma in children. Review of 16 cases given megavoltage radiation therapy. Childs Brain 1979;5:459–66.

264. Bynke H, Kagstrom E, Tjernstrom K. Aspects on the treatment of gliomas of the anterior visual pathway. Acta Ophthalmol 1977;55:269–80.
265. Miller NR, Iliff WJ, Green WR. Evaluation and management of gliomas of the anterior visual pathways. Brain 1974;97:743–54.
266. Jenken D, Angyalfi S, Becker L, et al. Optic glioma in children: surveillance, resection, or irradiation? Int J Radiat Oncol Biol Phys 1993;25:215–25.
267. Marquardt MD, Zimmerman LE. Histopathology of meningiomas and gliomas of the optic nerve. Hum Pathol 1982;13:226–35.
268. Jiang GL, Tucker SL, Guttenberger R, et al. Radiation-induced injury to the visual pathway. Radiother Oncol 1994;30:17–25.
269. Goldsmith BJ, Rosenthal SA, Wara WM, Larson DA. Ophthalmopathy after irradiation of meningioma. Int J Radiat Oncol Biol Phys [Submitted]
270. Cibis GW, Whittaker CK, Wood WE. Intraocular extension of optic nerve meningioma in a case of neurofibromatosis. Arch Ophthalmol 1985;103:404–6.
271. Johnson TE, Weatherhead RG, Nasr AM, Siqueira EB. Ectopic (Extradural) menigioma of the orbit: a report of two cases in children. J Pediatr Ophthalmol Strabismus 1993;30:43–7.
272. Samii M, Ramina R, Koch G, Reusche E. Malignant teratoma of the optic nerve: case report. Neurosurgery 1985;16:696–700.
273. Spencer WH, Borit A. Diffuse hyperplasia of the optic nerve in von Recklinghausen's disease. Am J Ophthalmol 1967;64:638–42.
274. Bergin DJ, Johnson TE, Spencer WH, McCord CD. Ganglionoma of the optic nerve. Am J Ophthalmol 1988;105:146–9.
275. Nerad JA, Kersten RC, Anderson RL. Hemangioblastoma of the optic nerve. Ophthalmology 1988;95: 398–402.
276. Garrity JA, Trautmann JC, Bartley JB, et al. Optic nerve sheath meningoceles. Ophthalmology 1990; 97:1519–31.
277. Myer DR, Wobig JL. Bilateral localized orbital neurofibromas. Ophthalmology 1992;99:1313–7.
278. Wulc AE, Bergin DJ, Barnes D, et al. Orbital optic nerve glioma in adult life. Arch Ophthalmol 1989; 107:1013–6.
279. De Dios AMV, Bond JR, Shives T, et al. Aneurysmal bone cyst. Cancer 1992;69:2921–31.
280. Sigler SC, Wobig JL, Dierks EF, et al. Cementifying fibroma presenting as proptosis. Ophthal Plast Reconstr Surg 1997;13:265–76.
281. Fakadej A, Boynton JR. Juvenile ossifying fibroma of the orbit. Ophthal Plast Reconstr Surg 1996;12: 174–7.
282. Sweet C, Silbergleit R, Mehta B. Primary intraosseous hemangioma of the orbit. CT and MR appearance. Am J Neuroradial 1997;18:379–81.
283. Ferry AP. Brown tumors (fibro-osseus bone replacement and overgrowth) of the orbit in hyperparathyroidism. Metab Pediatr Ophthalmol 1979;3:67–75.
284. Parrish CM, O'Day DM. Brown tumor of the orbit. Case report and review of the literature. Arch Ophthalmol 1986;104:1199–1202.
285. Powell JO, Glaser JS. Aneurysmal bone cysts of the orbit. Arch Ophthalmol 1975;93:340–2.
286. Hunter JV, Yokoyama C, Moseley IF, Wright JE. Aneurysmal bone cyst of the sphenoid with orbital involvement. Br J Ophthalmol 1990;74:505–8.
287. Yee RD, Cogan DG, Thorp TR, Schut L. Optic nerve compression due to aneurysmal bone cyst. Arch Ophthalmol 1977;95:2176–9.
288. Hoopes PC, Anderson RL, Blodi FC. Giant cell (reparative) granuloma of the orbit. Ophthalmology 1981; 88:1361–6.
289. Gogl H. Psammo-osteioid-fibrom der Nase und ihrer Negenhohlen. Monatsschr Ohrenheilkd Laryngorhinol 1949;83:1–10.
290. Margo CE, Weiss A, Habal MB. Psammomatoid ossifying fibroma. Arch Ophthalmol 1986;104:1347–51.
291. Stern RM, Beauchamp GR, Berlin AJ. Ocular findings in juvenile nasopharyngeal angiofibroma. Ophthal Surg 1966;17:560–4.
292. Bonavolonta G, Villari G, de Rosa G, Sammartino A. Ocular complications of juvenile angiofibroma. Ophthalmologica 1980;181:334–9.
293. Katz BJ, Nerad JA. Ophthalmic manifestations of fibrous dysplasia. Ophthalmology 1998;105:2207–15.
294. Tellado MV, McLean IW, Specht CS, Varga J. Adenoid cystic carcinomas of the lacrimal gland in childhood and adolescent. Ophthalmology 1997;104:1622–5.
295. Faktorvich EG, Crawford JB, Kong C, Char DH. Benign mixed tumor (pleomorphic adenoma) of the lacrimal gland in a six-year old boy. Am J Ophthalmol 1996:122:446–7.
296. Slavin ML, Glaser JS. Acute severe irreversible visual loss with sphenoethmoiditis—"posterior" orbital cellulitis. Arch phthalmol 1987;105:345–8.

17

Intraconal Tumors

The intraconal space (the volume surrounded by the extraocular muscles) is a common site of orbital neoplasms. Cavernous hemangioma is the most common adult intraconal tumor. Less frequently, other benign mesenchymal tumors, primary optic nerve neoplasms, metastases, benign lymphoid proliferations, and many less uncommon peripheral nerve and fibrous lesions can involve this area of the orbit, as can some rarer primary malignancies.

ORBITAL CAVERNOUS HEMANGIOMA

Cavernous hemangioma accounts for between 3 and 7 percent of orbital mass lesions and occurs most often in middle-aged women.[1–3] Proptosis is the most common presenting sign (Figure 17–1); however, diminished vision, an afferent pupil defect, visual field defects, lid swelling, a palpable mass, and diplopia can occur. The proptosis is usually axial, but the clinical appearance is not diagnostic.

Few large clinical series have been reported. Ruchman and Flanagan reported 12 cases, Wright 10, and Harris and Jakobiec reviewed 66 cases, which had been managed by Reese and others over a 60-year period at Columbia.[4–6] In the latter series, 70 percent of patients were females, and the mean age was 42 years.[6] McNab reported on the London experience of 85 patients managed between 1968 and 1988. In that report, cavernous hemangiomas accounted for approximately 7 percent of orbital cases.[7]

The author has managed about 35 orbital cavernous hemangiomas. Most patients were female; the mean patient age was 52 years (range 15 to 78 years). The interval between symptoms and diagnosis averaged 3.8 years with a range of 2 months to 10 years. All but one patient had a unilateral orbital lesion, and one had bilateral cavernous hemangiomas.

Usually, these tumors occur in the intraconal space; in approximately 20 percent, they are either both intra- and extraconal or entirely extraconal in location (Figure 17–2). Less commonly, this tumor involves the orbital apex, the optic nerve canal, or

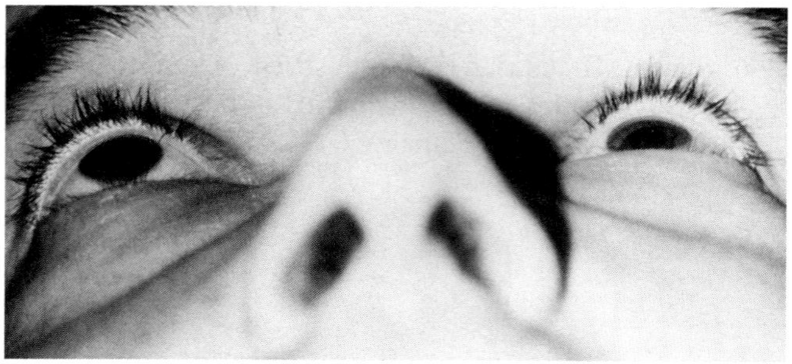

Figure 17–1. Patient with axial proptosis secondary to intraconal cavernous hemangioma.

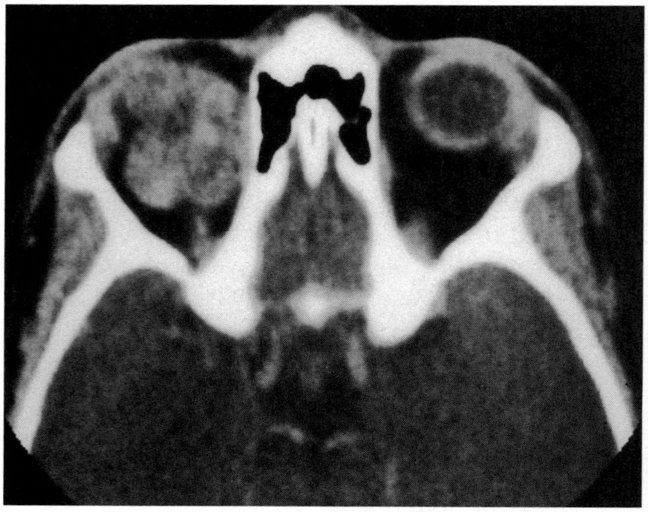

Figure 17–2. Axial CT demonstrates a cavernous hemangioma with both intraconal and extraconal involvement.

both and may present with profound loss of vision (Figure 17–3). Extraconal tumors are discussed in the next few chapters.

Visual acuity and color vision were diminished in more than one-half of the cases I have operated on. In a few patients, the initial symptoms were loss of peripheral visual field. Several patients had limitations of extraocular muscle movement.

Fundus abnormalities consisting of choroidal folds and/or disc edema occur in about one-half of patients with large tumors. Figure 17–4 demonstrates a typical pattern of horizontal choroidal folds. Figure 17–5 shows marked disc edema associated with a hemangioma compressing the optic nerve; neither finding is diagnostic for hemangioma. Almost all patients have some degree of proptosis ranging from 0.5 to 8 mm; in a minority of patients, it was ≥ 6 mm. Occasionally, the location of the tumor relative to the optic nerve can result in decreased vision on medial or lateral gaze (Figure 17–6).

All cavernous hemangiomas had a number of common characteristics identifiable on computed tomography (CT) or magnetic resonance imaging (MRI) scans. Lesions are rounded, homogeneous, encapsulated, and usually do not involve the orbital apex (Figure 17–7).[8,9] Most commonly they involve the temporal aspect of the intraconal space. One of our patients had bilateral cavernous hemangiomas (Figure 17–8).[10] Others have reported bilateral tumors in association with Maffucci's syndrome.[11]

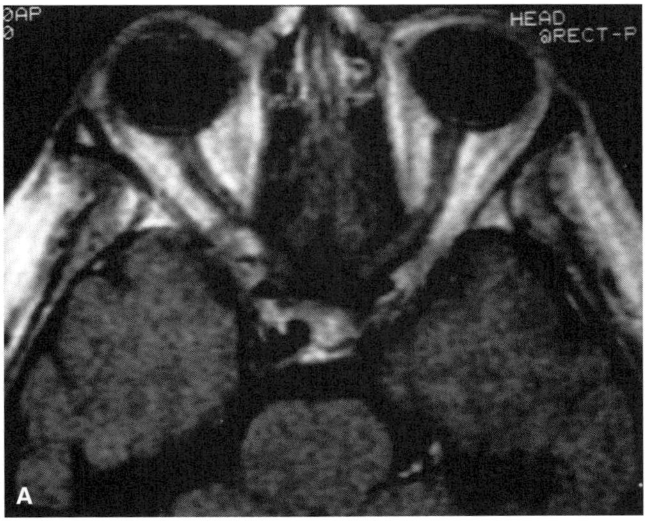

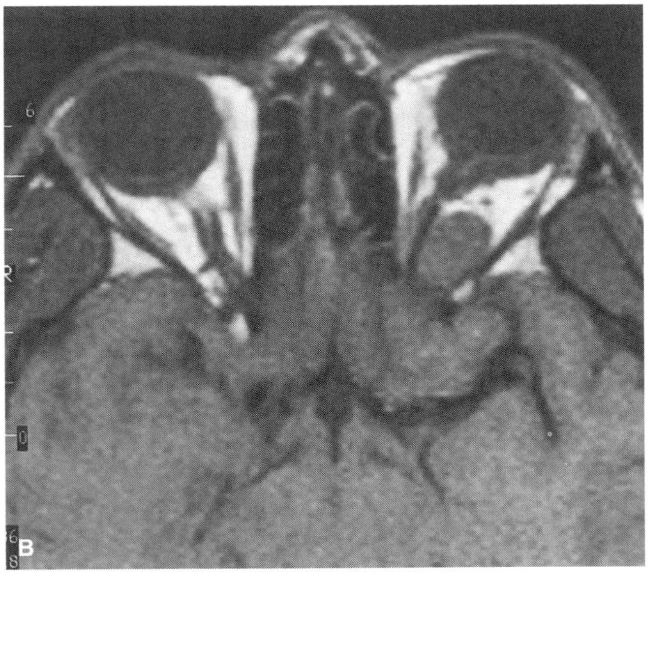

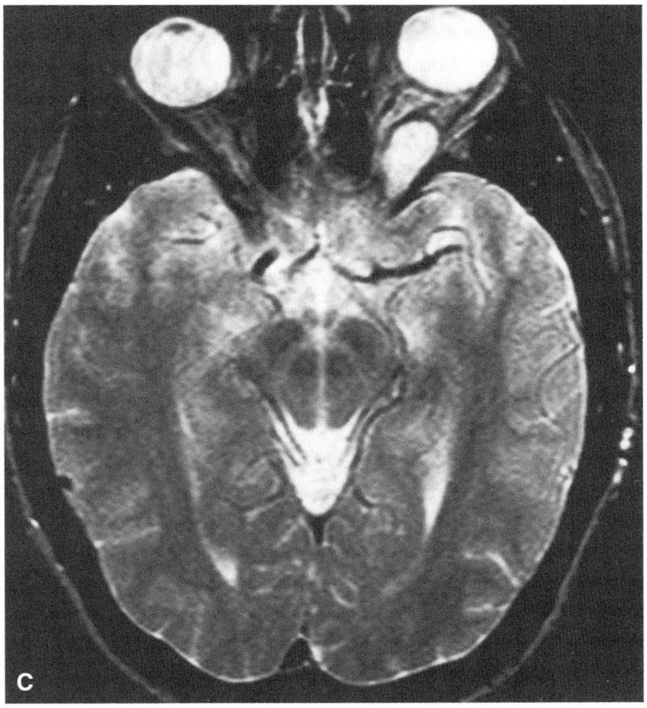

Figure 17–3. *A,* Orbital cavernous hemangioma uncommonly involves the optic canal, but is shown in Figure 17–3A to have a small cavernous hemangioma in the canal, which can cause profound visual loss. It was excised with a combined neurosurgery-ocular oncology procedure. *B* and *C,* Another cavernous hemangioma that involved the orbital apex and canal. Postoperatively, vision was good but the patient required strabismus surgery. Figure 17–3B demonstrates the lesion in a T_1-weighted axial scan. Figure 17–3C is a T_2-weighted scan. Typically hemangiomas are dark on T_1 and bright on T_2 scans. They also enhance with gadolinium.

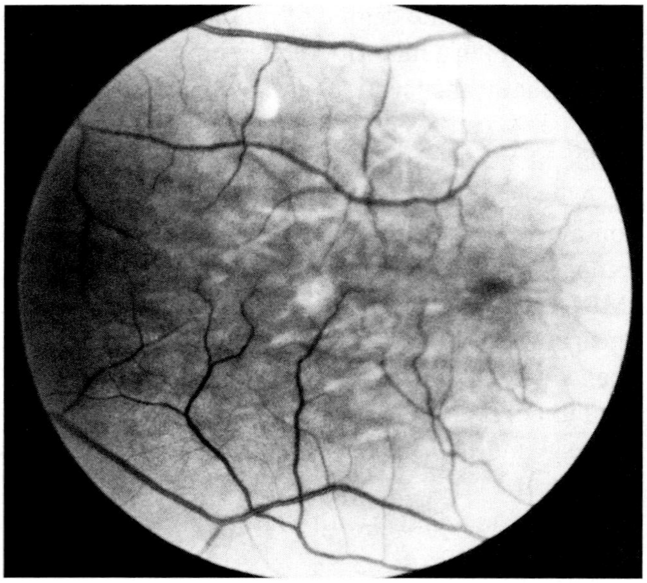

Figure 17–4. Choroidal folds in a patient with cavernous hemangioma.

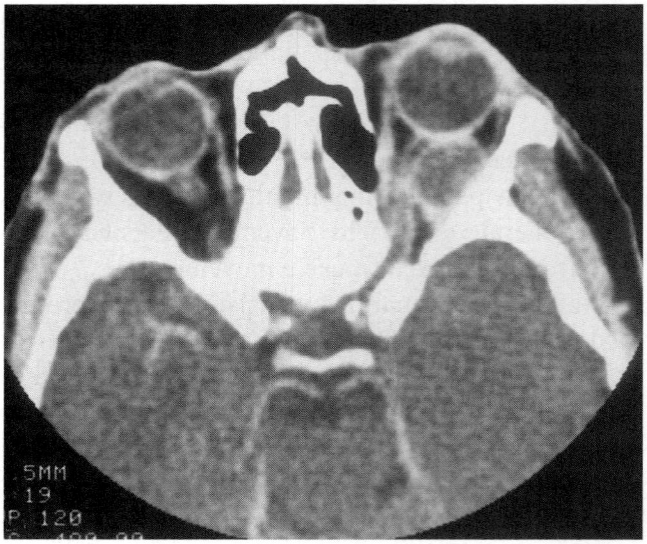

Figure 17–6. Axial CT with an intraconal hemangioma lateral to the optic nerve that produced positionally decreased vision on abduction due to optic nerve compression.

On thin-section MRI performed on a 1.5 Tesla unit, the MR pattern of cavernous hemangioma is typical.[9,12] The lesions were hypointense compared to brain and contrasted sharply to orbital fat on T_1-weighted images and are either isointense or hyperintense on T_2–weighted scans (Figure 17–9). Unfortunately, these T_1 and T_2 patterns are shared by a number of other benign and malignant orbital tumors (including neurofibroma, neurilemmoma, solitary fibrous tumor, rare metastases, and hemangiopericytomas). In the minority of cases, these tumors were not confined to the intraconal space, and some had both intraconal and extraconal involvement (see Figure 17–2). In one report, using the serial dynamic MRI technique, a cavernous hemangioma feeder vessel was visualized.[13] Surgically, the author's experience is that feeder vessels are usually not seen.

A number of lesions can simulate a cavernous hemangioma. In over 1,000 previous orbital biopsies, approximately 25 patients had tumors that mimicked the clinical or radiologic (CT or MRI)

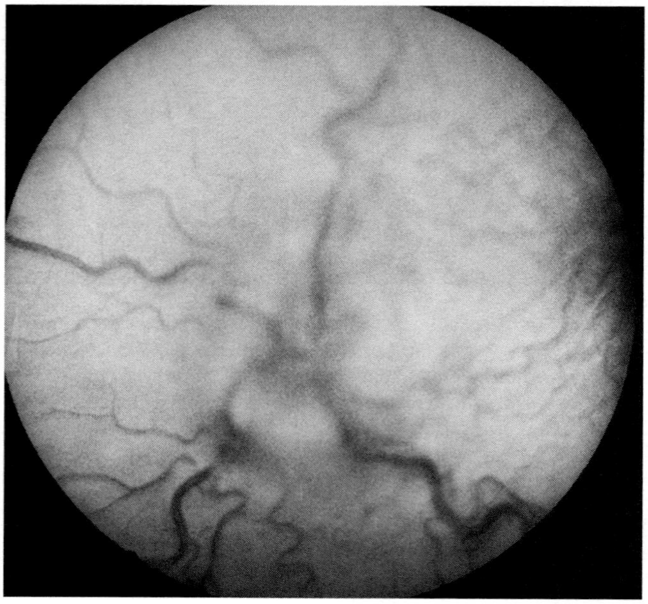

Figure 17–5. Optic disc changes associated with pressure from a cavernous hemangioma. Often, these alterations can take a few months to dissipate.

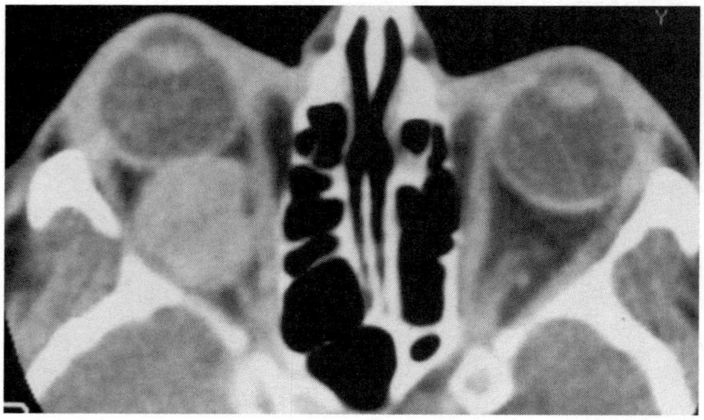

Figure 17–7. Axial CT demonstrates a typical cavernous hemangioma, which is a smooth, rounded, discrete homogeneous mass in an intraconal location with sparing of the orbital apex.

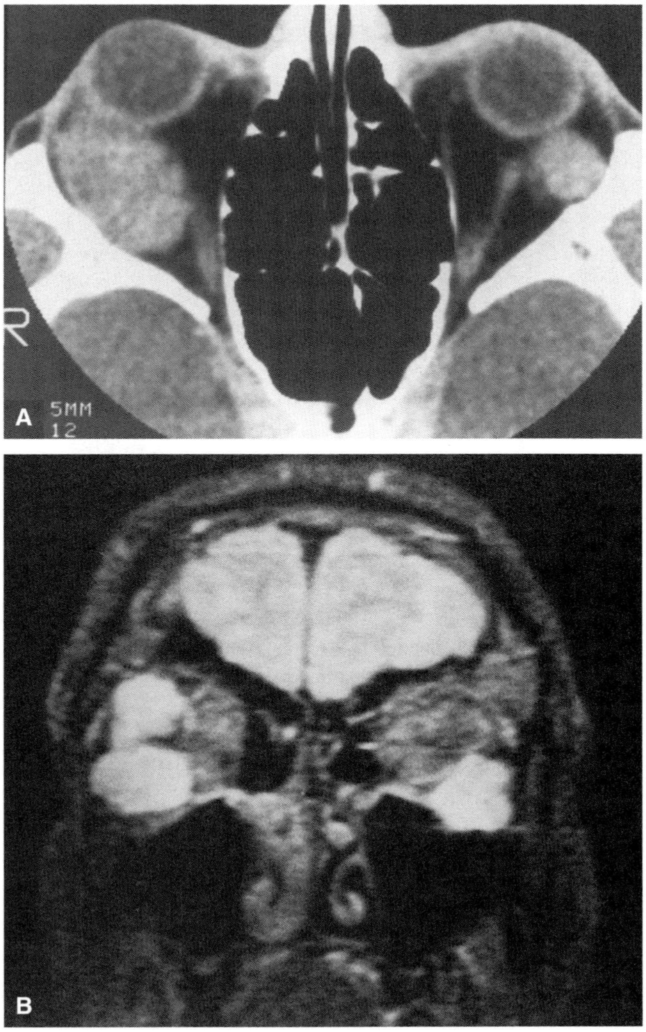

Figure 17–8. *A,* Axial CT scan of bilateral cavernous hemangiomas. *B,* MRI (T_2-weighted) coronal scan demonstrates bilateral cavernous hemangioma.

pattern of cavernous hemangioma.[14–18] The mean age of these patients was 37 years (range 8 months to 90 years). Proptosis was present in all cases; 6 had ≥ 6 mm of proptosis. Several were intraconal, some were extraconal, and a minority involved both compartments. As shown in Figures 17–10 to 17–18, lesions other than cavernous hemangioma can simulate the rounded homogenous mass on CT, ultrasonography, or MRI. In 5 of these cases, the history and clinical presentation was sufficient to rule out a cavernous hemangioma. Patients with an arteriovenous malformation or venous varix had proptosis which changed with the Valsalva maneuver; this is not a feature of cavernous hemangioma.[19,20] The patients with congenital inclusion cyst (see Figure 17–9) and focal lymphangioma (see Figure 17–11) were under age 5 years at the time of diagnosis. The patients with a metastatic uveal melanoma to the contralateral orbit (see Figure 17–12), a traumatic conjunctival inclusion cyst (see Figure 17–13), and recurrent malignant fibrous histiocytoma (see Figure 17–14), could be correctly diagnosed on the basis of history.

Some lesions cannot always be differentiated, either clinically or on imaging studies, from a cavernous hemangioma. These include alveolar soft part sarcoma (see Figures 19–13 and 19–14), orbital rhabdomyosarcoma, hemangiopericytoma (Figure 17–19), neurilemmoma (see Figure 17–16), neurofibroma, benign fibrous histiocytoma (see Figure 17–18) and extradural meningioma.[8,16,21–27]

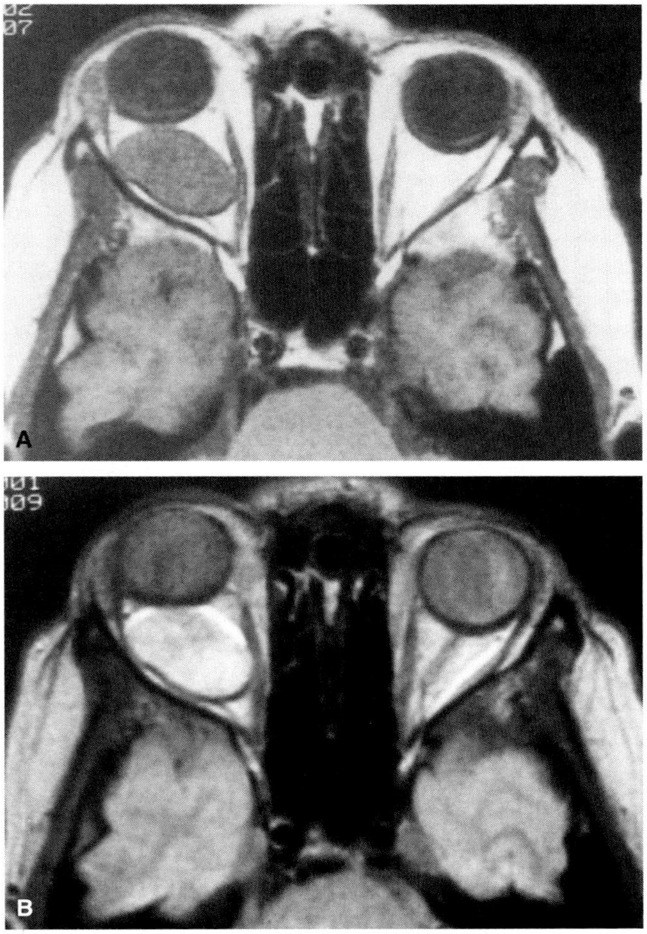

Figure 17–9. *A,* MRI scan demonstrates anatomic pattern of typical cavernous hemangioma. On T_1-weighted image the tumor is hypointense with respect to brain. *B,* T_2- weighted MRI scan demonstrates that the lesion in Figure 17–9A is either isointense or hyperintense with respect to the brain.

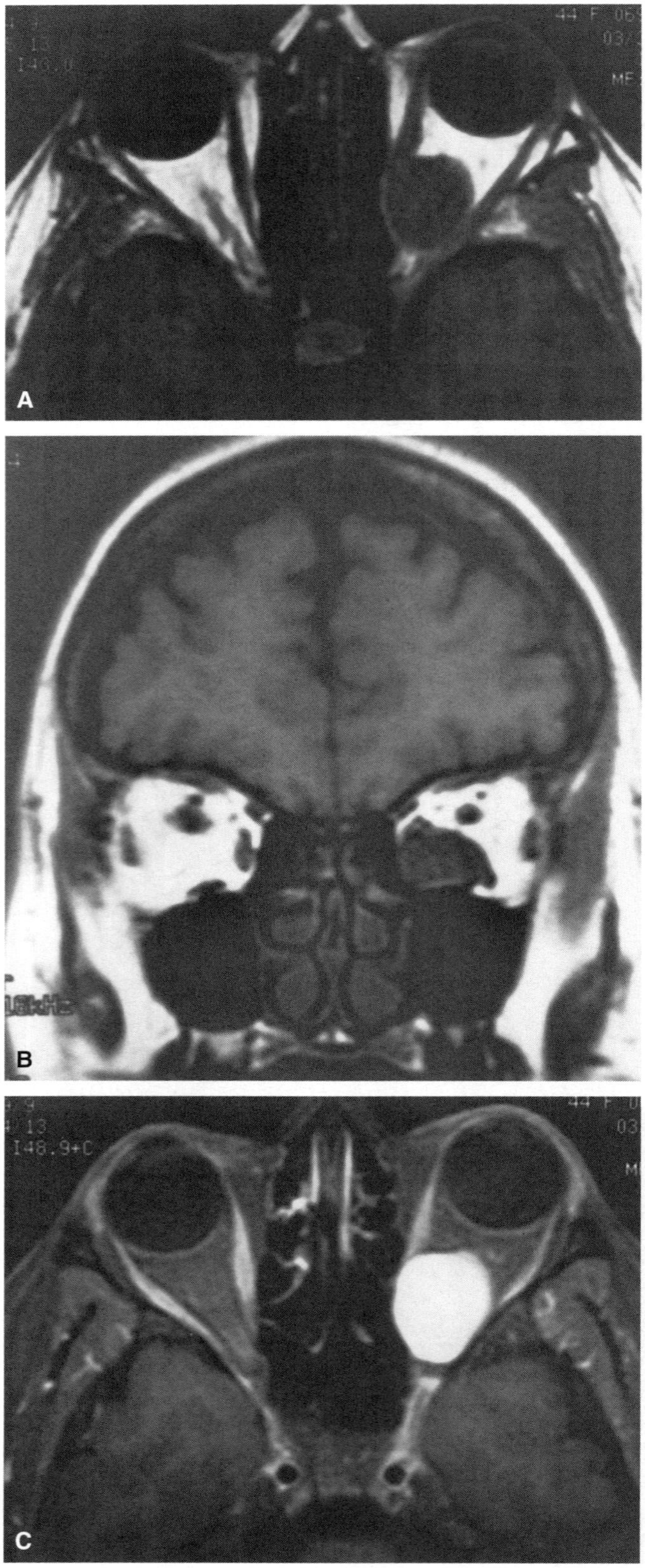

Figure 17–10. *A,* Neurilemmoma on T_1-weighted axial scan is intraconal and spares the apex. *B,* On a T_1–weighted coronal scan, the lesion is both intraconal and extraconal and is not as rounded as a cavernous hemangioma. *C,* On T_2-weighted image, this lesion is more hyperintense than most hemangiomas.

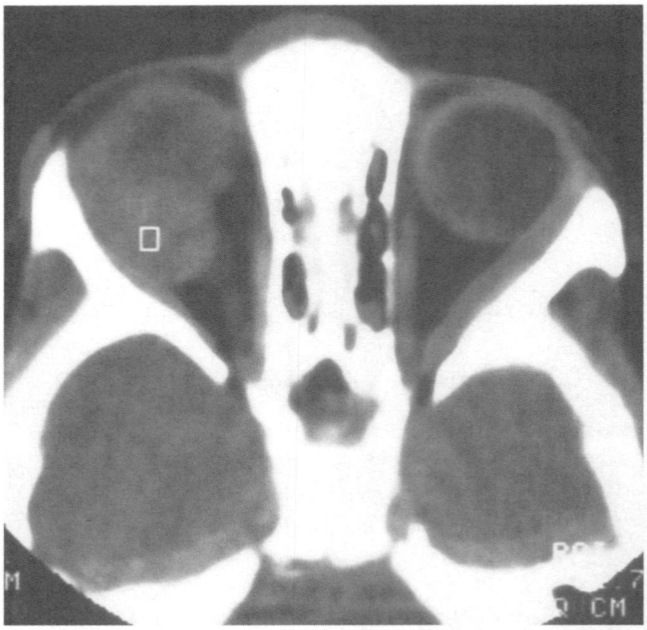

Figure 17–11. CT scan of solitary lymphangioma in a young child. Usually, this lesion is more diffuse.

While a mixed cell tumor of the lacrimal gland can simulate the ultrasonographic pattern of cavernous hemangioma, the clinical presentations are usually sufficiently disparate to allow easy differentiation of these two entities.[23] In one study, in which 11 patients with unilateral proptosis were felt to have cavernous hemangiomas on B-scan ultrasonography, this diagnosis was only confirmed histologically in 6.[25] Simi-

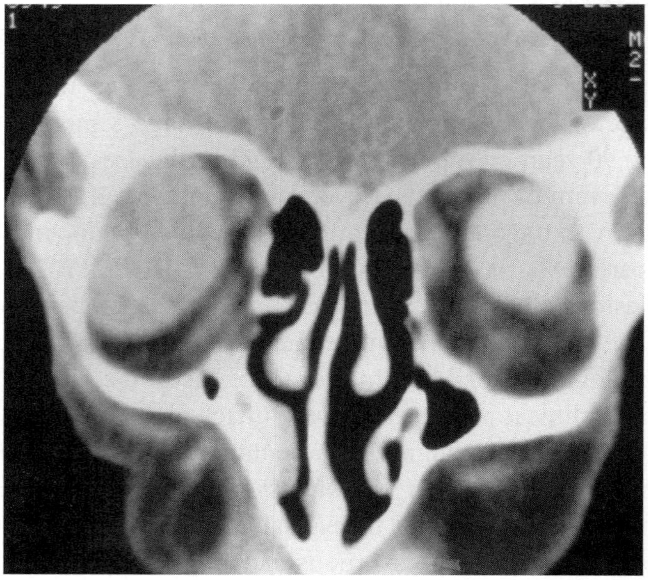

Figure 17–12. Uveal melanoma metastatic to contralateral orbit.

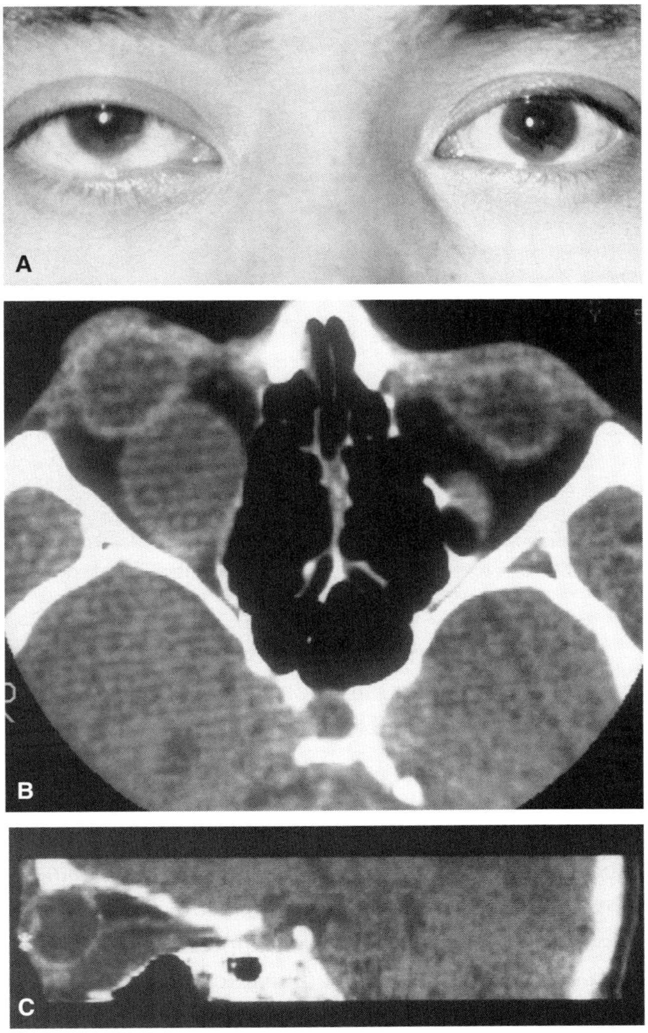

Figure 17–13. *A,* Clinical photograph demonstrates axial proptosis in a patient with traumatic conjunctival inclusion cyst. *B,* Axial CT scan of traumatic conjunctival inclusion cyst. *C,* Parasagittal reformation of the scan.

larly, a liposarcoma can simulate hemangioma on ultrasonography, but this confusion is not likely on CT or MRI.[28–30] Sometimes, cavernous hemangiomas can simulate other tumors. The patient shown in Figure 17–20 was followed up elsewhere for years with a presumed optic nerve tumor. While on axial scan this tumor appeared to involve the optic nerve, on direct coronal T_1-weighted scan the tumor can be seen to be inferior to the nerve (see Figures 17–20A to C). It was resected with some visual return. Figure 17–20D and E shows a tumor that was an extradural meningioma that produced a similar imaging pattern.

A varix can sometimes also simulate a cavernous hemangioma, and it has been one of the few lesions

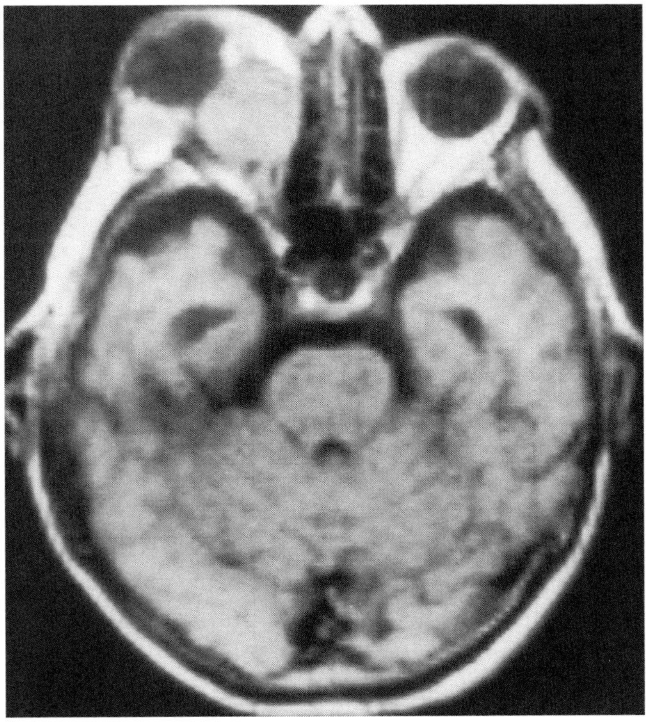

Figure 17–14. Axial T_1-weighted MRI scan of malignant fibrous histiocytoma. The tumor appears to be discrete and encapsulated, but that was not noted at surgery.

that we have found for which CT is a more useful adjuvant than MRI for diagnosis. On MR scan, often the pattern on T_1- and T_2–weighted scans show a heterogeneous pattern consistent with hemorrhage (Figure 17–21). The ability to perform a Valsalva maneu-

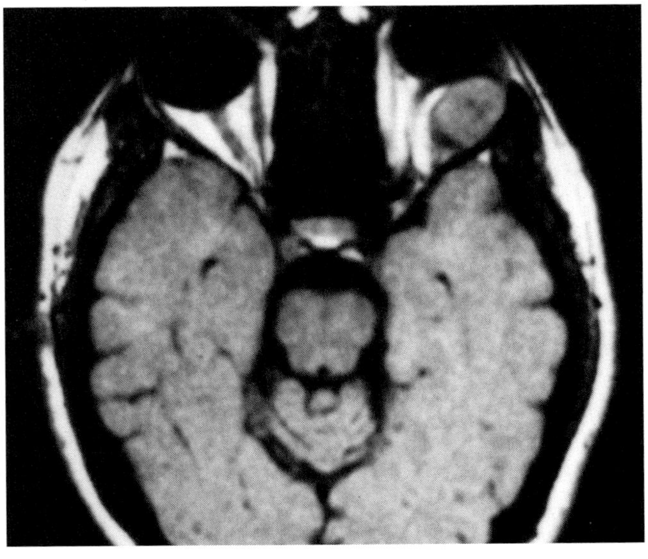

Figure 17–15. Axial T_1-weighted MRI of a benign fibrous histiocytoma.

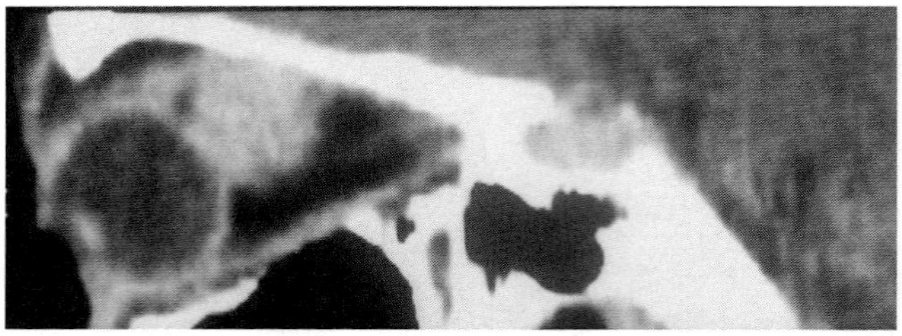

Figure 17–16. Parasagittal reformatted CT scan demonstrating neurilemmoma.

ver with greater ease, given the relative rapidity of helical CT versus MRI scans, is useful in these cases. Figures 17–22A and B show a case of an orbital varix, referred as a unilateral intraconal tumor, that was shown on CT with Valsalva to be a bilateral orbital varix.[28] Usually, these varices will spontaneously present with proptosis, pain, and diplopia; some will spontaneously close and we have had to either embolize or surgically clip the others.[31–36] Alternatively, Rootman and colleagues have advocated the use of cyanoacrylate glue intraoperative venography to control outflow and thrombose the lesion so that it can be more easily removed.[37] A more extensive orbital varix which required surgical intervention is shown in Figures 17–23A and B.

Rarely, cavernous hemangiomas can produce intracranial involvement. The patient shown in Figures 17–24A and B had such a lesion, with no vision. Orbital hemangiomas have rarely been reported in association with other diseases including the blue rubber nevus syndrome.[38]

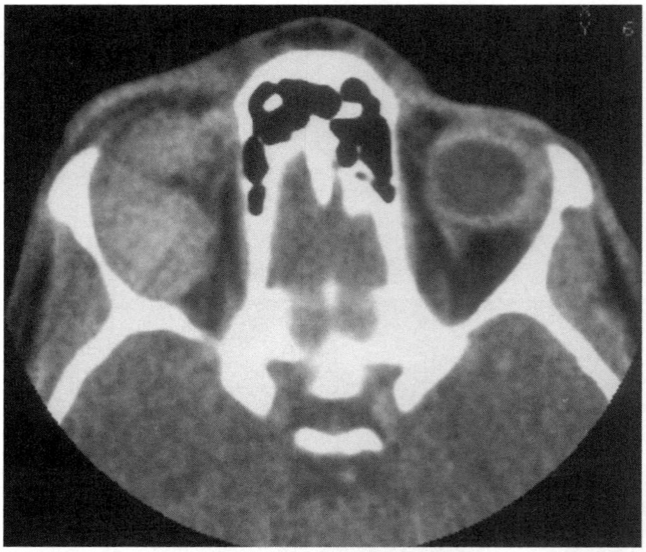

Figure 17–18. Axial CT of biopsy-proven benign fibrous histiocytoma.

The management of cavernous hemangiomas of the orbit is usually straightforward. If a lesion is not causing symptoms and is noted either serendipitously or, as in our bilateral case, as a small, second tumor, no treatment is indicated (Figure 17–25). There is an extremely small likelihood that a rounded, encapsulated, intraconal lesion could be a malignant hemangiopericytoma. Larger tumors can be removed through a number of different approaches, although most commonly, the size and position of these lesions require lateral orbitotomy.[39,40] The appearance of a cavernous hemangioma at surgery is quite characteristic (Figure 17–26). The lesion is a discrete, reddish,

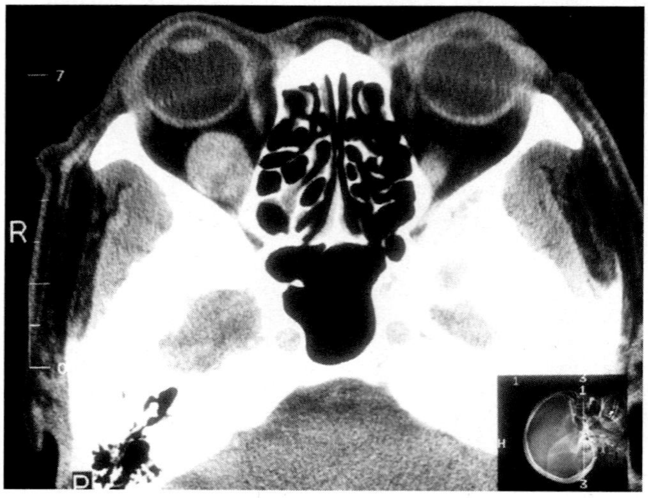

Figure 17–17. Metastatic sarcoma on axial CT simulates imaging characteristic of a cavernous hemangioma.

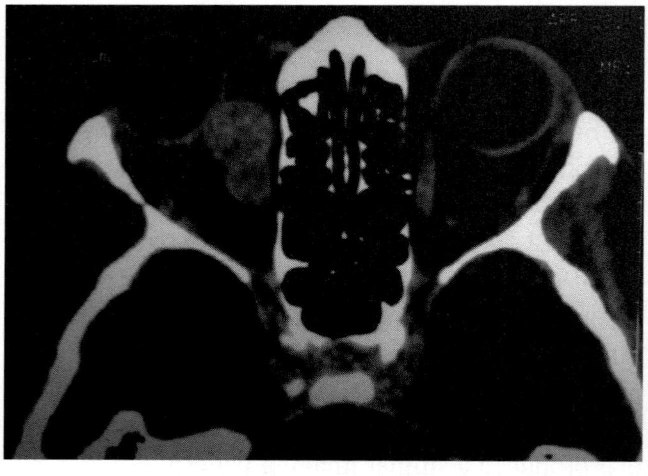

Figure 17–19. Hemangiopericytoma on axial CT. We have managed a few of these lesions, and they can simulate hemangiomas on both CT and MRI.

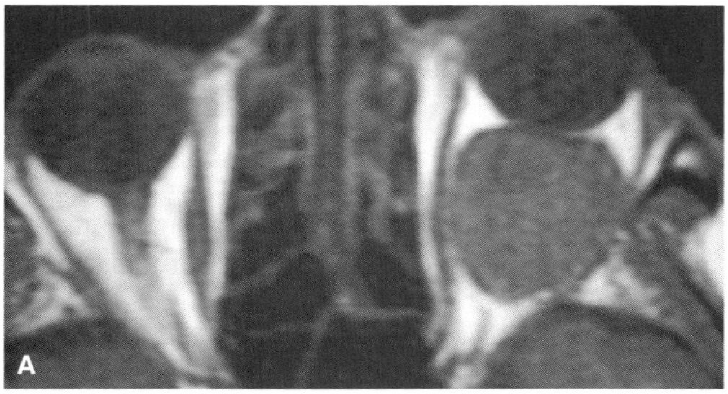

Figure 17–20. *A,* Patient followed up at another center for a presumed optic nerve tumor. T_1-weighted axial scan does not show a delineation between the nerve and the tumor. *B,* T_2-weighted axial scan of the above tumor. *C,* Direct coronal T_1-weighted MRI scan showing that the lesion from *A* and *B* is a cavernous hemangioma inferior to the optic nerve. *D,* An optic nerve sheath meningioma that is predominantly extradural simulating a cavernous hemangioma. *E,* Coronal T_2 image of lesion shown in Figure 17–20D.

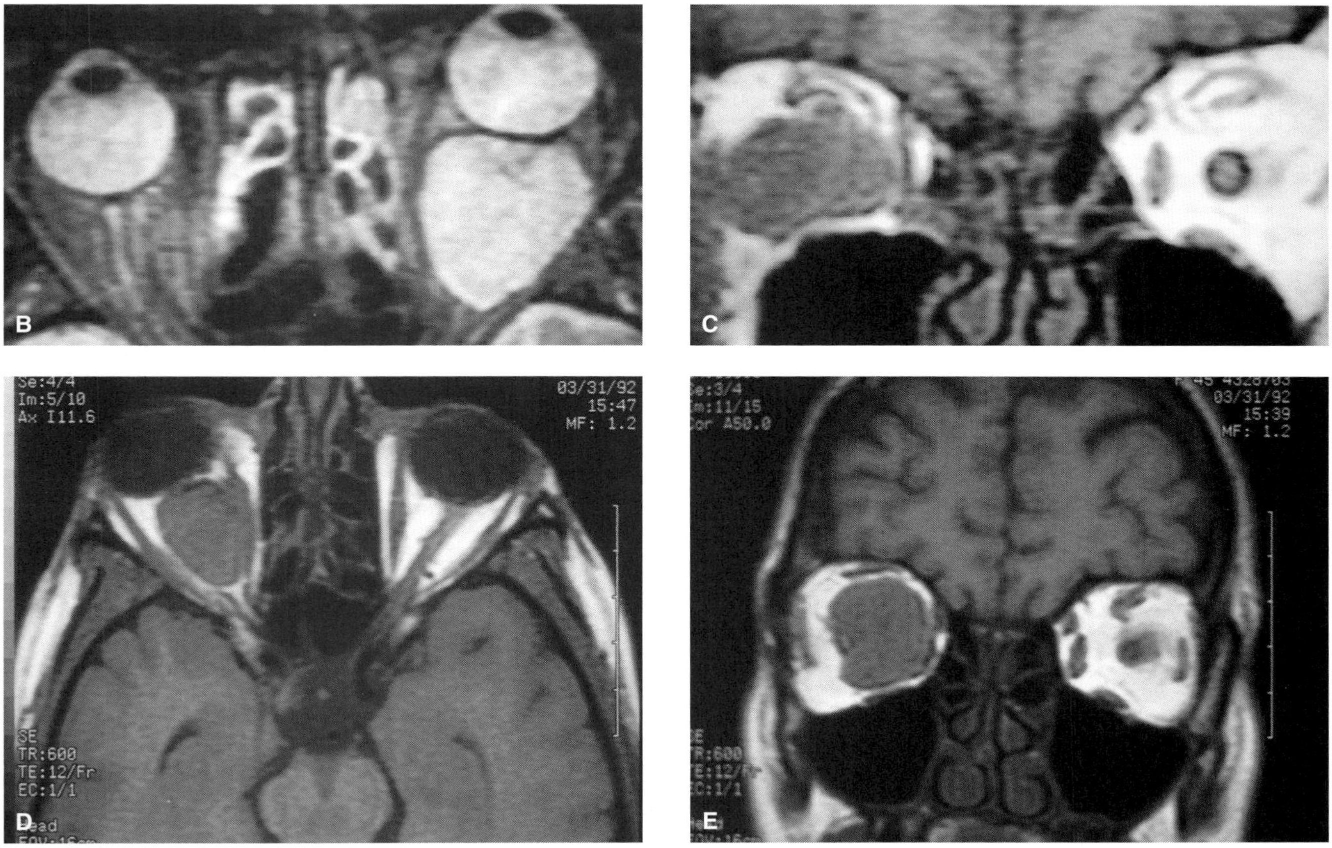

encapsulated, molded mass without feeder vessels. Fortunately, as our series documents, with newer surgical techniques, most cavernous hemangiomas can be safely removed without loss of vision.[41] This represents an improvement, compared with historic results in which as many as 25 percent of patients had diminished acuity after surgery.[6,7] Occasionally, a cavernous hemangioma can be removed through a conjunctival incision.[40] In our experience, this is a good approach for an inferior, extraconal lesion (Figure 17–27). As described by Henderson and colleagues, Wright, and others, the effect of partial resection of this neoplasm is unclear, but most do not recur in that setting.[7,41]

In small apical cavernous hemangiomas which are symptomatic, a number of approaches have been used to reach this area with less morbidity than a lateral orbitotomy.[42–46] At the very apex of the orbit, if the lesion is superior, we have reached it through a combined neurosurgical approach. If the lesion is quite small, symptomatic, and inferior to the nerve, we have often gone through the sinuses. In some of the latter cases, we have actually not removed the tumor but merely opened up the medial inferior wall along with the periorbita to allow decompression and alleviate the symptoms (unpublished data).

NEURILEMMOMA

Neurilemmomas or schwannomas account for approximately 1 percent of orbital tumors. In an analysis of several series with approximately 2,500 orbital tumors, 30 schwannomas were noted.[47–50]

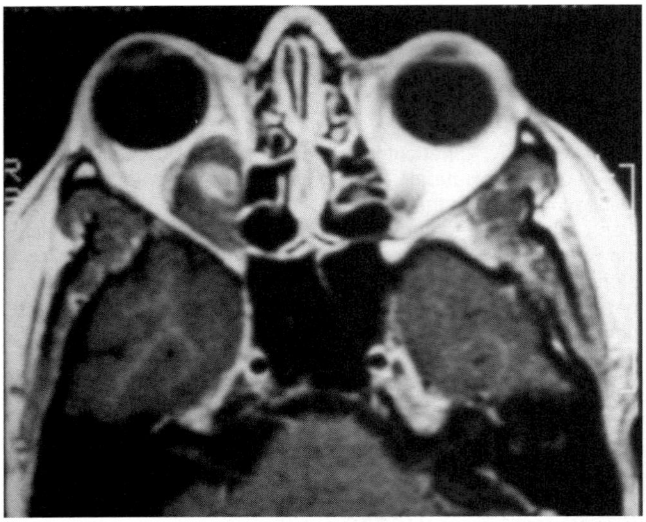

Figure 17–21. T_1-weighted axial MRI of a venous varix. Proptosis markedly increased with a Valsalva maneuver.

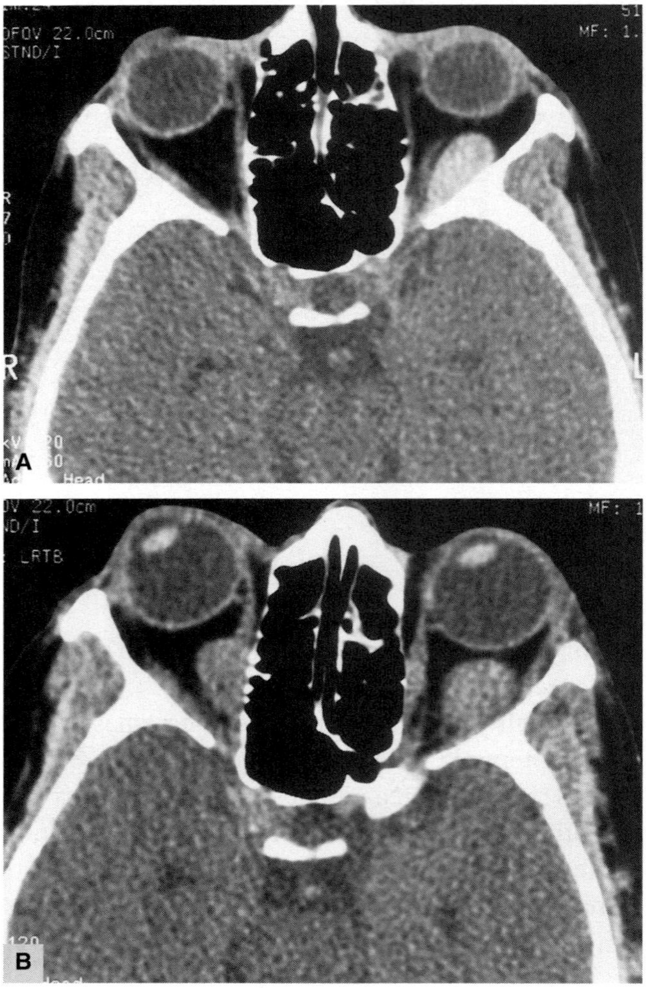

Figure 17–22. *A,* CT scan shows a unilateral orbital mass. *B,* CT scan with Valsalva maneuver demonstrates enlargement of the varix, with bilateral involvement in the same case.

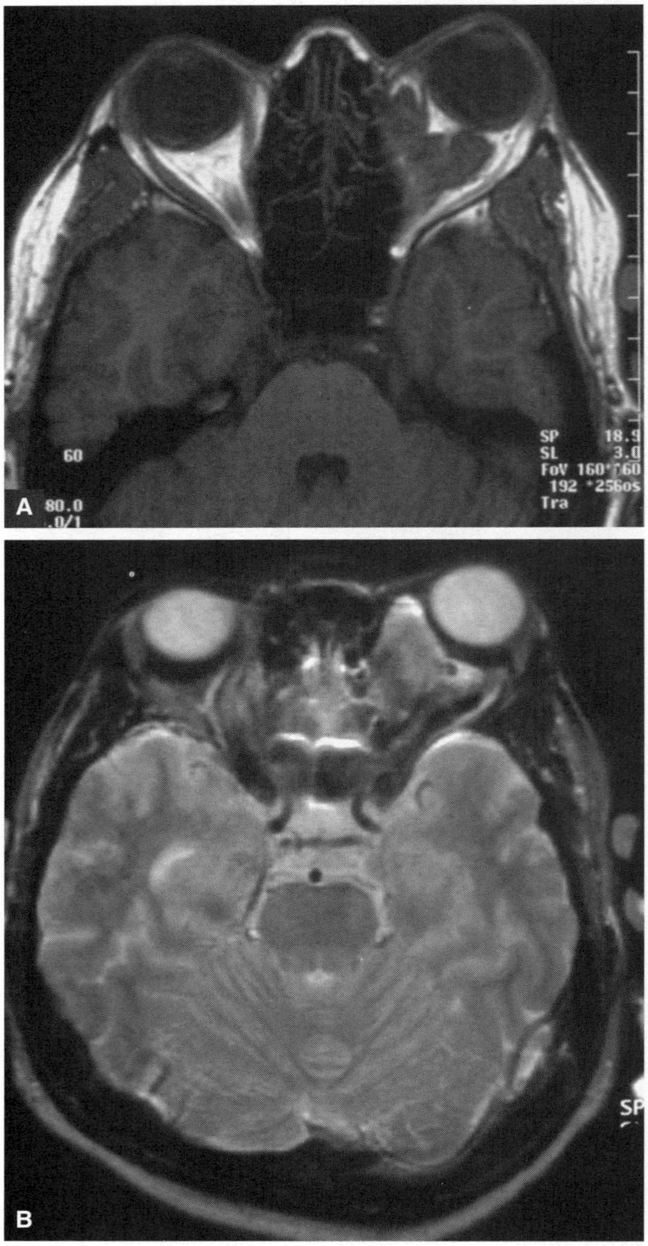

Figure 17–23. *A,* Orbital varix with a significant hemorrhage that required intraoperative intervention. Orbital venous varix on a T_1-weighted axial scan. The same lesion shown on T_2-weighted axial scan.

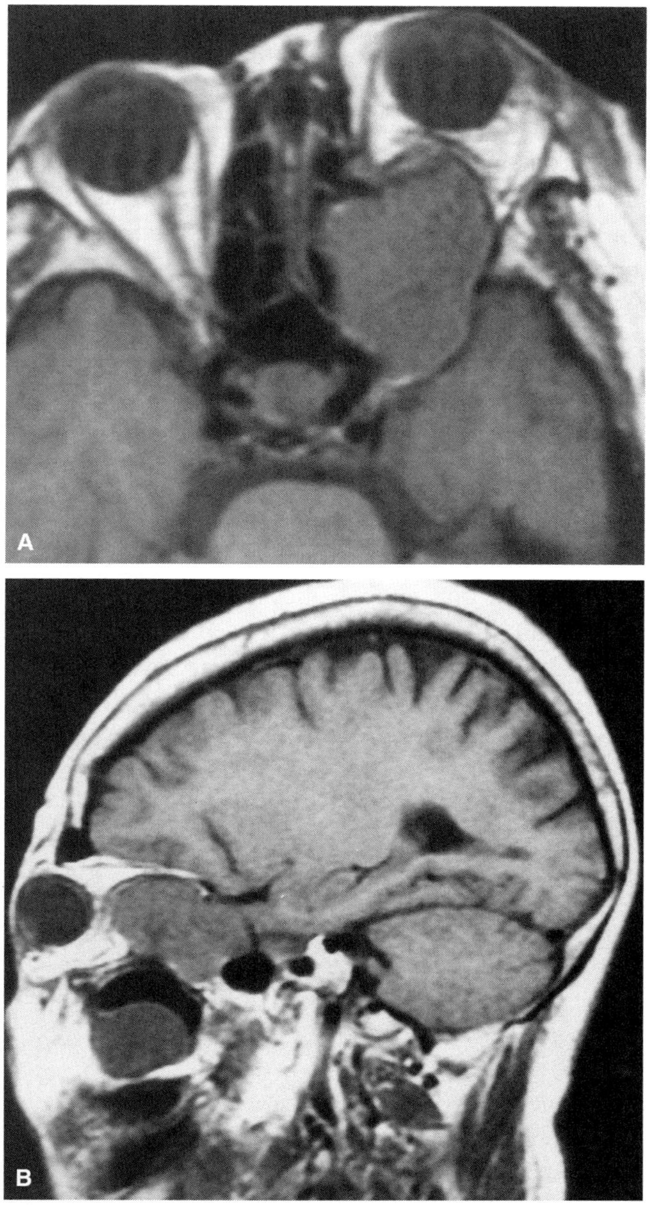

Figure 17–24. *A,* Axial T_1-weighted MRI scan of a massive cavernous hemangioma. *B,* Lesion shown in Figure 17–24A on T_1-weighted parasagittal scan.

Unfortunately, a neurilemmoma or extradural meningioma can almost perfectly simulate a cavernous hemangioma on imaging studies.[16,51] A CT scan of a neurilemmoma is shown in Figure 17–16. The MRI appearance in Figure 17–10 led the author preoperatively to believe this was most likely neurilemmoma, on the basis of the configuration of the anterior and posterior margins of the tumor; however, this was perhaps more of a "roundsmenship ploy" than a statement based on definitive data.

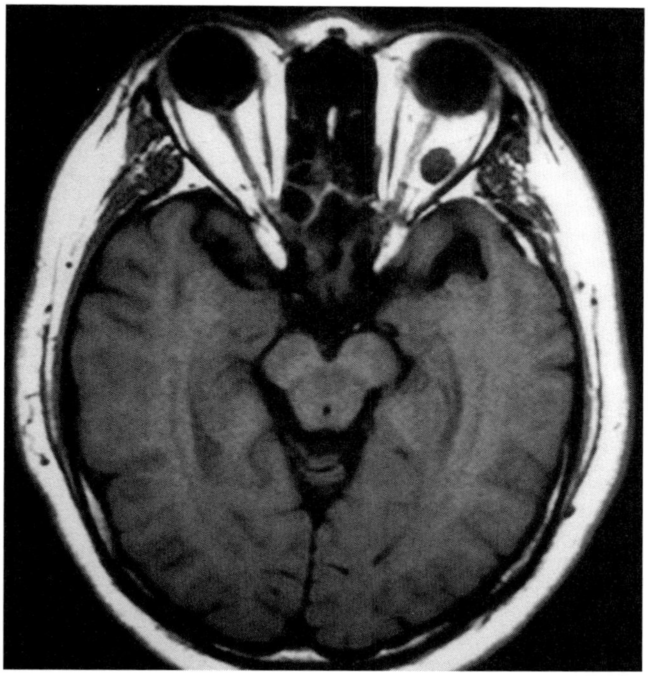

Figure 17–25. Axial T_1-weighted MRI scan shows a lesion detected when imaging was performed for headache. This mass is unchanged with over 10 years of follow-up.

Figure 17–28 shows a more cystic-appearing neurilemmoma on CT. The treatment of neurilemmomas is surgical excision. Usually, these tumors can be removed in toto. Occasionally, they can be adjacent to the nerve, and careful microdissection is necessary. Less commonly, they involve the superior orbital tissue.[50,52] Incomplete excision of a neurilemmoma has a very small but finite chance of producing malignant transformation of the remnant.[49,53] In

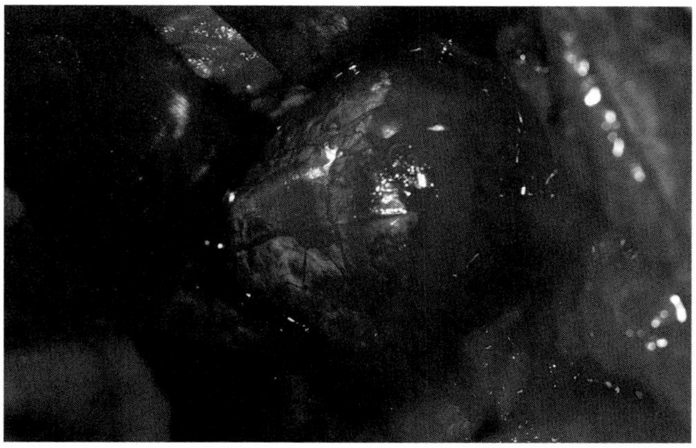

Figure 17–26. Photograph of a cavernous hemangioma at the time of surgical excision. This tumor has a characteristic appearance as a reddish, encapsulated, usually smooth mass.

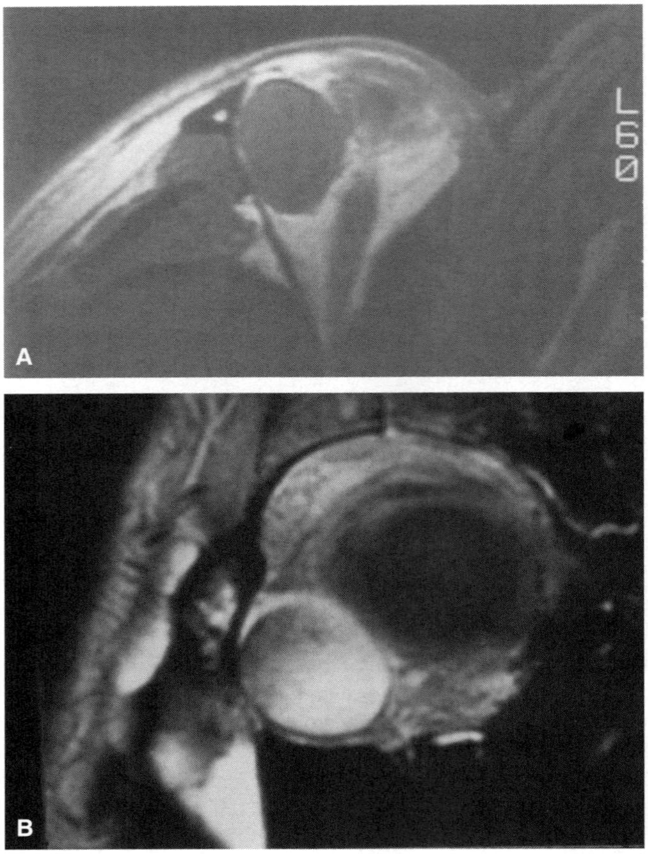

Figure 17–27. *A,* Extraconal, inferior-lateral cavernous hemangioma on T_1-weighted axial scan. The lesion was removed through a conjunctival incision. *B,* Lesion shown on a T_2-weighted coronal scan.

one case, an orbital neurilemmoma was the presenting finding of neurofibromatosis, type 1 (NF1).[52]

FIBROUS HISTIOCYTOMA

Fibrous histiocytomas of the orbit are not rare; Font and Hidayat reported on 150 cases from the Armed Forces Institute of Pathology.[54] Orbital involvement by this neoplasm was not recognized until the early 1960s. A number of terms have been used to describe benign and malignant forms of this process, including sclerosing hemangioma, dermatofibrosarcoma, and giant cell tumor.[55,56]

Usually, patients with fibrous histiocytomas present in middle age, although the reported age range is 4 to 85 years. These lesions can be difficult to diagnose, and a number of cases have been misdiagnosed as hemangiomas. Both benign (see Figures 17–14 and 15) and malignant fibrous histiocytomas have CT and MRI characteristics that may sometimes simulate cavernous hemangioma. Similarly, on histologic evaluation, some fibrous histiocytomas have initially been misdiagnosed as vascular tumors.

Fibrous histiocytomas have a tendency to involve the superior and superomedial orbit. Proptosis, a palpable mass, and decreased vision are the most common presenting findings. Generally, benign fibrous histiocytomas are smaller and have a longer disease course than their malignant counterparts. Surgical removal is sufficient for benign lesions; however, 31 percent of lesions have been found to recur, probably because many were initially incompletely excised. These lesions often have indistinct borders without a surgical capsule. Making the correct diagnosis of a recurrent fibrous histocytoma can be difficult. We had biopsied one patient once before because of a suspicious imaging finding for recurrence; that biopsy was negative. The patient was asymptomatic

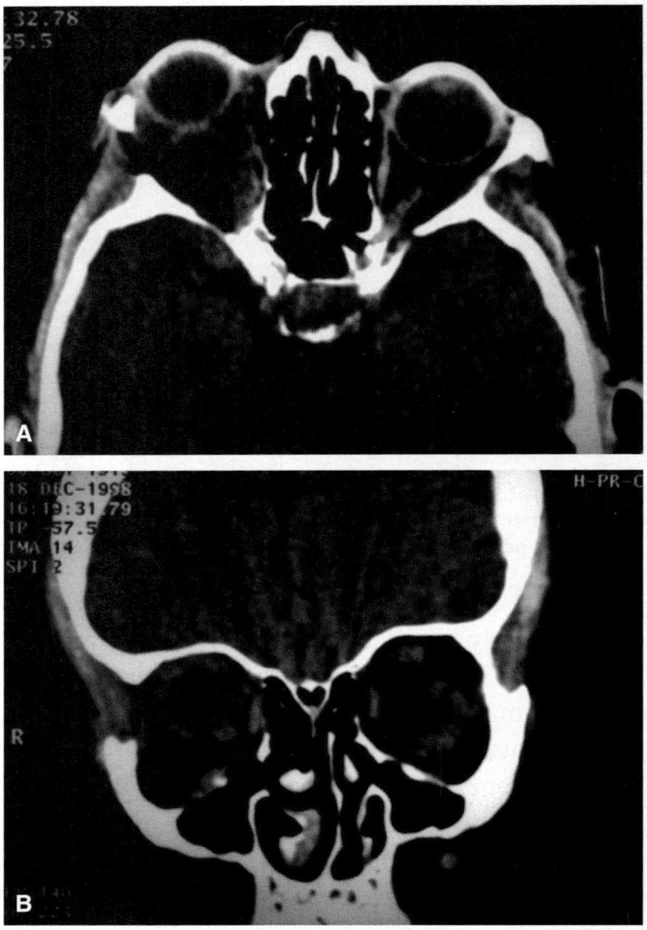

Figures 17–28. *A* and B, Cystic neurilemmoma on axial (*A*) and coronal (*B*) CT scans.

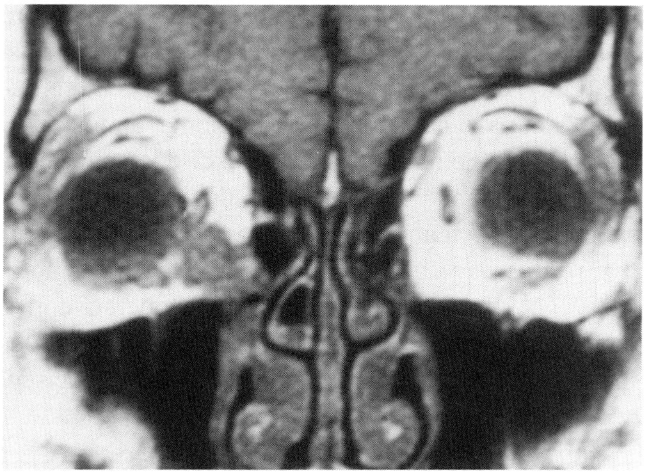

Figure 17–29. Coronal MRI scan shows a possible recurrence of fibrous histiocytoma.

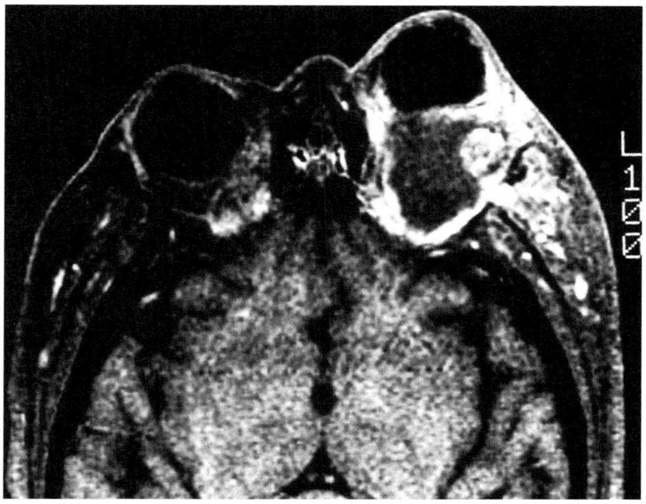

Figure 17–31. Malignant fibrous histiocytoma with early metastasis.

but had the MRI pattern shown in Figure 17–29. A positron emission tomography (PET) scan was felt to be diagnostic for recurrence (Figure 17–30), and the recurrent tumor was removed in an open biopsy.

The role of radiation treatment for fibrous histiocytoma is difficult to determine since no large series has been reported. In the clinicopathologic series reported by Font and Hidayat, in 13 of 18 irradiated cases, the tumor recurred; however, the radiation parameters in these cases were not well defined.[54]

Some of these tumors are initially benign but recur and undergo malignant degeneration. The patient shown in Figure 17–14 initially had three surgical resections for a recurrent benign tumor and eventually required exenteration after recurrence of a malignant transformation from the benign fibrous histiocytoma, despite surgery and irradiation. Figure 17–31 shows another patient with malignant histiocytoma with widespread disease who died within 3 months. Of 14 patients with orbital malignant fibrous histiocytoma in the series of Font and Hidayat, 6 died from either local extension or metastases. Exenteration is the treatment of choice.[54,57,58]

Solitary Fibrous Tumor

Among a group of tumors that had previously been characterized under the ruberic of fibrous histiocytomas are solitary fibrous tumors.[59] There have been approximately 10 cases involving the orbit. Figure

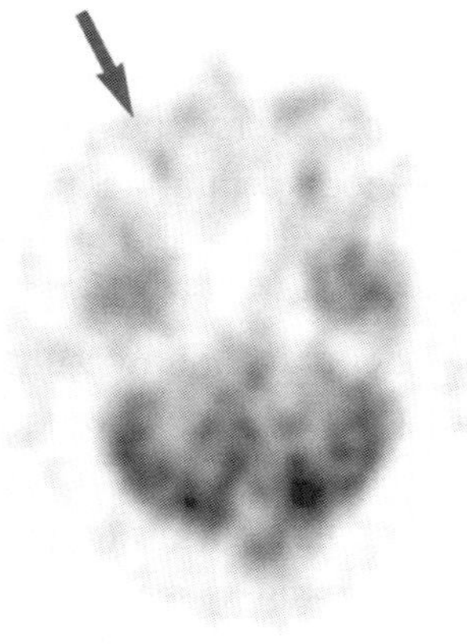

Figure 17–30. PET scan demonstrates marked asymmetry and was felt to be diagnostic for recurrence, and this was confirmed histologically.

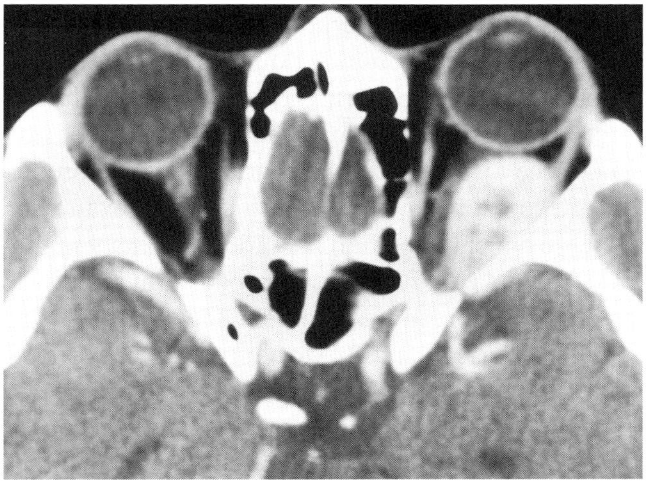

Figure 17–32. Solitary fibrous histiocytoma involving the orbit.

17–32 demonstrates such an intraconal lesion. On MRI, this was hypointense to brain on T_1 and hyperintense on T_2 (not shown). The management of these lesions is surgical removal.

NEUROFIBROMA

Isolated neurofibromas often occur in the intraconal space. In contrast to orbital cavernous hemangiomas, which are usually smaller and do not involve the orbital apex, neurofibromas (like neurilemmomas) commonly expand through the superior orbital fissure. Krohel and colleagues reported on 9 patients with localized orbital neurofibromas; 1 case was associated with neurofibromatosis.[60] In 5 patients, there were multiple tumors, and 4 had a pedicle extending from the superior orbital fissure. In 3 of 5 cases, neither CT nor ultrasonography demonstrated the multiple tumors that were present.

Usually, neurofibromas involve the superior orbit. The patient in Figure 17–33A demonstrates such a case. The eye has been displaced downward. On both axial reconstructed CT (Figures 17–33B to D) and direct coronal MRI (Figures 17–33E and F), a large mass going into the superior orbital fissure was found. We were able to resect this mass, using a lateral orbitotomy, as discussed in the chapter on orbital management.

HEMANGIOPERICYTOMA

Hemangiopericytoma can simulate the MRI, CT or ultrasonographic pattern of an intraconal cavernous hemangioma. Like cavernous hemangiomas, the T_1 pattern on MRI is often hypointense to CNS tissue with a variable T_2 pattern.[61] Both benign and malignant hemangiopericytomas can occur, and unfortunately, the histologic findings are not a good predictor of clinical behavior.[62] In a study by Croxatto and Font, 16 appeared benign, 5 borderline, and 9 malignant.[62] Four of 27 cases with long-term follow-up died of widespread metastases. Others have noted a similar disease course.[61] Mortality did not correlate with histologic type; 5-year actuarial survival was 89 percent.[62] Henderson and Farrow described 13 cases, which represented 1.7 percent of the orbital tumors examined.[63] Most patients were middle-aged; no hemangiopericytomas occurred in children. There was progressive proptosis. In almost all the patients, the tumor involved the superior orbit but could clinically simulate cavernous hemangioma almost perfectly.[62,63] If the tumors were not excised, recurrences were common.[63,65] The role of radiation in the management of hemangiopericytoma is uncertain. Positive results have been observed in some other body sites.[61,66,67] In our experience, with postoperative irradiation in a few cases, we have obtained tumor control, when the lesion has not been completely excised.

INFILTRATIVE INTRACONAL LESIONS

Pseudotumors occasionally involve the intraconal space but are not discrete. Twenty percent of orbital metastases involve the intraconal space. Usually, the intraconal orbital metastases either are diffuse, simulating pseudotumor or involve the contiguous muscle (Figure 17–34). The diffuse quality of both the pseudotumor and metastases in this area makes their delineation from cavernous hemangioma, hemangiopericytoma, or isolated neurofibromas relatively straightforward. Rarely, metastic tumors can be quite focal, however, as shown in Figure 17–35. Lymphoid tumors rarely occur as discrete intraconal masses (see Figure 26–11). Metastases and lymphoid lesions are discussed in separate chapters. Intraocular tumors can also spread contiguously to involve the intraconal area, but this is rare in the United States. Figure 17–36 shows a direct parasagittal MR image of a patient with an intraocular-orbital metastatic carcinoid tumor. Similarly, both melanoma and retinoblastoma can either contiguously involve the ipsilateral intraconal space or, occasionally, the contralateral orbit (see Figure 17–12). Adult optic nerve neoplasms are described separately. Childhood orbital neoplasms are described in the chapter on pediatric orbital tumors.

A number of rare intraconal neoplasms can occur. A liposarcoma is shown clinically in Figure 17–37A and the CT with reconstruction and MRI are shown in Figures 17–37B to D.[28,30,68] Similarly, we have seen one case of a chondrosarcoma which involved the intraconal space (Figure 17–38).

As discussed under orbital surgery, the optimal approach for tumors in the anterior or midintraconal space is via a lateral orbitotomy. Precise visualiza-

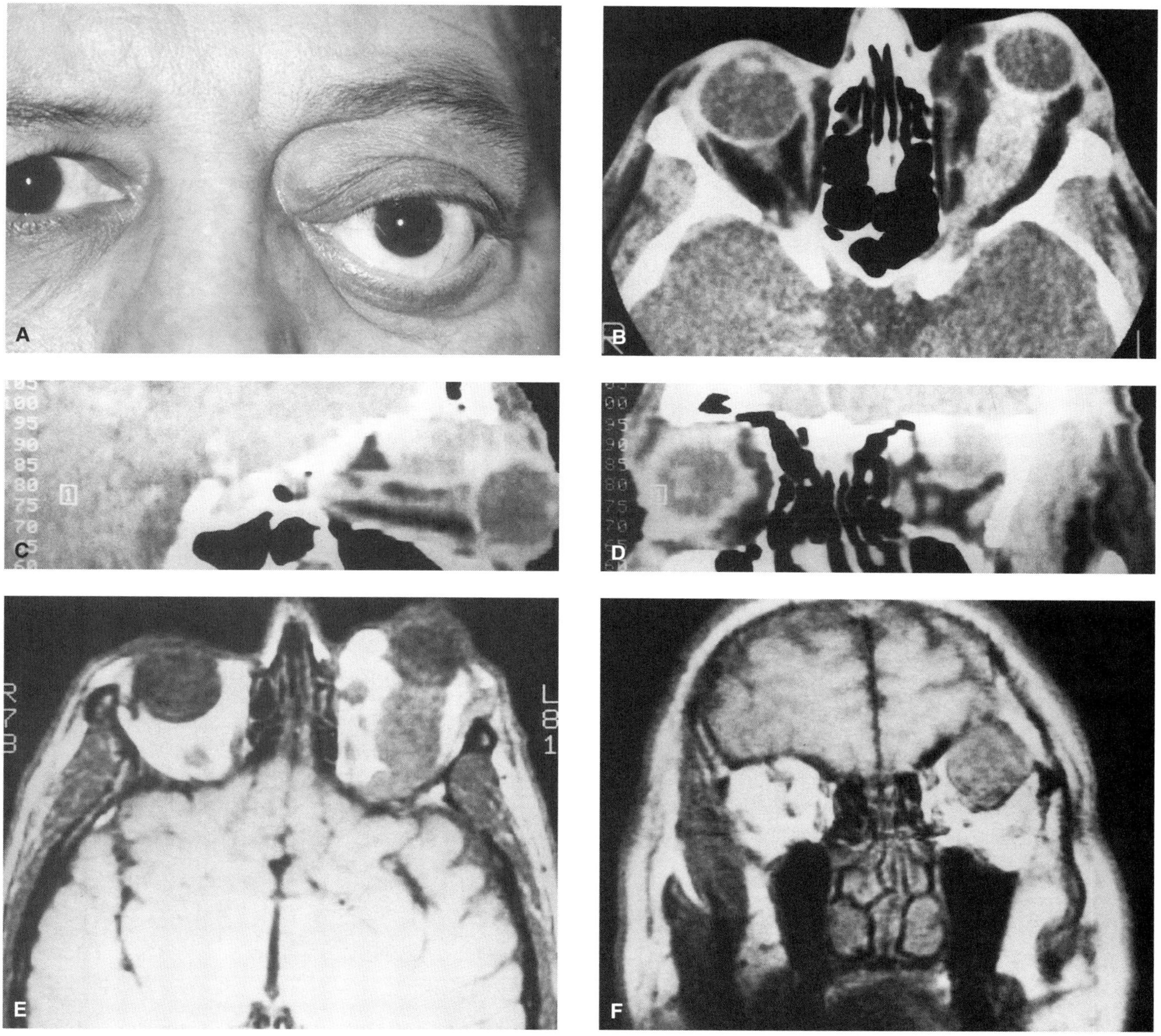

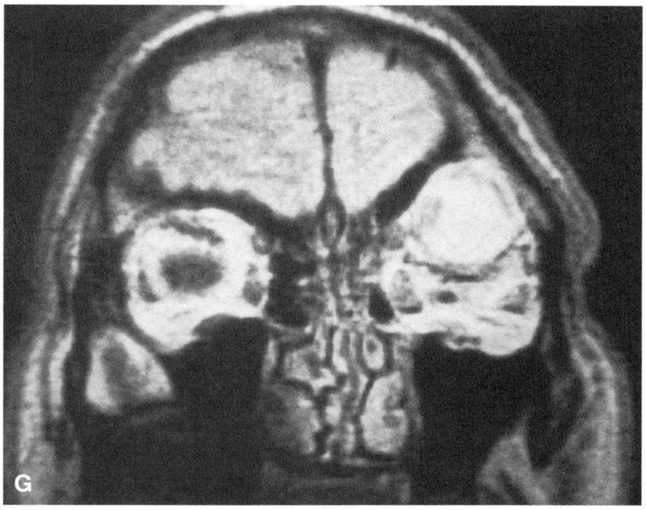

Figure 17–33. *A,* Clinical photograph of orbital neurofibroma. *B,* Axial CT scan. *C,* Parasagittal CT scan. *D,* Coronal reformated CT. *E,* Axial T_1-weighted MRI scan showing superior orbital mass isodense with muscle. *F,* Direct coronal T_1-weighted MRI scan showing hyperintense lesion in relation to brain. *G,* Direct T_1-weighted coronal MRI scan with gadolinium.

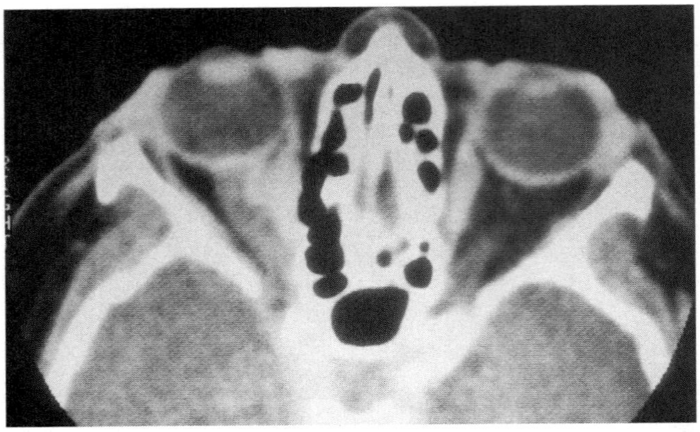

Figure 17–34. Metastatic intraconal tumor with involvement of contiguous extraocular muscle.

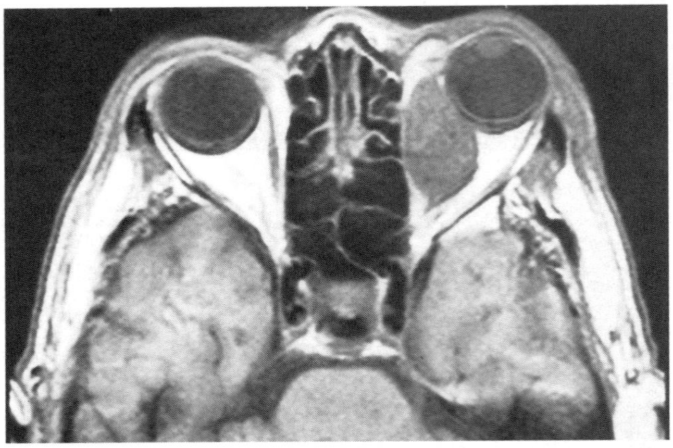

Figure 17–35. Focal metastases on an axial T_1-weighted MRI scan.

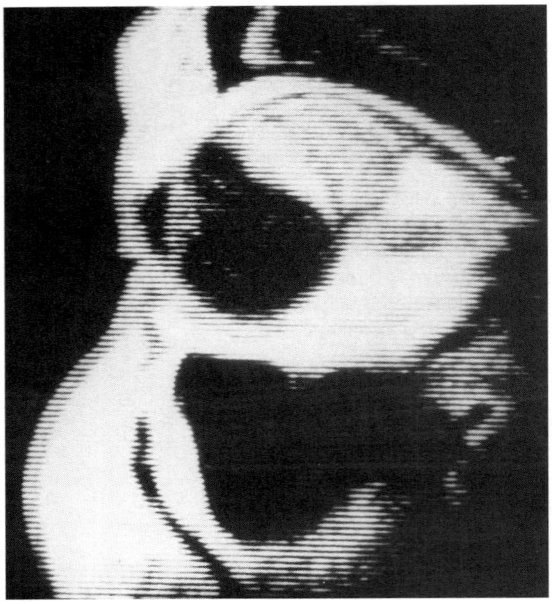

Figure 17–36. Carcinoid metastatic to the eye and intraconal space shown on direct parasagittal T_1-weighted MRI scan.

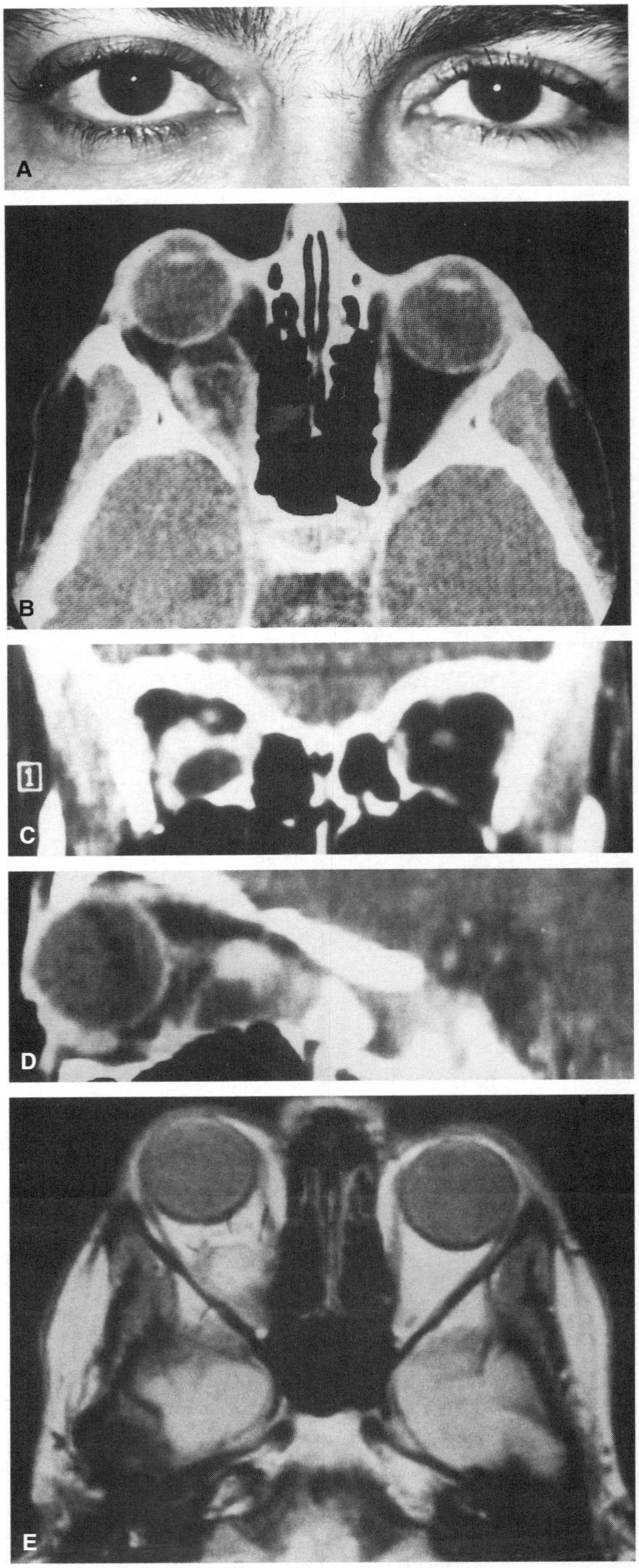

Figure 17–37. *A,* Clinical photograph of a patient with liposarcoma. *B,* Orbital CT with computer re-formation, showing a liposarcoma with an apparent cystic component. *C* and *D,* Parasagittal and coronal re-formation of the orbital CT scan. *E,* Axial T_1-weighted MRI scan.

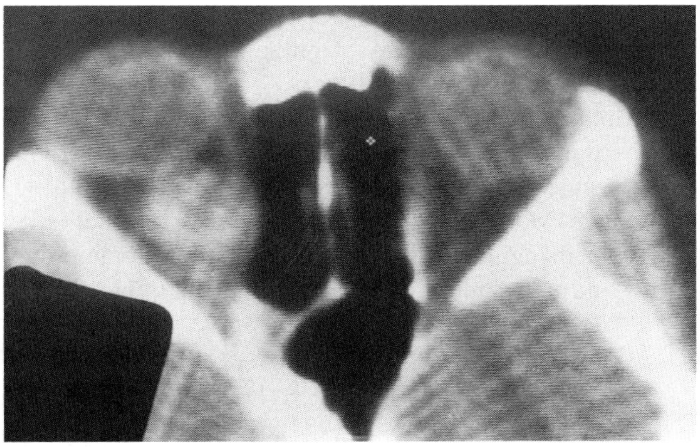

Figure 17–38. Axial CT scan of biopsy-proven intraconal chondrosarcoma.

tion during surgery is vital to avoid damage to contiguous vessels and nerves, and in most of these cases, surgery is carried out using hypotensive anesthesia and a microscope. Rarely, conjunctival cysts can produce an intraconal tumor, and we have seen two of those.[69,70] These lesions can occur without a history of trauma, although in the author's experience, it is more common after a sharp instrument has gone through the eyelid.

REFERENCES

1. Reese AB. Expanding lesions of the orbit. Trans Ophthalmol 1971;91:85–104.
2. Shields JA, Bakewell B, Augsburger JJ, Flanagan JC. Classification and incidence of space-occupying lesions of the orbit. Arch Ophthalmol 1984;102: 1606–11.
3. Savoiardo M, Strada L, Passerini A. Cavernous hemangiomas of the orbit: value of CT, angiography and phlebography. Am J Neuroradiol 1983;4:741–4.
4. Ruchman MC, Flanagan J. Cavernous hemangiomas of the orbit. Ophthalmology 1983;90:1328–36.
5. Wright JE. Symposium on orbital tumors. Trans Ophthalmol Soc UK 1979;99:216–9.
6. Harris GJ, Jakobiec FA. Cavernous hemangioma of the orbit. J Neurosurg 1979;51:219–20.
7. McNab AA, Wright JE. Cavernous hemangiomas of the orbit. Austral NZ J Ophthalmol 1989;17:337–45.
8. Char DH. The use of computed tomography and ultrasonography in the evaluation of orbital masses. Surv Ophthalmol 1982;27:49–63.
9. Fries PD, Char DH, Norman D. MR imaging of orbital cavernous hemangioma. J Comput Assist Tomogr 1987;11:418–21.
10. Fries PD, Char DH. Bilateral cavernous hemangiomas. Br J Ophthalmol 1988;72:871–3.
11. Johnson TE, Nasr AM, Nalbandian RM, Cappelen-Smith J. Enchondromatosis and hemangioma (Maffucci's syndrome) with orbital involvement. Am J Ophthalmol 1990;100:153–9.
12. Thorn-Kany, M, Arrue P, Delisle MB, et al. Cavernous hemangiomas of the orbit: MR imaging. J Neuroradiol 1999;26:79–86.
13. Ohtsuka K, Hashimoto M, Akiba H. Serial dynamic magnetic resonance imaging of orbital cavernous hamangioma. Am J Ophthalmol 1997;123:396–8.
14. Johnson LN, Sexton M, Goldberg SH. Poorly differentiated primary orbital sarcoma (presumed malignant rhabdoid tumor). Arch Ophthalmol 1991;109: 1275–8.
15. Shields JA, Shields CL, Eagle RCJ, et al. Necrotic orbital melanoma arising de novo. Br J Ophthalmol 1994;77:187–9.
16. Carrier DA, Mawad ME, Kirkpatrick JB. MR appearance of an orbital leiomyoma. Am J Neuroradiol 1993;14:473–474.
17. Neufeld M, Pe'er J, Rosenman E, Lazar M. Intraorbital glomus cell tumor. Am J Ophthalmol 1994;117: 539–40.
18. Bednar MM, Trainer TD, Aitken PA, et al. Orbital paraganglioma: case report and review of the literature. Br J Ophthalmol 1992;76:83–5.
19. Moss HM. Expanding lesions of the orbit. A clinical study of 230 cases. Am J Ophthalmol 1962;54: 761–70.
20. Kopelow SM, Foos RY, Straatsma BR, et al. Cavernous hemangioma of the orbit. Int Ophthalmol Clin 1971; 11:113–25.
21. Unsold R, Hoyt WF, Newton TH. Criteria of orbital hemangiomas and their importance in differential diagnosis of intraconal tumors. Klin Monatsbl Augenheilkd 1979;175:773–85.
22. Brown GC, Shields JA. Amaurosis fugax secondary to presumed cavernous hemangioma of the orbit. Ann Ophthalmol 1981;13:1205–9.
23. Ossoinig KC, Keenan TP, Bigar F. Cavernous hemangioma of the orbit: Ultrasonography in Ophthalmology. Bibl Ophthal 1975;83:236–44.
24. Coleman DJ, Jack RL, Franzen LA. Hemangiomas of the orbit. Arch Ophthalmol 1972;88:368–74.
25. Cappaert WE, Kiprov RV, Frank KE. Sector B-scan ultrasonographic hemangioma-like pattern. Arch Ophthalmol 1983;1983:101.
26. Char DH, Stone RD, Irvine AR, Unsold R. Orbital melanoma. Ann Ophthalmol 1981;13:911–3.
27. Shen WC, Yang DY, Ho WL, Lee SK. Neurilemmoma of the oculomotor nerve presenting as an orbital

mass: MR findings. Am J Neuroradiol 1993;14: 1253–4.

28. Nasr AM, Ossoinig KC, Kersten RF, Blodi FC. Standardized echographic-histopathologic correlations in liposarcoma. Am J Ophthalmol 1985;99:193–200.
29. Sklar EL, Quencer RM, Byrne SF, Sklar VEF. Correlative study of the computed tomographic, ultrasonographic, and pathological characteristics of cavernous versus capillary hemangiomas of the orbit. J Clin Neuroophthalmol 1986;6:14–21.
30. Jakobiec FA, Rini F, Char DH, et al. Primary liposarcoma of the orbit: problems in the diagnosis and management of five cases. Ophthalmology 1989; 96:180–91.
31. Cohen JA, Char DH, Norman D. Bilateral orbital varices associated with habitual bending. Arch Ophthalmol 1995;113:1360–2.
32. Bullock JD, Goldberg SH, Connelly PJ. Orbital varix thrombosis. Ophthalmology 1990;97:251–6.
33. Fourman S. Acute closed-angle glaucoma after arteriovenous fistulas. Am J Ophthalmol 1989;107:156–9.
34. Leib WE, Merton DA, Shields JA, et al. Colour doppler imaging in the demonstration of an orbital varix. Br J Ophthalmol 1990;74:305–8.
35. Hanneken AM, Miller NR, Debrun GM, Nauta HJW. Treatment of carotid-cavernous sinus fistulas using a detachable balloon catheter through the superior ophthalmic vein. Arch Ophthalmol 1989;107:87–92.
36. Christi DB, Kwon YH, Choi I, et al. Sequential embolization and excision of an orbital arteriovenous malformation. Arch Ophthalmol 1994;112:1377–9.
37. Lacey B, Rootman J, Marotta TR. Distensible venous malformations of the orbit: clinical and hemodynamic features and a new technique of management. Ophthalmology 1999;106:1197–209.
38. Mojon D, Odel JG, Rios R, Hirano M. Presumed orbital hemangioma associated with blue rubber bleb nevus syndrome. Arch Ophthalmol 1996;114:618–9.
39. Wolter JR. No need for cutting of the lateral rectus muscle: in the transconjunctival approach to the muscle cone of the orbit. J Pediatr Ophthalmol Strabismus 1980;17:40–3.
40. Hassler W, Schaller C, Farghaly F, Rohde V. Transconjunctival approach to a large cavernoma of the orbit. Neurosurgery 1994;34:859–62.
41. Henderson JW, Farro GM, Garrity JA. Clinical course of an incompletely removed cavernous hemangioma of the orbit. Ophthalmology 1990;97:625–8.
42. Carta F, Siccardi D, Cossu M, et al. Removal of tumors of the orbital apex via a postero-lateral orbitotomy. J Neurosurg Sci 1998;42:185–8.
43. Sethi DS, Lau DP. Endoscopic management of orbital apex lesions. Am J Rhinol 1997;11:449–55.
44. Kennerdell JS, Maroon JC, Celin SE. The posterior inferior orbitotomy. Ophthalmol Plast Reconstr Surg 1998;14:277–80.
45. Goldberg RA, Shorr N, Arnold AC, Garcia GH. Deep transorbital approach to the apex and cavernous sinus. Ophthal Plast Reconstr Surg 1998;14:336–41.
46. Maus M, Goldman HW. Removal of orbital apex hemangioma using new transorbital craniotomy through suprabrow approach. Ophthal Plast Reconstr Surg 1999;15:166–70.
47. Dahl I, Hagmar B, Idvall I. Benign solitary neurilemmoma (schwannoma). Acta Pathol Microbiol Immunol Scan Sec A 1984;92:91–101.
48. Konrad EA, Thiel HJ. Schwannoma of the orbit. Ophthalmologica 1984;188:118–27.
49. Schatz H. Benign orbital neurilemmoma: sarcomatous transformation in Von Recklinghausen's disease. Arch Ophthalmol 1971;86:268–73.
50. Rootman J, Goldberg C, Robertson W. Primary orbital schwannomas. Br J Ophthalmol 1982;66:194–204.
51. Lloyd GAS. CT scanning in the diagnosis of orbital disease. J Comput Assist Tomography 1979;3:227–39.
52. Bickler-Bluth ME, Custer PL, Smith ME. Neurilemoma as a presenting feature of neurofibromatosis. Arch Ophthalmol 1988;106:665–7.
53. Chisholm LA, Polyzoidis K. Recurrence of benign orbital neurilemmoma (schwannoma) after 22 years. Can J Ophthalmol 1982;17:271–3.
54. Font RL, Hidayat AA. Fibrous histiocytoma of the orbit: a clinicopathologic study of 150 cases. Hum Pathol 1982;13:199–209.
55. Verity MA, Ebert JT, Hepler RS. Atypical fibrous histiocytoma of the orbit: an electromicroscopic study. Ophthalmologica 1977;175:73–9.
56. Jakobiec FA, Howard GM, Jones IS, Tannenbaum M. Fibrous histiocytomas of the orbit. Am J Ophthalmol 1974;77:333–45.
57. Rodrigues MM, Furgiuele FP, Weinreb S. Malignant fibrous histiocytoma of the orbit. Arch Ophthalmol 1977;95:2025–8.
58. Weiss SW, Enzinger FM. Malignant fibrous histiocytoma. an analysis of 200 cases. Cancer 1978;41: 2250–66.
59. Char DH, Weidner N, Ahn J, Harbour J. Solitary fibrous tumor of the orbit. Orbit 1997;6:1–5.
60. Krohel JB, Rosenberg PN, Wright JE, Smith RS. Localized orbital neurofibromas. Am J Ophthalmol 1985;100:458–64.
61. Darcioglu ZA, Nsr AM, Haik BG. Orbital hemangiopericytoma: clinical and morphologic features. Am J Ophthalmol 1997;124:661–72.
62. Croxatto JO, Font RL. Hemangiopericytoma of the orbit: a clinicopathologic study of 30 cases. Hum Pathol 1982;13:1210–8.

63. Henderson JW, Farrow GM. Primary orbital hemangiopericytoma: an aggressive and potential malignant neoplasm. Arch Ophthalmol 1978;986:666–73.
64. Jakobiec FA, Howard GM, Jones IS. Hemangiopericytoma of the orbit. Am J Ophthalmol 1974;78:816–34.
65. Rice CD, Kersten RC, Mrak RE. An orbital hemangiopericytoma recurrent after 33 years. Arch Ophthalmol 1989;107:552–6.
66. Stetzkorn RK, Lee DJ. Hemangiopericytoma of the orbit treated with conservative surgery and radiotherapy. Arch Ophthalmol 1987;105:1103–5.
67. Mira JG, Chu FCH, Fortner JG. The role of radiotherapy in the management of malignant hemangiopericytyoma. Cancer 1977;39:1254–9.
68. Naeser P, Mostrom U. Liposarcomas of the orbit: a clinicopathological case report. Br J Ophthalmol 1982;66:190–3.
69. Schlote T, Nagel G, Vecsei PV, et al. Conjunctival cysts of the orbits: clinical aspects and histology in 4 patients. Klin Monatsbl Augenheilkd 1998;213:117–20.
70. Goldstein MH, Soparkar CN, Kersten RC, et al. Conjunctival cysts of the orbit. Ophthalmology 1998;105:2056–60.

18

Adult Optic Nerve Tumors

There are no clinical findings that are pathognomonic for optic nerve tumors. In adults without intraocular or central nervous system (CNS) pathology, mild proptosis and the presence of an afferent pupillary defect, marked visual loss with minimal proptosis, optic atrophy (with or without optociliary shunt vessels), chronic disc edema, or unexplained central visual field loss are consistent with the presence of an intraorbital optic nerve tumor.

A number of entities can produce enlargement of the adult optic nerve, including optic nerve sheath meningioma, optic nerve glioma, neurofibroma, hemangioblastoma, vascular insults, metastases, leukemia, lymphoma (Figure 18–1), neuritis, sarcoid (Figure 18–2), trauma, thyroid compressive neuropathy (Figure 18–3), idiopathic inflammation (Figure 18–4), contiguous infection, and drusen.[1–4] History and review of systems is usually sufficient to correctly categorize many of these lesions. Most of the patients with optic nerve infiltration by leukemias, lymphomas, or metastases have known systemic malignancy, although ocular metastases can be the first sign of a primary neoplasm (see Chapter 5). Similarly, it is usually straightforward to distinguish sarcoid, trauma, and hemangioblastoma from other optic nerve tumefactions on the basis of history, physical findings, fluorescein angiography, or laboratory tests.[5] The differentiation of a small optic canal tumor from retrobulbar optic neuritis, AION contiguous apical inflammation, infection or a cyst can be difficult.[6]

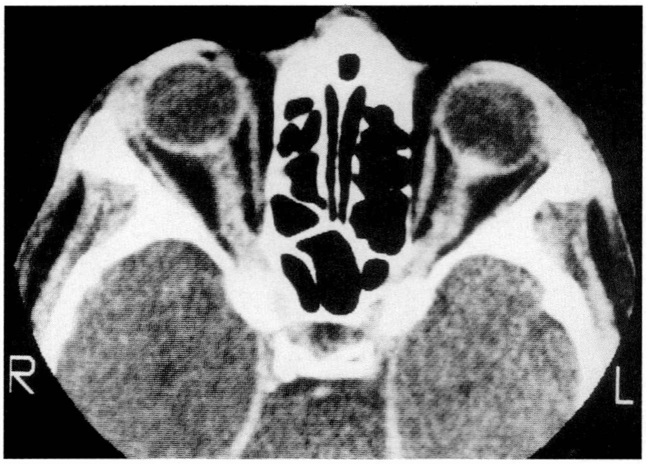

Figure 18–1. Biopsy-proven lymphoma infiltrating the optic nerve sheath, producing enlargement of the optic nerve on axial CT.

MENINGIOMA

The most common adult primary optic nerve sheath tumors are meningiomas; they account for approxi-

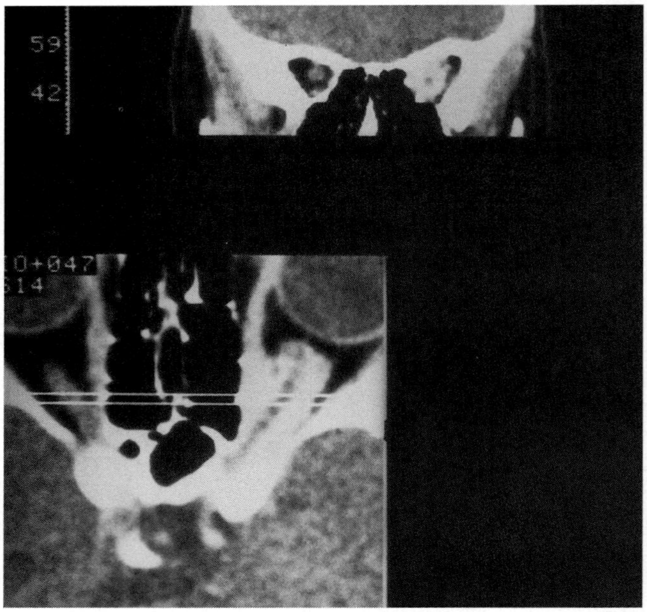

Figure 18–2. Sarcoidosis producing enlarged optic nerve.

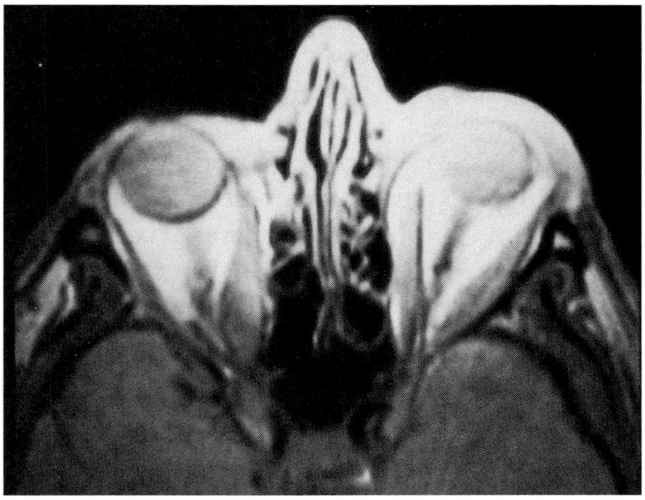

Figure 18–3. Thyroid optic neuropathy on axial MRI scan; usually the nerve is compressed.

mately 2 to 5 percent of orbital tumors. Meningiomas are responsible for approximately one-fifth of CNS tumors, and < 15 percent secondarily involve the orbit. Orbital involvement by meningiomas can occur as a result of a primary intraorbital neoplasm, almost always arising from the optic nerve sheath, or secondarily from a meningioma that involves the orbit by contiguous spread from the CNS often in the sphenoid wing. Rarely, a solitary orbital, nonoptic nerve sheath meningioma is found in association with neurofibromatosis.[7] Orbital involvement, either primarily or secondarily by meningiomas occur more frequently in females.[8] In five series of orbital meningiomas, 140 of 181 patients were women (77%).[9–13] In a series from the Mayo Clinic, 139 of 1,376 orbital biopsies (10%) were shown to be meningiomas, and over 66 percent initially arose from the sphenoid ridge; in less than one-third (42 of 139 cases), the meningioma arose in the orbits.[10]

The etiology of meningiomas is uncertain. Loss of heterozygosity at chromosome 22a due to mutations of the *NF2* gene (and secondary loss of merlin expression) occur in about one-half of the cases.[14] A number of other multistep genomic changes occur, especially in more aggressive meningioma tumors.[15,16]

The vast majority of primary orbital meningiomas arise either from the optic nerve sheath or the bony foramen of the canal. Very rarely, intraorbital, nonbony meningiomas have been reported.[7,17–19] Hyperplastic meningothelial cells are often associated with optic nerve gliomas, and some gliomas have been histologically misdiagnosed as meningiomas on the basis of this finding.[20] Most optic nerve meningiomas that have been reported in children without neurofibromatosis were probably optic nerve gliomas. In patients with neurofibromatosis (probably < 10% of total cases), bilateral optic nerve sheath meningiomas rarely occur.[21–23]

The location of an optic nerve sheath meningioma is a major factor in duration of symptoms, amount of visual loss, and degree of proptosis at the time of diagnosis. As examples, a very small, enlarging meningioma in the optic nerve canal will produce rapid visual loss without significant proptosis; rarely, a large optic nerve sheath meningioma grows through the dura and produces proptosis before visual loss (Figure 18–5). If the meningioma arises just posterior to the globe, the first symptoms may be the onset of unilateral hyperopia due to compression of the globe.

It is difficult to accurately assess the frequency of primary orbital meningiomas in various locations.

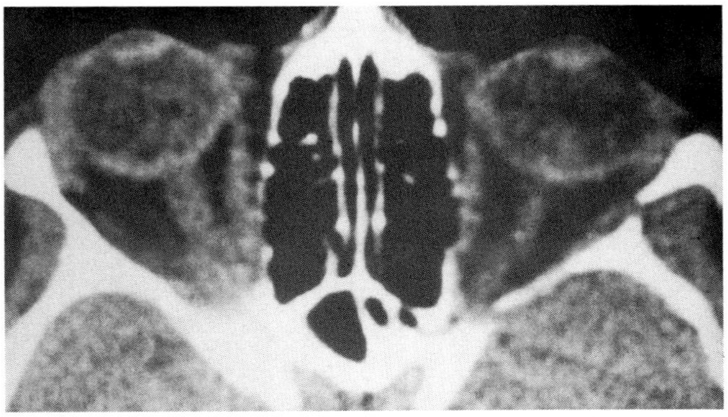

Figure 18–4. Optic neuritis associated with idiopathic diffuse orbital inflammation (pseudotumor).

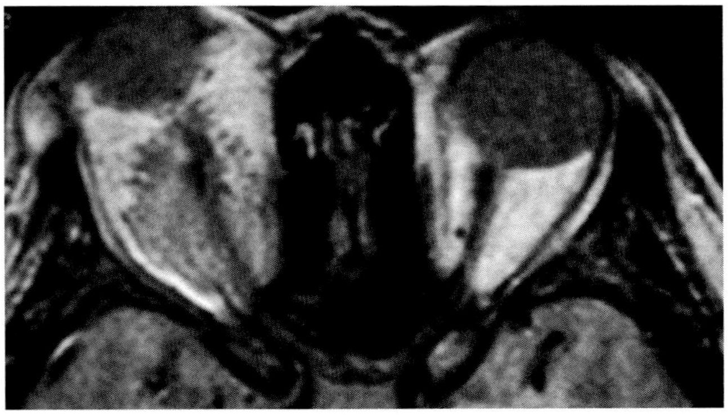

Figure 18–5. A large meningioma that grew through the dura and produced proptosis with minimal visual loss.

Intracanalicular meningiomas are approximately one-third as frequent as those involving the intraorbital optic nerve sheath.[9,12,18,19,24–29] Most commonly, optic nerve sheath meningiomas are not entirely confined to the orbit even when they clinically appear to be.

Most frequently, optic nerve sheath meningiomas present in middle-aged women with < 3 mm of axial proptosis and markedly decreased vision (Figure 18–6A). Other signs and symptoms include optic disc pallor, disc edema, headache, diplopia, loss of color vision, afferent pupil abnormality, opticociliary shunt vessels (Figures 18–6B and C) or intraocular invasion.[30] Usually, optic disc edema precedes the development of opticociliary shunt vessels by several years, and patients with greater amounts of proptosis have a longer history prior to the discovery of the optic nerve tumor.[31] In a middle-aged woman with chronic, profound unilateral "optic neuritis," subsequent optic atrophy, and minimal proptosis, this tumor should be ruled out with appropriate imaging studies (see below).

The pattern of an intrinsic orbital optic nerve tumor is usually different from a non-neoplastic simulating lesion on either computed tomography (CT) or magnetic resonance imaging (MRI).[5,32] There is some overlap in the CT imaging characteristics of the two most common primary optic nerve tumors: optic nerve sheath meningioma and optic nerve glioma.[33] The most useful characteristics that distinguish these two processes are the older age of presentation with meningiomas, calcifications in 25 percent of meningiomas versus almost none in gliomas, occasional outgrowth of meningiomas through the optic nerve sheath to involve other orbital structures, and the different patterns of posterior CNS extension. Posterior involvement of the optic nerve glioma usually involves visual pathways, while CNS extension of meningiomas involves the sphenoid bone. Meningiomas frequently produce pneumosinus dilation of the anterior clinoid and ethmoid air cells.

The most common radiologic finding associated with any type of meningioma is alteration of the

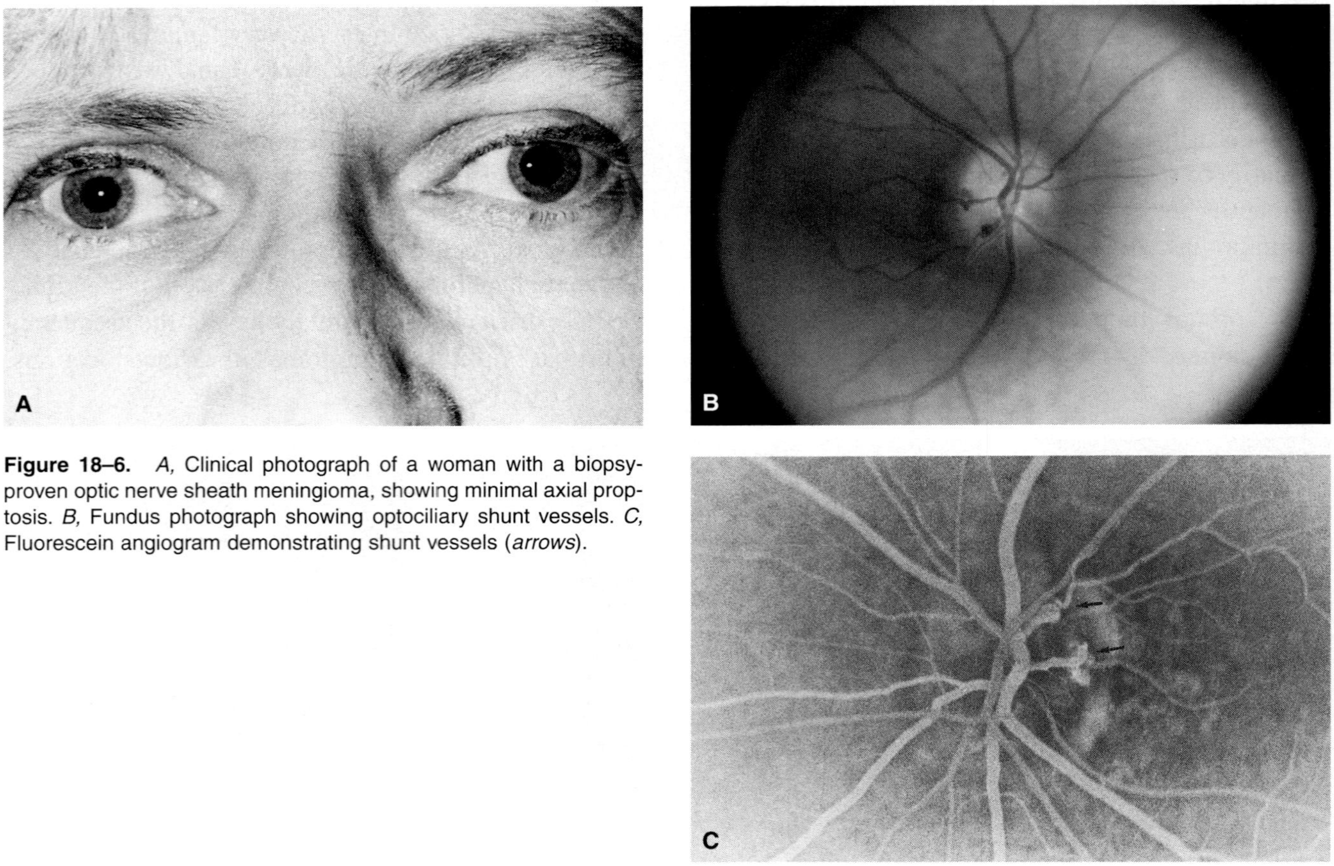

Figure 18–6. *A,* Clinical photograph of a woman with a biopsy-proven optic nerve sheath meningioma, showing minimal axial proptosis. *B,* Fundus photograph showing optociliary shunt vessels. *C,* Fluorescein angiogram demonstrating shunt vessels (*arrows*).

contiguous bone, often producing hyperostotic changes. If the optic canal is involved, usually the foramen is enlarged with irregular demineralization and hyperostosis.

The CT pattern of optic nerve sheath meningioma reflects the various growth patterns and calcification of the tumor. The nerve sheath can be enlarged in a tubular pattern (approximately two-thirds of cases, (Figure 18–7), a fusiform pattern (approximately one-third of cases, Figure 18–8), or, less commonly, an excrescent pattern (Figure 18–9). The tumors typically enhance with intravenous contrast. An excrescent tumor enlargement is relatively specific for a nerve sheath meningioma.[34] While central lucency (tram-track sign) is characteristic of an optic nerve sheath meningioma, it is also associated with other lesions.[32,33] This finding is noted in about 25 percent of cases.[37] Intratumor calcification can be diffuse, punctate, or psammomatous.[38]

MRI is the optimal technique to detect optic nerve sheath meningiomas.[39] CT has limited sensitivity for small posterior orbital meningiomas or those with subtle intracranial extension.[40] The use of fat saturation with gadolinium-DTPA significantly increases the sensitivity of detection of these lesions and their extent (Figures 18–10 and 18–11).[41,42] In some cases, fine-needle aspiration biopsies (FNABs) have been diagnostic.[43,44] While we have used this diagnostic modality in many orbital diseases (see Chapter 15), we have not found it necessary in most primary optic nerve tumors except atypical apical lesions.

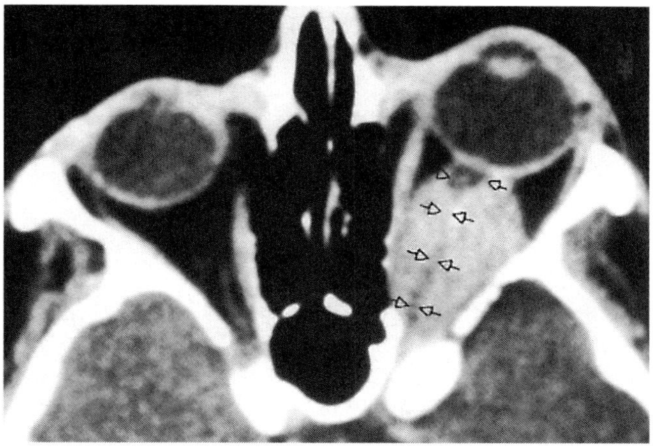

Figure 18–8. Optic nerve sheath meningioma with a fusiform enlargement. On a contrast-enhanced CT scan, the optic nerve (*arrows*) appears to be encased by tumor. (From Char et al.,[70] with permission)

Treatment of CNS meningiomas is the realm of the neurosurgeon.[45,46] Early treatment of CNS meningiomas that involve the anterior visual pathways may improve visual prognosis.[37,47] Most patients with optic nerve sheath meningiomas have poor vision at the time of presentation, and the neoplasm completely surrounds the optic nerve. Historically, we have followed most optic nerve sheath meningioma patients, if the tumor is confined to the orbit and proptosis was minimal. Often, visual acuity remained stationary for long periods, and there are reports of spontaneous visual improvements.[48] If the proptosis associated with an isolated optic nerve sheath meningioma becomes cosmetically unacceptable and the eye is blind, we have resected the orbital

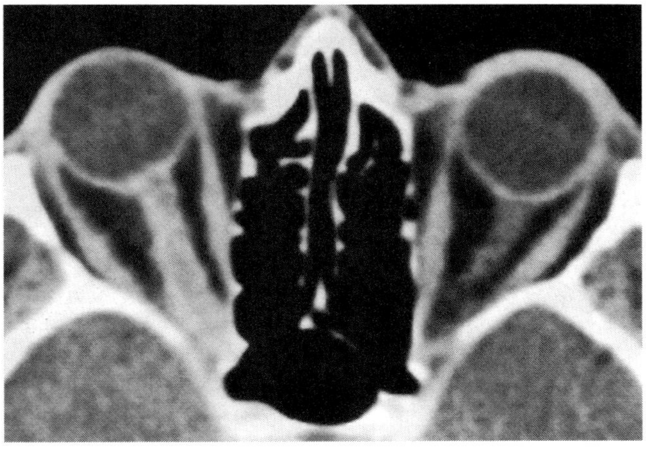

Figure 18–7. Axial contrast-enhanced CT scan demonstrating tubular enlargement of the optic nerve secondary to a nerve sheath meningioma. (From Char et al,[70] with permission)

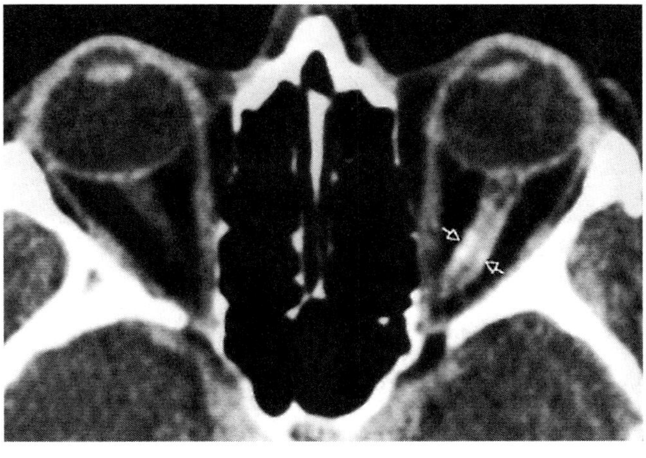

Figure 18–9. Optic nerve enlargement due to an excrescent calcifying optic nerve sheath meningioma. (From Char et al.,[70] with permission)

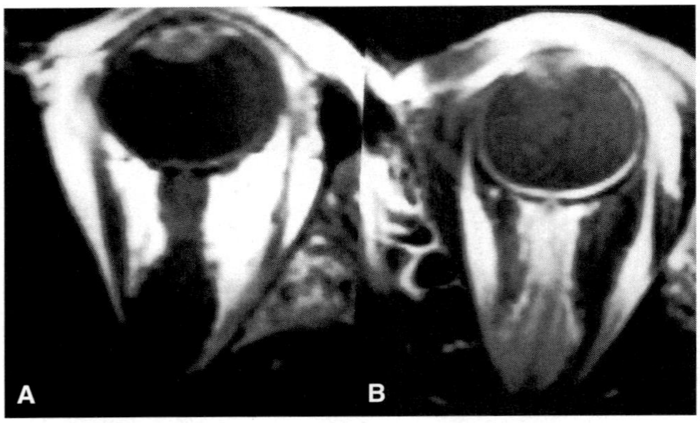

Figure 18–10. Comparison of T_1-weighted MRI scan (*A*) and T_1 fat saturation gadolinium scan (*B*) in the same case.

portion of the nerve through a lateral orbitotomy, leaving an intact eye (Figure 18–12).

Seven cases that have been classified by the reporting authors as optic nerve sheath meningiomas have been resected, with improved vision after surgery.[37] Probably some of these tumors were meningiomas that did not involve the nerve sheath, although one or two may have been very small lesions picked up just posterior to the globe.[14,19,37,49,50] In our experience, we have not seen a patient with an optic nerve sheath meningioma that could be removed with the preservation of good vision. Virtually all patients who have been operated on with optic nerve sheath tumors have had marked reduction of visual acuity.[37]

Patients with nonoptic nerve sheath meningiomas generally have a better visual outcome, and neither group of orbital meningioma patients has significant tumor-related mortality. Less than 2 percent of optic nerve sheath meningioma patients have died as a direct result of tumor, but a number of studies have demonstrated a higher tumor-related mortality in children.[12,51]

We have had good results with sphenoid wing-orbital meningiomas, using orbital resection and a combination of neurologic and ophthalmologic surgeons, with the addition of postoperative radiation.[52,53]

OTHER OPTIC NERVE TUMORS AND SIMULATING LESIONS

As previously mentioned, a number of lymphoid tumors can involve the optic nerve either primarily or secondarily. A systemic lymphoma with unknown CNS and optic nerve involvement is shown in Figure 18–1. This is one of the few areas in which orbital ultrasonography may be both as accurate as either CT or MRI and more cost effective at differentiating inflammation from an optic nerve tumor. Often, a "T sign" is produced on B-scan as a result of fluid in the sub-Tenon's space (Figure 26–23). Almost all these patients have other findings of lymphoid tumor in the orbit, often including a diffuse mass surrounding the nerve. Occasionally, the idiopathic benign lymphoid lesions can be difficult to differentiate from other inflammatory lesions as an isolated retrobulbar sarcoid inflammatory process.[54,55] The MRI findings in such cases are not always diagnostic.[5,56] An axial CT scan demonstrating biopsy-proven sarcoidosis surrounding the optic nerve is shown in Figure 18–2. The patient also had an elevated serum angiotensin converting enzyme

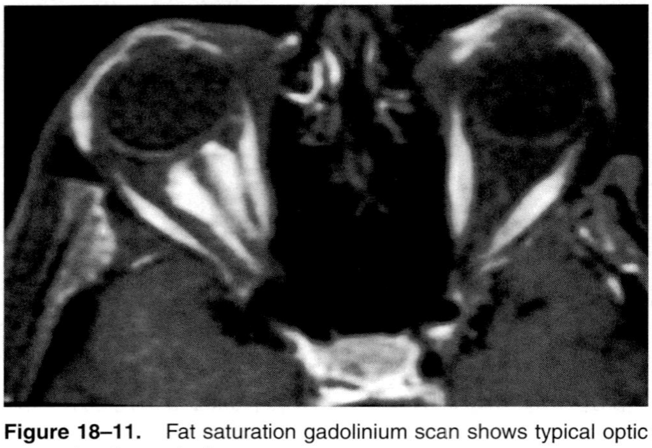

Figure 18–11. Fat saturation gadolinium scan shows typical optic nerve sheath meningioma.

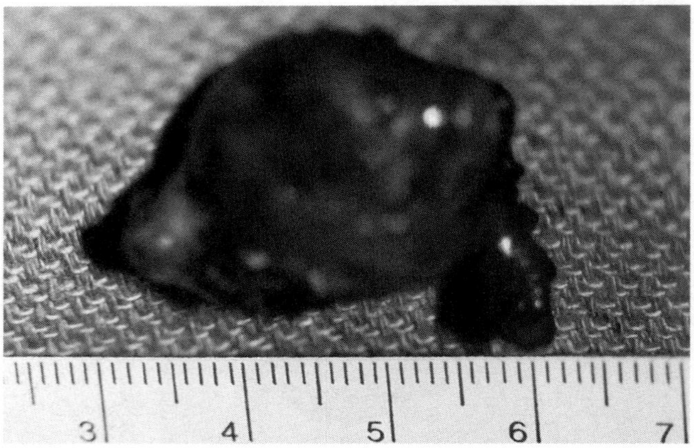

Figure 18–12. In patients with cosmetic defects from proptosis who have no light perception (NLP) vision, we have resected the intraorbital meningiomas.

(ACE) level and a positive limited gallium scan (see Figure 20–14) but was otherwise asymptomatic.

An idiopathic optic neuritis usually produces a smooth, diffuse enlargement of the nerve; in multiple sclerosis, MRI can often detect nonsymptomatic CNS plaques.[57,58]

An asymmetric enlarged inferior rectus muscle in thyroid eye disease can simulate an optic nerve tumor (Figure 18–13). While this was a problem with the first generation of CT scans, image reformation almost eliminated this misdiagnosis.[59] More recently, however, this problem has resurfaced. We have seen two cases in which axial MRI scans were thought to represent optic nerve tumors.

Metastases confined to the optic nerve are uncommon.[29,60–63] We have rarely observed these in association with either breast or lung carcinoma. Usually, the intraocular portion of the nerve is involved, and acute anterior ischemic optic neuropathy must be considered in the differential diagnosis. Occasionally, with prostate metastases to the area of the bony canal, compression neuropathy occurs. These lesions will often respond to corticosteroids and radiation. Optic nerve involvement by a peripapillary uveal melanoma or a retinoblastoma is readily apparent on fundus examination and has been observed much more frequently than distant metastases to this site.[61]

A number of rarer optic nerve tumors can occur in adults. Hoyt described malignant optic nerve gliomas with very high tumor-related mortality.[64] Paraganglioma can mimic an optic nerve sheath meningioma.[65] Usually, paragangliomas arise in the carotid body; and much less commonly, they can involve the larynx or sinuses. Approximately 30 cases of paragangliomas in the orbit have been described. About 40 percent of patients with orbital disease have died as a result of the tumor.[65,66] Amputation neuromas can also occur, and several cases have been reported after enucleation or severance of various intraorbital nerves.[67] Other rare tumors in the realm of the neuro-ophthalmologist include hemangioblastoma of the optic nerve, choristomas and arachnoid cysts of the optic nerve, and arteriovenous malformation.[57,68–70] The latter entity, also known as Wyburn-Mason syndrome, often has a typical fundus pattern and is discussed under retinal tumors (see Chapter 11).

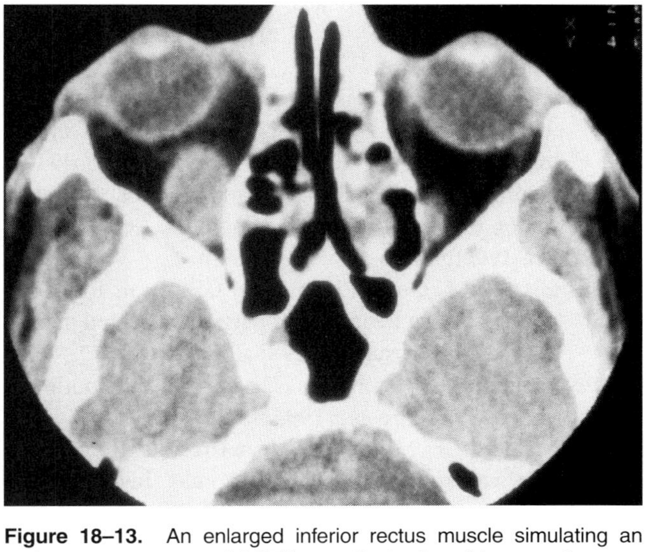

Figure 18–13. An enlarged inferior rectus muscle simulating an optic nerve tumor on axial CT in a patient referred for an optic nerve tumor. Reformatted images demonstrated the true nature of the lesion.

REFERENCES

1. Dutton JJ, Anderson RL. Idiopathic inflammatory perioptic neuritis simulating optic nerve sheath meningioma. Am J Ophthalmol 1985;100:424–30.
2. Li WW, Pettit TH, Zakka KA. Intraocular invasion by papillary squamous cell carcinoma of the conjunctiva. Am J Ophthalmol 1980;90:697–701.
3. Bullock JD, Yawes B, Kelly M, McDonald LW. Non-Hodgkin's lymphoma involving the optic nerve. Ann Ophthalmol 1979;11:1477–80.
4. Zappia RJ, Smith ME, Gay AJ. Prostatic carcinoma metastatic to optic nerve and choroid arch. Ophthalmology 1972;87:642–5.
5. Ing EB, Garrity JA, Cross SA, Ebersold MJ. Sarcoid masquerading as optic nerve sheath meningioma. Mayo Clin Proc 1997;72:38–43.
6. Leventer DB, Merriam JC, Defendini R, et al. Enterogenous cyst of the orbital apex and superior orbital fissure. Ophthalmology 1994;101:1614–21.
7. Johnson TE, Weatherhead RG, Nasr AM, Siqueria EB. Ectopic (extradural) meningioma of the orbit: a report of two cases in children. J Pediatr Ophthalmol Strabismus 1993;30:43–7.
8. Longstreth WT, Dennis LK, McGuire VM, et al. Epidemiology of intracranial meningioma. Cancer 1993;72:639–48.
9. Craig WMcK, Gogela LJ. Intraorbital meningiomas: a clinicopathologic study. Am J Ophthalmol 1949;32:1663–80.
10. Henderson JW. Orbital tumors, 3rd ed. New York, NY: Raven Press; 1994.

11. Wright JE. Primary optic nerve meningiomas: clinical presentation and management. Trans Am Acad Ophthalmol Otolaryngol 1977;83:617–25.
12. Karp LA, Zimmerman LE, Borit A, et al. Primary intraorbital meningiomas. Arch Ophthalmol 1974; 91:24–8.
13. Reese AB. Expanding lesions of the orbit. Trans Ophthalmol Soc UK 1971;91:85–104.
14. Ueki K, Wen-Bin C, Narita Y, et al. Tight association of loss of merlin expression with loss of heterozygosity at chromosome 22q in sporadic meningiomas. Cancer Res 1999;59:5995–8.
15. Tse JY, Ng HK, Lau KM, et al. Loss of heterozygosity of chromosome 14q in low- and high-grade meningiomas. Hum Pathol 1997;28:779–85.
16. Leone PE, Bello MJ, de Campos JM, et al. NF2 gene mutations and allelic status of 1p, 14q and 22q in sporadic meningiomas. Oncogene 1999;1:2231–9.
17. Wolter JR, Benz SC. Ectopic meningioma of the superior orbital rim. Arch Ophthalmol 1976;94:1920–2.
18. Tan KK, Lim SM. Primary extradural intraorbital meningioma in a Chinese girl. Br J Ophthalmol 1965;49:377–80.
19. Macmichael IM, Cullen JF. Primary intraorbital meningioma. Br J Ophthalmol 1969;53:169–73.
20. Cooling RJ, Wright JE. Arachnoid hyperplasia in optic nerve glioma: confusion with orbital meningioma. Br J Ophthalmol 1979;63:596–9.
21. Hart WM Jr, Burde RM, Klingele TG, Perlmutter JC. Bilateral optic nerve sheath meningiomas. Arch Ophthalmol 1980;98:149–51.
22. Liano H, Garcia-Alix C, Lousa M, et al. Bilateral optic nerve meningioma: case report. Eur Neurol 1982; 21:102–6.
23. Trobe JD, Glaser JS, Post JD, Page LK. Bilateral optic canal meningiomas: a case report. Neurosurgery 1978;3:68–74.
24. Kennerdell J, Maroon J. Intracanalicular meningioma with chronic optic disc edema. Ann Ophthalmol 1975;7:507–12.
25. Als E. Intraorbital meningiomas encasing the optic nerve: a report of two cases. Acta Ophthalmol 1969; 47:900.
26. Hannesson OB. Primary meningioma of the orbit invading the choroid: report of a case. Acta Ophthalmol 1971;49:627.
27. Walsh FB. Selected optic neuropathies. Japan J Ophthalmol 1974;18:1.
28. Mandelcorn MS, Shea M. Primary orbital perioptic meningioma. Can J Ophthalmol 1971;6:293.
29. Sanders M, Falconer MA. Optic nerve compression by an intracanalicular meningioma. Br J Ophthalmol 1964;48:13.
30. Henderson JW, Campbell RJ. Primary intraorbital meningioma with intraocular extension. Mayo Clin Proc 1977;52:504–8.
31. Imes RK, Schatz H, Hoyt WF, et al. Evolution of opticociliary veins in optic nerve sheath meningioma. Arch Ophthalmol 1985;103:59–60.
32. Backhouse O, Simmons I, Frank A, Cassels-Brown A. Optic nerve breast metastasis mimicking meningioma. Aust NZJ Ophthalmol 1998;26:247–9.
33. Jakobiec FA, Depot MJ, Kennerdell JS, et al. Combined clinical and computed tomographic diagnosis of orbital glioma and meningioma. Ophthalmology 1984;91:137–55.
34. Rotfus WE, Curtin HD, Slamovits TL, Kennerdell JS. Optic nerve sheath enlargement. Radiology 1984; 150:409–15.
35. Johns TT, Citrin CM, Black J, Sherman JL. CT evaluation of perineural orbital lesions: evaluation of the "tram-track" sign. Am J Neuroradiol 1984;5:587–90.
36. Peyster RG, Hoover ED, Hershey BL, Haskin ME. High resolution CT of lesions of the optic nerve. AJR Am J Roentgenol 1983;140:869–74.
37. Dutton JJ. Optic nerve sheath meningiomas. Surv Ophthalmol 1992;37:167–83.
38. Sibony PA, Kennerdell JS, Slamovits TL, et al. Intrapapillary refractile bodies in optic nerve sheath meningioma. Arch Ophthalmol 1985;103:383–5.
39. Daniels DL, Herfkins R, Gager WE, et al. Magnetic resonance imaging of the optic nerves and chiasm. Radiology 1984;152:79–83.
40. Alper MG, Sherman JL. Gadolinium enhanced magnetic resonance imaging in the diagnosis of anterior visual pathway meningiomas. Trans Am Ophthalmol Soc 1989;87:384–419.
41. Lindblom B, Truwit CL, Hoyt WF. Optic nerve sheath meningioma. Ophthalmology 1992;99:560–6.
42. Nadalo LA, Easterbrook J, McArdle CB, et al. The neuroradiology of visual disturbances. Neurol Clin 1991;9:1–33.
43. Kennerdell JS, Dubois PJ, Dekkeer A, Johnson BL. CT-guided fine needle aspiration biopsy of orbital optic nerve tumors. Ophthalmology 1980;87:491–6.
44. Cristallini EG, Bolis GB, Ottaviano P. Fine needle aspiration biopsy of orbital meningioma. Acta Cytologica 1990;34:236–8.
45. Barbaro NM, Gutin PH, Wilson CB, et al. Radiation therapy in the treatment of partially resected meningiomas. Neurosurgery 1987;20:5625–8.
46. Newmann SA. Meningiomas: a quest for the optimum therapy. J Neurosurg 1994;80:191–4.
47. Rosenberg LF, Miller NR. Visual results after microsurgical removal of meningiomas involving the anterior visual system. Arch Ophthalmol 1984;102: 1019–23.
48. Pless M, Lessell S. Spontaneous visual improvement in

orbital apex tumors. Arch Ophthalmol 1996;114: 704–6.
49. Mark LE, Kennerdell JS, Maroon JC, et al. Microsurgical removal of a primary intraorbital meningioma. Am J Ophthalmol 1978;86:704–9.
50. Kennerdell JS, Maroon JC, Malton M, Warren FA. The management of optic nerve sheath meningiomas. Am J Ophthalmol 1988;106:450–7.
51. Alper MG. Management of primary optic nerve meningioma: current status-therapy in controversy. J Clin Neuro-ophthalmol 1981;1:101–17.
52. Goldsmith BJ, Rosenthal SA, Wara WM, Larson DA. Optic neuropathy after radiation of meningioma. Radiology 1992;185:71.
53. Goldsmith BJ, Wara WM, Wilson CB, Larson DA. Postoperative irradiation of sub-totally receptive meningiomas: a retrospective analysis of 140 patients treated from 1967–1990. J Neurosurg 1994;80: 195–201.
54. Kelley JS, Green WR. Sarcoidosis involving the optic nerve head. Arch Ophthalmol 1973;89:486–8.
55. Som PM, Sacher M, Weitzner I Jr, et al. Sarcoidosis of the optic nerve. J Comput Assist Tomogr 1982;6: 614–6.
56. Carmody RF, Mafee MF, Goodwin JA, et al. Orbital and optic pathway sarcoidosis: MR findings. Am J Neuroradial 1994;15:775–83.
57. Howard CW, Osher RH, Tomsak RL. Computed tomographic features in optic neuritis. Am J Ophthalmol 1980;89:699–702.
58. Jacobs L, Kinkel PR, Kinkel WR. Silent brain lesions in patients with isolated idiopathic optic neuritis: a clinical and nuclear magnetic resonance imaging study. Arch Neurol 1986;43:452–5.
59. Char DH, Norman D. The use of computed tomography and ultrasonography in the evaluation of orbital masses. Surv Ophthalmol 1982;27:49–63.
60. Arnold AC, Hepler RS, Badr MA, et al. Metastasis of adenocarcinoma of the lung to optic nerve sheath meningioma. Arch Ophthalmol 1995;113:346–51.
61. Christmas NJ, Mead MD, Richardson EP, Albert DM. Secondary optic nerve tumors. Surv Ophthalmol 1991;36:196–206.
62. Sung JU, Lam BL, Curtin VT, Tse DT. Metastatic gastric carcinoma to the optic nerve. Arch Ophthalmol 1998;116:692–3.
63. Kattah JC, Chrousos GC, Roberts J, et al. Metastatic prostate cancer of the optic canal. Ophthalmology 1993;100:1711–5.
64. Hoyt WF, Meshel LG, Lessell S, et al. Malignant optic glioma of adulthood. Brain 1973;96:121–32
65. Amemiya T, Kadoya M. Paraganglioma in the orbit. J Cancer Res Clin Oncol 1980;96:169–79.
66. Bednar MM, Trainer TD, Aitken PA, et al. Orbital paraganglioma: case report and review of the literature. Br J Ophthalmol 1992;76:183–5.
67. Messmer EP, Camara J, Boniuk M, Font RL. Amputation neuroma of the orbit: report of two cases and review of the literature. Ophthalmology 1984;91: 1420–3.
68. Zimmerman LE, Arkfeld DL, Schenken JB, et al. A rare choristoma of the optic nerve and chiasm. Arch Ophthalmol 1983;101:766–70.
69. Lauten GJ, Eatherly JB, Ramirez A. Hemangioblastoma of the optic nerve: radiographic and pathologic features. Am J Neuroradiol 1981;2:96–9.
70. Char DH, Unsold R. Ocular and orbital pathology: clinical aspects. In: Newton TH, Bilaniuk LT, editors. Radiology of the eye and orbit. Raven Press; 1990 p. 9–1 –9.64.

19

Extraconal Tumors: Extraocular Muscle Enlargement

The extraconal space is defined as the extraocular muscles and the orbital volume outside the muscle cone. Intraconal tumors usually produce axial proptosis; extraconal tumors, depending on their location, more often displace the globe downward, laterally, medially, or upward. The duration of symptoms, history of systemic illness, tumor location, computed tomography (CT) or magnetic resonance imaging (MRI) are extremely important parameters in establishing a differential diagnosis for a patient.

Histologically identical tumors can occur in multiple or different orbital areas. We have arbitrarily divided our discussion of extraconal orbital tumors into those that most commonly involve the extraocular muscles, orbital bone, lacrimal fossa, and adjacent areas. Orbital lymphoid lesions are the most frequent extraconal adult tumors. In general, medial orbital tumors are frequently caused by sinus-related lesions. Lymphoid or epithelial lesions most commonly involve the lacrimal gland. Superior masses most frequently are either lymphoid/pseudotumors or metastases. Inferior orbital tumors are relatively uncommon.

EXTRAOCULAR MUSCLES

Extraocular muscle involvement is most often due to idiopathic inflammation, thyroid myopathy, or metastases, although a number of other entities can produce extraocular muscle enlargement (Table 19–1).[1]

An accurate history is crucial to establishing the correct diagnosis in these cases; the CT or MRI pattern is often characteristic for a given entity.[2,3] As discussed in the chapter on lymphoid lesions, idiopathic orbital myositis is most common in patients in the first three decades of life.[4–6] The clinical presentation is the rapid onset of discomfort and/or pain on extraocular movement. Usually, a single, unilateral muscle is involved. Limitation of movement is most common in the field of action of the involved muscle. Most commonly, single or multiple recti muscles are involved, although in about 20 percent of cases, the oblique muscles are infiltrated by lymphocytes.[7,8] Figure 19–1 shows a typical orbital MRI pattern of an idiopathic myositis that involves the entire muscle, including the tendon. Patients show a dramatic response to 80 mg of oral prednisone given for 7 to 10 days; in about 80 percent of cases, there is a complete resolution of symptoms with no recurrence.

Table 19–1. DIFFERENTIAL DIAGNOSIS OF ENLARGED EXTRAOCULAR MUSCLES: CT AND MRI SCANS
Graves' disease
Vascular (carotid-cavernous fistula or arteriovenous malformation): enlarged superior ophthalmic vein
Acute orbital myositis: irregular muscle enlargement
Orbital pseudotumor
Malignant lymphoid tumor
Metastatic breast carcinoma
Metastatic cutaneous melanoma
Metastatic neuroblastoma
Metastatic lung carcinoma
Metastatic carcinoid
Metastatic pancreatic carcinoma
Metastatic seminoma
Leukemia
Cysticercosis
Wegener's granulomatosis
Eosinophilic granuloma of soft tissue
Angioma
Rhabdomyosarcoma
Acromegaly
Malignant nonchromaffin paraganglioma
Mesodermal dysplasia
Trichinosis

(From Char[1], with permission)

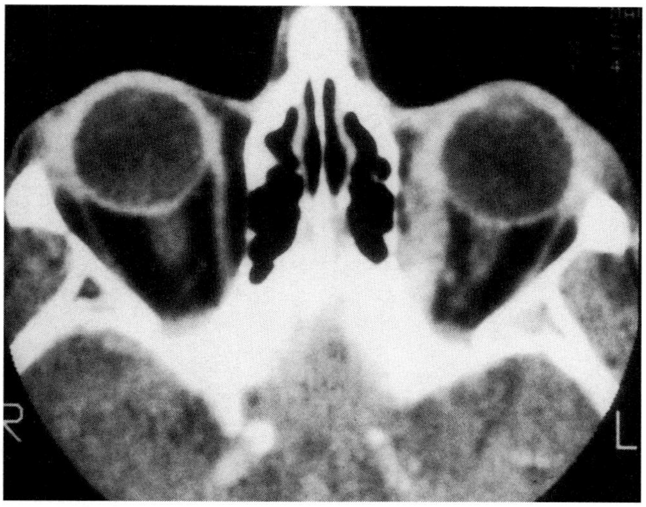

Figure 19–1. CT pattern of idiopathic orbital myositis. The entire length of the muscle and tendon is involved, in contrast to thyroid myopathy, which spares the tendon.

Extraocular muscle lymphoid lesions are less common in older patients, and there are often fewer symptoms in these cases. We have managed a number of patients, in their fifth through eighth decades of life, who presented with either benign or malignant lymphoid lesions involving the recti, oblique, or levator muscles and who had minimal evidence of muscle dysfunction (Figure 19–2).[9] Probably, the differences in clinical pattern between older and younger patient groups is partly due to different patterns of inflammatory cells. Younger patients with acutely symptomatic idiopathic orbital myositis have more acute inflammatory cells than are found in a neoplastic lymphocytic infiltration seen in older, relatively less symptomatic patients. Occasionally, lymphomas that involve the extraocular muscle can be acutely symptomatic. Figure 19–3 shows a lymphoma in the superior oblique muscle in a patient who presented with pain and diplopia. The patient developed nonophthalmic lymphoma and was treated with chemotherapy.

In approximately 80 percent of patients with thyroid orbitopathy, there is a history of systemic Graves' disease. Figure 19–4 shows a patient who had consulted three excellent ophthalmologists about a proptosis of uncertain etiology. Unfortunately, the obvious swelling of the neck had not been noted.

Although bilateral proptosis with scleral show is almost pathognomonic for thyroid-related eye disease, many patients referred to an ophthalmologist with unilateral proptosis have neither a known history of Graves' disease nor these signs. In the author's experience, < 60 percent of these patients have had appropriate studies that would have demonstrated one of the following: either an abnormal serum thyroid stimulating hormone (TSH) or thyroid antibodies prior to their initial referral.[1]

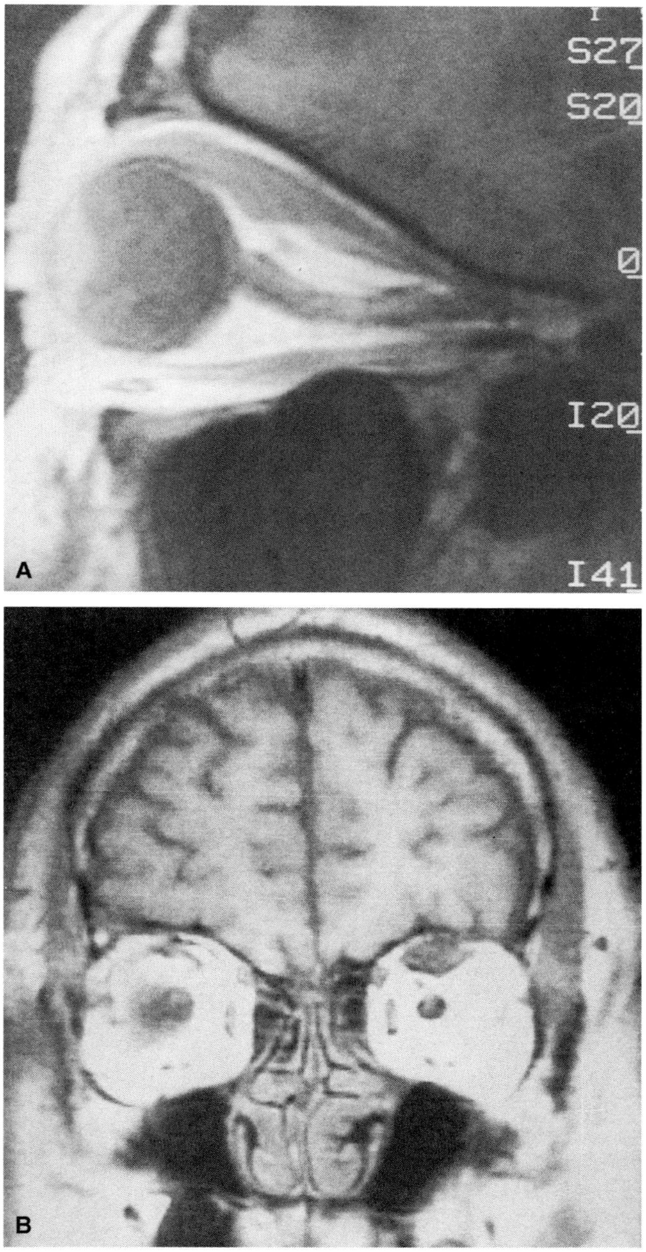

Figure 19–2. *A*, Monoclonal lymphoid lesion involving the superior rectus and levator. Direct parasagittal T_1-weighted MRI scan. *B*, Direct coronal T_1-weighted MRI scan; note enlargement of the left superior rectus and levator muscles.

A sequential systemic laboratory evaluation is indicated for a patient with proptosis who has enlarged extraocular muscles but no orbital mass (Table 19–2). It is often difficult to clinically differentiate idiopathic myositis from thyroid myopathy (see chapter on orbital lymphoid tumors). Figure 19–5 shows typical thyroid extraocular muscle involvement on axial CT. The tendon is spared, and there is enlargement of only the extraocular muscle belly. Often, patients with thyroid orbitopathy have asymmetric disease. They may have unilateral involvement of only a single muscle, which gives a pattern on either direct axial MRI or CT, without computer re-formation, that can simulate an apical orbital tumor (Figure 19–6). Thyroid-related orbitopathy can be ruled out if an orbital mass is present on imaging studies. Rarely, however, two processes can be concurrently present. Dabbs and Kline presented a patient who had bilateral optic nerve sheath meningiomas and thyroid ophthalmopathy.[10] Patients with myopathy, no mass, and negative thyroid tests may have "euthyroid ophthalmopathy" and up to 40 percent of those patients will develop thyroid disease on long-term follow-up.[2] If an extensive experimental laboratory evaluation is

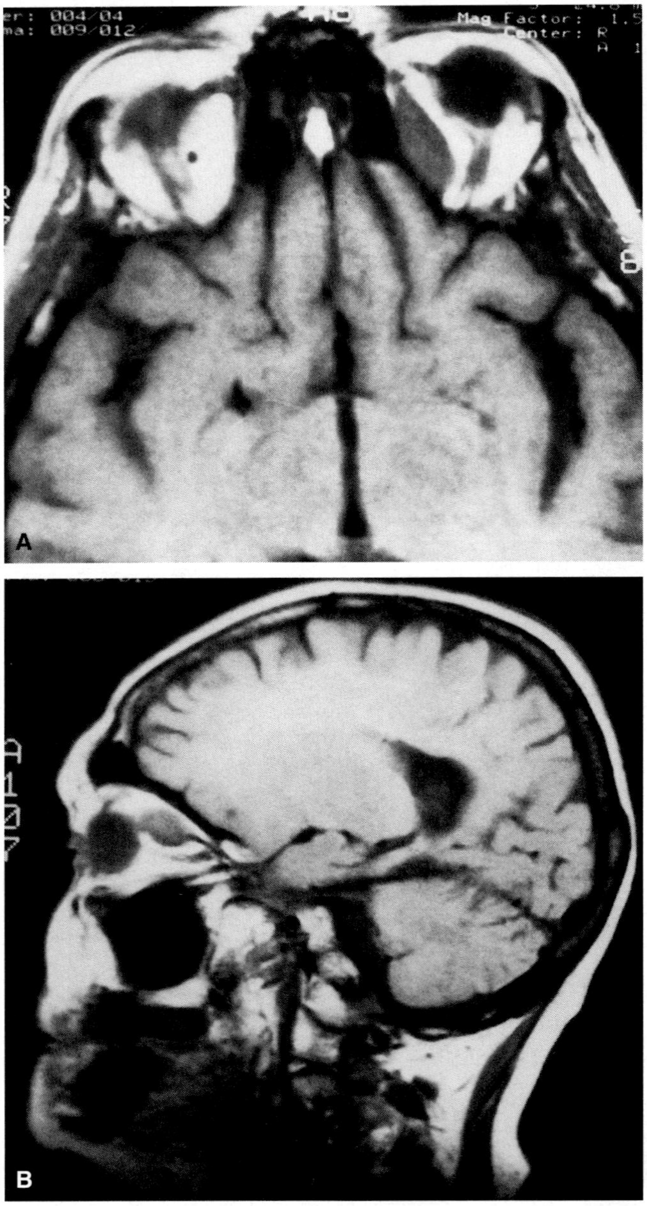

Figure 19–3. *A*, Lymphoma involving the superior oblique muscle. Direct T_1-weighted axial MRI scan. *B*, Direct T_1-weighted parasagittal MRI scan. The patient later developed widespread disease.

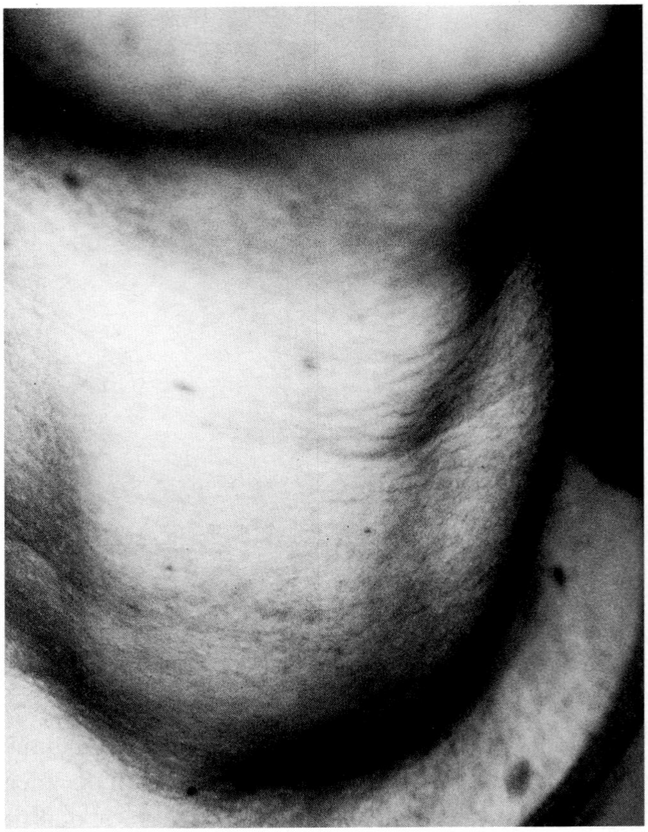

Figure 19–4. Enlarged thyroid gland in a patient who presented with orbitopathy.

Table 19–2. SEQUENTIAL LABORATORY EVALUATION TO DIAGNOSE THYROID ORBITOPATHY
1. Serum thyroid stimulating hormone (TSH), thyrotropin
2. Serum thyroid stimulating immunoglobulin antibodies (TSI)
3. Antimicrosomal and antithyroglobulin antibodies

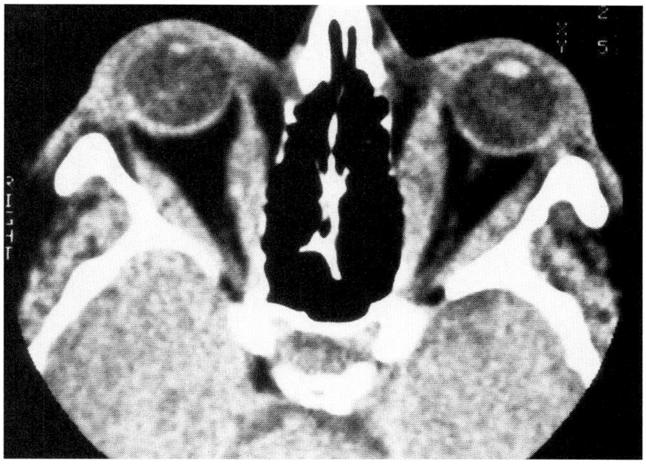

Figure 19–5. Axial CT scan of an enlarged extraocular muscle in thyroid orbitopathy with sparing of the tendons.

performed on all these patients, thyroid abnormalities are detectable, although with routine laboratory studies, this group still has a 10 percent false-negative rate.[1,6]

In thyroid ophthalmopathy, fibrosis and inflammation of the muscle usually produce restriction, with limitation of movement away from a muscle's field of action. Idiopathic myositis patients often have diffuse episcleral and scleral vascular engorgement. Thyroid eye disease, in contrast to idiopathic myositis, often has discrete dilated vessels over the insertions of the extraocular muscles (Figure 19–7). A number of less common causes of enlarged extraocular muscles are reviewed in reference 1.

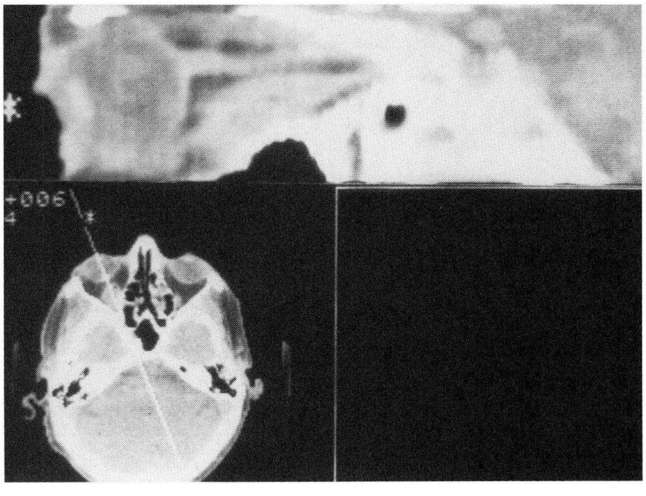

Figure 19–6. Asymmetric muscle involvement is not uncommon in thyroid orbitopathy. A direct axial MRI or CT scan without reconstruction can often simulate an orbital tumor.

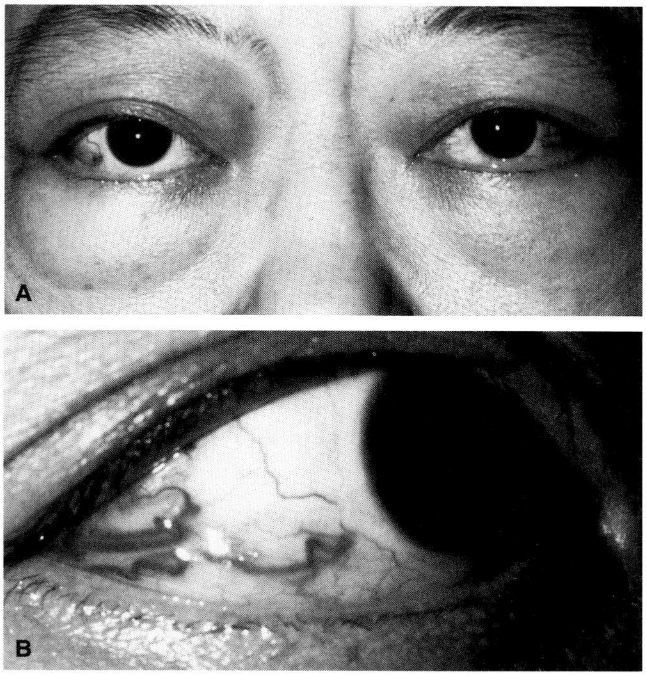

Figures 19–7. *A* and *B*, Dilated vessels over the insertion of the extraocular muscles in thyroid orbitopathy. (From Char,[1] with permission)

All patients but one with metastatic tumors to the extraocular muscles whom the author has managed presented with a known history of widespread disease.[11,12] In metastatic tumors to the extraocular muscles, three clinical and imaging patterns are common.

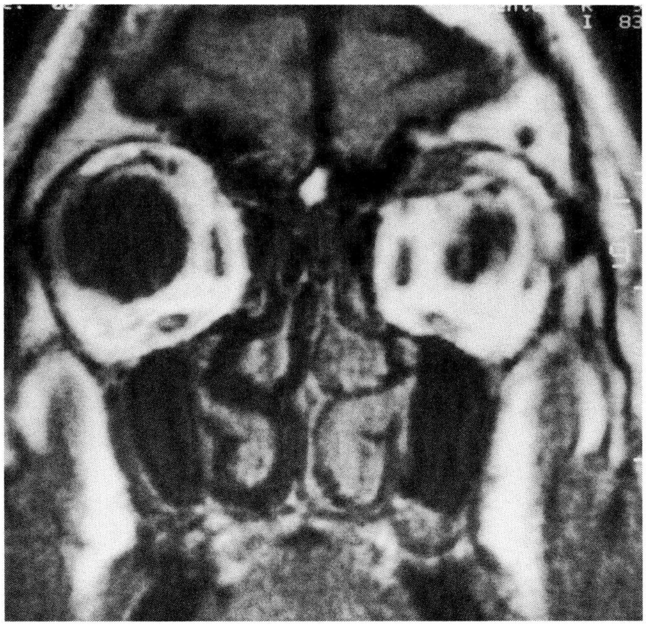

Figure 19–8. Adenocarcinoma metastatic to the superior muscle complex on direct coronal T_1-weighted image.

First, a single muscle may be involved by metastasis.[13–15] Figure 19–8 shows an adenocarcinoma metastatic to the superior muscle complex; a similar presentation in the medial rectus is seen in Figure 25–4. Second, there can be diffuse involvement of the extraocular muscles by a metastatic tumor (Figure 19–9). While this pattern can occasionally simulate thyroid orbitopathy, muscle enlargement is more uniform in thyroid orbitopathy and more patchy in metastases. Third, metastases can involve both the extraocular muscle and contiguous structures (Figure 19–10); this pattern allows easy differentiation of metastases from either idiopathic myositis or thyroid myopathy.

Other processes, such as a reaction to a foreign body, can simulate orbital myositis. The CT scan and fine-needle biopsy shown in Figure 19–11A and B were produced by a foreign body that responded to intralesional steroids.

Occasionally, other imaging findings may be important in ascertaining the correct etiology of extraocular muscle enlargement. Figures 19–12A and B show axial CT scans of a patient managed elsewhere with high-dose steroids for thyroid orbitopathy. An axial CT scan of the superior orbit demonstrates asymmetric enlargement of the superior ophthalmic vein. This pattern, in combination with arterialization of the conjunctiva (Figure 19–12C), is virtually pathognomonic for either a dural shunt or a carotid cavernous fistula.[16] Figure 19–13 shows a coronal CT scan of an alveolar soft

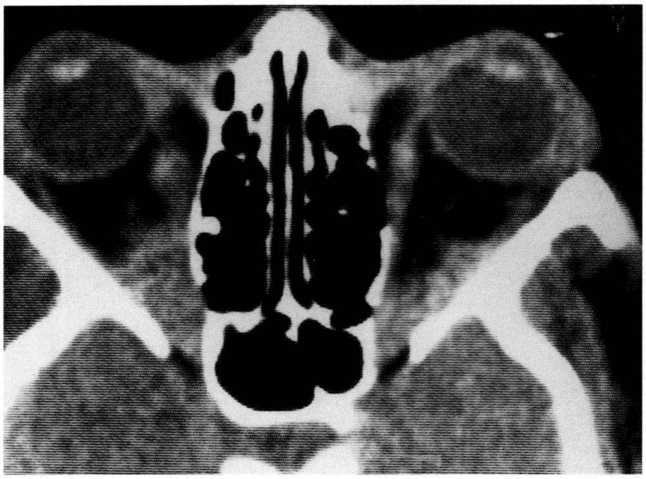

Figure 19–9. Metastases involving extraocular muscles and simulating apical compressive thyroid optic neuropathy. Note that the muscles are not as regularly enlarged as in thyroid myopathy.

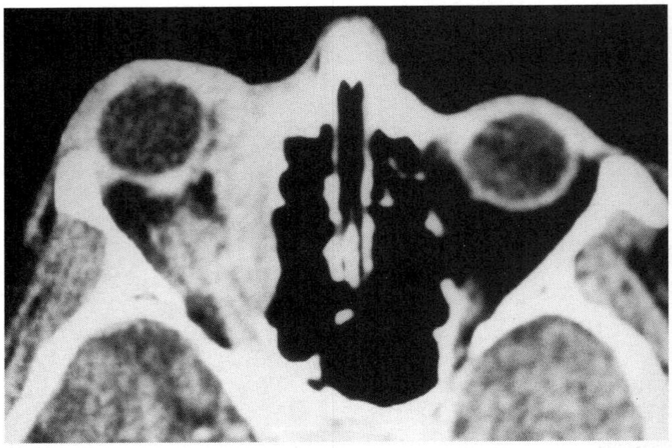

Figure 19–10. Metastasis to extraocular muscles and contiguous orbit on axial CT scan.

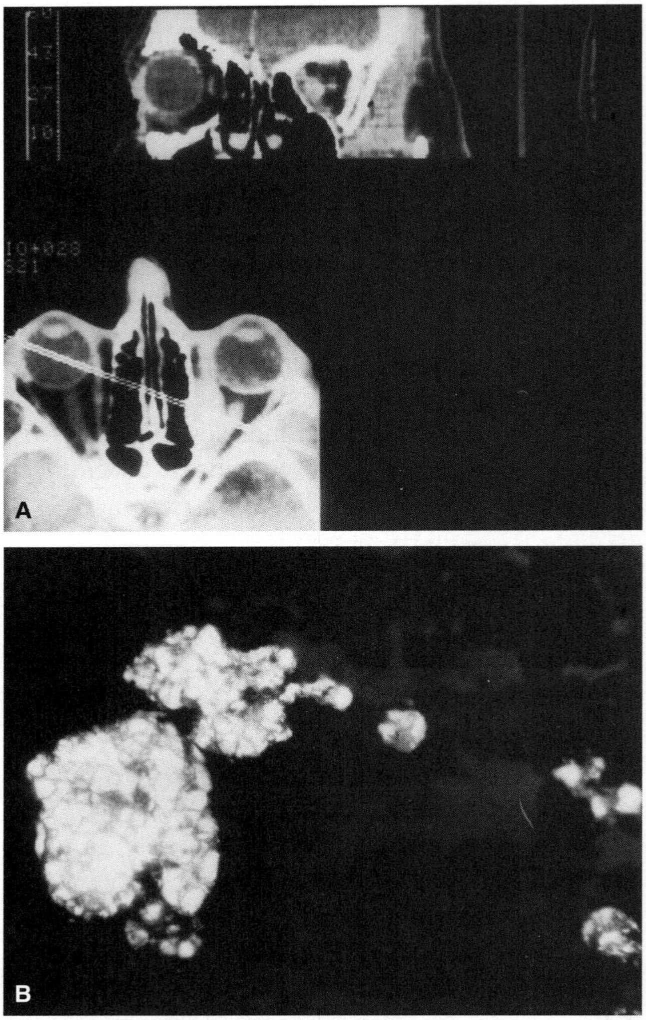

Figure 19–11. *A*, Axial CT scan with coronal re-formation demonstrates unsuspected foreign body mass involving medial rectus. *B*, Fine-needle biopsy shows polarizing foreign body; other areas of slide demonstrated numerous inflammatory cells. Symptoms resolved after periocular injection of steroids at the time of biopsy.

part sarcoma involving the lateral rectus muscle; this tumor sometimes produces markedly enlarged overlying vessels (Figure 19–14). Rarely, other lesions, such as intramuscular dermoid cysts, have been reported.[17] Hakim and colleagues have reported three cases of spontaneous intramuscle hemorrhage that simulates the appearance of thyroid myopathy.[18] In approximately 40 to 50 percent of patients with orbital cysticercosis, there is a cystic enlargement of an extraocular muscle.[19,20]

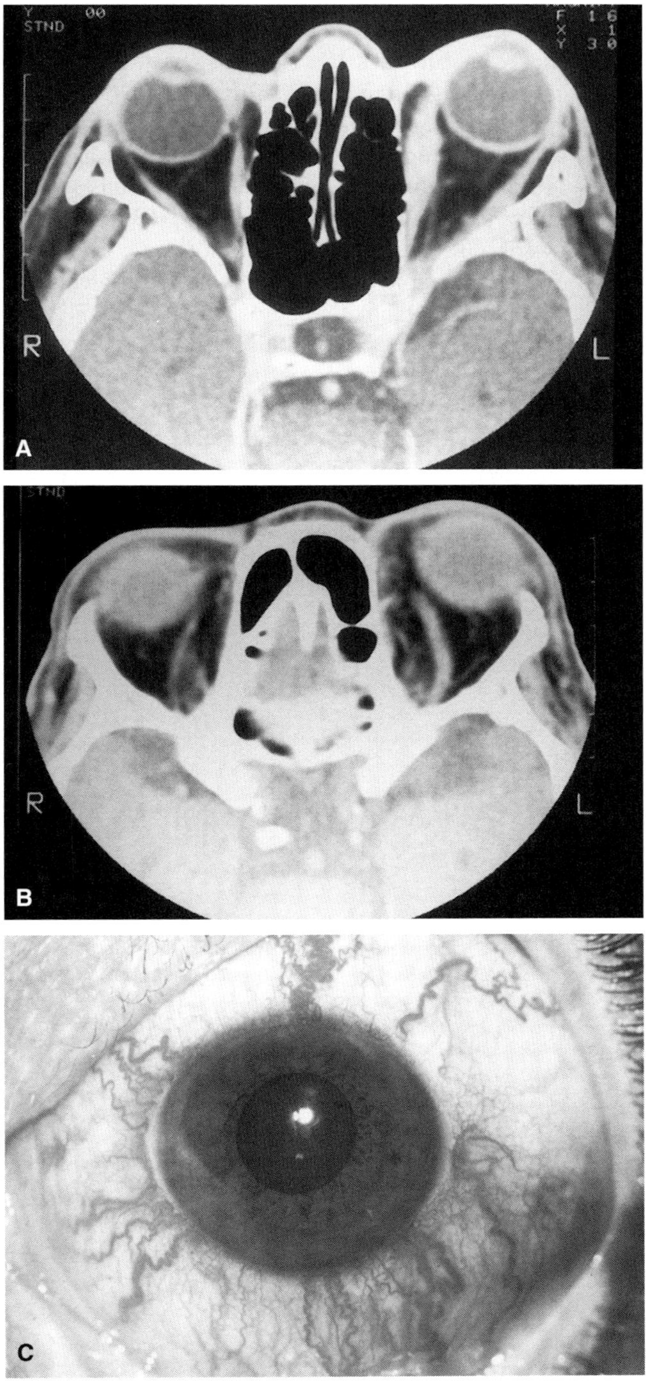

Figure 19–12. *A*, Axial CT scan shows unilateral enlargement of extraocular muscles in a pattern consistent with thyroid orbitopathy. *B*, Axial CT scan of the superior orbit shows marked asymmetry in the superior ophthalmic vein due to carotid-cavernous fistula. *C*, Clinical photograph shows arterialization of the conjunctival vessels that is almost pathognomonic for a carotid-cavernous or dural fistula.

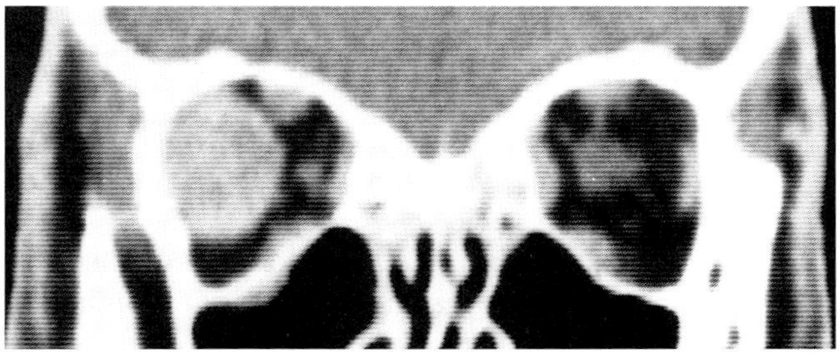

Figure 19–13. Alveolar soft part sarcoma involving the lateral rectus muscle on coronal CT scan.

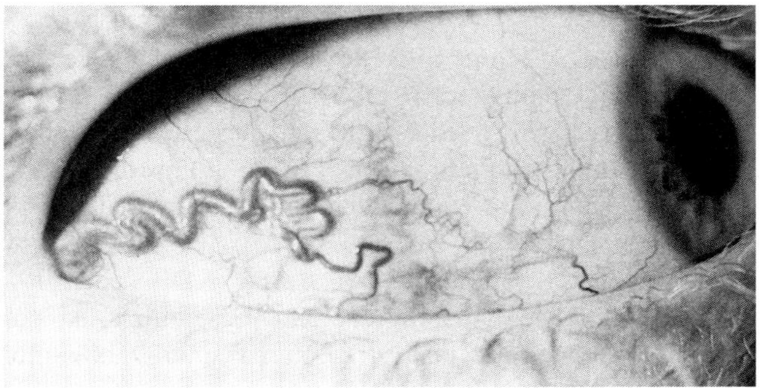

Figure 19–14. Enlargement of superficial vessels overlying an alveolar soft part sarcoma.

REFERENCES

1. Char DH. Thyroid eye disease, 3rd ed. Boston, MA: Butterworth-Heinemann Inc.; 1997.
2. Char DH, Norman D. The use of computed tomography and ultrasonography in the evaluation of orbital masses. Surv Ophthalmology 1982;27:49–63.
3. Char DH, Unsold R. Ocular and orbital pathology: clinical aspects. In: Newton TH, Hasso AN, Killon WP, editors. Modern neuroradiology, Vol 3: Computed tomography of the head and neck. New York, NY: Clavadel Press; 1988.
4. Slavin ML, Glaser JS. Idiopathic orbital myositis: report of six cases. Arch Ophthalmol 1982;100:1261–5.
5. Weinstein GS, Dresner SC, Slamovits TL, Kennerdell JS. Acute and subacute orbital myositis. Am J Ophthalmol 1983;96:209–17.

6. Siatokowski RM, Capo H, Byrne SF, et al. Clinical and echographic findings in idiopathic orbital myositis. Am J Ophthalmol 1994;118:343–50.
7. Wan WL, Cano MR, Green RL. Orbital myositis involving the oblique muscles: an echographic study. Ophthalmology 1988;95:1522–8.
8. Patrinely CR, Osborn AG, Anderson RL, Whiting AS. Computed tomographic features of nonthyroid extraocular muscle enlargement. Ophthalmology 1989;96:1038–47.
9. Hornblass A, Jakobiec FA, Reifler DM, Mines J. Orbital lymphoid tumors located predominantly within extraocular muscles. Ophthalmology 1987; 94:688–97.
10. Dabbs CB, Kline LB. Big muscles and big nerves. Surv Ophthalmol 1997;42:247–54.
11. DiBernardo C, Pacheco EM, Hughes JR, et al. Echographic evaluation and findings in metastatic melanoma to extraocular muscles. Ophthalmology 1996;103:1794–7.
12. Simpson JL, Alford MA, Carter KD, Keech RV. Metastatic rhabdomyosarcoma presenting as an isolated lateral rectus restriction. J Pediatr Ophthalmol Strabismus 1999;36:90–1.
13. Bedford PD, Daniel PM. Discrete carcinomatous metastases in the extrinsic ocular muscles: a case of carcinoma of the breast with exophthalmic ophthalmoplegia. Am J Ophthalmol 1960;49:723–6.
14. Ashton N, Morgan G. Discrete carcinomatous metastases in the extraocular muscles. Br J Ophthalmol 1974;58:112–7.
15. Jiang N-S, Fairbanks VF, Hay ID. Assay for thyroid-stimulating immunoglobulin. Mayo Clin Proc 1986;61:753–5.
16. Halbach VV, Higashida RT, Hieshima GB, et al. Dural fistulas involving the cavernous sinus: results of treatment in 30 patients. Radiology 1987;163:437–42.
17. Howard GR, Nerad JS, Bonavolonta G, Tranfa F. Orbital dermoid cysts located within the lateral rectus muscle. Ophthalmology 1994;101:767–71.
18. Hakim KN, McNab AA, Sullivan TJ. Spontaneous hemorrhage within the rectus muscle. Ophthalmology 1994;101:1631–4.
19. Sekhar GC, Lemke BN. Orbital cysticercosis. Ophthalmology 1997;14:1599–604.
20. Sekhar GC, Lemke BN, Singh SK. Cystic lesions of the extraocular muscles. Ophthal Plast Reconstr Surg 1996;12:199–205.

20

Lacrimal Gland Tumors

Perhaps the greatest degree of orbital neoplastic diversity occurs in the region of the lacrimal gland. The marked variation in tumor patterns and their behavior makes the evaluation and treatment of lacrimal gland masses a challenge. In adults, infection, inflammation, benign and malignant epithelial or lymphoid tumors, and metastatic disease can all present in the lacrimal fossa.[1–4] A number of other less common processes can also involve the lacrimal fossa.[5–10]

A number of symptoms and both clinical and radiographic signs are helpful to delineate the nature of different lacrimal processes. Any enlarging lacrimal mass can produce proptosis, and often the eye is displaced both medially and inferiorly. As a lacrimal gland mass enlarges, it often produces a characteristic "S-shaped" lid (Figure 20–1).

Age is not a useful parameter to differentiate benign from malignant processes. Malignancies of the lacrimal gland can occur at any age, except that they are very rare in children under 10 years old. Laterality, chronicity, dry eye symptoms, and pain are clinical findings that are sometimes helpful in differentiating disease processes. Bilateral involvement excludes an epithelial lacrimal gland neoplasm. Involvement of both lacrimal glands is most consistent with infection, inflammation, or lymphoma. As Gass and Blodi noted, a significant percentage of patients with bilateral lacrimal gland enlargement have an associated systemic process (see chapter on orbital pseudotumors).[11] Esoteric systemic processes can present first to the ophthalmologist with lacrimal fossa symptoms. A magnetic resonance imaging (MRI) scan from a patient with bilateral lacrimal gland enlargement secondary to syphilis is shown in Figure 20–2. Lacrimal gland enlargement in a patient with systemic lupus erythematosus is shown in Figure 20–3. The coronal MRI scan in Figure 20–4 shows bilateral lacrimal gland enlargement in Wegner's granulomatosis.

Epithelial malignancies of the lacrimal gland most commonly have pain and more rapid progression than benign epithelial neoplasms. Usually, patients with benign mixed tumors (pleomorphic adenomas) have

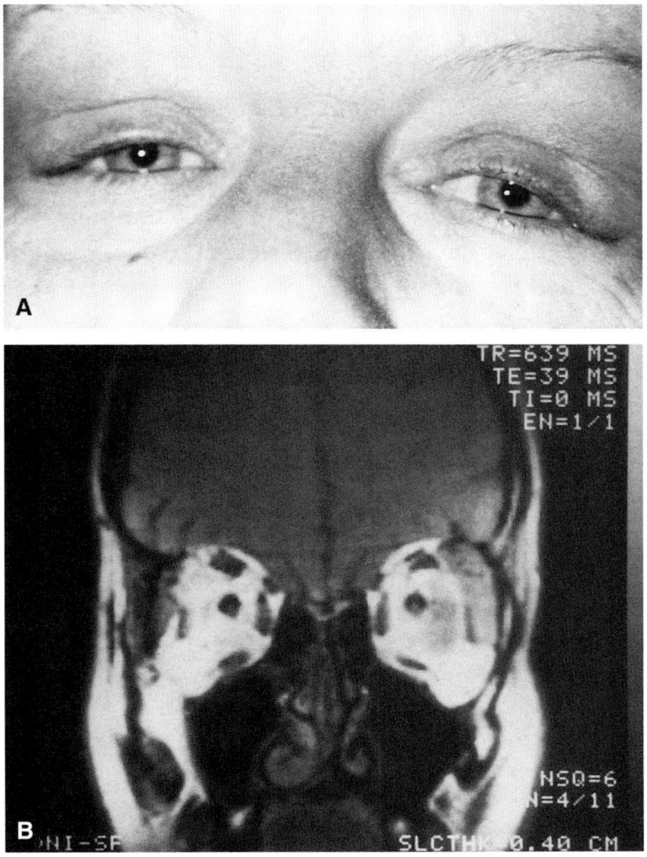

Figure 20–1. *A*, Lacrimal gland lymphoma as a presenting sign of systemic disease. The "S-shaped eyelid" is typical for lacrimal gland enlargement. *B*, Direct coronal MRI scan of biopsy-proven lesion. Bone marrow biopsies were also positive for lymphoma.

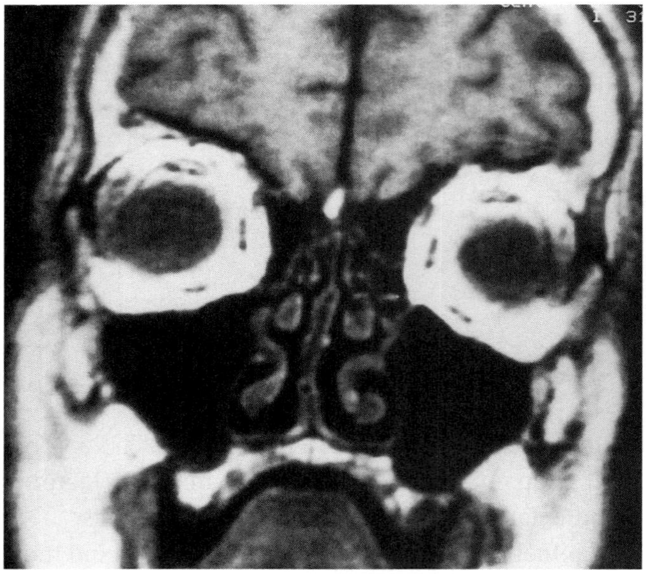

Figure 20–2. Coronal MRI scan of syphilitic involvement of the lacrimal glands.

an insidious onset and chronic symptoms; but these findings are neither specific nor diagnostic.[1] This author has never seen a patient with a lacrimal gland malignancy present with dry eye symptoms, although some have absent tear function on testing.

The presence and pattern of bone involvement noted on plain radiography, computed tomography (CT), or MRI are often useful in determining the nature of a lacrimal fossa lesion. Most benign

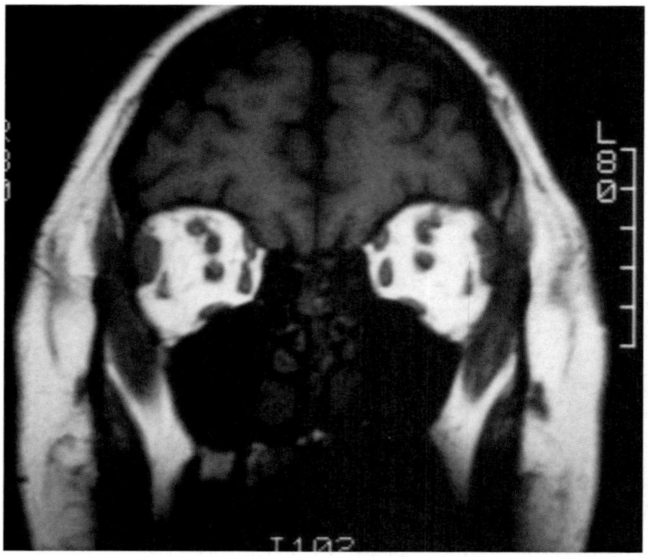

Figure 20–3. T_1-weighted MRI scan demonstrates bilateral lacrimal gland enlargement in a patient with systemic lupus erythematosus. FNAB was positive for benign nfiltrate.

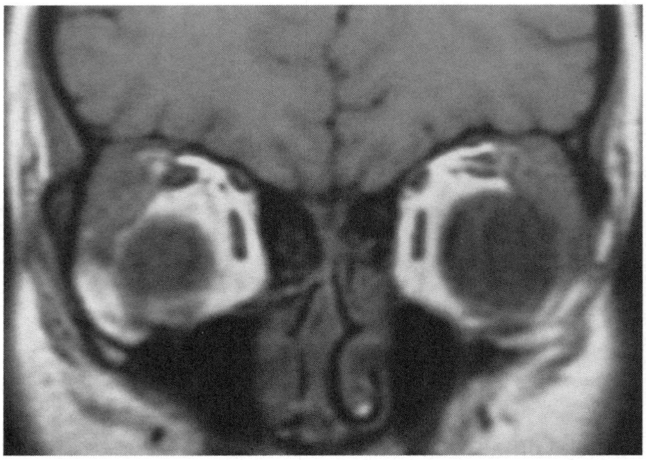

Figure 20–4. T_1-weighted coronal MRI shows bilateral lacrimal gland enlargement in Wegner's granulomatosis.

processes either do not involve the bones of the lacrimal fossa, or if they do, there is diffuse noninvasive fossa enlargement, without sclerosis. Generalized expansion of the orbit can occur in young patients with chronic lesions.[12] In adults, longstanding processes can result in localized, smooth enlargement of the fossa, and this pattern has been noted with benign epithelial lesions (mixed tumors or pleomorphic adenoma), pseudotumors, and rarely lymphomas. Dermoid cysts have a propensity to involve the lacrimal fossa in adults, and usually, they produce a rounded, nonsclerotic bone defect (Figure 20–5). Rarely, a dumbbell-shaped dermoid will break through the lateral orbital wall, as shown in Figure 20–6. Lacrimal fossa bone changes can occur in histiocytosis syndromes, as discussed in the chapter on pediatric orbital tumors. Rarely, traumatic hematic cysts (organized hematomas) can involve the lacrimal fossa (Figure 20–7). Sometimes these post-traumatic

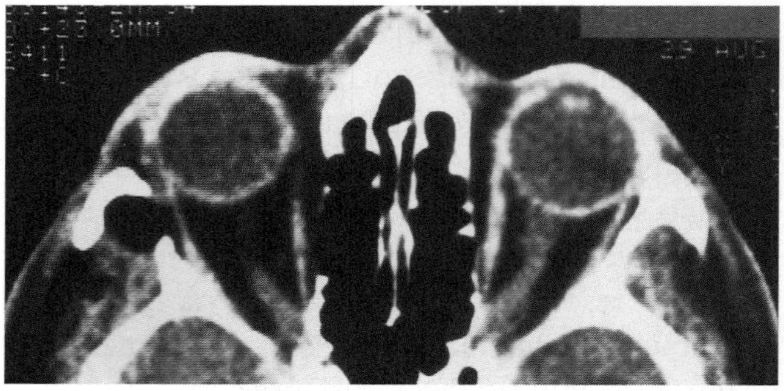

Figure 20–5. Axial CT scan demonstrating evenly rounded bone defect in the lacrimal fossa typical of dermoid cyst.

hematic cysts can simulate an epithelial malignancy with apparent bone invasion as shown in Figure 20–8.[13–15] Frank bone invasion is diagnostic of either a primary or metastatic malignancy. An adenoid cystic carcinoma of the lacrimal gland with bone involvement is shown in Figure 20–9A. This lesion was diagnosed by fine-needle aspiration biopsy (FNAB) (Figure 20–9B). Both the CT and MRI scans reveal a jagged, serrated invasion of the bone. Often, there is contiguous spread to adjacent structures as shown in Figures 20–9A, C, and 20–10B. These malignancies may be calcified and can also cause bone sclerosis.[16] Adjacent bone sclerosis is usually a sign of malignancy, although we have intragland calcification with amyeloid involvement of the lacrimal gland (Figure 20–11).[17] Bone sclerosis can occur in irradiated histiocytosis patients, and those with fibrous dysplasia, meningioma, or rarely sarcoid.[18]

Epithelial tumors of the lacrimal gland are a major diagnostic and clinical problem for the orbital

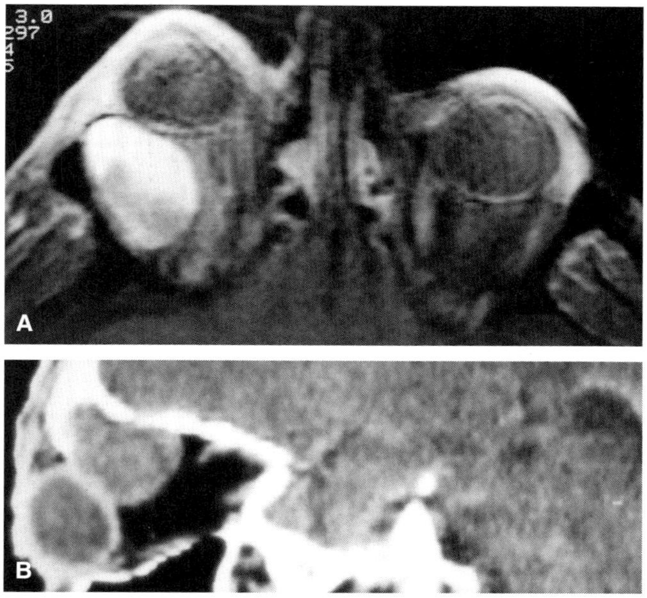

Figure 20–7. *A,* Axial MRI scan shows a biopsy-proven hematic cyst (organized hematoma) that mimics a dermoid. *B,* Computer reformatted parasagittal CT shows lesion shown in Figure 20–7A.

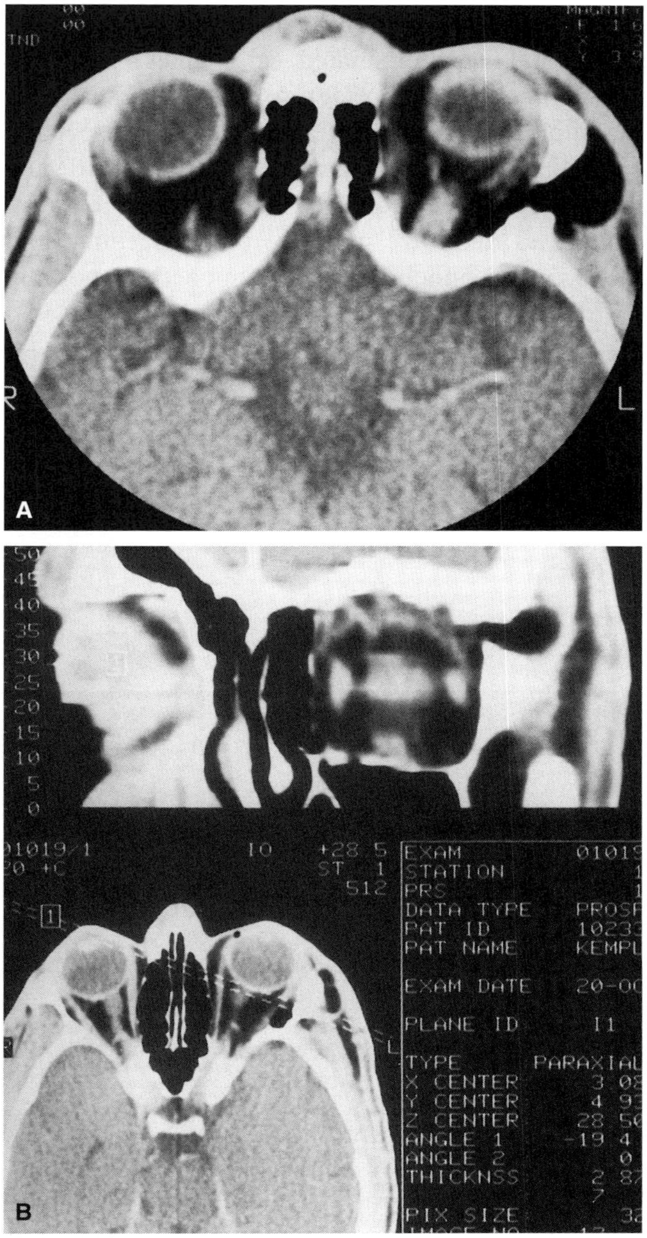

Figure 20–6. *A* and *B,* Axial CT scan with computed reformation of a dumbbell-shaped dermoid that involved both the orbit and temporalis fossa.

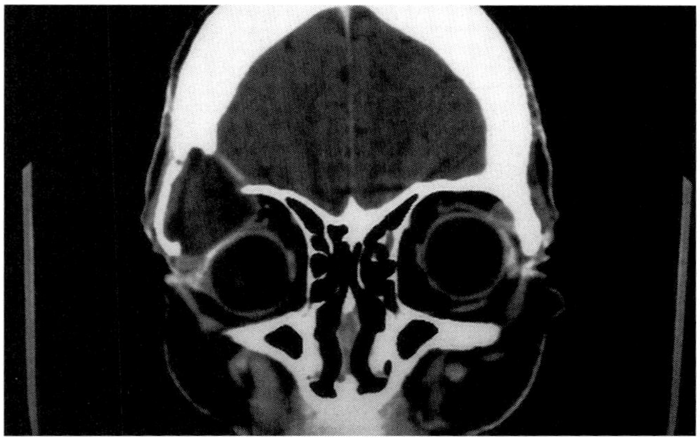

Figure 20–8. Direct coronal CT scan with coronal reconstruction demonstrating bone alterations in the lacrimal fossa. The lesion simulated an epithelial neoplasm on both CT and ultrasonography but was actually a hematic cyst secondary to trauma

surgeon for three major reasons: (1) histologic studies have demonstrated that approximately 50 percent of lacrimal masses are epithelial, and one-half of these are malignant. Despite some clinical and radiographic signs it can often be difficult to distinguish benign from malignant epithelial tumors.[19] Some authors believe that calcification or a dense surround with a more lucent center is typical for a malignancy, but others have not found that these patterns are reliable;[20] (2) the malignant epithelial tumors (adenoid cystic carcinoma, malignant mixed tumor, mucoepidermoid carcinoma, adenocarcinoma, and undifferentiated carcinomas) have 10-year tumor-related mortality of > 80 percent.[19,21,22] Incomplete excision of a potentially resectable epithelial malignancy has a fatal prognosis. All such lesions must be recognized and operated on in a manner to minimize potential tumor seeding; and (3) benign epithelial mixed tumor (pleomorphic

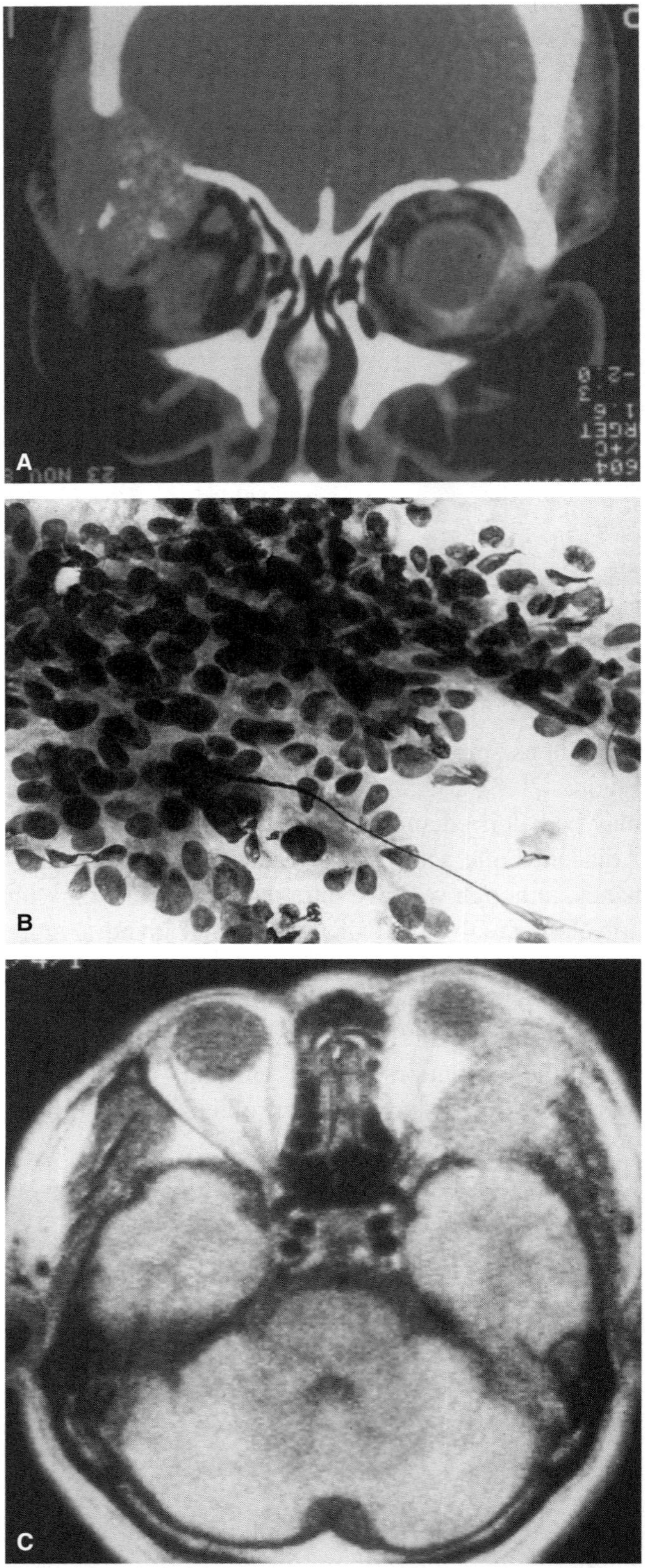

Figure 20–9. *A,* Invasion of bone by an adenoid cystic carcinoma of the lacrimal gland demonstrated on CT. *B,* Fine-needle aspiration biopsy reveals typical adenoid cystic carcinoma. *C,* MRI scan demonstrates invasion of bone, manifested as loss of normal bone signal void.

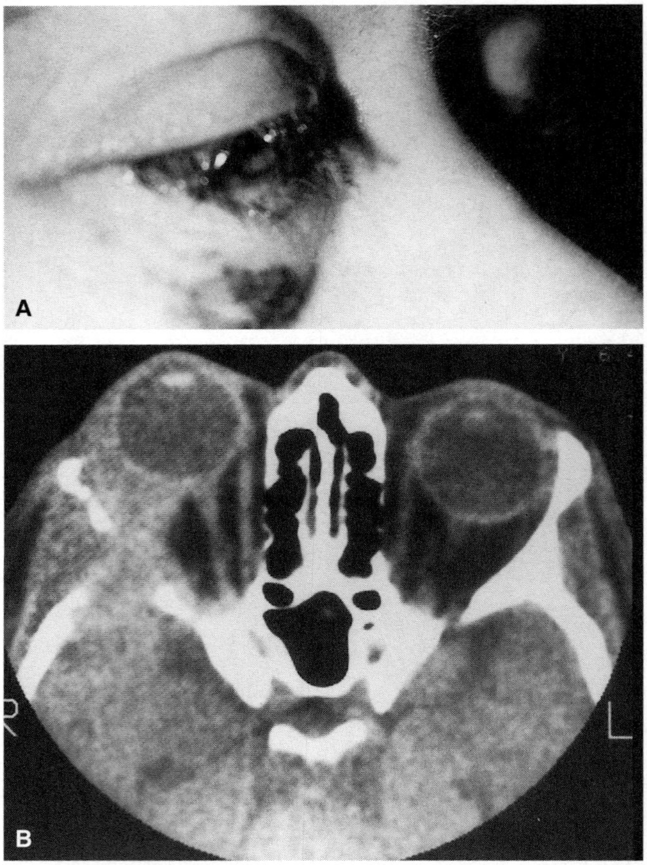

Figure 20–10. *A,* This adenoid cystic carcinoma patient's CT scan demonstrated contiguous involvement of the central nervous system. *B,* Follow-up CT scan 5 years after radiation treatment; usually, this fatal disease takes many years to kill the patient.

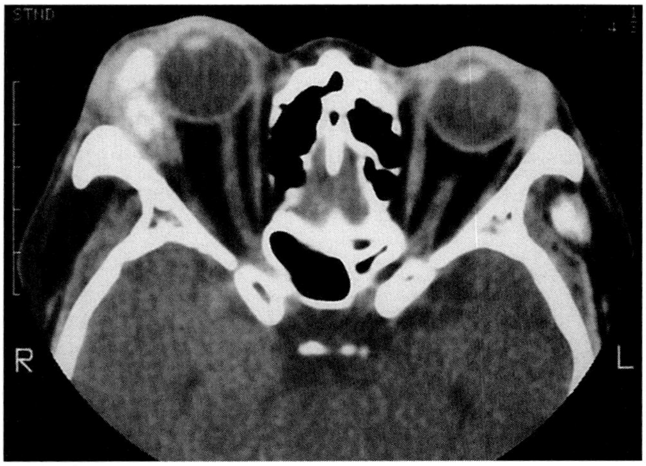

Figure 20–11. Intragland calcification in amyeloid.

adenoma) has a 20 percent malignant transformation rate, and recurrence occurs in at least 25 percent of incompletely resected lesions.[19]

DIAGNOSIS

A schema for diagnostic decisions based on the clinical presentation of patients with lacrimal gland lesions is shown in Table 20–1. Patients can be separated into those with and those without inflammatory symptoms and signs. Patients with acute swelling, periorbital pain, scleritis, painful eye movements, or an erythematous, indurated lid most likely have an inflammatory process. The evaluation of orbital inflammatory disease is a multidisciplinary problem. Infectious diseases can involve the lacrimal gland, and a review of systems with emphasis on recent respiratory or generalized infections should be sought. In children and teenagers, there is a history of a prodromal viral syndrome (see chapter on pediatric orbital tumors). As shown in Figure 20–1 lacrimal gland inflammation often gives an S-shaped, swollen, red lid. A number of acute and chronic infectious diseases can involve the lacrimal gland.[23] Sarcoidosis is one of many inflammatory lesions that can involve the lacrimal gland.[24] Figure 20–12 shows a bilateral case of sarcoidosis, while Figure 20–13 shows a patient who also had biopsy confirmation but who presented with a unilateral lacrimal gland mass with a negative systemic work-up for sarcoid.[13] These patients may have a history of systemic

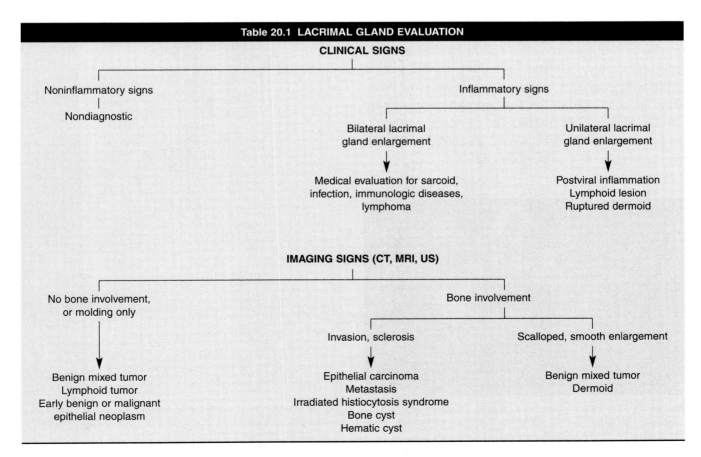

Table 20.1 LACRIMAL GLAND EVALUATION

CLINICAL SIGNS

- Noninflammatory signs
  - Nondiagnostic
- Inflammatory signs
  - Bilateral lacrimal gland enlargement
    - → Medical evaluation for sarcoid, infection, immunologic diseases, lymphoma
  - Unilateral lacrimal gland enlargement
    - → Postviral inflammation; Lymphoid lesion; Ruptured dermoid

IMAGING SIGNS (CT, MRI, US)

- No bone involvement, or molding only
  - → Benign mixed tumor; Lymphoid tumor; Early benign or malignant epithelial neoplasm
- Bone involvement
  - Invasion, sclerosis
    - → Epithelial carcinoma; Metastasis; Irradiated histiocytosis syndrome; Bone cyst; Hematic cyst
  - Scalloped, smooth enlargement
    - → Benign mixed tumor; Dermoid

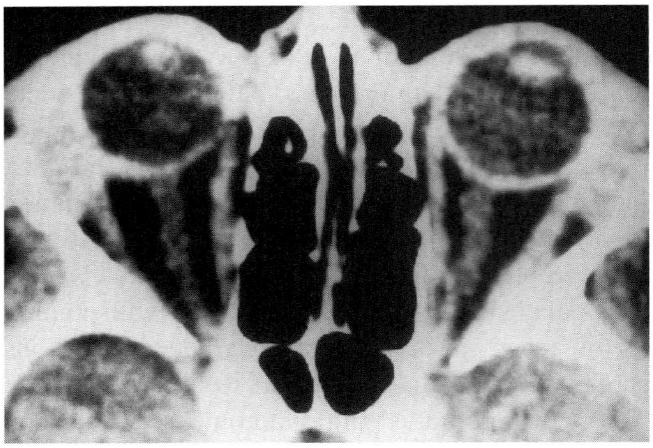

Figure 20–12. Bilateral lacrimal gland involvement as a manifestation of sarcoidosis.

sarcoidosis, respiratory problems, skin rashes, or joint symptoms.[24] In equivocal cases, serum angiotensin converting enzyme (ACE), lysozyme assays, and limited gallium scans (Figure 20–14) are useful.[25,26,27] Rarely, sarcoid can present in a very confusing manner. Peterson and colleagues reported on two older Caucasian women, ages 72 and 87 years, who presented with orbital soft tissue involvement outside the lacrimal fossa.[28] Mikalicz's syndrome with swelling of the lacrimal and salivary glands (Figure 20–15) can be caused by sarcoid as well as by several other entities. Rarely, bilateral herniation of the orbital septa with marked prolapse of fat can simulate bilateral lacrimal gland masses as shown in Figure 20–16. This patient, because of cosmetic concerns, had removal of fat with a good cosmetic result and no discernable tear system damage.

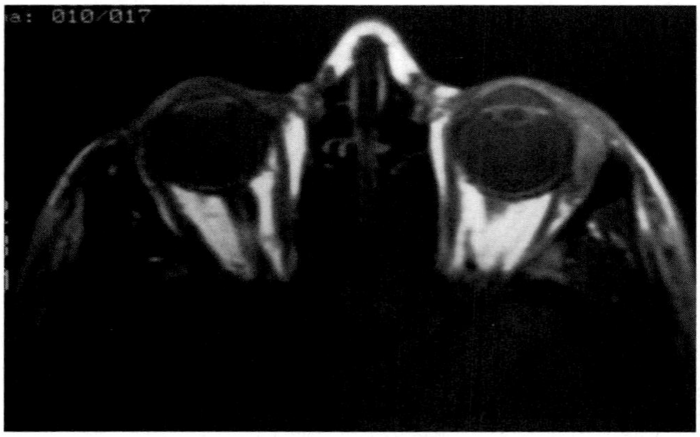

Figure 20–13. Patient had biopsy-proven sarcoid involving only one lacrimal gland with a negative systemic evaluation. Axial T_1–weighted MRI scan shows unilateral involvement.

Orbital lymphoid lesions are another common cause of lacrimal gland swelling.[29] This diagnostic group includes pseudotumor, lymphoid hyperplasia, and lymphoma. These diseases have a unique set of diagnostic and therapeutic challenges and often involve multiple orbital structures. They are separately

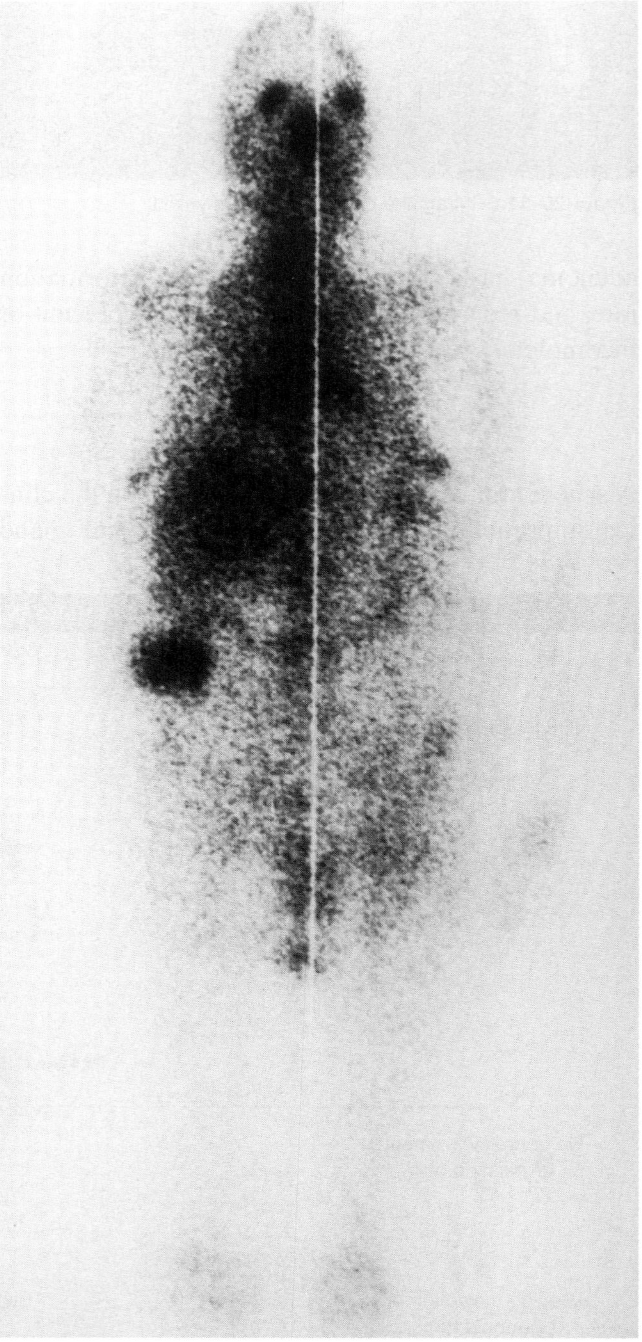

Figure 20–14. Hilar adenopathy and lacrimal gland uptake on a limited gallium scan are helpful to confirm the diagnosis of sarcoid in a patient not receiving corticosteroids.

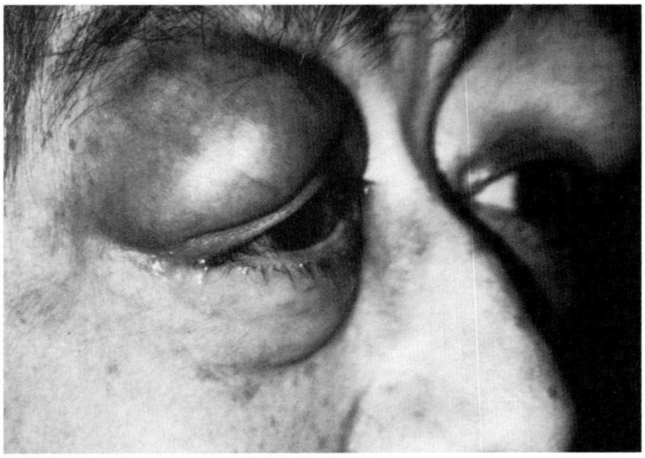

Figure 20–15. Clinical photograph of a patient with benign fibrolymphoid proliferation of lacrimal and salivary glands

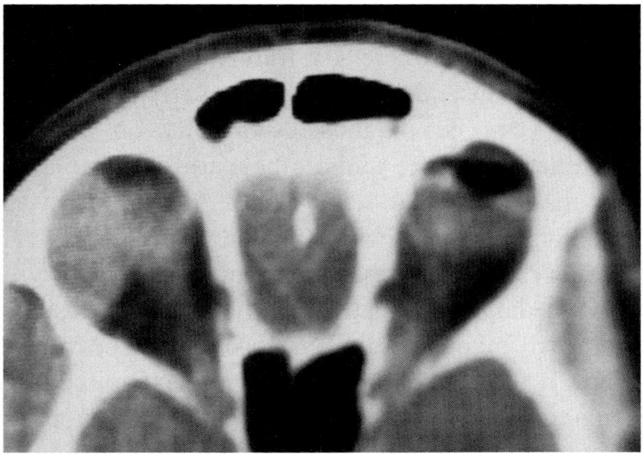

Figure 20–17. Axial CT scan of a biopsy-proven lymphoma presenting in the lacrimal gland.

covered in the chapter on orbital pseudotumors. Usually, lymphomas occur in a slightly older population than do epithelial lacrimal gland malignancies. Lloyd noted the mean age for lymphoma patients to be 63 years and for pseudotumor patients to be 43 years.[16] Benign or malignant lymphoid tumors can expand the lacrimal fossa (Figure 20–17), and can often be bilateral (see Figure 20–1B).[16] They usually contiguously involve muscle and fat, with irregular margins (Figure 20–18). Neither benign nor malignant lymphoid lacrimal gland masses usually invade bone.[30]

As discussed above, patients with bilateral lacrimal gland lesions most commonly have a systemic disease associated with inflammation (sarcoid, collagen vascular disease), infection (tuberculosis, lues, mumps), or lymphoma.[11] These patients should have an extensive medical evaluation prior to or simultaneous with the ocular evaluation. Depending on the patient's findings, complete blood count, urine analysis and urine sediment, urine for Bence-Jones protein, sedimentation rate, luetic serologies, serum ACE, lysozyme, serum protein electrophoresis, antinuclear antibody, anti-DNA antibodies, Sjögren antibodies, C3, blood urea nitrogen (BUN), creatinine, gallium scan, chest radiography, antineutrophil cytoplasmic antibody (ANCA) and skin tests may be indicated. A patient with Waldenstrom's macroglobulinemia with lacrimal gland involvement is shown in Figure 20–19.

The most difficult patients to correctly diagnose are those without inflammatory signs who present with a unilateral lacrimal gland mass. Unfortunately, the differential diagnosis includes many of the above mentioned entities, especially lymphoid

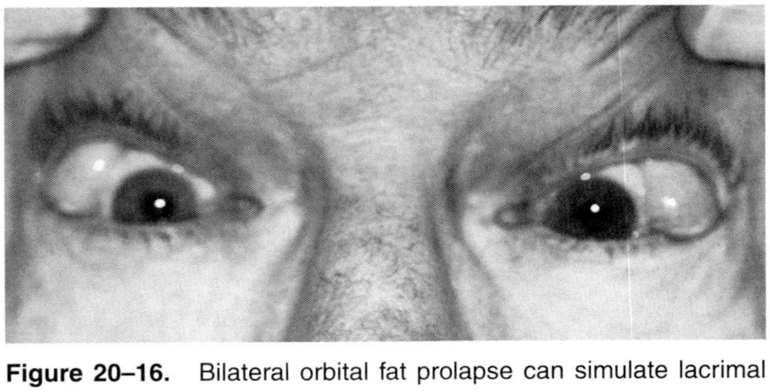

Figure 20–16. Bilateral orbital fat prolapse can simulate lacrimal gland tumors.

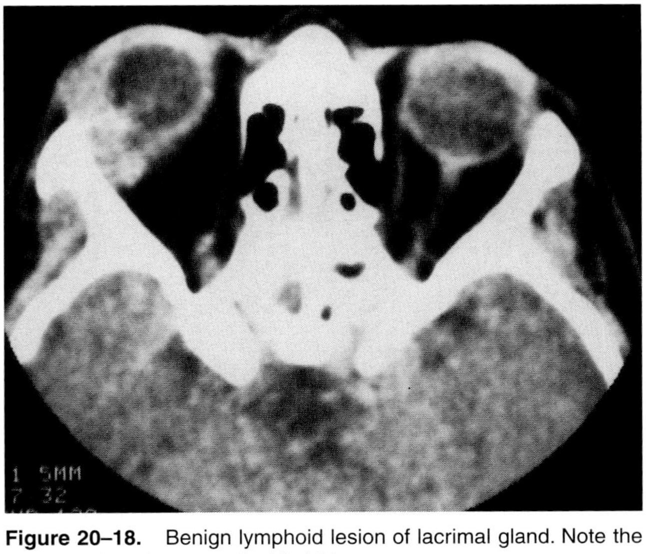

Figure 20–18. Benign lymphoid lesion of lacrimal gland. Note the "spill over" involvement of orbital fat.

lesions, plus epithelial tumors, mesenchymal neoplasms, and dermoid cysts. Rarely, some other simulating lesions, such as a lacrimal dacryops (Figure 20–20), can be diagnosed correctly on clinical examination alone, and if they are symptomatic, they may be excised.[31] In one case, this finding was noted in association with a benign mixed tumor.[32] A number of rarer causes of lacrimal fossa tumors will only be diagnosed histologically. Reported lesions included myoepithelium, fibrous histiocytoma, Warthin tumor, solitary fibrous tumor, epithelioid hemangoma, hemangiopericytoma, and Kimura's disease.[33–39]

Usually, patients with benign mixed tumors (pleomorphic adenomas) have a long history and minimal pain. In a series reported from London, 13 of 14 benign tumors were present for 1 year prior to surgery and only 1 patient had pain. Rarely, this tumor can present in children, as shown in a 5-year-old boy (Figure 20–21). On axial MRI scans, these are usually relatively discrete; commonly, they enhance with gadolinium (Figure 20–22). On CT, MRI, and plain film radiography, often there is smooth molding of the bone in patients with benign mixed tumors (Figure 20–23).[16] The diagnosis of a benign pleomorphic adenoma can be confusing. Wharton and O'Donnell reported a case where there was a hemorrhagic cyst that developed in association with this tumor, leading to diagnostic confusion.[40] Rarely, these tumors can develop in the palpebral lobe of the lacrimal gland.[41,42]

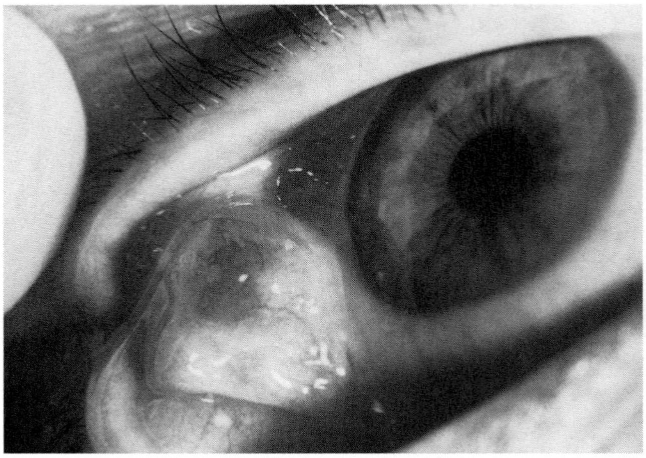

Figure 20–20. Lacrimal dacryops.

In contrast to benign epithelial lacrimal gland tumors, 12 of 17 patients with malignant epithelial tumors had pain.[43] In another large retrospective pathology series, neuronal involvement was noted in 11 percent of benign and 31 percent of malignant epithelial lacrimal gland neoplasms.[19] The patient shown in Figure 20–10A presented with pain and upper lateral quadrant swelling. At diagnosis, CT demonstrated extraorbital disease (see Figure 20–10B). While most lacrimal gland epithelial

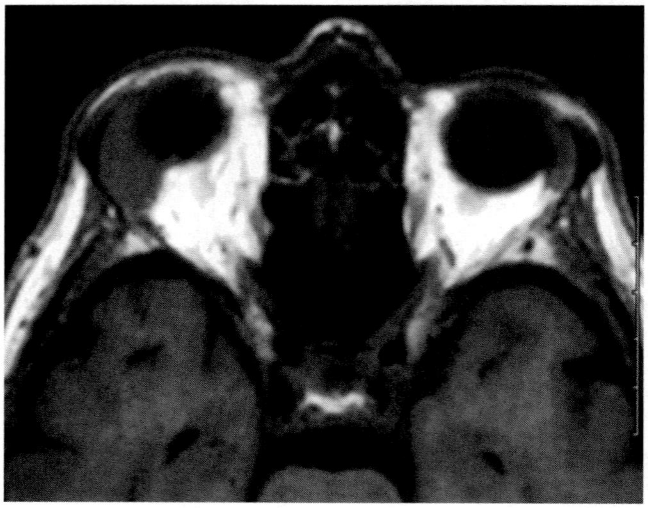

Figure 20–19. MRI scan of a patient with lacrimal gland involvement from Waldenstrom's macroglobulinemia.

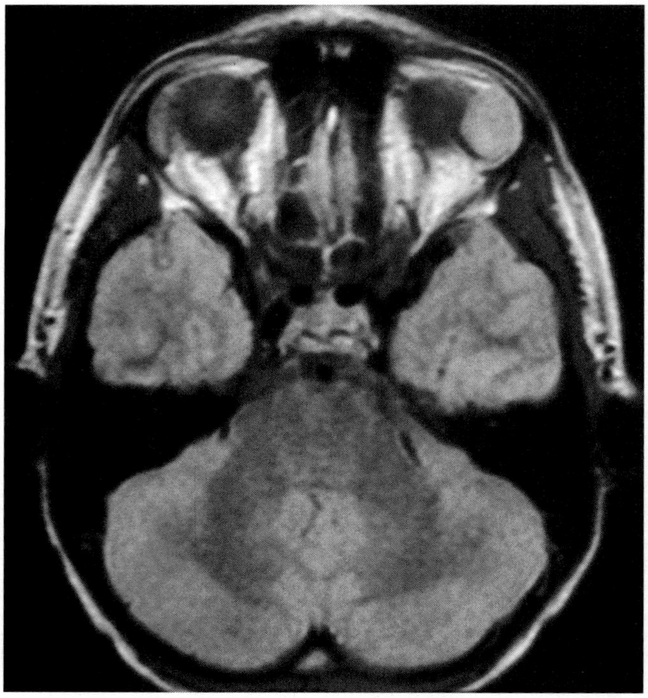

Figure 20–21. Benign mixed tumor in a 5-year-old shown on T_1-weighted MRI scan.

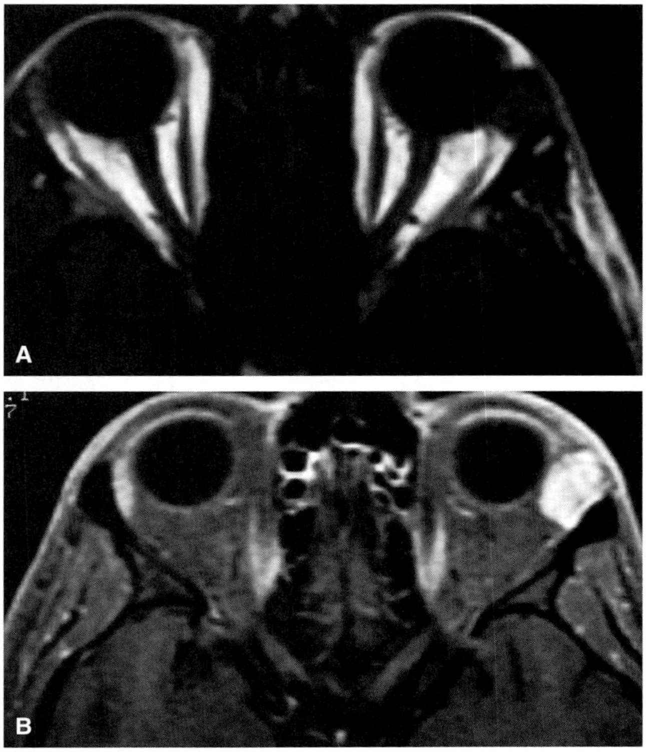

Figure 20–22. *A* and *B*, Benign mixed tumors are relatively discrete (*A*) and enhance with gadolinium (*B*).

malignancies arise in the main body, 17 percent in one series arose from the palpebral lobe.[42]

Dermoid cysts most often present as painless proptosis or patient awareness of a mass along the lateral orbital rim. Sathananthan reported 70 patients with dermoid cysts in the lateral canthus. Thirty-seven percent were mainly intraorbital, and 20 percent were mainly extraorbital. The bone in the lateral wall was found to be abnormal and bony damage is common.[44] Rarely, these patients initially present when the cyst breaks, and an inflammatory reaction has developed.[45] Even less frequently, dermoids can appear to invade the lateral rectus muscle.[46] Metastatic disease to the lacrimal gland, like metastases elsewhere in the orbit, can be the initial presenting sign of a primary tumor.[47] Rarely, a metastasis can simulate a malignant lacrimal epithelial tumor.[48] Sebaceous neoplasia from the conjunctiva surface can on rare occasions invade the lacrimal gland.[49]

There are no pathognomonic signs that separate a small adenoid cystic carcinoma from benign mixed tumors. Figure 20–24A demonstrates a small adenoid cystic carcinoma without bone involvement in a 14-year-old female. As such lesions enlarge, they may only demonstrate bone molding without invasion, as in the 17-year-old shown in Figure 20–25. Figure 20–26 shows a 9-year-old girl who presented to me with what we felt was a solitary benign tumor, which was an adenoid cystic carcinoma. At the time of diagnosis, larger adenoid cystic carcinomas have an irregular posterior extension, usually with bone involvement and frequently with central nervous system (CNS) extension (see Figures 20–9 and 20–10). CT evaluation, using bone window programs, is probably the most sensitive method to detect bone involvement associated with a lacrimal gland tumor.[50,51] We recently reviewed our results with MRI in lacrimal lesions and did not find that the use of this technique led to more accurate diagnosis than that with CT.[51–53] Some early studies demonstrated that ultrasonography was more accurate than early generation, thick-section CT. In the author's experience, this is not the case with high-resolution, thin-section (1.5 or 2 mm) CT or MRI.[53,54] Further, while ultrasonography has been listed in other reports as being quite accurate, the broad diagnostic groups used in that study were sufficiently diffuse to limit their value.[55] As an example, knowing that a lesion is

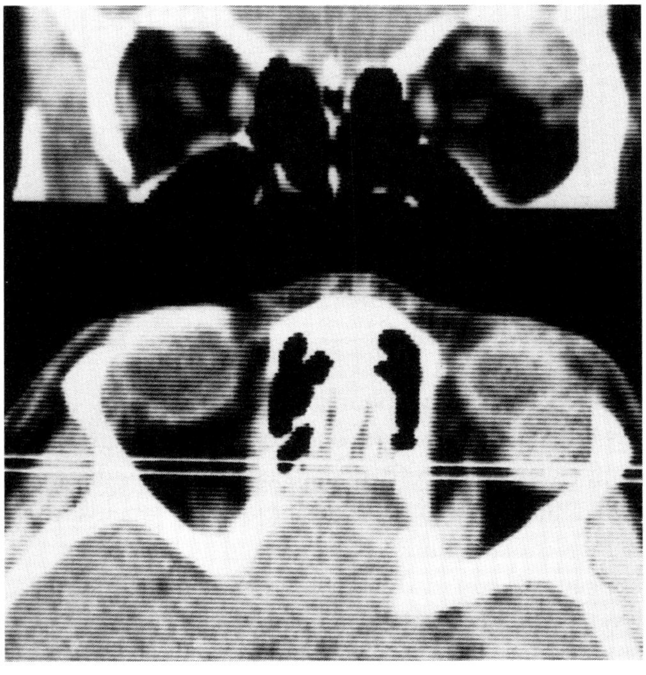

Figure 20–23. CT demonstrating expansion of the lacrimal fossa with molding of bone, secondary to a benign mixed tumor of the lacrimal gland.

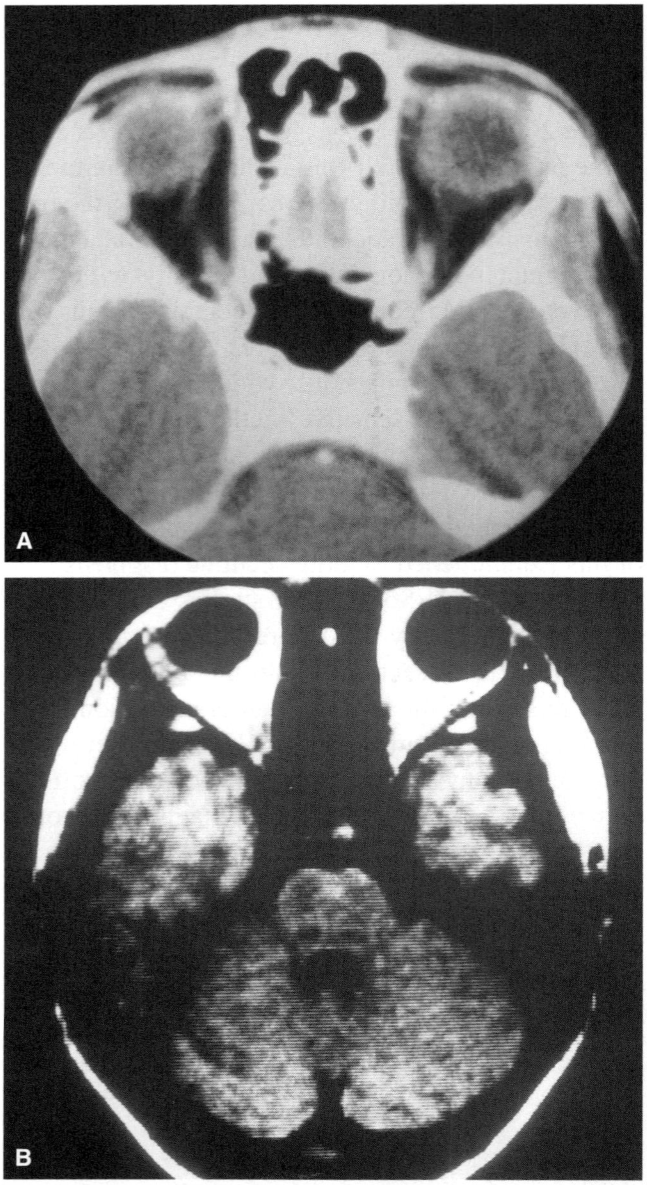

Figures 20–24. *A* and *B,* Small adenoid cystic carcinoma without evidence of bone involvement on axial CT (*A*). Another small tumor of the same histiologic cell type is shown on axial MRI in another young patient (*B*).

in the sarcoma/lymphoma/metastatic group is not extremely helpful.[55] In one series, a benign mixed tumor was incorrectly diagnosed with echography as a hemangioma, and a dermoid was labeled as a benign mixed tumor.[55] A diagnosis based on CT appearance can also be deceiving, since a traumatic blood cyst, both radiographically and on quantitative echography, can be consistent with an epithelial tumor. The MRI pattern of these degenerative blood lesions is usually typical.

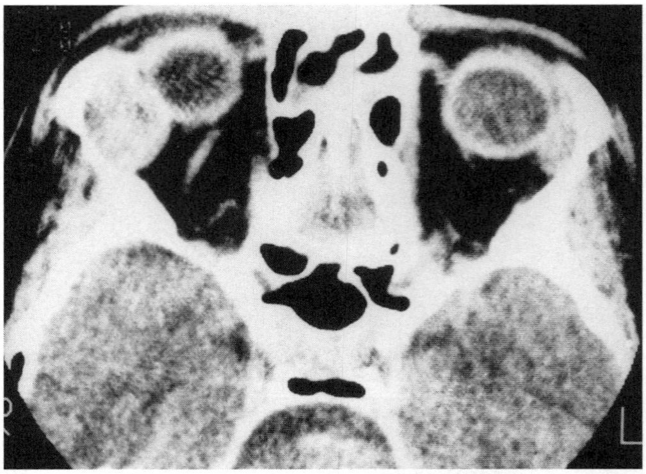

Figure 20–25. Early adenoid cystic carcinoma with bone enlargement without apparent invasion on axial CT scan.

We have used clinical examination combined with thin-section, high-resolution CT or MRI to establish a preliminary diagnosis in all lacrimal cases. As discussed in the chapter on diagnosis and management of orbital tumors, we do not use ultrasonography in the diagnosis of orbital tumors, since it does not add to the information available from CT or MRI, and it is neither as effective in delineating extraorbital spread nor as useful as CT or MRI in

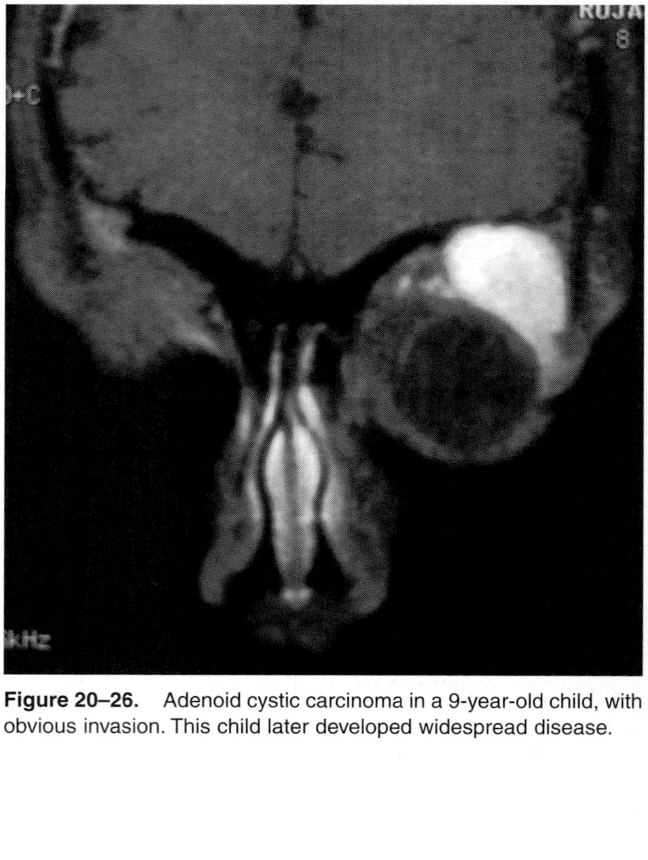

Figure 20–26. Adenoid cystic carcinoma in a 9-year-old child, with obvious invasion. This child later developed widespread disease.

treatment planning. If there is a unilateral lacrimal gland mass that has invaded bone, FNAB (see Chapter 15) is an excellent method to diagnose the nature of the lesion. Figure 20–9B shows the diagnostic FNAB of an adenoid cystic carcinoma. There are fewer than five cases reported in the medical literature of any human tumor spread by FNAB using a 23-gauge or smaller needle.

In unilateral lacrimal fossa lesions that do not have inflammatory signs associated with them, we assume (often a false-positive assumption) that the lesion may be an epithelial tumor and plan to remove it en bloc.

As discussed above, while the CT or MRI pattern of dermoid cysts is almost pathognomonic, with the rounded, scalloped bone loss, and a cystic mass (Figures 20–4 and 20–27), it is often difficult to differentiate small malignant neoplasms, benign mixed tumors, and less common lacrimal gland malignancies with noninvasive techniques. The surgical approach to these lesions is discussed in the chapter on orbital therapy.

THERAPY

The management of nonepithelial neoplasms of the lacrimal gland is relatively straightforward. Prior to any form of therapy, we obtain a Schirmer test to document tear production by the lacrimal gland. Dermoid cysts are removed surgically (see chapter on orbital surgery). If the capsule is ruptured prior to or during surgery, the lesion is removed piecemeal, the bony fossa is curetted, and 40 mg of long-acting steroid is injected into the area to decrease the inflammatory response.

The management of both benign and malignant lymphoid lesions is discussed in the chapter on lymphoid lesions. All these patients require a medical oncologic evaluation to rule out systemic lymphoma (physical examination, chest-abdominal CT, urine for Bence-Jones proteins, serum protein electrophoresis, complete blood count [CBC], and bone marrow biopsies). Benign lesions can often be effectively treated with short-term steroids or low-dose irradiation. Lymphomas require 35 to 40 gray (Gy) of photon irradiation, if the orbit is the only site of tumor involvement.

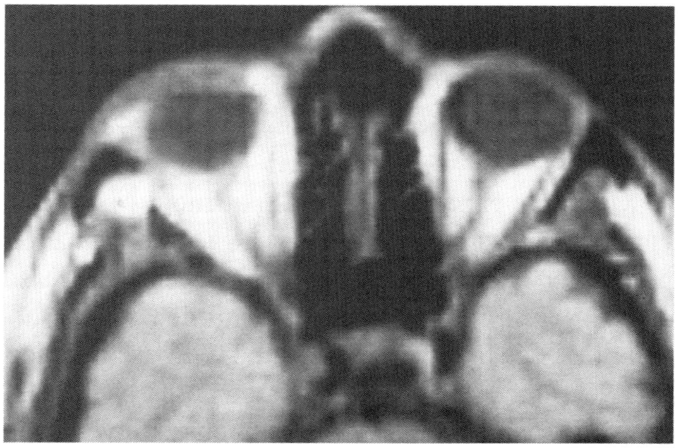

Figure 20–27. Typical axial T_1-weighted MRI pattern of a dermoid cyst in the lacrimal fossa.

The treatment for localized epithelial neoplasms is surgical.[56] Benign mixed tumors are usually encapsulated; if the entire neoplasm is not removed, there is a 20 to 28 percent recurrence rate, and approximately 20 percent of reported pleomorphic adenomas have undergone malignant degeneration.[19,20] If a benign mixed tumor is inadvertently incised, contiguous spread can occur in the orbit, bone, and adjacent areas. Completely resected pleomorphic adenomas have less than a 3 percent recurrence rate.[19] We attempt to resect any tumor localized in the lacrimal fossa area using careful dissection and isolation of both the orbital periosteum and periorbita. Sometimes, this is not possible. Wright noted that 6 of 26 benign mixed tumors had erosion of orbital bone through to the dura.[57]

It is difficult to make definitive statements regarding the management of malignant epithelial tumors of the lacrimal gland for three reasons: (1) there is a paucity of reported cases, and no controlled treatment trials; (2) most of the reported irradiated patients did not receive what is now felt to be optimal radiation;[58–60] and (3) while this group of tumors has a very high rate of metastases, often the interval between treatment and metastatic disease is very prolonged.[19]

Adenoid cystic carcinoma is the most frequent epithelial lacrimal gland malignancy, and it accounts for approximately 1.6 percent of all orbital tumors, and 29 percent of epithelial neoplasms of the lacrimal gland.[61,62] Usually, these patients present with proptosis and often have pain. Most patients are not candidates for local resection. Wright noted that only 4 of 24 adenoid cystic carcinoma patients had apparently localized intraorbital tumors at the time of presurgical evaluation. At orbitotomy, only 2 of these 4 lesions (8%) were confined to the orbit.[57] The Mayo Clinic experience with 26 adenoid cystic carcinomas was similarly dismal, and neither radiation nor surgery appeared to markedly affect the disease course.[61] In a retrospective uncontrolled study, survival in cases that were not treated with exenteration was 9 years, while the exenterated cases had a 6.7-year life span.[21] Only 3 of 26 remained alive at the completion of that study, most having died from contiguous spread to the CNS, lung (5 of 13), or lymph node (3 of 13) metastases.[61] Other sites of metastatic adenoid cystic carcinoma include the skeletal system and liver; widespread dissemination can become apparent even in the presence of local disease control.[63] Overall, 15-year survival with this tumor is < 10 percent.[64] Six long-term survivors have been reported; we have two additional patients.[65] In a histologic study, Gamel and Font noted that the presence of a basaloid histologic pattern was correlated with poor prognosis. If this pattern was present, 5-year survival was 21 percent; and if it was absent, it was 71 percent.[66]

Prognosis in patients 18 years of age and younger seems to be somewhat better. Eleven cases that met that inclusion criterion were reported from the Armed Forces Institute of Pathology. Eight with long-term follow-up survived. Probably, this reflected that the tumors had less aggressive histologic features.[67,68]

There have been no large series using radiation therapy to treat adenoid cystic carcinomas of the lacrimal gland. Brada and Henk reported their results with irradiation of 33 malignant epithelial lacrimal gland tumors.[69] They noted that adjunctive radiation after incomplete tumor excision was effective in only 1 of 13 patients with adenocarcinoma, undifferentiated carcinoma, or malignant mixed tumors. In 7 of 13 adenoid cystic carcinoma patients with residual local disease, they achieved good control and felt that > 60 Gy was best for tumor control.[70] Unfortunately, it is not clear in their study what surgical procedures were done to the patients before irradiation. It is therefore difficult to determine the exact effect of radiation in contrast to surgery on tumor-related mortality.[71,72]

Similarly, while our follow-up is < 10 years, we have obtained good palliation in lesions that have local disease and contiguous extraorbital spread with 60 Gy of photon radiation. Examples of pretreatment clinical photographs (see Figure 20–10A) and 5-year follow-up CTs (see Figure 20–10B) of a patient who initially presented with CNS extension of an orbital adenoid cystic carcinoma are shown. As Simpson and colleagues stressed, this tumor requires a higher radiation dose than previously thought.[58] Our limited experience with charged particle beam irradiation in this malignancy has emphasized the point that often tumor spread is underestimated, and we have observed late marginal recurrences with that modality. Probably, optimal treatment is with wide-field photon irradiation to approximately 70 Gy intensity-modulated conformal. The adjunct use of a charged particle beam may also allow more dose to the tumor with less morbidity to contiguous structures. As discussed in other chapters, the use of intensity-modulated conformal therapy may allow us to deliver more dose with less morbidity than currently possible. Other workers have used brachytherapy, but there are minimal data to support that approach.

Meldrun and colleagues reported the use of intracarotid chemotherapy for advanced disease in addition to radiation in a few patients with short-term follow-up.[70] Unfortunately, in the author's experience, often such patients will survive for up to 10 years, with locally extensive neoplasms before developing tumor-related mortality.

Gormley and colleagues presented 16 cases with intracranial extension of adenoid cystic carcinoma that involve the salivary glands. Their report was optimistic, but the caveat is that one really needs 15 years of follow-up to be certain of a cure.[71]

The optimal management of localized adenoid cystic carcinoma that has not invaded the orbital bones is uncertain. Surgical resection is usually not possible, as most of these carcinomas have bone and CNS involvement at presentation. Most long-term survivors underwent radical exenteration. The patient shown in Figure 20–25 is such a case.[57,61,64] The author would still advocate radical orbitectomy in a young patient, since some irradiated patients have been seen to have good tumor control for up to 7 years but then relapse. In an older patient with this disease, irradiation may be a reasonable primary therapy option.

Too few cases of other types of primary epithelial malignancies of the lacrimal gland have been reported to draw significant conclusions regarding treatment, and we treat all such patients in the same way as for adenoid cystic carcinomas.[72–78] In the largest report of primary adenocarcinomas of the lacrimal gland from several centers, the authors concluded, on the basis of 13 cases, that exenteration plus radiation was the most efficacious treatment.[79] In some cases of adenoid cystic carcinomas elsewhere, combination chemotherapy has had up to a 25 percent response rate.[80]

REFERENCES

1. Wright JE, Stewart WB, Krohel GB. Clinical presentation and management of lacrimal gland tumours. Br J Ophthalmol 1979;63:600–6.
2. Knochel JQ, Osborn AG, Wing SD. Differential diagnosis of lateral orbital masses. CT 1981;5:11–5.
3. Zimmerman LE, Sanders TE, Ackerman LV. Epithelial tumors of the lacrimal gland: prognostic and therapeutic significance of histologic types. Intl Ophthalmol Clin 1962;2:38–67.
4. Forrest AW. Pathologic criteria for effective management of epithelial lacrimal gland tumors. Am J Ophthalmol 1971;71:178–92.
5. Conlon MR, Chapman WB, Burt WL, et al. Primary localized amyloidosis of the lacrimal glands. Ophthalmology 1991;98:1556–9.
6. Redmon RM, Manor GE, Garner A, Rose GE. Lacrimal gland hemangiopericytoma. Am J Ophthalmol 1995;119:99–100.
7. Niffenegger JH, Jakobiec FA, Shore JW, Albert DM. Adult extrarenal rhabdoid tumor of the lacrimal gland. Ophthalmology 1992;99:567–74.
8. Cook HT, Stafford ND. Angiolymphoid hyperplasia with eosinophilia involving the lacrimal gland: case report. Br J Ophthalmol 1988;72:710–2.
9. Klein B, Couch J, Thompson J. Ocular infections associated with *Eikenella corrodens*. Am J Ophthalmol 1990;109:127–31.
10. Ostrowski M, Font RL, Halpern J, et al. Clear cell epithelial-myoepithelial carcinoma arising in pleomorphic adenoma of the lacrimal gland. Ophthalmology 1994;101:925–30.
11. Blodi FC, Gass JDM. Inflammatory pseudotumor of the orbit. Trans Am Acad Ophthalmol Otolaryngol 1963;71:303–23.
12. Lallemand DP, Brasch RC, Char DH, Norman D. Computed tomographic characterization of orbital tumors in children. Radiology 1984;151:85–8.
13. Bergin DJ, McCord CD, Dutton JJ, Garrett SN. Chronic hematic cyst of the orbit. Ophthal Plast Reconstr Surg 1988;4:131–6.
14. Kersten RC, Kersten JL, Bloom HR, Kulwin DR. Chronic hematic cysts of the orbit. Ophthalmology 1988;95:1549–53.
15. Ronner HJ, Jones IS. Aneurysmal bone cysts of the orbit: a review. Ann Ophthalmol 1983;15:626–9.
16. Lloyd GAS. Lacrimal gland tumours: the role of CT and conventional radiology. Br J Radiol 1981;54: 1034–8.
17. Massry GG, Harrison W, Hornblass A. Clinical and computed tomographic characteristics of amyloid tumor of the lacrimal gland. Ophthalmology 1996; 103:1233–6.
18. Newton TH. Roentgen appearance of lacrimal gland tumors. Radiology 1962;79:598–605.
19. Font RL, Gamel JW. Epithelial tumors of the lacrimal gland: an analysis of 265 cases. In: Jakobiec FA, editor. Ocular and adnexal tumors, Birmingham, AL: Aesculapius; 1978. p. 87–805.
20. Font RL, Patipa M, Rosenbaum PS, et al. Correlation of computer tomographic and histopathologic features in malignant transformation of benign mixed tumor of lacrimal gland. Surv Ophthalmol 1990;34:449–52.
21. Polito E, Leccisotti A. Epithelial malignancies of the lacrimal gland: survival rates after extensive and conservative therapy. Ann Ophthalmol 1993;25:422–6.
22. Bloche C, Lloyd DM, Izbicki JR, et al. Successful surgical treatment of liver and kidney metastases 25 years after a primary lacrimal gland tumor. Eur J Surg Oncol 1993;19:569–72.
23. Duke-Elder S, MacFaul P. The ocular adnexa. In: Duke-Elder S, MacFaul P, editors. System of ophthalmology, Vol. 13. St Louis, MO: CV Mosby; 1974. p. 595.
24. Collison JMT, Miller NR, Green WR. Involvement of orbital tissues by sarcoid. Am J Ophthalmol 1986;102:302–7.
25. Sacher M, Lanzieri CF, Sobel LI, Som PM. Computed tomography of bilateral lacrimal gland sarcoidosis. J Comp Assist Tomogr 1984;8:213–5.
26. Lowder CY, Char DH. Uveitis: a review. Western Med 1984;140:421–32.
27. Khan JA, Hoover DL, Giangiacomo J, Singsen BH. Orbital and childhood sarcoidosis. J Pediatr Ophthalmol Strabismus 1986;23:190–4.
28. Peterson EA, Hymas DC, Pratt DV, et al. Sarcoidosis with orbital tumor outside the lacrimal gland: initial

manifestation in two elderly white women. Arch Ophthalmol 1998;116:804–6.

29. Harris GJ, Dixon TA, Haughton VM. Expansion of the lacrimal gland fossa by a lymphoid tumor. Am J Ophthalmol 1983;96:546–7.
30. Monbaerts I, Schlingeman RO, Goldschmeding RN, et al. The surgical management of lacrimal gland pseudotumors. Ophthalmology 1996;103:1619–27.
31. Brownstein S, Belin MW, Krohel GB, et al. Orbital dacryops. Ophthalmology 1984;91:1424–8.
32. Christie DB, Woog JJ, Lahav M. Combined dacryops with underlying benign mixed cell tumor of the lacrimal gland. Am J Ophthalmol 1995;119:97–9.
33. Grossniklaus HE, Wojno TH, Wilson ME, Someren AO. Myoepithelioma of the lacrimal gland. Arch Ophthalmol 1997;115:1588–90.
34. al-Hazzaa SA, Specht CS, McLean IW, et al. Benign orbital fibrous histiocytoma simulating a lacrimal gland tumor. Ophthal Surg Lasers 1996;27:140–2.
35. Bonavolonta G, Tranfa F, Staibano S, et al. Warthin tumor of the lacrimal gland. Am J Ophthalmol 1997;124:857–8.
36. Scott IU, Tanenbaum M, Rubin D, Lores E. Solitary fibrous tumor of the lacrimal gland fossa. Ophthalmology 1996;103:1613–8.
37. Coombes AG, Manners RM, Ellison DW, Evans BT. Lacrimal gland epithelioid haemangioma. Br J Ophthalmol 1997;81:1020.
38. Kodama T, Kawamoto K. Kimura's disease of the lacrimal gland. Acta Ophthalmol Scand 1998; 76:374–7.
39. Burnsteine MA, Morton AB, Font MB, et al. Lacrimal gland hemangiopericytoma. Orbit 1998;17.
40. Wharton JA, O'Donnell BA. Unusual presentations of pleomorphic adenoma and adenoid cystic carcinoma of the lacrimal gland. Aust NZ J Ophthalmol 1999;27:145–8.
41. Yamada T, Kato T, Hayasaka S, et al. Benign pleomorphic adenoma arising from the palpebral lobe of the lacrimal gland associated with elevated intraocular pressure. Ophthalmologica 1999;213:269–72.
42. Vangveeravong S, Katz SE, Rootman J, White V. Tumors arising in the palpebral lobe of the lacrimal gland. Ophthalmology 1996;103:1606–12.
43. Stewart WB, Krohel GB, Wright JE. Lacrimal gland and fossa lesions: an approach to diagnosis and management. Ophthalmology 1979;86:886–95.
44. Sathananthan N, Moseley IF, Rose GE, Wright JE. The frequency and clinical significance of bone involvement in outer canthus dermoid cysts. Br J Ophthalmol 1993;77:789–94.
45. Sherman RP, Rootman J, Lapointe JS. Orbital dermoids. Clinical presentation and management. Br J Ophthalmol 1984;68:642–52.
46. Howard GR, Narad JS, Bonabolonta G, Tranfa F. Orbital dermoid cysts located within the lateral rectus muscle. Ophthalmology 1994;101:760–71.
47. Font RL, Ferry AP. Carcinoma metastatic to the eye and orbit. Cancer 1976;38:1326–35.
48. Bernstein-Lipschitz L, Lahav M, Chen V, et al. Metastatic thyroid carcinoma masquerading as lacrimal gland tumor. Graefes Arch Clin Exp Ophthalmol 1990;228:112–5.
49. Mooy CM. Intraepithelial sebaceous neoplasia invading the lacrimal gland. Br J Ophthalmol 1997;81: 612–3.
50. Norman D, Char DH, Newton TH. Imaging techniques in orbital disease. In: Littleton JT, Durizsch MC, editors. Sectional imaging methods: a comparison. Baltimore, MD: University Park Press; 1983.
51. Char DH, Sobel D, Kelly WM, et al. Magnetic resonance scanning in orbital and intraocular tumor diagnosis. Ophthalmology 1985;92:1305–10.
52. Jakobiec FA, Yeo JH, Trokel SL, et al. Combined clinical and computed tomographic diagnosis of primary lacrimal fossa lesions. Am J Ophthalmol 1982;94:785–807.
53. Polito E, Leccisotti A. CT and MRI features of lacrimal fossa tumors. Orbit 1993; 25–38.
54. Hesselink JR, Davis KR, Dallow RL, et al. Computed tomography of masses in the lacrimal gland region. Radiology 1979;131:143–7.
55. Balchunas WR, Quencer RM, Byrne SF. Lacrimal gland fossa masses: evaluation by computed tomography and A-mode echography. Radiology 1983; 149:751–8.
56. Janecka I, Housepian E, Trokel S, et al. Surgical management of malignant tumors of the lacrimal gland. Am J Surg 1984;148:539–41.
57. Wright JE. Factors affecting the survival of patients with lacrimal gland tumours. Can J Ophthalmol 1982;17:3–9.
58. Simpson JR, Thawley SE, Matsuba HM. Adenoid cystic salivary gland carcinoma: treatment with irradiation and surgery. Radiology 1984;151:509–12.
59. Sidrys LA, Fritz KJ, Variakojis D. Fast neutron therapy for orbital adenoid cystic carcinoma. Ann Ophthalmol 1982;14:42–5.
60. Sealy R, Buret E, Cleminshaw H, et al. Progress in the use of iodine therapy for tumors of the eye. Br J Radiol 1980;635:1052–60.
61. Lee DA, Campbell RJ, Waller RR, Ilstrup DM. A clinical pathologic study of primary adenoid cystic carcinoma of the lacrimal gland. Ophthalmology 1985;92:128–34.
62. Font RL, Smith SL, Bryan RG. Malignant epithelial tumors of the lacrimal gland: a clincopathologic study of 21 cases. Arch Ophthalmol 1998;116:613–6.

63. Byers RM, Berkeley RG, Luna M, Jesse RH. Combined therapeutic approach to malignant lacrimal gland tumors. Am J Ophthalmol 1975;79:53–5.
64. Marsh JL, Wise DM, Smith M, Schwartz H. Lacrimal gland adenoid cystic carcinoma: intracranial and extracranial en bloc resection. Plast Reconstr Surg 1981;68:577–85.
65. Naugle T Jr, Tepper DJ, Haik BG. Adenoid cystic carcinoma of the lacrimal gland: a case report. Ophthal Reconstr Surg 1994;10:45–8.
66. Gamel JW, Font RL. Adenoid cystic carcinoma of the lacrimal gland: the clinical significance of a basaloid histologic pattern. Hum Pathol 1982;13:219–25.
67. Tellado MV, McLean IW, Specht CS, Varga J. Adenoid cystic carcinomas of the lacrimal gland in childhood and adolescence. Ophthalmology 1997;104:1622–5.
68. Shields JA, Shields CL, Eagle RC, et al. Adenoid cystic carcinoma of the lacrimal gland simulating a dermoid cyst in a nine year old boy. Arch Ophthalmol 1998;116:1673–6.
69. Brada M, Henk JM. Radiotherapy for lacrimal gland tumours. Radiother Oncol 1987;9:175–83.
70. Meldrum L, Tse DT, Benedetto P. Neoadjuvant intracarotid chemotherapy for treatment of advanced adenocystic carcinoma of the lacrimal gland. Arch Ophthalmol 1998;116:315–21.
71. Gormley WB, Sekhar LN, Wright DC, et al. Management and long-term outcome of adenoid cystic carcinoma with intracranial extension: a neurosurgical perspective. Neurosurgery 1996;38:1105–13.
72. Wagoner MD, Chuo N, Gonder JR, et al. Mucoepidermoid carcinoma of the lacrimal gland. Ann Ophthalmol 1982;14:383–91.
73. Witschel H, Zimmerman LE. Malignant mixed tumor of the lacrimal gland. Albrecht Von Graffes Arch Klin Ophthalmol 1981;216:327–37.
74. Perzin KH, Jakobiec FA, Clivolsi VA, Desjardins L. Lacrimal gland malignant mixed tumors (carcinomas arising in benign mixed tumors): a clinicopathologic study. Cancer 1980;45:2593–2606.
75. Henderson JW, Farrow GM. Primary malignant mixed tumors of the lacrimal gland. Ophthalmology 1985;87:466–75.
76. Ni C, Wagoner MD, Wang WJ, et al. Mucoepidermoid carcinomas of the lacrimal sac. Arch Ophthalmol 1983;101:1572–4.
77. Beskid M, Zarzycka M. A case of onkocytoma of the lacrimal gland. Klin Oczna 1959;29:311–5.
78. Konrad EA, Thiel HJ. Adenocarcinoma of the lacrimal gland with sebaceous differentiation. A clinical study using light and electronmicroscopy. Graefes Arch Clin Exp Ophthalmol 1983;221:81–5.
79. Heaps RS, Miller NR, Albert DM, et al. Primary adenocarcinoma of the lacrimal gland. A retrospective study. Ophthalmology 1993;100:1856–60.
80. Dimery IW, Legha SS, Shirinian M, Hong WK. Fluorouracil, doxorubicin, cyclophosphamide and cisplatin combination chemotherapy in advanced or recurrent salivary gland carcinoma. J Clin Oncol 1990;8:1056–62.

21

Lacrimal Sac Tumors

Tumors of the lacrimal sac are uncommon. Approximately 400 cases have been reported in the literature, and a little more than one-half were malignant.[1–4] As evidence of the rarity of this neoplasm, only 10 cases were observed at the Institute of Ophthalmology in London between 1948 and 1967.[2] The clinical presentation of a lacrimal sac neoplasm is similar to that of chronic dacryocystitis; however, lacrimal sac tumors often involve the area both below and above the medial canthal tendon, whereas in chronic dacryocystitis, the swelling is usually limited to the area inferior to the tendon. Patients develop epiphora and a small medial canthus mass as the lesion expands (Figure 21–1). Spontaneous retrocanalicular bleeding associated with epiphora is a classic finding with a malignant lacrimal sac tumor, although it can also occur with inflammation. In a series of 117 cases from the Armed Forces Institute of Pathology, approximately 50 percent of lacrimal sac neoplasms presented with epiphora, 38 percent with dacryocystitis, and 36 percent with a mass.[5]

A number of different malignant processes can involve the lacrimal sac, and polyps in this location can undergo malignant degeneration.[6] Carcinoma generally occurs in older patients and is associated with pain or epiphora or both. Deaths from metastasis of lacrimal sac tumors are uncommon and are usually due to local extension.

Squamous cell carcinoma can involve the lacrimal sac or the canaliculi as either a primary tumor or as a result of contiguous spread from the eyelids, conjunctiva, or sinuses.[7,8] There are a few reports, similar to conjunctival squamous cell carcinoma, of human papilloma virus (HPV) positivity.[9] Mucoepidermoid carcinomas can involve the conjunctiva, lacrimal gland, or the sac.[10–12] Approximately 29 cases of lacrimal sac malignant melanomas have been reported; as with other malignancies in this area, symptoms are consistent with a chronic dacryocystitis.[4–13] As discussed in Chapter 4, in less than 4 percent of conjunctival melanomas, involvement of the lacrimal drainage system can occur.[14] A number of less common neoplasms have involved the lacrimal sac, including oxyphil cell adenoma, leukemia, sinus histiocytosis, hemangiopericytoma, mucoepidermoid

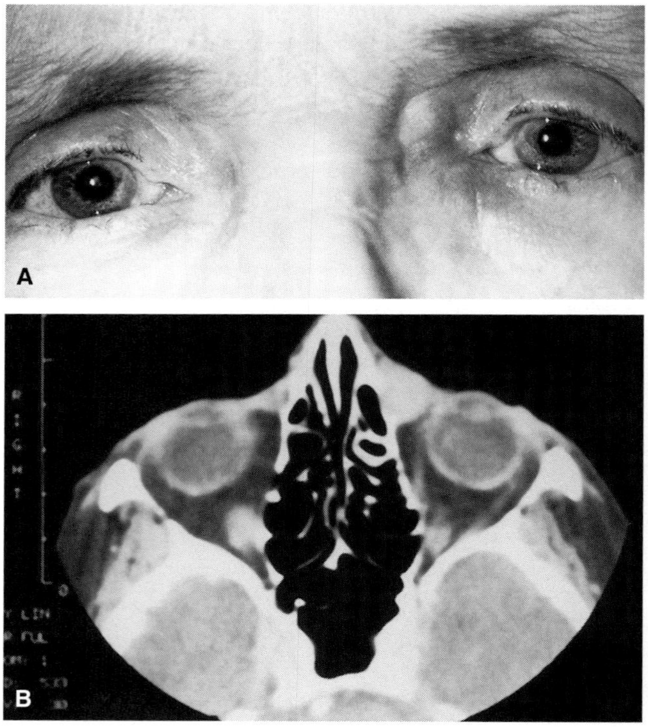

Figure 21–1. *A,* Lacrimal sac plasmacytoma that has produced a mass both above and below the medial canthal tendon. Growth superior to the medial canthal tendon is more consistent with a tumor than with dacryocystitis. This is its clinical appearance. *B,* Axial CT scan of the same case demonstrates a mass with bone molding.

carcinoma, cavernous hemangioma, adenoid cystic carcinoma, inverted papilloma (Figure 21–2), fibrous histiocytoma, fibroma, solitary fibrous tumors, angiofibroma, metastasis, contiguous extension of sinus carcinoma, juvenile xanthogranuloma, oncocytic hyperplasia, oncolytic adenocarcinomas, and lymphoid lesions including lymphoma and leukemia.[15–44] Figure 21–2A shows a lymphoid lesion that involved the lacrimal sac.

Sarcoidosis has also been reported in the lacrimal sac. Chest radiographs can be negative; either serum angiotensin converting enzyme (ACE) assays or limited gallium scans are usually positive.[45] Rarely, inflammatory sinus disease, such as Wegener's granulomatosis, can also involve the lacrimal drainage system.[46] Usually, Wegener's granulomatosis patients have positive serum antineutrophil cytoplasmic antibody (ANCA) levels and cutaneous ulceration.

The treatment of lacrimal sac neoplasms depends on the time of diagnosis (preoperative, intraoperative, or postoperative) and the nature of the tumor. Most cases are not suspected prior to surgery and are discovered either during or after performing a dacryocystohinostomy (DCR). Patients with a bloody canalicular discharge should have an evaluation with computed tomography (CT), using bone windows, and magnetic resonance imaging (MRI) prior to surgery (Figure 21–3). Some patients may have regional adenopathy involving the preauricular, submaxillary or cervical nodes. These later suspicious areas should be evaluated with fine-needle aspiration biopsy (FNAB) prior to surgery. Unlike chronic dacryocystitis, lacrimal sac malignancies often extend downward, with swelling developing above the medial canthal tendon. If a suspicious mass is noted at the time of a DCR, frozen-section biopsy should be performed.

The management of lacrimal sac tumor depends on its histology. While some benign tumors, such as fibrous histiocytomas, can recur, wide local excision, followed by intubation of the canalicular remnants with silicone tubes to retain patency of the nasal lacrimal drainage system, is often adequate treatment.

Only rarely has death by local extension of primary lacrimal sac neoplasms been reported. If a primary epithelial malignancy or melanoma is present and appropriate evaluations for contiguous extension (orbit, brain, and sinus imaging studies) and metastatic disease (chest and abdominal CT, complete blood count, lactate dehydrogenase, glutamyl

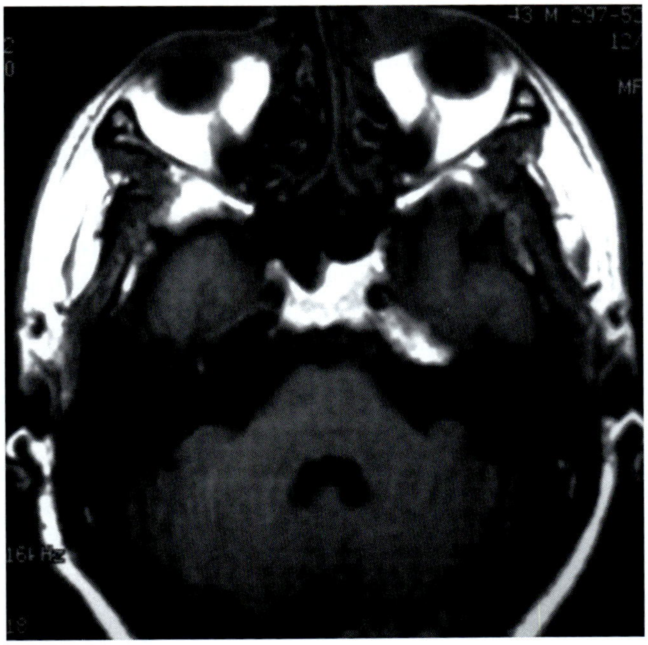

Figure 21–2. MR of an inverted papilloma of the lacrimal sac.

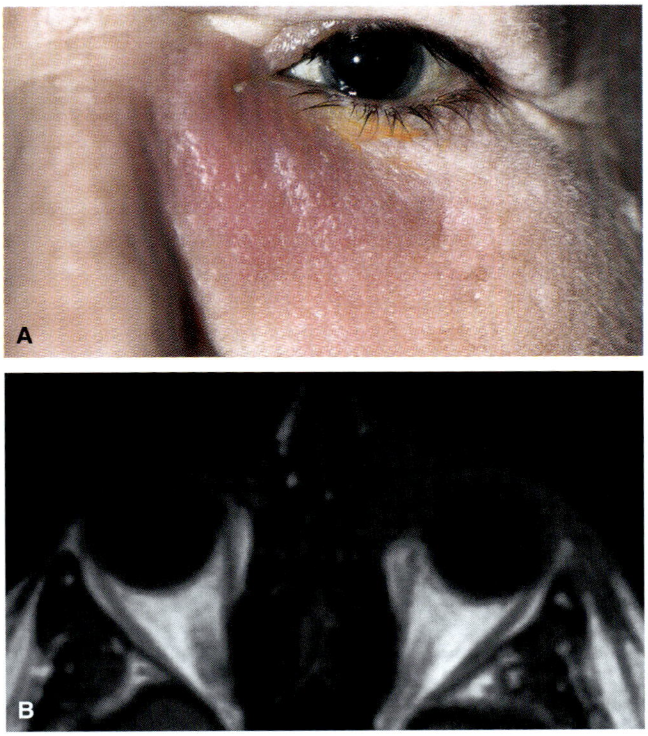

Figure 21–3. *A*, Lymphoid lesion that involved the lacrimal sac. *B*, Demonstrates the lesion from the patient shown in 3A on axial T_1–weighted MRI scan.

transpeptidase, carcinoembryonic antigen [CEA], alkaline phosphatase) are negative, exenteration is sometimes indicated. Some tumors, however, can be controlled with wide excision and wide-field photon irradiation.[8,30] Occasionally, radical combined orbital-sinus exenteration with postoperative irradiation has been performed.[20]

REFERENCES

1. Schenck NL, Ogura JH, Pratt LL. Cancer of the lacrimal sac. Presentation of 5 cases and review of the literature. Ann Otol Rhinol Laryngol 1973;82: 153–61.
2. Harry J, Ashton N. The pathology of tumours of the lacrimal sac. Trans Ophthalmol Soc UK 1969;88: 19–35.
3. Radnot M, Gall J. Tumors of the lacrimal sac. Ophthalmologica 1966;151:2–22.
4. Pe'er JJ, Stefanyszyn M, Hidayat AA. Nonepithelial tumors of the lacrimal sac. Am J Ophthalmol 1994; 118:650–8.
5. Stefanyszyn M, Hidayat AA, Pe'er JJ, Flanagan JC. Lacrimal sac tumors. Ophthal Plast Reconstr Surg 1994;10:169–84.
6. Ryan SJ, Font RL. Primary epithelial neoplasms of the lacrimal sac. Am J Ophthalmol 1973;76:73–88.
7. Kohn R, Nofsinger K, Freedman SI. Rapid recurrence of papillary squamous cell carcinoma of the canaliculus. Am J Ophthalmol 1981;92:363–7.
8. Bonder D, Fischer MJ, Levine MR. Squamous cell carcinoma of the lacrimal sac. Ophthalmology 1983; 90:1133–5.
9. Nakamura Y, Mashima Y, Kameyama K, et al. Detection of human papillomavirus infection in squmaous tumours of the conjunctiva and lacrimal sac by immunohistochemistry, in situ hybridisation, and polymerase chain reaction. Br J Ophthalmol 1997; 81:308–13.
10. Ni C, Wagoner MD, Wang WJ, et al. Mucoepidermoid carcinomas of the lacrimal sac. Arch Ophthalmol 1983;101:1572–4.
11. Blake J, Mullaney J, Gillan J. Lacrimal sac mucoepidermoid carcinoma. Br J Ophthalmol 1986;70:681–5.
12. Bambirra EA, Miranda D, Rayes A. Mucoepidermoid tumor of the lacrimal sac. Aruch Ophthalmol 1981;99:2149–50.
13. Yamade S, Kitagawa A. Malignant melanoma of the lacrimal sac. Ophthalmologica 1978;177:30–3.
14. McNab AA, McKelvie P. Malignant melanoma of the lacrimal sac complicating primary acquired melanosis of the conjunctiva. Ophthalmic Surg Lasers 1997;28: 501–4.
15. Lamping KA, Albert DM, Ni C, Fournier G. Oxyphil cell adenomas. Three case reports. Arch Ophthalmol 1984;102:263–5.
16. Peretz WL, Ettinghausen SE, Gray GF. Oncocytic adenocarcinoma of the lacrimal sac. Arch Ophthalmol 1978;96:303–4.
17. Benger RS, Frueh BR. Lacrimal drainage obstruction from lacrimal sac infiltration by lymphocytic neoplasia. Am J Ophthalmol 1986;101:242–5.
18. Marback RL, Kincaid MC, Green WR, Iliff WJ. Fibrous histiocytoma of the lacrimal sac. Am J Ophthalmol 1982;93:511–7.
19. Cole SH, Ferry AP. Fibrous histiocytoma of (fibrous xanthoma) the lacrimal sac. Arch Ophthalmol 1978; 96:1647–9.
20. Flanagan JC, Stokes DP. Lacrimal sac tumors. Ophthalmologica 1978;85:1282–7.
21. Domanski H, Ljungber O, Andersson LO, Schele B. Oxyphil cell adenoma (oncocytoma) of the lacrimal sac. Acta Ophthalmologica 1994;72:393–6.
22. Geiger K, Witschel H. Haemangiopericytoma of the lacrimal sac. Orbit 1994;13:91–6.
23. Kheterpal S, Chan SY, Batch A, Karkby GR. Previously undiagnosed lymphoma presenting as recurrent dacrocystitis. Arch Ophthalmol 1994;112:519–20.
24. Carnevali L, Trimarchi F, Rosso R, Stringa M. Haemangiopericytoma of the lacrimal sac: a case report. Br J Ophthalmol 1998;72:782–5.
25. Roth SI, August CZ, Lissner GS, O'Grady RB. Hemangiopericytoma of the lacrimal sac. Ophthalmology 1991;98:925–7.
26. Dolman PJ, Harris GJ, Weiland LH. Sinus histiocytosis involving the lacrimal sac and duct. A clinicopathologic case report. Arch Ophthalmol 1991;109:1582–4.
27. Karesh JW, Perman AI, Rodrigues MM. Dacrocystitis associated with malignant lymphoma of the lacrimal sac. Ophthalmology 1993;100:669–73.
28. Kincaid MC, Meis JM, Lee MW. Adenoid cystic carcinoma of the lacrimal sac. Ophthalmology 1989;96: 1655–8.
29. Ferry AP, Kaltreider SA. Cavernous hemangioma of the lacrimal sac. Am J Ophthalmol 1990;110:316–8.
30. Khan JA, Sutula FC, Pilch BZ, Joseph MP. Mucoepidermoid carcinoma involving the lacrimal sac. Ophthalmic Plast Reconstr Surg 1988;4:153–7.
31. Wirostko WJ, Garcia GH, Cory S, Harris GJ. Acute dacryocystitis as a presenting sign of pediatric leukemia. Am J Ophthalmol 1999;127:734–6.
32. Chen LJ, Liao SL, Kao SC, et al. Oncocytic adenomatous hyperplasia of the lacrimal sac: a case report and review of the literature. Ophthal Plast Reconstr Surg 1998;14:436–40.
33. Schnick B, Kind M, Draf W, et al. Extranasopharyngeal angiofibroma in a 15-month-old child. Int J Pediatr Otorhinolaryngol 1997;10:135–40.

34. Choi G, Lee U, Won NH. Fibrous histiocytoma of the lacrimal sac. Head Neck 1997;19:72–5.
35. Charles NC, Palu RN, Jagirdar JS. Hemangiopericytoma of the lacrimal sac. Arch Ophthalmol 1998; 116:1677–80.
36. Mrythyunjaya P, Meyer DR. Juvenile xanthogranuloma of the lacrimal sac fossa. Am J Ophthalmol 1997; 123:400–2.
37. Chan LJ, Lial SL, Kalscswu CT, et al. Oncocytic adenomatous hyperplasia of the lacrimal sac: case report and review of literature. Ophthal Plast Reconstr Surg 1998;14:436–40.
38. Nakamura K, Uehara S, Omagari J, et al. Primary non-Hodgkin's lymphoma of the lacrimal sac: a case report and a review of the literature. Cancer 1997; 80:2151–5.
39. Brosig J, Warzok R, Clemens S. Primary high malignancy B-cell lymphoma of the lacrimal sac. Klin Monatsbl Augenheilkd 1998;212:473–5.
40. Spielmann AC, Debell L, Lederlin P, et al. Massive bone destruction: an atypical sign of orbital lymphoma. J Fr Ophthalmol 1998;21:769–72.
41. Harris GJ, Williams GA, Clarke GP. Sarcoidosis of the lacrimal sac. Arch Ophthalmol 1981;99:1198–201.
42. Woo KI, Sun VL, Kim YD. Solitary fibrous tumor of the lacrimal sac. Ophthal Plast Reconstr Surg 1999; 15:450–3.
43. Charles NC, Palu RN, Jagirtar JS. Hemangiopericytoma of the lacrimal sac. Arch Ophthalmol 1998; 116:1677–80.
44. Chen LJ, Liao SL, Kao SC, et al. Oncocytic adenomatous hyperplasia of the lacrimal sac: a case report and review of the literature. Ophthal Plast Reconstr Surg 1998;14:436–44.
45. Kuchar A, Novak P, Steinkogler FJ. Manifestation of Wegener's granulomatosis as lacrimal sac tumor. Klin Monatsbl Augenhilkd 1998;212:59–60.
46. Friedman DP, Rao MV, Flanders AE. Lesions causing a mass in the medial canthus of the orbit: CT and MR features. AJR Am J Roentgenol 1993;160:1095–9.

22

Orbital Sinus Lesions

A number of benign and malignant sinus processes can contiguously involve the adult orbit. These include infections and their sequelae, immunologically mediated diseases, idiopathic isolated inflammations, and both benign and malignant neoplasms.[1] Sinusitis with contiguous infectious extension into the orbit is less common in adults than in children, unless the patient has an acquired immunodeficiency.

MUCOCELE

In adults, the most common orbital sinus problem is mucocele, generally arising from either the ethmoid or frontal sinus.[2–5] In the current era, most patients with mucoceles have a history of either midface bone trauma or severe sinusitis since childhood. Usually, the patients present with a history of recurrent nose and sinus disease and the onset of unilateral proptosis (Figure 22–1). Figure 22–2A shows a typical ethmoid mucocele on axial computed tomography (CT) and coronal T_1-weighted magnetic resonance imaging (MRI) (Figure 22–2B). The scans show a cystic lesion arising from the sinus which has destroyed the lamina papyracea and invaded the orbit. A dermoid cyst arising in the medial orbit can appear clinically similar to a mucocele (Figure 22–3), but dermoid cysts leave the medial orbital wall intact (Figure

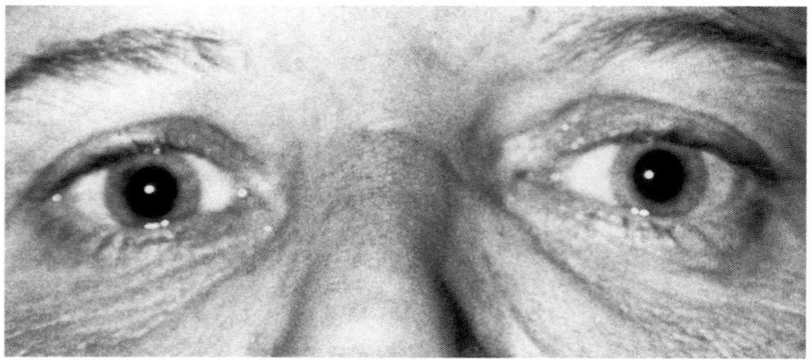

Figure 22–1. Patient with slight anterior and lateral proptosis due to sinus mucocele.

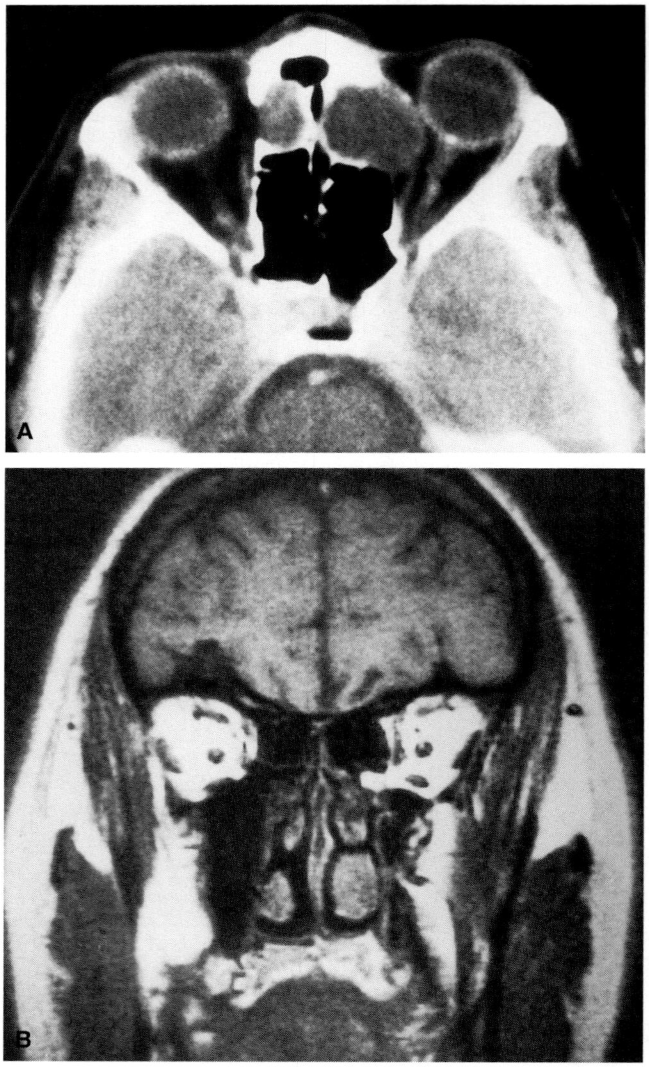

Figure 22–2. *A,* Axial CT demonstrating mucocele arising from the ethmoid sinus. *B,* T_1-weighted direct coronal MRI scan.

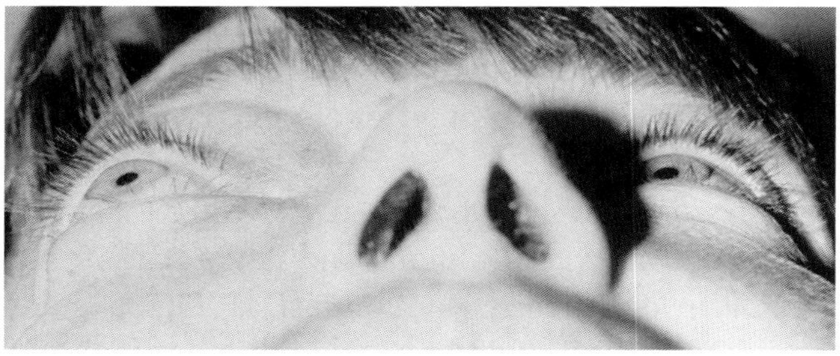

Figure 22–3. Clinical picture of a medial dermoid is similar to that of an ethmoid mucocele.

22–4), whereas with a mucocele the orbital bone is breached (see Figure 22–2). Occasionally, with frontal mucoceles, there is sufficient bony erosion so that the mucocele can markedly depress the globe (Figure 22–5) or even involve both the orbit and the extradural central nervous system (CNS) space (Figure 22–6).

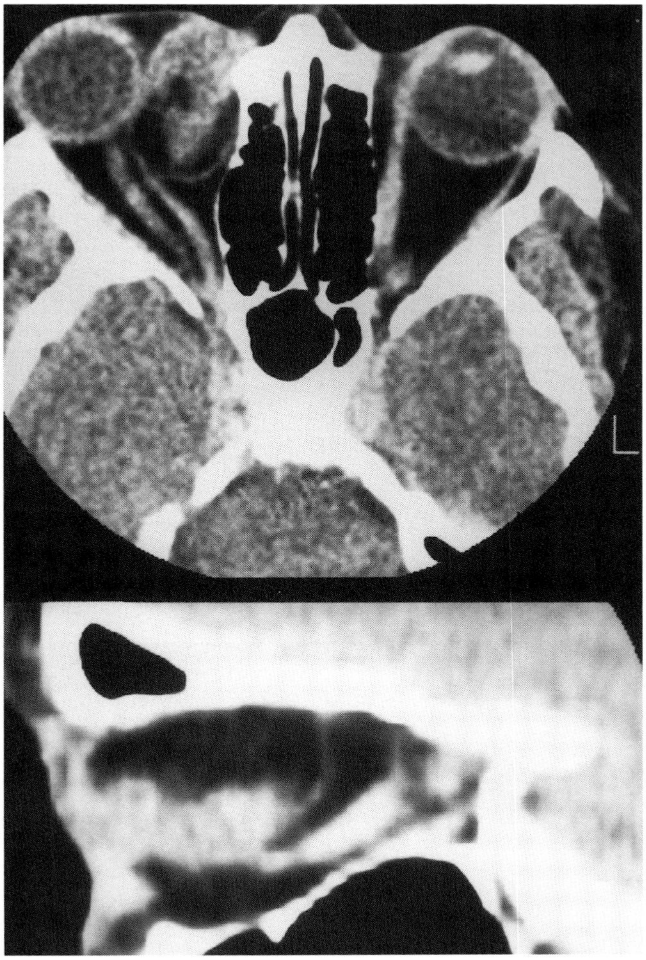

Figure 22–4. Axial CT with parasagittal re-formation of orbital dermoid cyst. Note that in contrast to Figure 22–2, the medial wall of the orbit is intact.

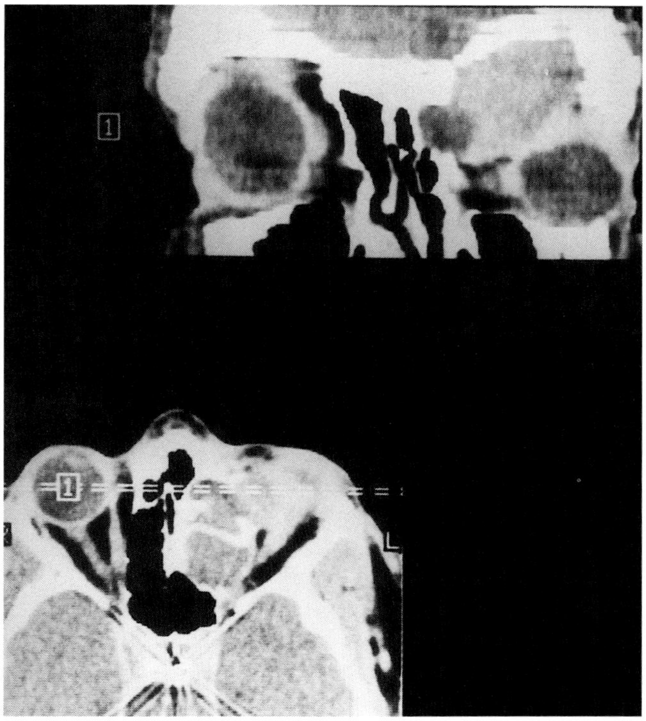

Figure 22–5. Large frontal-ethmoid mucocele depressing globe.

There are a number of ophthalmic manifestations of mucocele. Often, patients present with headache, proptosis, and a disturbance in extraocular motility.[6] Especially with sphenoid mucoceles, vision loss is not infrequent.[7] Occasionally, enophthalmos can be a presenting sign of a maxillary sinus mucocele.[5] Mucoceles can become infected. Weaver and Bartley describe 7 patients with both a mucocele and a malignancy arising in the same sinus.[8,9]

The surgical management of mucoceles that invade the orbit is discussed in Chapter 27. In addition to removing the mucocele, a permanent drainage pathway must be established in the altered sinus area to avoid a recurrent problem. We have used either the lining of the mucocele or a remnant of normal nasal mucosa to establish drainage into the nasal atrium. Figure 22–7 shows a coronal CT scan and both preoperative and postoperative photographs of a patient with a large multiple sinus mucocele that involved the sinuses, orbit, and CNS.

SINUS CARCINOMA

The second most common sinus process that involves the adult orbit is malignant squamous cell

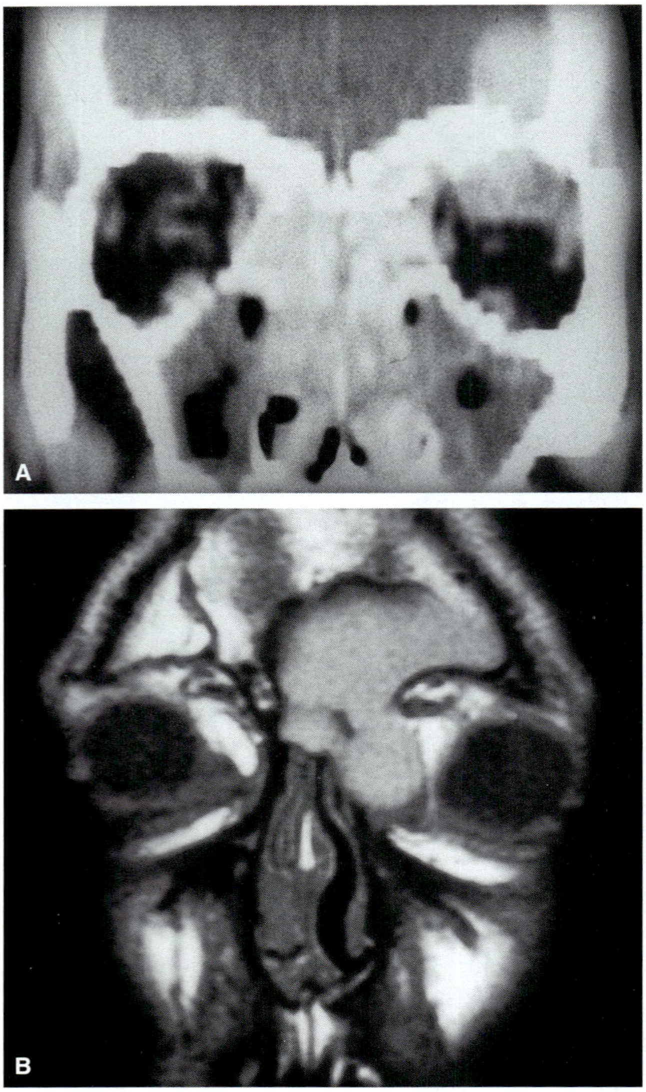

Figure 22–6. *A,* Coronal reformatted CT scan demonstrating extradural extension of a mucocele. *B,* Direct coronal MRI demonstrates a process similar to the one shown in Figure 22–10A and in other patients.

carcinoma with contiguous spread.[10–14] Epidemiologic studies have demonstrated that a number of environmental toxins, including nickel, chrome pigments, mustard gas, radium, and dust are associated with an increased risk of sinus cancer.[15] Squamous or undifferentiated carcinomas account for more than 70 percent of all sinus cancer.[15,16] Most of these malignancies are not localized to the sinuses at the time of diagnosis.[17] Approximately 20 to 45 percent have orbital invasion, and 80 percent have cranial nerve involvement when they are first seen by a physician.[10,11,18] The patient shown in Figure 22–8 presented with diplopia and vision loss as her chief complaint from an undiagnosed sinus carcinoma. Figure 22–9 shows a sinus carcinoma including the orbit on axial CT.

Johnson and co-workers reviewed 79 patients with sinus and nasal tumors, and noted that 47 had orbital involvement.[19] In contrast, a Dutch study noted that only 5 of 22 patients with ethmoidal cancers had orbital spread documented at diagnosis.[11,20,21] Orbital involvement by a sinus carcinoma has an extremely poor prognosis. Historically, the 10-

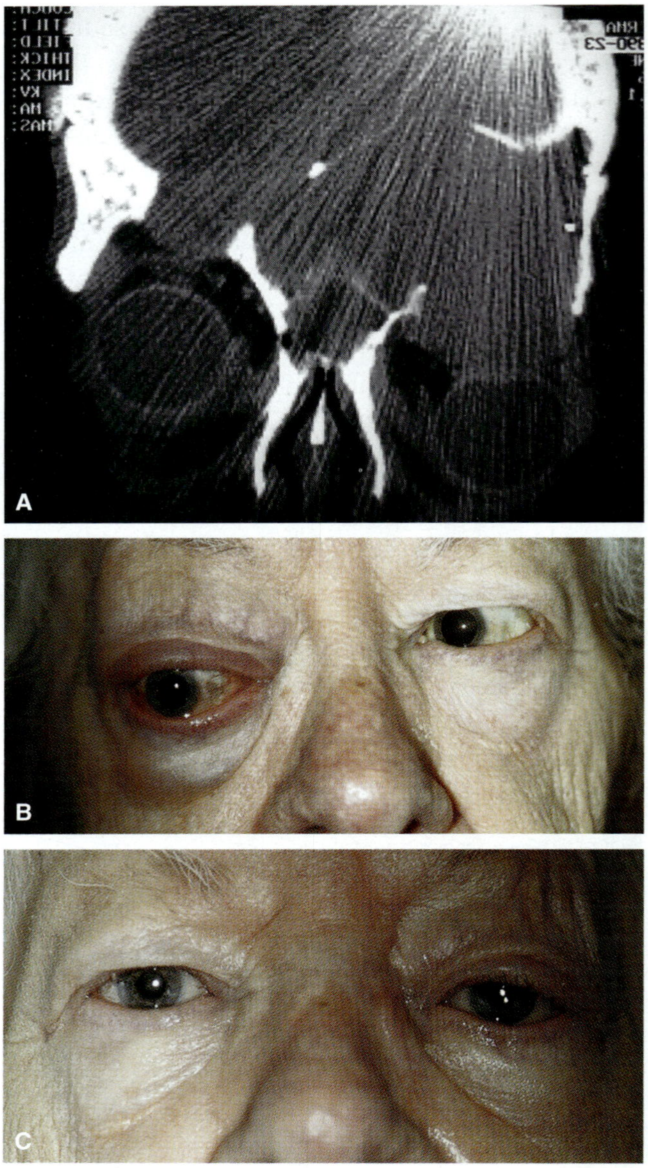

Figure 22–7. *A,* Coronal CT of large multiple sinus, orbit, and CNS mucocele. *B,* Preoperative photographs of Figure 22–7A. *C,* Postoperative photographs of Figure 22–7A.

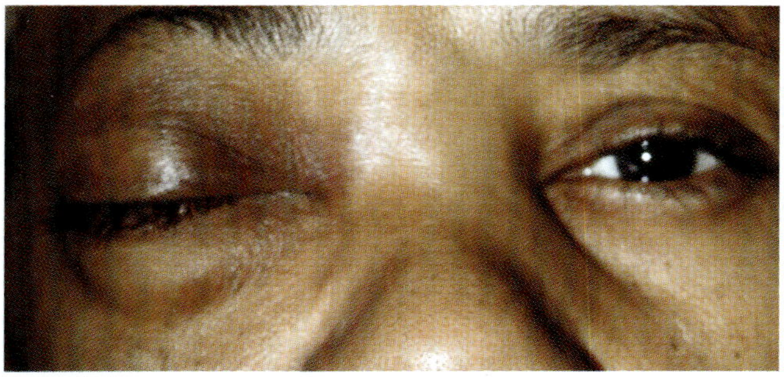

Figure 22–8. Large sinus carcinoma in a patient whose initial symptoms were diplopia and visual loss.

year survival is less than 2 percent.[22] Treatment consists of surgery, radiotherapy, and chemotherapy.[22–25]

Newer approaches have improved survival and decreased morbidity. Itami and colleagues reported on 37 patients with large maxillary sinus tumors that had a local recurrence-free survival of 59 percent at 5 years. Unfortunately, historically there was a significant incidence of visually destructive radiation retinopathy in survivors.[26–33] In one series from Japan, 8 of 25 patients who were irradiated had significant ocular complications within 2 years of treatment.[34] The use of intensity-modulated conformal therapy should probably diminish the incidence of radiation damage to the eyes and orbits.[35] Figure 22–10A and B demonstrate the conformal treatment plan, which shows that while the sinuses have received high-dose radiation, there is relative sparing of the eye and visually important structures.

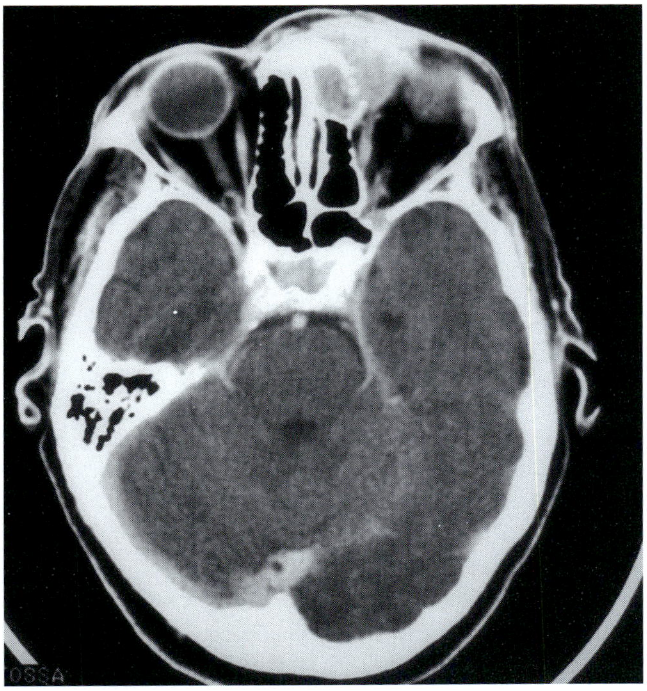

Figure 22–9. Axial CT shows sinus carcinoma invasion of the orbit.

MISCELLANEOUS LESIONS

A variety of other malignant sinus tumors can involve the orbit, including osteosarcoma, adenocarcinoma, adenoid cystic carcinoma, chondrosarcoma, mucoepidermoid carcinoma, rhabdomyosarcoma, esthesioneuroblastoma, and fibrosarcoma. The MRI

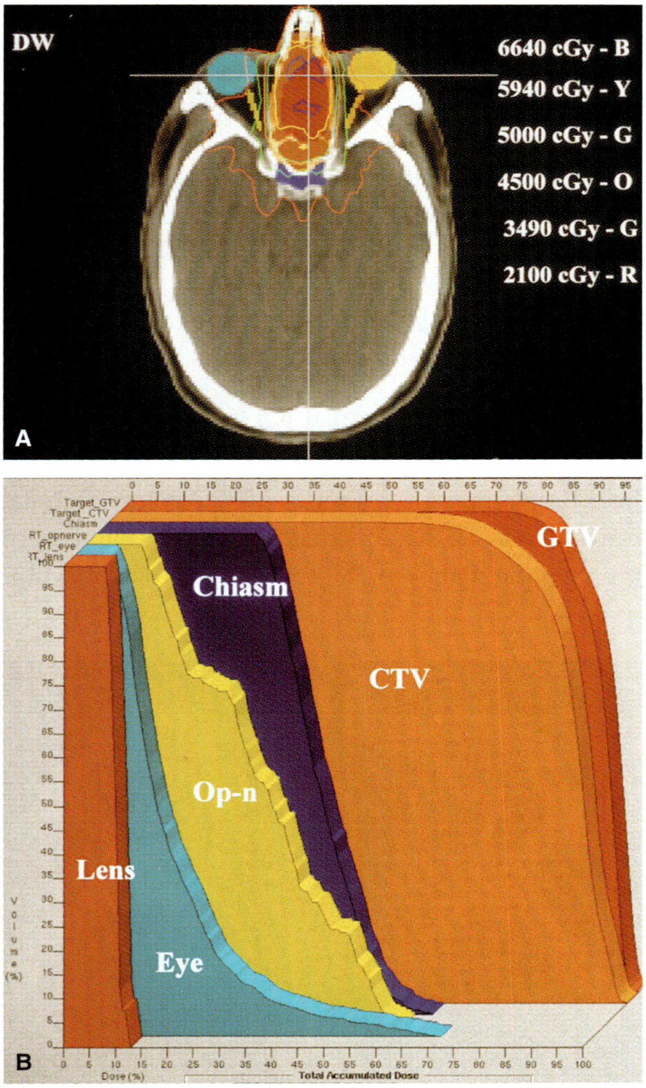

Figure 22–10. *A* and *B*, Intensity-modulated conformal therapy demonstrating a marked reduction of radiation to the eye, nerve, and visual pathways using this newer technique. This lateral approach should markedly diminish radiation complications associated with high-dose treatment for sinus carcinoma.

patterns of both orbital and sinus lymphomas is typical; usually, these lesions are hypointense on T_1 and hyperintense with gadolinium enhancement.[36] Rarely, a CNS tumor can invade both the sinuses and the orbit.[37] Figure 22–11 demonstrates a young woman with an apical involvement of the orbit and painful ophthalmoplegia secondary to an inapparent adenoid cystic carcinoma arising from the sinus. A fine needle is visible in the apical tumor; the fine-needle aspiration biopsy (FNAB) was used to establish a diagnosis. Retrospective analysis of the CT shows a small focus of sinus origin. Figure 22–12 shows a nasopharyngeal carcinoma with orbital involvement in a 25-year-old Asian male. Orbital invasion from a nasopharyngeal carcinoma is relatively rare, and in a series of 562 cases, only 18 had orbital involvement, 4 being bilateral.[38] We have also rarely managed lymphomas that arose in the sinuses and secondarily involved the orbit as shown in Figure 22–13.

Figure 22–14 shows a poorly differentiated sarcoma arising from a maxillary antrum and involving the orbit. This patient had a history of Wegener's granulomatosis that was quiescent at that time.

Esthesioneuroblastoma is a variant of neuroblastoma that arises in the sinuses, most commonly in young men (Figure 16–4). Approximately 250 cases have been reported. In a series of 38 patients from the Mayo Clinic, 28 had ophthalmic signs at the time of presentation with 5 of 38 (13%) having ocular symptoms, such as pain, proptosis, or epiphora as their initial complaint.[39] In one case report, the initial presentation of this tumor was with unilateral blindness.[40] Approximately 50 percent of patients survive.

Occasionally, an infectious process can simulate a sinus carcinoma with apical involvement.[41] Figure 22–15 shows a clinical photograph and axial CT of an 80-year-old otherwise healthy woman with rapid

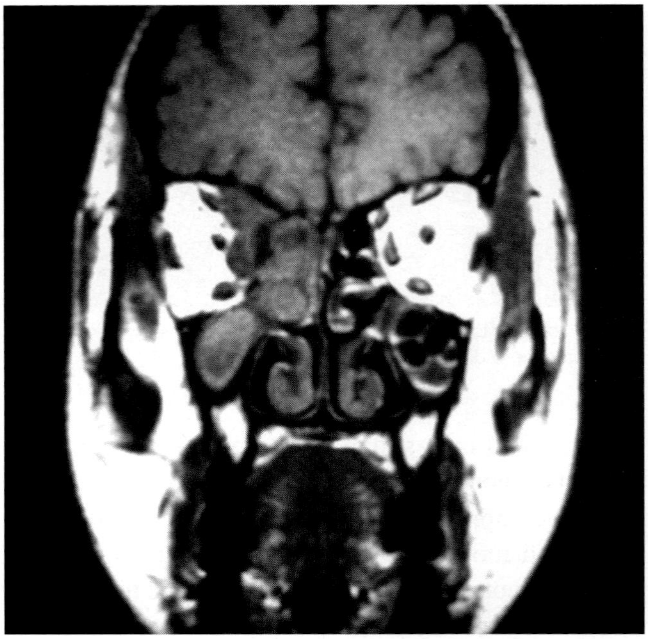

Figure 22–12. Nasopharyngeal carcinoma is more common in Asians. On direct coronal T_1-weighted MRI scan, this lesion involved the sinuses and orbit.

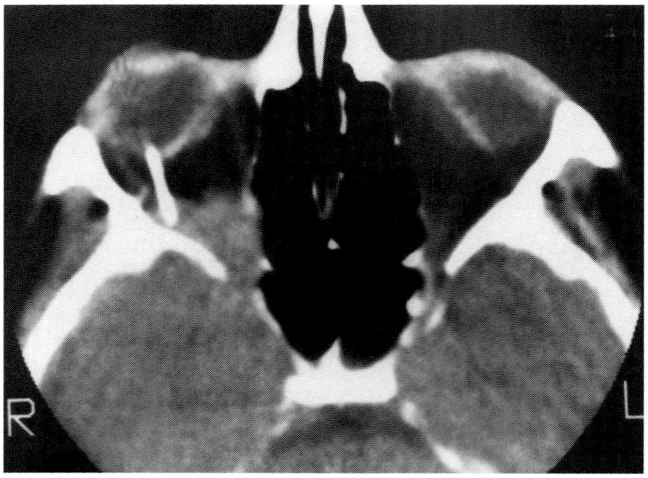

Figure 22–11. Apical involvement from an adenoid cystic carcinoma of the sinus. Fine-needle aspiration biopsy scout film demonstrates the needle in correct position.

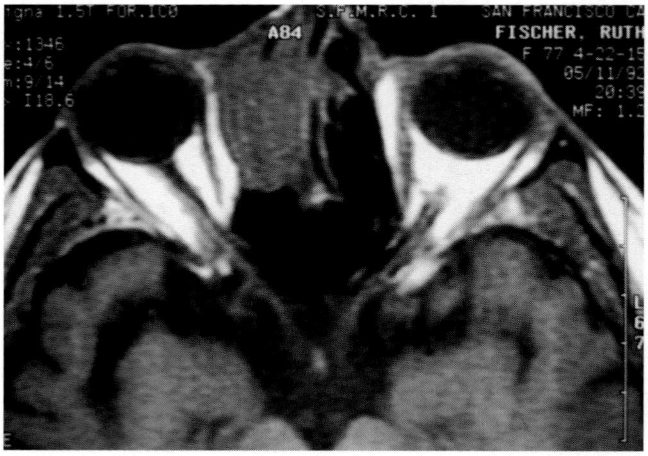

Figure 22–13. Sinus lymphoma with secondary orbital involvement. Patient presented with an initial complaint of epiphora. On axial T_1-weighted MRI scans, an ethmoidal mass was seen; on biopsy, this tumor was a large cell lymphoma.

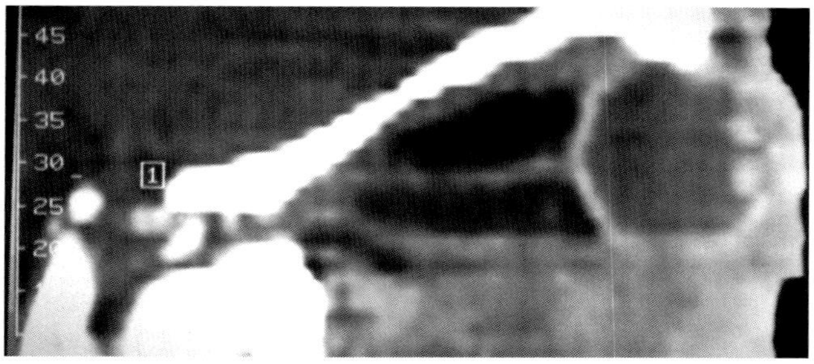

Figure 22–14. CT-reconstructed parasagittal scan shows a maxillary mass secondarily involving the orbit. The patient had been treated for longstanding Wegener's granulomatosis. The mass was a poorly differentiated sarcoma.

onset of ophthalmoplegia and vision loss secondary to an apparent sinus carcinoma with secondary involvement of the orbital apex. At biopsy *Aspergillus* was found in the ethmoid and sphenoid sinuses, without underlying tumor.

Inverted sinus papillomas are uncommon benign tumors that account for < 5 percent of sinus neoplasms.[42] Most commonly they occur in middle-aged males and are locally quite aggressive.[43] Such a case is shown in Chapter 21. In a recent report of 10 cases that invaded the orbit, 8 had recurrences after their initial resection, and 3 had spread into the brain.[44] Rarely, they can involve the orbit or metastasize.[43–46] Incomplete excision usually results in a high recurrence rate, estimated between 30 and 70 percent.[46]

Cemento-ossifying fibromas of the ethmoid sinuses can involve either the pediatric or adult orbit.[47] Juvenile nasopharyngeal angiofibromas usually occur in male teenagers and can cause death by either CNS extension or hemorrhage. These occasionally involve the orbit and may recur with or without radiation. It is uncertain whether surgery with embolization and/or radiation is more efficacious.[48]

Benign or malignant lymphoid lesions of the sinuses (see Figure 22–13) can involve the orbit.[49] While orbital pseudotumor involving the sinuses is rare, it can occur.[50] Wegener's granulomatosis will often present with sinus disease and secondarily produce either ocular or orbital findings (Figure 22–16).[51–54] Occasionally, the disease can be limited to just sinus and lung without renal involvement.[54] Ophthalmic involvement has the same frequency in both the limited and complete forms of Wegener's granulomatosis.[55]

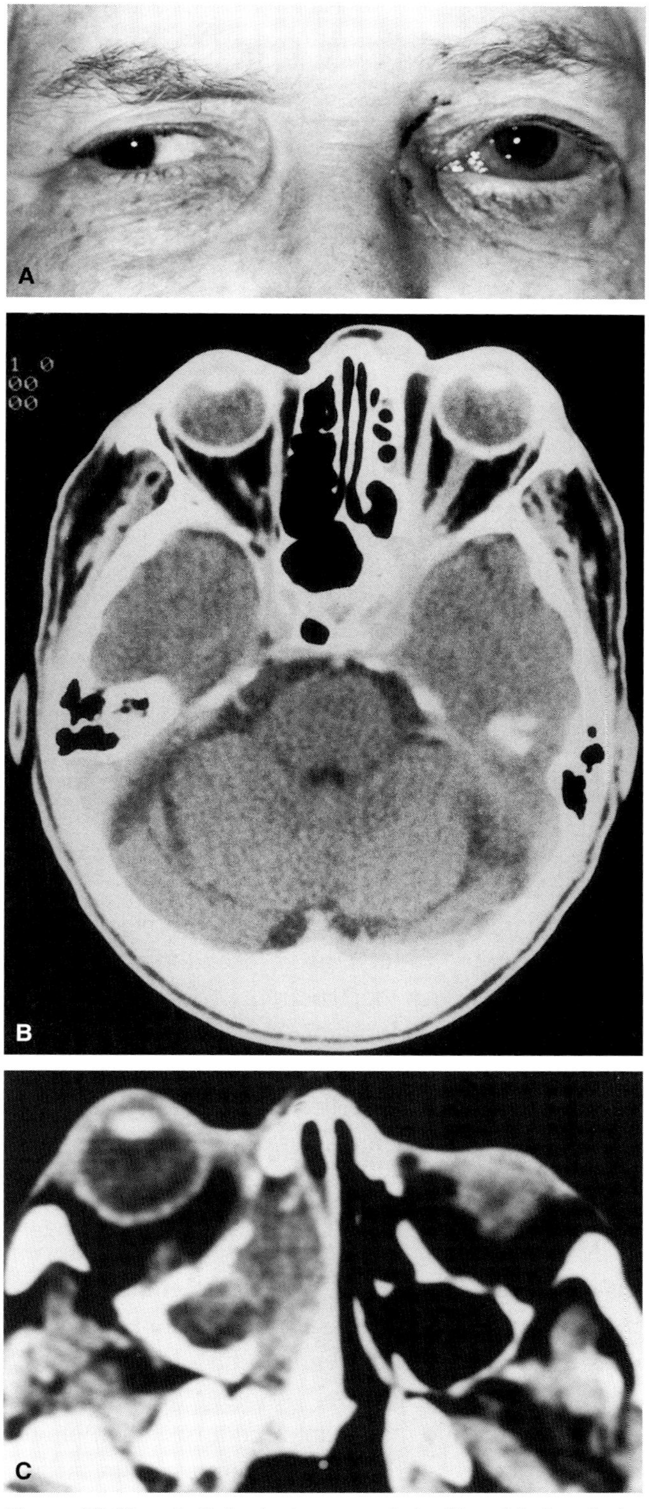

Figure 22–15. *A,* Patient who presented with ophthalmoplegia, pain, and loss of vision due to aspergillosis of the ethmoid sinus. The clinical appearance is suggestive of a sinus carcinoma. *B,* Axial CT scan showing apical involvement with bone loss secondary to aspergillosis. This pattern simulated a sinus carcinoma with secondary spread. A similar case of an actual sinus carcinoma is shown in Figure 22–15C. *C,* Axial CT scan demonstrating sinus carcinoma with secondary orbital involvement.

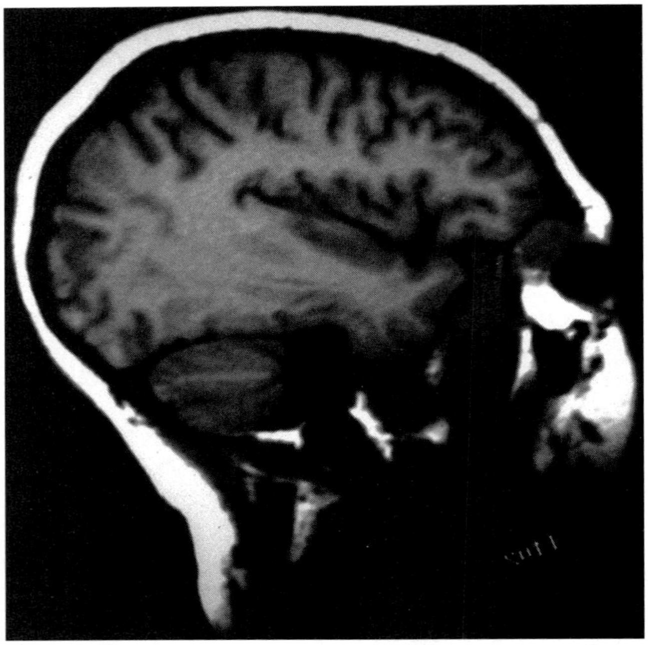

Figure 22–16. Wegener's granulomatosis with orbital involvement. ANCA tests were positive.

Historically, establishing the correct diagnosis in Wegener's granulomatosis was difficult. In one series, only 7 of 13 orbital biopsies had the classic triad of vasculitis, granuloma, and necrosis.[56] Occasionally, this disease can produce unusual ophthalmic findings, such as a pseudomelanoma or nasolacrimal duct obstruction.[57–58] As discussed under orbital pseudotumor, the commercial availability of the antineutrophil cytoplasmic antibody (ANCA) test has made the diagnosis of Wegener's granulomatosis much easier, even in the limited form of the disease.[59] Most cases of ophthalmic involvement have had positive antibodies.

Midline lethal granuloma may clinically appear histologically similar to Wegener's granulomatosis but it does not involve tissues below the neck.[60] It is often difficult to differentiate histologically from other types of lymphoma. Another variant of this process is midline malignant reticulosis, a lymphoma often difficult to differentiate from a benign inflammatory process.[60–63] An example of a midline lethal granuloma eventually diagnosed as a lymphoma is shown in Figure 22–17. Rhinoscleroma is another rare benign granulomatous disease. This is endemic in the developing countries but is quite rare in the United States.[63]

Occasionally, an osteoma arising from the sinus involves the orbit and produces proptosis, limitation of ductions, and pain.[64] A patient with an orbital osteoma is shown in Figure 22–18A. Either a plain x-ray film (Figure 22–18B) or a CT scan (Figure 22–18C) is diagnostic.

Orbital osteoma was first described by Veiga in 1856.[65] There are three theories of origin of osteomas: developmental, infection, or trauma.[65–68] Twelve cases of orbital osteomas were reported from the Mayo Clinic. Nine of the 12 had proptosis, and 3 had limitation of extraocular movement. There has been 1 case of amaurosis fugax as a result of a secondary osteoma.[69] Occasionally, these tumors are seen in association with Gardner's syndrome, an autosomal-dominant condition characterized by intestinal polyposis, skin and soft tissue tumors, and osteomas.[70] In the 5 cases that the author managed, all presented with proptosis, ocular pain, and motil-

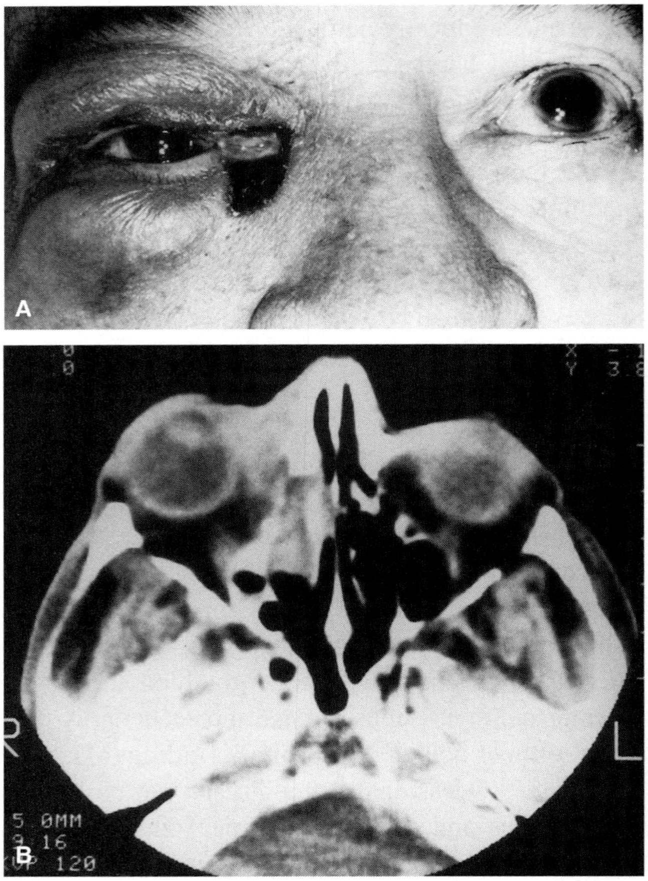

Figure 22–17. *A,* Clinical appearance of lethal midline granuloma of the orbit (Courtesy of D. Goodman, MD, San Francisco, CA). *B,* CT scan of patient shown in Figure 22–17A.

ity disturbances. The clinical pattern is not diagnostic, although usually, the eye is pushed laterally and downward (see Figure 22–18A). As pointed out by Ciappetta and co-workers, orbital involvement occurs in < 5 percent of cranial osteomas, and there is a higher incidence of surgical complications in this location.[71]

If removal of an osteoma is planned, CT with bone windows is useful. A coronal reformatted CT scan (see Figure 22–18C) shows that the tumor, which, on axial CT, appeared to arise from the medial orbital wall, actually arose in the area of the cribriform plate. The author removed this lesion with a dental burr (Figure 22–18D); lesions in less strategic areas can be broken off with a towel clip, or a dental burr may be used. Osteomas almost never recur or undergo malignant degeneration.

More recently, the use of computer assisted resection techniques using a three-dimensional CT technology can be an important adjuvant.[72] While the author has used the former technique for sphenoid wing mengiomas, there has not yet been a need to use it for an osteoma. Unfortunately, in cases in which the surgeon is not familiar with orbital osteomas, significant morbidity can occur. The patient shown in Figure 22–19 had a large osteoma with a preoperative vision of 20/20 and a postoperative vision of light perception after an incomplete resection. I was able to remove the tumor and restore vision to 20/50, but with only a small central island of vision.

Finally, we have examined a few patients from the airline industry who presented with enophthalmos as a result of barotrauma when a cabin depres-

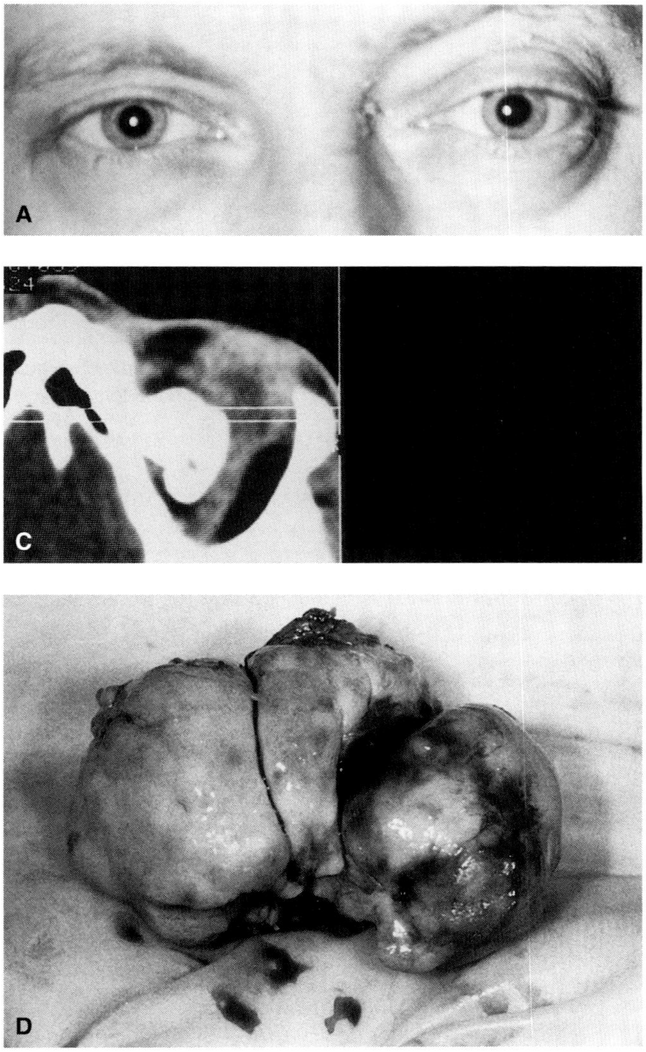

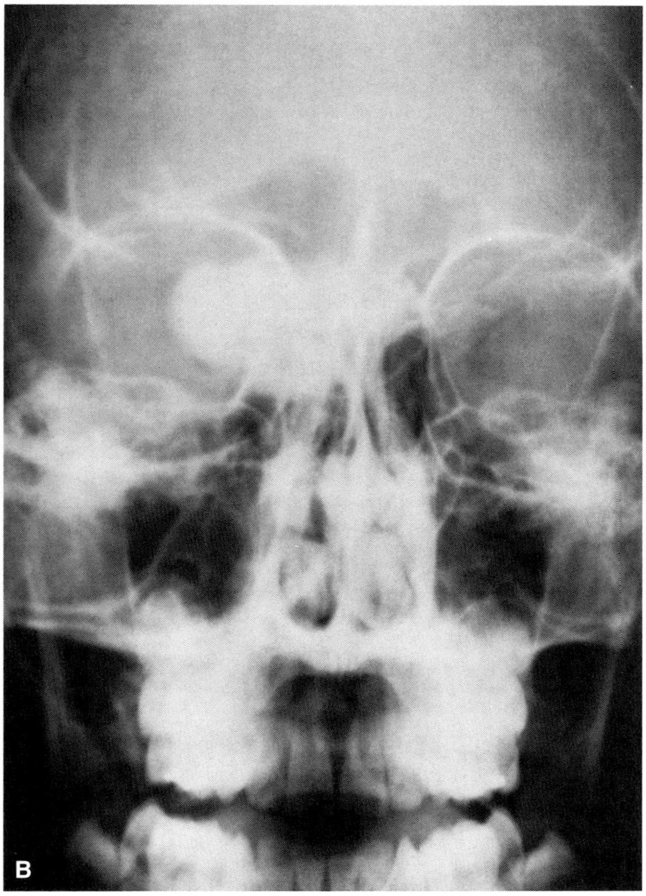

Figure 22–18. *A,* Clinical appearance of patient with frontal-ethmoid-orbital osteoma. *B,* Plain radiograph; the pattern is pathognomonic. *C,* Axial CT scans shows the osteoma apparently arising from the medial orbital wall. The coronal reformatted image demonstrates that the origin is actually near the lamina cribrosa. *D,* Lesion after removal with dental burr.

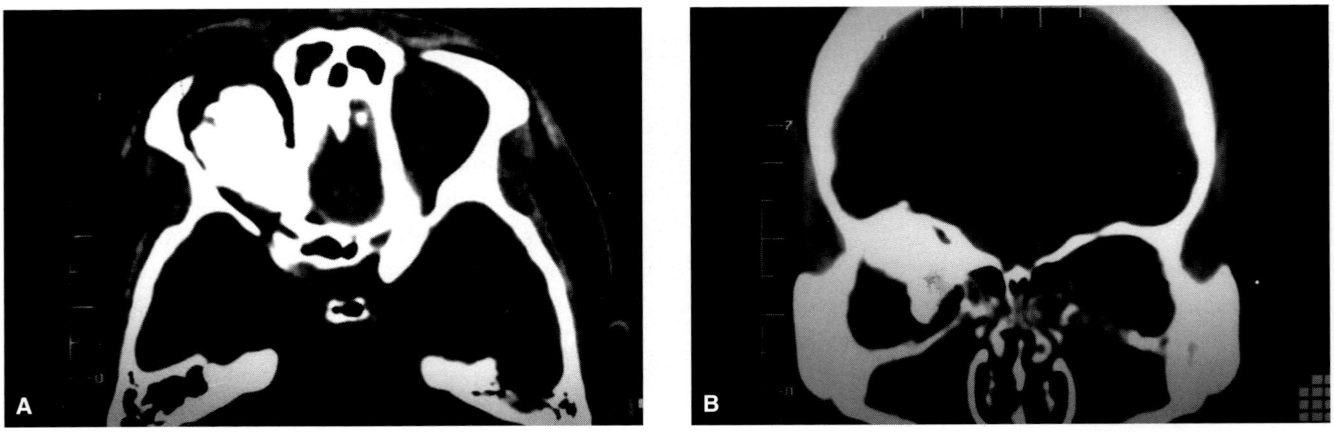

Figure 22–19. *A,* Axial CT of a large osteoma that involved the orbit. *B,* Same case in Figure 22–19A on direct coronal CT scan.

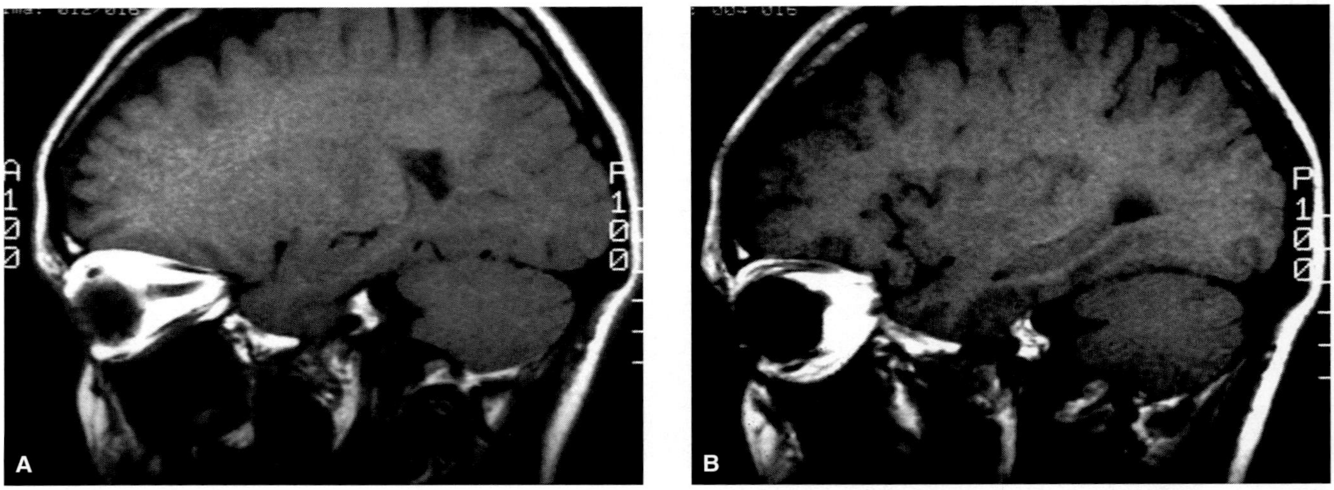

Figure 22–20. *A* and *B,* Barotrauma, from airplane decompression, has imploded the left maxillary antrum producing enophthalmos. Figure 22–20A shows the normal side on a T_1-weighted parasagital MRI scan. Figure 22–20B shows the collapsed orbital floor on the left side.

surized. Figures 22–20A and B show the normal (see Figure 22–20A) and imploded (see Figure 22–20B) maxillary antrums.

REFERENCES

1. Som PM. CT of the paranasal sinuses. Neuroradiology 1985;27:189–201.
2. Som PM, Shugar JMA. The CT classification of ethmoid mucoceles. J Comput Assist Tomogr 1980;4:199–203.
3. Avery G, Tang RA, Close LG. Ophthalmic manifestations of mucoceles. Ann Ophthalmol 1983;15:734–7.
4. Abrahamson RA Jr, Lobaluyot ST, Tew JM Jr, Sciovile G. Frontal sinus mucocele. Ann Ophthalmol 1979;11:173–8.
5. Traustason OI, Feldon SE. Cause of enophthalmos secondary to maxillary sinus mucocele. Am J Ophthalmol 1983;95:838–40.
6. Sethi DS, Lau DP, Chan C. Sphenoid sinus mucocoele presenting with isolated oculomotor nerve palsy. J Laryngol Otol 1997;111:471–3.
7. Nugent GR, Sprinkle P, Bloor BM. Sphenoid sinus mucoceles. J Neurosurg 1970;32:443–51.
8. Stankiewicz JA, Newell DJ, Park AH. Complications of inflammatory disease of the sinuses. Otolaryngol Clin North Am 1993;26(4):639–55.
9. Weaver DT, Bartley GB. Malignant neoplasia of the paranasal sinuses associated with mucocele. Ophthalmology 1991;98:342–6.
10. Graamans K, Slootweg PJ. Orbital exenteration and surgery of malignant neoplasm of the paranasal sinuses. Arch Otolaryngol 1989;115:977–80.
11. Dilhuydy JM, Lagarde P, Allal AS, et al. Ethmoidal

cancers: a retrospective study of 22 cases. Rad Oncol 1992;24:113–6.
12. Ascaso FJ, Adiego MI, Garcia J, et al. Sinonasal undifferentiated carcinoma invading the orbit. Eur J Ophthalmol 1994;4:234–6.
13. Raveh J, Turk JB, Ladrach K, et al. Extended anterior subcranial approach for skull base tumors: long-term results. J Neurosurg 1995;82:1002–10.
14. Hayasaka S, Sekimoto M, Shibasaki H, et al. Ophthalmic complications in patients with malignant tumors of the nose and paranasal sinuses. Ann Ophthalmol 1992;24:429–33.
15. Redmond CK, Sass RE, Roush GC. Nasal cavity and paranasal sinuses. In: Schottenfeld D, Fraumeni JF Jr, editors. Cancer epidemiology and prevention. Philadelphia, PA: WB Saunders Company; 1982. p. 519–35.
16. Sisson GA, Becker SP. Cancer of the nasal cavity and paranasal sinuses. In: Suen JY, Myers RN, editors. Cancer of the head and neck. New York, NY: Churchill Livingstone; 1981. p. 242–79.
17. Gullane PJ, Conley J. Carcinoma of the maxillary sinus. J Otolaryngol 1983;12:141–5.
18. Kenady DE. Cancer of the paranasal sinuses. Surg Clin North Am 1986;60:119–31.
19. Johnson LN, Krohel GB, Yeon EB, Parnes SM. Sinus tumours invading the orbit. Ophthalmol 1984;91: 209–17.
20. Seregard S, Kock E. Orbital presentation of ethmoid sinus adenocarcinoma. Acta Ophthalmol Scand 1995;73:457–9.
21. Curtin HD, Rabinov JD. Extension to the orbit from paraorbital disease. The sinuses. Radiol Clin North Am 1998;36:1201–13.
22. Terz JJ, Young HF, Lawrence W. Combined craniofacial resection for locally advanced carcinoma of the head and neck. Am J Surg 1980;140:618–24.
23. Robin PE, Powell DJ. Treatment of carcinoma of the nasal cavity and paranasal sinuses. Clin Otolaryngol 1981;6:401–14.
24. Shibuya H, Horiuchi J, Suzuki S, et al. Maxillary sinus carcinoma: result of radiation therapy. Int J Radiat Oncol Biol Phys 1984;10:1021–6.
25. McCary WS, Levine PA. Management of the eye in the treatment of sinonasal cancers. Otolaryngol Clin North Am 1995;28:1231–8.
26. Thompson GM, Migdal CS, Whittle RJM. Radiation retinopathy following treatment of posterior nasal space carcinoma. Br J Ophthalmol 1983;67:609–14.
27. de Schryver A, Wachtmeister L, Baryd I. Ophthalmologic observations on long-term survivors after radiotherapy for nasopharyngeal tumours. Acta Radiol (Ther) (Stockh) 1971;10:193–209.
28. Perrers-Taylor M, Brinkley D, Reynolds T. Choroido-retinal damage as a complication of radiotherapy. Acta Radiol (Ther) (Stockh) 1965;3:431–40.
29. Shukowsky LJ, Fletcher GH. Retinal and optic nerve complications in a high dose-irradiation technique of ethmoid sinus and nasal cavity. Radiology 1972;104:629–34.
30. Ellingwood KE, Milton RR. Cancer of the nasal cavity and ethmoid/sphenoid sinuses. Cancer 1979;43: 1517–26.
31. Morita K, Kawabe Y. Late effects on the eye of conformation radiotherapy for carcinoma of the paranasal sinuses and nasal cavity. Radiology 1979;130: 227–32.
32. Nakissa N, Rubin P, Strohl R, Keys H. Ocular and orbital complications following radiation therapy of paranasal sinus malignancies and review of the literature. Cancer 1983;51:980–6.
33. Dilhuydy JM, Lagarde P, Allal AS, et al. Ethmoidal cancers: a retrospective study of 22 cases. Int J Radiat Oncol Biol Phys 1993;25:113–6.
34. Takeda A, Shigematsu N, Suzuki S, et al. Late retinal complications of radiation therapy for nasal and paranasal malignancies: relationship between irradiation-dose area and severity. Int J Radiat Oncol Biol Phys 199;44:599–605.
35. Itami J, Uno T, Aruga M, Ode S. Squamous cell carcinoma of the maxillary sinus treated with radiation therapy and conservative surgery. Cancer 1998;82: 104–7.
36. Gufler H, Laubenberger J, Gerling J, et al. MRI of lymphomas of the orbits and the paranasal sinuses. J Comput Assist Tomogr 1997;21:887–91.
37. Brandes A, Carollo C, Gardiman M, et al. Unusual nasal and orbital involvement of glioblastoma multiforme: a case report and review of the literature. J Neuro-oncol 1998;36:179–83.
38. Luo CB, Teng MM, Chen SS, et al. Orbital invasion in nasopharyngeal carcinoma: evaluation with computed tomography and magnetic resonance imaging. Chung Hua I Hsueh Tsa Chih (Taipei) 1998;61: 382–8.
39. Rakes SM, Yeatts RP, Campbell RJ. Ophthalmic manifestations of esthesioneuroblastoma. Ophthalmology 1985;92:1749–50.
40. Berman EL, Chu A, Wirtschafter JD, et al. Esthesioneuroblastoma presenting as sudden unilateral blindness. Histopathologic confirmation of optic nerve demyelination. J Clin Neuro-Ophthalmol 1992;12:31–6.
41. Weber AL, Mikulis DK. Inflammatory disorders of the paraorbital sinuses and their complications. Radiol Clin North Am 1987;25:615–30.
42. Bosley CE, Pruet CW. Inverted sinonasal papillomas. Ear Nose Throat J 1984;63:509–13.

43. Schoub L, Timme AH, Uys CJ. A well differentiated inverted papilloma of the nasal space associated with lymphnode metastasis. SAFR Med J 1973;47: 1663–5.
44. Elner VM, Burnstine MA, Goodman ML, Dortzbach RK. Inverted papillomas that invade the orbit. Arch Ophthalmol 1995;113:1178–83.
45. Lawton AW, Karesh JW, Gray WC. Proptosis from maxillary sinus inverted papilloma with malignant transformation. Arch Ophthalmol 1986;104:874–7.
46. Karcioglu ZA, Wesley RE, Greenidge KC, McCord CD Jr. Proptosis and pseudocyst formation from inverted papilloma. Ann Ophthalmol 1982;14:443–8.
47. Cohn HC, MacPherson TA, Barnes L, Kennerdell JS. Cemento-ossifying fibroma of the ethmoidal sinus manifesting as proptosis. Ann Ophthalmol 1982;14: 173–5.
48. Fields JN, Haverson KJ, Devineni VR, et al. Juvenile nasopharyngeal angiofibroma: efficacy of radiation therapy. Radiology 1990;176:263–5.
49. Font RL, Laucirica R, Patrinely JR. Immunoblastic B-cell malignant lymphoma involving the orbit and maxillary sinus in acquired immune deficiency syndrome. Ophthalmology 1993;100:966–70.
50. Som PM, Brandwein MS, Maldjian C, et al. Inflammatory pseudotumor of the maxillary sinus: CT and MR findings in six cases. AJR Am J Roentgenol 1994;163:689–92.
51. Coutu RE, Klein M, Lessell S, et al. Limited form of Wegener granulomatosis. JAMA 1975;233:868–71.
52. Fauci AS, Haynes BF, Katz P, Wolff SM. Wegener's granulomatosis: prospective clinical and therapeutic experience with 85 patients for 21 years. Ann Intern Med 1983;98:76–85.
53. Wolff SM, Fauci AS, Horn RG, Dale DC. Wegener's granulomatosis. Ann Intern Med 1974;81:513–25.
54. Spalton DJ, Graham EM, Page NGR, Sanders MD. Ocular changes in limited forms of Wegener's granulomatosis. Br J Ophthalmol 1981;65:553–63.
55. Stavrou P, Deutsch J, Rene D, et al. Ocular manifestations of classical and limited Wegener's granulomatosis. Quart J Med 1993;86:719–25.
56. Kalina PH, Lie JT, Campbell RJ, Garrity JA. Diagnostic value limitations of orbital biopsy in Wegener's granulomatosis. Ophthalmology 1992;99:120–4.
57. Hardwig PW, Bartley GB, Garrity JA. Surgical management of nasolacrimal duct obstruction in patients with Wegener's granulomatosis. Ophthalmology 1992;99:133–9.
58. Janknecht P, Mittelviefhaaus H, Loffler KU. Sclerochoroidal granuloma in Wegener's granulomatosis simulating an uveal melanoma. Retina 1995;15(2): 150–3.
59. Soukiasian SH, Foster CS, Niles JL, Raizman MB. Diagnostic value of anti-neutrophil cytoplasmic antibodies in scleritis associated with Wegener's granulomatosis. Ophthalmology 1992;99:125–32.
60. Kay MC, McCrary JA. Multiple cranial nerve palsies in late metastases of midline malignant reticulosis. Am J Ophthalmol 1979;88:1087–90.
61. Simonis-Blumenfrucht S, Mestdagh C, Lustman F, et al. Le granulome malin centro-facial. Dermatologica 1979;158:153–62.
62. Spalton DJ, O'Donnell PJ, Graham EM. Lethal midline lymphoma causing acute dacryocystitis. Br J Ophthalmol 1981;65:503–6.
63. Lubin JR, Jallow SE, Wilson WR, et al. Rhinoscleroma exophthalmos: a case report. Br J Ophthalmol 1981; 65:14–7.
64. Mansour AM, Salti H, Uwaydat S, et al. Ethmoid sinus osteoma presenting as ipiphora and orbital cellulitis: case report and literature review. Surv Ophthalmol 1999;43:413–26.
65. Teed RW. Primary osteoma of the frontal sinus. Arch Otolaryngol 1941;33:255–92.
66. Arnold J. Zwei Osteome der Stirnhohlen. Virchow's Arch Pathol Anat 1873;57:145.
67. Ersner MS, Saltzman M. Osteoma of the sinuses. Laryngoscope 1938;48:29.
68. Rawlins AG. Osteoma of the maxillary sinus. Ann Otol Rhinol Laryngol 1938;47:735.
69. Wilkes SR, Traumann JC, DeSanto LW, Campbell RJ. Osteoma: an unusual cause of amaurosis fugax. Mayo Clin Proc 1979;54:258–60.
70. Whitson WE, Orcutt JC, Walkinshaw MD. Orbital osteoma in Gardner's syndrome. Am J Ophthalmol 1986;101:236–41.
71. Ciappetta P, Delfini R, Inanneti G, et al. Surgical strategies in the treatment of symptomatic osteomas of the orbital walls. Neurosurgery 1992;31:628–35.
72. Senior BA, Lanza DC, Kennedy DW, Weinstein GS. Computer-assisted resection of benign sinonasal tumors with skull base and orbital extension. Arch Otolaryngol Head Neck Surg 1997;123:706–11.

23

Bony Orbital Tumors

Bony orbital involvement can be due to infection, reparative processes, benign neoplasms, malignant primary tumors, and metastases. Metastases to the orbit are the most common tumors that involve the orbital bones, but unlike primary bone lesions, they almost always also invade adjacent structures. As discussed in the chapter on orbital metastases, breast, lung, renal, and gastrointestinal carcinomas can often invade the orbit with secondary bony involvement. The pattern of orbital metastases that involve bone is fairly typical, and as shown in Figure 23–1, these lesions may also invade contiguous structures. In prostate metastases, they may either have that pattern or predominantly produce an osteoblastic lesion (Figure 23–2). In children, neuroblastoma metastases are the most common malignancy to affect the bony orbit, although Wilms' tumor and Ewing's sarcoma can also produce this pattern (see chapter on pediatric orbital cancer). Histiocytosis syndromes and infantile myofibromatosis can also involve the orbit.[1]

A number of other lesions can involve the bony orbital walls. Dermoid cysts in the lacrimal fossa (Figure 23–3) typically create a smooth, scalloped bone defect. Similarly, the pattern of sclerotic bone involvement in unifocal eosinophilic granuloma, part of the Langerhan's cell histiocytosis syndrome is fairly characteristic (see Figures 16–41A, B and 16–42).

Malignant epithelial lacrimal gland tumors, most commonly adenoid cystic carcinomas, invade bone and have a pattern similar to bony metastases, except that the location in the lacrimal fossa region makes the former diagnosis much more likely (see Figure 20–24). Metastases with bone invasion of the orbit rarely involve the lacrimal fossa.

Hematic orbital cysts, especially those in a subperiosteal position, can simulate a bony lesion (Figure 23–4). The six orbital cases that the author treated all occurred in the superior orbit, although some have been reported in other locations.[2–11] The magnetic resonance imaging (MRI) pattern of a chronic hematoma is hyperintense on both T_1- and

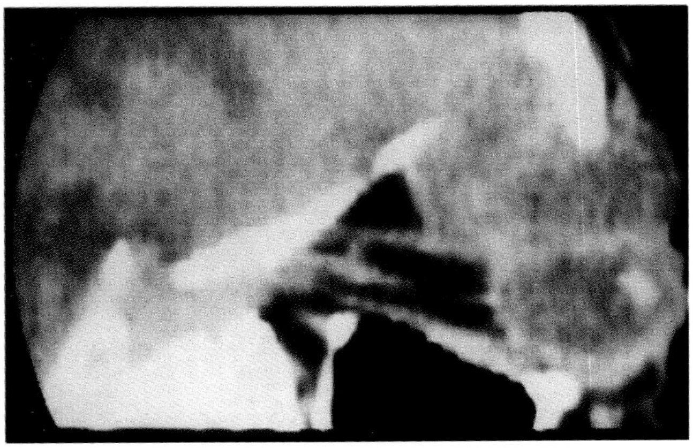

Figure 23–1. Lung carcinoma metastases to orbital bone and contiguous structures.

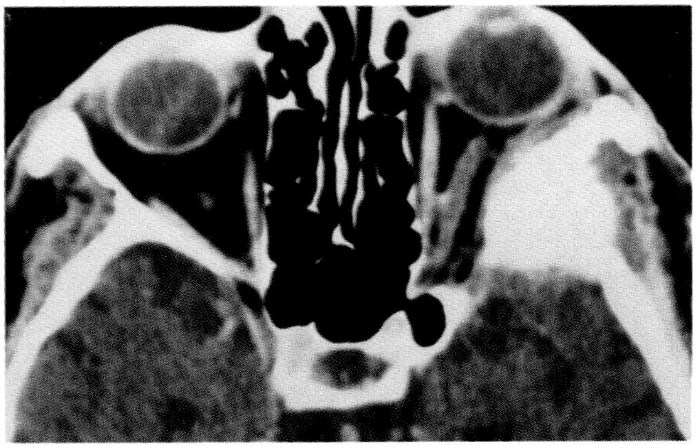

Figure 23–2. Axial CT shows a prostate metastasis with an osteoblastic response.

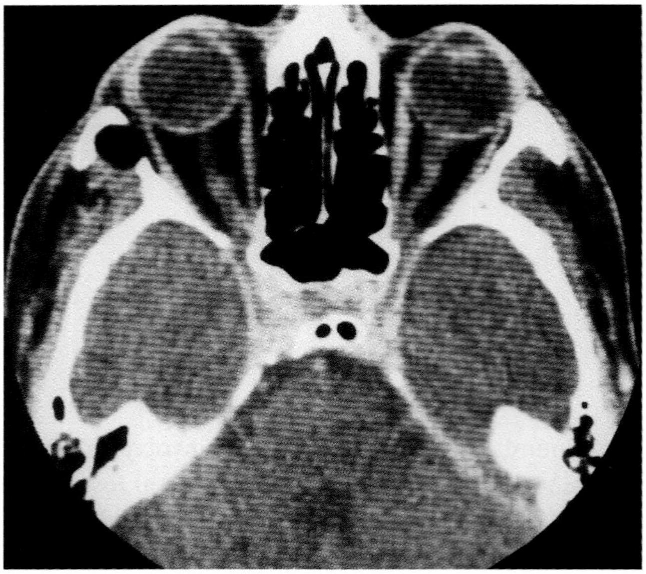

Figure 23–3. Axial CT scan showing smooth bone defect secondary to an enlarging dermoid cyst.

T_2-weighted images, and this is virtually diagnostic of this process.[12]

A number of expansile benign orbital tumefactions can mold the orbital bone but do not invade it. In very young children with diffuse orbital tumors, the orbital cavity can show generalized enlargement (see Figure 16–26).

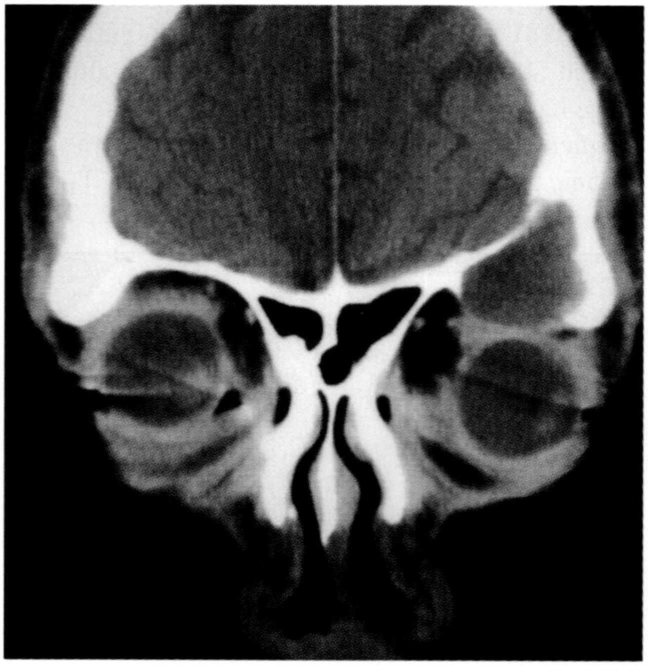

Figure 23–4. Traumatic hematic cyst simulating bony invasion by a malignant tumor.

Approximately 200 cases of fibrous dysplasia of the orbit have been described.[12] A number of synonyms have been used for this disease including juvenile Paget's fibrocystic disease and osteogenesis imperfecta tarda. Most patients present with orbital involvement with decreased vision, diplopia or proptosis. Usually, the proptosis is axial, and the globe is displaced downward.[8] The bone on plain x-ray films has a ground-glass appearance. The computed tomography (CT) pattern is more typical, with an amorphous ground-glass texture and thickening (Figure 23–5).[13,14] The MRI of these lesions is neither diagnostic nor more helpful than CT data. Occasionally, there can be optic nerve compression from fibrous dysplasia, and in such cases, decompression has been done.[14] Molecular biologic studies have demonstrated that an oncogene, *c-fos*, may be important in the development of these bone lesions.[15–17] Rarely, malignant degeneration can occur, as was documented in a recent case report of a 78-year-old woman.[18]

Osteomas involve the orbit secondarily (see chapter on orbital sinus lesions). Most arise as a result of developmental defects, trauma, or infection in the ethmoid or frontal sinuses.[17] Occasionally, orbital osteomas can occur in association with the autosomal dominant Gardner's syndrome and osteoma patients require a complete medical evaluation (physical examination, blood studies, gastrointestinal radiologic studies) to rule out this possibility.[19–21] Orbital osteomas are associated with more operative compli-

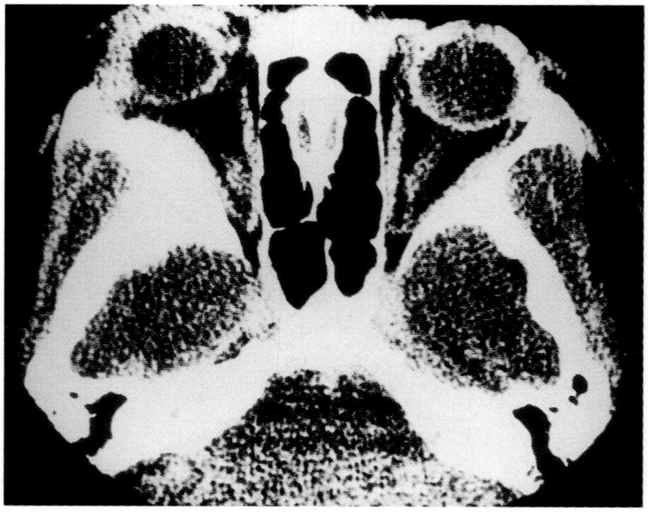

Figure 23–5. Axial CT scan showing amorphous ground-glass texture and thickening typical of fibrous dysplasia involving the orbit.

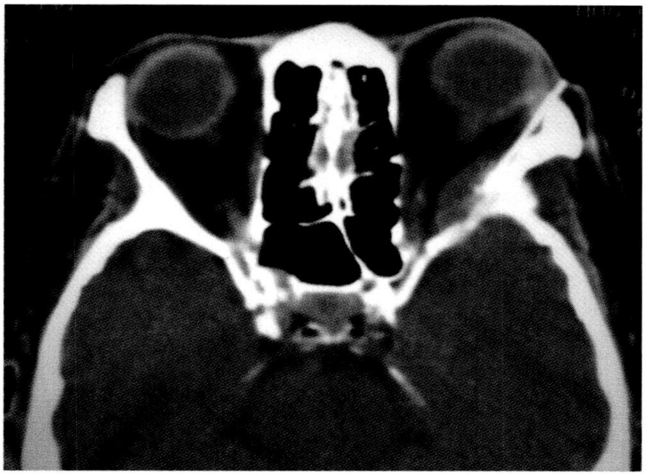

Figure 23–6. CT shows a small lateral extraconal mass with a minor degree of bone alteration.

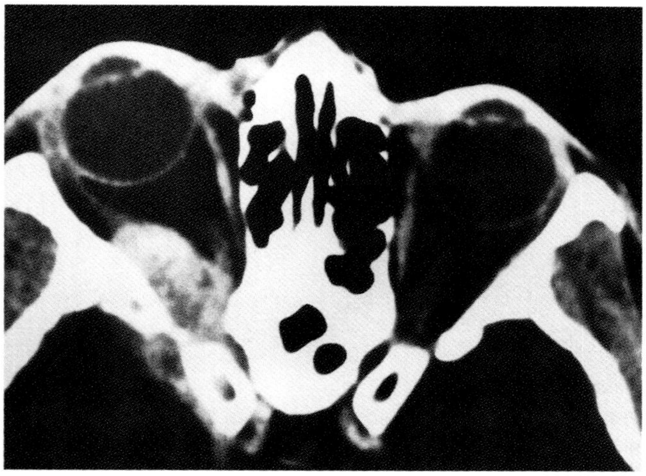

Figure 23–7. Orbital CT scan showing a meningioma secondarily involving the orbit. Note the hyperostosis and invasion of the sphenoid wing.

cations than these tumors in other body sites.[22] Rarely, these tumors can provide confusion, such as a recent case report of a patient with a Ewing's cell sarcoma of the fibula who was noted on bone scan to have an orbital lesion which was due to an osteoma.[20]

Meningiomas that secondarily involve the orbit can be difficult to diagnose (Figure 23–6). They involve the sphenoid wing in the posterior lateral orbit predominantly, are usually not palpable, and can grow en plaque with few signs or symptoms, until either a vessel or nerve is compromised.[21] These tumors are much more common than optic nerve sheath meningiomas.[22] Some meningiomas have an early effect on bone, and the presence of hyperostosis on radiologic studies aids in making the correct diagnosis (Figure 23–7). They may have orbital, bone, and central nervous system (CNS) changes at presentation (Figure 23–8). Advanced CNS meningiomas that invade the orbit may produce proptosis, lid swelling, conjunctival chemosis, or a temporal fossa mass (Figure 23–9). Lid and conjunctival edema is probably due to obstruction of venous return. Usually, these meningiomas have an indolent course and present with either proptosis or decreased vision. Occasionally, compression by the tumor may produce central retinal artery occlusion.[22] We have diagnosed some of these lesions with CT-directed fine-needle biopsy (Figure 23–10). Historically, most patients developed some evidence of optic nerve dysfunction, with impaired direct and consensual pupillary reaction, a positive Marcus-Gunn pupil, unilaterally decreased color vision and perception of brightness, and central or paracentral visual field defects. As discussed in Chapter 18, survival with meningioma is excellent.[23,24]

The management of orbital meningiomas is in flux.[25–26] We currently try to grossly remove the entire neoplasm and irradiate the area; with reasonable follow-up, we have had > 95 percent control using this approach.[27] A skull-based surgical approach using a team of neurosurgical and ophthalmological surgeons yields good results.[28] In some cases, the author has found the CO_2 laser quite useful to ablate the intraor-

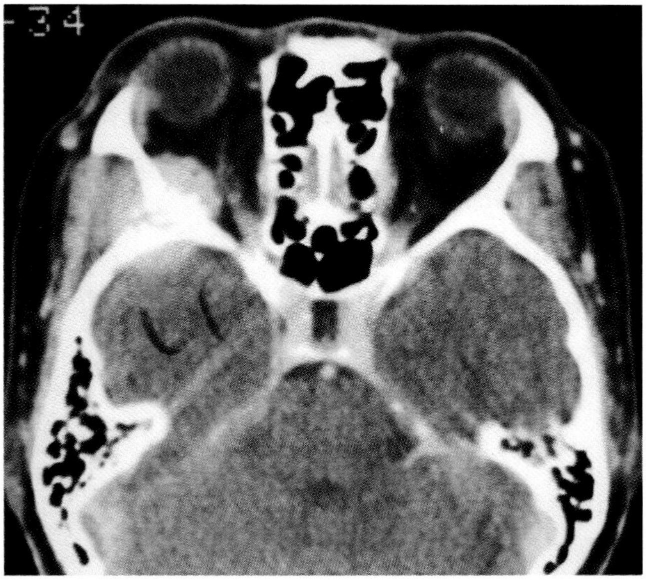

Figure 23–8. Axial CT demonstrates a sphenoid wing meningioma that invaded both the orbit and CNS at the time of presentation.

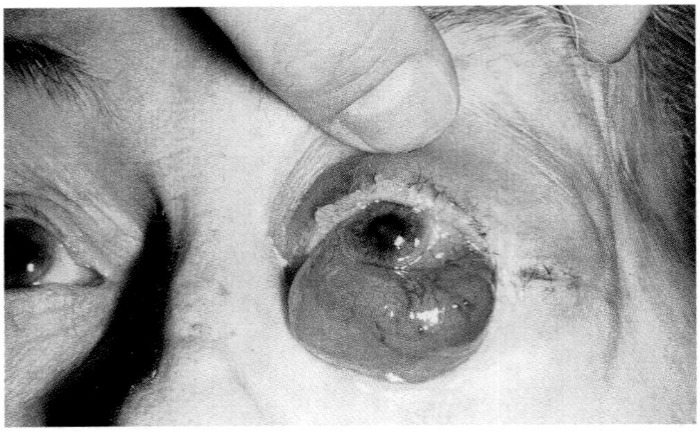

Figure 23–9. Obstruction of venous return by a large CNS meningioma invading the orbit. The patient has lid swelling and chemosis.

bital and orbital bone meningioma component of this lesion (see Chapter 27). Figures 23–11 and 23–12 show a lesion prior to and after its removal with a CO_2 laser. The patient was then treated with photon radiation. Intraoperative CT localization can be useful in minimizing morbidity in lesions of the sphenoid wing. In the case shown in Figure 23–13, we used this approach to safely remove gross tumor, without damaging the intraorbital contents.[29]

Giant cell granulomas of the orbit can occur after surgery. When they become a problem, they can be curetted.[30] Usually, these are expansive lytic lesions, but are quite rare.[31] Similarly, subperiosteal orbital abscesses can simulate a tumor in bone and often require drainage.[32] These lesions are usually a response to acute sinus inflammation and require management on an emergency basis. In one case, blindness occurred within a few hours of the onset

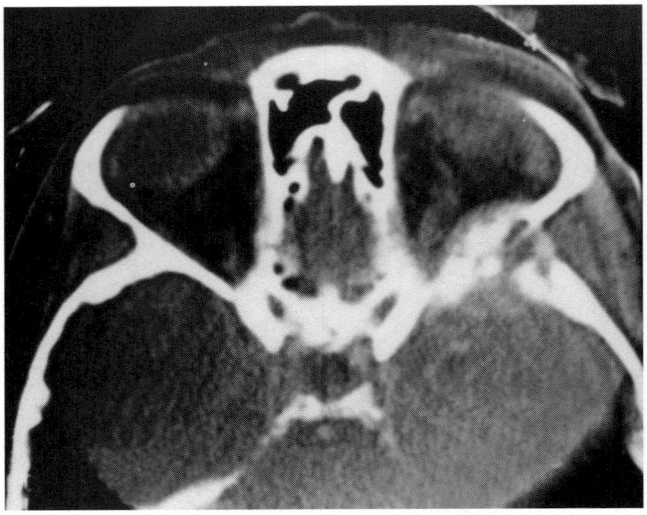

Figure 23–11. Axial CT shows sphenoid wing meningioma prior to surgery.

of symptoms. Most commonly, there is a history of a recent upper respiratory tract infection with the rapid development of eye edema, proptosis, and pain. Usually, it is difficult to distinguish subperiosteal abscess from other forms of sinusitis with contiguous orbital involvement.

Rarely, hemangiomas may arise in bone; they account for approximately 1 percent of primary bone tumors in other areas of the body (Figure 23–14).[33] There have been fewer than 20 case reports of intraosseous hemangiomas of the orbit. Occasionally, hemangiomas can simulate meningioma, since they have areas of bone density on CT, but an area of round or oval rarefaction of bone is almost pathognomonic.[34] Unlike meningioma, the

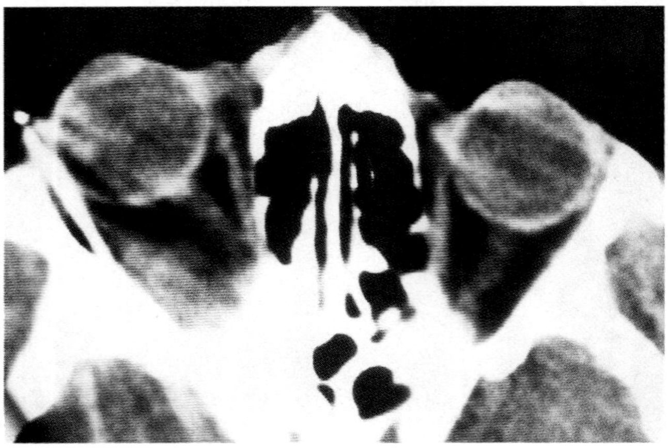

Figure 23–10. CT-directed fine-needle biopsy shows needle in a meningioma.

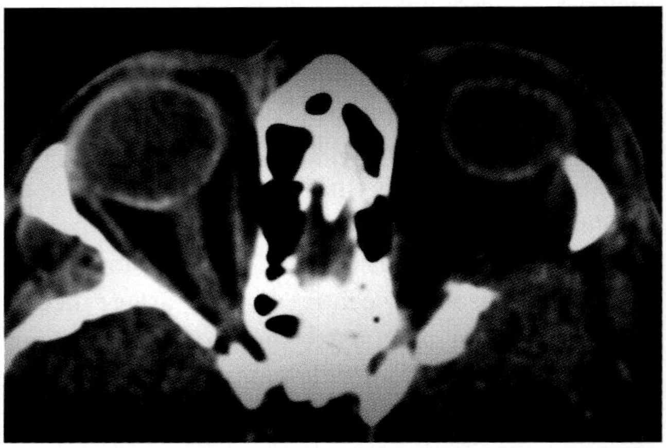

Figure 23–12. Axial CT shows area after removal of tumor with a CO_2 laser. The patient received postoperative photon radiation.

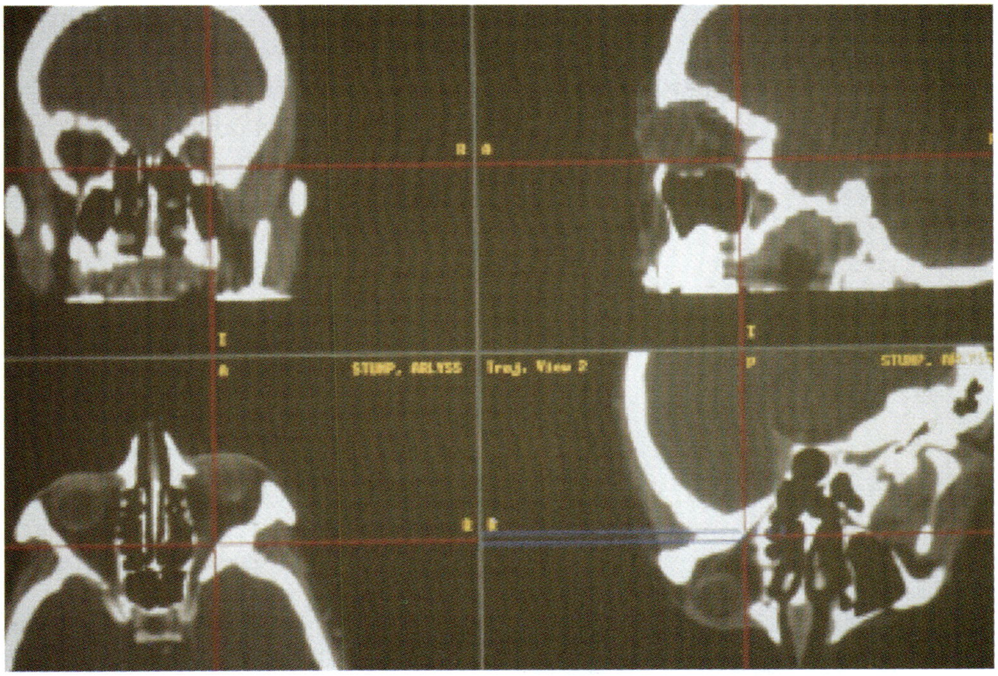

Figure 23–13. Stealth localization system for intraoperative use with optimum resolution of a posterior lateral orbital meningioma.

striations and stippled effect are vertical and parallel. These lesions are usually encapsulated and are best treated surgically.[35,36] Some will not recur even after a partial excision.[34] Rarely, multiple lesions have been reported.[37]

Brown tumors are secondary tumors of orbital bone that represent focal bone lesions of hyperparathyroidism.[38] The bone in these cases is replaced by proliferating fibrous tissue. This lesion can be occasionally confused with a fibrous dysplasia or a mucocele on imaging studies.[39] However, these patients usually have a history of either primary hyperparathyroidism or hyperparathyroidism in association with renal failure. Sometimes these tumors are quite vascular, and some clinicians embolize them prior to surgery.[40]

Osteoblastoma, another rare condition affecting the bony orbit, usually arises from the orbital portion of the frontal bone. It may involve the sinuses, and most commonly occurs in children.[41] It is managed by neurosurgery.[42]

Osteogenic sarcoma can also rarely involve the orbit either as a primary neoplasm or following treatment of bilateral retinoblastoma patients.[43–45] In any child who has survived bilateral retinoblastoma, the incidence of secondary osteogenic sarcoma is approximately 400-fold that in normals. These children should be evaluated with yearly bone scans, and any sign of an orbital tumor should mandate prompt

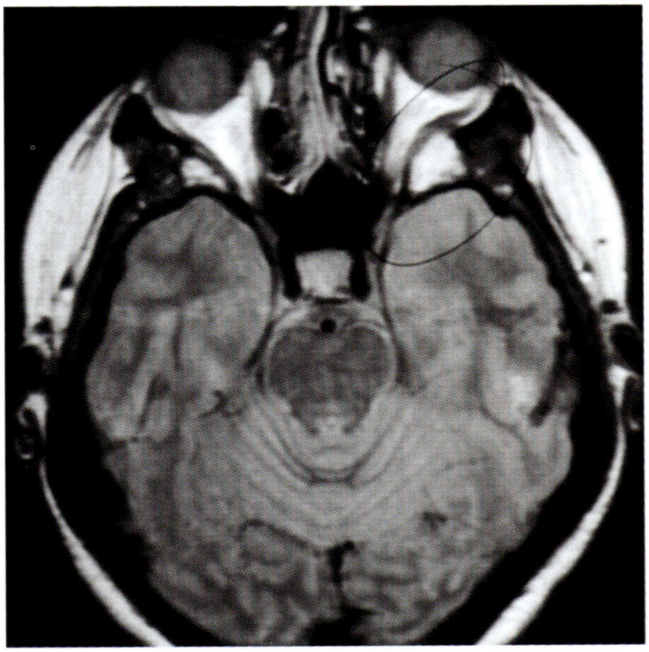

Figure 23–14. T_1-weighted axial MRI scan of an intradiploic hemangioma.

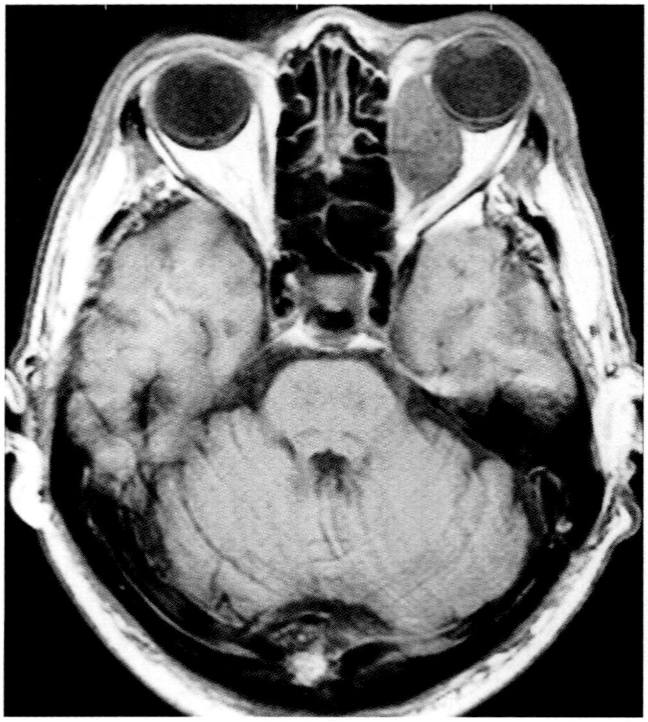

Figure 23–15. Chordoma metastatic to an extraocular muscle on T_1-weighted axial MRI scan.

biopsy. The management of orbital osteogenic sarcoma is local surgical debulking and chemotherapy.

Chondrosarcoma is a similar neoplasm arising from cartilage[46] (see Figure 17–38). Approximately 10 orbital cases have been reported.[47,48] The preferred treatment is surgical excision. The tumor is characterized by progressive slow recurrence without distant metastases. Death can occur as a result of contiguous spread into the CNS.

Chordomas, usually arising either in the CNS in the region of the dorsum sellae or clivus or arising from the sinuses, can secondarily involve the orbit. They are quite rare and the author has not managed such a case.[49,50] We did manage a metastatic chordoma that secondarily involved extraocular muscle (Figure 23–15).

Aneurysmal bone cysts are discussed in the chapter on pediatric orbital tumors. These usually are multisystem vascular lesions, and often patients have other bone abnormalities.[51,52]

Several other benign and malignant processes can involve the orbital bones. Approximately 30 cases of epidermoid cysts of the orbital bones have been reported.[53,54] On MRI scans, these are usually hypointense on T_1-weighted and hyperintense on T_2-weighted scans and do not enhance with gadollinium.[55] The histologic patterns of these lesions is distinct from an orbital dermoid, and these epidermoid lesions usually are in the intradiploic space.[53–56] Rarely, a necrotizing vasculitis has been reported to destroy a portion of the orbital wall.[57] A benign myxoma of the orbital wall can also destroy orbital bone.[58]

Giant cell tumors are approximately twice as frequent as aneurysmal bone cysts.[59,60] The management of the giant cell bone tumors is excision. Postoperative radiation in one series resulted in a local control rate in 19 of 21 cases in all body sites. The two failures were ultimately salvaged.[59]

REFERENCES

1. Duffy MT, Harris M, Hornblass A. Infantile myofibromatosis of the orbital bone. A case report with computed tomography, magnetic resonance imaging, and histologic findings. Ophthalmology 1997;104:1471–4.
2. Milne HL III, Leone CR, Kincaid MC, Brennan MW. Chronic hematic cyst of the orbit. Ophthalmology 1987;94:271–7.
3. Shapiro A, Tso MOM, Putterman AM, Goldberg MF. A clinicopathologic study of hematic cysts of the orbit. Am J Ophthalmol 1986;102:237–41.
4. Mund ML. Subperiosteal hematic cyst of the orbit. Ophthalmology 1981;88:992–6.
5. Roberts W. Hematoma of the orbit: Report of two cases. Am J Ophthalmol 1955;40:215–9.
6. Sevel D, Rosales A. Orbital blood cyst. Br J Ophthalmol 1978;62:571–4.
7. Goldberg SH, Sassan JW, Parnes A. Traumatic intraconal hematic cyst of the orbit. Arch Ophthalmol 1992;110:378–80.
8. Loeffler M, Hornblass A. Hematic cyst of the orbit. Arch Ophthalmol 1990;108:886–7.
9. Amrith S, Baratham G, Khoo CY, et al. Spontaneous hematic cysts of the orbit presenting with acute proptosis. A report of three cases. Ophthalmic Plast Reconstr Surg 1990;6:273–7.
10. Bergin DJ, McCord CD, Dutton JJ, Garrett SN. Chronic hematic cyst of the orbit. Ophthal Plast Reconstr Surg 1988;4:131–6.
11. Kersten RC, Kersten JL, Bloom HR, Kulwin DR. Chronic hematic cysts of the orbit. Ophthalmology 1988;95:1549–53.
12. Moore RT. Fibrous dysplasia of the orbit. Surv Ophthalmol 1969;15:321–34.

13. Daffner RH, Kirks DR, Gehweiler JA Jr, Heaston DK. Computed tomography of fibrous dysplasia. AJR Am J Roentgenol 1982;139:943–8.
14. Donoso LA, Magargal LE, Eiferman RA. Fibrous dysplasia of the orbit with optic nerve compression. Ann Ophthalmol 1982;14:80–3.
15. Candeliere GA, Glorieux FH, Prud'Homme J, St. Arnaud R. Increased expression of the c-fos protooncogene in bone from patients with fibrous dysplasia. N Engl J Med 1955;332:1546–51.
16. Epley DK, Lasky JB, Karesh JW. Osteosarcoma of the orbit associated with Paget disease. Ophthal Plast Reconstr Surg 1998;14:62–6.
17. Wilkes SR, Traumann JC, DeSanto LW, Campbell RJ. Osteoma. An unusual cause of amaurosis fugax. Mayo Clin Proc 1979;54:258–60.
18. Whitson WE, Forcett JC, Walkinshaw MD. Orbital osteoma and Gardner's syndrome. Am J Ophthalmol 1986;101:236–41.
19. Ciappetta P, Delfini R, Iannetti G, et al. Surgical strategies in the treatment of symptomatic osteomas of the orbital walls. Neurosurgery 1992;31:628–35.
20. Chynn EW, Rubin PA. Metastatic Ewing cell sarcoma of the sinus and osteoid osteoma of the orbit. Am J Ophthalmol 1997;123:565–7.
21. Quest DO. Meningiomas: an update. Neurosurgery 1978;3:219–25.
22. Maroon JC, Kennerdell JS, Vidovich DV, et al. Recurrent spheno-orbital meningioma. J Neurosurg 1994;80:202–8.
23. Barbaro NM, Gutin PH, Wilson CB, et al. Radiation therapy in the treatment of partially resected meningiomas. Neurosurgery 1987;20:525–8.
24. Dutton JJ. Optic nerve sheath meningiomas. Surv Ophthalmol 1992;37:167–83.
25. Newmann SA. Meningiomas: a quest for the optimum therapy. J Neurosurg 1994;80:191–4.
26. Carrizo A, Basso A. Current surgical treatment for sphenoorbital meningiomas. Surg Neurol 1998;50: 574–8.
27. Goldsmith BJ, Wara WM, Wilson CB, Larson DA. Post-operative irradiation of sub-totally resected meningioma. A retrospective analysis of 140 patients treated from 1967 to 1990. J Neurosurg 1994;80:195–201.
28. McDermott MW, Durity FA, Rootman J, Woodhurst WB. Combined frontotemporal-orbitozygomatic approach for tumors of the sphenoid wing and orbit. Neurosurgery 1990;26:107–16.
29. Senior BA, Lanza DC, Char DH, et al. Computer assisted resection of benign sinonasal tumors with skull base and orbital extensions. Arch Otolaryngol Head Neck Surg 1997;123:706–11.
30. Hoopes PC, Anderson RL, Blodi SC. Giant cell (reparative) granuloma of the orbit. Ophthalmol 1981;88: 1361–6.
31. Vernet O, Ducrey N, Deruaz J-P, De Tribolet N. Giant cell tumor of the orbit. Neurosurgery 1993;32: 848–51.
32. Harris GJ. Subperiosteal abscess of the orbit. Arch Ophthalmol 1983;101:751–7.
33. Dahlin DC. Bone tumors. General aspects and an analysis of 2,276 cases. Springfield, Mass: Charles C. Thomas; 1957.
34. Relf SJ, Bartley GB, Unni KK. Primary orbital intraosseous hemangioma. Ophthalmology 1991; 98:541–7.
35. Gross HJ, Roth AM. Intraosseous hemangioma of the orbital roof. Am J Ophthalmol 1978;86:565–9.
36. Lyon DB, Tang TT, Kidder TM. Epithelioid hemangioendothelioma of the orbital bones. Ophthalmology 1992;99:1773–8.
37. Kiratli H, Orhan M. Multiple orbital intraosseous hemangiomas. Ophthal Plast Reconstr Surg 1998; 14:348–8.
38. Slem G, Varinli S, Koker F. Brown tumor of the orbit. Ann Ophthalmol 1983;15:811–2.
39. Levine MR, Chu A, Abdul-Karim FW. Brown tumor and secondary hyperparathyroidism. Arch Ophthalmol 1991;109:847–9.
40. Park K, Mannor GE, Wolfley DE. Preoperative embolization of an orbital brown tumor. Am J Ophthalmol 1994;117:679–80.
41. Leone CR Jr, Lawton AW, Leone RT. Benign osteoblastoma of the orbit. Ophthalmology 1988; 95:1554–8.
42. Scott M, Peale AR, Croissant PD. Intracranial midline anterior fossae ossifying fibroma invading orbits (paranasal sinuses) and right maxillary antrum. J Neurosurg 1971;34:827–31.
43. Blodi FC. Unusual orbital neoplasms. Am J Ophthalmol 1969;68:407–12.
44. Mortada A. Exophthalmos in rare tumors of the orbital bones. Am J Ophthalmol 1964;57:270–5.
45. Sagerman R, Cassady J, Trotter P et al. Radiation-induced neoplasia following external beam therapy for children with retinoblastoma. Am J Roentgenol Radium Ther Nucl Med 1966;105:529–35.
46. Holand MG, Allen JH, Ichinose H. Chondrosarcoma of the orbit. Trans Am Acad Ophthalmol Otolaryngol 1961;65:898–905.
47. Bagchi M, Husain N, Goel MM, et al. Extraskeletal mesenchymal chondrosarcoma of the orbit. Cancer 1993;72:2224–6.
48. Potts MJ, Rose GE, Milroy C, Wright JE. Dedifferentiated chondrosarcoma arising in the orbit. Br J Ophthalmol 1992;76:49–51.

49. Binkhorst CD, Schierbeek P, Petten GJW. Neoplasms of the notochord: report of a case of basilar chordoma with nasal and bilateral orbital in involvement. Ophthalmologica 1955;133:12–22.
50. Crickelair GF, McDonald JJ. Nasopharyngeal chordoma. Plast Reconstr Surg 1955;16:138–44.
51. Dailey R, Gilliland G, McCoy GB. Orbital aneurysmal bone cyst in a patient with renal cell carcinoma. Am J Ophthalmol 1994;117:643–6.
52. Bealer LA, Cibis GW, Barker BF, et al. Aneurysmal bone cyst: report of a case mimicking orbital tumor. J Pediatr Ophthalmol Strabismus 1993;30:199–200.
53. Eijpe AA, Koornneef L, Verbeeten B Jr, et al. Intradiploic epidermoid cysts of the bony orbit. Ophthalmology 1991;98:1737–43.
54. Bitar SR, Selhorst JB, Archer CR. Epidermoid-induced pulsating eye. Ann Ophthalmol 1993;25:45–9.
55. Rumelt S, Harsh GR 4th, Rubin PAD. Giant epidermoid involving 3 cranial bones. Arch Ophthalmol 1997;115:922–4.
56. Sathananthan N, Moseley IF, Rose GE, Wright JE. The frequency and clinical significance of bone involvement in outer canthus dermoid cysts. Br J Ophthalmol 1993;77:789–94.
57. Whyte IF, Kemp EG. Orbital inflammatory disease and bone destruction. Eye 1992;6:662–6.
58. Candy EJ, Miller NR, Carson BS. Myxoma of bone involving the orbit. Arch Ophthalmol 1991;109: 919–20.
59. Malone S, O'Sullivan B, Catton C, et al. Long-term follow-up of efficacy and safety of megavoltage radiotherapy in high-risk giant cell tumors of bone. Int J Radiat Oncol Biol Phys 1995;33 :689–94.
60. De Dois AMV, Bond JR, Shives T, et al. Aneurysmal bone cyst. Cancer 1992;69:2921–31.

24

Fibrous Orbital Tumors

Symptomatic fibrous orbital tumefactions are relatively uncommon; they occur either as a result of a primary fibrous tumor or as a secondary reactive process. These lesions most frequently involve extraconal areas of the orbit. Most commonly, fibrous orbital processes occur as part of a spectrum of changes associated with orbital pseudotumors (see Chapter 26) or thyroid orbitopathy.[1] A computed tomography (CT) scan of a patient with Graves' disease, thyroid orbitopathy, and orbital fibrosis is shown in Figure 24–1. On CT, orbital detail is obliterated by this fibrous process.

For most orbital tumefactions, imaging studies are quite diagnostic; for fibrous lesions, their accuracy is limited.[2,3] There is a great deal of overlap, which can result in misdiagnoses. Generally, benign fibrous tumors tend to be well circumscribed, while aggressive malignant lesions infiltrate and destroy bone. Similarly, on magnetic resonance imaging (MRI) the benign lesions are more likely to be homogeneous, while the malignant tumors can change their pattern of homogeneity between T_1- and T_2-weighted images.[2]

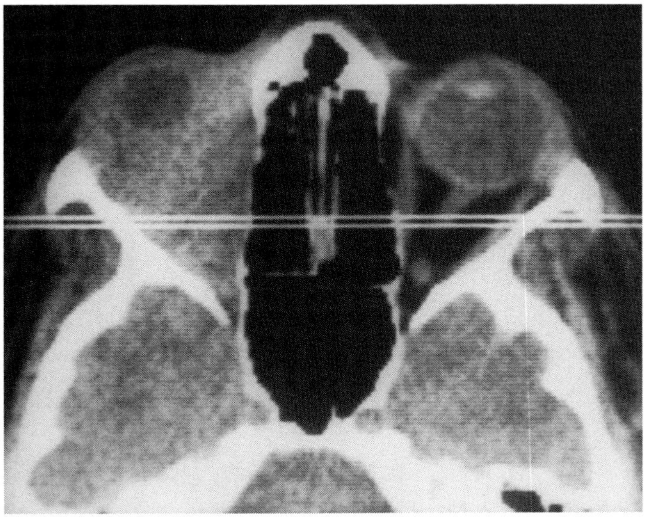

Figure 24–1. "Orbital wipeout syndrome"; secondary fibrosis as a result of thyroid orbitopathy.

Both benign and malignant fibrous histiocytomas can involve all areas of the orbit.[4–8] In the author's experience they have a predilection for the intraconal space, and they are therefore discussed in Chapter 17. Fibrous histiocytomas appear to have a loss of chromosome 13 as their most frequent genomic alteration, suggesting there may be a tumor suppressor gene in that location.[9] Neurofibromas, either multiple or plexiform, as part of the neurofibromatosis syndrome, as an isolated finding, or after enucleation, can occur in an intra- or extraconal location (Figure 24–2).[10] Fibroma can also occur as a consequence of trauma or surgery.[11]

Nodular fasciitis was first described in 1955, and there have been over 1,000 cases reported.[12] It can often be difficult to histologically differentiate this lesion from other tumors, especially sarcomas.[12,13] One case of an ophthalmic nodular fasciitis, diagnosed with fine-needle aspiration biopsy, has been reported.[13] Font and Zimmerman described 10 patients with ophthalmic findings: 5 involving the lids, 2 the periorbita, 1 the brow, 1 subconjunctivally, and 1 the limbus.[14] Generally, these lesions were nonencapsulated, round, oval tumors. I have seen one such orbital case. As shown in Figure 24–3, this patient had a lesion of the orbital floor with elevation of the globe. Both clinically and histologically, it is difficult to differentiate such a lesion from a fibrosarcoma, myxoma, neurofibroma, neurilemmoma, or sarcoma.[13,15]

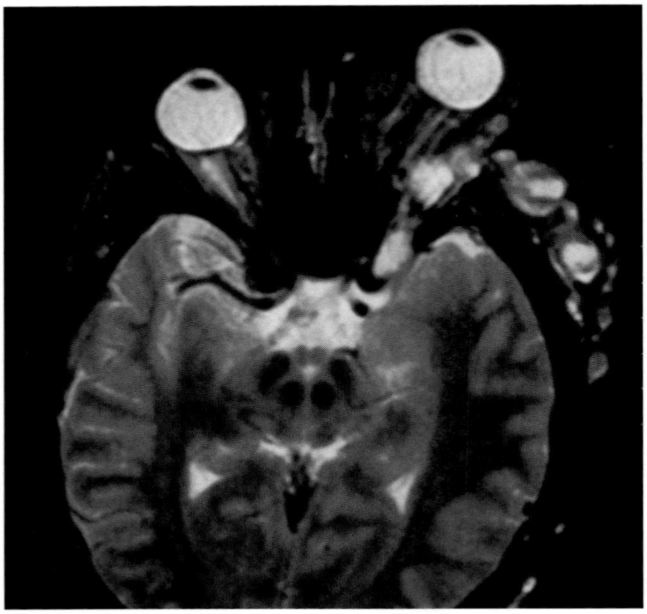

Figure 24–2. Axial MRI scan demonstrates a number of neurofibromas both inside and lateral to the orbit in a young man with NF1.

Amyloid tumors can produce orbital fibrosis. Approximately 20 cases of orbital amyloid have been reported. Most often, these are hard, irregular, nontender masses in the superior extraconal space.[16] Figure 24–4 demonstrates amyloidosis in the lacrimal fossa on axial CT. This case is interesting, in that it points out that although calcification in the lacrimal fossa has been felt by some to be almost diagnostic of malignancy, it is not necessarily so. Most patients have been between 25 and 80 years of age; 4 cases have been bilateral. Most patients with amyloid tumors of the orbit do not have systemic amyloidosis.[17] In a minority of cases, there is systemic involvement with hematologic abnormalities, including hypergammaglobulinemia, and Bence-Jones proteins in the urine.

Less commonly, other processes can produce orbital fibrosis. Congenital orbital fibrosis can occur as an idiopathic, isolated orbital disease (Figure 24–5). Fibrous dysplasia of the orbit is a bony lesion usually seen in young people; it is discussed in Chapter 23. Lesions arising from the sinuses produce fibrosis; they are discussed in Chapter 22. Many other reactive processes with widely varied etiologies can produce orbital fibrosis. In three cases, we have even observed localized orbital fibrosis from migrated contact lenses.[18]

Several less common fibrotic tumors can involve the orbit. As described under bone lesions, brown tumors secondary to hyperparathyroidism can have a fibrotic component, but mainly they involve the bone.[19] Various adult sarcomas, either primary or as a result of the retinoblastoma cancer diathesis (see Chapter 13), can be quite fibrotic: these include fibrous histiocytoma, fibrosarcoma, leiomyosarcoma, and other less common mesenchymal malignancies.[20,21]

Occasionally, fibrous tumors present asymptomatically or are discovered as a result of studies for other problems. An ossifying fibroma of the orbital

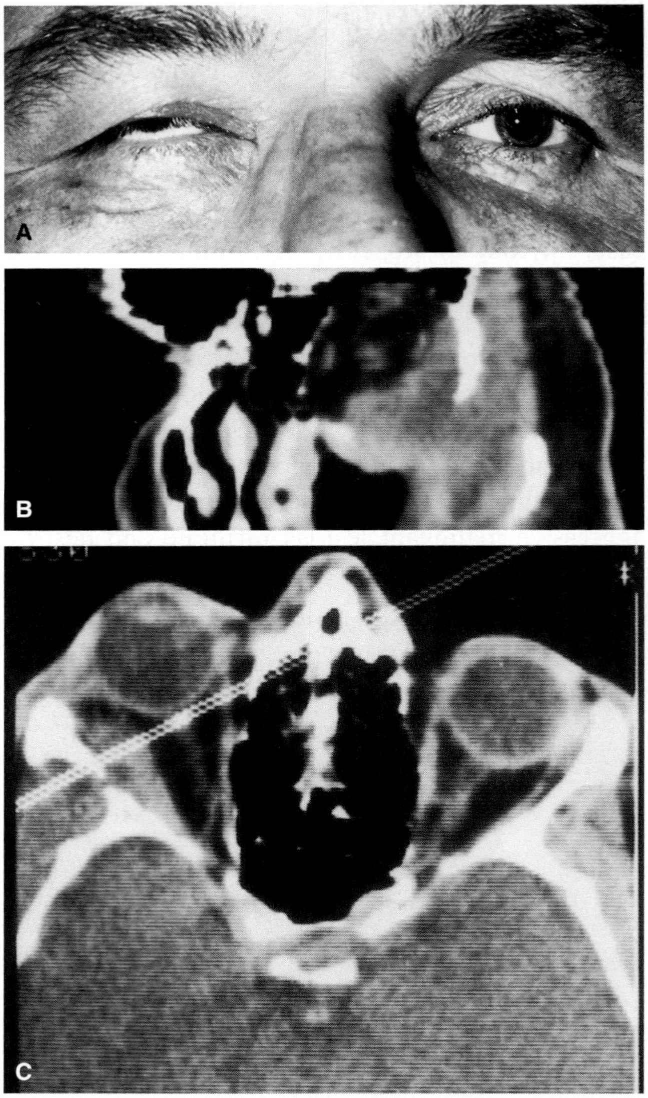

Figure 24–3. *A,* Nodular fasciitis with the globe displaced superiorly. *B,* CT with computer reformation of the case shown in Figure 24–3A with nodular fasciitis.

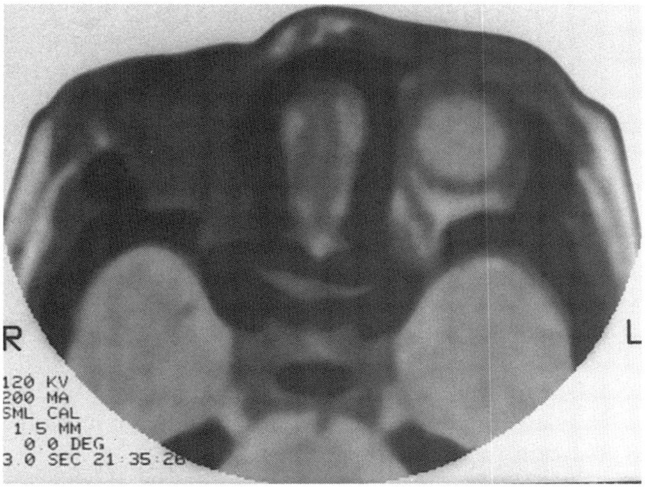

Figure 24–4. Orbital amyloid localized in the lacrimal fossa. This patient was initially referred as a probable malignant lacrimal gland tumor because of the calcification noted.

wall was detected by us and resected because of a history of malignancy (Figure 24–6).

The confusion regarding the pathology of fibrous tumors has led to an evolution in the nomenclature. Approximately 10 cases of solitary fibrous tumors of the orbit have been reported.[22–24] In the differential diagnosis with solitary fibrous tumor or giant cell fibroblastoma and giant cell angiofibromas, approximately 15 such cases involving the orbit have been described.[25–27] Usually, these lesions behave in a benign manner, although recurrences can develop.[25] Psammonatoid ossified fibromas of the orbit should be completely excised, which is a curative procedure.[28] Rarely, an orbital leiomyosarcoma can ossify and be somewhat confusing histologically.[29]

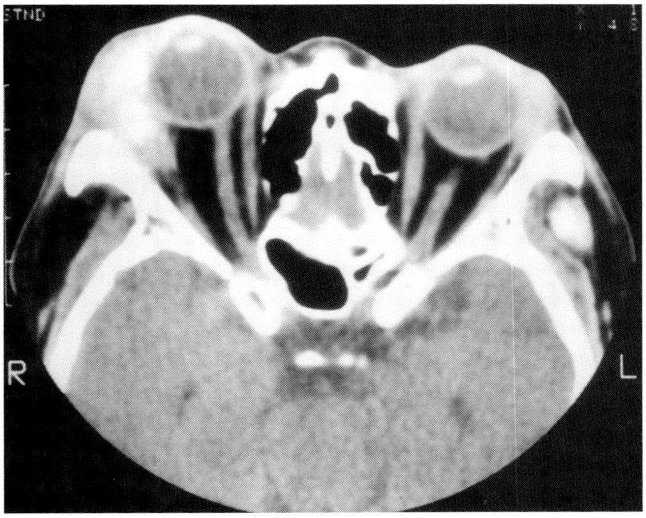

Figure 24–5. Congenital orbital fibrosis in a neonate with no history of family or in utero problems.

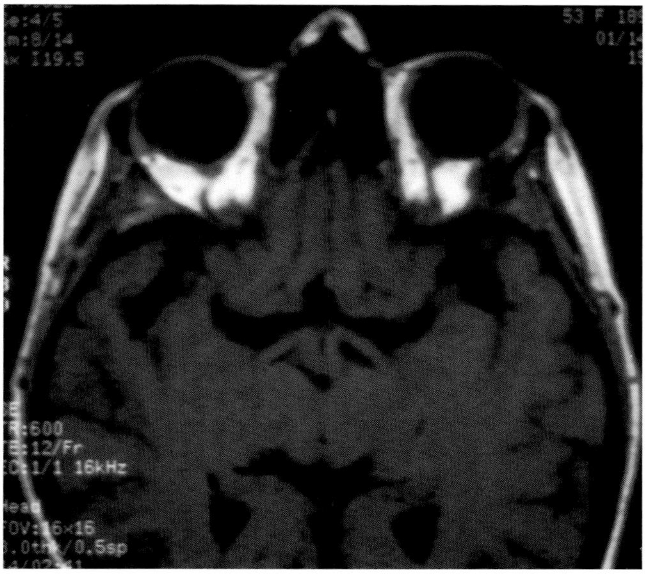

Figure 24–6. Ossifying fibroma of the orbital wall.

The use of cosmetic silicone injections and of paraffin products in some dressings used for sinus surgery have resulted in a small number of reports of localized or diffuse orbital fibrosis. In patients with orbital fibrosis who have had cosmetic silicone injections or sinus surgery, history is crucial because it points out the necessity for specialized histologic stains to establish the diagnosis.[30,31]

REFERENCES

1. Char DH. Thyroid eye disease, 2nd ed. New York, NY: Churchill Livingstone Inc.; 1989.
2. Dalley RW. Fibrous histiocytoma and fibrous tissue tumor of the orbit. Radiol Clin North Am 1999;37:185–94.
3. Wenig BM, Mafee MF, Ghosh L. Fibro-osseous, osseous, and cartilaginous lesions of the orbit and paraorbital region. Correlative clinicopathologic and radiographic features, including the diagnostic role of CT and MR imaging. Radiol Clin North Am 1998;36:1241–51.
4. Font RL, Hidayat AA. Fibrous histiocytoma of the orbit. Hum Pathol 1982;13:199–209.
5. Verity MA, Ebert JT, Hepler RS. Atypical fibrous histiocytoma of the orbit: an electromicroscopic study. Ophthalmologica 1977;175:73–9.
6. Jakobiec FA, Howard JM, Jones IS, Tannenbaum M. Fibrous histiocytomas of the orbit. Am J Ophthalmol 1974;77:333–45.

7. Rodrigues MM, Furgiuele FP, Weinreb S. Malignant fibrous histiocytoma of the orbit. Arch Ophthalmol 1977;95:2025–8.
8. Weiss SW, Enzinger FM. Malignant fibrous histiocytoma: an analysis of 200 cases. Cancer 1978;41: 2250–66.
9. Mairal A, Terrier P, Chibon F, et al. Loss of chromosome 13 is the most frequent genomic imbalance in malignant fibrosis histiocytoma. Cancer Genet Cytogenet 1999;111:134–8.
10. Myer DR, Wobig JL. Bilateral localized orbital neurofibromas. Ophthalmology 1992;99:1313–7.
11. Tricoulis D, Davaris P, Sarafianos K, Economou N. Fibroma of the orbital wall after dacryocystectomy: a case report. Ann Ophthalmol 1981;13:1167–8.
12. Allen PW. Nodular fasciitis. Pathology 1972;4:920–6.
13. Font RL, Zimmerman LE. Nodular fasciitis of the eye and adnexa. Arch Ophthalmol 1966;75:475–81.
14. Kaw YT, Ruesta RA. Nodular fasciitis of the orbit diagnosed by fine needle aspiration cytology. Acta Cytologica 1993;37:957–60.
15. Meacham CT. Pseudosarcomatous fasciitis. Am J Ophthalmol 1974;77:747–9.
16. Nehen JH. Primary localized orbital amyloidosis. Acta Ophthalmolgica 1979;57:287–95.
17. Cohen MN, Lessell S. Amyloid tumor of the orbit. Neuroradiol 1979;18:157–9.
18. Nocolitz E, Flanagan JC. Orbital mass as a complication of contact lens wear. Arch Ophthalmol 1978; 96:2238–9.
19. Levine MR, Chu A, Abdul-Karim FW. Brown tumor and secondary hyperparathyroidism. Arch Ophthalmol 1991;109:847–9.
20. Johnson LN, Sexton M, Goldberg SH. Poorly differentiated primary orbital sarcoma (presumed malignant rhabdoid tumor). Arch Ophthalmol 1991;109:1275–8.
21. White VA, Heathcote JG, Hurwitz JJ, et al. Epithelioid sarcoma of the orbit. Ophthalmology 1994;101: 1680–7.
22. Char DH, Caputo G, Miller T. Orbital fibrous histiocytomas. Orbit 2000 [in press].
23. Ing EG, Kennerdell JS, Olson PR, et al. Solitary fibrous tumor of the orbit. Ophthal Plast Reconstr Surg 1998;14:57–61.
24. Heathcote JG. Pathology update: solitary fibrous tumour of the orbit. Can J Ophthalmol 1997;32: 432–5.
25. Dei Tos AP, Seregard S, Calonje E, et al. Giant cell angiofibroma. A distinctive orbital tumor in adults. Am J Surg Pathol 1995;19:1286–93.
26. Wiebe BM, Gottlieb JO, Holch S. Extraorbital giant cell angiofibroma. APMIS 1999;107:695–8.
27. Hayashi N, Borodic G, Karesh JW, et al. Giant cell angiofibroma of the orbit and eyelid. Ophthalmology 1999;106:1223–9.
28. Hartstein ME, Grove AS Jr, Woog JJ, et al. The multidisciplinary management of psammomatoid ossifying fibroma of the orbit. Ophthalmology 1998;105: 591–5.
29. Wiechens B, Werner JA, Luttges J, et al. Primary orbital leiomyoma and leiomyosarcoma. Ophthalmogica 1999;213:159–64.
30. Raszewski R, Guyuron B, Lash RH, et al. A severe fibrotic reaction after cosmetic liquid silicone injection: a case report. J Cranio-Maxillo-Facial Surg 1990;18:225–8.
31. Hintschich GR, Beyer-Machule CK, Stefani FH. Paraffinoma of the periorbit: a challenge for the oculoplastic surgeon. Ophthalmic Plast Reconstr Surg 1995;11:39–43.

25

Metastases

Metastases to the orbit are uncommon but can simulate primary orbital tumors, thyroid orbitopathy, or idiopathic orbital inflammation. There is little data on the molecular biology of orbital metastases. Heartstein and co-workers queried whether different integrin subunits might be important for the tendency of tumors to metastasize to the orbit, but data in support of this concept is tenuous.[1]

Metastases can involve single or multiple orbital areas. In two large surgical series, the incidence of orbital metastases was 3 percent and 7 percent.[2] Metastatic tumors can involve extraocular muscles, the intraconal space, the globe and contiguous orbit (see Figure 17–18), the orbital bones, and the orbit and adjacent brain and sinuses.[3–8] Atypical orbital metastatic presentations include cystic tumors, diffuse extraocular muscle enlargement, bone production, enophthalmos, and pulsatile tumors.[9–12]

The orbit is a much less common site of metastases than the eye. Two series have noted that between 11 and 14 percent of ophthalmic metastases involve the orbit; one series reported a 32 percent incidence.[1,7,12–14] Similar to patients with ocular metastases, approximately 50 percent of those with orbital metastases present to the ophthalmologist prior to the discovery of the primary neoplasm.[7]

In adult men and children, ophthalmic involvement is often the first sign of malignancy.[15–19] In contrast, metastases to the orbit in adult women are most often from breast carcinoma; these patients have usually had treatment for the primary breast malignancy prior to the discovery of the orbital metastases.[7] A number of rarer causes of orbital metastases include pancreatic carcinoma, hepatocellular carcinoma, pheochromocytoma, testicular carcinoma, prostate cancer, bladder carcinoma, seminoma, cardiac myxoma, bile duct carcinoma, cervical carcinoma, male breast cancer carcinoid, mycosis fungoides, gastrinoma (Zollinger-Ellison syndrome), pleural mesothelioma, liposarcoma, thymus carcinoma, Ewing's sarcoma, and squamous cell carcinoma.[7,8,14,20–47]

A complete history is the most important component of the clinical evaluation of patients with possible orbital metastases. In over 60 percent of cases, a known history of primary malignancy can be obtained, especially in breast cancer cases.[48] I surveyed our orbital tumor files and noted that one-third of the patients were referred without a history of known malignancy and eventually were diagnosed as having orbital metastases. In most of these patients, a thorough history did not reveal the true nature of the orbital process.

In some metastatic tumors, there can be a very long latency between the primary neoplasm and the discovery of metastatic disease. In breast carcinoma, melanoma, and renal cell carcinoma, this interval has been as long as 30 years.[49]

The clinical and computed tomography (CT) or magnetic resonance imaging (MRI) patterns of orbital metastases in adults are varied. Often, the superior, extraconal orbit is involved with contiguous bone lesions. Frequently, the eye is proptotic and displaced inferiorly (Figure 25–1). In orbital lesions that are neither in the lacrimal fossa nor adjacent to the sinuses, bony destruction is most commonly due to a metastatic tumor (Figure 25–2). Other causes of bone destruction include mucocele, infection, Wegener's granuloma, midline lethal granuloma, a type of angiocentral T-cell lymphoma, Langerhans' histocytosis syndromes, sarcomas, hematic cysts

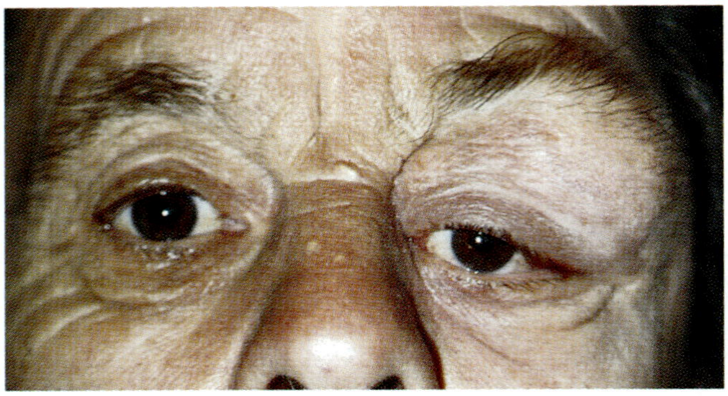

Figure 25–1. Often metastases involve the superior, extraconal orbit with proptosis and inferior displacement of the globe.

(organized hematomas), epithelial lacrimal malignancies, and lymphoid lesions.[50]

In older patients, a diffuse orbital involvement simulating a pseudotumor may be a presentation of metastatic disease.[51] Figure 25–3A shows a patient with axial proptosis secondary to a diffuse intraconal tumor metastasis (Figure 25–3B). The diagnosis was established as adenocarcinoma on the basis of a fine-needle aspiration biopsy (FNAB) (Figure 25–3C).

Metastases can also simulate a benign extraocular muscle process, for example, idiopathic myosis (Figures 25–4A and B), intramuscular hemangioma,

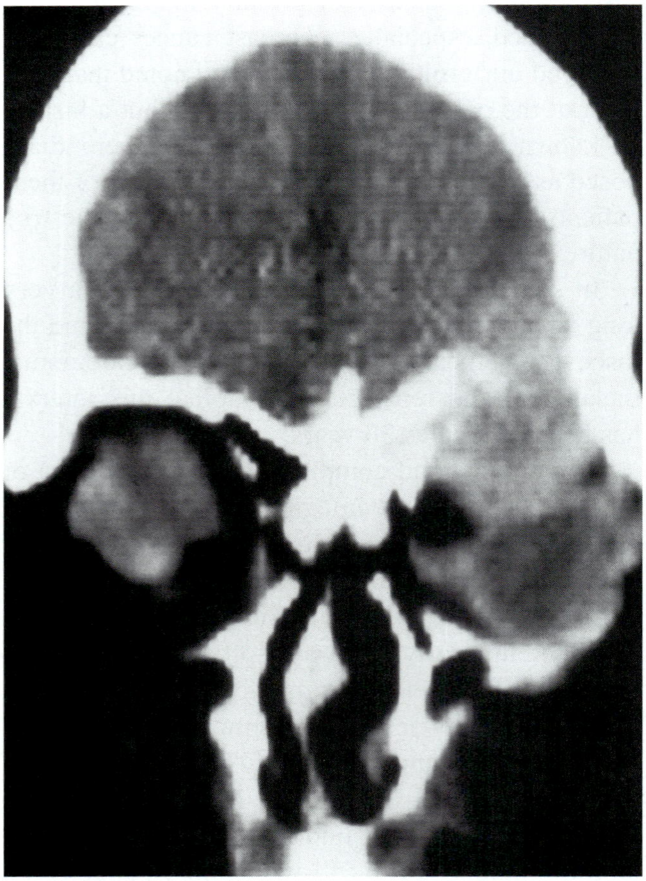

Figure 25–2. Direct coronal scan demonstrating metastatic renal carcinoma causing destruction of the orbital roof.

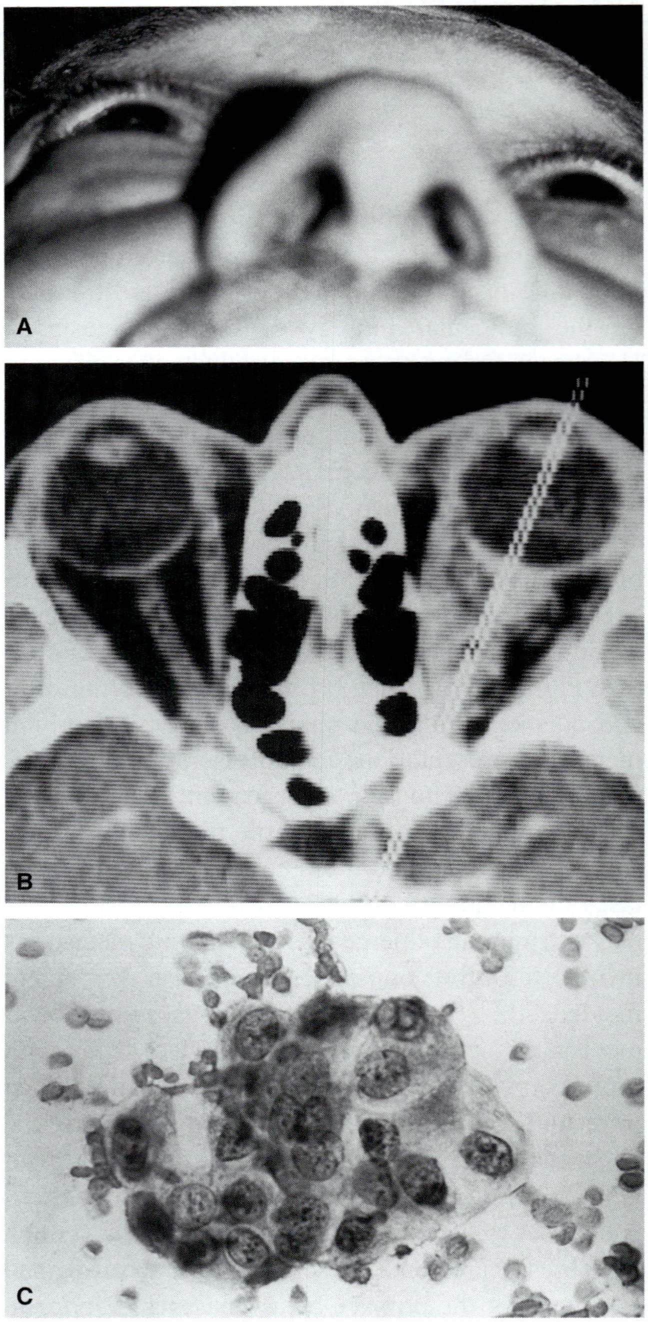

Figure 25–3. *A,* Patient who presented with axial proptosis and ophthalmoplegia. History and laboratory evaluation were negative for malignancy; diagnosis was established by FNAB. *B,* Axial CT scan demonstrates intraconal diffuse metastasis. *C,* FNAB shows the presence of an adenocarcinoma of unknown origin.

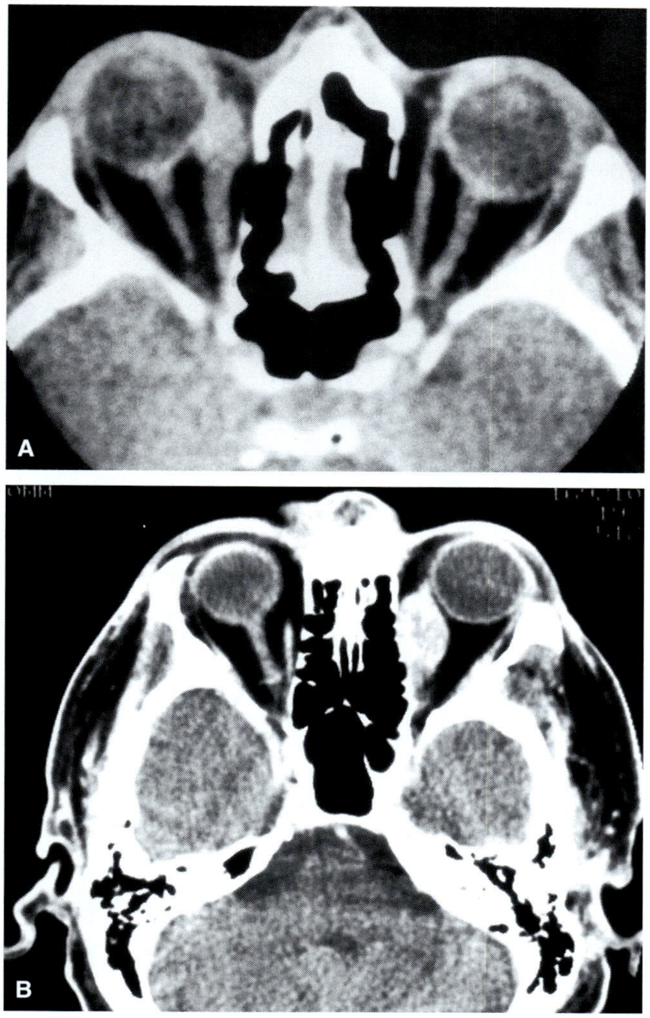

Figure 25–4. *A* and *B*, Metastatic cutaneous melanomas simulating a unifocal medial rectus enlargement. Diagnosis in both cases was confirmed with FNAB.

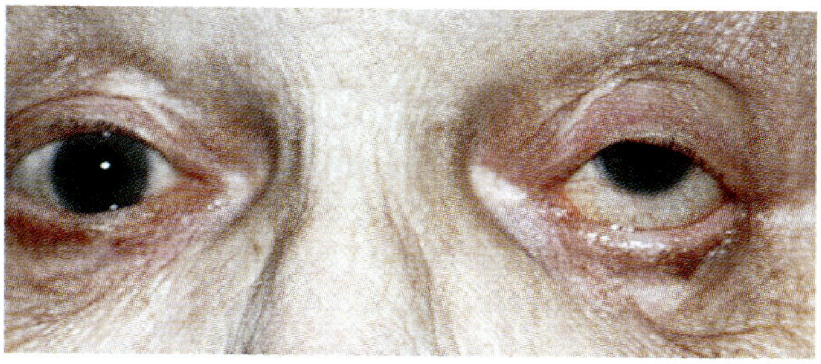

Figure 25–5. Clinical photograph of a patient with metastatic scirrhous breast carcinoma to the orbit.

or thyroid orbitopathy (see Figure 19–5). Unlike thyroid orbitopathy, which usually involves only the muscle belly, metastatic deposits in the extraocular muscles are usually less regular and often involve both the muscle belly and its tendon.

Most orbital metastases are unilateral; endophthalmos is an uncommon presentation (mainly with scirrhous breast or gastric carcinoma) (Figure 25–5).[52] Restriction of extraocular motility is frequent, and in our experience with outpatients, 50 percent presented with this symptom. The location of orbital metastases on the basis of imaging studies demonstrates that over 50 percent are extraconal, 20 percent are intraconal, and 20 percent involve both locations.[50,53] Approximately 50 percent of metastatic orbital foci involve bone; this finding is more common in patients who present with the orbital lesion prior to the discovery of the primary malignancy.[7] Figure 25–6 shows a carcinoma metastatic to the orbital bone producing an osteoblastic pattern. CT and MRI are more useful than ultrasonography in the evaluation and management of patients with suspected orbital metastases.[54,55] Often, in older patients with unsuspected orbital metastases, the differential diagnosis is between a pseudotumor and a metastasis; ultrasonography cannot differentiate these two entities.[56] The diagnostic category used by some ultrasonographers that lumps pseudotumor and metastases together is of questionable utility, since it includes the two most common diagnostic entities. We retrospectively observed that CT and MRI were more accurate than ultrasonography for diagnosing orbital metastases, and the delineation of bone, sinus, or brain involvement on MRI or CT were also superior. In some cases the T_1 and T_2 patterns of inflammation and metastases are different, but this is not

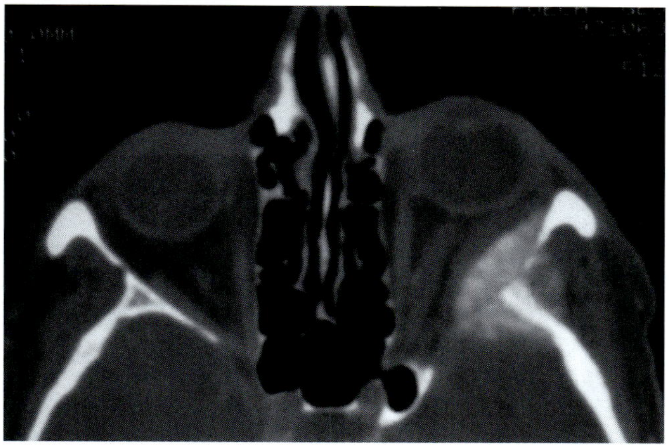

Figure 25–6. Prostate carcinoma metastatic to orbital bone. A PSA was markedly elevated.

reliable (see Table 15–2).[54] In addition, if radiation is going to be used for treatment, it is imperative to be certain that there are no occult frontal lobe metastases. The imaging techniques should be used to assess areas contiguous to the orbit.

FNAB is an excellent ancillary diagnostic modality in patients suspected of having ocular metastasis.[52,57] Figure 25–7 shows two metastatic orbital tumors diagnosed using FNAB. Figure 25–8A shows a case of scirrhous carcinoma metastatic to the orbit. The author performed multiple fine-needle biopsies under CT control, but only obtained fibrous material. An open biopsy established the correct diagnosis (Figure 25–8B). Fibrous scirrhous metastases often cannot be correctly diagnosed with this technique.[58]

In some cases, imaging studies demonstrate an indiscrete or focal lesion, and subjective findings are negative for malignancy. Figures 25–9 to 25–12

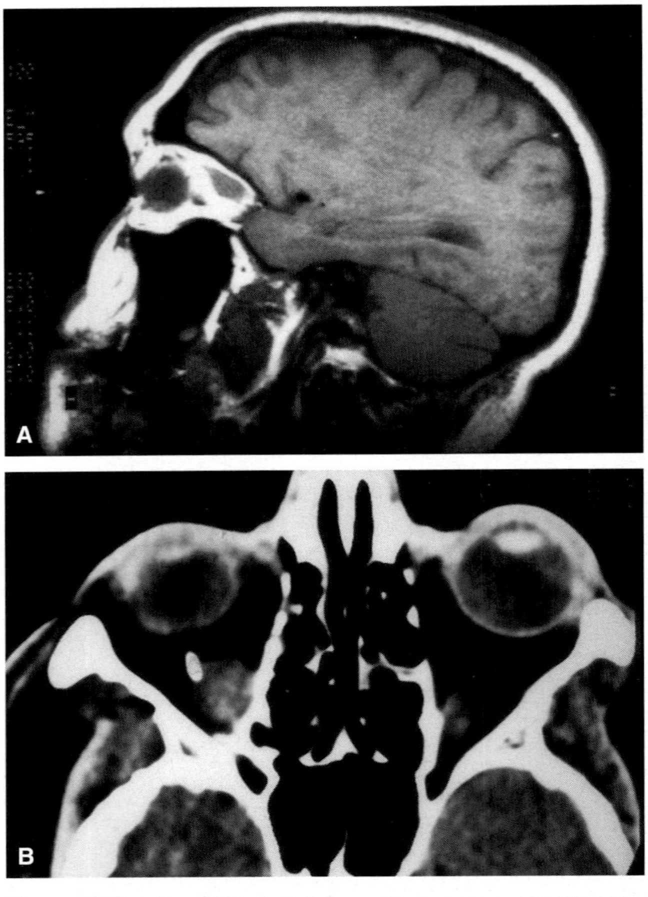

Figure 25–7. *A* and *B,* In both these patients, a diagnosis of metastases could be established with FNAB, under CT control. This biopsy technique has much lower morbidity than open surgical procedure.

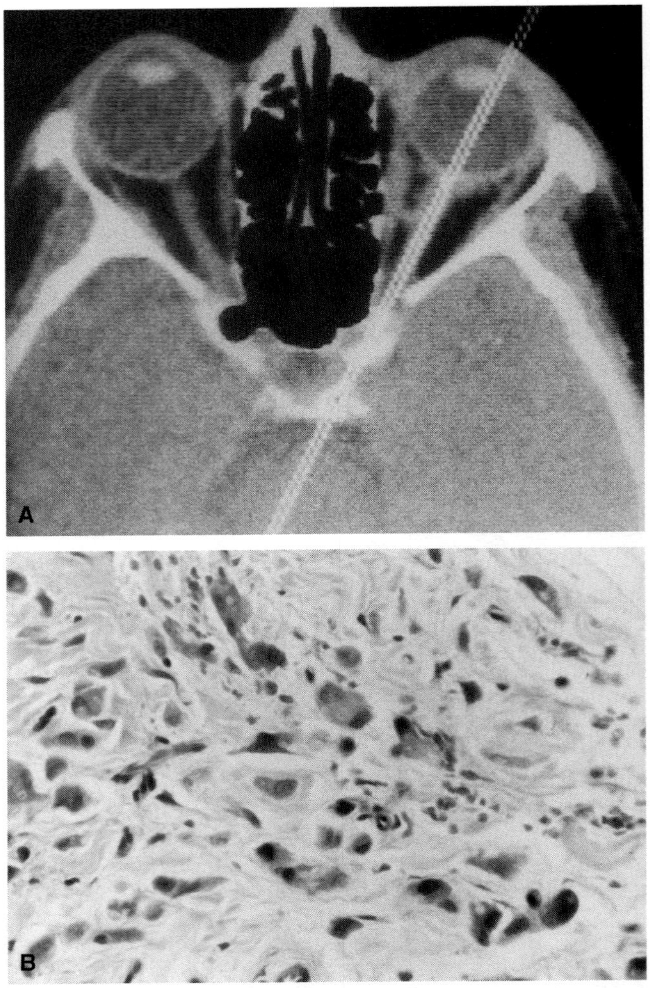

Figure 25–8. Scirrhous carcinoma metastasis into the orbit. This lesion could not be diagnosed with FNAB despite numerous attempts.

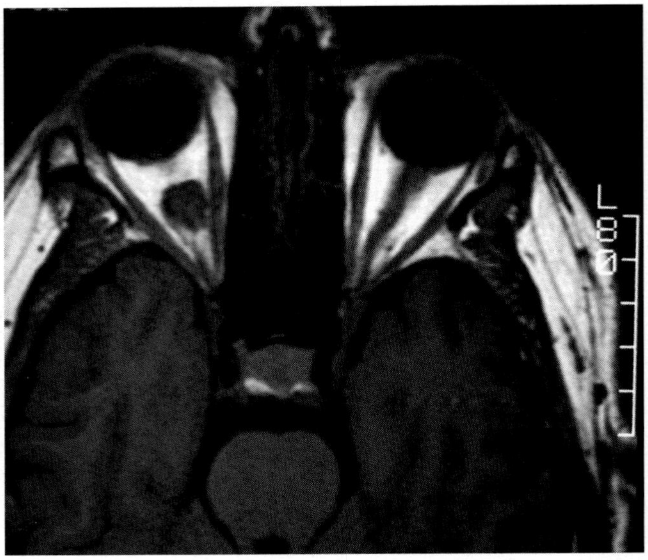

Figure 25–9. Solitary discrete orbital metastasis in a patient with no history of systemic malignancy.

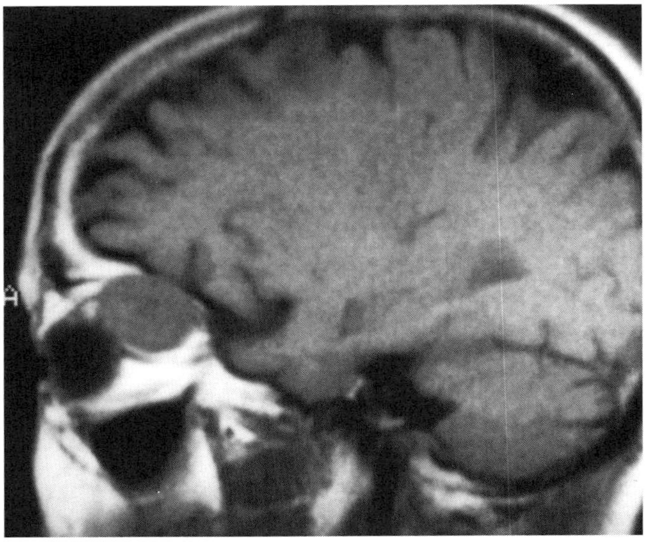

Figure 25–10. Solitary orbital lesion in a patient with a history of breast carcinoma, but no other evidence of metastatic disease.

show atypical metastatic lesions that we thought were primary orbital tumors prior to biopsy.

Palliative therapy is indicated for most orbital metastases. In one study of breast metastases to ocular structures, those to the orbit were associated with a worse prognosis than those to the choroid (2 versus 6 months survival), although data on this point are sparse.[59] In our experience with approximately 30 cases, the mean survival was < 1.3 years and < 30 percent of patients survived beyond 2 years.[1]

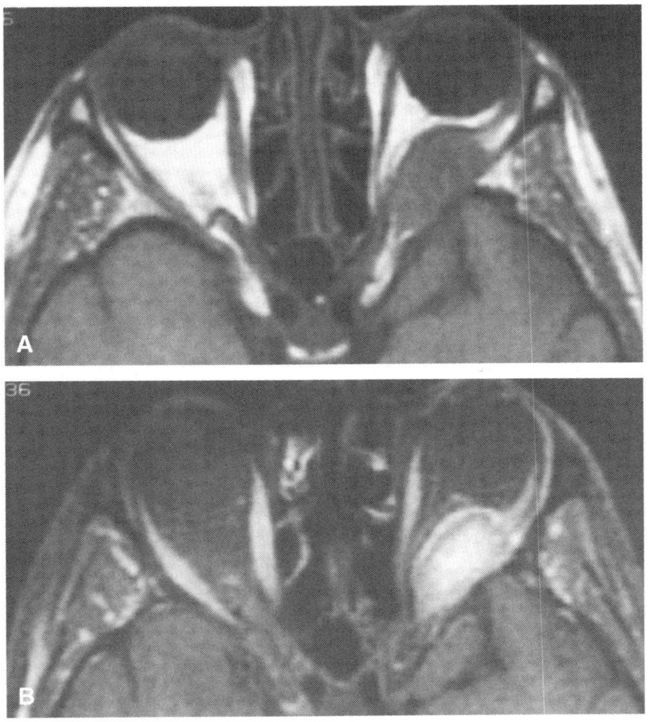

Figure 25–11. *A,* Patient with discrete lateral extraconal tumor on axial T_1-weighted MRI scan. *B,* While this tumor, like many metastases, enhanced with gadolinium, a number of other benign and malignant tumors also have this imaging pattern.

Orbital metastases are treated in four general ways. If a focal symptomatic lesion is found, it is removed (see Figure 17–12). As an example, we and others have removed uveal melanomas that have metastasized to the other orbit when they have impinged upon the remaining optic nerve, causing visual loss.[60,61] Figure 25–13 shows such a lesion compressing the optic nerve. After its removal, vision returned to 20/20. More commonly, visual loss is due to a nonresectable metastatic lesion, as this breast metastasis that compressed the optic nerve at the orbital apex (Figure 25–14). Usually, patients

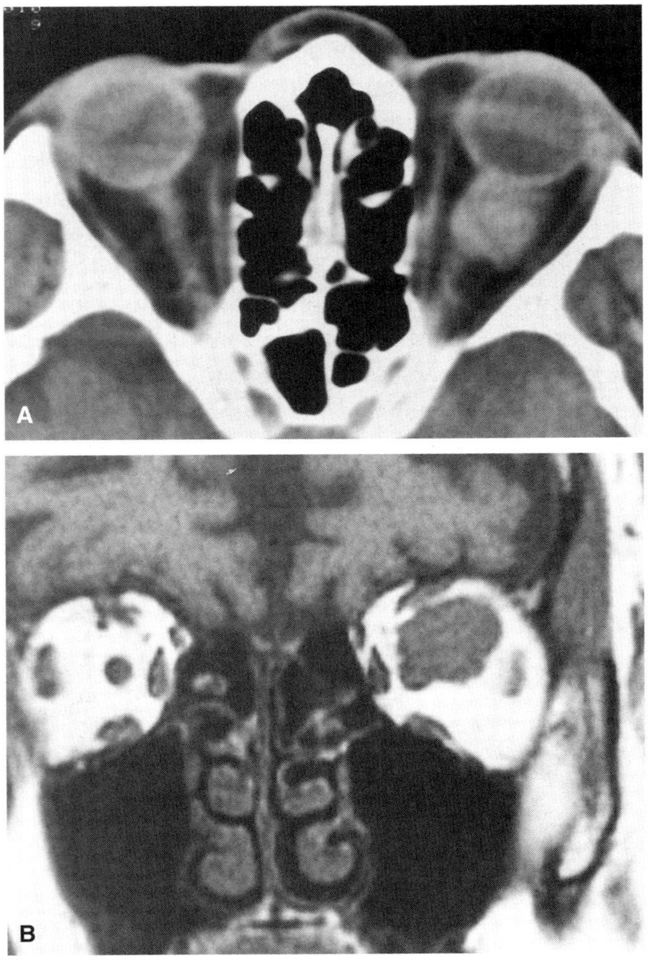

Figure 25–12. *A,* Axial CT scan shows discrete intraconal mass with a negative medical history. Biopsy showed it to be metastatic. *B,* Coronal T_1-weighted MRI scan of case shown in Figure 25–12A.

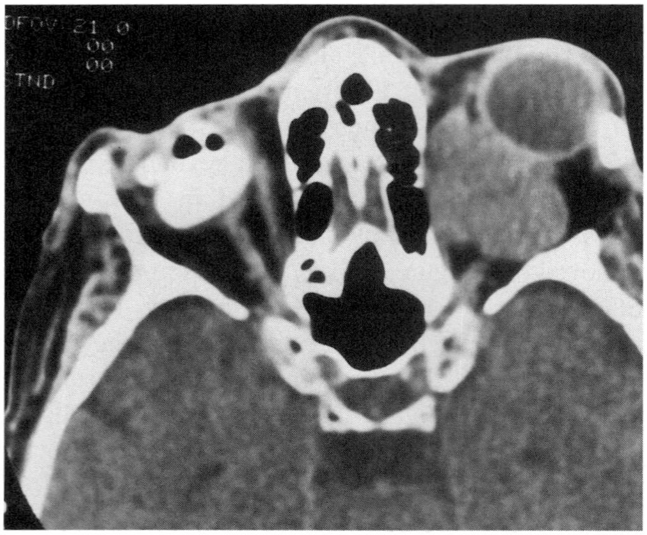

Figure 25–13. Metastatic uveal melanoma compresses the contralateral optic nerve, producing visual loss. Resection of tumor produced return of vision.

have either diffuse orbital involvement or a lesion that can only be partially debulked, due to either its location or its association with vital structures. Some of these patients respond to chemotherapy; if a new lesion is present and other systemic disease is noted, this is an excellent therapeutic option. As others have noted, many metastatic orbital foci will respond to radiation therapy.[4,13,59–67] Often, we use a total of 40 gray of external beam photon irradiation for diffuse orbital metastases, for lesions that cannot be removed in toto without damage to vision, and for lesions not responsive to chemotherapy. Most patients with orbital metastases whom we have treated with radiation and chemotherapy had a good orbital response. Some authors have noted that patients with orbital carcinoid, which produces 5-hydroxyindoleacetic acid (5-HIAA), appear not to respond well to this treatment; but that was not our experience in 4 patients. Patients with cutaneous melanoma metastatic to the orbit were not responsive to either photon or charged particle radiation.[47,48]

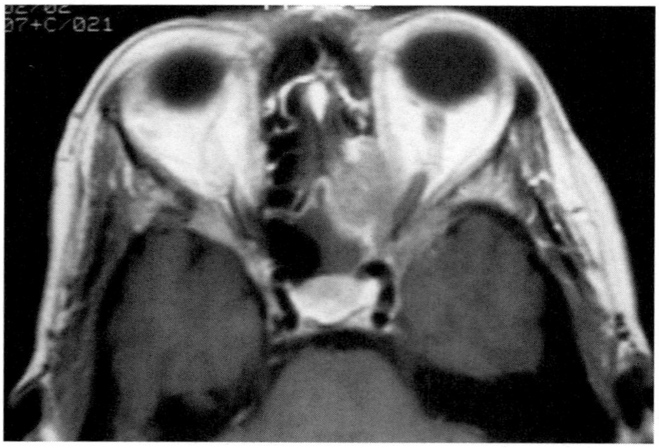

Figure 25–14. T_1-weighted axial MRI scan shows optic nerve compression by a breast metastasis to the orbital apex. This responded nicely to irradiation.

As others have observed, patients with orbital metastases have a limited life expectancy. In our experience, the mean survival is 1.3 years, which is similar to that reported in some other series.

REFERENCES

1. Char DH, Miller T, Kroll S. Orbital metastases: diagnosis and course. Br J Ophthalmol 1997;81:586–90.
2. Henderson JW. Metastatic carcinoma. In: Orbital tumors. New York, NY: Raven Press; 1994. p. 361–76.
3. Bedford PD, Daniel PM. Discrete carcinomatous metastases in the extrinsic ocular muscles: a case of carcinoma of the breast with exophthalmic ophthalmoplegia. Am J Ophthalmol 1960;49:723–6.
4. Ashton N, Morgan G. Discrete carcinomatous metastases in the extraocular muscles. Br J Ophthalmol 1974;58:112–7.
5. Cuttone JM, Litvin J, McDonald JE. Carcinoma metastatic to an extraocular muscle. Ann Ophthalmol 1981;13:213–6.
6. Hesselink JR, Davis KR, Weber AL, et al. Radiological evaluation of orbital metastasis with emphasis on computed tomography. Radiology 1980;137:363–6.
7. Font RL, Ferry AP. Carcinoma metastatic to the eye and orbit: III. A clinicopathologic study of 28 cases metastatic to the orbit. Cancer 1976;38:1326–35.
8. Healy JF. Computed tomographic evaluation of metastasis to the orbit. Ann Ophthalmol 1983;15:1026–9.
9. Wolter JR, Hendrix RC. Osteoblastic prostate carcinoma metastatic to the orbit. Am J Ophthalmol 1981;91:648–51.
10. Griffith DG, Passmore JW, Penner R. Ultrasonographic discovery of cyst formation in metastatic neuroblastoma. Am J Ophthalmol 1967;63:313–6.
11. Cline RA, Rootman J. Enophthalmos: a clinical review. Ophthalmology 1984;91:229–37.
12. Howard GM, Jakobiec FA, Trokel SL, et al. Pulsating metastatic tumor of the orbit. Am J Ophthalmol 1978;85:767–71.
13. Hart WM. Metastatic carcinoma to the eye and orbit. Int Ophthalmol Clin 1962;2:465–82.
14. Hutchinson DS, Smith TR. Ocular and orbital metastatic carcinoma. Ann Ophthalmol 1979;11:869–73.

15. Fratkin JD, Purcell JJ, Krachmer JH, Taylor JC. Wilms' tumor metastatic to the orbit. JAMA 1977;238: 1841–2.
16. Clark WC. Adrenal neuroblastoma with particular reference to metastasis to the orbit: report of a case and notes on 2 other cases. Arch Ophthalmol 1939;22: 575–80.
17. Kindermann WR, Shields JA, Eiferman RA, et al. Metastatic renal cell carcinoma to the eye and adnexae. A report of 3 cases and a review of the literature. Ophthalmology 1981;88:1347–50.
18. Ferry AP, Naghdi MR. Bronchogenic carcinoma metastatic to the orbit. Arch Ophthalmol 1967;77: 214–6.
19. Albert DM, Rubenstein RA, Scheie HG. Tumor metastasis to the eye: II. Clinical study in infants and children. Am J Ophthalmol 1967;63:727–32.
20. Krauss HR, Slamovits TL, Sibony PA, et al. Orbital metastasis of bladder carcinoma. Am J Ophthalmol 1982;94:265–7.
21. Harris AL, Montgomery A, Reyes RR, et al. Carcinoid tumour presenting as an orbital metastasis. Clin Oncol 1981;7:365–72.
22. Reifler DM, Kini SR, Liu D, Littleton RH. Orbital metastasis from prostatic carcinoma: identification by immunocytology. Arch Ophthalmol 1984;102:292–5.
23. Sniderman HR, Neel WV. Orbital metastasis from tumor of the pancreas; report of 2 cases with necropsy findings. Am J Ophthalmol 1942;25:1215–21.
24. Winkler CF, Goodman GK, Eiferman RA, Yam LT. Orbital metastasis from prostatic carcinoma: identification by an immunoperoxidase technique. Arch Ophthalmol 1981;99:1406–8.
25. Divine RD, Anderson RL, Ossoinig KC. Metastatic carcinoid unresponsive to radiation therapy presenting as a lacrimal fossa mass. Ophthalmology 1982; 89:516–20.
26. Bullock JD, Straughen WJ. Carcinoma of the common bile duct metastatic to the orbit. Ann Ophthalmol 1981;13:619–21.
27. Zubler MA, Rivera R, Lane M. Hepatoma presenting as a retro-orbital metastasis. Cancer 1981;48:1883–5.
28. Khan AU, Greene LF, Neault RW. Orbital metastasis from prostatic carcinoma. Int Surg 1977;62:465–7.
29. Scharf Y, Ben Arieh Y, Gellei B. Orbital metastases from extra-adrenal pheochromocytoma. Am J Ophthalmol 1970;69:638–40.
30. Lubin JR, Grove AS Jr, Zakov ZN, Albert DM. Hepatoma metastatic to the orbit. Am J Ophthalmol 1980;89:268–73.
31. Usui T, Ishibe T, Nihira H. Orbital metastasis from prostatic carcinoma. Br J Urol 1975;47:458.
32. Harris AL, Montgomery A. Orbital carcinoid tumor. Am J Ophthalmol 1980;90:875–7.
33. Carriere VM, Karcioglu ZA, Apple DJ, Insler MS. A case of prostate carcinoma with bilateral orbital metastases, and review of the literature. Ophthalmology 1982;89:402–6.
34. Zucker JL, Doyle MF. Mycosis fungoides metastatic to the orbit. Arch Ophthalmol 1991;109:688–91.
35. Liu GT, Schatz NJ, Curtin VT, Tse DT. Bilateral extraocular muscle metastases in Zollinger-Ellison syndrome. Arch Ophthalmol 1994;112:451–2.
36. Feinmesser M, Hurwitz JJ, Heathcote JG. Pleural malignant mesothelioma metastatic to the orbit. Can J Ophthalmol 1994;29:193–7.
37. Fan JT, Buettner H, Bartley GB, Bolling JP. Clinical features and treatment of seven patients with carcinoid tumor metastatic to the eye and orbit. Am J Ophthalmol 1995;119:211–8.
38. Van Gelderen WFC. Gastric carcinoma metastases to extraocular muscles. J Comput Assist Tomogr 1993; 17:499–500.
39. Hartstein ME, Grove AS Jr, Woog JJ. The role of the integrin family of adhesion molecules in the development of tumors metastatic to the orbit. Ophthal Plast Reconstr Surg 1997;13:227–38.
40. Font RL, Maturi RK, Small RG, Garcia-Rojas M. Hepatocellular carcinoma metastatic to the orbit. Arch Ophthalmol 1998;116:942–5.
41. Feeza J, Sinard J. Metastatic liposarcoma to the orbit. Am J Ophthalmol 1997;123:271–2.
42. Gunalp I, Gunduz K. Secondary orbital tumors. Ophthal Plast Reconstr Surg 1997;13:31–5.
43. Stockl FA, Tucker N, Burnier M. Thymic carcinoma metastatic to the orbit. Am J Ophthalmol 1997;124: 401–3.
44. Chynn EW, Rubin PAD. Metastatic Ewing cell sarcoma of the sinus and osteoid osteoma of the orbit. Am J Ophthalmol 1997;123:565–7.
45. Garcia GH, Weinberg DA, Glasgow BJ, et al. Carcinoma of the male breast metastatic to both orbits. Ophthal Plast Reconstr Surg 1998;14:130–3.
46. Lee HM, Choo CT, Poh WT. Orbital metastasis from carcinoma of the cerivx. Br J Ophthalmol 1997; 81:330–1.
47. Geetha N, Chandralekha B, Kumar A, et al. Carcinoma of the pancreas presenting as an orbital tumor: a case report. Am J Clin Oncol 1998;21:532–3.
48. Bullock JD, Yanes B. Ophthalmic manifestations of metastatic breast cancer. Ophthalmology 1980;87: 961–73.
49. Rosenkranz L, Schroeder C. Recurrent malignant melanoma following a 46 year disease-free interval. NY State J Med 1985;85:95.
50. Norman D, Char DH. Current concepts in imaging of the orbit. In: Margulis AR, Goodling CA, editors.

Diagnostic radiology. San Francisco, CA: Radiological Research and Education Foundation; 1984. p. 321.
51. Toller KK, Gigantelli JW, Spalding MJ. Bilateral orbital metastases from breast carcinoma. A case of false pseudotumor. Ophthalmology 1998;105:1897–901.
52. Logrono R, Inhorn SL, Dortzbach RK, Kurtycz DF. Leiomyosarcoma metastatic to the orbit: diagnosis of fine-needle aspiration. Diagn Cytopathol 1997;17:369–73.
53. Balchunas WR, Quencer RM, Byrne SF. Lacrimal gland and fossa masses: evaluation by computed tomography and A-mode echography. Radiology 1983;149:751–8.
54. Char DH, Sobel D, Kelly WM, et al. Magnetic resonance scanning in orbital tumor diagnosis. Ophthalmology 1985;92:1305–10.
55. DiBernardo C, Pacheco EM, Hughes FR, et al. Echographic evaluation and findings in metastatic melanoma to extraocular muscles. Ophthalmology 1996;103:1794–7.
56. Kennerdell JS. Discussion. Ophthalmology 1985;92: 669–70.
57. Cangiarella JF, Cajigas A, Savala E, et al. Fine-needle aspiration cytology of orbital masses. Acta Cytol 1996;40:1205–11.
58. Mottow-Lippa L, Jakobiec FA, Iwamoto T. Pseudoinflammatory metastatic breast carcinoma of the orbit and lids. Ophthalmology 1981;88:575–80.
59. Ratanatharathorn V, Powers WE, Grimm J, et al. Eye metastasis from carcinoma of the breast: diagnosis, radiation treatment and results. Cancer Treat Rev 1991;18:261–76.
60. Orcutt JC, Char DH. Melanoma metastatic to the orbit. Ophthalmology 1988;95:1033–7.
61. Hutchinson BM, Damato BE, Kyle PM, Harnett AN. Choroidal melanoma metastatic to the contralateral orbit. Orbit 1994;13:85–9.
62. Apple DJ. Metastatic orbital neuroblastoma originating in the cervical sympathetic ganglionic chain. Am J Ophthalmol 1969;68:1093–5.
63. Heckemann R, Schmitt G. Ergebnisse der Strahlentherapie metastatischer Orbitatumoren. Strahlentherapie 1978;154:179–81.
64. Hih SH, Nisce LZ, Simpson LD, Chu FCH. Value of radiation therapy in the treatment of orbital metastasis. Am J Roentgenol Radium Ther Nucl Med 1974;120:589–94.
65. Musarella MA, Chan HS, DeBoer G, Gallie BL. Ocular involvement in neuroblastoma: prognostic implications. Ophthalmology 1984;91:936–40.
66. Burmeister BH, Benjamin CS, Childs WJ. The management of metastases to eye and orbit from carcinoma of the breast. Austral NZ J Ophthalmol 1990; 18:187–90.
67. Goldberg RA, Rootman J, Cline RA. Tumors metastatic to the orbit: a changing picture. Surv Ophthalmol 1990;35:1–24.

26

Orbital Lymphoid Lesions and Orbital Pseudotumors

Orbital pseudotumor was first described by Birch-Hirschfield in 1905. As in idiopathic inflammations of other body sites, a number of pathogenic theories have been proposed, but the etiology of orbital pseudotumor is still unknown and lacks an animal model.[1–4] Orbital pseudotumor remains a diagnosis of exclusion.

Histologically, these lesions usually consist of either a monoclonal or heterogenous lymphoid proliferation or an inflammatory-fibrotic process; occasionally, vasculitis or a combination of these types is present. Several classifications have been proposed; some authors separate lymphoid lesions from other inflammatory and fibrotic processes.[5] Others have grouped all these idiopathic lesions together under the same rubric of orbital pseudotumor. This chapter includes all these entities. They have not been separated for three reasons: (1) the etiologies are uncertain. While it is likely that several of the entities are distinct and have a different pathogenesis and natural history, until we have better understanding of the nature of these processes, there is no point in having an artificial classification system; (2) often, these lesions can have an overlapping set of symptoms and presentations; and (3) many of these orbital pseudotumors are treated in a similar manner.

The choice between one all-inclusive system or separate systems of classification is, at present, semantic. As we develop a better understanding of the pathogenesis and pathophysiology of these processes, a classification system based on those parameters will be developed. A major point, which will be discussed in detail below, is that in the patient with idiopathic, apparently benign, lymphoid lesions (even those which are heterogenous on flow cytometry or DNA Southern blots) there is a significant risk for the development of systemic lymphoma. In patients with pure inflammatory and fibrotic processes, this risk is not present.

The differential diagnosis of inflammatory pseudotumor includes numerous conditions, a list of which is found in Table 26–1.[3]

Fungal and parasitic infections can involve the orbit and simulate pseudotumors; such entities include aspergillosis, mucormycosis, actinomycosis,

Table 26–1. DIFFERENTIAL DIAGNOSIS OF PSEUDOTUMOR
Benign systemic diseases with associated orbital inflammation
Systemic lupus erythematosus
Polyarteritis nodosa
Sarcoidosis
Lipidosis
Pseudotumor with sclerosing cholangitis
Langerhans' cell proliferations (histiocytosis syndromes)
Pseudorheumatoid nodule
Necrobiotic xanthogranuloma
Erdheim-Chester disease
Wegener's granulomatosis
Sinusitis with contiguous orbital inflammation
Malignant lymphoid lesions
Lymphoma
Leukemia
Plasmacytoma
Midline lethal granuloma
Mycosis fungoides
Infectious processes
Fungus (aspergillosis, mucormycosis, actinomycosis, histoplasmosis, coccidiodomycosis, parasitic echinococcosis, cysticercosis, dirofilariasis, bilharziasis, ascariasis, onchocerciasis)
Bacteria
Miscellaneous processes
Ruptured dermoid
Retained orbital foreign body
Amyloidosis
Nodular fasciitis
Metastasis

histoplasmosis, coccidiomycosis, echinococcosis, cysticercosis, dirofilarisasis, bilharzia, ascariasis, and onchocerciasis.[3] In acquired immune deficiency syndrome (AIDS) and with more sophisticated means of salvaging patients with advanced systemic malignancies using agents which may cause further immunosuppression, other rare infectious agents have been shown to produce orbital involvement.

Orbital lymphoid lesions and idiopathic orbital pseudotumors are common; they account for 11 to 20 percent of orbital biopsies.[6,7] Orbital malignant lymphoid lesions usually present as an isolated neoplasm; in < 15 percent of these cases, there is either a history of systemic lymphoma or the simultaneous onset of orbital and widespread disease. Generally, pain is a less common presenting symptom in malignant than in benign lymphoid lesions.

DIAGNOSIS

The clinical presentation of orbital pseudotumors is varied and depends on the pattern of orbital and ocular involvement. Inflammation can be isolated to single or multiple extraocular muscles (idiopathic orbital myositis) (Figures 26–1 to 26–4), or it can diffusely involve the orbit and globe (Figure 26–5). Inflammation may present as a lacrimal gland mass (Figure 26–6) and have diffuse infiltration of orbital fat, mus-

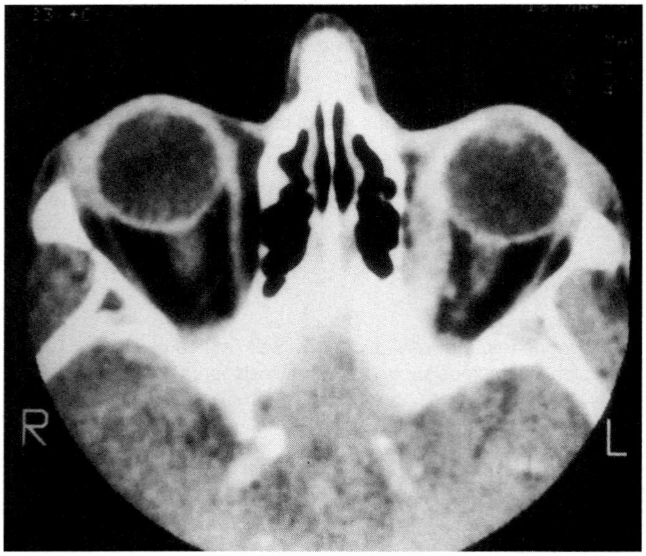

Figure 26–1. Axial CT scan shows idiopathic myositis. This case responded completely to high-dose oral steroids. Note: unlike thyroid myopathy, both the muscle and its tendon are involved.

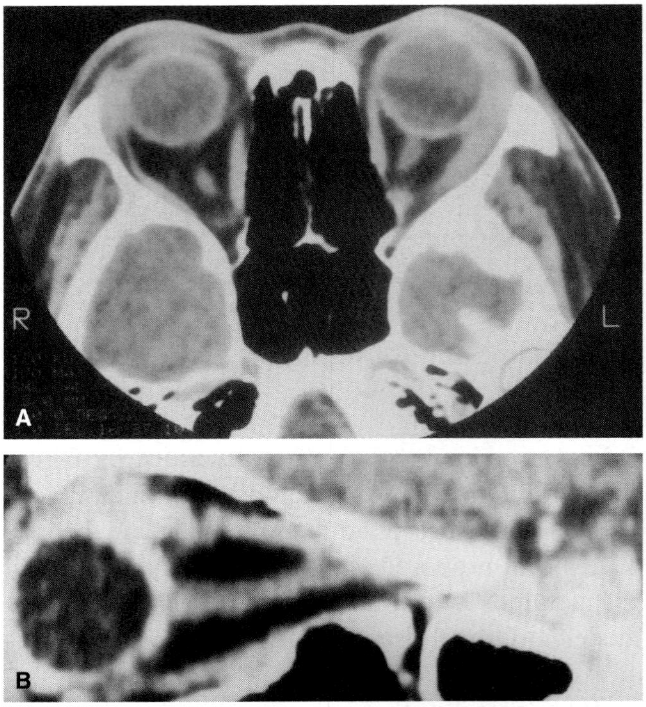

Figure 26–2. *A,* Axial CT scan of a patient with lateral rectus myositis. *B,* Parasagittal reconstruction of a CT scan of a different patient with idiopathic myositis involving the superior rectus complex.

cle, sclera, and nerve (Figure 26–7 and 26–8), or it may focally affect the orbital apex and cavernous sinus area (Tolosa-Hunt syndrome) (Figures 26–8A and B).[8–10] Rarely, it can even present with intraocular signs, such as cystoid macular edema.[11] If inflammation is limited to the orbital apex, pain, ptosis, and ophthalmoplegia are present; often the pupil is spared.[12–14] Any age group may develop orbital lymphoid lesions, but idiopathic myositis appears to be more common in young adults, while other forms of orbital pseudotumors or lymphomas are more common in older patients.[15–17]

Orbital pseudotumor patients usually present with the history of sudden onset of deep orbital pain and periocular redness. If there is anterior inflammation, an associated diffuse scleritis is usually seen (Figure 26–9), along with lid swelling (Figure 26–10). In cases of posterior orbital inflammation or isolated mass lesions, scleritis may not be visible. Pain is less common in patients who present with an isolated lymphoid mass lesion (Figure 26–11).

Idiopathic orbital myositis is a relatively uncommon form of orbital pseudotumor, and it is more common in young patients (see Figures 26–1 to 26–4).[16,17]

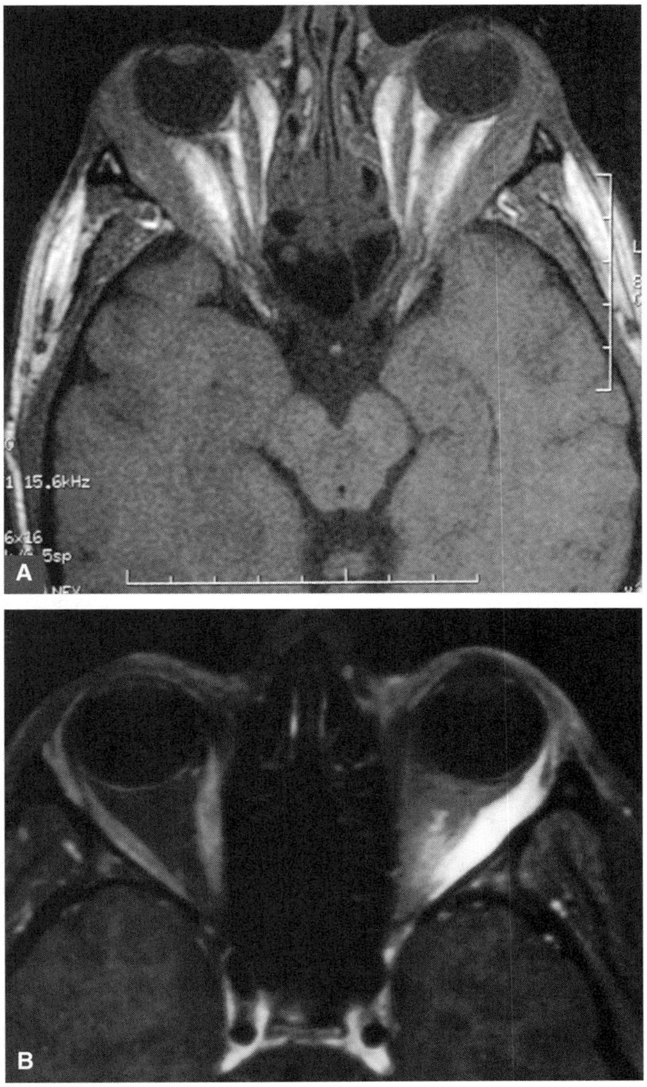

Figure 26–3. *A,* T_1-weighted axial MRI scan of a patient with lateral rectus myositis. *B,* Usually, with gadolinium, there is enhancement of the inflammatory mass. This process completely resolved on a 1-week course of high-dose oral corticosteroids.

If it is present, there is usually painful limitation of the muscle, especially toward its field of action. This pattern is usually distinct from that observed in thyroid orbitopathy. In thyroid eye disease, if the inferior rectus is involved, the patient can look down but is restricted in upgaze. In contrast, with idiopathic myositis, if the inferior rectus is involved, usually, the patient can look up but has problems looking down. This pattern is not always the case and during the natural history of this disease alterations can occur. In one series, 13 of the 15 reported cases involved patients between the ages of 18 and 30 years.[18,19] These patients have acute onset of pain, double

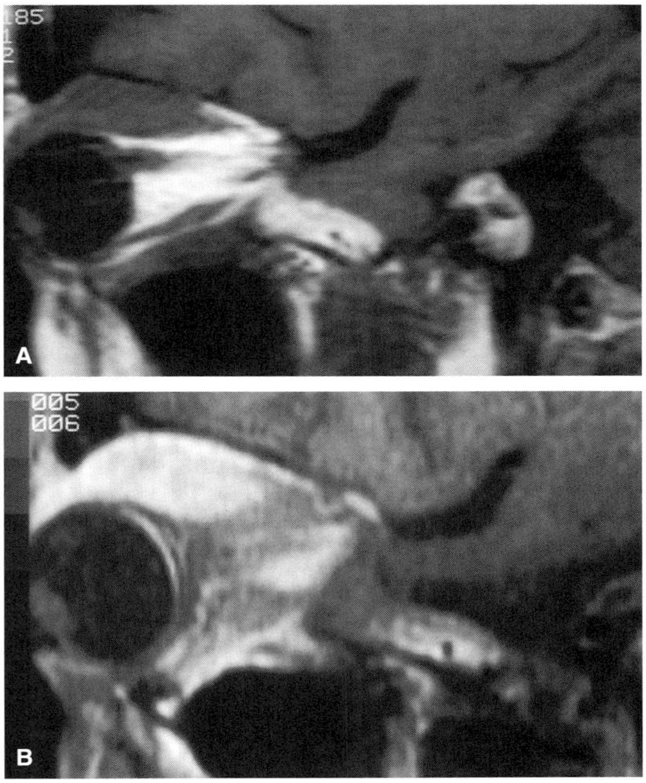

Figure 26–4. *A,* Direct parasagittal MRI scan of a lymphoid lesion of the superior muscle complex. *B,* Gadolinium of the lesion shown in Figure 26–4A.

vision, and eyelid swelling. They are extremely responsive to short-term systemic steroids.[20,21] In retrospective analysis, one group noted that a solitary muscle was involved in 68 percent of cases.[18] The two most common muscles involved are the medial and lateral recti. In about one-third of cases, there was

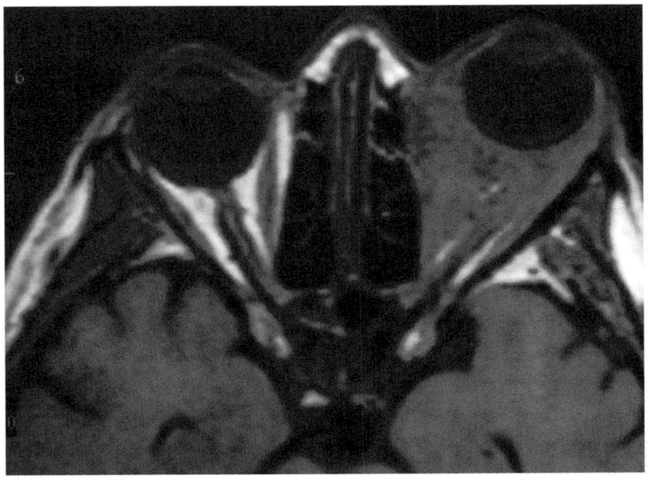

Figure 26–5. Axial MRI scan demonstrating diffuse orbital inflammation of biopsy-proven pseudotumor.

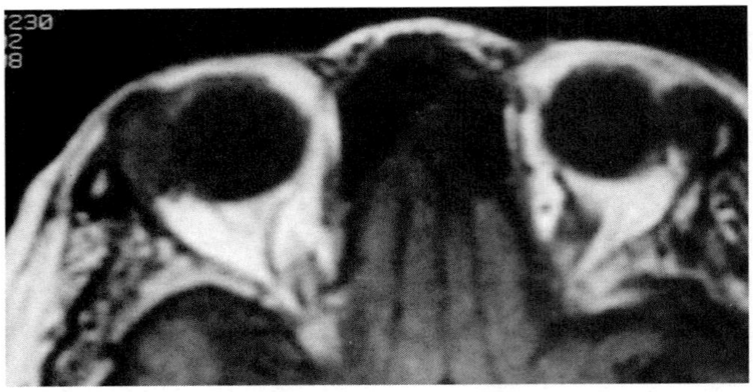

Figure 26–6. Axial MRI scan shows a pseudotumor arising bilaterally in the region of the lacrimal glands.

coexistent scleritis.[18] In that study, 68 percent responded to oral steroids, but 20 percent had one or more recurrences. In a series of 26 patients in a report from London, 6 had recurrent disease, and factors associated with recurrence were male gender, lack of proptosis, eyelid retraction, and bilateral involvement. Eighty-five percent of patients responded to a 3-week course of nonsteroidal medications. Nine of the 26 who did not respond to this had a good response to midrange oral prednisone, although 23 percent of these patients had recurrences.

A small minority of these patients with idiopathic myositis have later been diagnosed with thyroid orbitopathy. Rarely, the strabismus due to orbital myositis does not resolve, and a few patients have been treated with botulinum injection. In one series, 3 of 5 had a reasonable response.[22]

In addition to the marked difference in symptoms between idiopathic orbital myositis and thyroid orbitopathy, either magnetic resonance imaging

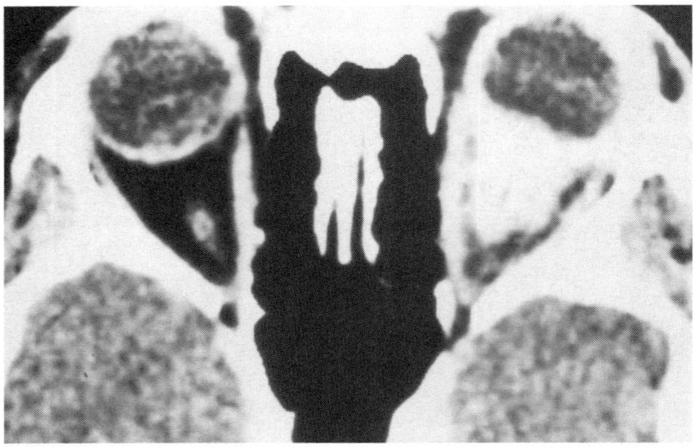

Figure 26–7. Axial CT scan shows the pseudotumor that involves the sclera, optic nerve, and the orbit diffusely.

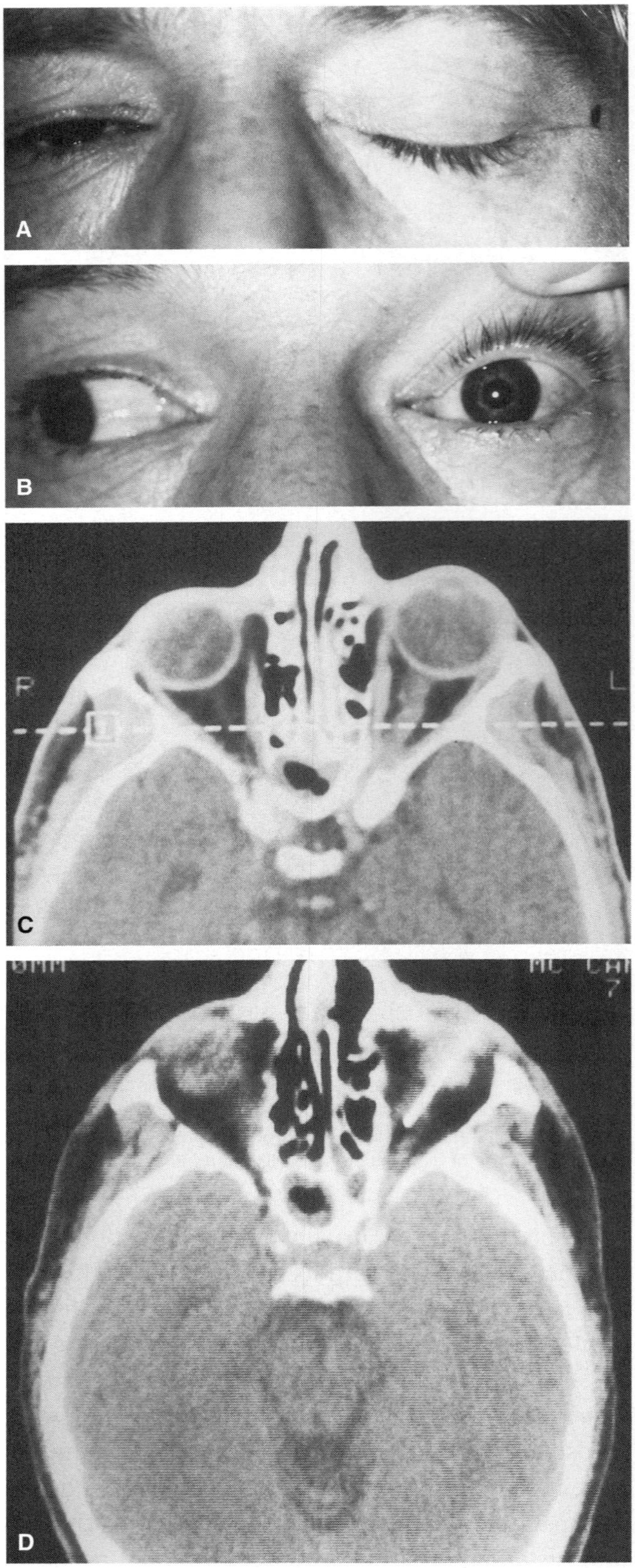

Figure 26–8. *A* and *B,* Tolosa-Hunt syndrome: clinical photographs of a patient who presented with ophthalmoplegia. *C,* Axial CT scan with coronal reconstruction showing apical and cavernous sinus inflammation. *D,* Fine-needle aspiration biopsy confirming diagnosis.

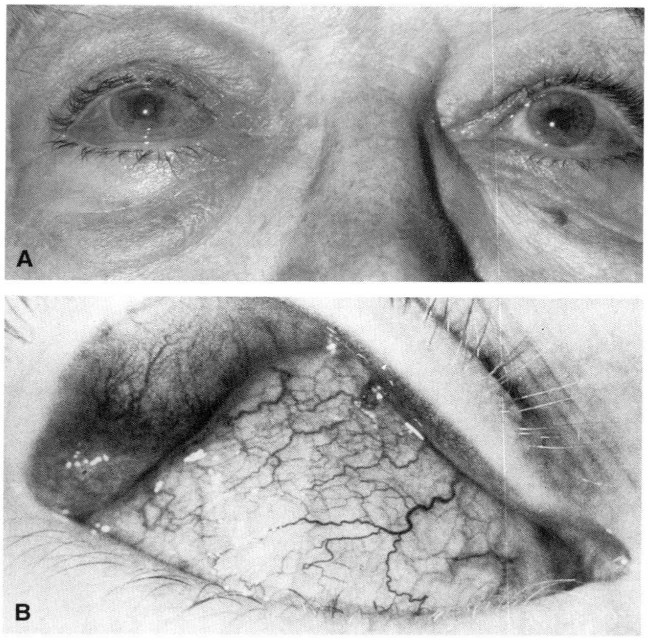

Figure 26–9. Clinical photographs of scleritis in a patient with orbital pseudotumor. (From Char et al.,[25] with permission).

(MRI) or computed tomography (CT) usually shows sparing of the tendinous portion of the muscle in thyroid myopathy versus the involvement of the entire muscle in orbital myositis (see Figures 26–1 to 26–4).[17] In older patients, lymphoid lesions can involve the extraocular muscles (see Figures 19–2 and 19–3), but often, there are less dramatic muscular symptoms associated with those processes.

A paucity of associated systemic signs or symptoms accompanies orbital pseudotumor; the presence of other nonocular signs or symptoms or bilateral orbital inflammation suggests a systemic disease process.[23] Blodi and Gass noted that the incidence of systemic disease was significantly higher in patients with bilateral orbital inflammation.[23] Orbital inflammation is more prevalent in the middle or superior orbit than in the inferior orbital area. Some authors feel that there is a higher predilection for lymphoid lesions in the anterior orbit while pseudotumor is more likely to have posterior involvement. My experience and the experience of most others have not mirrored this.[24–26]

A number of less common findings have been reported with orbital pseudotumor, including optic neuritis, which can simulate a meningioma, posterior scleritis, which can simulate a melanoma, and uveitis (see Figure 26–7).[27,28] The uveitis associated with orbital pseudotumor is variable. If there is predominantly anterior inflammation, it is more common to see an iridocyclitis; in diffuse orbital disease, diffuse (anterior and posterior) uveal inflammation is more prevalent. Extraorbital extension of orbital pseudotumor is rare. We believe that unless proven otherwise with a representative biopsy, extraorbital extension suggests malignant disease. Nevertheless, central nervous system (CNS) (Figure 26–12) and contiguous sinus involvement (Figure 26–13) have both been reported with orbital pseudotumors.[29–34] Rarely, idiopathic inflammation can involve a single nerve, as shown in Figure 26–14. Orbital pseudotumors can rarely be a presenting sign of temporal arteritis.[35] Other findings that are helpful to establish the diagnosis of temporal arteritis are jaw claudication, neck pain, elevated erythrocyte sedimentation rate (ESR), and elevated cross-reactive protein.[36]

Sclerosing orbital pseudotumors have been described since the 1960s and account for around 20

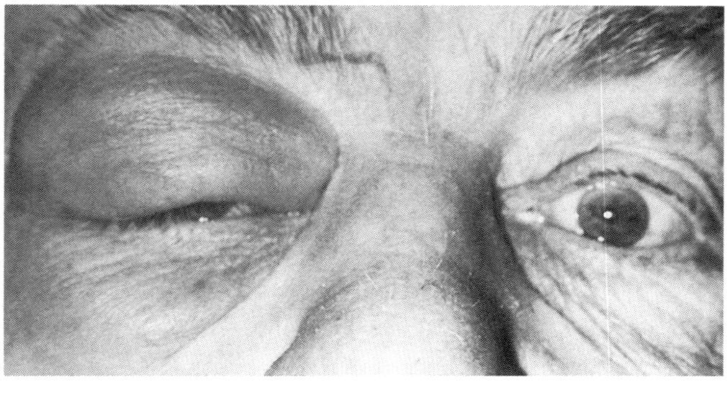

Figure 26–10. Clinical photograph of a patient presenting with lacrimal gland orbital pseudotumor and extensive anterior segment inflammation.

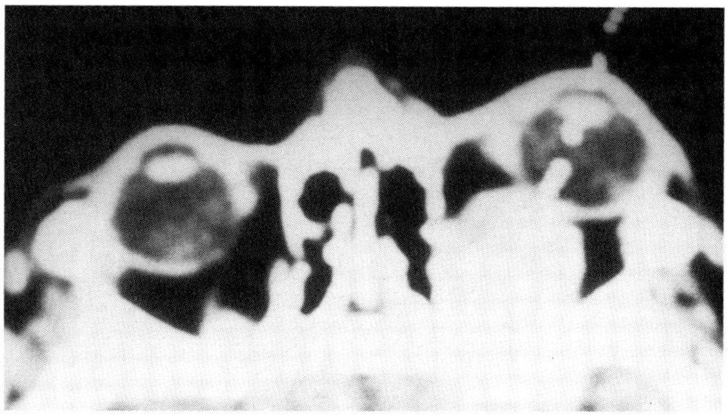

Figure 26–11. Axial CT scan with parasagittal reconstruction of an orbital lymphoid lesion.

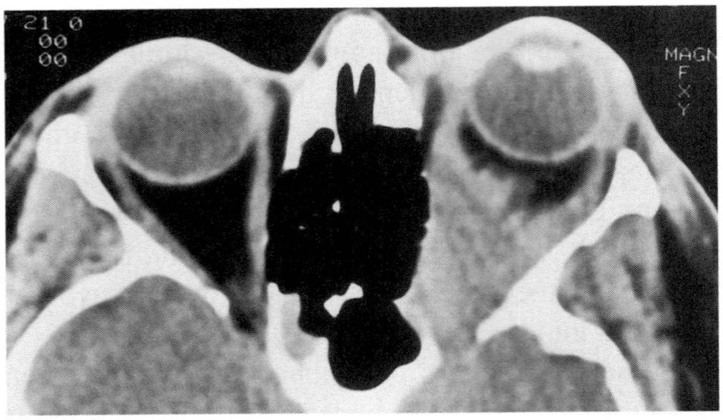

Figure 26–12. Axial CT scan demonstrates biopsy-proven orbital pseudotumor with involvement of the contiguous central nervous system.

percent of orbital pseudotumors.[37–39] Several investigators have commented on the possibility that this reflects a systemic process, and that often these will respond to cytotoxic agents.[38,39]

Wegener's granulomatosis can simulate orbital pseudotumor.[40–42] Ocular involvement is common; in one series, the eye and adnexa were involved in 58 percent of the cases. This entity is characterized by necrotizing granulomas of the respiratory tract and both necrotizing granulomas and angiitis of the sinuses, kidney, and orbit. Ocular involvement usually coincides with sinus disease but may include scleritis, marginal keratitis, and isolated involvement of the extraocular muscles, cranial nerves, or lacrimal gland.[43] In a series of 13 cases with orbital involvement, all eventually developed sinus disease.[44] Iris neovascularization can also occur. A limited form of Wegener's granulomatosis has been described with pulmonary, but not renal, involve-

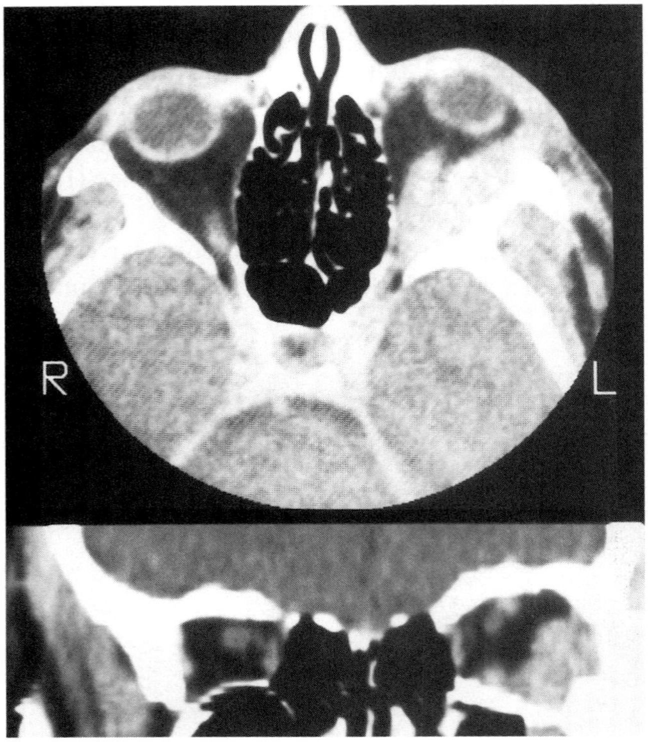

Figure 26–13. Orbital pseudotumor on axial CT scan with coronal reconstruction demonstrating involvement of the maxillary sinus.

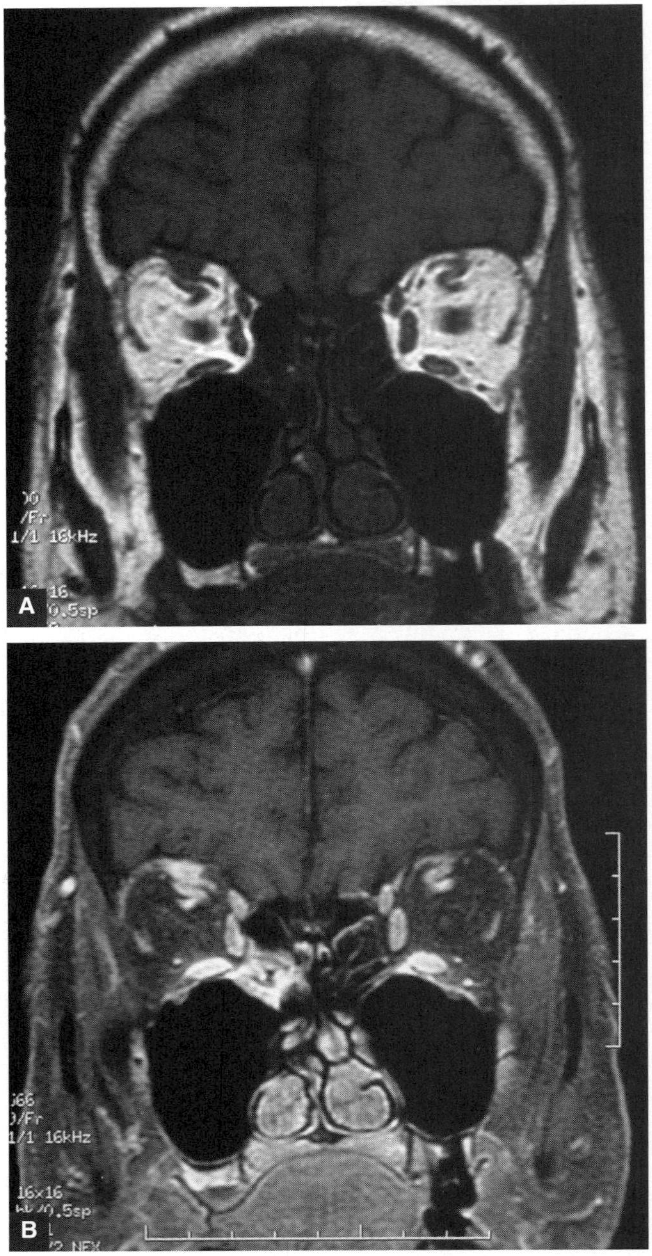

Figure 26–14. *A,* Direct T_1-weighted coronal MRI scan of idiopathic inflammation of an orbital nerve. *B,* Gadolinium-enhanced biopsy shows only inflammation.

ment. The ocular findings are similar to the generalized disease.[45] The CT or MRI pattern of orbital disease in Wegener's granulomatosis is nondiagnostic; many cases have shown diffuse orbital inflammation (Figure 26–15).[46] An orbital biopsy is not always diagnostic. In one series of 13 cases, giant cells were very rarely seen. In only 7 of the 13 was the classic triad of vascularitis, necrosis and granulomas noted.[47,48] As part of the standard laboratory work-up, tests for antinuclear antibody (ANA), blood urea nitrogen (BUN), and creatinine should be done; urinalysis should include examination of sediment. A chest radiograph should be obtained to help exclude pulmonary involvement from Wegener's granulomatosis. The development of an antineutrophil cytoplasmic antibody (ANCA) test has made the diagnosis of Wegener's granulomatosis easier. A subset of the ANCA, antimyeloperoxidase (AMPO), and antiproteinase 3(PR3) are possibly more specific for Wegener's granulamatosis, and these antibody studies often correlate with disease status.[49–52] Unfortunately, with greater experience, the false negatives associated with ANCA tests can be seen to be at least 30 percent.[53] In a prospective study from Duke University, the specificity of the c-ANCA was 96 percent, and the sensitivity was 28 percent.[54]

The treatment of Wegener's granulomatosis is outside the purview of this book. Most patients receive intravenous cyclophosphamide, although modifications of that approach have been reported.[55] Other options have also been used, including antithymocyte globulin for orbital Wegener's granulomatosis.[56]

Several rare processes can also simulate orbital pseudotumor. In contrast to Wegeners granulomatosis, midline lethal granuloma does not involve areas below to the cervical region; malignant histiocytosis or lymphoma can also simulate this entity.[57–59] Rarely, a sino-orbital giant cell granuloma can give a medial canthal mass with an osteolytic expansile lesion that also involves the sinuses; it is a less common idiopathic inflammatory disease that involves the orbit.[60] Langerhans' cell histocytosis is discussed in the chapter of pediatric orbital tumors, and there has been a marked alteration in both our understanding of the disease and its management.[61,62]

Erdheim-Chester disease often will present with bilateral exophthalamos and can simulate orbital

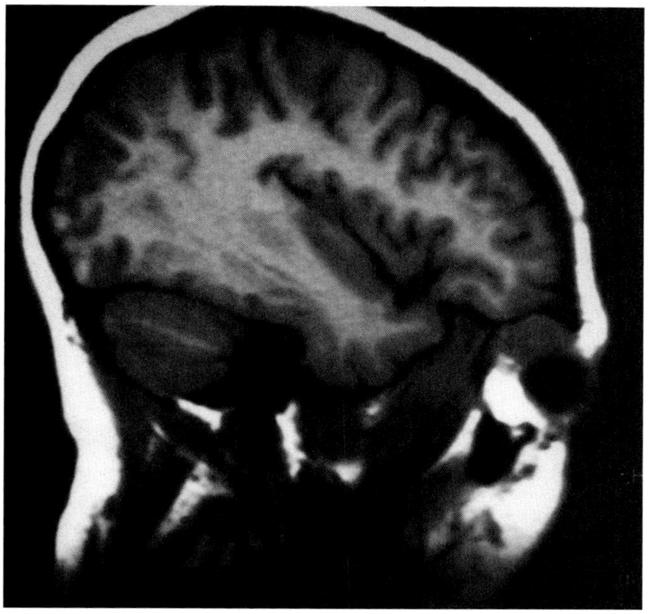

Figure 26–15. MRI scan demonstrates a lesion in a patient with Wegener's granulomatosis. Imaging findings are not diagnostic in this entity, although often the sinuses are involved.

pseudotumor.[63,64] There have been approximately 15 cases reported since 1983, and usually these patients die of either cardiovascular or renal carcinoma. The classic hallmark of Erdheim-Chester disease is infiltration with multinucleated Touton giant cells.[64]

Similarly, rare patients with sarcoidosis can present in an atypical manner, such as those > 70 years old with a confusing clinical picture.[65] Kimura's disease, which is lymphoid hyperplasia with a plasma cell infiltrate can involve the sinuses and orbit in both younger and older patients; this has been more common among the Japanese.[66,67] Castleman's disease can also produce the pseudotumor pattern.[68] Roseai-Dorfman disease can present with orbital disease as well, although this finding is described in only about 10 percent of patients. It is an idiopathic histoproliferative disorder, associated with cervical adenopathy, fever, and weight loss.[69]

Orbital tuberculosis and orbital luetic diseases are much less common today than previously. An MRI scan in a case of orbital luetic disease is shown in Figure 26–16. A chest radiograph, purified protein derivative of tuberculin (PDT) skin test, serum venereal disease research laboratories (VDRL or RPR) test, and fluorescence *Treponema* antibodies (FTA-ABS) should be obtained to rule out other

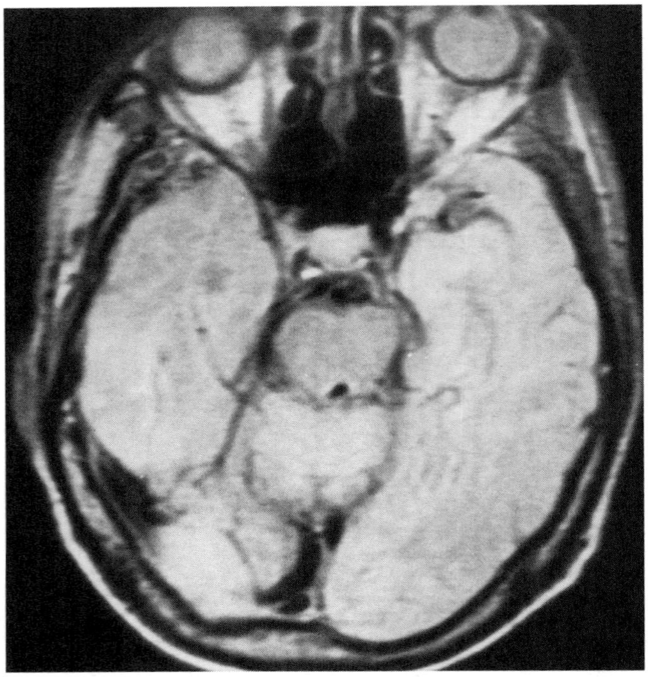

Figure 26–16. Axial MRI scan demonstrating luetic involvement of both lacrimal glands.

causes of orbital inflammation. Orbital tuberculosis can occasionally present as a mass with both lytic and blastic involvement of the orbital bones. In the United States, most of the patients are immigrants with pulmonary disease, and the chest radiographs are positive. Such patients will usually respond to antituberculous therapy.[70]

In the evaluation of a patient with a suspected orbital pseudotumor, active orbital infection, lymphoma, and systemic disease processes should be ruled out. A review of systems should include questions regarding sinus disease, arthritis, primary malignancies, respiratory problems, and changes in renal function.

Other processes that can simulate orbital pseudotumor should be suspected, if there are either signs or symptoms of systemic disease or bilateral orbital involvement (see Table 26–1).

Chest radiography is useful to detect tuberculosis or possible hilar adenopathy associated with sarcoidosis. Usually, the latter condition presents with bilateral lacrimal gland inflammation, although other patterns of orbital involvement occur (Figure 26–17).[71] A limited gallium scan, along with serum angiotensin converting enzymes (ACE), has approximately 95 percent sensitivity in detecting sarcoidosis, if the patient is not on systemic steroids. A typical example of this is illustrated in Figure 20–14.

To determine whether orbital inflammation is associated with systemic vasculitis, such as polyarteritis nodosa or with systemic lupus eyrthematosus (SLE), a complete blood count (CBC), erythrocyte sedimentation rate (ESR), platelet levels, ANCA, serum ANA, complement levels, immune complex titers, and liver function tests should be obtained. SLE with involvement of the lacrimal glands is shown in Figure 26–18. To rule out Sjögren's syndrome in a patient with xerostomia or dry eye and bilateral lacrimal gland inflammation, a labial biopsy should be obtained, since the various antibody titers are only positive in approximately 60 percent of primary Sjögren's syndrome patients and are often negative in patients with Sjögren's disease secondary to other processes.

Rheumatoid scleritis can simulate pseudotumor; occasionally, patients will present with a pseudorheumatoid nodule.[72] The CT pattern of orbital inflammation associated with rheumatoid disease is similarly nondiagnostic.

Mixed collagen vascular disease and necrobiotic xanthogranuloma (Figure 26–19) are rarer systemic processes that can also produce orbital inflammation.[73–76] The spectrum of these processes can vary widely but usually there is some systemic involvement.[77,78]

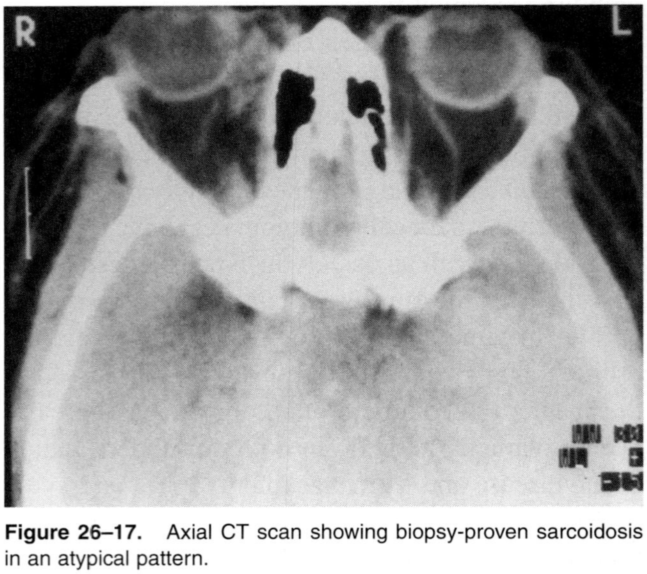

Figure 26–17. Axial CT scan showing biopsy-proven sarcoidosis in an atypical pattern.

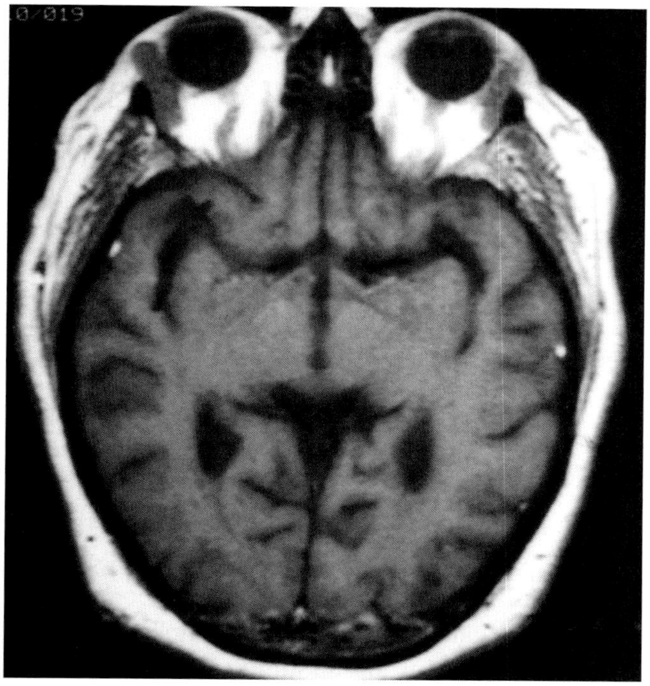

Figure 26–18. SLE shown on an axial T_1-weighted MRI scan, with involvement of both lacrimal glands.

One of the two more recently described syndromes include an orbital myositis as a variant of perineoplastic syndrome. In this case, the patient presented with a pattern that appeared to simulate thyroid eye disease on imaging. The patient had a high-grade lymphoma with other neuropathies, and on biopsy, there was extensive destruction of the muscles.[79] Lyme disease can also produce an orbital myositis. Leib and colleagues reported a case of a patient who had another pattern that on imaging appeared to simulate thyroid disease but who also had a giant cell myocarditis. There have been three reports of this entity, and all patients had poor outcomes due to cardiac disease.[80] A number of the histiocytoses can involve the orbit, and there is often involvement in the orbit with fever and systemic manifestations.[81]

Sinus histiocytosis has an associated cervical lymphadenopathy, low-grade fever, anemia, leukocytosis, and elevated immunoglobulin G (IgG) levels.[81,82] Orbital cellulitis, from either hematogenous spread or contiguous sinus disease, should manifest itself with significant systemic symptoms of infection.

Histiocytic disorders of the orbit are rare, and account for < 1 percent of orbital biopsies.[83,84] Most of the benign and malignant histiocytosis syndromes are due to abnormal Langerhans' cell proliferation.[83] Unlike orbital pseudotumor, patients with unifocal or multifocal eosinophilic granuloma have marked orbital bone changes apparent on clinical and radiographic examination (see Figures 16–41 and 16–42). These histiocytic processes range from obviously benign to frankly malignant; in cases of multifocal eosinophilic granuloma and diffuse histiocytosis, other body systems are involved. Usually, patients with widespread disease are younger than most patients with idiopathic orbital pseudotumor. Rarely, patients with malignant histiocytosis have orbital involvement, as shown in Figure 26–20.

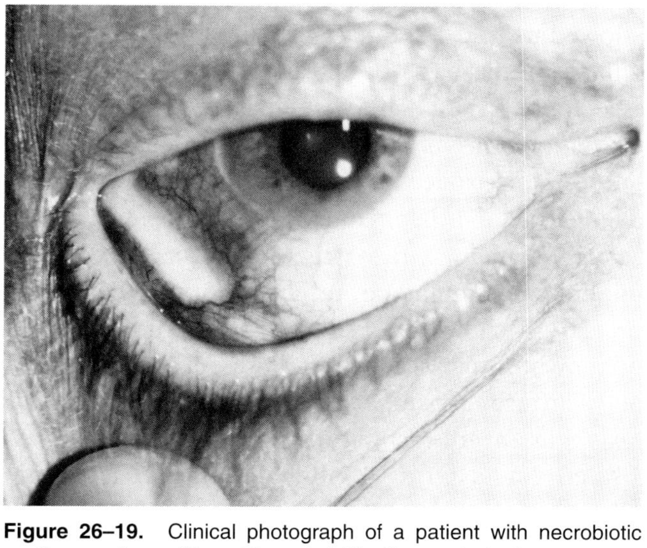

Figure 26–19. Clinical photograph of a patient with necrobiotic xanthogranuloma. (From Char et al.,[73] with permission)

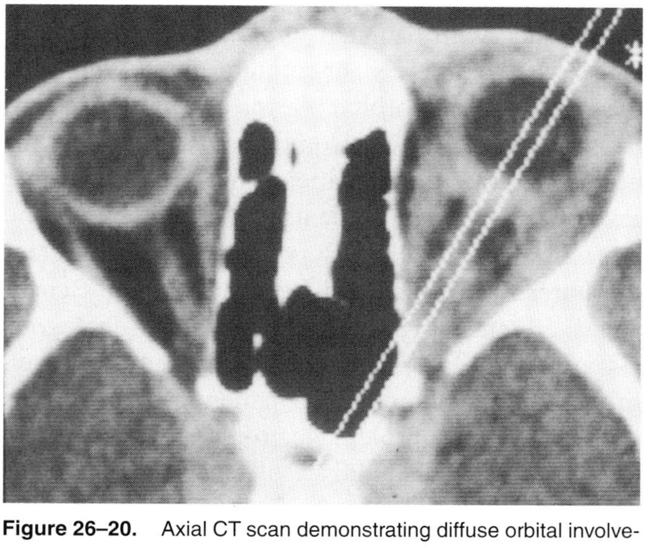

Figure 26–20. Axial CT scan demonstrating diffuse orbital involvement and malignant histiocytosis.

There is a cooperative study under the auspices of the Histiocytosis Society, using newer chemotherapeutic agents, including etoposide, with promising results for systemic histiocytosis syndrome.[85]

Nodular fasciitis can simulate orbital pseudotumor. At surgery, this process appears very similar to the fibrotic form of pseudotumor. Approximately 10 percent of pseudotumors are predominantly fibrotic.[86–88] A CT scan of such a case is shown in Figure 24–3. The histologic differential diagnosis in the case of nodular fasciitis is between benign and malignant fibrotic lesions.

Rarely, an orbital pseudotumor-like picture can be produced by a drug. Two different calcium antagonists have been implicated in this process.[89] As previously discussed, infectious agents can simulate orbital myositis, and several cases have been reported as either a myositis or a diffuse pseudotumor with a viral or fungal etiology.[90,91]

The most important differential diagnosis in patients suspected of having a lymphoid variant of orbital pseudotumor is differentiation between this benign condition and orbital lymphoma. Pain is more common in pseudotumor than in lymphoma, but it is not a useful differentiating feature. Even histologically, it can be difficult to differentiate these two conditions. As in other body sites, lymphoid proliferations can occur in a spectrum from obviously benign to frankly malignant.[92,93] Rarely, some other neoplasms, such as an infiltrating granular cell tumor, can simulate a sclerosing pseudotumor.[94]

An atypical subgroup in this lymphoid spectrum is patients with isolated orbital plasmacytomas. These are extremely uncommon, with approximately 50 cases of orbital plasma cell tumors having been reported.[95,14] Approximately 25 percent of orbital plasmacytoma patients developed multiple myeloma.[96–98] Such patients should have a bone marrow biopsy, skeletal survey, and a protein electrophoresis; urine should be analyzed for Bence-Jones proteins. Figure 26–21 compares analogous CT and MRI scans in a patient with a biopsy-proven orbital plasmacytoma. This patient had a gamma globulin spike on protein electrophoresis but no evidence of widespread disease. Occasionally, these patients present with orbital myositis.[99] Waldenstrom's macroglobulinemia can involve the orbit.[100] Figure 26–22 shows a case that was proven on biopsy. The pattern is certainly not diagnostic.

There are few pathognomonic findings on ultrasonography, CT, or MRI scans, which allow the differentiation of idiopathic orbital pseudotumor from other causes of orbital inflammation or from either lymphoma or tumors metastatic to the orbit.[26,101] The advantage of either CT or MRI over ultrasonography is spatial resolution, anatomic detail, improved diagnostic orbital accuracy, and their ability to better demonstrate sinus abnormalities and detect small foreign bodies. In pseudotumors which produce fluid in the sub-Tenon's space, the "T" sign on immersion B-scan is a finding which is specific for inflammation and is helpful in the differential diagnosis (Figure 26–23).[102–104] Usually, neither lymphoma nor pseudotumor invades orbital bone. While some investigators have felt that lymphoma can be differentiated from pseudotumor on both CT or ultrasonography, most experienced ophthalmic oncologists do not believe this differentiation is possible.[101,105,106] Usually, on T_1- and T_2-weighted images, lymphoid lesions are hypointense, although many will become hyperintense with gadolinium.[100] Some authors have felt that the relative homogeneity of the lesion on CT is suggestive of a lymphoma. In one series, this was noted in 75 percent of lymphomas versus 23 percent of orbital pseudotumors.[107] The streaky appearance of orbital fat is similarly nondiagnostic to distinguish a benign lymphoid process, metastatic orbital tumor, and a primary lymphoma.[108] Our experience has not allowed us to differentiate pseudotumors from lymphoma on the basis of T_1- and T_2-weighted images (see Table 15–2). A T_1-weighted image of a biopsy-proven orbital lymphoma is shown in Figure 26–22; the lesion is isodense with brain. Sinus disease producing orbital inflammation is readily apparent on CT scans or plain x-ray films.[109] Metastatic orbital tumors can simulate an inflammatory process. Figure 26–24 shows the CT scan of a patient with an unknown primary tumor who presented with apparently diffuse myositis that was shown to be a metastasis. Fine-needle aspiration biopsy (FNAB) demonstrated metastatic tumor. Similarly, leukemic involvement of the extraocular muscles is not diagnostic on imaging studies (Figure 26–25).

In lacrimal gland lesions, it is especially important to differentiate lymphoid tumors from primary epithelial cancers; the latter group of malignancies has over 90 percent tumor-related mortality.[110] Epithelial lacrimal tumors in their benign form commonly produce expansion of the fossa, whereas malignant processes are associated with bone invasion. Bone destruction, however, is not uniformly present in malignant epithelial lacrimal tumors.[111] Wright and co-workers have stressed the use of an incisional biopsy of lacrimal gland lesions to avoid penetrating the periosteum, which can be a barrier to malignant spread. The author routinely uses a lateral orbitotomy to approach these isolated lacrimal gland lymphoid lesions but carefully isolates the area and tags the cut edges of periosteum with a 4-0 silk suture. A frozen section is obtained during the operation to determine whether there is an adequate sample and also to make sure that this is not a malignant epithelial tumor. If it is a malignant epithelial tumor,

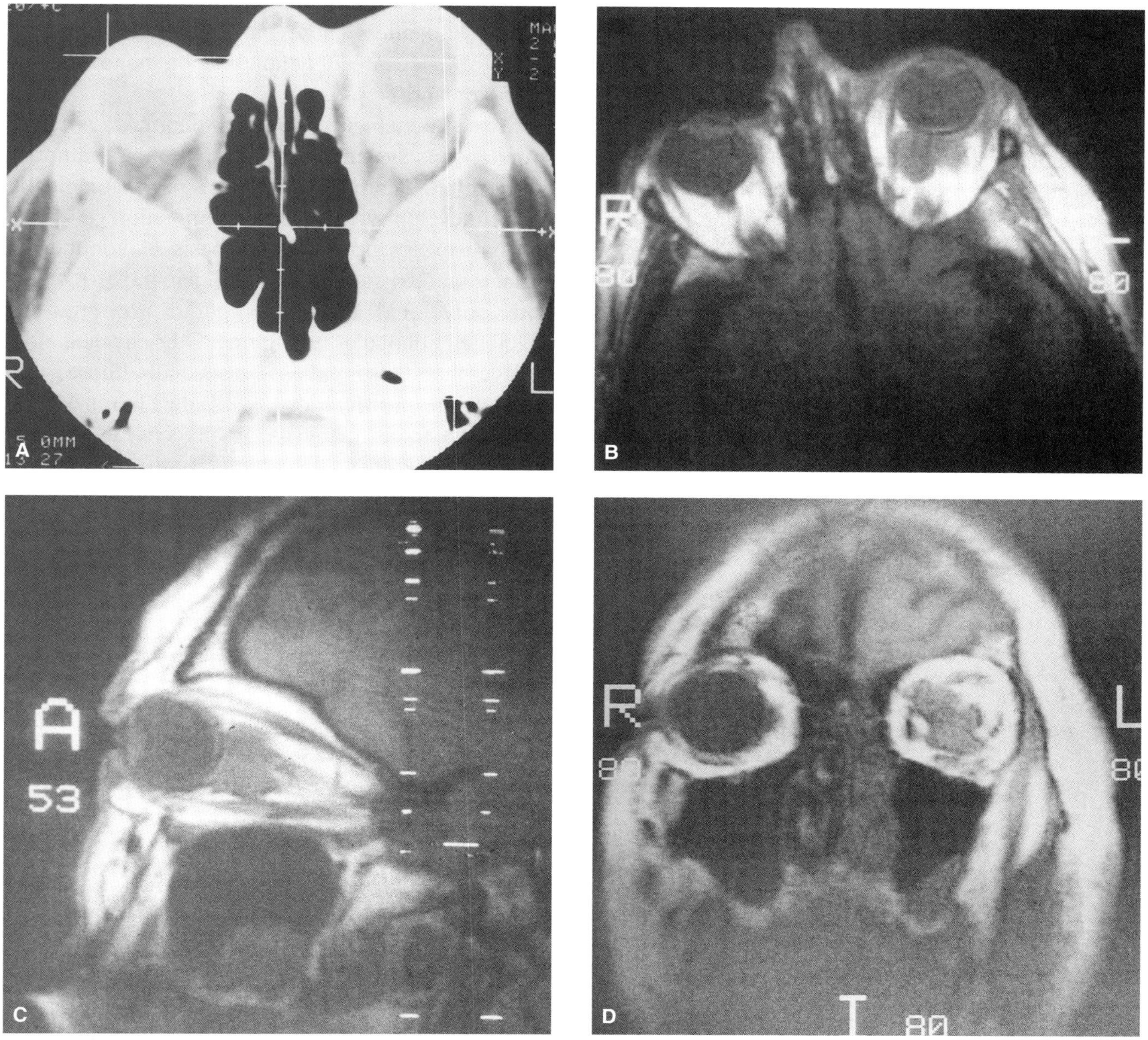

Figure 26–21. *A,* Case of plasmacytoma demonstrated by axial CT scan. *B,* Case of plasmacytoma demonstrated by axial MRI scan. *C,* Case of plasmacytoma demonstrated by direct parasagittal T_1-weighted MRI scan. *D,* Case of plasmacytoma demonstrated by direct coronal T_1-weighted MRI scan.

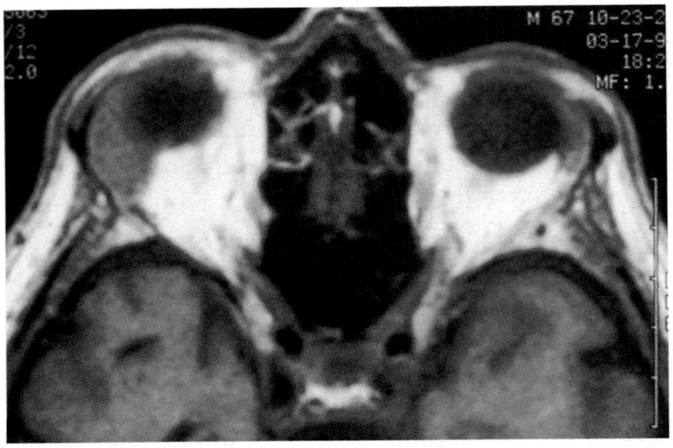

Figure 26–22. Axial MRI scan showing an orbital lymphoid lesion that was shown to be a Waldenstrom's macroglobulinemia.

an en bloc resection with periosteum is performed at the time of surgery (see Chapter 20).

Rarely, lymphoma predominantly involves extraocular muscles, as shown in Figures 19–2 and 19–3.[112]

In our experience, only 10 percent of orbital lymphomas have known systemic spread at the time the patient is examined. In most series, the orbit is involved in about 2 percent of lymphoma patients.[113] Most patients with known systemic lymphoma secondarily involving the orbit or those with simultaneous ophthalmic and systemic presentation of lymphomas have a history of chills, weight loss, and lymphadenopathy. These patients often have evidence of widespread lymphoma on bone marrow aspiration and biopsy.

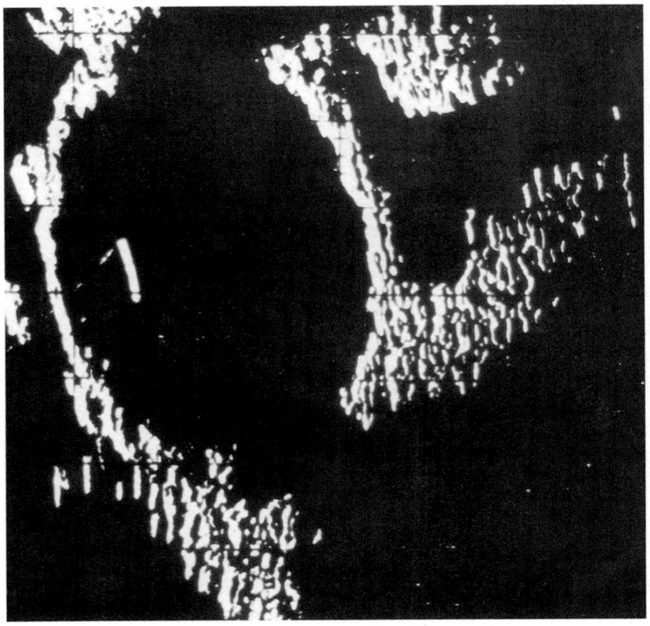

Figure 26–23. "T" sign of fluid in sub-Tenon's space is characteristic of an orbital pseudotumor that involves the posterior sclera.

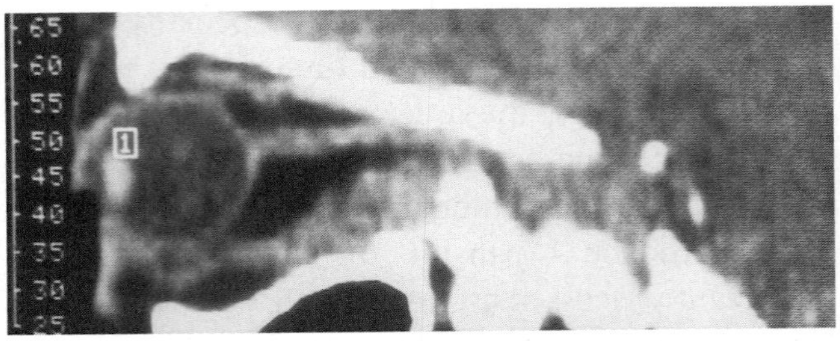

Figure 26–24. Parasagittal reformatted CT scan demonstrating involvement of the rectus muscles by an adenocarcinoma of unknown origin.

Most patients with orbital lymphoma do not have simultaneous systemic disease, and only a minority of those in whom this diagnosis is histologically proven develop widespread dissemination. Jakobiec and co-workers noted, on the basis of lymphocyte surface marker studies, that 29 percent of patients with polyclonal orbital lymphoid proliferations developed nonocular lymphoma. Other investigators believe that these patients, especially those with monoclonal proliferations, will develop systemic lymphoma in as many as 50 percent of cases.[114] Forty-five percent of patients with monoclonal B-cell proliferations in the orbit developed systemic lymphoma, as did 67 percent of patients with histo-

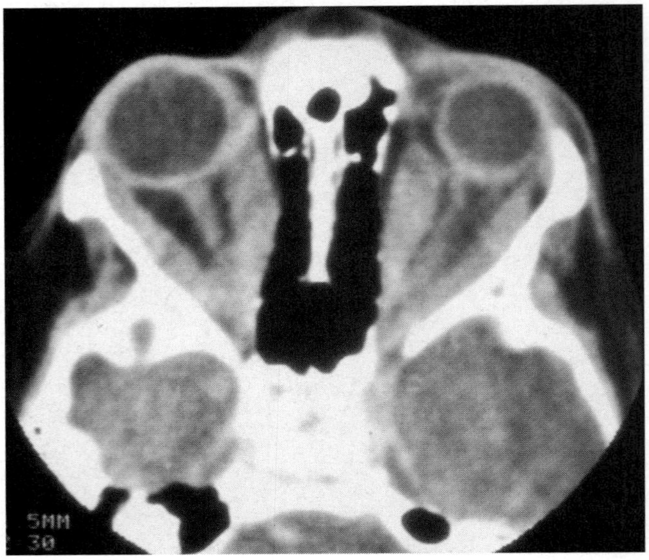

Figure 26–25. Axial CT scan shows diffuse extraocular muscle involvement in leukemia.

logically poorly differentiated orbital lymphoid lesions.[35,115] Generally, there was a lower incidence of systemic spread in patients with disease confined to the conjunctiva (24%) than in patients with orbital disease (21 of 53 [40%]) or lid involvement (4 of 5).[35,115] In a series of 112 cases from Glascow and Berlin, there was an equal incidence of malignant lymphoma with systemic spread in the conjunctiva, compared with those with orbital and lid involvement.[116] In that study, all patients with diffuse large B-cell lymphoma and T-cell lymphoma were more likely to have systemic spread, as were those with greater proliferation rates.[116] The patient shown in Figure 20–1 had simultaneous orbital and systemic lymphoma. Figures 26–26 and 26–27 show two biopsy-proven orbital lymphomas on axial and direct coronal CT scans. The vast majority of orbital lymphomas are non–Hodgkin's, although rarely nodular sclerosis of the Hodgkin's type has been described.[117,118] Approximately 20 percent of orbital lymphomas have bilateral involvement.[118,119] Orbital involvement is more commonly noted in systemic lymphomas that are high-grade disease.[120]

The optimal histologic classification of all lymphoid lesions, but especially those in the orbit, remains uncertain. There have been a number of different histologic classifications and working formulations for lymphoma, including those described by Rappaport, Lukes, and Collins, and the group in Kiel, the working formulation, Revised European American Lymphoma (REAL), and the World Health Organization (WHO) classifications.[121–127] The lymphoma classification continues to evolve. The newer classifications contain over 20 distinct lymphoid neoplasms and incorporate histology as well as immunology and molecular biologic alterations.[121,128] In mucosal associated lymphomas (MALT), which often involve the orbit, approximately one-third will have an obvious molecular alteration.[129] In one study of ophthalmic lymphoid tumors, over 70 percent exhibited at least one gene rearrangement, and in that series, 53 percent developed systemic disease.[130] Unfortunately, even the newer molecular analyses have a number of diagnostic pitfalls.[131,132]

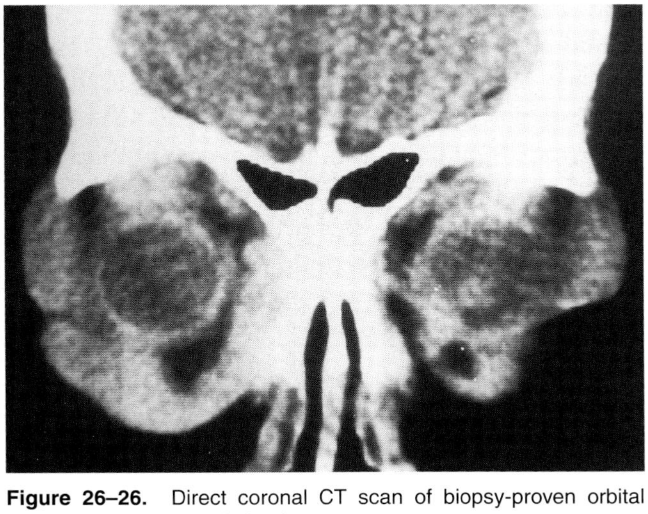

Figure 26–26. Direct coronal CT scan of biopsy-proven orbital lymphoma with systemic involvement.

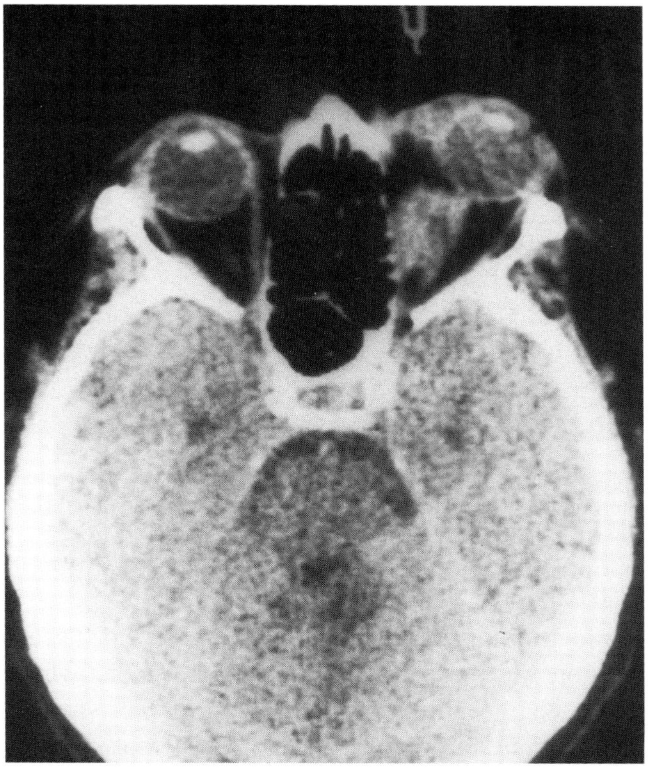

Figure 26–27. Axial CT scan of orbital lymphoma. The diagnosis was confirmed by bone marrow biopsy as well as fine-needle biopsy of the orbit. The axial CT scan shows the needle in correct position.

As expected, since CNS lymphoma is markedly increased in the immunocompromised population, several reports have described orbital lymphoma involvement in patients with AIDS.[133–138] Sometimes subjective findings make the differentiation between benign and malignant lymphoid lesions more difficult. The patient whose axial and coronal MRI scans are shown in Figure 26–28 had a history

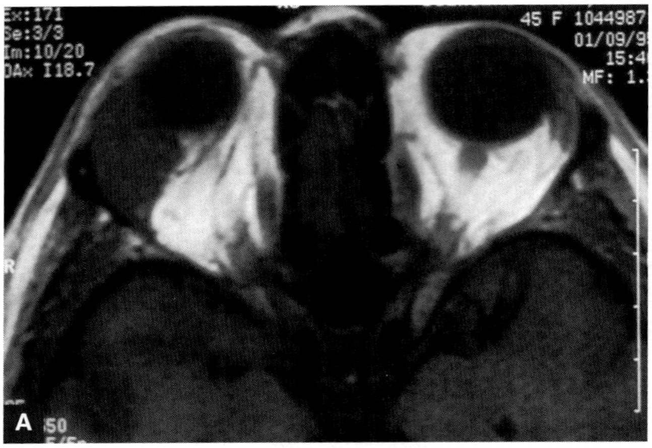

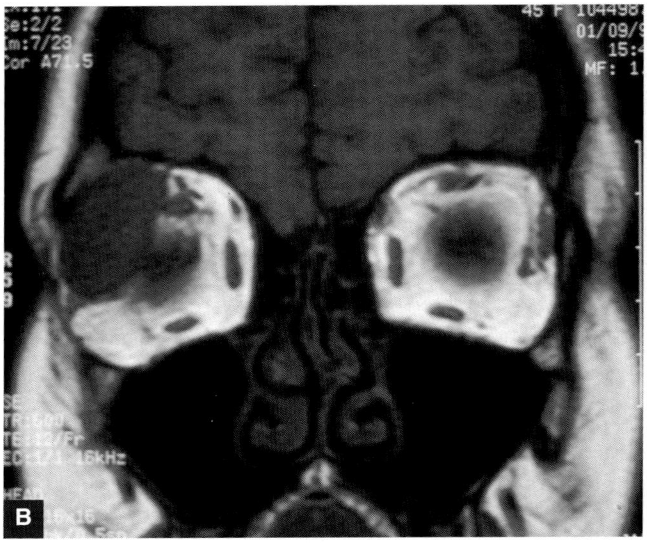

Figure 26–28. *A,* Axial MRI scan demonstrates a benign lymphoid lesion in a patient with a history of Hodgkin's lymphoma treated 20 years previously. *B,* Coronal scan of Figure 26–28A.

of radiation of a Hodgkin's lymphoma over 20 years previously. She presented with this lesion, which was a benign lymphoid process on marker studies, and she had no other evidence of systemic involvement. On the other hand, a patient with a history of lymphoma who presents with an orbital problem should be assumed to have that process until proven otherwise. The patient shown in Figure 26–29A was initially treated for a viral illness and was only referred when the eye went blind. A needle biopsy demonstrated recurrent lymphoma, which responded quite dramatically after the first radiation session with 200 cGy of photons (Figure 26–29B).

MANAGEMENT

Orbital Pseudotumor

The management of orbital pseudotumor varies, depending on its presentation. In a young patient presenting with painful ophthalmoplegia, ptosis, and mild proptosis along with an orbital CT pattern showing only myositis (see Figures 26–1 to 26–4), we administer 80 mg of oral prednisone every morning at 8 a.m. for 1 week and then stop the medication. In the majority of cases, a short-term course of steroids (< 10 days) will produce disease resolution, and this approach will not produce pituitary-adrenal suppression. The author would rather re-treat these patients than produce the complications associated with long-term steroids.[139,140] Unlike the British experience described earlier, the author has not had as good results with nonsteroidal therapy. While metastatic orbital tumors can involve the extraocular muscles, these are relatively uncommon in young patients, are more focal on CT or MRI, and usually do not produce similar symptoms.

Young patients with orbital apex syndrome (Tolosa-Hunt syndrome) are also treated with high-dose systemic steroids without biopsy.[8–14] In older patients who present with a Tolosa-Hunt-like picture, the probability of another cause is likely. Figure 26–30 shows such a case in an older man who was treated as having Tolosa-Hunt syndrome, when, in fact, he had a carcinoma. We have seen a few patients who had infections, metastatic tumors to the orbital apex, or contiguous sinus carcinoma involving that region, and were misdiagnosed as having Tolosa-Hunt syndrome (see Figure 22–15). In the last group of patients, pain was not a common symptom, and FNAB under CT control usually allowed the correct diagnosis to be made. In Tolosa-Hunt syndrome, high-dose steroids must often be continued for longer periods of time to obtain a remission of signs and symptoms.[8–10] Some of these patients require oral steroids for several months.

A biopsy should be performed on all other patients with possible orbital pseudotumor, especially those who present with an isolated mass. We have found that FNAB appears to be as efficacious

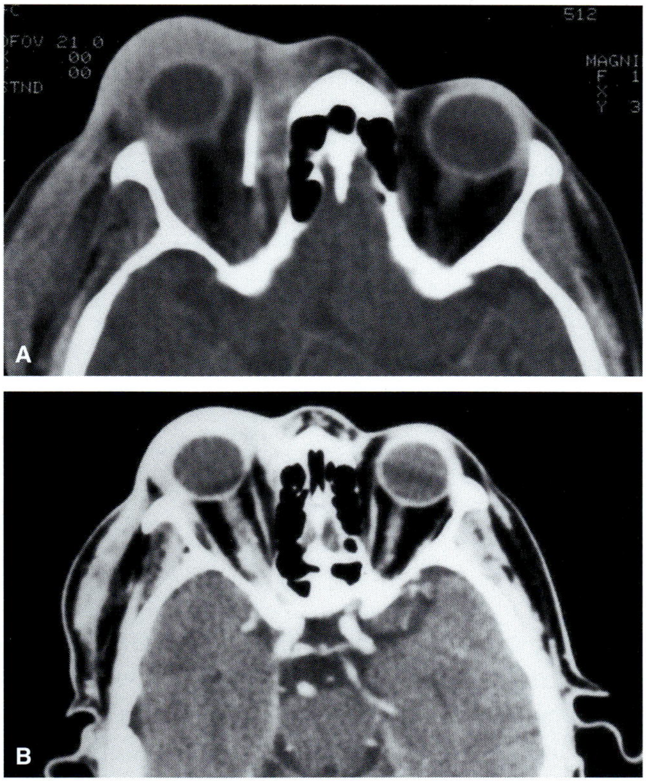

Figure 26–29. *A,* Axial CT scan with placement of FNAB. The patient had a history of systemic lymphoma treated 3 years previously. An incorrect diagnosis of a viral problem led to delay in treatment. *B,* Shows the patient 1 day later, after the first fraction of 200 cGy of photons.

as an open biopsy in the management of most orbital pseudotumor patients. We have been able to differentiate most benign simulating lesions as well as lymphomas from orbital pseudotumors on the basis of standard cytopathology interpretation as well as ancillary studies. Others have used cytologic techniques and have reported a good correlation with the working formulation classification of lymphoma.[141] The availability in many laboratories of flow cytometry that can be performed on fine-needle aspirates has also markedly improved the ability to delineate these processes. From a single or multiple fine-needle aspirate, as many as 10^7 cells can be obtained; these cells can be individually labeled with monoclonal antibodies, and this pattern can be detected by the laser, as the cells individually pass it in the flow cytometer.[28] In several centers, FNAB with flow cytometry has been used in this setting with promising results.[141–146] Figure 26–31 shows flow cytometry printouts of a benign heterogeneous collection of lymphocytes, compared with a monotonous, monoclonal malignant lymphoma from the orbit. Some cases of inaccurate biopsies have been reported, and we noted a 10 percent false-negative rate.[25,147]

If FNAB does not yield sufficient cells or if the result is ambiguous, an open biopsy should be obtained. At surgery, a number of different patterns of orbital pseudotumor can be observed. Sometimes the preoperative CT or MRI pattern demonstrates the fibrotic or cellular nature of the lesion. Figure 26–32 shows a case in which the orbit was almost entirely replaced by fibrosis, obscuring all intraorbital detail. This degree of fibrosis is rare; at surgery, these fibrotic tumors are found have a somewhat gritty nature and usually do not involve bone. We routinely obtain a frozen section biopsy at the time of surgery. This is not done to establish a definitive diagnosis but to ensure that an adequate, representative biopsy has been obtained. At the time of orbital biopsy, if lymphoma is suspected on frozen section, we do bilateral bone marrow biopsies and later obtain chest-abdominal scans.

There are a number of histologic classifications of orbital pseudotumors, but few findings which correlate with either response to therapy or prognosis. Reese initially divided pseudotumors into five histologic groups: (1) those with lymphoid follicles, (2) follicular and perivascular lymphocytic infiltration, (3) diffuse inflammation, (4) early fibrosis, and (5) inflammation with a pre-existing vascular lesion. Farrow classified pseudotumors into those with vasculitis and necrosis versus those with generalized lymphocytic infiltration.[7] As Garner has pointed out,

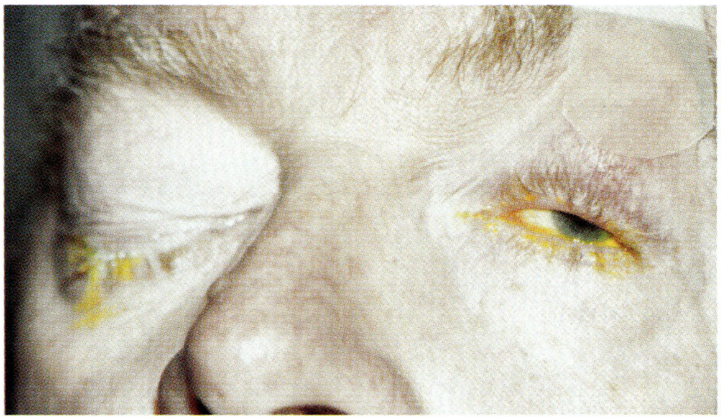

Figure 26–30. Tolosa-Hunt syndrome in older patients should be biopsied. This patient was managed for 2 years with progressive cranial nerve problems, and carcinoma was finally diagnosed on biopsy.

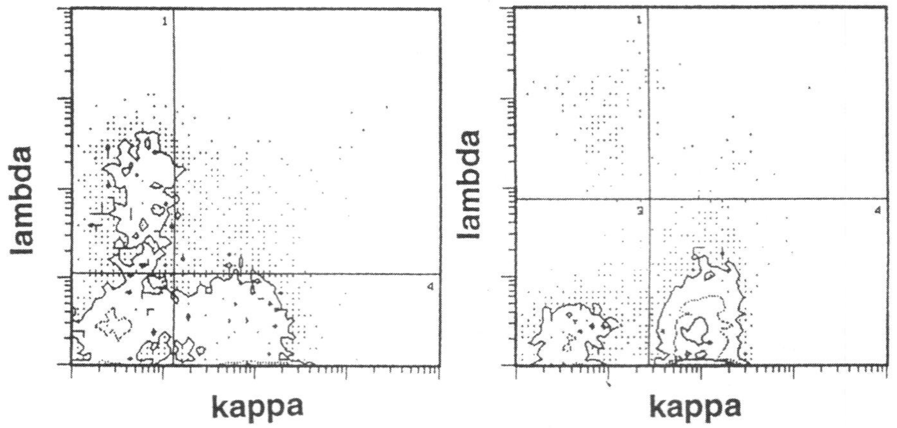

Figure 26–31. Dual-color fluorescence plots of kappa-FITC versus lambda-PE from a reactive lymphoid infiltrate (A) and a B-lineage non-Hodgkin lymphoma (B). The reactive infiltrate shows a polytypic pattern of light chain staining, with a kappa/lambda ratio of 1.8:1. The lymphoma cells show a monotypic staining pattern and a light chain ratio of 40:1, indicating the presence of a monoclonal B-cell population.

there is marked similarity between the orbital lymphoid lesions and those that are mucosa associated in the intestine.[148]

The lack of normal lymph node architecture precludes the use of capsular invasion as one of the diagnostic criteria which can be used to differentiate a lymphoma from a benign lymphoid proliferation. Germinal follicles, mixed cell populations, and intranuclear lymphocyte inclusions are more common in benign lymphoid proliferations. Histologic differentiation between benign and malignant lymphoid lesions is difficult. As Morgan and Harry first noted, the histologic differentiation of lymphoma from pseudotumor has an error rate which can approach 50 percent in difficult cases.[149] Similar long-term retrospective studies from the Armed Forces Institute of Pathology (AFIP) have demonstrated up to a 40 percent error rate in the differentiation of lymphoma from pseudotumor.[150]

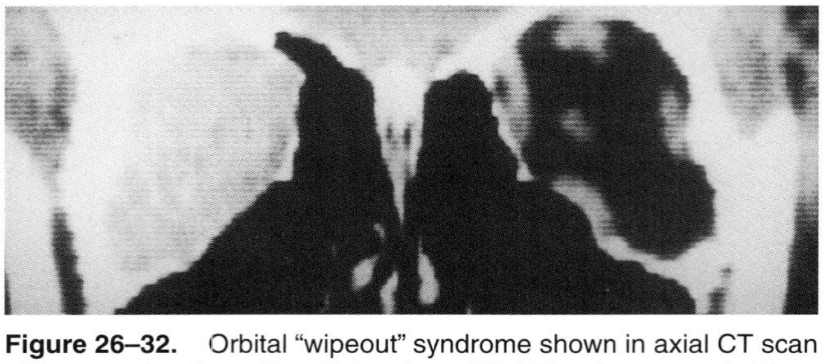

Figure 26–32. Orbital "wipeout" syndrome shown in axial CT scan with coronal re-formation. Extensive orbital fibrosis occurred. (From Char,[152] with permission).

A number of different approaches have been tried to improve the ability to differentiate lymphomas from benign orbital lymphoid lesions. Immunohistologic and DNA hybridization approaches appear to be the most promising, utilizing both monoclonal antibodies against lymphocyte subset surface markers and Southern blot techniques. These approaches are based on the premise that lymphomas are a monotonous proliferation of a monoclonal population of malignant lymphocytes. In contrast, pseudotumors are a heterogenous proliferation of cells. An individual B lymphocyte produces a single class of either lambda or kappa light chains. Normal B cells consist of mixed populations with a predominance of cells having surface kappa light chains. The individual gene arrangement for a given B cell's immunoglobulin (or a T-cell's immune receptor) and its progeny is unique.[151]

A number of groups, including our own, have used various techniques to attempt to differentiate lymphoma from pseudotumor on the basis of enumeration of subsets of T and B cells.[106,152,153] These early studies were performed using functional assays to distinguish lymphocyte monoclonality on the basis of subset analysis. A number of workers have demonstrated that orbital lymphomas are predominantly malignant B-cell proliferations.[106,143,152–159] Unfortunately, a significant number of T cells can either infiltrate or surround a B-cell lymphoma, making diagnosis using monoclonal antibodies difficult.[160] A number of theoretical and technical problems have limited the accuracy of these monoclonal antibody techniques in the differentiation of pseudotumor from lymphoma.[161,162] Some lymphomas have been demonstrated to be polyclonal in nature, and some benign diseases have been demonstrated to have monoclonal proliferations.[160,163–165]

Immunoglobulin gene rearrangements, as unique clonal markers of human lymphoid neoplasms, can be detected with Southern blot techniques and were hoped to be a more sensitive and accurate method to diagnose malignant versus benign lymphoid lesions.[143,146] A polyclonal population of either T or B cells shows no single immunoglobulin gene rearrangement by the Southern blot technique. As discussed in a series of publications by Jakobiec and Knowles, the initial optimism that this technique would allow better separation of lymphoma from benign lymphoid proliferation has not been borne out. A major conclusion is that approximately 25 percent of patients with benign lymphoid lesions, despite the type of technique used to identify them, will go on to develop lymphoma. The implication of that finding is that any patient with an orbital lymphoid lesion, regardless of morphology, needs sequential medical oncologic follow-up.[166]

An unsolved dilemma centers on the nature of those orbital lymphoid monoclonal B-cell proliferations that have not disseminated after 10 years of follow-up.[165] These may be akin to the pseudolymphoma in Sjögren's syndrome, in which some progress to full-blown lymphoma. There have been a few reports of malignant lymphomas of the orbit in association with the benign lymphoepithelial lesions of the parotid glands.[167] Since only approximately one-half of histologically clear-cut lymphomas spread outside the orbit, most of the cases of monoclonal proliferations that have not been shown to disseminate on long-term follow-up may or may not be true lymphomas.[106,159] Longer follow-up of these cases is necessary to answer this question.

As previously described, we do not biopsy and we empirically initiate high-dose, short-term, systemic steroid therapy for most young patients with the orbital apex syndrome or for those with inflammation isolated to the extraocular muscles. The effect of steroids on these lesions is dramatic; often, there is marked or complete resolution within 1 week. Unfortunately, as others have noted, in some series over half of these cases will recur after steroids are discontinued.[168]

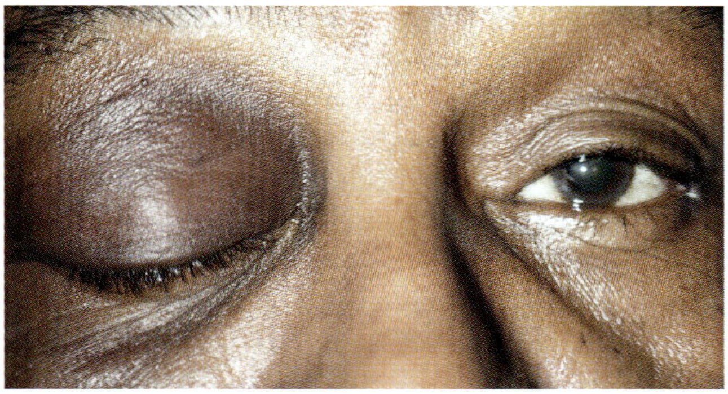

Figure 26–33. Focal inflammatory mass prior to surgery.

If a localized inflammatory mass is present that can be completely excised (this represents only a minority of orbital pseudotumors), surgery is performed. Figures 26–33 and 26–34 show such a patient prior to and after surgical extripation of the inflammatory mass.[169] In diffuse lesions or those which involve vital structures, we use high-dose, short-term steroids as our initial form of therapy. We have observed no significant complications when 100 mg of oral prednisone is administered daily for 7 to 10 days and then abruptly discontinued. While some investigators, including ourselves, have noted that response to steroids does not have a complete correlation with response to radiation, generally those patients who have a partial steroid response will do very well with radiotherapy.[170,171] Experience from a number of centers shows that approximately 50 percent of patients treated with either local or systemic steroids will have resolution of the

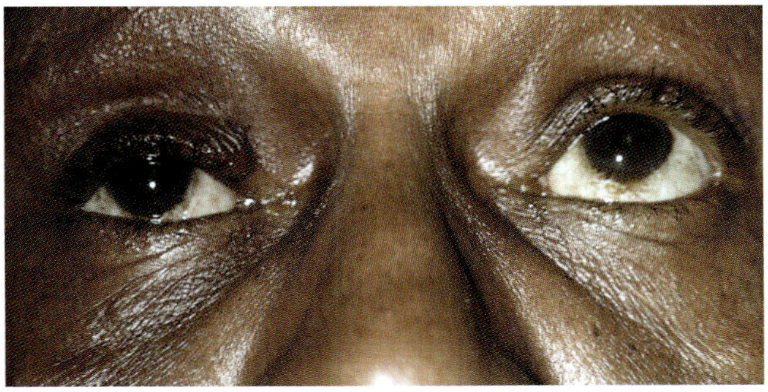

Figure 26–34. Patient shown in Figure 26–33 after surgical resection of a relatively focal inflammatory mass.

pseudotumor. In a series from London, 27 of 55 cases had a good response to steroids; lesions with germinal follicles or extensive eosinophils seemed to do best with this medicine.[172] We retrospectively analyzed the natural history of 81 patients with orbital pseudotumors treated at some point in their course at our unit. In 49, there were essentially complete remissions. The response to therapy was difficult to assess due to five important caveats in our study: (1) it was retrospective and many of the initial treatments were done at other centers and would not have been our treatment of choice; (2) there is no reproducible scoring system either for disease-associated morbidity or response to therapy; (3) in some orbital pseudotumors, spontaneous remission can occur; (4) some patients were obviously treated with multiple modalities; and (5) in some cases, while we recommended radiation, it was done in centers that did not have experience with that approach.[23]

In the 42 patients who received high-dose steroids, there was a complete and lasting remission in 24 percent and nearly a complete remission in an additional 7 percent of cases. Figures 26–35 to 26–38 show an excellent response to a 1-week course of oral corticosteroids. Patients who had a myositis or marked inflammation did significantly better than those with fibrotic lesions ($p < .04$). A poor steroid response was observed in 10 of 11 patients who had mass lesions. Some investigators have found that the use of bone-sparing agents, such as Etidronate, may decrease bone resorption, especially in the elderly on steroids.[173] In a series of 32 patients with orbital pseudotumors (20 with histologic confirmation), 27 received systemic steroids, and 21 had an initially good response. Unfortunately, only 10 (31%) were cured, while 11 (34%) had recurrences.[174] As discussed below, fibrotic tumors respond poorly to steroids or irradiation; the fibrotic nature of these lesions is apparent at surgery. In patients who had fibrous mass lesions, surgery alone was effective in 19 of 25.[69]

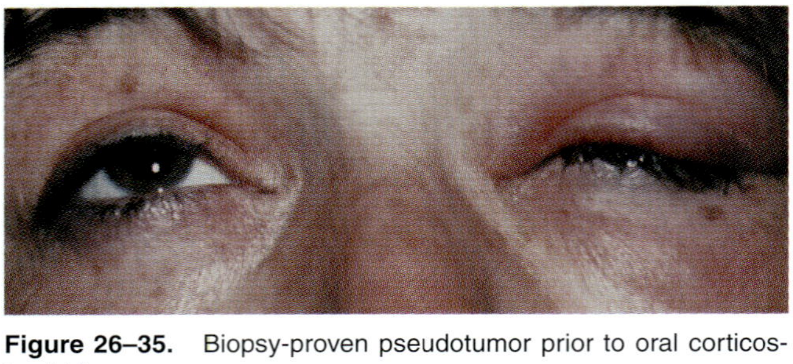

Figure 26–35. Biopsy-proven pseudotumor prior to oral corticosteroid therapy.

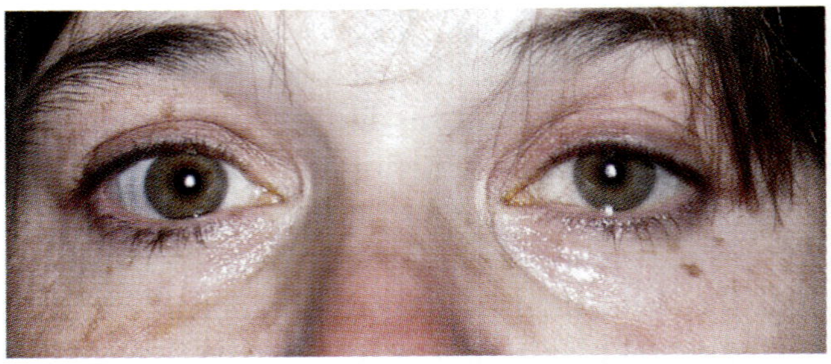

Figure 26–36. Patient shown in Figure 26–35 after 1 week of high-dose oral corticosteroids.

We have also observed a few patients who have had sufficient orbital fibrosis to produce visual loss from optic nerve compression. Unlike orbital decompression surgery in compressive thyroid optic neuropathy, we have had to actually remove the fibrotic tissue up to the optic nerve.[175] Rarely, more aggressive surgery is indicated in patients with orbital pseudotumor. We have managed a few patients who developed intractable proptosis and pain that were unresponsive to analgesics, nerve blocks, steroids, and irradiation. Very rarely, patients such as these require exenteration.

Orbital pseudotumors that are predominantly lymphoid have the most rapid and complete response to radiation or steroids. Pseudotumors which have an extensive vasculitis component are less responsive to these modalities.[170]

Radiation therapy has been used in the management of orbital pseudotumor for a number of years, but there is a paucity of reports on irradiated orbital pseudotumor patients in the literature.[172,173,176] Most have previously received steroids but had either an incomplete or no response to them. Approximately 75 percent of irradiated patients had a complete response to orbital irradiation.[176–184] Figure 26–39 shows an excellent response to 20 gray (Gy) of photon irradiation. The most recent series from Stanford University noted that 15 of 20 orbital pseudotumors treated with 20 Gy of photon irradiation had good resolution.[183] In our retrospective review, radiation was effective in 64 percent of patients. We noted that radiation response was significantly better in nonfibrotic lesions, in those with a shorter interval

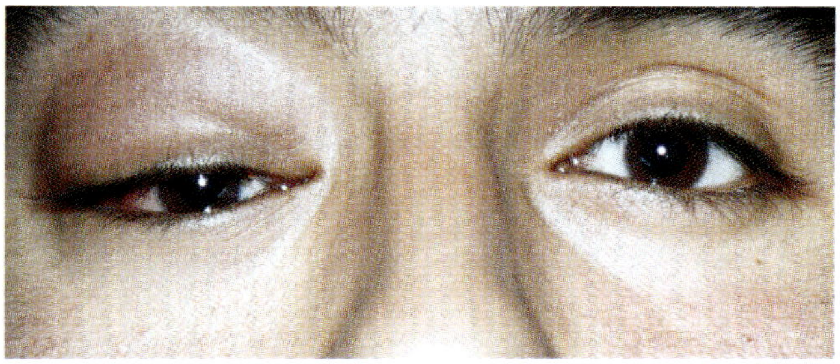

Figure 26–37. Pseudotumor prior to steroids.

between diagnosis and treatment, and in those who had erythema on presentation ($p < 0.05$).[23] In the Stanford University experience, poorer responses were noted in younger and female patients. Patients with orbital vasculitis appeared to be slightly less responsive, as did those with diplopia.[183] Other studies have shown similar results.[184,185] Intriguingly, in one study of 65 patients, there was no difference in local or systemic recurrence rates among those patients who had benign lymphoid hyperplasia, those who had definite lymphomas, and those who had indeterminate lymphoid lesions.[185]

One problem in attempting to interpret the literature on irradiation of orbital pseudotumor is that it is unclear how many of these patients may have had lymphoma. In those series with a longer post-treatment follow-up, some patients who were initially felt to have had orbital pseudotumor have developed extraorbital lymphoma.[177,179,185] A few patients treated with orbital irradiation for thyroid orbitopathy developed retinopathy. However, on re-examination, it was apparent that the fractionation, dose, and beam calculations had been improper.[176]

We are unaware of significant ocular complications at 20 Gy of orbital irradiation. Specifically, no lens opacities or clinically apparent radiation vasculopathies have been produced.

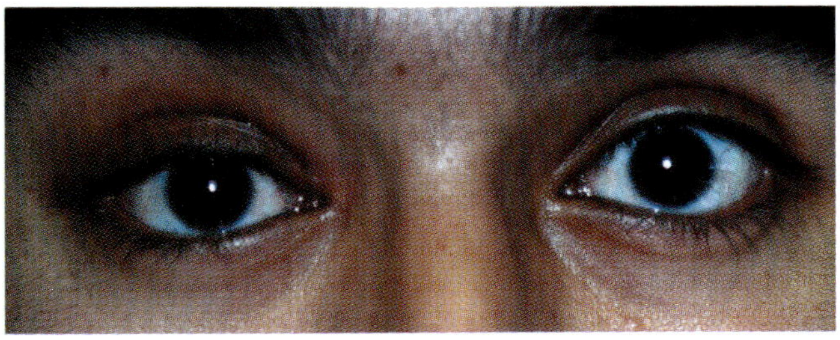

Figure 26–38. Case shown in Figure 26–37 after 1 week of high-dose steroids.

Orbital Lymphoma

The management of orbital lymphoma is predicated on the systemic status of the patient. If, at the time of orbital biopsy, the frozen section of the lesion is not pathognomonic for a benign orbital pseudotumor versus a lymphoma, we obtain bilateral bone marrow aspirations and biopsies while the patient is under general anesthesia. If the malignant lymphoid disease is confined to the orbit, as evidenced by negative chest and abdominal scans, patients receive 30 Gy of photon irradiation. At this dose, we have had approximately 95 percent success in controlling the orbital involvement.[178] In most other series, orbital radiation has been curative for local disease, although systemic disease development has occurred in about a quarter of these patients.[55,186,187] Donaldson feels that higher grade tumors may require combination radiation and systemic chemotherapy and also may do better at a slightly higher radiation dose.[188] Figure 26–40 shows an excellent orbital response to 40 Gy of photon irradiation of an anterior orbital lymphoma. Approximately 50 percent of patients with orbital lymphoma have extraorbital dis-

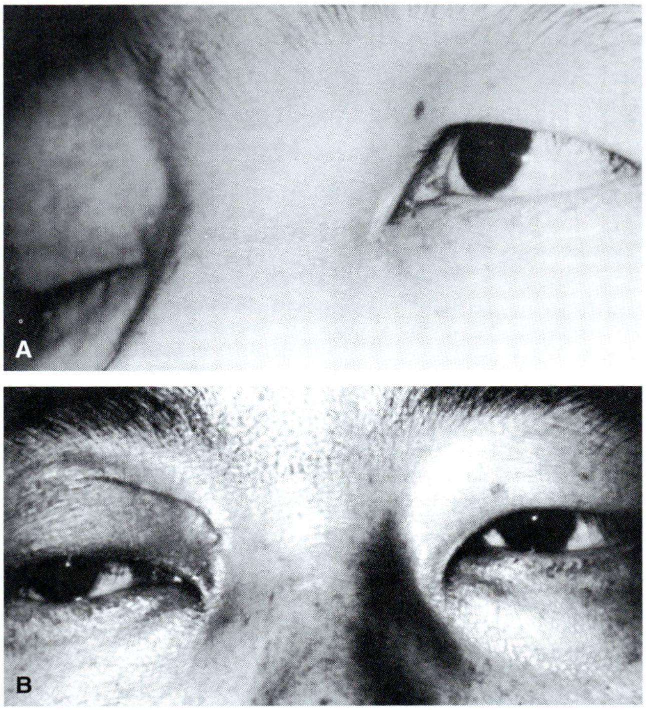

Figure 26–39. *A,* Orbital pseudotumor involving the superior orbit prior to 20 Gy of photon irradiation. *B,* Clinical photograph after irradiation.

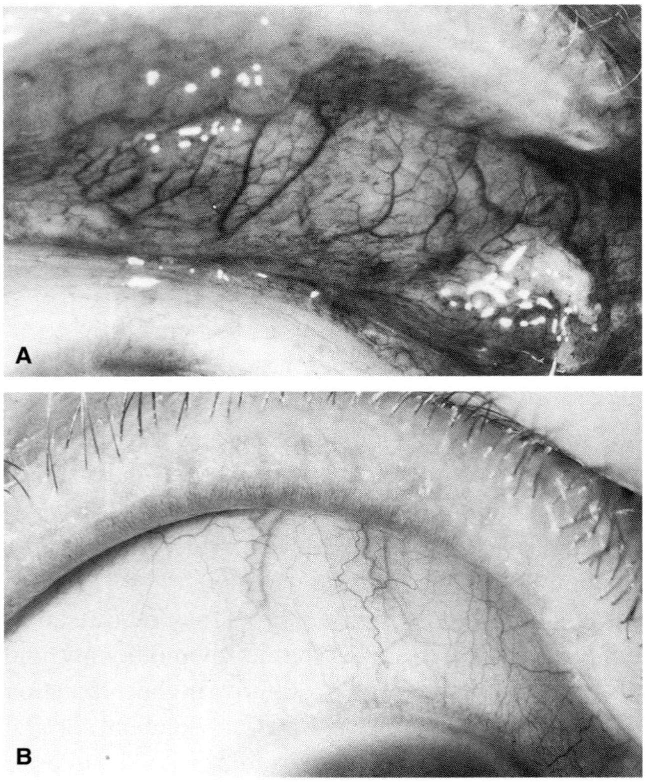

Figure 26–40. *A*, Biopsy-proven orbital lymphoma prior to irradiation. *B*, Clinical photograph after 40 Gy of orbital photon irradiation.

semination discovered within 5 years of the orbital presentation. Twenty percent of patients initially present with widespread lymphoma and later develop orbital disease. An additional 10 percent of cases present with orbital proptosis without known systemic lymphoma but, on evaluation, are shown to have simultaneous orbital and widespread lymphoma. Management of patients with disseminated lymphoma is outside the scope of this book. As would be expected, patients with high-grade lymphomas have a poorer prognosis.[189] At doses used to irradiate the orbit for lymphoma, there is a significant incidence of cataract. Generally, if the lens receives 16.5 Gy in fractionated photons, in almost all cases, opacities develop[190] Our experience has been that if vision is eliminated for more than 72 hours by orbital compression, the chance of obtaining a useful return of vision is extremely limited.[191] In one report, however, Moshfeghi and colleagues noted a patient who had no light perception for over a month, and after radiation, vision was restored to 20/40.[192]

REFERENCES

1. Birch-Hirshfeld A. Zur Diagnostik und Pathologie der Orbitaltumeren. Ber Dtsch Ophthalmol Ges 1905; 32:127–35.
2. Goodner EK, Aronson SB. Experimental immunogenic orbital inflammation. Arch Ophthalmol 1974;91: 303–7.
3. Garner A. Pathology of "pseudotumors" of the orbit: A review. J Clin Oncol 1973;26:639–48.
4. Atabay C, Tyutyunikov A, Scalise D, et al. Serum antibodies reactive with eye muscle membrane antigens are detected in patients with nonspecific orbital inflammation. Ophthalmology 1995;102:145–53.
5. Mombaerts I, Goldschmeding R, Schlingemann RO, Koorneef L. What is orbital pseudotumor? Surv Ophthalmol 1996;41:66–78.
6. Shields JA, Bakewell B, Augsburger JJ, Flannagan JC. Classification and incidence of space-occupying lesions of the orbit. A survey of 645 biopsies. Arch Ophthalmol 1984;102:1606–11.
7. Henderson JW Lymphocytic inflammatory pseudotumor. In: Orbital Tumors. New York, NY: Raven Press; 1980. p. 391.
8. Hunt WE. Tolosa-Hunt syndrome: one cause of painful ophthalmoplegia. J Neurosurg 1976;44:544–9.
9. Dornan TL, Espir ML, Gale EA, et al. Remittent painful ophthalmoplegia: the Tolosa-Hunt syndrome: a report of seven cases and a review of the literature. J Neurol Neurosurg Psychiatry 1979;42:270–5.
10. Mathew NT, Chandy J. Painful ophthalmoplegia. J Neurol Sci 1970;11:243–56.
11. Igarashi H, Igarashi S, Ishiko S, et al. Cystoid macular edema as an initial symptom of orbital pseudotumor. Arch Ophthalmologica 1997;211:236–41.
12. Kline LB. The Tolosa-Hunt syndrome. Surv Ophthalmol 1982;27:79–95.
13. Campbell RJ, Okazaki H. Painful ophthalmoplegia (Tolosa-Hunt variant): autopsy findings in a patient with necrotizing intracavernous carotid vasculitis and inflammatory disease of the orbit. Mayo Clin Proc 1987;62:520–6.
14. Kansu T, Us O, Sarpel G, Arac N. Recurrent multiple cranial nerve palsies (Tolosa-Hunt plus?). J Clin Neuro Ophthalmol 1983;3:263–6.
15. Sekhar GC, Mandal AK, Vyas P. Nonspecific orbital inflammatory diseases. Doc Ophthalmologic 1993; 84:155–70.
16. Grouteau E, Chaix Y, Armbruster V, et al. Acute orbital myositis and idiopathic inflammatory pseudotumor in children: three cases. Arch Pediatr 1998;5:153–8.
17. Mannor GE, Rose GE, Moseley IF, Wright JE. Outcome of orbital myositis. Clinical features associated with recurrence. Ophthalmology 1997;104: 409–14.
18. Siatkowski RM, Capo H, Byrne SF, et al. Clinical and

echographic findings in idiopathic orbital myositis. Am J Ophthalmol 1994;118:343–50.
19. Bullen CL, Younge BR. Chronic orbital myositis. Arch Ophthalmol 1982;100:1749–51.
20. Slavin ML, Glaser JS. Idiopathic orbital myositis: report of six cases. Arch Ophthalmol 1982;100:1261–5.
21. Weinstein GS, Dresner SC, Slamovits TL, Kennerdell JS. Acute and subacute orbital myositis. Am J Ophthalmol 1983;96:209–17.
22. Bessant DAR, Lee JP. Management of strabismus due to orbital myositis. Eye 1995;9:558–63.
23. Blodi FC, Gass JD. Inflammatory pseudotumor of the orbit. Trans Am Acad Ophthalmol Otolaryngol 1967;71:303–23.
24. Hosten N, Schorner W, Zwicker C, et al. Lymphozytare infiltrationen der orbita in MRT und CT. Forschr Rontgenstr 1991;155:445–51.
25. Char DH, Miller T. Orbital pseudotumor: fine-needle aspiration biopsy and response to therapy. Ophthalmology 1993;100:1702–10.
26. Polito E, Galieni P, Leccisotti A. Clinical and radiological presentation of 95 orbital lymphoid tumors. Graefes Arch Clin Exp Ophthalmol 1996;234:504–9.
27. Ryan SJ, Zimmerman LE, King FM. Reactive lymphoid hyperplasia. An unusual form of intraocular pseudotumor. Trans Am Acad Ophthalmol Otolaryngol 1972;76:652–71.
28. Zhang TL, Shao SF, Zhang T, et al. Idiopathic inflammation of the optic nerve simulating optic nerve sheath meningioma: CT demonstration. J Comput Assist Tomogr 1987;11:360–1.
29. Frohman LP, Kupersmith MJ, Lang J, et al. Intracranial extension and bone destruction in orbital pseudotumor. Arch Ophthalmol 1986;104:380–4.
30. Eshaghian J, Anderson RL. Sinus involvement in inflammatory orbital pseudotumor. Arch Ophthalmol 1981;99:627–30.
31. Bencherif B, Zouaoui A, Chedid G, et al. Intracranial extension of the idiopathic orbital inflammatory pseudotumor. Am J Neuroradiol 1993;14:181–4.
32. Som PM, Brandwein MS, Maldjian C, et al. Inflammatory pseudotumor of the maxillary sinus: CT and MRI findings in six cases. Am J Roentgenol 1994; 163:689–92.
33. Whyte IF, Young JD, Guthrie W, Kemp EG. Orbital inflammatory disease and bone destruction. Eye 1992;6:662–4.
34. Wild T, Strotzer M, Volk M, Feuerbach S. Idiopathic hypertrophic cranial pachymeningitis associated with an orbital pseudotumor. Eur Radiol 1999;9:1401–3.
35. Nassai S, Cocito L, Arcuri T, Favale E. Orbital pseudotumor as a presenting sign of temporal arteritis. Clin Exp Rheumatol 1995;13:367–9.
36. Hayreh SS, Podhajsky PA, Raman R, Zimmerman B. Giant cell arteritis: validity and reliability of various diagnostic criteria. Am J Ophthal 1997;123:285–96.
37. Weissler MC, Miller E, Fortune MA. Sclerosing orbital pseudotumor: a unique clinical pathologic entity. Ann Otolrhinol Laryngol 1989;98:496–501.
38. Rootman J, McCarthy M, White V, et al. Idiopathic sclerosing inflammation of the orbit. A distinct clinicopathological entity. Ophthalmology 1994;101: 570–84.
39. Friling R, Monos T, Lifshitz T, et al. Sclerosing pseudotumor of the orbit. Orbit 1994;13:199–202.
40. Haynes BF, Fishman ML, Fauci AS, Wolff SM. The ocular manifestations of Wegener's granulomatosis. Fifteen years experience and review of the literature. Am J Med 1977;63:131–41.
41. Straatsma BR. Ocular manifestations of Wegener's granulomatosis. Am J Ophthalmol 1957;44:789–799.
42. Fauci AS, Haynes BF, Katz P, Wolff SM. Wegener's granulomatosis: prospective clinical and therapeutic experience with 85 patients for 21 years. Ann Intern Med 1983;98:76–85.
43. Coutu RE, Klein M, Lessel S, et al. Limited form of Wegener granulomatosis. Eye involvement as a major sign. JAMA 1975;233:868–71.
44. Perry SR, Rootman J, White VA. Clinical and pathologic constellations of Wegener granulomatosis of the orbit. Ophthalmology 1997;104:683–94.
45. Spalton DJ, Graham EM, Page NG, Sanders MD. Ocular changes in limited forms of Wegener's granulomatosis. Br J Ophthalmol 1981;65:553–63.
46. Provenzale JM, Allen NB. Wegener granulomatosis: CT and MR findings. Am J Neuroradiol 1996;17: 875–92.
47. Kalina PH, Lie JT, Campbell RJ, Garrity JA. Diagnostic value limitations of orbital biopsy in Wegener's granulomatosis. Ophthalmology 1992;99:120–4.
48. Courcoutasakis NA, Langford CA, Sneller MC, et al. Orbital involvement in Wegener granulomatosis: MR findings in 12 patients. J Comput Assist Tomogr 1997;21:452–8.
49. Trocme SD, Bartley GB, Campbell RJ, et al. Eosinophil and neutrophil degranulation in ophthalmic lesions of Wegener's granulomatosis. Arch Ophthalmol 1991;109:1585–9.
50. Soukiasian SH, Foster CS, Niles JL, Raizman MB. Diagnostic value of anti-neutrophil cytoplasmic antibodies in scleritis associated with Wegener's granulomatosis. Ophthalmology 1992;99:125–32.
51. Power WJ, Rodriguez A, Neves RA, et al. Disease relapse in patients with ocular manifestations of Wegener granulomatosis. Ophthalmology 1995; 102:154–60.
52. Kallenberg CGM, Brouwer E, Mulder AHL, et al. ANCA-pathophysiology revisited. Clin Exp Immunol 1995;100:1–3.
53. Bajema IM, Hagen EC, Van Der Woude FK, Bruijn JA. Wegener's granulomatosis: a meta-analysis of 349 literary case reports. J Lab Clin Med 1997;129:17–22.

54. Rao JK, Allen N, Feussner JR, Weinberger M. A prospective study of antineutrophil cytoplasmic antibody (c-ANCA) and a clinical criteria in diagnosing Wegener's granulmoatosis. Lancet 1995;346 (II):926–31.
55. Guillevin L, Cordier JF, Lhote F, et al. A prospective multi-centered randomized trial comparing steroids and pulse cyclophosphamide versus steroids and oral cyclophosphamide in the treatment of generalized Wegener's granulomatosis. Arthritis Rheum 1997;40:2187–98.
56. Kool J, De Keizer RJW, Siegert CEH. Antithymocyte globulin treatment of orbital Wegener granulomatosis: a follow-up study. Am J Ophthalmol 1999;127: 738–9.
57. Simonis-Blumenfrucht A, Mestdagh C, Lustman F, et al. Lethal midline granuloma. A case report. Dermatologica 1979;158:153–62.
58. Spalton DJ, O'Donnell PJ, Graham EM. Lethal midline lymphoma causing acute dacryocystitis. Br J Ophthalmol 1981;65:503–6.
59. Meyer JH, Scharf B, Gerling J. Midline granuloma presenting as orbital cellulitis. Graefes Arch Clin Exp Ophthalmol 1996;234:137–9.
60. Hyver SW, Ellis DS, Stewart WB, et al. Sino-orbital giant cell reparative granuloma. Ophthal Plast Reconstr Surg 1998;14:178–81.
61. Arceci RJ, Brenner MK, Pritchard J. Controversies and new approaches to treatment of Langerhan's cell histiocytosis. Hematol Oncol Clin North Am 1998; 12:339–57.
62. Lampert F. Langerhans cell histiocytosis. Hematol Oncol Clin North Am 1998;12:213–9.
63. Valmaggia C, Neuweiler J, Fretz C, Gottlog I. A case of Erdheim-Chester disease with orbital involvement. Arch Ophthalmol 1997;115:1467–98.
64. De Palma P, Ravalli L, Grisanti F, et al. Bilateral orbital involvement in Erdheim-Chester disease. Orbit 1998;17:97–105.
65. Peterson EA, Hymas DC, Pratt DV, et al. Sarcoidosis with orbital tumor outside the lacrimal gland. Arch Ophthalmol 1998;116:804–6.
66. Mulhern M, Power N, Kennedy S, Moriarty P. Bilateral orbital Kimura's disease. Orbit 1996;15:91–6.
67. Kanazawan S, Gong H, Kitaoka T, Amemiya T. Eosinophilic granuloma (Kimura's disease) of the orbit: a case report. Graefes Arch Clin Exp Ophthalmol 1999;237:518–21.
68. Kurokawa T, Suguki S, Kawaguchi K, et al. Castleman's disease presenting with ophthalmic signs and symptoms. Am J Ophthalmol 1999;128:114–6.
69. Resnick DK, Johnson BL, Lovely TJ. Rosai-Dorfman disease presenting with multiple orbital and intracranial masses. Acta Neuropathol 1996;91:554–7.
70. Sheridan PH, Edman JB, Starr SE. Tuberculosis presenting as an orbital mass. Pediatrics 1981;67:874–5.
71. Snead JW, Seidenstein L, Knific RJ, et al. Isolated orbital sarcoidosis as a cause of blepharoptosis. Am J Ophthalmol 1991;112:739–40.
72. Barr CC, Davis H, Culbertson WW. Rheumatoid scleritis. Ophthalmology 1981;88:1269–73.
73. Char DH, LeBoit PE, Ljung BM, Wara W. Radiation therapy for ocular necrobiotic xanthogranuloma. Arch Ophthalmol 1987;105:174–5.
74. Miller RL, Sheeler LR, Bauer TW, Bukowski RM. Erdheim-Chester disease. Case report and review of the literature. Am J Med 1986;80:1230–6.
75. Bankhurst AD, Carlow TJ, Reidy RW. Exophthalmos in systemic lupus erythematosus. Ann Ophthalmol 1984;16:669–71.
76. Rozenberg I, Wechsler J, Koenig F, et al. Erdheim-Chester disease presenting as malignant exophthalmos. Br J Radiol 1986;59:173–7.
77. Shields JA, Karcioglu ZA, Shields CL, et al. Orbital and eyelid involvement with Erdheim-Chester disease. Arch Ophthalmol 1991;109:850–4.
78. Cornblath WT, Dotan SA, Trobe JD, Headington JT. Varied clinical spectrum of necrobiotic xanthogranuloma. Ophthalmology 1992;99:103–7.
79. Harris GJ, Murphy ML, Schmidt EW, et al. Orbital myositis as a perineoplastic syndrome. Arch Ophthalmol 1994;112:380–6.
80. Leib ML, Odel JG, Cooney MJ. Orbital polymyositis and giant cell myocarditis. Ophthalmology 1994; 101:950–4.
81. Gonzalez CL, Jaffe ES. The histiocytoses: clinical presentation and differential diagnosis. Oncology 1990;4:47–60.
82. Friendly DS, Font RL, Rao NA. Orbital involvement in sinus histocytosis. A report of four cases. Arch Ophthalmol 1977;95:2006–11.
83. Char DH, Ablin A, Beckstead J. Histiocytic disorders of the orbit. Ann Ophthalmol 1984;16:867–73.
84. Trocme SD, Baker RH, Bartley GB, et al. Extracellular deposition of eosinophil major basic protein orbital histiocytosis X. Ophthalmology 1991;98:353–6.
85. Ladisch S, Gadner H. Treatment of Langerhans cell histiocytosis-evolution in current approaches. Br J Cancer 1994;23:S41–6.
86. Perry RH, Ramani PS, McAllister V, et al. Nodular fasciitis causing unilateral proptosis. Br Ophthalmol 1975;59:404–8.
87. Font RI, Zimmerman LE. Nodular fasciitis of the eye and adnexa. A report of ten cases. Arch Ophthalmol 1966;75:475–81.
88. Abramovitz JN, Kasdon DL, Sutula F, et al. Sclerosing orbital pseudotumor. Neurosurgery 1983;12:463–8.
89. Friedland S, Kaplan S, Lahav M, Shapiro A. Proptosis and periorbital edema due to diltiazem treatment. Arch Ophthalmol 1993;111:1027–8.
90. Slavin ML. Primary aspergillosis of the orbital apex. Arch Ophthalmol 1991;109:1502–3.

91. Volpe NJ, Shore JW. Orbital myositis associated with herpes zoster. Arch Ophthalmol 1991;109:471–2.
92. Rootman J, Patel S, Jewell L. Polyclonal orbital and systemic infiltrates. Ophthalmology 1984;91:1112–7.
93. Fishleder A, Tubbs R, Hesse B, Levine H. Uniform detection of immunoglobulin-gene rearrangement in benign lymphoepithelial lesions. N Engl J Med 1987;316:1118–21.
94. Dolman PJ, Rootman J, Dolman CL. Infiltrating orbital granular cell tumor: a case report and literature review. Br J Ophthalmol 1987;71:47–53.
95. Jonasson F. Orbital plasma cell tumours. Ophthalmologica 1978;177:152–7.
96. Clarke E. Plasma cell myeloma of the orbit. Br J Ophthalmol 1953;37:543–54.
97. Rodman HI, Font RL. Orbital involvement in multiple myeloma. Review of the literature and report of three cases. Arch Ophthalmol 1972;87:30–5.
98. Gonnering RS. Bilateral primary extramedullary orbital plasmacytomas. Ophthalmology 1987;94:267–70.
99. de Smet MD, Rootman J. Orbital manifestations of plasmacytic lymphoproliferations. Ophthalmology 1987;94:995–1003.
100. Ettl AR, Birbamer GG, Philipp W. Orbital involvement in Waldenstrom's acroglobulinemia: ultrasound, computed tomography and magnetic resonance findings. Ophthalmologica 1992;205:40–5.
101. Cytryn AS, Putterman AM, Schneck GL, et al. Predictability of magnetic resonance imaging in differentiation of orbital lymphoma for orbital inflammatory syndrome. Ophthal Plast Reconstr Surg 1997;11:129–34.
102. Harr DL, Quencer RM, Abrams GW. Computed tomography and ultrasound in the evaluation of orbital infection and pseudotumor. Radiology 1982; 142:395–401.
103. Coleman DJ, Jack RL, Jones IS, Franzen LA. Ultrasonography. VI. Pseudotumors of the orbit. Arch Ophthalmol 1972;88:472–80.
104. Arnold AC, LaMasters DL. Foraminal expansion by malignant retro-orbital lymphoma: CT findings. J Comput Assist Tomogr 1987;11:730–2.
105. Schroeder W. Zur Topographie Orbitaler Lymphome. Klin Monatsbl Augenheilk 1979;174:157–65.
106. Knowles DM II, Jakobiec FA. Orbital lymphoid neoplasms: a clinicopathologic study of 60 patients. Cancer 1980;46:576–89.
107. Westacott S, Garner A, Moseley IF, Wright JE. Orbital lymphoma versus reactive lymphoid hyperplasia: an analysis of the use of computed tomography in differential diagnosis. Br J Ophthalmol 1991;75:722–5.
108. Yeo JH, Jakobiec FA, Abbott GF, Trokel SL. Combined clinical and computer tomographic diagnosis of orbital lymphoid tumors. Am J Ophthalmol 1982; 94:235–45.
109. Krohel GB, Krauss HR, Winnick J. Orbital abscess: presentation, diagnosis, therapy, and sequelae. Ophthalmology 1982;89:492–8.
110. Gamel JW, Font RL. Adenoid cystic carcinoma of the lacrimal gland: the clinical significance of a basaloid histologic pattern. Hum Pathol 1982;13:219–25.
111. Jakobiec FA, Yeo JH, Trokel SL, et al. Combined clinical and computed tomographic diagnosis of primary lacrimal fossa lesions. Am J Ophthalmol 1982;94:785–807.
112. Hornblass A, Jakobiec FA, Reifler DM, Mines J. Orbital lymphoid tumors located predominantly within extraocular muscles. Ophthalmology 1987; 94:688–97.
113. Liang R, Loke SL, Chiu E. A clinico-pathological analysis of 17 cases of non-Hodgkin's lymphoma involving the orbit. Acta Oncologica 1991;30:335–8.
114. White VA, Gascoyne RD, McNeil BK, et al. Histologica findings and frequency of clonality detected by the polymerase chain reaction in ocular adnexal lymphoproliferative lesions. Mod Pathol 1996;9:1052–61.
115. Jakobiec FA, Neri A, Knowles DM II. Genotypic monoclonality in immunophenotypically polyclonal orbital lymphoid tumors. Ophthalmology 1987;94:980–94.
116. Coupland SE, Kraus L, Delecluse H-J, et al. Lymphoproliferative lesions of the ocular adnexa: analysis of 112 cases. Ophthalmology 1998;105:1430–41.
117. Kielar RA. Orbital granuloma in Hodgkin's disease. Ann Ophthalmol 1981;13:1197–9.
118. Nikaido H, Mishima HK, Kiuchi Y, Nanba K. Primary orbital malignant lymphoma: a clinicopathology study of 17 cases. Graefes Arch Clin Exp Ophthalmol 1991;229:206–9.
119. Jackson A, Kwartz J, Noble JL, Reagan MJ. Case report: multiple myeloma presenting as bilateral orbital masses: CT and MR appearances. Br J Radiol 1993;66:266–8.
120. Bairey O, Kremer I, Rakowsky E, et al. Orbital and adnexal involvement in systemic non-Hodgkin's lymphoma. Cancer 1994;73:2395–9.
121. Harris NL, Jaffe ES, Armitage JO, Ship, M. Lymphoma classification: from REAL to WHO and beyond. Principles Prac Oncol 1999;13:1–14.
122. Ellis JH, Banks PM, Campbell RJ, Liesegang TJ. Lymphoid tumors of the ocular adnexa. Clinical correlation with the working formulation classification and immunoperoxidase staining of paraffin sections. Ophthalmology 1985;92:1311–24.
123. Nabholtz JM, Friedman S, Collin F, Guerrin J. Modification of Kiel and working formulation classifications for improved survival prediction in non-Hodgkin's lymphoma. J Clin Oncol 1987;5:1634–9.
124. National Cancer Institute sponsored study of classifications of non-Hodgkin's lymphomas. Summary and description of a working formulation for clinical usage. Cancer 1982;49:2112–35.

125. Rappaport H. Tumors of the hematopoietic system. Atlas of tumor pathology, Section 3, Fasc., 8. Washington, DC: U.S. Armed Forces Institute of Pathology; 1966. p. 97–161.
126. Lukes RJ, Collins RD. Lukes-Collins classification and its significance. Cancer Treat Rep 1977;61:971–9.
127. Dorfman RF, Kim H. Relationship of histology to site in the non-Hodgkin's lymphomata: a study based on surgical staging procedures. Br J Cancer 1975;31: 217–20.
128. Campo E, Jaffe ES. Mantle cell lymphoma: accurate diagnosis yields new clniical insights. Arch Pathol Lab Med 1996;120:12–4.
129. Auer IA, Gascoyne RD, Conors JM, et al. T(11;18)(q21;q21) is the most common translocation in MALT lymphomas. Ann Oncol 1997;8:979–85.
130. Johnson TE, Tse DT, Byrne GE, et al. Ocular-adnexal lymphoid tumors: a clinicopathologic and molecular genetic study of 77 patients. Ophthal Plast Reconstr Surg 1999;15:171–9.
131. Collins RD. Clonality equivalent to malignancy: specifically is immunoglobulin gene rearrangement diagnostic of lymphoma? Hum Pathol 1997;2817: 57–9.
132. Lust JA. Molecular genetics and lymphoproliferative disorders. J Clin Lab Anal 1996;10:359–67.
133. Park KL, Goins KM. Hodgkin's lymphoma of the orbit associated with acquired immune deficiency syndrome. Am J Ophthalmol 1993;116:111–2.
134. Font RL, Laucirica R, Patrinely JR. Immunoblastic B-cell malignant lymphoma involving the orbit and maxillary sinus in acquired immune deficiency syndrome. Ophthalmology 1993;100:966–70.
135. Turok DI, Meyer DR. Orbital lymphoma associated with acquired immune deficiency syndrome. Arch Ophthalmol 1992;110:610–1.
136. Karp JE, Broder S. Acquired immunodeficiency syndrome and non-Hodgkin's lymphomas. Cancer Res 1991;51:4743–56.
137. Matzkin DC, Slamovits TL, Rosenbaum PS. Simultaneous intraocular and orbital non-Hodgkin's lymphoma in the acquired immune deficiency syndrome. Ophthalmology 1994;101:850–5.
138. Logani S, Logani SC, Ali BH, Goldberg RA. Bilateral, intraconal non-Hodgkin's lymphoma in a patient with acquired immunodeficiency syndrome. Am J Ophthalmol 1994;118:401–2.
139. Fujikawa LS, Meisler DM, Nozik RA. Hyperosmolar hyperglycemic nonketotic coma. A complication of short-term systemic corticosteroid use. Ophthalmology 1983;90:1239–42.
140. Chamberlain P, Meyer WJ III. Management of pituitary-adrenal suppression secondary to corticosteroid therapy. Pediatrics 1981;67:245–51.
141. Shabb N, Katz R, Ordonez N, et al. Fine-needle aspiration evalulation of lymphoproliferative lesions in human immunodeficiency virus-positive patients. Cancer 1991;67:1008–18.
142. Fleisher TA. Immunophenotyping of lymphocytes by flow cytometry. Immunol Allergy Clin North Am 1994;14:225–40.
143. Knowles DM. Immunophenotypic and immunogenotypic approaches useful in distinguishing benign and malignant lymphoid proliferations. Semin Oncol 1993;20:583–610.
144. Skoog L, Lowhagen T, Astarita RW, et al. Fine-needle aspiration cytology and immunocytochemistry of ocular adnexal lymphoid tumors. Orbit [In press]
145. Sneige N, Dekmezian RH, Katz RL, et al. Morphologic and immunocytochemical evaluation of 220 fine needle aspirates of malignant lymphoma and lymphoid hyperplasia. Acta Cytologica 1990;34:311–22.
146. Joensuu H, Alanen K, Klemi PJ. Prognosis of lymphoma from a fine-needle aspirate. Eur J Cancer 1993;291:29–33.
147. Tijl JWM, Koornneef L. Fine-needle aspiration biopsy in orbital tumours. Br J Ophthalmol 1991;75:491–2.
148. Garner A. Orbital lymphoproliferative disorders. Br J Ophthalmol 1992;76:47–8.
149. Morgan G, Harry J. Lymphocytic tumours of indeterminant nature: a 5-year follow-up of 98 conjunctival and orbital lesions. Br J Ophthalmol 1978;62:381–3.
150. Jakobiec FA, McLean I, Font RL. Clinicopathologic characteristics of orbital lymphoid hyperplasia. Ophthalmology 1979;86:948–66.
151. Waldmann TA, Korsmeyer SJ, Bakhshi A, et al. Molecular genetic analysis of human lymphoid neoplasms. Immunoglobulin genes and the c-myc oncogene. Ann Intern Med 1985;102:497–510.
152. Char DH. Orbital tumor diagnosis: lymphoma versus pseudotumor. Trans Pacific Coast Oto-Ophthalmol Soc 1980;60:21–5.
153. Char DH. Immunology of uveitis and ocular tumors. New York, NY: Grune and Stratton; 1978.
154. Garner A, Rahi AH, Wright JE. Lymphoproliferative disorders of the orbit: an immunological approach to diagnosis and pathogenesis. Br J Ophthalmol 1983;67:561–9.
155. Aisenberg AC. Current concepts in immunology: cell-surface markers in lymphoproliferative disease. N Engl J Med 1981;304:331–6.
156. Stein RS, Cousar J, Flexner JM, Collins RD. Correlations between immunologic markers and histopathologic classifications: clinical implications. Semin Oncol 1980;7:244–54.
157. Harmon DC, Aisenberg AC, Harris NL, et al. Lymphocyte surface markers in orbital lymphoid neoplasms. J Clin Oncol 1984;2:856–60.
158. Knowles DM II, Jakobiec FA. Identification of T lymphocytes in ocular adenexal neoplasms by hybridoma monoclonal antibodies. Am J Ophthalmol 1983; 95:233–42.

159. van der Gaag R, Koornneef L, van Heerde P, et al. Lymphoid proliferations in the orbit: malignant or benign? Br J Ophthalmol 1984;68:892–900.
160. Arnold A, Cossman J, Bakhshi A, et al. Immunoglobulin-gene rearrangements as unique clonal markers in human lymphoid neoplasms. N Engl J Med 1983;309:1593–9.
161. Warnke RA, Rouse RV. Limitations encountered in the application of tissue section, immunodiagnosis to the study of lymphomas and related disorders. Hum Pathol 1985;16:326–31.
162. Wick MR. Immunocytochemical markers of benignancy and malignancy. Do they exist? Arch Pathol Lab Med 1986;110:180–1.
163. Cleary ML, Sklar J. Lymphoproliferative disorders in cardiac transplant recipients of multiclonal lymphomas. Lancet 1984;2:489–93.
164. Lucas DR, Knox F, Davies S. Apparent monoclonal origin of lymphocytes and plasma cells infiltrating ocular adnexal amyloid deposits: report of 2 cases. Br J Ophthalmol 1982;66:600–6.
165. McNally L, Jakobiec FA, Knowles DM II. Clinical, morphologic, immunophenotypic, and molecular genetic analysis of bilateral ocular adnexal lymphoid neoplasms in 17 patients. Am J Ophthalmol 1987;103:555–68.
166. Jakobiec FA, Knowles DM. An overview of ocular adnexal lymphoid tumors. Tr Am Ophthalmol Soc 1989;87:420–42.
167. Font RL, Laucirica R, Rosenbaum PS, et al. Malignant lymphoma of the ocular adnexa associated with the benign lymphoepithelial lesion of the parotid glands. Report of two cases. Ophthalmology 1992; 99:1582–7.
168. Mombaerts I, Koornneef L. Current status in the treatment of orbital myositis. Ophthalmology 1997;104: 402–8.
169. Mombaerts I, Schlingemann RO, Goldschmeding R, et al. The surgical management of lacrimal gland pseudotumors. Ophthalmology 1996;103:1619–27.
170. Donaldson SS, McDougall IR, Egbert PR, et al. Treatment of orbital pseudotumor (idiopathic orbital inflammation) by radiation therapy. Int J Radiat Oncol Biol Phys 1980;6:79–86.
171. Hurbli T, Char DH, Harris J, et al. Radiation therapy for thyroid eye disease. Am J Ophthalmol 1985;99: 633–7.
172. Chavis RM, Garner A, Wright JE. Inflammatory orbital pseudotumor. A clinicopathologic study. Arch Ophthalmol 1978;96:1817–22.
173. Reid IR. Preventing glucocorticoid-induced osteoporosis. N Eng J Med 1997;337:420–1.
174. Mombaerts I, Schlingemann RO, Goldschmeding R, Koornneef L. Are systemic corticosteroids useful in the management of orbital pseudotumors. Ophthalmology 1996;103:521–8.
175. Kinyoun JL, Kalina RE, Brower SA, et al. Radiation retinopathy after orbital irradiation for Graves' ophthalmopathy. Arch Ophthalmol 1984;102:1473–6.
176. Coop ME. Pseudotumour of the orbit. A clinical and pathological study of 47 cases. Br J Ophthalmol 1961;45:513–42.
177. Fitzpatrick PJ, Macko S. Lymphoreticular tumors of the orbit. Int J Radiat Oncol Biol Phys 1984;10: 333–40.
178. Sergott RC, Glaser JS, Charyulu K. Radiotherapy for idiopathic inflammatory orbital pseudotumor: indications and results. Arch Ophthalmol 1981;99:853–6.
179. Jereb B, Lee H, Jakobiec FA, Kutcher J. Radiation therapy of conjunctival and orbital lymphoid tumors. Int J Radiat Oncol Biol Phys 1984;10:1013–9.
180. Kennerdell JS, Johnson BL, Deutsch M. Radiation treatment of orbital lymphoid hyperplasia. Ophthalmology 1979;86:942–7.
181. Kim RY, Roth RE. Radiotherapy of orbital pseudotumor. Radiology 1978;127:507–9.
182. Orcutt JC, Garner A, Henk JM, Wright JE. Treatment of idiopathic inflammatory orbital pseudotumors by radiotherapy. Br J Ophthalmol 1983;67:570–4.
183. Austin-Seymour MM, Donaldson SS, Egbert PR, et al. Radiotherapy of lymphoid diseases of the orbit. Int J Radiat Oncol Biol Phys 1985;11:371–9.
184. Lanciano R, Fowble B, Sergott RC, et al. The results of radiotherapy for orbital pseudotumor. Int J Radiat Oncol Biol Phys 1990;18:407–11.
185. Keleti D, Flickinger JC, Hobson SR, Mittal BB. Radiotherapy of lymphoproliferative diseases of the orbit. Am J Clin Oncol 1992;15:422–7.
186. Bolek TW, Moyses HM, Marculs RB Jr, et al. Radiotherapy in the management of orbital lymphoma. Int J Radiat Oncol Biol Phys 1999;44:31–6.
187. Yaghouti F, Nouri M, Mannor GE. Ocular adnexal granulocytic sarcoma as the first sign of acute myelogenous leukemia relapse. Am J Ophthalmol 1999;127:361–3.
188. Smitt MC, Donaldson SS. Radiotherapy is successful treatment for orbital lymphoma. Int J Radiat Oncol Biol Phys 1993;26:59–66.
189. Platanias LC, Putterman AN, Vijayakumar S, et al. Treatment and prognosis of orbital non-Hodgkin's lymphomas. Am J Clin Oncol 1992;15:79–83.
190. Henk JM, Whitelocke RAF, Warrington AP, Bessell EM. Radiation dose to the lens and cataract formation. Int J Radiat Oncol Biol Phys 1993;25: 815–20.
191. McCartney DL, Char DH. Return of vision following orbital decompression after 36 hours of postoperative blindness. Am J Ophthalmol 1985;100:602–4.
192. Moshfeghi DM, Finger PT, Cohen RB, et al. Visual recovery after radiation therapy of orbital lymphoma. Am J Ophthalmol 1992;114:645–6.

27

Orbital Therapy

Management options in the treatment of orbital neoplasms are limited by the bony constraints of the orbital cavity, the plethora of important nerves and small vessels that course through it, the eye, and the vital nature of contiguous structures. Given these constraints, it is usually impossible to resect a malignant neoplasm with both adequate margins and retention of visual function. Similarly, some benign and malignant apical tumors cannot be excised without doing irreparable harm to ophthalmic or central nervous system (CNS) function, and many benign processes are sufficiently diffuse to make complete removal fraught with ocular complications.

As discussed in other sections, almost any orbital lesion can be biopsied with either a fine-needle or standard surgical technique. Most orbital neoplasms should be biopsied with the possible exception of typical, stationary intraorbital optic nerve sheath meningiomas and pediatric optic nerve gliomas. I follow many of these lesions without intervention, if they are asymptomatic, until growth is documented; their imaging patterns are usually sufficiently characteristic to obviate the need for biopsy. Many focal encapsulated benign neoplasms can be removed in toto. Some malignant neoplasms can be removed with minimal margins, and in some cases, debulking with adjunctive radiation and chemotherapy has significantly improved survival.

Therapy for most malignant orbital neoplasms is predicated on the tumor's radiation and chemotherapy sensitivity versus the need, in nonresponsive malignancies, to perform an exenteration. The standard exenteration technique is discussed under treatment of posterior uveal tumors. Modification of this technique to include a temporalis skin flap or an anterior exenteration is discussed in Chapter 4.

Malignancies that are sensitive to either chemotherapy, radiation, or both usually can be biopsied, debulked, and given adjunctive therapy. This approach has decreased the tumor-related mortality associated with orbital rhabdomyosarcoma from approximately 50 percent to < 5 percent. If there is a tumor metastatic to the orbit, radiation or chemotherapy alone is often sufficient palliative therapy (see chapter on orbital metastases). Unfortunately, the radiation sensitivity of some primary and metastatic tumors is not well established, since only a few cases have been followed up for a sufficient time since the development of modern radiotherapy.

RADIATION THERAPY

Radiation therapy has been used to treat orbital neoplasms since the first decade of the 20th century.[1] Table 27–1 (see p. 466) lists various orbital conditions that have been treated with radiation.

The advent of multiple types of megavoltage radiation (photons, electrons, and particles), the use of computer simulation, newer delivery systems (including protons and intensity-modulated conformal therapy), and recent data on radiobiologic effects on neural tissue have changed many approaches to the radiation of eye and orbital malignancies. Four radiation parameters are of paramount importance in minimizing damage to normal ocular tissue: radiation equipment, fraction size, fractionation schedule, and total dose.[1] A number of investigators have shown that using daily radiation fractions < 225 centigrays (cGy) (225 rads) substantially decreases radiation-induced morbidity.[2] Similarly the length of time between radiation fractions can markedly influence normal tissue damage, as can total dose. Generally, with the above fractionation schedule (< 225 cGy/d), significant radiation vasculopathy of the retina or optic nerve usually does not occur at < 50 Gy of total dosage.[2] Unfortunately, for most adult primary orbital malignancies, total radiation doses between 55 and 60 Gy are necessary for a possible cure, and these historically produced marked ocular complications.[3–9]

The quality of radiation therapy is highly dependent on the radiation treatment planning capacity of the institution, including both computer simulation and radiation physics, plus the age and sophistication of the radiation equipment.[10] We have been able to diminish ocular morbidity with the use of computer simulation and a combination of different radiation therapies, including electrons, photons, intensity-modulated conformal therapy, and charged particles. Treatment with obsolescent radiotherapy equipment results in more complications than when modern techniques are used. Optimal orbital irradiation occasionally requires extremely sophisticated radiation treatment planning, as shown schematically in Figure 27–1. Here, multiple radiation fields were used to optimize therapy.[11] Treatment planning based on computed tomagraphy (CT) is imperative for good radiotherapy; absence of this modality can result in as little as 60 percent of the planned dose being delivered to the tumor.[12]

Conventional treatment of both orbits with lateral radiation ports for either thyroid bilateral orbitopathy or pseudotumor is schematically shown in Figure 27–2.[10,13] The isodose distribution for the split-beam technique used to treat bilateral orbital lymphomas is shown in Figure 27–3[14,15] while the oblique-field isocentric technique used to treat a unilateral orbital tumor is shown in Figure 27–4.[14–16]

Newer radiation delivery approaches to precisely encompass the treatment field but avoid contiguous structures, and therefore lessen morbidity, have been developed. The two major new approaches that impact ophthalmologic oncology are the use of the Gamma Knife and intensity-modulated conformal therapy. There is little ophthalmic data available for either of these approaches. Gamma Knives have been used with great success to treat CNS lesions generally < 1 cm^3 in volume. The technology is such that treatment of larger lesions results in much less precise

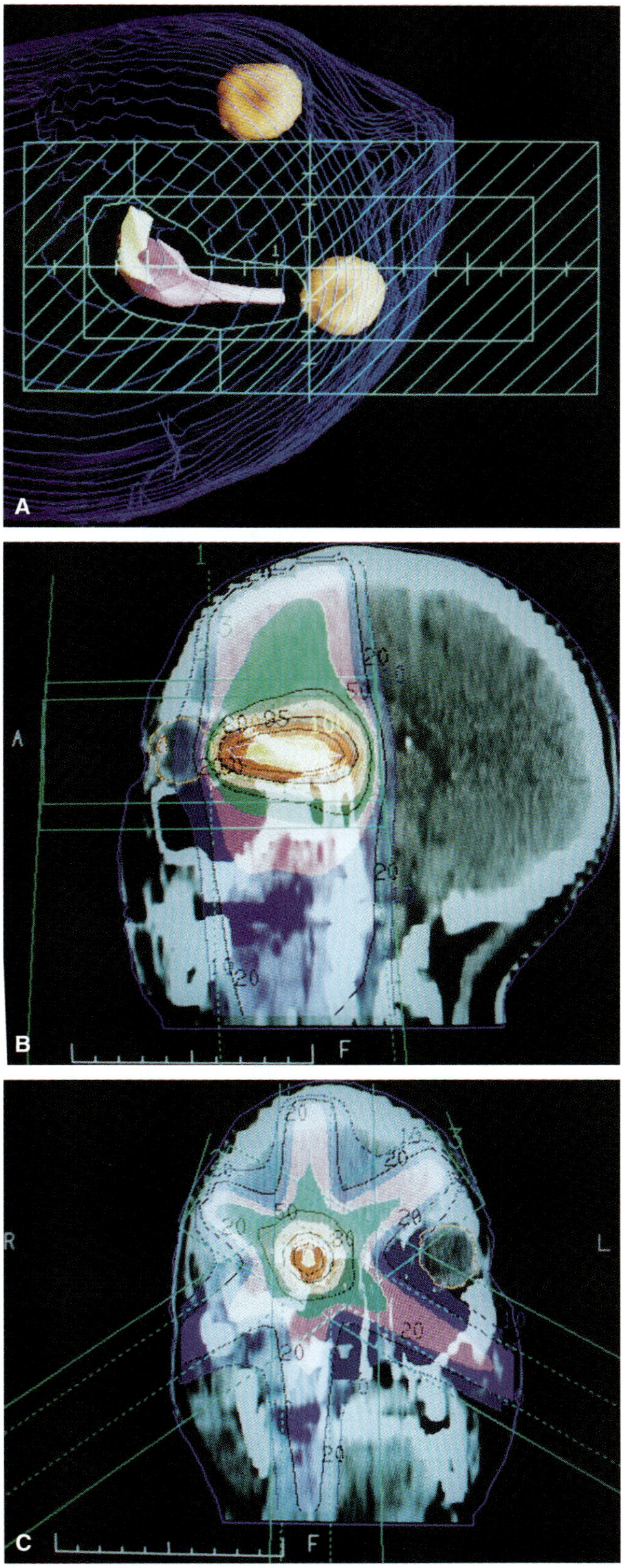

Figure 27–1. Complex treatment planning and use of multiple radiation fields to treat a unilateral orbital tumor. (From Harisadis et al., with permission.)

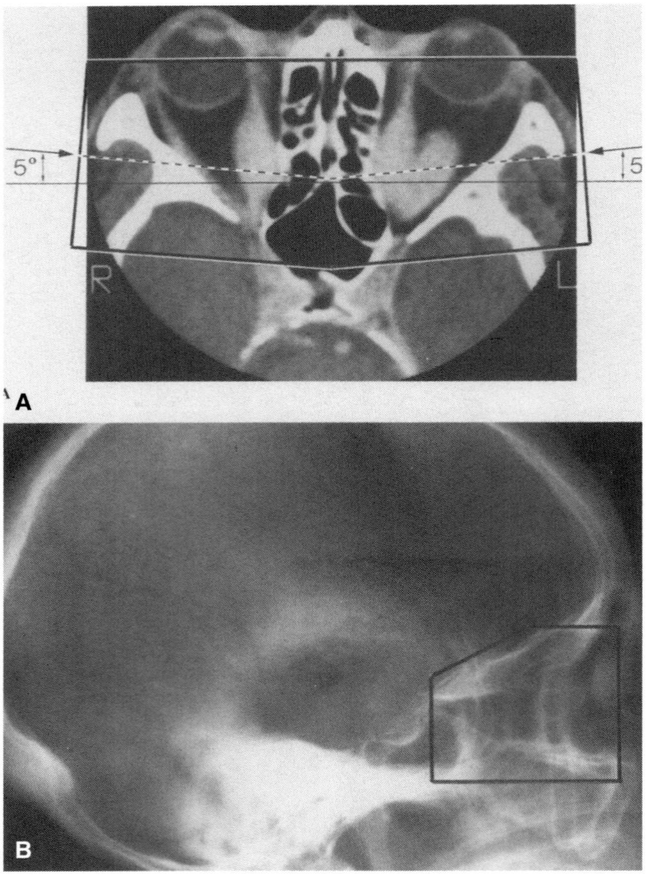

Figure 27–2. *A,* Radiation field used for treatment of bilateral thyroid orbitopathy or pseudotumor. *B,* CT simulation of treatment in Figure 27–2A (From Char,[42] with permission.)

radiation delivery than is available with other approaches. Gamma Knife radiation is discussed in the chapters on uveal melanoma and retinal tumors. Intensity-modulated conformal therapy has been shown to decrease morbidity with excellent disease control, in other body sites.[17] As shown in the chapter on orbital sinus lesions, conformal therapy can deliver a high dose of radiation to the area in question, with sparing of uninvolved orbital structures. There are limited long-term data demonstrating the efficacy of this technique to prevent ophthalmic morbidity, but I believe it is highly likely that this will come. The downside of intensity-modulated conformal therapy is that it is extremely time consuming, the equipment is expensive, and the technique is in evolution. Figure

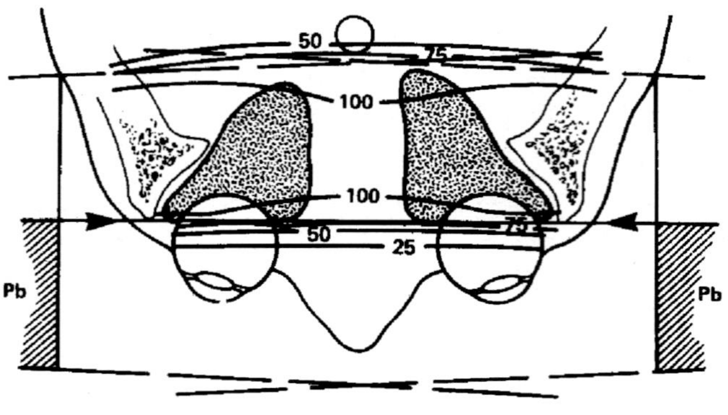

Figure 27–3. Isodose distribution for orbital radiation using lateral fields (From Donaldson et al.,[14] with permission.)

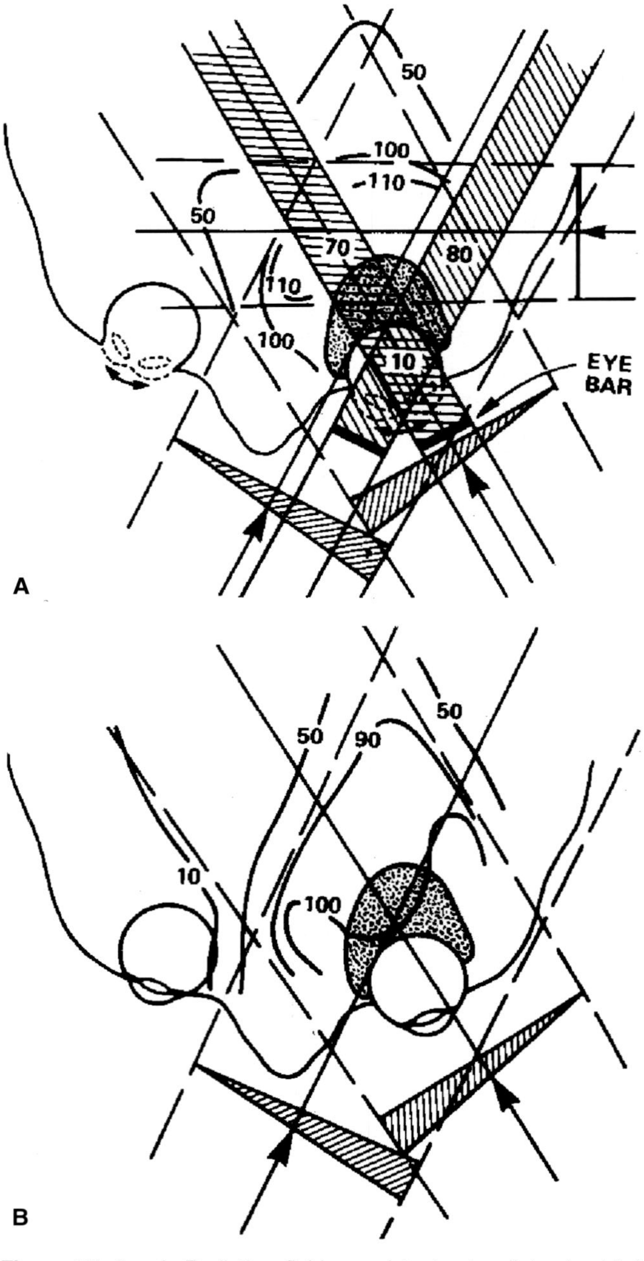

Figure 27–4. *A,* Radiation fields used to treat unilateral orbital process, with eye bars. *B,* Without eye bars. (From Donaldson et al.,[14] with permission)

27–5 shows a patient with metastatic lung cancer to the orbit treated with conformal therapy. Note that the isodose delivery to the eye demonstrates much lower radiation to ocular structures than possible with conventional forms of therapy.

Some authors have advocated the use of brachytherapy for orbital tumors.[18,19] The author believes that the use of intensity-modulated conformal therapy has obviated the use of this, except in cases where exenteration has been performed and one is using radiation as an adjunctive treatment or in those centers that do not have the capacity to provide intensity-modulated conformal therapy.

ORBITAL SURGERY

Surgical Approaches

There are a number of surgical approaches into the orbit. The choice of approach is predicated primarily on tumor location but is also affected by the type of orbital surgery anticipated (incisional or excisional biopsy), tumor size, and involvement of contiguous structures (sinuses, CNS, or bone). The advent of ophthalmic orbital surgery is relatively recent; Kroenlein's initial procedure was first described in the early part of the 20th century.[20] Five major surgical techniques are described in this chapter. Most orbital tumor surgery is performed in the lateral, superior, or medial orbit; inferior tumors are less common, and they are approached in an analagous manner with minor modifications.

A few general principles are germane to all types of orbital tumor surgery. As discussed in the chapter on diagnosis and management of orbital tumors, the use of high-resolution CT with computer re-formation or direct multiplanar magnetic resonance imaging (MRI) is very useful prior to surgery to optimize the surgeon's knowledge of the tumor's relationship to normal orbital, CNS, or sinus stuctures. In a number of cases, excellent imaging data resulted in the choice of a better and different orbital surgical approach than would have been anticipated prior to obtaining those studies. We do not dilate the pupil

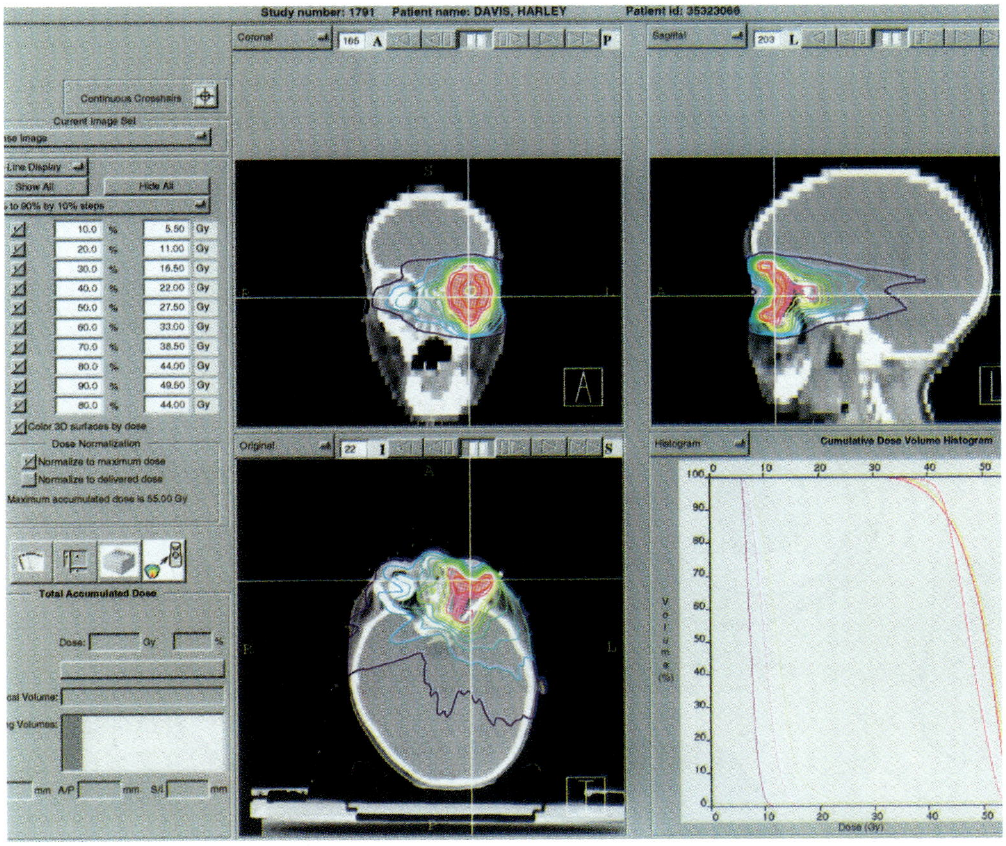

Figure 27–5. Intensity-modulated conformal therapy to treat a lung carcinoma metastatic to the orbit.

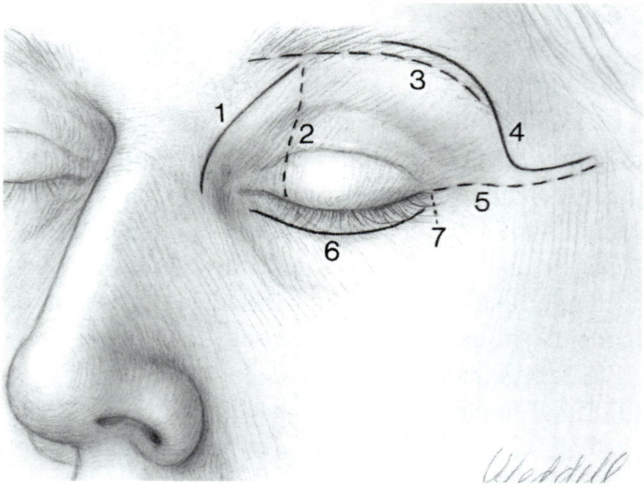

Figure 27–6. Orbital Incisions: (1) Lynch incision used to reach tumors that involve the ethmoid/frontal sinuses and the medial orbit. (2) Byron Smith incision for superior nasal orbital tumors. (3) Benedict's incision used to biopsy superior orbital lesions. (4) Modified Wright's incision for lateral and intraconal biopsies. (5) Berke incision, which was used historically and was modified from the Kroenlein incision to enter the lateral orbit. (6) Subciliary lower eyelid incision. (7) and (8) (not shown) Conjunctival or caruncle incisions.

prior to orbital surgery. Nonpharmacologic pupillary dilation during an orbital procedure indicates either pressure on the optic nerve or trauma, traction, or pressure on the ciliary ganglion. Consequently, not dilating the pupil provides a useful means of monitoring potential damage to these structures. We often use intravenous steroids during orbital surgery for benign inflammatory lesions, especially those in the intraconal space. Historically, such cases often had pronounced postoperative inflammatory rebound; the use of these medications has diminished its occurrence. Figure 27–6 outlines in a schematic manner various surgical approaches to the orbit.

Lateral Orbitotomy

The major indication for a lateral orbitotomy is to gain access to the lateral or intraconal orbital area to resect or biopsy a mass (Figure 27–7). This approach is occasionally used as an adjunct to decompress thyroid orbitopathy or to create space to remove a large medial neoplasm; lateral displacement of the globe facilitates removal of a large tumor from the superior medial, medial, or inferior orbit.

There have been a number of modifications to lateral orbitotomy techniques since Kroenlein's initial description in 1913.[20–24] For access to the lateral or intraconal orbital spaces, the author prefers a modified Stallard-Wright lateral orbitotomy to the original Kroenlein procedure or Berke's modification.[22–24] There are three major advantages to the modified approach: (1) it affords greater exposure than the Berke procedure, in which the orbit is entered via a canthal incision directly posterior into the temporalis fossa; (2) there is a lower incidence of cosmetic complications, since the lateral canthus is left intact; and (3) closure after a modified Stallard-

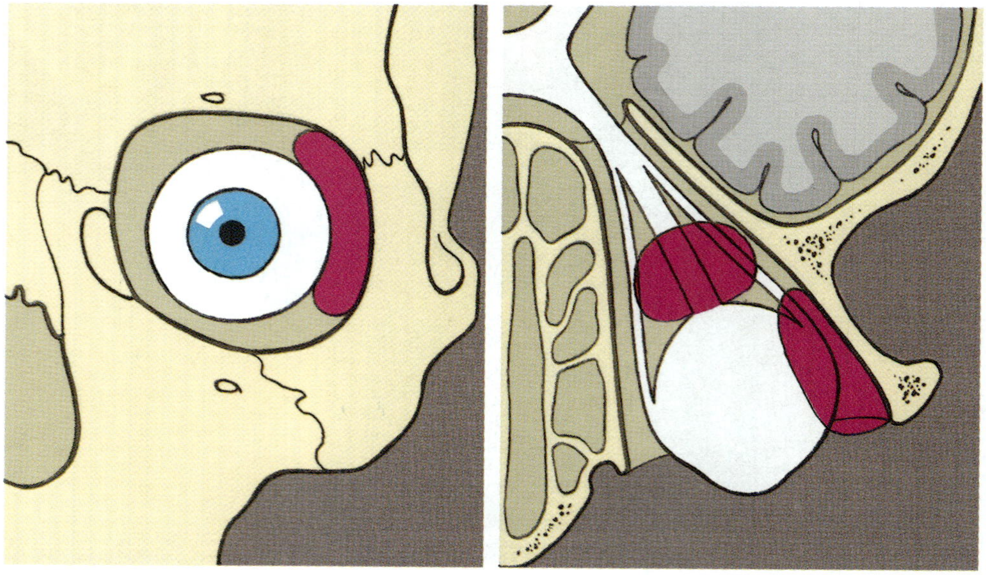

Figure 27–7. Schematic representation of tumors optimally approached through a lateral orbitotomy.

Wright orbitotomy is more rapid than when the canthus has to be reconstructed.

The major limitation of the Stallard-Wright approach is that the lateral rectus muscle is not as easy to identify as when it can be traced directly from its insertion posteriorly into the orbit.[25] This minor problem can be overcome, if there is a potential question, by isolation of the intraorbital portion of the lateral rectus muscle with 2-0 silk sutures. A second limitation is the presence of a tumor in the inferior portion of the intraconal space. In those cases, we combine a Wright's incision with a lateral canthotomy and disinsert the lower crus of the lateral canthal tendon to gain additional access through the opening of the lateral lower lid. The author does not believe that a scalp (bifrontal coronal flap) incision affords significant cosmetic advantage, especially in males with the potential for alopecia. As discussed later, closure of a Wright's incision with subcuticular nylon produces a minimal scar.

A basic orbital surgery set is shown in Figure 27–8. The author does not shave the lateral half of the eyebrow and is unaware of any case in which eyebrow hair did not grow back after orbitotomy. The incision for a Stallard-Wright orbitotomy is through the brow (Figure 27–9). It is curved approximately 5 mm posterior to the lateral orbital rim until it is just posterior to the lateral canthus; it is then directed posteriorly in one of the horizontal skin lines just inferior to the lateral canthus.

After the dermis has been incised with a scalpel, a cutting Bovie set at approximately 30 is used to

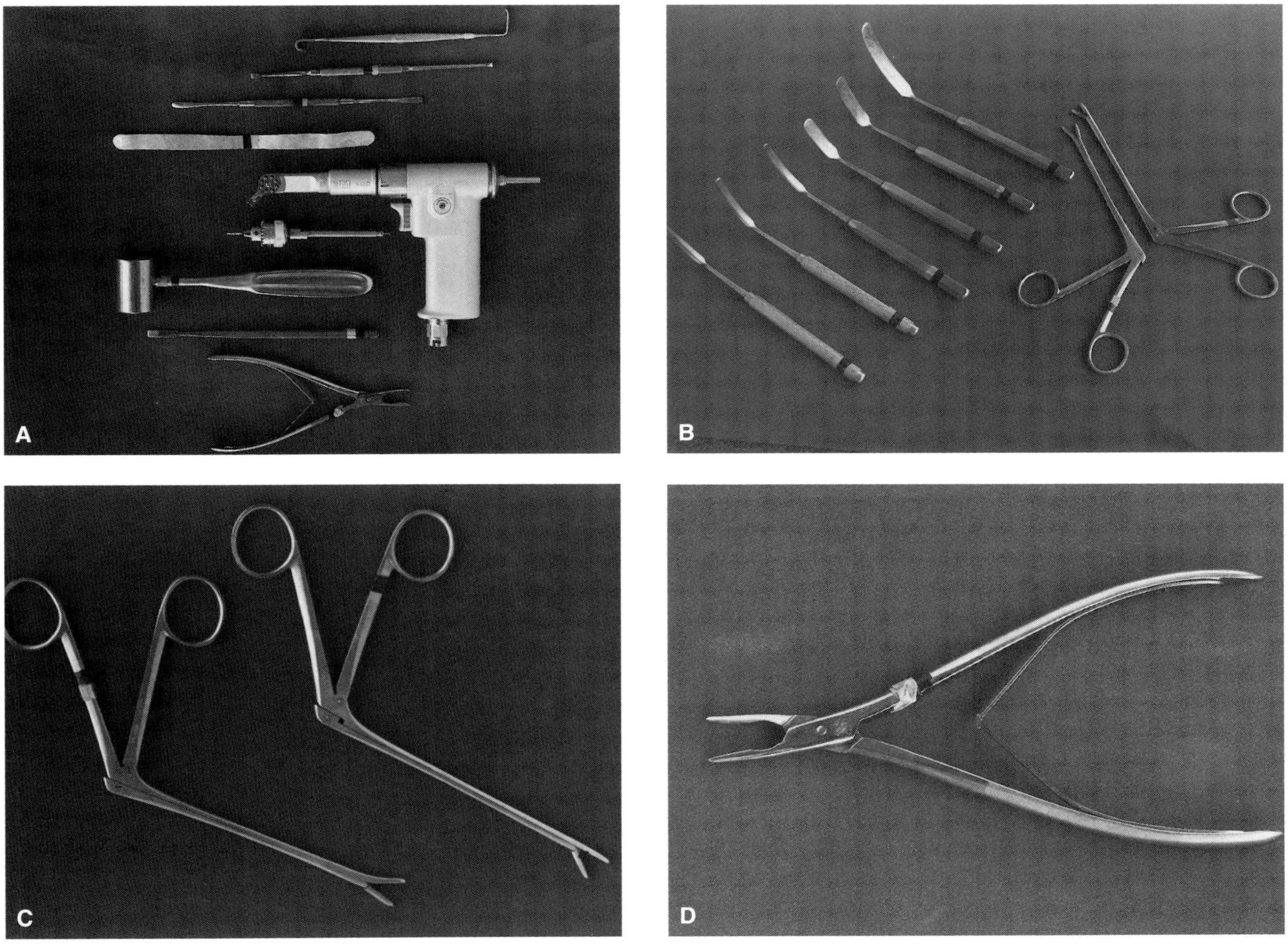

Figure 27–8. *A,* Basic orbital surgical set used by the author. Minidriver combination saw and drill and other instruments used to enter the orbit. The minidriver allows more control than a Stryker saw. *B,* Six Soule retractors and two Takahashi forceps. *C,* Close-up view of Takahashi forceps. *D,* Lempert rongeur.

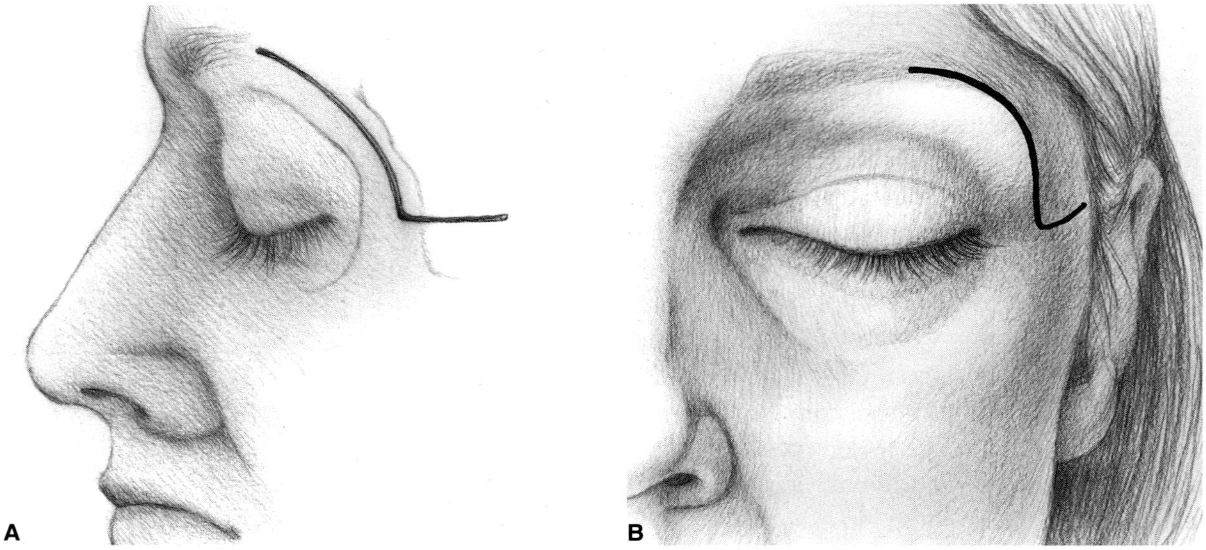

Figure 27–9. Anterior and lateral schematic views of the skin incision for a Stallard-Wright modification of lateral orbitotomy.

reach the periosteum. Hemostasis is achieved with the Bovie; small severed arterioles are first grasped with a snap and then coagulated. There are no arteries of sufficient size to require surgical ties.

A No. 15 Bard-Parker blade is used to incise the periosteum approximately 3 mm posterior to the lateral rim of the orbit, and a posteriorly hinged periosteal flap is created for the entire length of the skin incision (Figure 27–10). At each end of the periosteal incision, along the orbital rim, anterior-posterior cuts are made. It is important to position the periosteal incision slightly posterior to the orbital rim to avoid inadvertent penetration through the periorbita, especially if an epithelial lacrimal tumor is suspected. Sharp and dull Freer elevators are used to remove the periosteum from the bone. A single-edged sharp Freer elevator (see Figure 27–10) is used to create a plane between the periosteum and bone, especially at the bone sutures, and then a dull double-edged elevator is used to separate the periosteum from both the anterior and posterior surfaces of the orbital rim. The author prefers to remove the periosteum from the nonorbital surface of the bone first, to become familiar with the strength of its attachment, and then turns the attention to the orbital bone surface. Special care must be used to avoid inadvertent

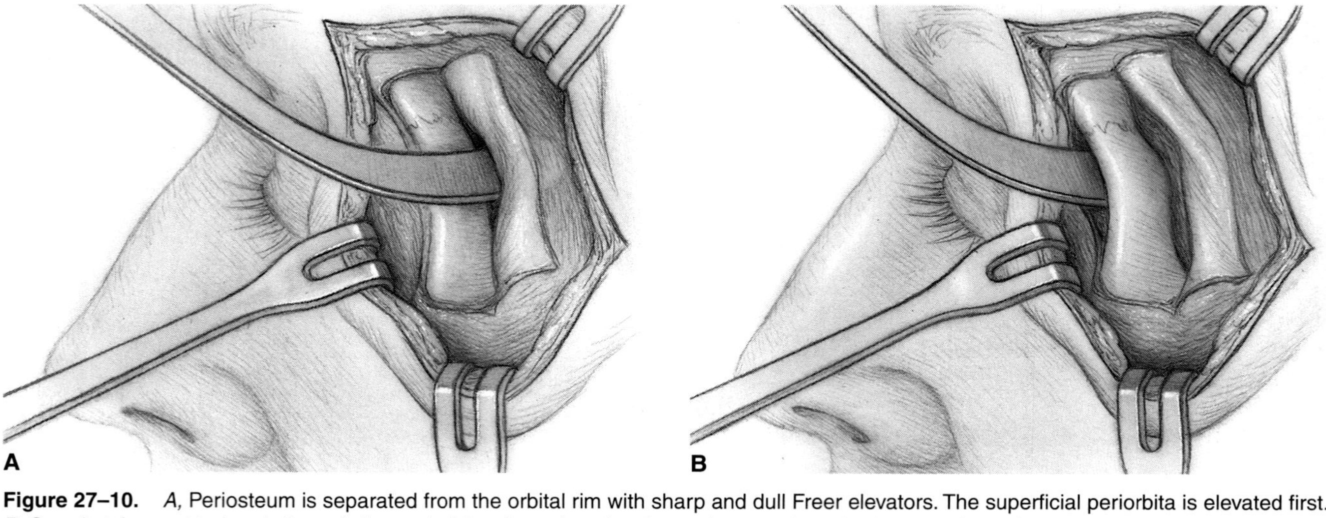

Figure 27–10. *A,* Periosteum is separated from the orbital rim with sharp and dull Freer elevators. The superficial periorbita is elevated first. *B,* Care is taken not to break through the periorbita when elevating the periosteum from the inner surface of the orbital rim.

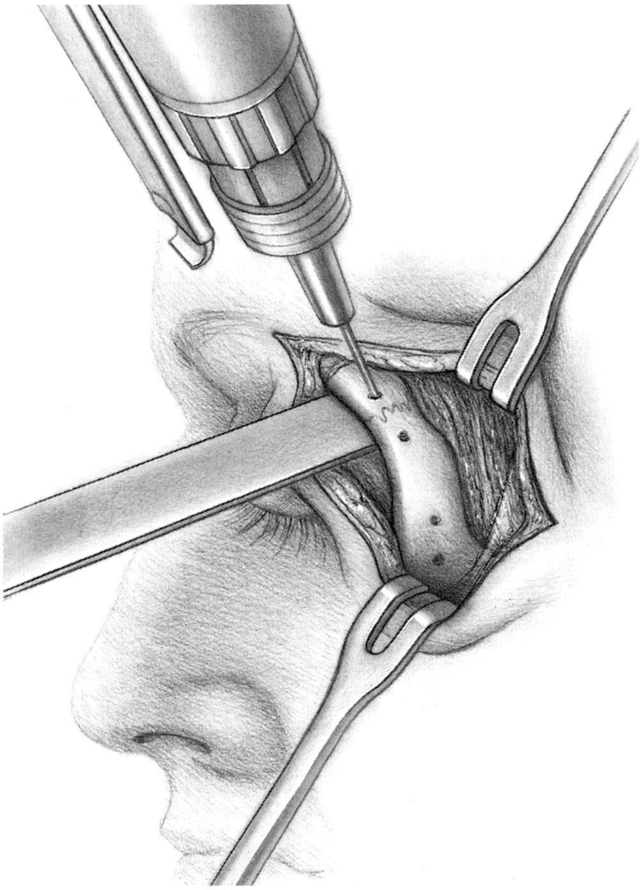

Figure 27–11. Bone holes are drilled on each side of the proposed sites of orbital bone incisions.

penetration through the periorbita as the periosteum is separated from the inner intraorbital surface of the bony rim; the instrument's tip is pressed laterally as the periosteum is removed from the anterior superficial and inner surfaces of the orbital rim.

The degree of periosteum removal from both the anterior and posterior surfaces of the orbital rim depends on the location of the orbital tumor and the orbital exposure required. In surgery for benign lacrimal gland tumors, such as orbital dermoid, we may not remove the lateral orbital rim, but merely hinge it with the periosteum attached posteriorly. In large or more posterior tumors, we often use the cutting Bovie to incise the temporalis muscle to gain greater exposure to the lateral orbital bones behind the rim.

Holes are drilled on each side of the proposed cuts in the orbital bones (Figure 27–11) so that after the orbitotomy, the bone segment can be secured

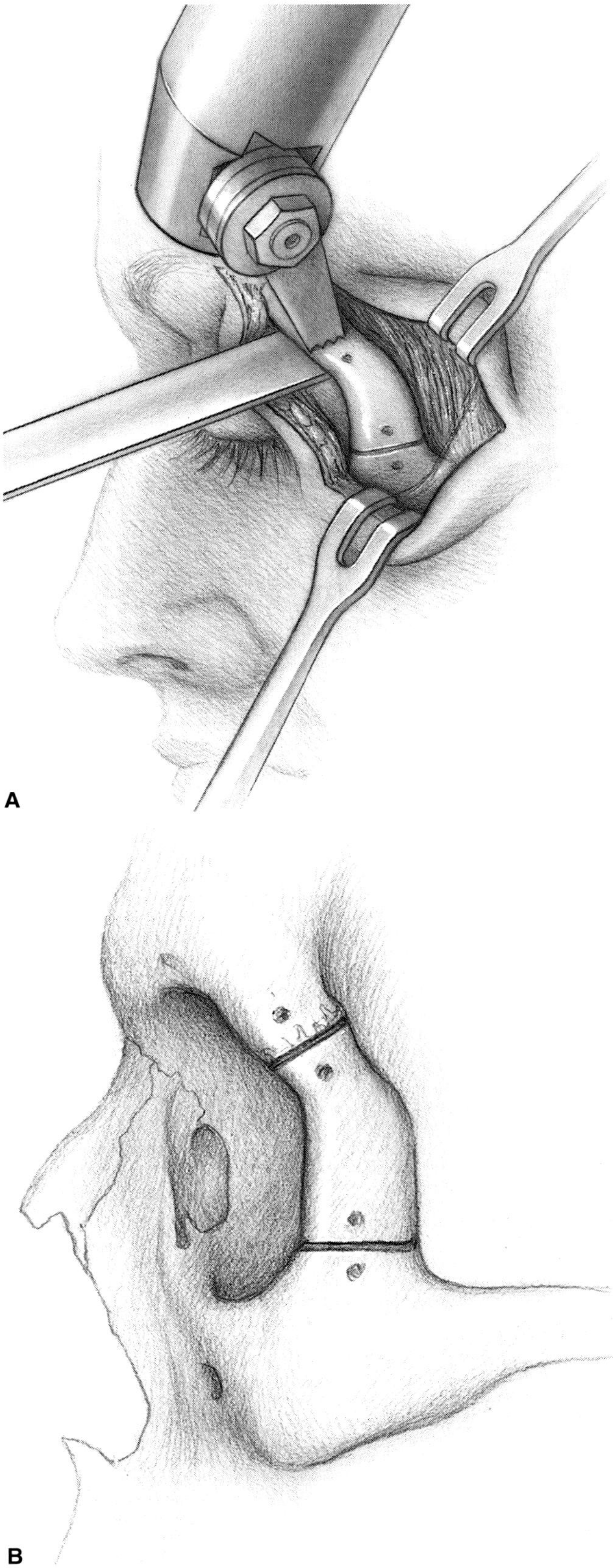

A

B

Figure 27–12. *A,* Bone cuts are performed with a bone saw. *B,* Position of cuts.

with 2-0 nylon. The author prefers this closure to wire, since it does not produce imaging artifacts if later MRI scans are required. A malleable retractor is placed between the lateral orbital wall and the periorbita to protect the orbit and globe while bone holes are drilled. It is often difficult for a novice to drill safely through bone, so the malleable retractor is positioned to protect the globe. After two holes have been completed inferiorly, the malleable retractor is placed at the superior edge of the incision, and two holes are drilled in that portion of the orbital wall.

A malleable retractor is placed between the rim and the orbital contents and the saw is used to make the cuts through the lateral orbital bone (Figure 27–12). Approximately 30 to 35 mm of orbital rim is removed; the bone incision is from the frontal process of the zygomatic bone at the upper edge of the zygomatic arch to above the frontozygomatic suture. The author prefers the more easily controlled minidriver made by Minnesota Mining and Manufacturing to a Stryker saw (see Figure 27–8A). There are now a number of other new combinations of saws and drills that have equal control. Approximately 85 percent of bone thickness is incised with the saw and the remaining 15 percent with hammer and chisel. After using the saw and chisel, the incised bony rim is grasped with a cross-action Lempert rongeur and broken away from the remainder of the orbital rim and posterior cancellous bone.

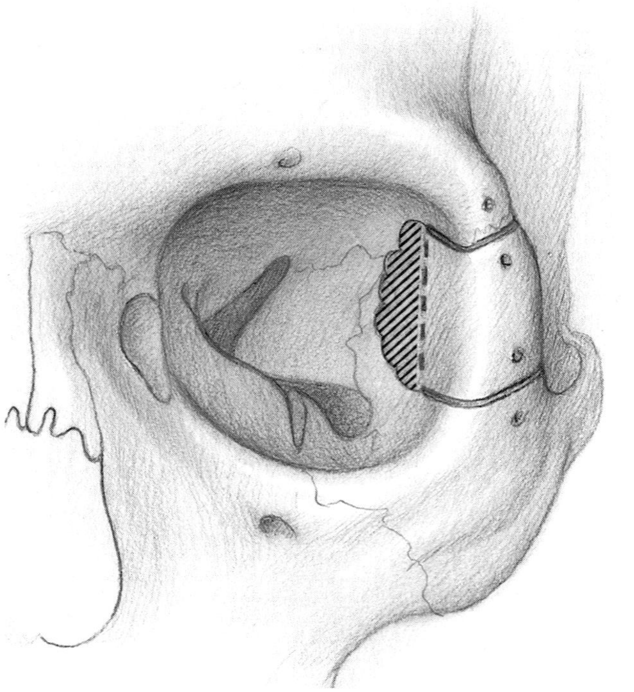

Figure 27–13. A Lempert ronguer is used to remove bone behind the orbital rim (*shaded area*) to gain greater access to the intraconal space.

The bone flap can be either removed or its connection with periosteum and muscle may be retained and the bone hinged posteriorly. If the bone is to be removed, scissors are used to remove the muscle attached to its posterior surface. The bone fragment is placed in a sterile, saline-soaked sponge on the nurses' stand, until it is repositioned in the bony defect at the completion of the procedure. In cases in which the tumor is in the intraconal space, it is advantageous to gain greater access by removing cancellous bone posterior to the orbital rim. After the bone flap is removed, a Lempert rongeur is used to remove the thin cancellous bone posteriorly (Figure 27–13). Occasionally, when orbital rim or cancellous bone is removed, there is sufficient bleeding from the inner table of bone to obscure visualization. This is tamponaded with bone wax applied with the end of a Freer elevator. While others have noted rare complications with bone wax, the author personally has never seen this.[26] Fortunately, bone wax is used in $<$ 10 percent of cases, although in very young children who still have bone marrow in this area, it is often necessary.

There are a number of different periorbital incisions, depending on the size and position of the tumor. If a lacrimal gland malignancy is suspected after either a fine-needle aspiration biopsy (FNAB) or frozen-section biopsy, we attempt to remove the lacrimal gland and the periorbita en bloc. In intraconal tumors, a "T" or "L" shaped incision is made in the periorbita (Figure 27–14). The normal lacrimal gland is visible directly under the periorbita (Figure 27–15), and blunt dissection by spreading Stevens scissors is used to separate and create a plane in the orbital fat either above or behind the lacrimal gland. Four Soule retractors (see Figure 27–7B) are then positioned to retract orbital fat from the capsule of the tumor. In most cases, the author has not found various self-retaining orbital retractors more effective, and they are rather cumbersome to handle.

A large neurosurgical paddy is placed over the bony orbital incision to absorb minor venous leakage from bone, temporalis muscle, or periorbita.

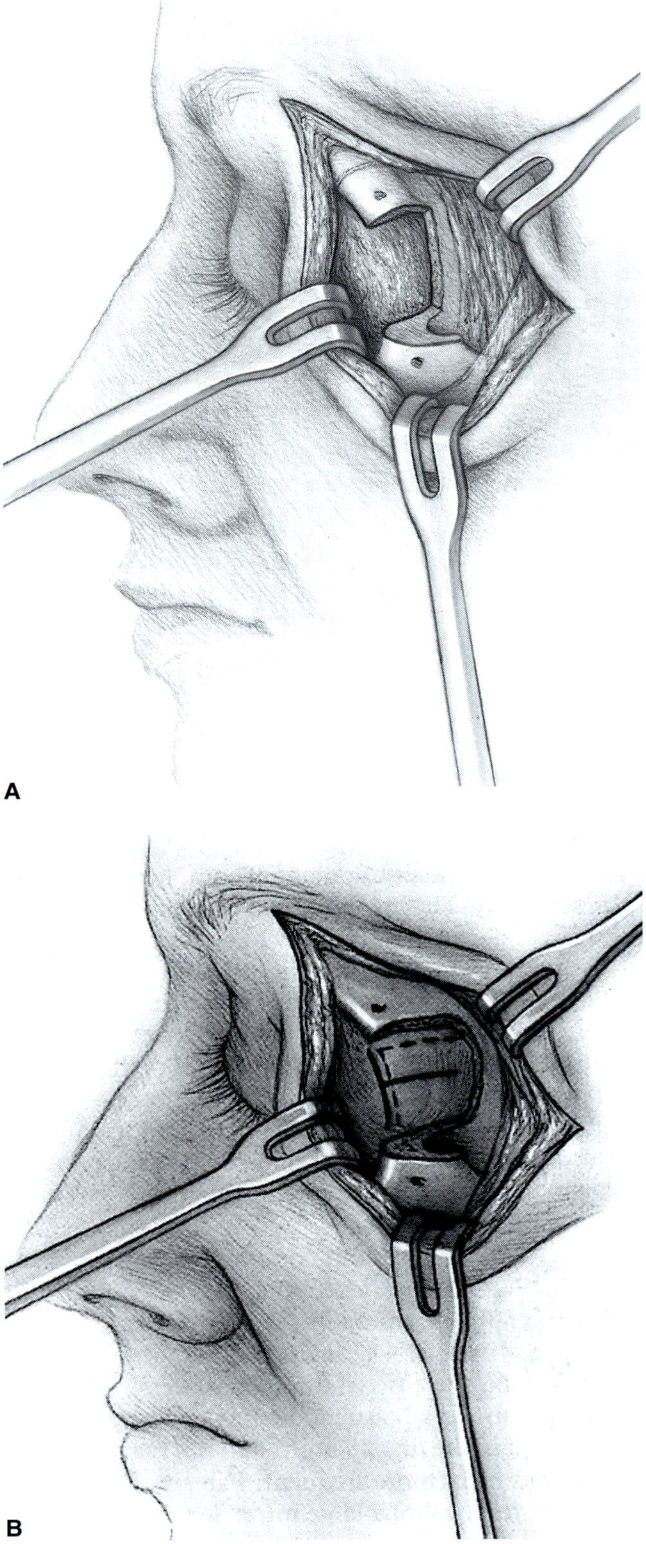

A

B

Figure 27–14. *A,* After removal of the lateral orbital rim, the periorbita is visible. Extreme care must be taken, in the case of a unilateral lacrimal gland tumor, not to breach this layer and inadvertantly invade the capsule of an epithelial lacrimal tumor. *B,* Two periorbita incisions: an "L-shaped" incision (dotted line) and a "T-shaped" incision (*solid line*).

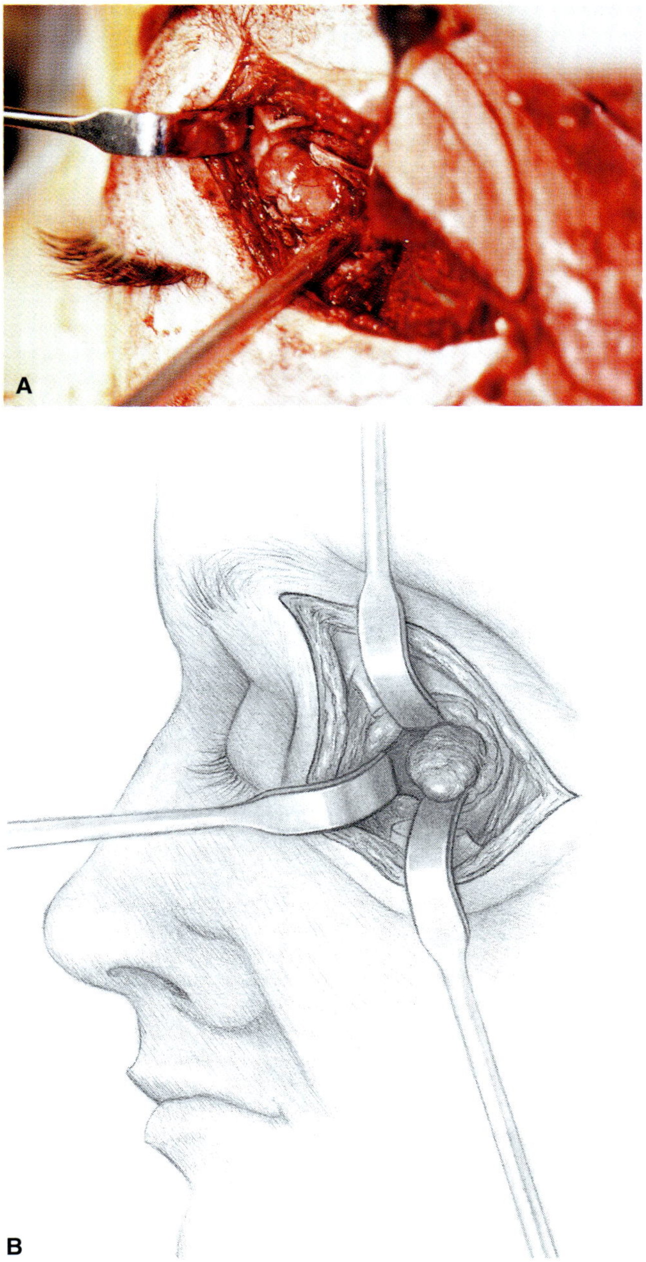

A

B

Figure 27–15. *A,* Normal lacrimal gland visible after the periorbita is opened. *B,* Contiguous retractors (either malleable or Soule) are required to displace fat and allow visualization of either an intraconal tumor or a mass next to the optic nerve.

Usually, when benign encapsulated tumors are removed, there is little bleeding. Occasionally, there is bleeding from incised periorbita, which is easily controlled with a point electrocautery set at 10 to 15. More recently, we have used a modified neurosurgical wet-field bipolar cautery and have found it to be a very useful instrument (Figure 27–16). The advantage of this instrument is that it produces much less

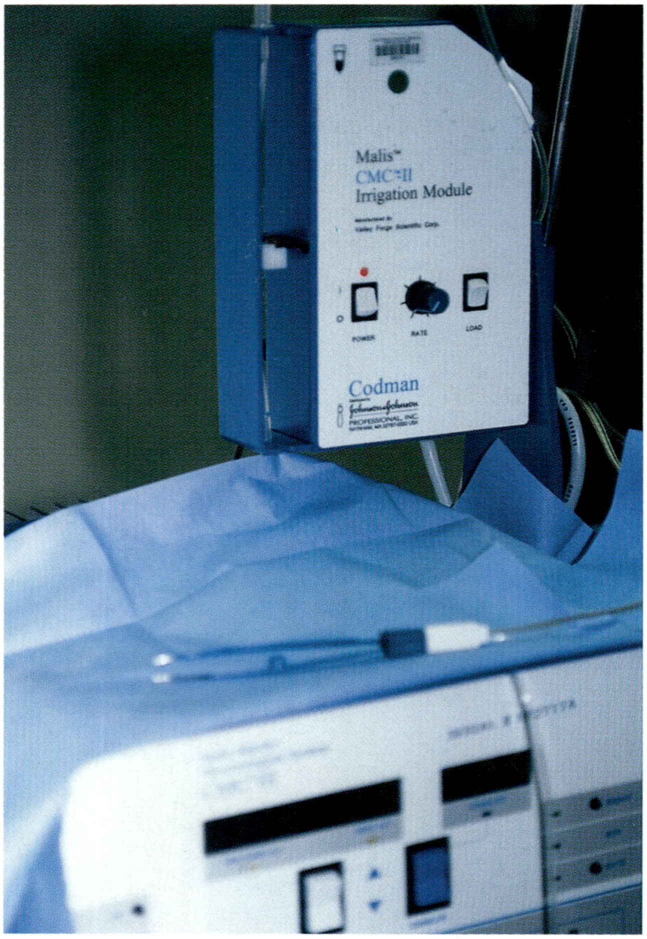

Figure 27–16. Wet-field bipolar cautery is used to produce less damage to normal tissue and more precise control of bleeding than older techniques.

damage to tissue than does the Bovie, and in some debulking procedures, it allows a much less bloody tumor removal.

Less commonly, when a large metastatic tumor or an inflammatory lesion is biopsied, significant hemorrhage occurs, and a suction electrocautery can be a useful adjunct. Similarly, since a significant orbital hemorrhage can always occur, we routinely set up two independent suction lines. In the surgical repair of arteriovenous malformations, the author has very rarely had to use vascular clips. Most of these, and some highly vascular tumors, are routinely embolized prior to surgery.[27–29]

Hypotensive anesthesia and an operating microscope are useful for intraconal tumors, especially those either adherent or contiguous to the optic nerve sheath. The use of these adjunctive manuevers allows a more precise surgical dissection in a relatively bloodless field.[30] We usually do not decrease the blood pressure until we are just about to enter the orbit and then keep the patient hypotensive only until the tumor is removed. It is useful to have the blood pressure restored to normal levels prior to closing an orbit so that any potential unseen bleeding vessel can be visualized and hemostasis achieved. We have not found these adjunctive options necessary in the management of most extraconal tumors. If the pupil begins to dilate while a tumor is being removed from around the nerve sheath, all attempts should be made to minimize optic nerve trauma.

We remove the entire tumor, whenever possible. If a discrete encapsulated tumor is present in the orbit, a cryoprobe is used to grasp the capsule and manipulate the mass (Figure 27–17).[31,32] A blunt Freer elevator is used to free the capsule from surrounding structures, and the mass is delivered through the orbital incision. There is a much lower incidence of tumor capsule breakage with a cryoprobe than with the forceps.

Some lesions require a representative open biopsy. In these cases, we use scissors and forceps, unless it is a very posterior lesion, in which case a front-biting Takahashi forceps can be used (see Figure 27–8C). We have used a carbon dioxide (CO_2) laser to debulk portions of tumors such as lymphangiomas, vascular metastases, and sphenoid wing meningiomas. This technique has the potential advantage of vaporizing tissue with good hemostasis. In practice, the author has not found the microscope-mounted CO_2 laser advantageous in most orbital dissections.

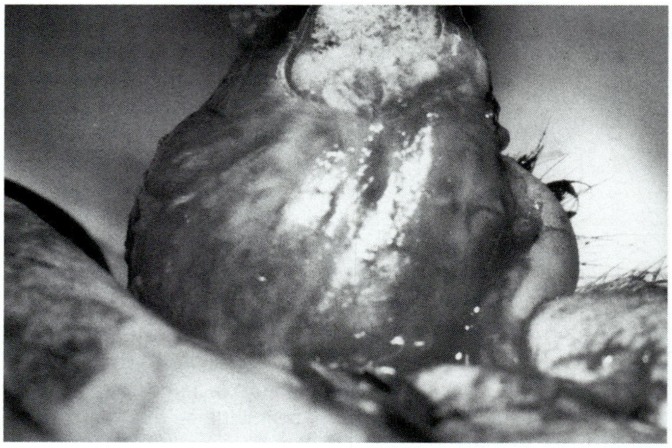

Figure 27–17. Cryoprobe used to grasp the capsule of a large tumor.

Almost always, the intraconal space is entered above the lateral rectus muscle. Usually, it is not difficult to separate the lateral rectus muscle from contiguous tumors, and the author has not accidentally damaged this muscle. If the CT or MRI studies suggest that the lateral rectus muscle may be incorporated in the tumor, the orbital portion of the lateral rectus muscle is isolated with a 2-0 suture. The eyelid is opened and toothed forceps are used to grasp the lateral limbus. The lateral rectus muscle is just inferior to the lacrimal gland and can be palpated as the globe is moved with the forceps in a medial and lateral direction.

In sphenoid wing meningiomas or other tumors that involve bone, newer intraoperative three-dimensional CT localization techniques are a useful adjunct. In cases where there is very abnormal bony anatomy, we have found that this technique allows us to more precisely drill and obliterate the bony portion of the tumor without damage to the intraorbital content.

At the completion of surgery, the orbit should be dry. The author places a thrombin-soaked sponge in the orbit for a few minutes. If there is no hemorrhage, it is closed without a drain. If the orbit has persistent venous leakage, a small Penrose drain is used. While Wright and others have strongly advocated the need for drains after all lateral orbitotomies, the author uses one only if the orbit is not dry at the end of surgery. In only 3 cases has vision diminished unexpectedly after surgery. In 2 of those patients, orbital surgery was for a regrowth of a tumor attached to the optic nerve after receiving photon irradiation; radiation vasculopathy plus surgical trauma to the delicate vessels around the nerve were the cause of vision loss. Unfortunately, in 1 patient from whom the author removed a medium-sized lacrimal fossa tumor, there were complications even though the patient had a dry orbit at the end of the case. The patient did not have enough pain during the afternoon or evening to contact a nurse, but the next morning when the dressing was changed, he had no light perception. An intraorbital hemorrhage was noted (Figure 27–18), and when the blood was evacuated, visual acuity did not return.

The periorbita can be either left open or closed with 6-0 gut. If the orbital rim was hinged posteriorly and the periosteum is intact, we often do not place nylon sutures through the bone, but merely close the periosteum around the bone and secure it with interrupted 4-0 vicryl sutures. If bone was removed from the orbital rim, it is brought together with 2-0 dermalon sutures. The ends of the suture are carefully placed through the bone holes; if the suture ends are left exposed, the patient may experience pain or suture extrusion. Periosteum is closed with interrupted 4-0 vicryl, and this suture is used to close subcutaneous tissues in two additional layers. The corner of the skin incision near the canthus is approximated at the outset of the second layer of closure, and the most superficial layer of 4-0 sutures is tied with buried interrupted knots. To minimize cosmetically unacceptable scars, subcutaneous closure with the above suture should make it appear such that skin closure almost seems unnecessary. The major cause of unsightly cutaneous scarring

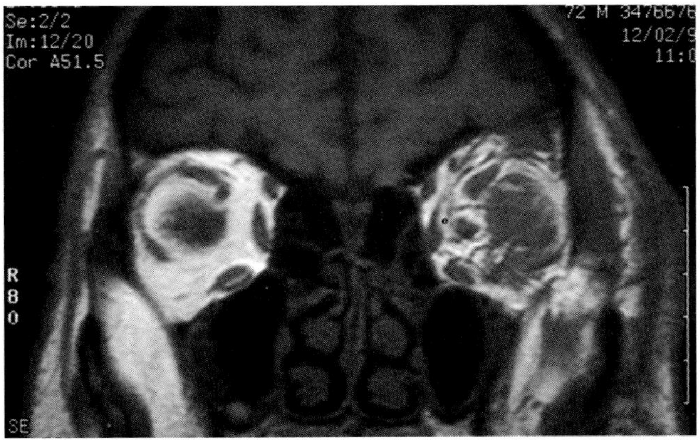

Figure 27–18. Postoperative hematoma after resection of a lacrimal fossa, without obvious complication.

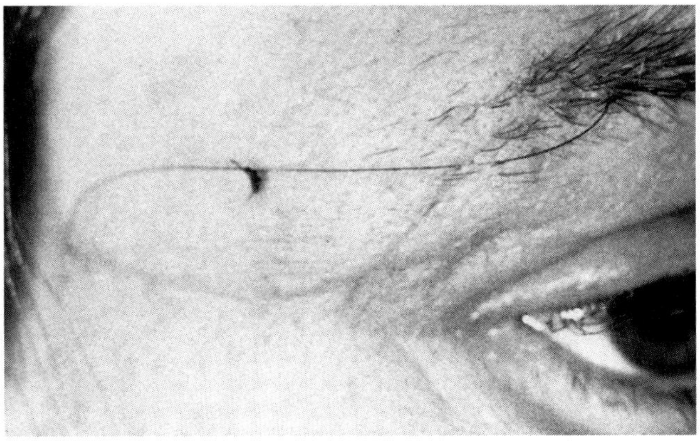

Figure 27–19. Lateral orbitotomies are closed with a subcuticular 6-0 dermalon.

after surgery is poor closure of subcutaneous tissues with late spreading in that layer.

The skin is closed with a running subcuticular 6-0 dermalon (Figure 27–19). The author prefers this closure over silk sutures for two reasons: (1) unlike lid skin, there is a greater tendency for the skin on the lateral aspect of the face to scar, and this is less likely with a subcuticular closure; and (2) if a malignancy that requires radiation is discovered at surgery, the subcuticular suture can be left in situ for months without cosmetic defect, and radiation can commence immediately.

We routinely tightly bandage a dry orbit for 24 to 48 hours, and then re-dress the area with a second pressure bandage for an additional 48 hours. If the orbit could not be closed dry, the initial dressing change, with drain advancement, is done at 24 hours after surgery. The drain is then advanced at 24-hour intervals, until removal on the second or third day.

There are a number of potential complications of lateral orbitotomy. The most serious is loss of vision, due to either direct damage to the optic nerve or damage to its vascular supply.[33] As mentioned previously, in approximately 1,000 orbitotomies, the author has had the latter complication on only three occasions. A second major complication can be inadvertent removal of the lacrimal gland, mistaking it for fat. Another severe complication is accidental severance of an extraocular muscle, most commonly the lateral rectus. These complications should not occur, if careful attention is paid to the anatomy.

The three most common complications after lateral orbitotomy are persistent postoperative lid edema, a

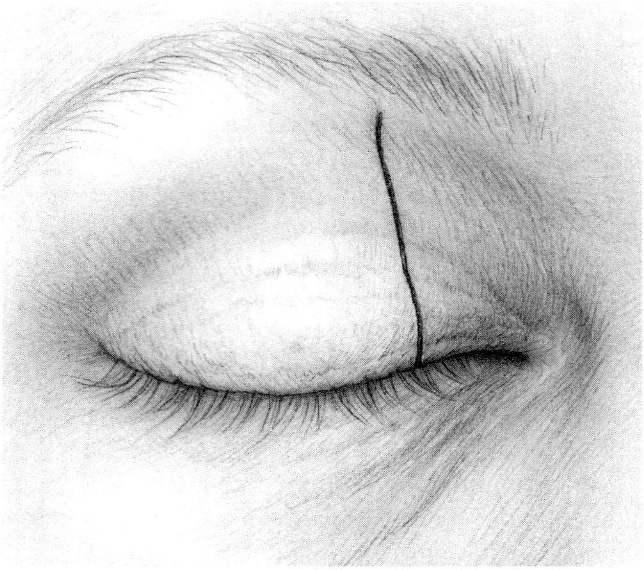

Figure 27–21. Byron Smith incision is used to reach tumors confined to the superior medial orbit.

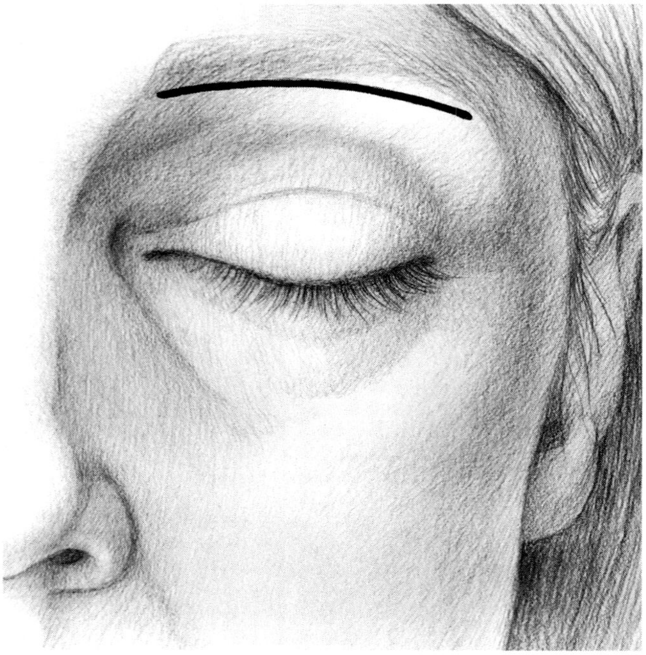

Figure 27–20. Benedict incision is used to approach extraconal superior orbital tumors.

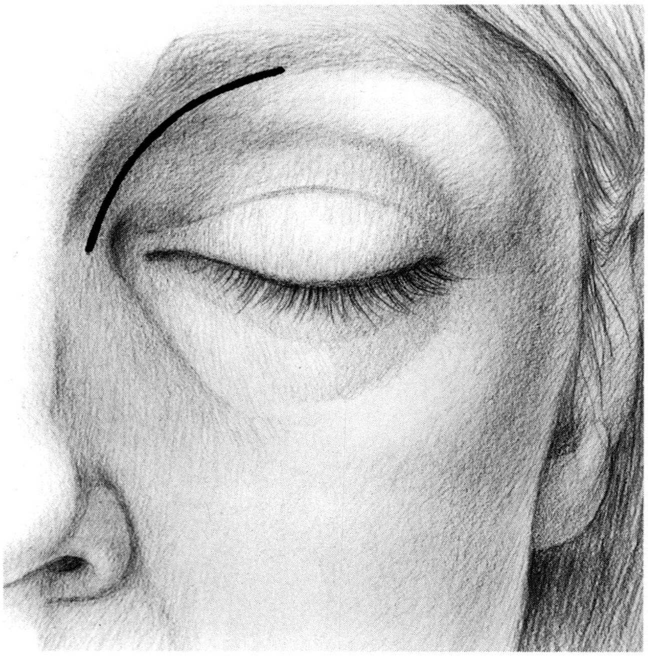

Figure 27–22. Lynch incision is useful to reach superior medial tumors that involve both the orbit and the sinus.

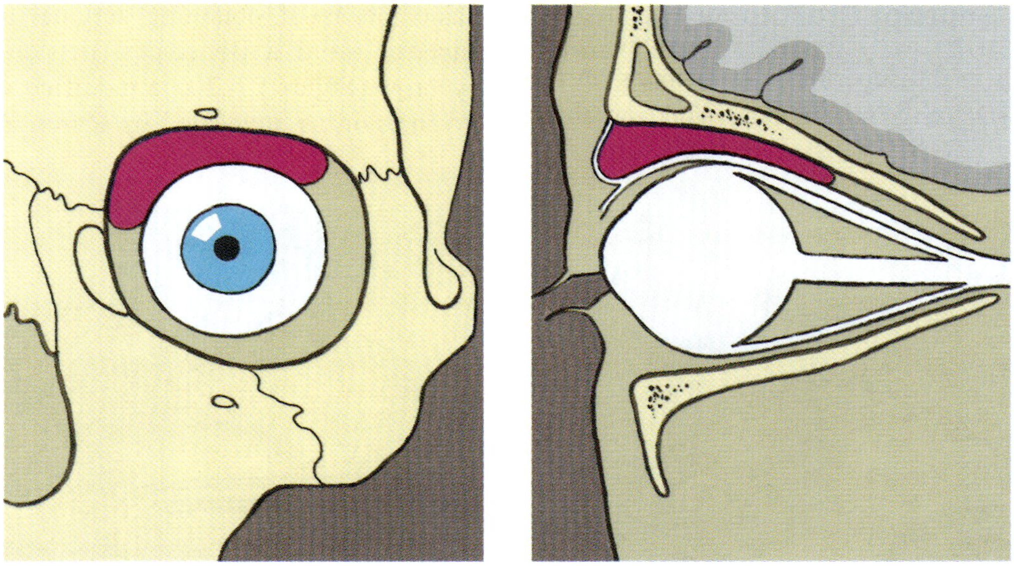

Figure 27–23. Orbital areas that can be explored through a Benedict incision.

small hematoma in the temporalis fossa, and lateral rectus paresis. The incidence and amount of lid swelling can be decreased if the orbit is pressure-patched as discussed above. When a moderate pressure dressing is discontinued in the first 48 hours and not reapplied, this problem has been more frequent. Paresis of the lateral rectus after removal of a large intraconal tumor is common. The muscle has been chronically stretched for months, and it usually takes 1 to 3 months for the muscle to regain correct tension. Temporalis muscle hematomas do not cause major problems; they usually spontaneously resolve in 14 to 21 days.

A number of rarer complications can occur. In intraconal surgery, damage to the ciliary ganglion will result in an enlarged pupil; the pupil may be eccentrically or completely dilated. Wound abscess is uncommon. The incisions in the temporalis muscle following posterior orbitotomy can produce some pain on movement of the jaw.

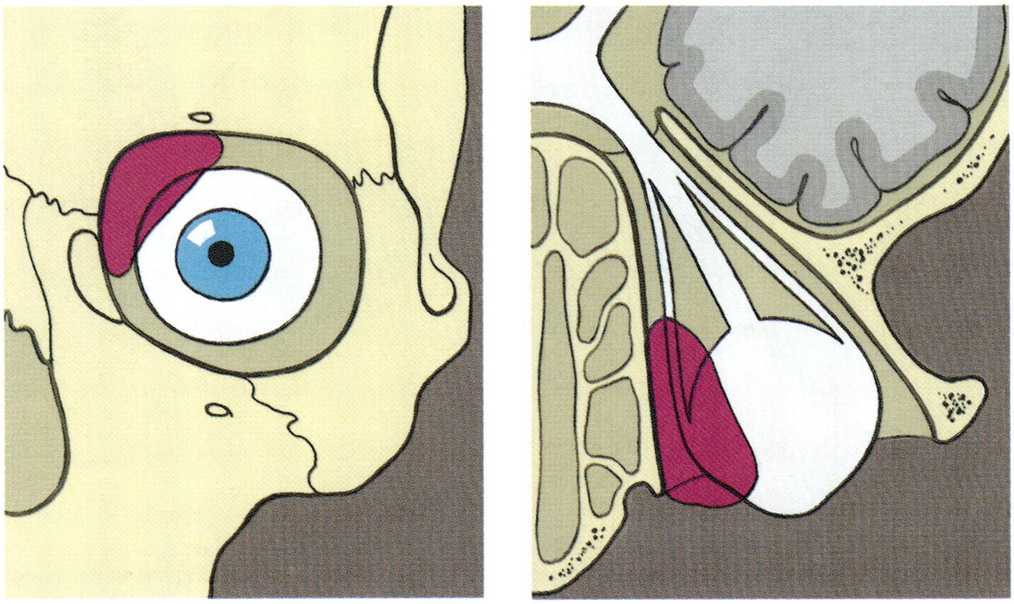

Figure 27–24. Locations of lesions approachable through a Byron Smith incision.

Superior Orbitotomy

The approach to the superior orbit depends on the position and size of the orbital mass. There are three basic means of obtaining surgical access to the superior orbit: a Benedict's incision through the eyebrow (Figure 27–20), a modified vertical upper lid incision as advocated by Byron Smith (Figure

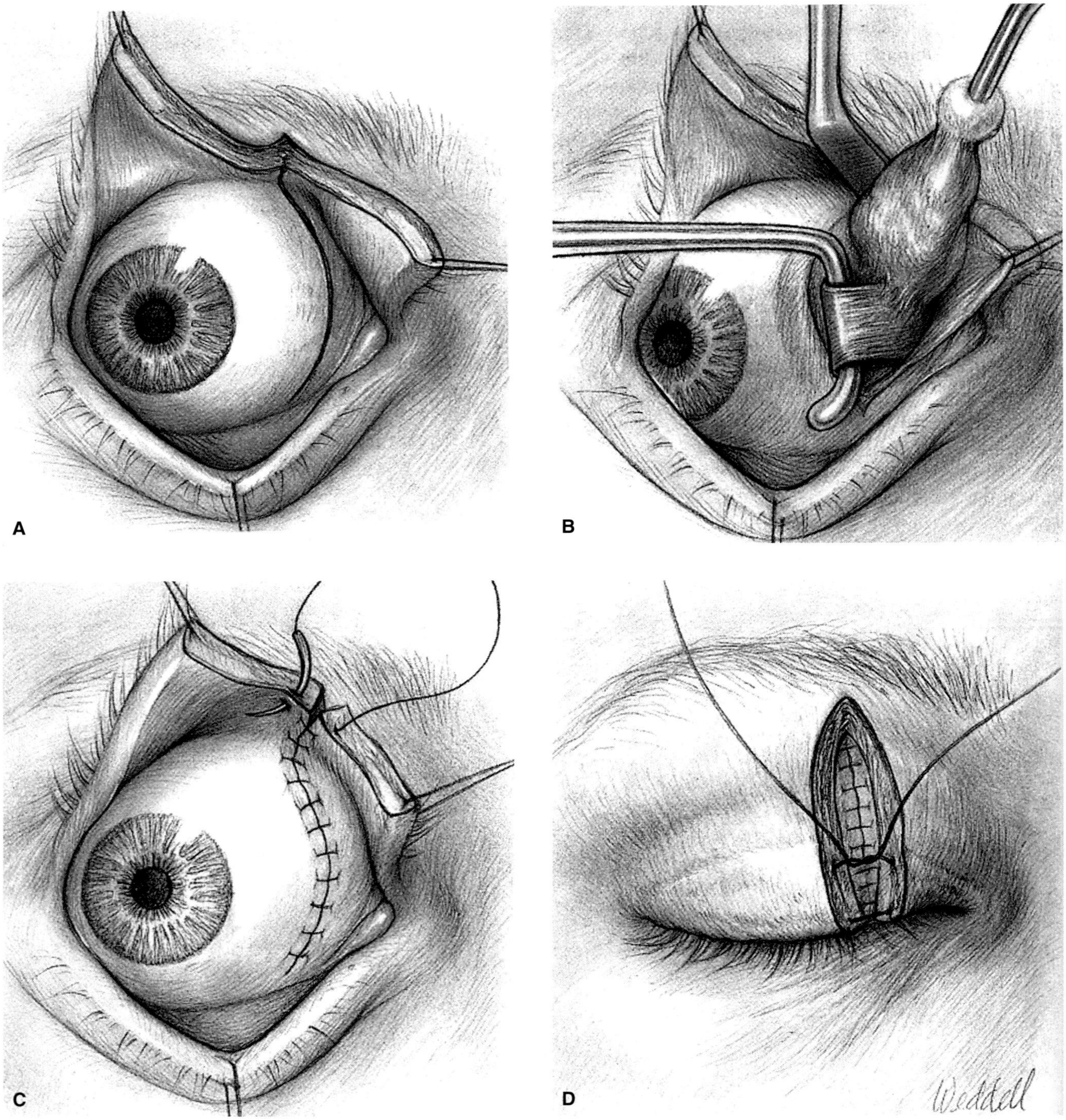

Figure 27–25. *A,* Byron Smith skin incision (see Figure 27–21) is taken through the entire lid just lateral to the superior punctum, and the palpebral conjunctival opening is extended onto the bulbar conjunctiva. *B,* A Soule retractor is placed in the superomedial orbit, the medial rectus muscle is isolated, and the tumor is removed with a cryoprobe. *C,* The incision is closed in layers: closure of the conjunctiva and correct apposition of the tarsus. *D,* Followed by closure of the palpebral conjunctiva and the subcutaneous and skin layers.

27–21), or a Lynch incision (Figure 27–22).[34–38] Occasionally, these procedures, especially the Lynch and Benedict's incisions, are combined.[38] Sometimes, the Lynch or vertical lid incision is performed in conjunction with a lateral orbitotomy to gain additional space to remove a medial or superiomedial tumor by deflecting the eye laterally.

In lesions which involve the extraconal superior orbit, a Benedict's incision (Figure 27–23) is made through the brow and carried down to the periosteum just superior to the orbital opening. This approach gives exposure for tumors in the orbital space above the extraocular muscles, as well as those which have transgressed the superior orbital periosteum (Figure 27–23). This approach does not allow adequate exposure for removal of a large mass and is best for an incisional biopsy or debulking of a superior orbital tumor, such as a metastasis or rhabdomyosarcoma. The tumor shown in Figures 27–23 and 27–26 could be biopsied through this approach.

Larger, encapsulated lesions confined to the superior or superior-medial orbit are best approached with a vertical incision through the upper lid (Figure 27–24).[35] Straight, sharp scissors are used to make a through- and-through lid incision 1 mm lateral to the superior punctum (see Figure 27–21). Stevens scissors are used to incise the conjunctiva from the superior edge of the lid incision to the limbus (Figure 27–25). Often a 90° limbal peritomy is fashioned. If the tumor has an intraconal component, the medial, superior recti, and sometimes the superior oblique muscles are slung with 2-0 sutures. This approach to the superior orbit gives more exposure than the Benedict's incision, especially if the tumor is more medial. The author has delivered large encapsulated tumors that extended to the orbital apex through this incision. Occasionally, a tumor is so large that an adjunctive lateral orbitotomy is required to move the globe laterally and create sufficient space to remove the neoplasm.

We close this vertical upper lid incision by reconstructing the conjunctiva with running 6-0 plain gut, and close deeper tissues after approximating the tarsus with interrupted 4-0 vicryl sutures. The lid incision is closed in a standard manner (see Chapter 3) with approximation of the tarsus first, followed by closure of the subcutaneous tissues and skin. Tumors in the superior medial orbit are less likely to be encapsulated benign lesions but are more commonly malignant masses, mucoceles, dermoid cysts, or inflammatory abscesses. Hemorrhage is more common in these lesions, so a small drain is sometimes brought out through the skin incision.

If a superior orbital tumor also involves the adjacent sinuses (Figure 27–26), a Lynch incision is used for biopsy or removal of the mass. This incision is

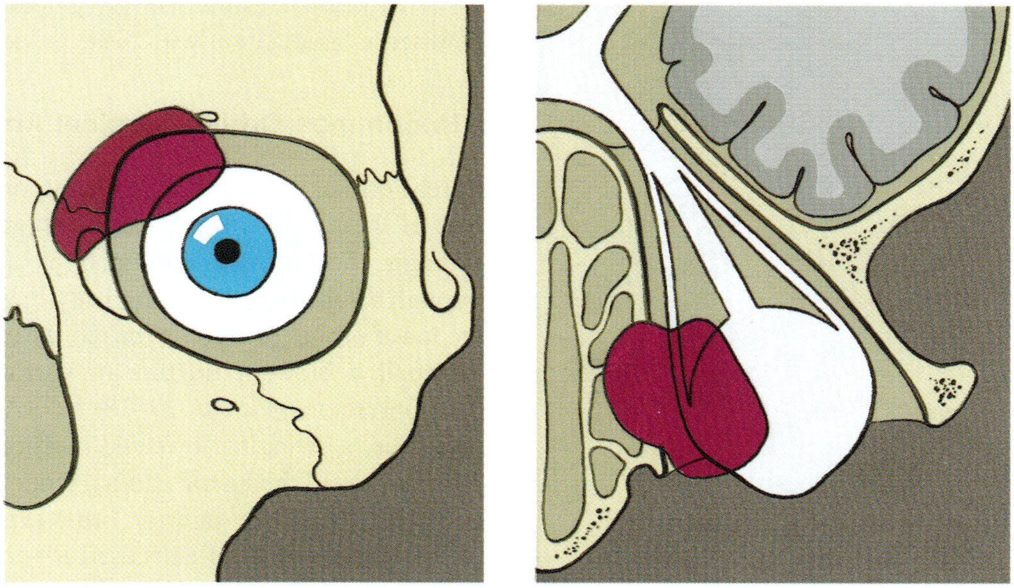

Figure 27–26. Superior medial tumors with adjacent sinus involvement (most often mucoceles) are approached through a Lynch-Benedict incision.

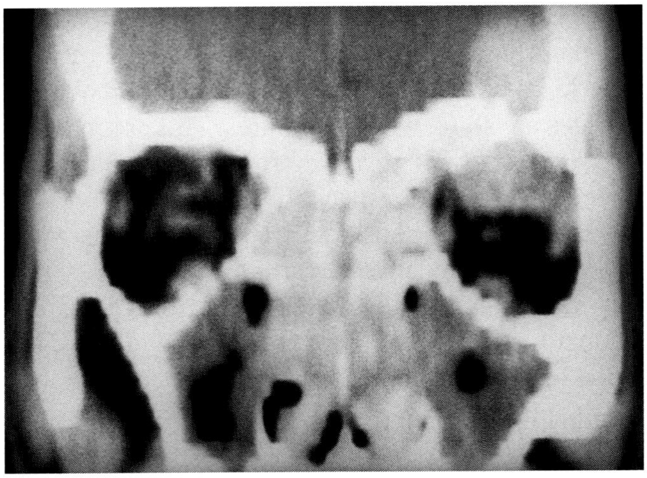

Figure 27–27. Mucocele has destroyed a portion of the orbital and frontal sinus roof.

similar to an opening for an extended dacryocystorhinostomy. If tumors or mucoceles involve both the orbital and the frontal and/or ethmoid sinuses, this incision may be combined with a Benedict's skin incision to obtain better exposure superiorly. The skin incision is brought down to the periosteum. The periosteum anterior to both the orbital rim and trochlea is incised with a scapel. Freer elevators are used to lift the periosteum from the underlying bone. As long as the trochlea is elevated in this manner, superior oblique tendon damage is unlikely.

Tumors or mucoceles involving both the orbit and sinuses are approached in conjunction with our otorhinolaryngology service. In the posterior ethmoid sinuses, the possibility of hemorrhage from a severed anterior or posterior ethmoidal artery or inadvertent penetration through the lamina cribrosa should be avoided. If a mucocele involving the orbit is removed, some of the mucocele's wall or sinus mucosa must be used to create and line a drainage opening into the nasal antrum. After combined orbital-sinus surgery, we pack the opening of the sinus-nasal passage with thrombin-soaked gel-foam and place the patient on a 7-day course of oral antibiotics.

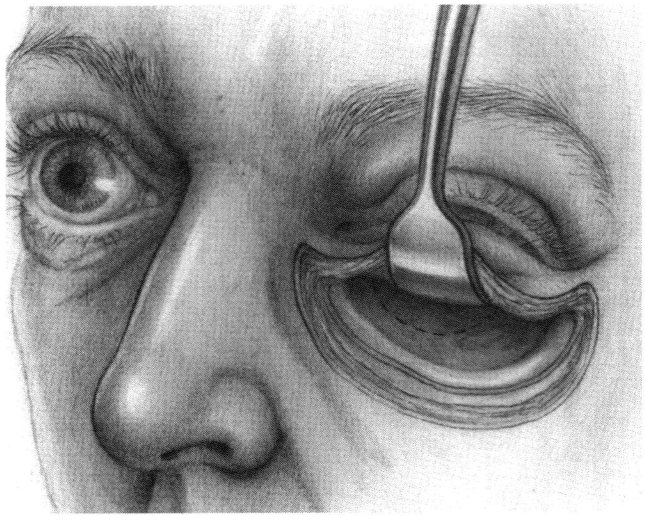

Figure 27–28. Approach to an orbital floor tumor by direct incision over the inferior rim, through the inferior conjunctival cul-de-sac, or through a subciliary lower lid incision.

Five distinct sets of complications occur with superior orbitotomies: (1) especially in biopsies of tumors which breach the orbital roof or with extensive frontal or ethmoid mucoceles (Figure 27–27), inadvertent perforation into the CNS can occur and must be avoided. In cases where there is a distinct possibility of a penetration through the meninges, the lateral aspect of the thigh is prepared and draped if a fascia lata graft is required during surgery. Histoacryl tissue glue is also available;[39] (2) especially in combined orbital-sinus surgery, the possibility of significant hemorrhage from the anterior and posterior ethmoidal arteries should be anticipated. We routinely include both a suction Bovie and two separate suction lines on our operative table for such cases; (3) as discussed above, it is easy to damage the tendon of the superior oblique muscle in any superior orbital surgery; (4) if the Lynch incision is too curved, a bowstring cosmetic deformity results; and (5) blindness has been reported in association with these procedures.[40]

Uncommon Orbital Surgical Approaches

Rarely, orbital tumors involve the inferior orbit or the roof of the maxilla. These can be approached either through the inferior conjunctival cul-de-sac or through a subciliary blepharoplasty incision to reach the lower orbital rim, analogous to the approach used to repair a blowout fracture or perform a thyroid decompression (Figure 27–28).[41,42] As previously discussed, a swinging lower lid incision, cutting the inferior crus of the lateral canthal tendon, also allows good access to the inferior orbit (Figure 27–29). Occasionally, we have also used a vertical incision through the lower lid just lateral to the inferior punctum. This procedure is analagous to one in the upper

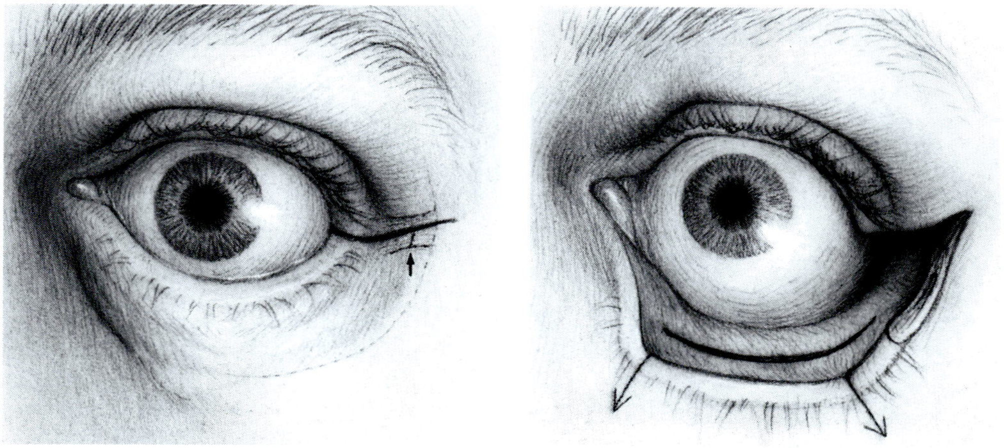

Figure 27–29. Swinging lower lid: surrounded incision severs the lateral canthal tendon to allow access to the orbital floor.

lid, except that the inferior oblique muscle must be carefully avoided to prevent secondary strabismus.

Tumors of the extreme posterior intraconal area and orbital apex present a difficult surgical challenge (Figure 27–30). This problem is even more difficult when a tumor involves the apex contiguous to the canal as shown in Figure 27–31. In such cases, a lateral orbitotomy provides poor visualization and exposure of the entire mass. We have managed such cases with two different approaches. If the tumor is in the superior apex or in the optic canal, removal is best accomplished with a combined neurosurgical-ophthalmologic team approach.[30,43–45] In such cases the neurosurgeons provide access through a craniotomy with unroofing of the canal, and we remove the tumor. This approach is more problematic if a portion of the posterior orbital optic nerve has to be moved (such as for a tumor just inferior to the nerve at the apex) since movement at the apex can produce severe morbidity.

If a benign lesion is inferior to the optic nerve at the apex and produces visual loss, we often decompress the area through a Caldwell-Luc approach with otorhinolaryngologists. A disadvantage of that approach is that it is sometimes not possible to remove a small (< 4 mm^3) lesion at the apex, since the optic nerve can-

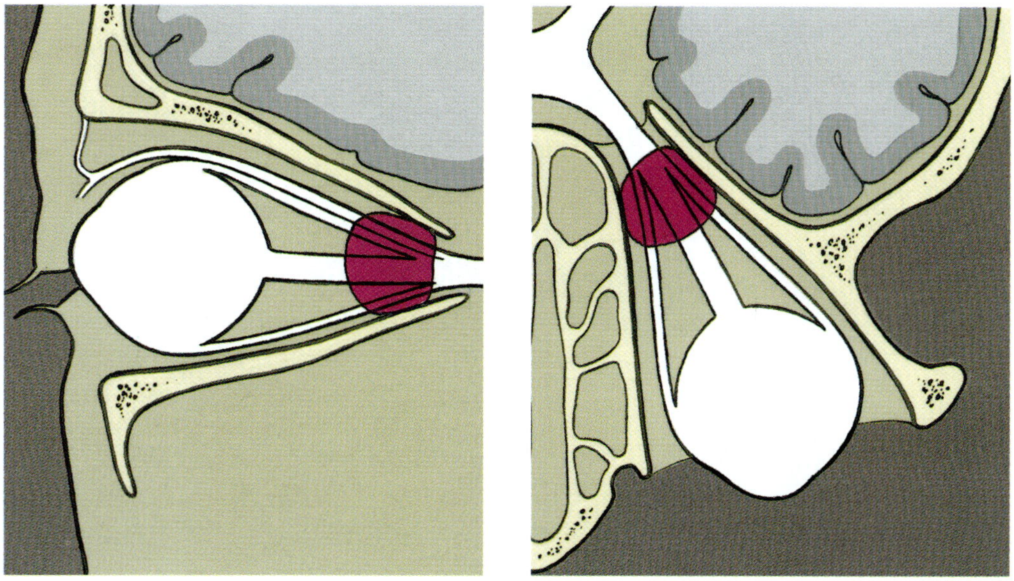

Figure 27–30. Orbital apex lesions are best approached with a combined neurosurgical-ophthalmic operation.

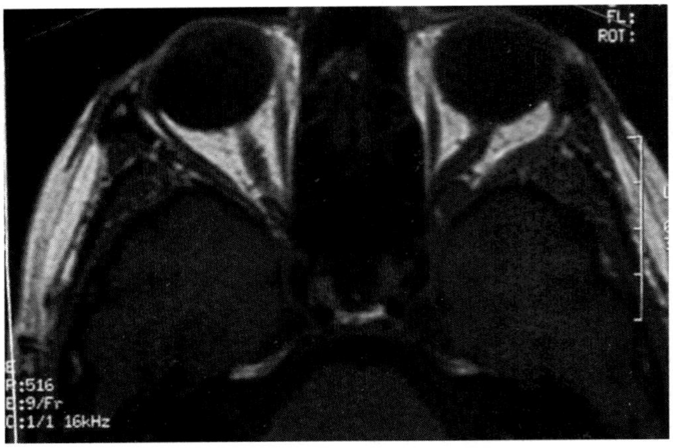

Figure 27–31. MRI scan demonstrates a posterior orbit tumor extrinsic to the optic nerve that has compressed that structure, producing loss of vision.

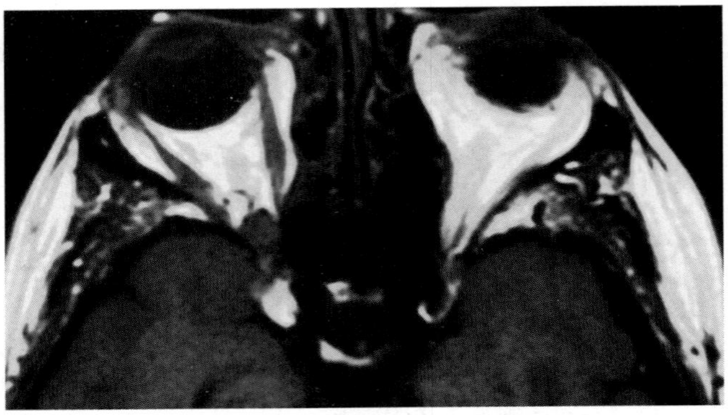

Figure 27–33. Small apical benign tumor producing marked visual symptoms. We were unable to remove this tumor, but the laminal papyracea was removed, orbital fat was prone to prolapse, and visual function returned to normal.

not be safely manipulated in this area and the orbital fat is difficult to retract in this confined space. More recently, we have used an endoscopic sinus approach to reach some of these tumors, especially those that are medial to the apical portion of the optic nerve. A standard sinus endoscopic approach done in conjunction with the ENT surgeons is performed (Figure 27–32). Simultaneously, the author also approaches the lesion through the orbit medially, either with or without removing the insertion of the medial rectus muscle from the globe. Several other authors have reported on this technique or variations of it.[46–50] In the author's experience, in a benign lesion if we are not able to safely remove the tumor, just decompressing the area around it will often improve vision, as in the case shown in Figure 27–33. In some of these settings, the use of a neurosurgical microscope is desirable, since it can be manipulated into an infinite number of planes. The microscope has the added advantage of allowing an assistant sufficient visualization to safely retract orbital fat.

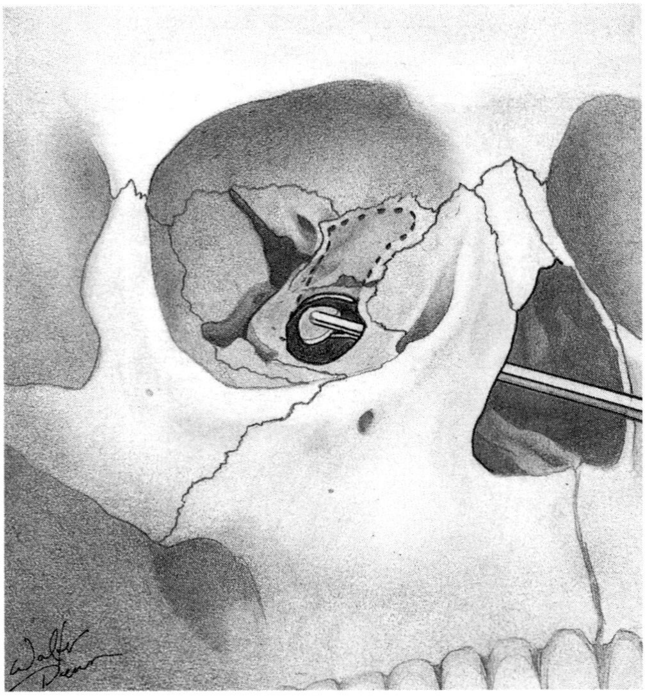

Figure 27–32. Schematic endoscopic approach to the sinuses through the nose.

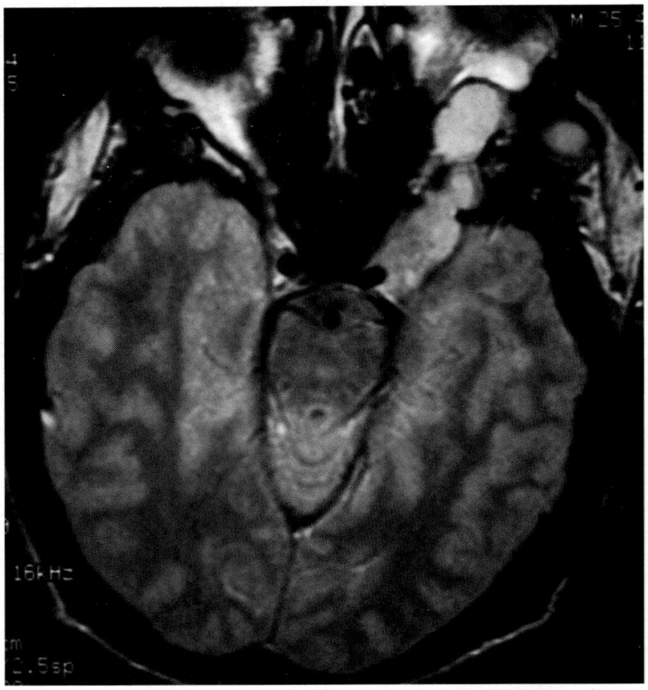

Figure 27–34. Orbital MRI scan shows multiple neurofibromas.

Ancillary Orbital Approaches

A conjunctival approach can be used to remove a small tumor immediately behind the globe or to biopsy the anterior optic nerve sheath.[25,51–53] If a nerve sheath biopsy or fenestration is required, we perform a 360° limbal periotomy. The medial rectus muscle is imbricated with a 5-0 Vicryl suture and detached with a generous stump left on the globe. A 4-0 silk traction suture is placed through the muscle stump, and a pair of Soule retractors are used to expose the orbit and move the globe laterally. While a number of self-retaining retractors have been developed for this purpose, they do not provide better exposure than Soule retractors, and they are more cumbersome to use. An inferior-temporal orbital tumor can also be removed in this manner. We similarly perform a periotomy, sling the recti muscles, then use Soule retractors to lift the globe away from the floor to reach the tumor. We have removed several cavernous hemangiomas in this manner. There are a few complications reported with this technique, the most common being a transient diplopia.[53]

A horizontal incision through the upper lid can be used to approach some anterior superior or central orbital tumors. Occasionally, a small dermoid in the lacrimal fossa can be removed through a curvilinear incision just anterior to the lateral orbital rim. The author has not biopsied lacrimal gland tumors through the upper lid to determine if they are malignant. As discussed previously, the author prefers to approach all lacrimal gland tumors as potentially malignant and isolate them at surgery, do an FNAB or frozen section, and remove them en bloc, if necessary.

We have approached more complex tumors using skull-based surgical techniques. This option combines the skills of neurosurgeons, head-neck surgeons, and ophthalmic surgeons. It is most useful either for tumors that involve several compartments (ie, orbit, sinus, and brain) or more diffuse lesions in the orbit for which the standard surgical approaches discussed above do not provide optimal exposure. As an example, in a case of multiple neurofibromas, as seen in Figure 27–34, this approach affords removal of multiple orbital and extraorbital lesions at one time. Similarly, we now approach most sphenoid wing meningiomas in this manner. In some diffuse benign intraorbital tumors, such as diffuse lymphangiomas, these approaches provide better exposure and the ability to remove a tumor more completely.[52–56] These techniques are outside of the realm of this book. The author's role in these procedures is viewed as joining a team to carry out the orbital portion of the procedure. Occasionally, in these procedures, a computer-assisted localization device, such as the Stealth localization system, can be helpful.[57] The main use of that device is in localization of deep CNS tumors.

The basic exenteration procedure is described in the chapter on treatment of posterior uveal tumors. Rarely, a cerebrospinal fluid leak can occur.[58] In such cases, either glue or a fascia lata graft may be appropriate. If a benign orbital process is exenterated and a flatter contour is optimal, a temporalis flap can be fashioned.[59] After the orbital contents have been removed, a skin incision with a No. 15 Bard-Parker blade is made from the lateral canthus horizontally into the temporalis fossa. The incision is curved down to orbital bone and temporalis muscle in a manner analogous to a lateral orbitotomy. The scalpel is used to incise the orbital periosteum at the anterior edge of the lateral orbital rim. A Freer elevator is used to remove the periosteum from the exterior surface of the orbital rim. A dental burr is used to drill through the lateral orbital wall. The temporalis muscle is exposed, and the proximal one-fourth is severed at its superior origin and mobilized (see Figure 8–75). Hemostasis is achieved with cautery.

The temporalis muscle flap is then positioned through the orbital wall and attached to remnants of the medial periosteum with interrupted 4-0 sutures (see Figure 8-76). We can place an 18-mm hydroxyapatite sphere posterior to the temporalis muscle. The subcutaneous incision on the lateral aspect of the face is closed with 4-0 sutures for the subcutaneous tissues, and a subcuticular 6-0 nylon monofilament suture for the skin.

The orbital closure over the temporalis flap is performed with advancement of the skin, if the lids are retained or with a split-thickness skin graft if the lids have been sacrificed (see Figure 8–77).

A temporalis muscle flap can be used in the closure of an exenteration to produce better cosmesis; this technique significantly reduces the concavity

Table 27–1. ORBITAL CONDITIONS THAT HAVE BEEN TREATED BY IRRADIATION

Benign disease
Orbital pseudotumor
Thyroid orbitopathy
Posterior scleritis
Langerhan's cell histiocytosis syndromes (eosinophilic granuloma, etc.)
Malignant disease
Primary orbital tumors
Orbital rhabdomyosarcoma
Primary orbital lymphoma
Malignant epithelial lacrimal gland tumors
Miscellaneous orbital sarcomas
Optic nerve glioma
Optic nerve sheath meningioma
Lacrimal sac malignancies
Secondary malignancies
Cutaneous basal cell carcinoma invading the orbit
Meibomian gland carcinoma invading the orbit
Sinus carcinoma with contiguous orbital extension
Tumors metastatic to the orbit
Orbital extension of uveal melanoma
Orbital extension of retinoblastoma
Systemic malignant lymphoid tumors (leukemia, lymphoma)

observed if only a split-thickness skin graft is used. However, the author does not employ this technique if there is a high likelihood of tumor recurrence. A temporalis muscle flap may be used when there is very little chance of recurrence, such as in cases of conjunctival squamous cell carcinoma that has involved the eye or superficial orbit, anterior orbital and ocular involvement from a skin neoplasm, or exenteration necessitated by radiation complications.

REFERENCES

1. Char DH. Radiation therapy in the management of ocular and adnexal tumors. In: Sears ML, Tarkkanen A, editors. Surgical pharmacology of the eye. New York, NY: Raven Press; 1985;523–39.
2. Harris JR, Levene MB. Visual complications following irradiation for pituitary adenomas and craniopharyngiomas. Radiology 1976;120:167–71.
3. Chan RC, Shukovsky LJ. Effects of irradiation on the eye. Radiology 1976;120:673–6.
4. Nakissa N, Rubin P, Strohl R, Keys H. Ocular and orbital complications following radiation therapy of paranasal sinus malignancies, and review of the literature. Cancer 1983;51:980–6.
5. Morita K, Kawabe Y. Late effects on the eye of conformation radiotherapy for carcinoma of the perinasal sinuses and nasal cavity. Radiology 1979;130: 227–32.
6. Shukobesky LJ, Fletcher GH. Retinal and optic nerve complications in a high-dose irradiation technique of ethmoid sinus and nasal cavity. Radiology 1972;104:629–34.
7. Ellingwood KE, Milton RR. Cancer of the nasal cavity and ethmoid/sphenoid sinuses. Cancer 1979;43: 1517–26.
8. Parsons JT, Fitzgerald CR, Hood CI, et al. The effects of irradiation on the eye and optic nerve. Int J Radiat Oncol Biol Phys 1983;9:609–22.
9. Merriam GR, Focht EF. A clinical study of radiation cataracts in relationship to dose. AJR Am J Roengenol 1957;77:759–85.
10. Hancock SL. Anterior eye protection with orbital neoplasia. Int J Radiat Oncol Biol Phys 1986;12:123–30.
11. Harisadis L, Misisco DJ, Schell MC, et al. Irradiation of bilateral orbital lymphoma: a non-coplanar technique with case reports. Radiother Oncol 1987;8: 123.
12. Rosenman J, Chaney EL, Sailer S, et al. Recent advances in radiotherapy treatment and planning. Cancer Invest 1991;9:465–81.
13. Hurbli T, Char DH, Harris J, et al. Radiation therapy of thyroid eye disease. Am J Ophthalmol 1985;99: 633–7.
14. Donaldson SS, McDougall IR, Egbert PR, et al. Treatment of orbital pseudotumor (idiopathic orbital inflammation) by radiation therapy. Int J Radiat Oncol Biol Phys 1980;6:79–86.
15. Kim RY, Roth RE. Radiotherapy of orbital pseudotumor. Radiol 1978;127:507–9.
16. Kim WH, Fayos JV. Primary orbital lymphoma: a radiotherapeutic experience. Int J Radiat Oncol Biol Phys 1976;1:1099–1105.
17. Dearnaly DP, Khoo VS, Norman AR, et al. Comparison of radiation side-effects of conformal and conventional radiotherapy in prostate cancer: a randomized trial. Lancet 1999;353:267–72.
18. Tyl JW, Blank LECM, Koornneef L. Brachytherapy in orbital tumors. Ophthalmology 1997;104:1475–9.
19. Bacskulin A, Ehrhardt M, Strietzel M, et al. An adjuvant afterloading brachytherapy device for use after orbital exenteration in patients with orbital malignancies. Gen J Ophthalmol 1996;5:484–8.
20. Krönlein RU. Die Traumatische Meningitis. In: Handbuch der Praktischen Chirurgie, Vol 4. Stuttgart, Germany: F. Enke; 1913.
21. De Takats G.: Surgery of the orbit. Arch Ophthalmol 1932;8:259–68.
22. Elschnig A. Operations for tumors of the orbit. Surg Gynecol Obstet 1927;45:65–73.
23. Berke RN. Modified Krönlein operation, AMA. Arch Ophthalmol 1954;51:609–32.

24. Dandy WE. Orbital tumors: results following the transcranial operative attack. New York, NY: Oskar Piest; 1941.
25. Wright JE. Surgical exploration of the orbit. Trans Ophthalmol Soc UK 1979;99:238–40.
26. Katz SE, Rootman J. Adverse effects of bone wax in surgery of the orbit. Ophthal Plast Reconstr Surg 1996;12:121–6.
27. Goldberg RA, Garcia GH, Duckwiler GR. Combined embolization and surgical treatment of arteriovenous malformation of the orbit. Am J Ophthalmol 1993;116:17–25.
28. Christi DB, Kwon YH, Choi I, et al. Sequential embolization and excision of an orbital arteriovenous malformation. Arch Ophthalmol 1994;112:1377–9.
29. Park K, Mannor GE, Wolfley DE. Preoperative embolization of an orbital brown tumor. Am J Ophthalmol 1994;117:679–80.
30. Housepian EM. Intraorbital tumors. In: Schmidek HH, Sweet WH, editors. Operative neurosurgical techniques, Vol. 1. New York, NY: Grune & Stratton; 1982. p. 227–44.
31. Putterman A, Goldberg MF. Retinal cryoprobe in orbital tumor management. Am J Ophthalmol 1975; 80:88.
32. Henderson JW, Neault RW. The use of the cryoprobe in the removal of posterior orbital tumors. Ophthal Surg 1976;7:45–7.
33. Long JC, Ellis PP. Total unilateral visual loss following orbital surgery. Am J Ophthalmol 1971;71:218–20.
34. Benedict WL. Surgical treatment of tumors and cysts of the orbit: eleventh de Schweinitz lecture. Am J Ophthalmol 1949;32:763–73.
35. Smith B. The anterior surgical approach to orbital tumors. Trans Am Acad Opthalmol Otolaryngol 1966;70:607–11.
36. Boniuk MP. Surgical approaches to orbital lesions. In: Transactions of the New Orleans Academy of Ophthalmology. Boniuk M, editor. St. Louis, MO: CV Mosby Company; 1982;30:15067.
37. Montgomery WW. The management of the orbit in surgery of the paranasal sinuses. Otolaryngol Clin North Am 1983;16(2):423–40.
38. Leone CR. Surgical approaches to the orbit. Ophthalmology 1979;86:930.
39. Tse DT, Panje WR, Anderson RL. Cyanoacrylate adhesive use to stop CSF leaks during orbital surgery. Arch Ophthalmol 1984;102:1337–9.
40. Maniglia HH, Chandler JR, Goodwin WJ Jr, Flynn J. Rare complications following ethmoidectomies: report of 11 cases. Laryngoscope 1981;91:1234–42.
41. Callahan A. Removal of orbital tumor through inferior route with Kuhnt-Szymanowski repair of ectropion. South Med J 1948;41:790–3.
42. Char DH. Thyroid eye disease, 3rd ed. Boston, MA: Butterworth-Heinemann Inc; 1997.
43. Housepian EM. Microsurgical anatomy of the orbital apex and principles of transcranial orbital exploration. Clin Neurosurg 1978;25:556.
44. Murray JE, Matson DM, Habal MB, et al. Regional cranio-orbital resection for recurrent tumors with delayed reconstruction. Surg Gynecol Obstet 1972; 134:437–47.
45. Schurmann K, Oppel O. Transfrontal orbitotomy as a method of operation in retrobulbar tumors. Klin Monatsbl Augenheilkd 1961;139:130–59.
46. Sethi DS, Lau DP. Endoscopic management of orbital apex lesions. Am J Rhinol 1997;11:449–55.
47. Asarai RH, Koay B, Elston JS, Bates GE. Endoscopic orbital decompression for thyroid eye disease. Eye 1998;12:990–5.
48. Dailey RA, Dierks E, Wilkins J, Wobig JL. LeFort I orbitotomy: a new approach to the inferonasal orbital apex. Ophthal Plast Reconstr Surg 1998;14:27–31.
49. Kennerdell JS, Maroon JC, Celin SE. The posterior inferior orbitotomy. Ophthal Plast Reconstr Surg 1998;14:277–80.
50. Mir-Salim PA, Berghaus A. Endonasal, microsurgical approach to the retrobulbar region exemplified by intraconal hemangioma. HNO 1999;47:192–5.
51. Polito E, Leccisotti A, Frezzotti R. A re-evaluation of the transconjunctival approach to orbital tumors. Orbit 1994;13:17–24.
52. Hassler W, Schaller C, Farghaly F, Rohde V. Transconjunctival approach to a large cavernoma of the orbit. Neurosurgery 1994;34:859–62.
53. Hejazi N, Hassler W. The transconjunctival microsurgical approach to the orbit: recent experience in 22 cases. Br J Neurosurg 1997;11:310–7.
54. Gabibov GA, Tcherekayev VA, Korshunov AG, Heboyan KA. Meningiomas of the anterior skull base expanding into the orbit, paranasal sinuses, nasopharynx, and oropharynx. J Craniofacial Surg 1993;4:124–7.
55. Lang DA, Neil-Dwyer G, Evans BT. A multidisciplinary approach to tumours involving the orbit: orbital re-construction, a 3-dimensional concept. Acta Neurochirurgica 1994;128:101–8.
56. Raveh J, Turk JB, Ladrach K, et al. Extended anterior subcranial approach for skull base tumors: long-term results. J Neurosurg 1995;82:1002–10.
57. Klimek L, Wenzel M, Mosges R. Computer-assisted orbital surgery. Ophthal Surg 1993;24:411–7.
58. Wulc AE, Adams JL, Dryden RM. Cerebrospinal fluid leakage complicating orbital exenteration. Arch Ophthalmol 1989;107:827–30.
59. Rose GE, Wright JE. Exenteration for benign orbital disease. Br J Ophthalmol 1994;78:14–8.

Index